Trauma

Contemporary Principles and Therapy

Trauma

Contemporary Principles and Therapy

EDITORS

▬ LEWIS FLINT, MD, FACS

Professor of Surgery,
University of South Florida College of Medicine,
Tampa, Florida

▬ J. WAYNE MEREDITH, MD, FACS

Richard T. Myers Professor and Chair, Department of Surgery,
Wake Forest University School of Medicine,
Chief of Surgery, Wake Forest University Baptist Medical Center,
Winston-Salem, North Carolina

▬ C. WILLIAM SCHWAB, MD, FACS

Professor of Surgery,
Department of Surgery,
University of Pennsylvania, School of Medicine;
Chief, Division of Traumatology and Surgical Critical Care,
Hospital of the University of Pennsylvania,
Philadelphia, Pennsylvania

▬ DONALD D. TRUNKEY, MD, FACS

Professor Emeritus of Surgery,
Department of Surgery,
Oregon Health Sciences University,
Portland, Oregon

▬ LORING W. RUE, III, MD, FACS

John H. Blue Professor of Surgery,
Vice Chair for Clinical Services,
Department of Surgery,
Senior Associate Dean for Clinical Affairs,
University of Alabama at Birmingham;
Chief, Trauma, Burns, and Surgical Critical Care,
University of Alabama at Birmingham Hospital,
Birmingham, Alabama

▬ PAUL A. TAHERI, MD

Professor,
Department of Surgery,
University of Vermont School of Medicine,
Burlington, Vermont

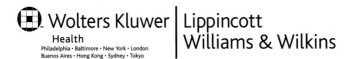

Wolters Kluwer
Health
Philadelphia · Baltimore · New York · London
Buenos Aires · Hong Kong · Sydney · Tokyo

Lippincott
Williams & Wilkins

Acquisitions Editor: Brian Brown
Senior Managing Editor: Julia Seto
Project Manager: Bridgett Dougherty
Manufacturing Manager: Kathleen Brown
Marketing Manager: Lisa Parry
Design Coordinator: Risa Clow
Production Services: Laserwords Private Limited, Chennai, India

© 2008 by LIPPINCOTT WILLIAMS & WILKINS, a Wolters Kluwer business

530 Walnut Street
Philadelphia, PA 19106 USA
LWW.com

Printed in the USA

Library of Congress Cataloging-in-Publication Data
Trauma : contemporary principles and therapy / editors, Lewis Flint . . . [et al.].
   p. ; cm.
  Includes bibliographical references and index.
  ISBN-13: 978-0-7817-5650-1
  ISBN-10: 0-7817-5650-2
  1. Wounds and injuries. 2. Emergency medicine. I. Flint, Lewis M.
  [DNLM: 1. Wounds and Injuries—therapy. 2. Critical Care—methods. 3. Trauma Centers—organization & administration. 4. Wounds and Injuries—prevention & control. WO 700 T77563 2008]
  RD93.T685 2008
  617.1—dc22

                                      2007043521

To purchase additional copies of this book, call our customer service department at (800) 638-3030 or fax orders to (301) 223-2320. International customers should call (301) 223-2300.

Visit Lippincott Williams & Wilkins on the Internet: at LWW.com. Lippincott Williams & Wilkins customer service representatives are available from 8:30 am to 6 pm, EST.

10 9 8 7 6 5 4 3 2 1

Contributors List

Michel B. Aboutanos, MD, MPH Division of Trauma, Critical Care and Emergency General Surgery and VCURES, Virginia Commonwealth University Medical Center, Richmond, Virginia

Jorge E. Alonso, Professor, Section of Orthopaedic Trauma, Division of Orthopaedic Surgery, University of Alabama at Birmingham, Birmingham, Alabama

Darwin Noel Ang, MD, PhD, MPH Fellow, Department of Surgery, University of Washington; Fellow, Department of Surgery, Harborview Medical Center Seattle, Washington

Saman Arbabi, MD, MPH, FACS Associate Professor of Surgery, Department of Surgery, University of Washington; Associate Professor of Surgery, Department of Surgery, Harborview Medical Center, Seattle, Washington

Nicholas Arredondo, MD Senior Resident in Neurosurgery, University of South Florida College of Medicine, Tampa, Florida

Juan A. Asensio, MD, FACS Professor and Chief, Division of Clinical Research in Trauma Surgery, Department of Surgery–Division of Trauma; Senior Attending Surgeon, University Hospital, University of Medicine and Dentistry of New Jersey at Newark, Newark, New Jersey

William Baugh, D. Min Director of Pastoral Care Services, Tampa General Hospital, Tampa, Florida

Paul D. Biddinger, MD Instructor in Surgery, Department of Surgery, Harvard Medical School; Director, Prehospital and Disaster Medicine, Department of Emergency Services, Massachusetts General Hospital, Boston, Massachusetts

Thane A. Blinman, MD Assistant Professor, Department of General and Thoracic Surgery, Children's Hospital of Philadelphia, Philadelphia, Pennsylvania

Ernest F.J. Block, MD, FACS, NREMT Trauma Medical Director, Orlando Regional Medical Center, Orlando, Florida

Charles C. Branas, PhD Associate Professor, Department of Biostatistics and Epidemiology, University of Pennsylvania, Philadelphia, Pennsylvania

Benjamin Braslow, MD Assistant Professor, Department of Surgery, University of Pennsylvania Medical School; Assistant Professor, Department of Surgery, Division of Traumatology/Surgical Critical Care, Hospital of the University of Pennsylvania, Philadelphia, Pennsylvania

James Forrest Calland, MD Assistant Professor, Department of Surgery, University of Virginia School of Medicine; Associate Trauma Director, Department of Surgery, University of Virginia Health System, Charlottesville, Virginia

Troy Caron, DO Orthopaedic Trauma Service, Tampa General Hospital, Florida Orthopaedic Institute, University of South Florida, Tampa, Florida

Brendan G. Carr, MD, MA Clinical Scholar, The Robert Wood Johnson Clinical Scholars Program, University of Pennsylvania School of Medicine; Instructor, Department of Emergency Medicine, Hospital of the University of Pennsylvania, Philadelphia, Pennsylvania

Eddy H. Carrillo, MD, FACS Assistant Clinical Professor of Surgery, Department of Surgery, University of Miami, Miami, Florida; Chief of Trauma Services, Division of Trauma and Surgical Critical Care, Memorial Regional Hospital, Hollywood, Florida

Michael C. Chang, MD, FACS Professor of Surgery, Department of General Surgery, Wake Forest University School of Medicine; Director, Trauma/Burn Services, Department of General Surgery, Wake Forest University Baptist Medical Center, Winston-Salem, North Carolina

Onuma Chaiwat, MD Research Fellow, Department of Anesthesiology, The University of Washington; Research Fellow, Department of Anesthesiology, VA Puget Sound Healthcare System, Seattle, Washington

Rose A. Cheney, PhD Executive Director, Firearm and Injury Center at Penn, Adjunct Assistant Professor of Surgery, Department of Surgery, University of Pennsylvania, Philadelphia, Pennsylvania

William C. Chiu, MD Associate Professor, Department of Surgery, University of Maryland School of Medicine; Director, Surgical Critical Care Fellowship Program, R Adams Cowley Shock Trauma Center, University of Maryland Medical Center, Baltimore, Maryland

David Cho, MD Surgical Resident, Department of Surgery, Division of General Surgery, Trauma/Critical Care Section, Oregon Health & Science University, Portland, Oregon

Alasdair K.T. Conn, MD, FACS Associate Professor, Department of Surgery, Harvard Medical School; Chief, Department of Emergency Services, Massachusetts General Hospital, Boston, Massachusetts

Martin A. Croce, MD   Department of Surgery, University of Tennessee Health Science Center, Memphis, Tennessee

Brian M. Derby, MD   Resident, Institute for Plastic Surgery, Southern Illinois University School of Medicine, Springfield, Illinois

L. Christopher DeRosier, MD   Chief Resident, Department of Surgery, University of Alabama at Birmingham, Birmingham, Alabama

Thérèse M. Duane, MD   Assistant Professor of Surgery, Department of Surgery, Virginia Commonwealth University Medical Center, Richmond, Virginia

Justin N. Duke, MD   Research Fellow, Division of Orthopedic Surgery, University of Alabama at Birmingham, Birmingham, Alabama

Rodney M. Durham, MD, FACS   Professor of Surgery, University of South Florida College of Medicine, Tampa, Florida

Allan Durkin, MD   Fellow in Plastic and Reconstructive Surgery, University of South Florida College of Medicine, Tampa, Florida

Frederick W. Endorf, MD   Acting Instructor, Department of Surgery, University of Washington; Clinical Burn Fellow, Department of Surgery, Harborview Medical Center, Seattle, Washington

C. Kristian Enestvedt, MD   Research Fellow and Resident, Department of Surgery, Oregon Health & Sciences University, Portland, Oregon

Philip R. Fine, PhD, MSPH   Director, Injury Control Research Center, University of Alabama at Birmingham, Birmingham, Alabama

Mary Kate FitzPatrick, RN, MSN, CRNP   Clinical Director, Nursing Operations, Nursing Administration, Hospital of the University of Pennsylvania, Philadelphia, Pennsylvania

Phillip Jeffrey Foster, Jr., MPH   Program Manager, Department of Rheumatology, University of Alabama at Birmingham, Birmingham, Alabama

Eric R. Frykberg, MD, FACS   Professor of Surgery, Chief, Division of General Surgery, University of Florida-Shands Jacksonville Medical Center, Jacksonville, Florida

Luis M. García-Núñez, MD   International Visiting Scholar/Research Fellow, Trauma Surgery and Surgical Critical Care, Department of Surgery–Division of Trauma, University Hospital, University of Medicine and Dentistry of New Jersey at Newark, Newark, New Jersey

Arvin Chun-Yin Gee, MD, PhD   Fellow, Department of Surgical Trauma/Critical Care, Oregon Health & Science University, Portland, Oregon

Richard Leslie George, MD, MSPH   Assistant Professor, Department of Surgery, The University of Alabama at Birmingham, School of Medicine; Trauma, Burns, and Surgical Critical Care, Associate Director, UAB Burn Center, Department of Surgery, The University of Alabama at Birmingham, Medical Center, Birmingham, Alabama

Brian James Gestring, MS   Assistant Professor, Department of Chemistry/Forensic Science, Cedar Crest College, Allentown, Pennsylvania

Mark Lawrence Gestring, MD   Associate Professor, Department of Surgery, Emergency Medicine and Pediatrics, University of Rochester School of Medicine; Director, Adult Trauma, Department of Surgery, University of Rochester Medical Center, Rochester, New York

Laurent G. Glance, MD   Associate Professor, Department of Anesthesiology, University of Rochester School of Medicine and Dentistry, Rochester, New York

Vicente H. Gracias, MD, FACS, FCCP   Associate Professor of Surgery; Chief, Surgical Critical Care, Medical Director Critical Care, Hospital University of Pennsylvania School of Medicine, Philadelphia, Pennsylvania

M. Sean Grady, MD   Department of Surgery, Division of Trauma and Surgical Critical Care, University of Pennsylvania, Philadelphia, Pennsylvania

Fahim Habib, MD   Division of Trauma and Surgical Critical Care, Memorial Regional Hospital, Hollywood, Florida

David Halpern, MD   Division of Plastic and Reconstructive Surgery, University of South Florida College of Medicine, Tampa, Florida

Robbi Hartsock,   Hospital of the University of Pennsylvania, Philadelphia, Pennsylvania

Mark R. Hemmila, MD   Assistant Professor, Department of Surgery, University of Michigan Medical School; Attending Surgeon, Division of Trauma, Burn, and Critical Care, University of Michigan Health System, Ann Arbor, Michigan

James H. Holmes IV, MD   Assistant Professor of Surgery, Department of General Surgery, Wake Forest University School of Medicine; Director, Burn Center, Wake Forest University Baptist Medical Center, Winston-Salem, North Carolina

William Scott Hoff, MD, FACS   Clinical Associate Professor, Department of Surgery, University of Pennsylvania Medical Center, Philadelphia, Pennsylvania; Trauma Program Medical Director, Division of Trauma and Surgical Critical Care, St. Luke's Hospital, Bethlehem, Pennsylvania

Rao R. Ivatury, MD   Division of Trauma, Critical Care and Emergency General Surgery and VCURES, Virginia Commonwealth University Medical Center, Richmond, Virginia

Jay S. Jenoff, MD   Fellow, Division of Traumatology and Surgical Critical Care, University of Pennsylvania, School of Medicine, Philadelphia, Pennsylvania

Jeffrey D. Kerby, MD, PhD, FACS   Associate Professor, Section of Trauma, Burns, and Surgical Critical Care, University of Alabama at Birmingham School of Medicine; Trauma Surgeon, Department of Surgery, University of Alabama Hospital, Birmingham, Alabama

Paul Kerr, DO, FACS   Assistant Professor of Surgery, University of South Florida College of Medicine, Tampa, Florida

Patrick Kim, MD   Assistant Professor, Department of Surgery, Hospital of the University of Pennsylvania, Philadelphia, Pennsylvania

Edward Hal Kincaid, MD   Assistant Professor of Cardiothoracic Surgery, Cardiothoracic Surgery Department, Wake Forest University School of Medicine; Cardiothoracic Surgeon, Department of Cardiothoracic Surgery, Wake Forest University Baptist Medical Center, Winston-Salem, North Carolina

Richard D. Klein, MD   Division of Plastic and Reconstructive Surgery, Department of Surgery, University of South Florida College of Medicine, Tampa, Florida

George Joseph Koenig, Jr., DO, MS   Chief Surgical Resident, Department of Surgery, Mercy Catholic Medical Center, Darby, Pennsylvania

John D. Lang, Jr., MD   Associate Professor, Department of Anesthesiology, The University of Washington; Chief, Department of Anesthesiology, VA Puget Sound Health Care System, Seattle, Washington

Shawn Larson, MD   Senior Resident in Surgery, Department of Surgery, University of South Florida College of Medicine, Tampa, Florida

Peter D. LeRoux, MD   Associate Professor and Vice-Chairman, Department of Neurosurgery, University of Pennsylvania School of Medicine, Philadelphia, Pennsylvania

Erika M. Levin, MD   Assistant Professor, Department of Ophthalmology and Visual Sciences, Department of Pediatrics and Communicable Diseases, University of Michigan Medical School, Ann Arbor, Michigan

Arpan K. Limdi, MSBE   Associate Vice-President, Facilities and Capital Projects, University of Alabama Hospital, Birmingham, Alabama

Lawrence Lottenberg, MD, FACS   Associate Professor of Surgery and Anesthiology, Department of Surgery, University of Florida College of Medicine; Trauma Medical Director, Department of Surgery, Shands Hospital at the University of Florida, Gainesville, Florida

Matthew W. Lube, MD   Attending Surgeon, Associate Director, Department of Surgical Education, Orlando Regional Medical Center, Orlando, Florida

C. Wayne Maberry, D. Min   Director, Trauma/Critical Care Pastoral Services, Tampa General Hospital, Tampa, Florida

Paul A. MacLennan, PhD   Assistant Professor, Department of Surgery, University of Alabama at Birmingham, Birmingham, Alabama

Paul M. Maggio, MD   Assistant Professor, Department of Surgery, University of Michigan Health System, Ann Arbor, Michigan

Ajai K. Malhotra, MD   Division of Trauma, Critical Care and Emergency General Surgery and VCURES, Virginia Commonwealth University Medical Center, Richmond, Virginia

Neil R. Malhotra, MD   Chief Resident, Department of Neurosurgery, University of Pennsylvania, Philadelphia, Pennsylvania

Niels D. Martin, MD   Fellow, Department of Surgery, Division of Traumatology and Surgical Critical Care, University of Pennsylvania, Philadelphia, Pennsylvania

Donald B. McConnell, MD   Professor of Surgery, Department of Surgery, Oregon Health & Science University; Section Chief, Department of General Surgery, Portland VA Medical Center, Portland, Oregon

Gerald McGwin, Jr., MS, PhD   Professor, Department of Epidemiology, Surgery, Ophthalmology, University of Alabama at Birmingham, Birmingham, Alabama

Janet McMaster, RN, MHSA, CPHQ   Performance Improvement Coordinator, Department of Trauma, Hospital of the University of Pennsylvania, Philadelphia, Pennsylvania

J. Wayne Meredith, MD, FACS   Richard T. Myers Professor and Chair, Department of Surgery, Wake Forest University School of Medicine; Chief of Surgery, Wake Forest University Baptist Medical Center, Winston-Salem, North Carolina

Anthony A. Meyer, MD, PhD   Professor and Chair, Department of Surgery, University of North Carolina; Chief, Department of Surgery, University of North Carolina Health Care System, Chapel Hill, North Carolina

William J. Mileski, MD   Professor, Director of Surgery, The University of Texas Medical Branch at Galveston; Chief, Trauma Services, The University of Texas Medical Branch, Galveston, Texas

E. Lanette Milligan, MPH   Doctoral Student, Department of Health Services Administration, University of Alabama at Birmingham, Birmingham, Alabama

Joseph A. Molnar, MD, PhD   Associate Professor, Department of Plastic and Reconstructive Surgery, Wake Forest University School of Medicine

Allen F. Morey, MD, FACS   Professor, Department of Urology, The University of Texas Southwestern Medical Center at Dallas; Chief, Department of Urology, Parkland Health & Hospital System, Dallas, Texas

Melanie S. Morris, MD   Surgical Resident, Department of Surgery, Oregon Health & Science University, Portland, Oregon

Sherry Morris, RN, MHL, LHRM   Trauma Program Manager, Tampa General Hospital, Tampa, Florida

Michael L. Nance, MD   Associate Professor, Department of Surgery, University of Pennsylvania; Director, Pediatric Trauma Program, Department of Surgery, The Children's Hospital of Philadelphia, Philadelphia, Pennsylvania

Lucas P. Neff, MD   Department of General Surgery, Wake Forest University Baptist Medical Center, Medical Center Boulevard, Winston-Salem, North Carolina

Robert M. Nelson, Jr., MD, MS Professor and Chairman, Department of Pediatrics, University of South Florida, Tampa, Florida

Turner Osler, MD, MS, FACS, FAAST Research Professor of Surgery, Department of Surgery, University of Vermont School of Medicine, Burlington, Vermont

Christopher A. Park, MD Instructor, Department of Plastic and Reconstructive Surgery, Wake Forest University, Winston-Salem, North Carolina

Jose L. Pascual, MD, PhD, FRCS(C) Assistant Professor, Department of Surgery, University of Pennsylvania; Assistant Professor, Department of Surgery, University of Pennsylvania Health System, Philadelphia, Pennsylvania

Patrizio Petrone, MD Chief Research Fellow, Division of Trauma and Surgical Critical Care, University of Southern California, Los Angeles County Hospital and University of Southern California Medical Center, Los Angeles, California

John P. Pryor, MD Surgeon and Trauma Program Director, Division of Trauma and Surgical Critical Care, Hospital of the University of Pennsylvania, Philadelphia, Pennsylvania

Glenda G. Quan, MD Resident, General Surgery, Department of Surgery, Oregon Health & Science University, Portland, Oregon

Tarek Razek, MDCM, FACS, FRCSC Assistant Professor, Department of Surgery; Director, Trauma Program, McGill University Health Center, Montreal, Quebec

Donald A. Reiff, MD, FACS Assistant Professor, Director, Undergraduate Surgical Education, Department of Surgery, Section of Trauma, Burns and Critical Care, University of Alabama at Birmingham School of Medicine; Director, Trauma/Burns Intensive Care Unit, Department of Surgery, Section of Trauma, Burns and Critical Care, University of Alabama at Birmingham, Birmingham, Alabama

Patrick Reilly, MD Associate Professor, Department of Surgery, Division of Traumatology and Surgical Critical Care, University of Pennsylvania, Philadelphia, Pennsylvania

Therese S. Richmond, PhD, CRNP, FAAN Associate Professor, Biobehavioral and Health Systems, School of Nursing, University of Pennsylvania; Translational Nursing Research, Department of Nursing, Hospital of the University of Pennsylvania, Philadelphia, Pennsylvania

Andrew Rosenthal, MD, MBA Fellow, Department of Surgical Critical Care and Trauma, Emory University School of Medicine, Grady Memorial Hospital, Atlanta, Georgia

Grace S. Rozycki, MD, FACS Professor of Surgery, Emory University School of Medicine, Grady Memorial Hospital, Atlanta, Georgia

Loring W. Rue, III, MD, FACS John H. Blue Professor of Surgery, Vice Chair for Clinical Services, Department of Surgery, Senior Associate Dean for Clinical Affairs, University of Alabama at Birmingham; Chief, Trauma, Burns, and Surgical Critical Care, University of Alabama at Birmingham Hospital, Birmingham, Alabama

H. Claude Sagi, MD Assistant Clinical Professor, Department of Orthopaedic Surgery, University of South Florida; Orthopaedic Trauma Service, Tampa General Hospital, Tampa, Florida

Moises Salama, MD Division of Plastic and Reconstructive Surgery, Department of Surgery, University of South Florida College of Medicine, Tampa, Florida

Kelli D. Salter, MD, PhD Resident, Department of General Surgery, Oregon Health & Science University, Portland, Oregon

Richard A. Santucci, MD, FACS Specialist-in-Chief, Department of Urology, The Detroit Medical Center; Chief, Department of Urology, Detroit Receiving Hospital, Detroit, Michigan

Babak Sarani, MD Assistant Professor, Department of Surgery, Division of Traumatology and Surgical Critical Care, University of Pennsylvania, Philadelphia, Pennsylvania

Thomas M. Scalea, MD, FACS Francis X Kelly Professor of Trauma Surgery, Director, Program in Trauma, University of Maryland School of Medicine; Physician-in-Chief, R Adams Cowley Shock Trauma Center, Baltimore, Maryland

C. William Schwab, MD, FACS Professor of Surgery, Department of Surgery, University of Pennsylvania, School of Medicine; Chief, Division of Traumatology and Surgical Critical Care, Hospital of the University of Pennsylvania, Philadelphia, Pennsylvania

Bradford G. Scott, MD Assistant Professor of Surgery, General Surgery Division, Michael E. DeBakey Department of Surgery, Baylor College of Medicine, Houston, Texas

Donald A. Smith, MD Department of Neurosurgery, University of South Florida College of Medicine, Tampa, Florida

James P. Stannard, MD Professor of Surgery, Division of Orthopaedic Surgery; Chief, Department of Orthopaedic Trauma, University of Alabama at Birmingham, Birmingham, Alabama

S. Peter Stawicki, MD Fellow in Traumatology and Surgical Critical Care, Department of Surgery, Division of Traumatology and Surgical Critical Care, University of Pennsylvania School of Medicine, Philadelphia, Pennsylvania

Rena L. Stewart, MD, FRCS (C) Assistant Professor, Section of Orthopaedic Trauma, Division of Orthopaedic Surgery, University of Alabama at Birmingham, Birmingham, Alabama

Paul A. Taheri, MD Professor, Department of Surgery, University of Vermont School of Medicine, Burlington, Vermont

James J. Thomas, BS Medical Student, Department of Urology, The University of Texas Southwestern Medical Center at Dallas, Dallas, Texas

Peter G. Thomas, DO Assistant Clinical Professor of Surgery, Department of Surgery, Hospitals of the University of Pennsylvania, Philadelphia, Pennsylvania

Brandon H. Tieu, MD Surgery Resident, Department of Surgery, Oregon Health & Sciences University, Portland, Oregon

Glen H. Tinkoff, MD, FACS Clinical Associate Professor of Surgery, Department of Surgery, Thomas Jefferson University, Philadelphia, Pennsylvania; Medical Director of Trauma, Department of Surgery, Christiana Care Health Services, Newark, Delaware

Donald D. Trunkey, MD, FACS Professor Emeritus of Surgery, Department of Surgery, Oregon Health Science University, Portland, Oregon

Christopher R. Turner, MD, PhD, MBA Clinical Associate Professor, Department of Anesthesiology, University of Michigan; Department of Anesthesiology, University of Michigan Health System, Ann Arbor, Michigan

Andrea T. Underhill, MS, MPH Associate Director, University Transportation Center; Project Administrator, Injury Control Research Center, University of Alabama at Birmingham, Birmingham, Alabama

David A. Volgas, MD Associate Professor of Surgery, Division of Orthopedic Surgery, University of Alabama at Birmingham, Birmingham, Alabama

Wendy L. Wahl, MD Clinical Professor of Surgery, Director of Trauma Burn Critical Care Services, Department of Surgery, University of Michigan, Ann Arbor, Michigan

Matthew J. Wall, Jr., MD, FACS Professor, Michael E. DeBakey Department of Surgery, Baylor College of Medicine; Deputy Chief of Surgery, Chief of Cardiothoracic Surgery, Ben Taub General Hospital, Houstan, Texas

Jordan A. Weinberg, MD Assistant Professor, Department of Surgery, University of Alabama School of Medicine; Department of Surgery, University of Alabama at Birmingham Hospital, Birmingham, Alabama

Edmund M. Weisberg, MS Editor, Center for Clinical Epidemiology and Biostatistics, University of Pennsylvania School of Medicine, Philadelphia, Pennsylvania

Adrienne L. West, MD Assistant Professor, Department of Ophthalmology, University of Michigan Medical School, Ann Arbor, Michigan; Medical Director, University of Michigan Kellogg Eye Center in Brighton, University of Michigan Health System, Brighton, Michigan

Douglas J. Wiebe, PhD Assistant Professor, Department of Biostatistics and Epidemiology, School of Medicine; Assistant Professor of Epidemiology in Surgery, Department of Surgery, School of Medicine, University of Pennsylvania, Philadelphia, Pennsylvania

Tammy Zapalac, CST Chief Surgical Technologist, Department of Operative Services, Ben Taub General Hospital, Houston, Texas

Minhao Zhou, MD Department of Surgery, Oregon Health & Science University

Preface

As the senior editors began to consider the task of compiling this book, we reflected on the fact that death and disability due to physical force injury remains a leading public health challenge for our contemporary world. As sobering as this fact is, we are heartened by the enormous progress that has been made in injury control over the last 25 years. Consider primary prevention. The American automobile industry has learned that safety sells. Most state and municipal governments now invest significantly in roadway and intersection design and construction to improve safety. Moreover, we have concrete proof that trauma systems reduce mortality and return nearly half of the seriously injured patients to productive lives where they contribute positively to society. In this volume, we have sought to document the progress in injury control, illuminate the new challenges, and offer avenues for further improvement.

Trauma surgeons have led the effort to analyze the process of patient care within trauma centers and reports emerge, literally every day, in the medical literature documenting improved outcomes for the resuscitation, operative care, critical care and rehabilitation of the injured. Witness the fact that skin substitutes for coverage of burn wounds was once a dream but is now a reality visible on the clinical horizon. The frequency and mortality of the multiple systems organ failure syndrome has been cut by nearly half. As progress has been made, new challenges have emerged as evermore severely injured patients survive. We now know that infection remains an obstacle to patient recovery and that evermore powerful antibiotics often hurt as much as they help. Simple hygiene has emerged as an effective means of preventing infection in the critically ill. Meeting these challenges has renewed the excitement that comes with active participation in the care of the injured and reconfirmed the fulfillment that a career in trauma care offers to the surgeon. Achieving survival of a patient, against all odds, in the often chaotic, no excuses atmosphere of trauma care produces a level of professional satisfaction that is difficult to describe. It is our sincere hope that this book sends one clear message: trauma care is a spectacularly rewarding professional life!

Leadership is required to successfully manage the complex organization that is the modern trauma center. No longer is expertise in patient care enough to ensure that the benefits of the modern trauma system are available to patients. Today's trauma surgeons must tackle issues that were unusual, if not foreign, to our thinking 30 years ago. Coordinating the efforts of multiple medical specialists to produce excellent patient care requires a major investment of time and effort. Trauma nurses have become essential partners in producing excellent clinical outcomes. Trauma nursing produces high quality research that helps patient care. New, more formalized communication links have been required to ensure that the patient is the beneficiary from free exchange of information and viewpoints between trauma surgeons and trauma nurses. Pathways to rehabilitation must be identified within the first days of injury and the interval between injury and rehabilitation shortened. Physiatrists and physical therapists now become involved soon after resuscitation and the benefit to the patient is enormous. The hazards of the critical care environment for the immunologically challenged patient must be appreciated. The clinical pharmacist has become a daily source of information about multiple drug interactions in critically ill injured patients and a valuable resource, along with the nutritionist, in planning metabolic therapies.

Post-traumatic stress disorder has now been recognized as a major barrier to successful reintegration of the injured patient into society and the value of early, intelligent psychological support of the trauma patient has been recognized. We now know the importance of emotional care for the family and loved ones of the injured patient as effective family support has a major influence on overall outcome. Finally, the benefit to patients and families that is realized from having well-understood, culturally sensitive pastoral care and end-of-life care has been recognized. This volume describes our experiences with these approaches.

Trauma surgeons are now expected to lead efforts to organize an integrated response to mass casualty incidents. Natural and terrorist instigated disasters occur daily in our world and preparation is essential! Physical force injury is the most likely mass casualty event that will be faced by our global society and the special characteristics of injuries sustained due to terrorist actions has become a necessary part of the knowledge base for a trauma surgeon. The trauma system is the natural backbone of successful responses to these events whether the patients generated are victims of physical force injury, infection, or toxic exposure.

One of the main goals of this book is to describe the various parts of the clinically successful trauma center as well as the ways that these parts can be made into a functioning whole. We have sought to provide a sound scientific foundation for the methods that we, the senior editors, have often learned from harsh clinical experiences. Our hope is that we have combined our experience with the intelligence and knowledge offered by the many talented contributors to this book to provide you, the reader with a practical reference that will bring value to your daily practice. We have intentionally tried not to produce an encyclopedia of trauma care but a guidebook containing useful, easily accessible information. If this book helps the modern trauma surgeon become successful then that success is our success.

Contents

SECTION VI: CRITICAL CARE OF INJURED PATIENTS 661

The Trauma System

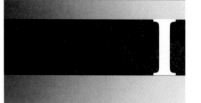

Trauma Care and Trauma Systems: Past, Present, and Future

Donald D. Trunkey

"What experience and history teach is this – that people and governments never have learned anything from history, or acted on principles deduced from it."
–George Wilhelm Friedrich Hegel (1832 Philosophy of History – Introduction)

THE PAST

According to Diamond (*"Guns, Germs and Steel"*) sometime after 13,000 BC, men began to domesticate animals and ceased to be hunter-gatherers in several parts of the northern temperate climate zones of the globe. The areas included China, India, the Middle East, the Mediterranean area, and meso-America. Accidents became common while working with domesticated animals and in building cities and settlements for people congregated together for protection and social amenities. As cultures developed and prospered, war became inevitable. This in turn led to the development of wound care. In this chapter, we will look primarily at those developments in our history, which led to present day trauma surgery. These include wound care, the concept of shock, resuscitation, analgesia/anesthesia, and antisepsis. As in medicine, the development of basic sciences in the last 500 years was also extremely important.

Trauma care antedates recorded history, and there are examples of anthropological findings showing trepanation of the skull dated to 10,000 BC. These skulls have been found in the Tigris-Euphrates Valley, along the shores of the Mediterranean, and in meso-America. It is most likely these operations were done for depressed skull fractures and possibly epidural hematomas. The surgery was most likely performed by priests or shamans within the various cultures. Some of the skulls show that the operation was

done more than once; and there is ample evidence that there was success because there was healing of the man-made hole. There is also evidence that they were able to treat fractures and dislocations successfully by knitting of the bones.

The first example in recorded history of care of the wounded comes from the Sumerians, who most likely invented writing. They were overrun by the Akkadians in 2600 BC. Their language was rich in description of wounds, and they also left us with two ways to treat wounds: those that were survivable and those that were not. These were set down in the 282 Laws of King Hammurabi's Code dating from about 1700 BC. Included in these codes are the laws concerning doctors. Interestingly, the code did not hold the physician responsible unless he used his knife. There is no mention of a "surgeon," and medicine was dispensed by an *"ashipu"* or sorcerer. There was reference to an *"asu"* or physician. Unfortunately, the former evolved into the primary practitioner. Knowledge of anatomy and physiology was essentially nil. The concept of shock did not exist, and wounds were treated with a bandage and soothing oil. There was a rudimentary understanding of inflammation and fever.

There was a commonality in early cultures to use poultices of various plant extracts, resins, and spices. Although this was probably used on an empiric basis, it may have had a serendipitous result. In 1943, around

2,300 species of medicinal plants belonging to 166 families were studied in Oxford. Plants of 28 families were active against *Staphylococcus aureus, Escherichia coli,* or both. Plants undoubtedly developed these components through evolution as protection to bacteria and fungus. Resins and spices were undoubtedly used on wounds to make them less malodorous.

Almost concomitant with the development of writing in Mesopotamia was the rise of culture in the Nile valley. The three medical papyri—Kahun Papyrus, Smith Papyrus, and Ebers Papyrus—are rich sources of Egyptian medicine. In addition, archeological findings show that fractured limbs were set by means of splints and bandages. Mass graves from 2000 BC show bodies of six soldiers, which are preserved well enough to show mace wounds, gaping wounds, and arrows still imbedded in the bone. Fractures were common with 1 out of every 32 individuals from 6,000 skeletons showing callous formation. Bites were common, including those from hippopotamus, lion, and crocodile. As near as can be determined, there was no word for "surgeon." The physician or *swnw* dispensed pharmaceuticals and occasionally would take to the knife.

Probably the most famous early writing is the Breasted interpretation of the Smith Papyrus. It is *the* most ancient medical text. One of the more interesting aspects of the Breasted rendition is that surgical cases are divided into three categories, depending on the chances of successful treatment—*an ailment which I will treat, an ailment which I will contend, and an ailment not to be treated.* Wounds were bandaged or held together by thorns and stitches. The use of the cautery was advocated for wounds of a vessel. Abscesses were treated by "fire-drill." Wounds were also treated with fats and oils, and fresh meat was used as a "poultice." Poultices were also made out of plants, including the leaves of a willow tree, which contain a small amount of salicin (aspirin). The Egyptian physician could also use the extract of the opium poppy to control pain. Green pigment was extracted from malachite and chrysocalla, which contains copper, and was used in wound dressings. Copper is a toxic bactericidal. Wounds were treated with lint, with honey and grease incorporated into the dressing. One of the interesting aspects of Egyptian "medicine" was that of embalming. It is most likely they buried the body under their all-purpose natural soda—natron. This is a mixture of sodium carbonate and bicarbonate, with a few impurities. When mixed with fats, natron acts as a mild detergent and is very effective in drying out the corpse.

The Greeks were the first to develop a trauma system. In Homer's Iliad, there are 147 recorded wounds, with an overall mortality of 77.6%. Thirty-one soldiers sustained wounds to the head, all of which were lethal. The Greek physicians recognized the need for a system of combat care, and the wounded were given care in special barracks, *klisiai,* or in nearby ships. Wound care was primitive; arrowheads were removed by enlarging the wound with a knife or by pushing the arrowhead through the wound. Drugs, usually derived from plants, were applied to these wounds, which were then bound, and hemostasis was treated by an *epaoide.* This meant that someone sang a song or recited a charm over the wound. Fractures were splinted, and the Greeks had nine methods of reducing dislocation of the upper and lower extremities. There is also evidence that the Greeks used opium to reduce pain and possibly for anesthesia.

In the Hippocratic Collection, there are numerous surgical treatments. The Greek language ignored the word *cheriorugos,* which meant "physician" including the verb *cheirugein,* which meant "to work with the hand." Hemorrhage was treated with a towel dipped in cold water and wrapped around the wound. After the hemorrhage was controlled, the wound was wrapped in a white bandage soaked in red wine. In addition, the juice of the fig tree was also used to stop bleeding. Another method that surely did not work was bleeding the patient. This was done usually by cutting a vein above the hemorrhage. In the Hippocratic Collection, it states, "Hemorrhage kills, but bleeding helps." Unfortunately, bleeding became a common treatment and persisted until just before the Civil War. It is interesting that the Hippocratic Collection also documents that ligature of bleeding vessels was not yet known, and the use of a tourniquet was condemned, which was reinforced by a Roman *Scribonius Largus,* who showed in experiments with a skin bag that if you tied a tourniquet around it, it forced more fluid out of the skin bag. The conclusion was that this made the bleeding worse. Drainage of abscesses was common, including empyema of the chest. Lacerations were treated by closing them with stitches threaded onto a bronze needle, and after the wound was closed, it was covered with a mixture of copper oxide and honey. Wounds to the head were bandaged if they did not involve the bone. The Greeks had at least three types of bone drills (*trypanon*). Trephination was used for fractures of the calvarium.

The Hippocratic Collection also puts forth their understanding of physiology, which were the four humors: blood, yellow bile, phlegm, and black bile. This was to persist for the next two millennia. They also felt that in nature everything is balanced. "Too much" or "too little" causes an imbalance, which is disease. The four humors were supposed to be harmoniously mixed, and disease ensues if they are unmixed or in wrong proportions. This also explained why the Greeks would bleed a patient even when they were hemorrhaging. They also thought that pus actually prevented more dangerous complications. In order to encourage the formation of pus they would, in some instances, insert greasy wool into the wound to help it suppurate. Paradoxically, they also understood that some wounds healed best if suppuration did not occur. Therefore, they would often put in powders of lead oxide and copper oxide to prevent suppuration. They also used moist solutions that had antiseptic properties, such as white vinegar, honey, sodium carbonate, and alum.

Some of the Greek pharmacy actually caused more harm than good. This included the side effects of poisoning with hellebore, which came from the Christmas rose. This would often raise blisters on the skin and invoke vomiting and diarrhea, and occasionally delirium, muscle cramps, and asphyxia. Purging the patient was considered necessary for them to survive.

There was undoubtedly intercourse between Greece and Egypt and exchange of medical ideas. Neither culture knew how to amputate. Wound dressings and suturing techniques were remarkably similar. Wine and honey were used in dressings. Vinegar was used as an antiseptic.

Several thousand miles to the east, in Asia, medicine was flourishing, but in quite a different way than that of Greece and Egypt. During the Chou Dynasty, which lasted from 1030 to 221 BC, several books, including the *Huang Ti Nei Ching*, the *I Ching*, were written; the latter was primarily a medical text. Surgery was discouraged, and physicians were admonished not to use medicines when "an illness occurred through no fault of your own." It was thought that such an illness would "pass of itself." Another medical text, Chou Li, is important because it further denigrates the status of surgery. It was thought that they were limited to a small group of "third-rate graduates." This is in direct contrast to China's neighbor, India, where surgery was a noble art. It is noteworthy that the practice of medicine was a tightly organized state system. Physicians were graded according to their achievement, which was followed by regular examinations. These objective techniques for measuring the ability of a candidate were devised as early as the fourth century BC and slowly diffused to the west through Baghdad and the Islamic world. The practice of examining physicians, required in Sicily under the statute of Roger II, the Norman in 1140, was in all likelihood a reflection of these Chinese standards.

Chinese medicine, like Greek medicine, had a simple explanation of disease, but there were only two factors, the yin and the yang, compared to the four humors of Greek medicine. Acupuncture was a common form of treatment. The *yang i* means "ulcer physician." The primary treatments were psychology (cure the spirit), diet, drugs, acupuncture, and clinical medicine (the latter being "treat the bowels, the viscera, the blood, and the breath"). Little is mentioned about surgery of wounds. Judicial castration was common, and these eunuchs often became members of the court, since they were unable to procreate. The Chinese also used dressings that contained resins and possibly derivatives from plants because these were very common in the medical pharmacopeia. There is no mention in these historical treatises about trauma systems. Shock must have been a concept because one of their herbs, *ma huang*, is the same compound as *ephedra* (ephedrine), which was used by the Romans. This treatment of shock may well have been passed from west to east or east to west along the Silk Road.

The Hindu culture arose approximately 1500 BC when the Aryans, who came from Persia, captured the original dark-skinned inhabitants of India. They brought with them a system of medicine that was eventually called Ayurveda or science life. As noted in the preceding text, in contrast to China, India treated surgery as a noble art. The Indus valley in the west was part of the Persian Empire, whereas the valley of the Ganges in the east was subdivided into many small kingdoms. Among the kingdoms of the east, Magadha was eventually to become the most powerful. The kings were allegedly converted to Buddhism by Buddha himself, and one of these was Ashoka III of the Maurya dynasty. It was Ashoka who developed a system of trauma care for his armies. Shortly after ascending the throne, Ashoka decided to invade Kalinga on his eastern border. During his conquest, he left behind a number of rock edicts, inscriptions carved into rock. One of these refers to hospitals and another edict refers to the "provision of comforts for men and animals." In addition to the rock edicts, there is also a book associated with Ashoka's dynasty: *The Artashastra*. This book clearly shows that Ashoka's army had an ambulance service, with well-equipped surgeons and women to prepare food and beverages, and assist in bandaging the wounded. Sushruta may have lived just before Ashoka, and he describes in detail the care of wounds. If a person was wounded by an arrow, he would not go to the internist (*rogahara*) nor the poison expert (*vishahara*), but instead would go to the *shalyahara*, which meant "arrow remover." This is the first historical mention of a doctor (*diadya*) who specialized in surgery. They had several ways of removing arrows, including pushing them on through, removing them in a reverse manner, or tying the arrow to a bent willow and then releasing the willow branch. The wounds were often plastered with a generous scoop of honey and ghee, and bandaged with a clean piece of linen. This was essentially the same as the salve of the Smith Papyrus. The *shalyahara* could also probe wounds when the arrow broke off, and for injured blood vessels they used the cautery. Like other medical practices, they also had to subdue demons, and they did so by burning incense sticks and making sacrifices of food. Postoperative nutrition was provided by giving barley powder in boiled water. Their understanding of physiology was hinged on the notion that 700 vessels originating in the umbilicus carried varying proportions of blood, wind, bile, and phlegm. For snake bites, the *vaidya* placed a ligature above the wound. He would then consecrate the wound with a mantra and might incise the wound with a knife.

The *shalyahara* was also an expert in reconstructive plastic surgery. Repair of ear lobes was common because of the placement of weighted earrings. Judicial removal of the nose, unfortunately, was also common, and Sushruta had a reconstructive method using a pedicle flap brought down from the forehead. The *shalyahara* also treated abscesses, including empyema of the chest. Fractures were common and were splinted, and wounds were sutured with thorns and an ingenious method was followed by using the pincers of ants, who once they clamped onto the wound were beheaded.

Initially, the Romans had no physicians at all. This was not due to ignorance, and Pliny explains it as, "It was not medicine itself that the forefathers condemned, but medicine as a profession...chiefly because they refused to pay fees to profiteers in order to save their own lives." Two hundred years before Christ, they slowly adopted Greek medicine in Pliny's *Historia Naturalis*. He details a number of folk remedies, some of which are still in use today. Fern is recommended for intestinal worms, and it is somewhat effective. Rennet, either from goat, hare, or deer is also used to coagulate or bind. It is Pliny who refers to ephedra, previously mentioned, used to staunch a patient's hemorrhage. It is noteworthy that other vasoconstrictive drugs were used for the treatment of shock until 1964.

Celsus was another great Roman doctor. One of the great finds of antiquity was a copy of his *De Medicina* that was discovered in 1427 at the Basilica of St. Ambrose in Milan. Most of this work is based on the Hippocratic books. There are extensive sections in his book on human vivisection using criminals and gladiators. He condemned such practices. Celsus' description of a surgeon captures the emotions of operating in an era of no anesthesia. "Now a surgeon should be youthful, or at any rate, nearer youth than age; with a strong and steady hand which never trembles, and ready to use the left hand, as well as the right; with vision sharp and clear, and spirit undaunted; filled with pity, so that he wishes to cure his patient, yet is not moved by his cries, to go too fast, or to cut less than is necessary; but he does everything just as if the cries of pain cause him no emotion." Surgical instruments were many and specialized. Many of these have been found in the remains of Pompeii. Surgical knives, probes, and dilators, were most likely used for extracting barbed arrows. Celsus also recognized that patients who were wounded "should not die from hemorrhage or inflammation." He treated hemorrhage by placing lint into the wound and then pressing down on the wound directly with his hand. If this did not check the hemorrhage, it was tried again, this time soaking the lint with vinegar. He also advocated ligature, and stated, "The veins that are pouring out blood are to be seized, and around the wounded spot, they are to be tied in two places." Pompeiian forceps are remarkably similar to the *bec de corbin* that Ambrose Paré invented 1,500 years later. Wounds were sutured shut or closed with metal pins (*fibulae*). Wound plasters were also used and often contained copper acetate or lead oxide and resins. Celsus also described the signs of acute inflammation: rubor, tumor, calor, and dolor. It is most likely that this was copied from either an Egyptian medical treatise or Greek writings. Celsus also drew extensively on Indian medicine in creating his treatise on medicine. One of the more unique aspects of Roman medicine was the reintroduction of a trauma system by the Roman Army. In the first and second century AD, Roman generals provided special quarters, called *valetudinaria*, for the sick and wounded. At least 25 archeological remains of these *valetudinaria* have

been found along the borders of the Roman Empire. Eleven of the trauma centers have been found in Roman Britannia, which is more than what currently exists (see Fig. 1). These hospitals for the wounded were very sophisticated. Open ventilation was stressed. Patient flow, including triage, was based on the seriousness of their wounds. Surgical instruments have been found in the remains, as well as unmistakable medicinal herbs. These include henbane (scopolamine) and dried poppies, which was undoubtedly used for pain management. The Roman army is known to have had surgeons because at least 85 army surgeons are recorded, mainly because they died and earned an epitaph. Some of their names are Greek: the majority is Latin.

A special mention has to be made about Galen because his writings would influence surgery for the next 1,500 years. Galen was a prodigious writer with 22 volumes still extant. At least one third of his writings have been lost. He was born in 130 AD in Pergamon, and at age 28, became surgeon to the gladiators. For 4 years, he cared for them, and according to his own writings, none of his gladiator patients died of their wounds. This is not true, because in his commentaries, he describes wounds of the heart. He stated, "They died faster if the wound reached into the left cavity. If the wound did not poke through, they could survive for up to 24 hours, and then they died of 'inflammation.'" He did not understand the concept of shock, nor did he really appreciate the circulation although he could view the beating human heart.

One of the things that distinguished Galen was his interest in dissection. Remarkably, he dissected apes, horses, asses, mules, cows, camels, sheep, lions, wolves, dogs, lynx, stags, bears, weasels, mice, snakes, a variety of fish and birds, and several elephants. Unfortunately, he was also guilty of vivisection, and his favorite animal was the Barbary ape. Using vivisection, he worked out the relationship of cutting the spinal cord and the type of paralysis that it produced. While he was vivisecting pigs, he worked out the two nerves that controlled squealing. He found that if he cut the two recurrent nerves in the throat, the pig could no longer squeal. He misinterpreted the course and purpose of the recurrent nerves and stated that it was tension on the nerves that caused the voice box to move and not the muscles they innervated. In treating the wounded gladiators, he was the first to describe suture of tendons and muscle.

One of the more vexing issues surrounding Galen was his way of controlling hemorrhage. He had opened live animal vessels and found that they contained blood, not air, but he still did not understand the cardiovascular system. He did control bleeding from vessels, primarily by pressure and dressings. He also knew that if a vessel was grasped with a forceps or hook, then twisted, this would often control the bleeding. He noted if the vessel was seized with a forceps, it could also be tied, and he used silk ligatures obtained from silk dresses that were in vogue in Rome. He was also

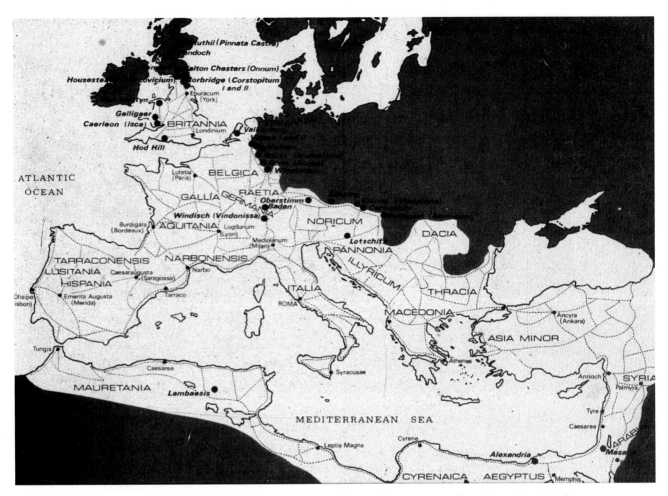

Figure 1 Each dot represents a Roman *valetudinaria* of trauma center found by archeological exploration or documented in the literature. Courtesy of Harvard University Press (From Majno G. *The healing hand: Man and wound in the ancient world.* Cambridge: Harvard University Press; 1975).

familiar with styptics and their ability to control superficial hemorrhage.

Following his time with the gladiators, he moved to Rome, where he spent 24 years and rose to the position of court physician to none other than Marcus Aurelius. This association was interesting because it was Aurelius who had sent a mission of merchants to China along the Old Silk Road, and this was how Chinese silk had been obtained.

As noted in the preceding text, Galen's theories and management of wounds persisted for the next 1,500 years. It was not until the Renaissance that the flaws in some of his anatomic dissections and management of wounds were challenged, and in some instances, ridiculed. This condemnation, in my opinion, was too harsh because it failed to recognize his genius in starting the basic science of anatomy. His failure to make salient observations on physiology, and in particular the circulation, remains a mystery, and may in fact, be due to the loss of almost one third of his writings. Nevertheless, Europe slumped into the Dark Ages and feudal times. It was an era of

itinerant surgery, quackery, and charlatans who practiced surgery with little or no training. It was also the time of burning of books, including the Egyptian alchemy books in Alexandria, which were burned by Diocletian in 292 AD. There was repeated destruction of the Alexandria library in 392 AD by Theodosius I and again in 640 AD.

Many historians have argued that during the Dark Ages, the art and science of surgery did not advance. There are exceptions to this indictment. One of the reasons that Greek medicine survived through this dark period is in no small part due to the Nestorian epic. In 431 AD at the Council of Ephesus, Nestorius, who was the patriarch of Constantinople, was excommunicated for heresy. Nestorius disagreed with the conclusions of the Council of Nicaea, and did not accept the Holy Trinity. Nestorius was exiled and fled to Egypt, where he died probably in 451 AD (see Fig. 2). He took with him a number of books, some of which were burned by Theodosius II. His followers continued the exile to Edessa in upper Mesopotamia. From there, they found permanent asylum at Jundi Shapur University in Persia. The books carried by his followers were then

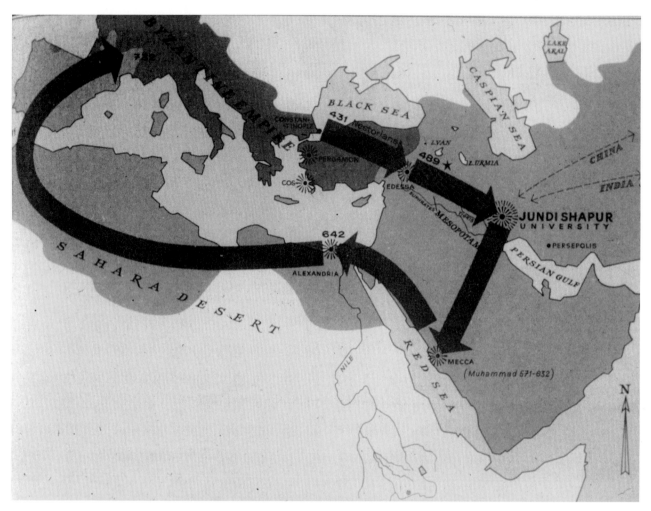

Figure 2   The Nestorian epic. Courtesy Harvard University Press (From Majno G. *The healing hand: Man and wound in the ancient world.* Cambridge: Harvard University Press; 1975).

translated into Arabic, and the university became a leading intellectual center, particularly in medicine. Ironically, most of the translations and scribing was done by Jewish scholars. The consequence of the Nestorian epic is that eventually these works made their way to Mecca, then back to Alexandria, and eventually across the crescent of North Africa into Spain, where the Moors reintroduced the historical record to the Byzantine empire. The second consequence was that Arab medicine reached a pinnacle during the years 700 to 900 AD, including the famous Arabic physicians Rahzes, Avicenna, and Albucasis. Unfortunately, the Arab physicians, like their Asian colleagues, looked down upon surgery as a second class of medicine. Using the books obtained from the Nestorians, they maintained Greek methodology and Galen's surgery. This included treatment of fractures, reduction of dislocations, and use of the cautery and wound dressings which essentially remained the same. An exception was Rahzes, who practiced in the ninth century, and described the use of catgut for suturing wounds.

Another advance made before the Renaissance was the credentialing of physicians, and in particular, surgeons. Beginning in the thirteenth century, the School of Solerno, a secular university, sparked a resurgence of medical education. As noted earlier, Roger II of Italy adopted the techniques from China, which required examination and a license to practice medicine. This was soon followed by Frederick II, Emperor of the Holy Roman Empire. Surgeons were still treated as second-class citizens compared to physicians. This is beautifully documented by the Barber Surgeons in England, which eventually evolved into the Royal College of Surgeons. Across the English Channel in Paris, the same discrimination was carried out at the College of St. Côme. Paré was probably the most famous surgeon of the sixteenth century. He was not allowed to join the College of St. Côme until he was 44 years of age. At that time, he was the court physician to King Henry II, but it was the friendship of Charles Etienne de la Riviere that made his membership possible. Etienne had been a dissector for the *Faculté de Médicine* and a Barber Surgeon. There were only two Barber Surgeons in the College of St. Côme when Paré was admitted. Ambrose Paré served four French kings during the time of the French-Spanish civil and religious wars. His major contributions toward treating penetrating trauma included his treatment of gunshot wounds, his use of ligature instead of cautery, and use of nutrition during the postinjury period. Paré was also much interested in prosthetic devices and designed a number of them for amputees.

A contemporary and acquaintance of Paré was Andreas Vesalius, who was to dramatically change surgery in the ensuing Renaissance. His dissections and interpretation corrected all of the mistakes that Galen had made. He also resurrected the treatment of empyema that had long been neglected. Paré and Vesalius attended to a very famous patient. Henri II was wounded on June 29, 1559 by a lance during a tournament. The lance struck the king above the right eye, and Paré was one of the surgeons in attendance. Vesalius was sent for from Brussels, but they were unable to ascertain the course of the splinters. The king died 11 days after the accident, and an autopsy showed a quantity of blood between the dura and the pia mater with early signs of infection.

It was in the seventeenth century that a major contribution to our understanding of the circulation was postulated by William Harvey. In 1628, Harvey published his seminal work, *De Motu Cordis*. Although one could surmise that the understanding of the circulation would lead to new concepts of shock, this did not occur until 290 years later. However, 28 years after Harvey's discovery, Christopher Wren demonstrated that medicines could be administered to animals by the intravenous route. Ten years after his observation, Lower showed that homologous blood could be directly transfused between animals. Attempts to use blood transfusion in humans met with very disappointing results, complications, and death. The routine use of blood would have to wait until World War I. Between 1700 and 1900, there were major advances in the basic sciences. Morgagni was instrumental in developing the science of cellular pathology. John Hunter refined dissection and made major contributions to management of the wounds of war. Anesthesia was to be one of the major contributions to the surgical discipline. Ether was demonstrated by Crawford Long in 1842 and by William Morton in 1846 to be no "humbug." A year after ether was introduced James Simpson demonstrated the effectiveness of chloroform, which became the primary anesthetic for the Confederates during the American Civil War. The nineteenth century was marked by the introduction of antiseptic surgery and the brilliant work of Louis Pasteur and Virchow were welcome additions to the basic sciences. Another major advance in the diagnosis of traumatic wounds was the invention of x-ray by Roentgen in 1895. Before this period, it was common to probe wounds. One reason to probe was to remove the missile if possible, the second was to determine the trajectory of the missile and predict what organs were injured. In many instances, probing caused more harm. X-rays essentially eliminated the need for probing wounds.

It was Dominique Larrey, Napoleon's surgeon, who addressed trauma from a systematic and organizational standpoint. Larrey introduced the concept of the "flying ambulance," the sole purpose of which was to provide rapid removal of the wounded from the battlefield. Larrey also introduced the concept of putting the hospital as close to the front lines as feasible in order to permit wound surgery as soon as possible (see Fig. 3). His primary intent was to operate during the period of "wound shock," when there was an element of analgesia, but also to reduce

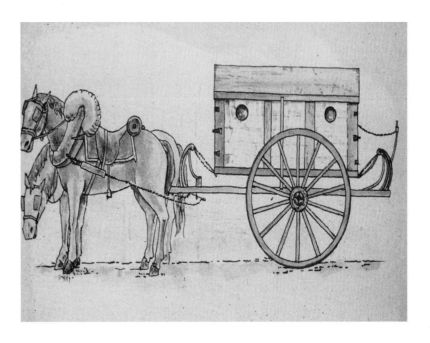

Figure 3 Larrey's Flying Ambulance.

infection in the postamputation period. He was a superb technical surgeon amputating the lower leg in 1.5 minutes and the upper arm in the same time.

Larrey had an understanding of problems that were unique to military surgery. Some of his contributions can best be appreciated by his efforts before Napoleon's Russian campaign. Larrey did not know which country Napoleon was planning to attack, and there was conjecture about an invasion of England. He left Paris on February 24, 1812, and was ordered to Mentz, Germany. Shortly thereafter, he went to Magdeburg and then on to Berlin, where he began preparations for the campaign, still not knowing precisely where the French army was headed. In his own words: "Previously to my departure from this capital, I organized six divisions of flying ambulances, each one consisting of eight surgeons. The surgeons-major exercised their divisions daily, according to my instructions, in the performance of operations, and the application of bandages. The greatest degree of emulation, and the strictest discipline, were prevalent among all the surgeons."

The nineteenth century may have been the century of enlightenment for surgical care in combat. This was partly because of better statistical reporting, but also because of major contributions of patient care, including the introduction of anesthesia. During the Crimean War (1853 to 1856), the English reported a mortality rate of 92.7% in cases of penetrating wounds of the abdomen, and the French a rate of 91.7%. During the American Civil War, there were 3,031 deaths among the 3,717 cases of abdominal penetrating wounds, a mortality of 87.2%.

The Crimean War was noteworthy in having been the conflict in which the French tested a number of local antiseptic agents. Ferrous chloride was found to be very effective against hospital-related gangrene, but the English avoided the use of antiseptics in wounds. It was also during the Crimean War that two further major contributions to combat medicine were introduced when Florence Nightingale emphasized sanitation and humane nursing care for combat casualties.

The Franco-Prussian War (1870 to 1874) was marked by terrible mortality and by the reluctance of some surgeons to use the wound antiseptics advocated by Lister. The mortality rate for thigh fractures was 65.8% in one series, and ranged from 54.2% to 91.7% in other series. Late in the conflict, surgeons finally accepted Lister's recommendations, and the mortality fell dramatically. Antiseptic surgery remains a major contribution of the nineteenth century.

During the Boer War (1899 to 1902), the British advised celiotomy in all cases of penetrating abdominal wounds. However, early results were abysmal, and a subsequent British military order called for conservative or expectant treatment.

Although Larrey was the first surgeon to introduce systematic principles in care of injured people during war, the American effort during the Civil War on the Union

TABLE 1	
CIVIL WAR DEATHS	
Union	
In battle	110,070
Disease	224,586
Accidents, suicides	24,872
Total	359,528
Confederacy	
In battle	94,000
Disease	164,000
Total	258,000
Total Union and Confederacy	617,528

and Confederate sides was remarkable. One of the most notable achievements was the publication of *The Medical and Surgical History of the War of the Rebellion* by the Union forces in six volumes. The only other national publications comparable with this were done by the French government in 1865 and the British government in 1854, 1855, and 1856 relating to the Crimean War (see Table 1). Although more soldiers died as a result of medical diseases than of penetrating injury, the overall death rate was staggering. The Union enlistments totaled 2,893,304 soldiers and the Confederacy enlistments were approximately between 1,277,890 and 1,406,180 soldiers. Of the 246,712 wounds resulting from weapons of war that were reported in the medical records, 245,790 were gunshot wounds and 922 were saber and bayonet wounds. The average Union mortality rate from gunshot wounds to the chest was 62% and for soldiers with abdominal wounds the mortality rate was 87%. Much of the organization for the Union effort is credited to Surgeon General William A. Hammond.

In one of the first reports of the war, Surgeon General Hammond showed that in a 4-month period (September to December 1862) soldiers with flesh wounds of the upper extremity had a very low mortality rate of 1.2% and soldiers with flesh wounds of the lower extremity had a mortality rate of 2%. In contrast, the mortality rate of soldiers with gunshot wounds of the humerus and upper arm was 30.7%; of the forearm, 21.9%; of the femur, 31.7%; and of the leg, 14.4%. These results were superior to those results reported for soldiers in the Franco-Prussian War, which was fought several years later. In addition to anesthesia, antiseptics were first used by Union medical officers predating Listerian surgery. There were at least three studies by Union surgeons during the Civil War documenting the effectiveness of antiseptics. In 1863, a study by Goldsmith showed that bromine reduced wound sepsis mortality to 2.6% in 308 patients with hospital gangrene. A comparable group of 30 patients in whom the antiseptic was not used had a 43.3% mortality rate. In 1864, Hackenberg reported to the Surgeon General that turpentine was effective in reducing hospital gangrene. In the third study by North in 1863, 60 patients with hospital gangrene had a mortality rate of

6.6%. North used "strong nitric acid." Unfortunately, these antiseptics were not used routinely and hospital gangrene was a major cause of death.

From a systems standpoint, hospitals were organized along Department of Army organization. For example, at Gettysburg almost every division had its own hospital grouped according to Army corps. These hospitals were located strategically near creeks to provide much needed water. When there were numerous regimental hospitals in one battle, they banded together to form a brigade hospital. The next level of care was the division hospital, and finally the general hospital. Many general hospitals, such as Carver, Stanton, and Campbell were located in or near Washington, DC. The south had one very large hospital, Chimborazo, located in Richmond. James B. McCaw was the medical director. The hospital had 6,000 beds and treated 76,000 patients during the war. The hospitals in Richmond included Windsor, which had 5,000 beds, and Jackson with 2,500 beds. According to the United States Sanitary Commission, Jackson Hospital was considered a model of excellent care.

There were numerous other accomplishments during the Civil War including treatment of open wounds. The Sanitary Commission of the US Army issued a directive "it is good practice to leave the wounds open to heal by granulation." Another accomplishment was the establishment of an ambulance corps. In September 1862, the Secretary of War, Stanton, directed Surgeon General William A. Hammond to form an ambulance corps. This was done under the guidance of Jonathan Letterman, who was at that time medical director of the Army of Potomac. One of the most important innovations during the Civil War was the introduction of nursing care modeled after that established by Florence Nightingale in the Crimean War. The Sanitary Commission was founded in 1861 primarily to assist the government in the care of the troops. The commission provided temporary shelters, clean bedding, wholesome food, and much needed nursing care. A leader in this movement was Clara Barton, who later founded the National Red Cross and the School of Nursing at Bellevue Hospital. In the South, Sally Louise Tompkins maintained the Robertson Hospital in Richmond, VA and was the only woman commissioned a Captain in the Confederate States Army.

The medical problems facing the surgeons of the Confederate States Army and Navy were not unique but were compounded by the lack of supplies and in some instances by poor administration. Similar to the surgeons of the Union Army, the surgeons of the Confederate Army had little or no training or experience in military medicine or surgery. The medical department of the regular Army of the new Confederate States of America was initiated by the provisional congress at Montgomery, AL on February 26, 1861. Unfortunately, the medical officers were indifferent toward the maintenance of surgical records and nothing comparable with the documentation of the Union Army exists. However, there is well-documented

data from the organization and administration of the Confederate Medical Department. For example, the original measure of the Provisional Congress provided for a medical department consisting of one surgeon general, four surgeons, and six assistant surgeons. The surgeon general would receive an annual salary of $3,000; whereas the surgeon's pay ranged from $162 to $200 per month and that of assistant surgeons ranged from $110 to $150 for the same period. Fleet surgeons received an annual stipend of $3,500, whereas a surgeon's remuneration for the first 5 years after the date of his commission was set at $2,200 or $2,000, depending on whether he was on sea duty. As noted in the preceding text, medical and surgical supplies were often difficult to obtain, particularly after the Union blockade was imposed on British ships bringing in such supplies. In many instances, surgical supplies were obtained when Union troops were captured.

In addition to the hospitals in Richmond, numerous principal hospitals were established in the Confederate states: these included Virginia (39 hospitals), North Carolina (21), South Carolina (12), Georgia (50), Alabama (23), Mississippi (three), Florida (four), and Tennessee (two). There were Naval hospitals in Richmond, Charleston, Wilmington, Savannah, and Mobile. The first surgeon general was David C. DeLeon. He was relieved of duty shortly after appointment and after a 2-week temporary replacement he was replaced by Samuel Preston Moore who served as surgeon general for the duration of the war. Moore had significant problems appointing and maintaining an efficient corps of medical officers. Nevertheless, the surgical results were equal to or better than those achieved in the Union army, which was far better supplied.

Hospital gangrene was as much a problem in the South as it was in the North. Wards and even entire hospitals were fumigated, but this did little to reduce the gangrene and erysipelas. Patients were given sesquichloride of iron and quinine by mouth. In some instances, wounds were treated with nitric acid, turpentine, alum, nitrate of silver, sulfate and chloride of zinc, tincture of iron, tincture of iodine, yellow wash, and Darby's solution. There was no unified treatment of wounds and the results varied from hospital to hospital. A particular blight on the confederate medical system was Andersonville prison, where hospital gangrene was rampant. The prison was established in 1864 to relieve some of the congestion associated with the prisons around the capitol of Richmond. There were only 13 doctors to care for 26,000 prisoners. Unfortunately, as Sherman and Grant began their stranglehold of Richmond and the march through Atlanta, the transportation and supply system deteriorated, which led to deprivation of food, medical supplies, and adequate housing for the prisoners. Of the 15,987 prisoners who were treated in Andersonville, 11,086 died.

The Union recognized the shortcomings of their organization of hospitals. The regimental hospital was not adequate to care for patients who were sick and injured. Furthermore, as the regiment moved on, they could not take the patients with them and it became necessary to establish independent hospitals that could receive the sick and wounded soldiers after the troops moved. These hospitals became known as general hospitals and were permanent. Furthermore, they provided an echelon of care where patients were evacuated from hospitals near the battle line back to safer areas and to hospitals that could provide additional definitive surgery and rehabilitation.

Between the Civil War and World War I there were very few advances in the development of trauma systems. The first report of civilian surgeons treating soldiers with gunshot wounds of the abdomen appeared as early as 1889 but represented cases (five patients of whom four survived) from 1881 to 1888. Nancrede reported three patients at the American Surgical Association meeting in 1887. Two of his patients died. Subsequent studies during the Spanish American War and the Boer War showed fairly abysmal results for surgical treatment of soldiers with abdominal gunshot wounds (see Table 2).

Relatively new technologic advances were designed and applied during World War I. Blood transfusions were used relatively extensively and to good advantage. Open treatment of contaminated wounds with delayed closure was accepted at the Inter-Allied Surgical Conference in March 1917. Motorized ambulances were employed, although care was often delayed by as many as 12 to 24 hours after injury. In this preantibiotic era, patients with wound sepsis were primarily treated with topical agents such as Dakin's solution. A commission was appointed to study shock and resuscitation and from these studies, Cannon published his classical work. As many as 8,538,315 soldiers were killed in action or died of wounds or disease. The US military force numbered 4,734,991 men. The number of American soldiers who died in battle was 53,402; this was exceeded by the number of deaths from disease, which was 63,114 (see Table 3).

As noted previously, the concept of shock was not articulated until 290 years after Harvey described the circulation. Seventeenth and eighteenth century surgeons thought of shock in very prosaic terms. LeDran defines shock as "reflections drawn from experiences with gunshot wounds." John Warren, another eighteenth century surgeon stated, "Shock is a momentary pause in the act of death"; and Samuel Gross thought that shock was "the manifestation of the rude unhinging of the machinery of life." The seminal work on shock came in 1918 when Walter B. Cannon, based on a 3-month study of casualties at Clearing Station 33 during World War I, provided a definition of shock that is applicable even today. He stated, "Wound shock occurs as a consequence of physical injury. It is characterized by a low venous pressure, a low or falling arterial pressure, a rapid, thready pulse, a diminished blood volume, a normal or increased erythrocyte count and hemoglobin percentage and peripheral blood (thereby differing from simple hemorrhage), a leukocytosis, an increased blood nitrogen, a reduced blood alkali, a lowered metabolism, a subnormal temperature, a cold skin moist with sweat, a pallid or grayish or slightly cyanotic appearance, also by this, by shallow and rapid respiration, often by vomiting and restlessness, by anxiety, changing usually to mental dullness, and by lessened

TABLE 3
SURGICAL MORTALITY FOR HEAD, CHEST, AND ABDOMINAL WOUNDS (US ARMY)

War	Head	Thorax	Abdomen
First World War cases	189	104	1,816
Percentage of mortality	40	37	67
Second World War cases	2,051	1,364	2,315
Percentage of mortality	14	10	23
Korean Conflict cases	673	158	384
Percentage of mortality	10	8	9
Vietnam Conflict cases	1,171	1,176	1,209
Percentage of mortality	10	7	9

TABLE 2
PERCENTAGE OF WOUNDED DYING OF WOUNDS (US ARMY)

War	Year	Number of Wounded	Percentage of Wounded Who Died of Wounds
Mexican War	1846–1848	3,400	15
American War between the States	1861–1865	318,200	14
Spanish-American War	1898	1,600	7
First World War (excluding gas)	1918	153,000	8
			8
Second World War	1942–1945	599,724	4.5
Korean Conflict	1950–1953	77,788	2.5
Vietnam Conflict	1965–1972	96,811	3.6

sensitivity." Cannon classified shock into three groups: compensated, partially compensated, and uncompensated. Cannon recognized that all organs autoregulate in response to a shock insult, and he thought that if the blood pressure could be kept above 80 mm Hg, that was all that was necessary, and the patient could be taken to the operating room, and the hemorrhage controlled. He recognized that delay in operation increased the mortality dramatically. His description of shock is matched only by his intellectual and sound approach to resuscitation. To understand from a historical perspective, we need to return to the work started by Wren and Lower. Following this work, it was in 1831 that W. B. O'Shaughnassy treated patients who had diarrhea with fluid and electrolyte solution. This work was confirmed in 1850 by Karl Schmidt, but all these authors were essentially ignored. Between 1880 and 1882, Sidney Ringer showed that potassium was a normal constituent of physiologic fluids. Nine years later, Rudolf Matas reported success with intravenous fluid administration again for diarrhea and cholera. In 1915, three pediatricians described the chemical composition of diarrhea fluid as compared with normal stools in infants. Thirteen years later, Alexis F. Hartmann, another pediatrician in St. Louis, described the chemical changes in the body as the result of certain diseases and developed fluid therapy based on the 1915 work. He could not dissolve bicarbonate, therefore gave lactate as a replacement. He gave this to seven medical students, and they had no undesirable side effects. Six years later, it was used in children suffering from cholera and dysentery, with a remarkable reduction in mortality from 60% to 10%. The next major hurdle was to use blood. Work by Nuttal, identified the blood groups. Arthus and Pages showed that calcium was necessary for clotting, and Hustin described citrate anticoagulation. It was Robinson who used citrated blood for combat casualties in World War I. The next major advance was the work by Shires in 1964, where he showed that in severe shock there was depletion of the extracellular space above and beyond the predicted and measured loss of blood in patients. This physiologic concept had been predicted by Cannon, but Shires' work showed conclusively with volume of distribution measurements the extent of the fluid loss.[1,2] Another pivotal clinical study was done during the World War II in northern Italy in 1943. In soldiers with severe shock, blood volumes were obtained showing a straight line relationship between the loss of blood and the degree of fall in blood pressure. The pulse rate did not correlate with the fall in blood volume; however, the quality of the pulse and pulse pressure did decrease. Unfortunately, modern resuscitation uses blood components and several crystalloid solutions. Normal saline has been shown to be harmful, and recent evidence in Iraq again reestablishes the principle that whole blood and judicious use of electrolytes is the optimal choice for resuscitation.

Between the Spanish American War and World War II surgeons in the United States began the foundations of modern trauma systems. In 1912, at a meeting of the American Surgical Association in Montreal, a committee of five was appointed to prepare a statement on the treatment of fractures. This led to a standing committee. One year later the American College of Surgeons (ACS) was founded, and in May 1922, the Board of Regents of the ACS started the first Committee on Fractures with Charles Scudder as chairman. This eventually became the Committee on Trauma. Another function begun by the College in 1918 was the Hospital Standardization Program, which evolved into the Joint Commission on Accreditation of Hospitals. One function of this Hospital Standardization Program was an embryonic start of a trauma registry with the acquisition of records of patients who were treated for fractures. In 1926, the Board of Industrial Medicine and Traumatic Surgery was formed. Therefore, it was the Hospital Standardization Program by the ACS, the Fracture Committee appointed by the ACS, the availability of patient records from the Hospital Standardization Program, and the new Board of Industrial Medicine and Traumatic Surgery that provided the seeds of a trauma system.

Between the two world wars, some significant advances were made in the development of trauma care for civilian patients. Böhler formed the first trauma care system for civilians in Austria in 1925. Although initially directed at work-related injury, it eventually expanded to include all accidents. Blood banking became routine and Fleming discovered penicillin in 1929. Unfortunately, excellent consistent trauma care remained elusive.

As with many wars, in World War II, lessons learned in previous conflicts had to be relearned. For example, it was necessary for Edward Churchill of Boston to go to the New York Times to publicize the shortage of blood before he could convince the War Department to provide blood in operating rooms (North Africa). In 1943, it was necessary for Major General Kirk to mandate that all military surgical personnel leave all amputation wounds open. Nevertheless, antibiotics made wound infections much less of a problem than in previous conflicts; finally Major General Ogilvie directed that all soldiers with colon injuries required colostomy. Transportation time for shifting the wounded soldiers from battalion aid stations to definitive care facilities was reduced to 4 to 6 hours with a subsequent reduction in mortality. Inadequately treated shock was still a problem and contributed to a high incidence of acute renal failure with attendant high mortality.

After World War II a serious attempt was made by the American Board of Surgery to form a new Board of Traumatic Surgery. This was mentioned in 1952, 2 years after the start of the Korean Conflict, and was considered at two subsequent meetings before it was abandoned.

Several advances in trauma system concepts were developed during the Korean Conflict. The introduction of air ambulances including helicopters reduced the time from injury to definitive surgical care to between 2 and 4 hours. Forward surgical hospitals (Mobile Army Surgical Hospital units) were introduced, which also reduced the time from injury to definitive surgical care. Vascular injuries were repaired, which reduced the number of amputations. Blood was used extensively, but unfortunately shock still remained a problem as did acute renal failure and the resulting high mortality.

Between the Korean Conflict and the Vietnam Conflict, many developments occurred that impacted heavily on the development of trauma care systems. The importance of ambulance services was addressed in a Scudder Oration by George Curry in 1958. Pioneer work by Moyer and Butcher, and Champion et al. led to the recognition that patients in shock lost more extravascular fluid into the intracellular space, explaining the high incidence of renal failure when not treated. This also confirmed the observations by Cannon during World War I.

The extensive use of helicopters in the Vietnam Conflict reduced the time from injury to definitive surgical care to <1 hour. By applying the resuscitation principles established by Shires, renal failure became an uncommon problem, but a new syndrome, *Da Nang lung*, became apparent. This reflected a misunderstanding of some of the principles espoused by Starling before World War I. Specifically, although crystalloid resuscitation was beneficial, overuse contributed to shock insult to the lung and reperfusion injury.

THE PRESENT

In order to set the stage for these next two sections, I would like to examine the impact of intentional and unintentional injuries on a worldwide basis. There is no better resource than the Global Burden of Disease Study by Murray and Lopez.[3] In their study, they divided the world into developed and developing regions, and subcategorized the world into eight distinct economic regions (see Fig. 4). In 1990, 5 million people worldwide were estimated to have died from intentional and unintentional injuries. The risk of injury death varies strongly by region, age, and sex. If one compares mortality from violent causes, in the European market economies, injuries caused approximately 6% of all deaths in 1990, compared with 9% to 11% in other regions. It is particularly striking and problematic in sub-Saharan Africa and Latin America where 12% to 13% of deaths are related to violence. It is primarily a problem in men, where it accounts for 16% to 17% of deaths. Worldwide, road traffic accidents are the number nine cause of death. In developed regions, road traffic accidents are the number eight cause of death, and self-inflicted injuries are the number nine. In developing regions of the world, road traffic accidents are number 10, and infectious diseases are number four, number six, number eight, and number nine (diarrheal diseases, tuberculosis, measles, and malaria).

In an attempt to quantify the burden of disease and injury of various human populations, Murray and Lopez have used the concept of Disability Adjusted Life Years

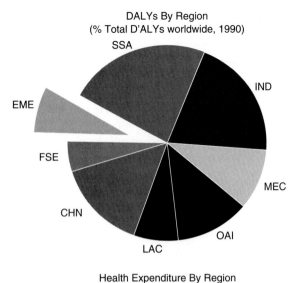

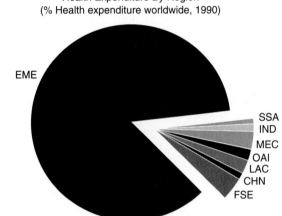

Figure 4 Results from the Global Burden of Disease Study. Courtesy of World Health Organization (Murray CJL, Lopez AD. *The global burden of disease*. Harvard University Press for the World Health Organization; 1996).

(DALY). A DALY is defined as the sum of life years lost due to premature mortality and years lived with disability adjusted for severity. This obviously gives us a different perspective of how injury impacts negatively on individual lives and societal costs. Worldwide in 1990, road traffic accidents were number nine as a cause of DALYs. In developed regions, the traffic accidents were the number four cause of DALYs, and self-inflicted injuries was number nine. In developing regions, road traffic accidents was number 11, war was number 16, violence was number 18, and self-inflicted injuries was number 19. Murray and Lopez conclude that injuries play a surprisingly large role in the burden of disease. Overall, it accounts for 14.5% of the burden in developed regions and 15.2% in developing regions. It is noteworthy that there is variability across the eight economic regions in the world (see Fig. 5).

The lessons learned in military conflicts of the twentieth century have been applied to trauma care of civilians. However, the evolution of trauma care systems for civilians

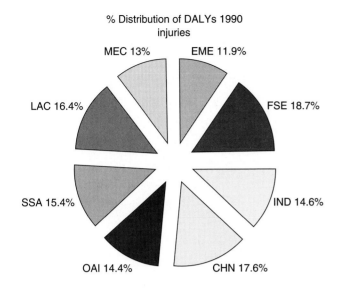

% Distribution of DALYs 1990
injuries

Regions G.B.D	
EME	Established Market Economies
FSE	Formerly Socialist Economies Europe
CHN	China
LAC	Latin America/Caribbean
OAI	Other Asia and Islands
MEC	Middle Eastern Crescent
IND	India
SSA	Sub-Saharan Africa

Figure 5 Distribution of DALYs 1990 within the eight economic regions of the Global Burden of Disease (Murray CJL, Lopez AD. *The global burden of disease.* Harvard University Press for the World Health Organization; 1996).

was accelerated in 1966, with the establishment of two trauma centers in the United States.[4] One of these trauma centers was started at San Francisco General Hospital under the leadership of William Blaisdell and the other was started at Cook County Hospital in Chicago under the leadership of Robert Freeark. The rationale for these two trauma centers was multiple. Titles 18 and 19 (Medicare and Medicaid) had just been introduced, and the old city and county hospitals were essentially without patients. At the same time, urban violence was on the rise, primarily as a consequence of the increase in urban ghettos and drug-related violence. The leaders of these two trauma centers recognized the need for a systematic approach to trauma care and the concept of a trauma center was pivotal to this overall need.

Shortly after these two centers were started, the political and administrative genius of R. Adams Cowley were combined when he established the Maryland system of trauma care, which eventually became a state-wide system. The most remarkable development of a state-wide trauma system occurred early in the 1970s in Germany.[5] At

that time, road traffic accidents accounted for 18,000 deaths annually. Since 1975, this has been reduced to approximately 7,000 (see Fig. 6).

One year later in 1976, the ACS Committee on Trauma developed a formal outline of injury care called Optimal Criteria for Care of the Injured Patient. Subsequently, task forces of the ACS Committee on Trauma met approximately every 4 years and updated their optimal criteria, which are now used extensively in establishing regional and state trauma systems. More recently, the ACS Committee on Trauma, working with the American College of Emergency Physicians, has developed some new guidelines for trauma care systems. Under the new model, the system of trauma care is inclusive rather than exclusive. In the old system, only patients who were injured severely were treated at a trauma center. Under the new system, all patients, including those with moderate and minor injuries, are part of the model trauma care plan. The model trauma care system cares for patients whether they are in an urban or a rural setting and the providers have been expanded to include teams and system management and prehospital care, trauma care facilities, and rehabilitation services. The components of this system include leadership; system development; legislation; finance; public information, education, and prevention; human resources; prehospital care with the subcomponents of communication; medical direction; triage and transport; definitive care, including the subcomponents of trauma facilities, interfacility transfer, and rehabilitation; and finally a quality improvement program that evaluates all of these components. Other contributions by the ACS Committee on Trauma include introduction of the advanced trauma life support (ATLS) courses, establishment of a national trauma registry (National Trauma Data Bank), and a national verification program. The latter is analogous to the old Hospital Standardization Program and verifies whether a hospital's trauma center meets the guidelines of the ACS.

Since 1984, more than 20 articles have been published showing that trauma systems benefit society by increasing the chances of survival when patients are treated in specialized centers.[6] In addition, two studies have shown that trauma systems also reduce trauma morbidity.[7,8] In 1988, a report card was issued on the current status and future challenges of trauma systems.[9] At that time an inventory was taken of all directors of state emergency medical services (EMSs) or directors of health departments who had responsibility over emergency and trauma planning. They were contacted by telephone in February 1987 and were asked eight specific questions on their state trauma system. Of the eight criteria, only two states, Maryland and Virginia, had all eight essential components of a regional trauma system. Nineteen states and Washington, DC, either had incomplete state-wide coverage or lacked essential components. Not limiting the

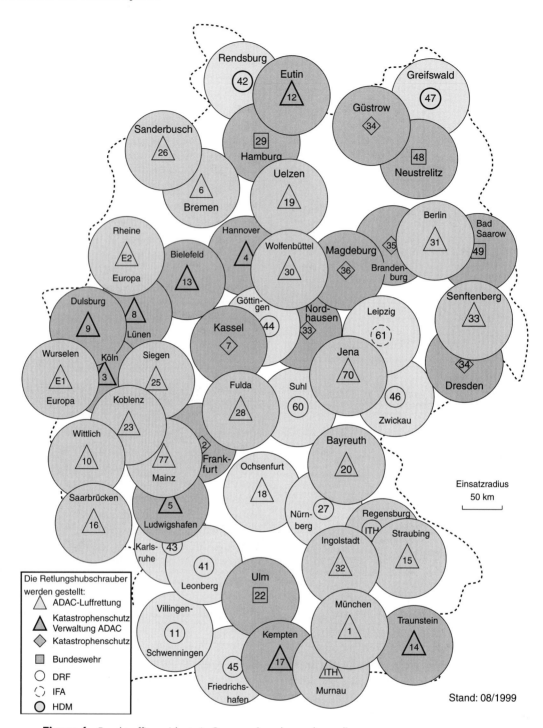

Figure 6 Road traffic accidents in Germany [need more legend].

number of trauma centers in a region was the most common deficient criterion.

In 1995, another report card was issued in the Journal of the American Medical Association.[10] This report card was an update on the progress and development of trauma systems since the 1988 report. It was a more sophisticated approach; it expanded the eight original trauma criteria and was more comprehensive. According to the 1995 report, five

states (Florida, Maryland, Nevada, New York, and Oregon) had all the components necessary for a state-wide system. Virginia no longer limited the number of designated trauma centers. An additional 15 states and Washington, DC had most of the components of a trauma system.

Bazzoli upgraded her 1995 report card at the Salishan Conference in 1998.[11,12] There are now 35 states that are actively engaged in meeting trauma system criteria. Many of these states have implemented their systems through Federal support of the Trauma Care Systems Planning and Development Act (Public Law 101-590). Although there has been constant growth and development of state-wide trauma systems, there are still underserved areas in the United States, particularly in the rural areas. This is unfortunate because one study has shown conclusively that a state-wide trauma center makes a major difference in trauma outcome in rural areas once a trauma system has been established. Finally in 2006, a more definitive study evaluating the efficacy of trauma center care on mortality showed that the mortality from trauma was 7.6% in designated trauma centers compared to 9.5% in hospitals that were not designated.[13] One year after discharge, the significance continued with a mortality of 10.4% versus 13.8%. This slight increase in the 1-year mortality most likely represents deaths in the elderly and late deaths from traumatic brain injury. Another study published in 2006 from Florida showed that in counties with a trauma center, the mean fatality rate was 50% less than in counties without a trauma center.[14] It can be seen from this data that the effectiveness of a trauma center is irrefutable as shown by these two recent studies and the data from Germany.

The centerpiece for the Canadian trauma system is represented by the 17 medical schools in the various provinces. Designation of trauma centers is up to the province, and in several instances, there is more than one trauma center per major metropolitan area. Like the United States, Canada has some very rural areas, particularly the plains of the provinces of Central Canada and the Rocky Mountain West. Prehospital care in these regions can be prolonged despite common 911 number and prehospital aircraft rescue systems.

There have been some studies from the Montreal McGill University regarding prehospital care, not only in Montreal but also extending from Quebec into Ontario provinces.[15,16] It was these studies that refuted the concept of trying to stabilize the patient at the scene and showed that physicians were not as effective as paramedics. At present, there is no country-wide designation and verification process. ATLS is taught to almost all eligible physicians, and critical care is provided both by surgeons and physicians.

A study from Mexico shows that 96% of seriously injured patients are transported to hospital by ambulance[17]. Fifty percent of the prehospital personnel are volunteers with little or no training; the remaining half has basic emergency medical technician training. In a 1999 study, it was shown that in some trauma centers in large cities that focused on care of the injured,[18] interestingly, only a few of the general surgeon attendings had taken ATLS courses, and essentially none of the residents had had ATLS training. In this particular article, it was pointed out that the primary problem in having functional and designated trauma centers was the lack of funding and resource commitments. More recently, a study has been done comparing trauma care delivery in three areas within

Mexico.[19] They used as their guidelines the World Health Organization (WHO)'s *Guidelines for Essential Trauma Care*.[3,4] The authors then did a study and evaluated these three areas by a "pre-review questionnaire" and a site-visit process. In total, five clinics, four small hospitals, and seven large hospitals were surveyed. The large hospitals averaged 1,000 to 9,000 trauma admissions annually. Using the WHO criteria, they showed that in the small hospitals, resources were extremely limited. They lacked pulse oximetry as an example. Large hospitals were fairly well supplied for acute resuscitation. However, most did report problems occasionally with blood supply. Using this study, which also looked at manpower, it was the intent of the investigators to show that the WHO criteria are reasonable, and using them would allow various Mexican states to improve trauma care. The WHO criteria will be discussed in more detail later in this section; nevertheless, some of the shortcomings are that the WHO lists specialists and tertiary care facilities in developing countries as "desirable" rather than as "essential". This might include image intensification and angiography. It is noteworthy that they found that quality improvement is mandated by the Secretariat of Health for the larger hospitals. The quality of these programs was not studied in detail in this particular paper and does represent a departure from the verification visits conducted by the ACS. The most positive thing about this study is that it shows that Mexico is addressing trauma as a serious public health problem, and physicians are addressing this from a systems standpoint, including human resources and equipment resources.

Costa Rica is a progressive country from the standpoint of health care.[22] In 1942, the *Caja Costarricense de Seguro Social* (CCSS) was passed into law. This is essentially a social health care system that covers 87.6% of the population and consists of 23 hospitals with 5,861 beds. Trauma is the fourth leading cause of death in Costa Rica, with both general surgeons and orthopaedic surgeons managing trauma patients. Because it is a social system, trauma care would be provided in one of the larger hospitals, but there are problems in the rural areas, prehospital care, and getting patients to these centers in a timely manner. Furthermore, there are only 154 general surgeons and 85 orthopaedic surgeons in the country. In the 2002 paper, it was admitted that the issue of surgical complications is difficult to analyze because statistics about this problem are underreported. A review of the literature does not catalog the number of surgeons who have taken ATLS training and critical care is somewhat fragmented among medical, anesthesia, and surgical specialties.

South America represents a very heterogeneous mix of trauma system and trauma care. One of the most violent areas in South America is Columbia. Trauma centers are present in Bogata, Medellín, Cali, and Cartagena. Violence is a particular problem secondary to drug trafficking, and the FARC (Revolutionary Armed Forces of Columbia) terrorize the eastern part of Columbia and contribute to the violence in the cities. Because of the differences in altitude and terrain it is extremely difficult to provide ambulance services to some of the more rural and remote parts of Columbia. Even within major cities, there is inconsistent ambulance service. At present, there is no state-wide trauma system.

In a recent study from Brazil, emergency care was assessed for victims of trauma.[23] This was a comparative study between two different periods before and after the introduction of modifications in prehospital care. The emergency unit of the University of Saõ Paulo is a hospital committed to trauma care. In addition to changing the prehospital system, they have also introduced ATLS. Despite these measures, the anticipated improvement in outcomes did not match that of the Major Trauma Outcome Study in North America. Nevertheless, it does show that with improvements in education and prehospital health care delivery, outcomes can be improved. Brazil is another country that has violence within the cities and a very large land mass with remote rural areas. There is no country-wide trauma system, and I believe it is fair to say that the universities within the major cities provide the bulk of trauma care. The same is true in Chili, where the economy has improved immensely within the last 30 years. Excellent trauma care is provided in the larger cities, particularly Santiago, but again, because of the geography with mountainous areas and a very long coastline, prehospital care is problematic.

In contrast to North America, the initial trauma care, resuscitation, and critical care in South America is not necessarily provided by general surgeons. Trauma surgeons are not recognized as a separate specialty except in Venezuela. Critical care is more often provided by adult intensivists trained in internal medicine. Many of the Latin American countries have also adopted ATLS and this is particularly true in Argentina. They have also introduced Prehospital Trauma Life Support.

Most of the countries in Latin America have embryonic or developing trauma systems, but the great majority of care is provided by university hospitals. In many instances, this is dependent on local leadership. In addition, the relatively recent organization, Pan American Trauma Society has fostered exchange of information and education between North America and South America.

The countries making up Europe also represent a potpourri of trauma care and trauma systems. Böhler formed the first civilian trauma system in Austria in 1925. The Birmingham Accident Hospital was founded in 1941. It continued to provide regional trauma care until recently. A study done by the Royal College of Surgeons in England showed that preventable death rate approached 33% of the 514 patients with major trauma admitted to hospital accident and emergency departments.[24] As a consequence, an experimental trauma center was started in Northwest Midland region.[25] The effectiveness of this regional trauma

system, in essence, failed. Multiple critiques were offered in the British Medical Journal on the reasons for this failure, including data analysis.[26-29] It was also pointed out in letters to the editor in British Medical Journal that in Glasgow, where 16% of all major trauma is penetrating injuries, the results approach those obtained in the United States. Similar results have been presented from Edinburgh.[30] More recently, trauma centers have been started in the London area, but there is no state trauma system in Great Britain.

One of the better trauma systems in Europe is the one that is found in Germany.[31-33] This system was established in 1975 and was based on the system that had been developed in Austria. This particular system has all four major components of acute care, including prehospital care, resuscitation units, critical care units, and rehabilitation units. The results are remarkable. The mortality has decreased by more than 50% since the establishment of this state-wide trauma system. Incorporation of East Germany into the German Republic has also shown an interesting comparison. The same decrease in mortality is now evident in the East German counties, despite an increase in the number of people injured because of increased use of automobiles. The German system also has a patient registry, and the patients are followed up from the time of injury until resolution of their care through rehabilitation.

Another excellent system in Europe is the one that is found in The Netherlands.[34] This system is based on 12 trauma centers that are geographically distributed across the country with both Level I and Level II centers. They have also focused on improvements in teaching, training (ATLS), regionalization, ambulance of care, mobile medical teams, trauma helicopters, categorization and designation of trauma centers, and rehabilitation. Like many trauma systems, the Dutch system is imperfect, but the physicians are addressing the shortage of intensive care beds and are trying to establish consistent and reasonable funding for their system.

Ari Leppäniemi has been a leader in studying trauma systems in Europe.[35] He points out that there are some major differences on how various countries have approached trauma as a public health and public policy problem. The French emergency system was developed primarily to respond to civilian, nontraumatic medical problems. As such, their prehospital care has a physician aboard the ambulances, and they attempt to stabilize the patient at the scene. This has not been a success with regard to trauma patients. The mortality within the French system is higher than it is in North America. A study that was done in Montreal, Canada, where the system was similar to the system in France, showed that prehospital outcomes were better when a paramedic transported the patient rapidly to the trauma center rather than try to stabilize the patient at the scene.[15] Leppäniemi has also cataloged the various European countries with regard to what constitutes a trauma surgeon and the countries that lack state mandated trauma systems. This has led to development of new systems in Sweden, Norway, Russia, Bosnia, and Herzegovina.

One of the major problems in Europe is there is not a concerted effort by the European Union (EU) to establish criteria for trauma systems nor to coordinate trauma care between countries within the EU.[36] Similarly, the EU does not have standards for prehospital care, nor is there a network of rehabilitation facilities that have standards and are peer reviewed. In theory, surgeons trained in one EU country should be able to cross the various national borders and practice surgery, including trauma care, within these different countries. Again, there is no standard for what constitutes a trauma surgeon, and in fact, trauma surgery is a potpourri of different models.[37] One model is exemplified by Austria, where trauma surgery is an independent specialty. Another model incorporates trauma surgical training into general surgery, and this includes France, Italy, The Netherlands, and Turkey. A third model is where most of the trauma training is given with orthopaedic surgery residency training. This would include Belgium[38] and Switzerland.[39] The largest model is where trauma surgery training is given to specific specialties without any single specialty having any major responsibility for trauma training, and this would include Denmark, Germany, Portugal, Estonia, Iceland, England, Norway, Finland, and Sweden. The differences in trauma systems, management, and education in Europe are highlighted in a report by Uranüs and Lennquist.[40] In their survey, they looked at trauma surgery as a specialty; helicopter transport, initial care of the patients, management in the emergency room (ER), management in the hospital, and availability of rehabilitation facilities. Surgical specialists' responses were also surveyed.

Between the Maghreb of Northern Africa and South Africa is a large expanse of land with several million people and essentially primitive trauma care. This part of the world may be the most challenging in regard to future development of trauma systems and trauma care.

The largest cities in Northern Africa are Cairo (7.5 million), Casablanca (3.5 million), Algiers (3.2 million), Rabat (1.3 million), and Tunis (1.9 million). These cities also have universities and large hospitals that do serve as trauma centers, but organized trauma systems are completely lacking, including prehospital care, particularly in remote areas.[41] In contrast, South Africa has seven well-established universities and several large hospitals in other metropolitan areas that serve essentially as Level I trauma centers. Their workload is extensive on a day-to-day basis because of the violence in this country. Resources to run these hospitals are increasingly difficult to obtain, and the system is susceptible to implosion. Rural trauma in South Africa is also problematic because of distances and allocation of resources. The land mass between South Africa and the Maghreb is essentially a developing part of the world where accidents, civil unrest, and civil war are a daily part of life.

Mock has done extensive study on sub-Saharan Africa and the resources available for trauma care.[42–44] Working with the WHO, he has come up with *Guidelines for Essential Trauma Care*. The strength of the publication is that it sets forth 14 core essential trauma care services that can reasonably be provided to every injured person in every country (see Table 4). Modeled after the Optimal Criteria document of the ACS, it looks at prehospital care, acute care, critical care, and rehabilitation possibilities in low income and middle income countries. In one of his studies, he looked at patients in Ghana with Injury Severity Scores >9 who were transported for care within the city of Kumasi[45–47]. Fifty-eight percent arrived by taxi, 22% by private car, 7% by bus, 2% by police, and 11% by unspecified means. None was transported by ambulance. For patients who lived in rural areas 100 miles from Kumasi, it was found that only 41% of the patients arrived at the hospital within 24 hours of their injury, 44% between 1 and 7 days, and 15% after 1 week. Similar data has been shown in Nigeria.[48–49] In Lagos, 55% of injured persons are transported in public vehicles, 35% are conveyed in private cars, and only 6% are moved in ambulances. Not surprisingly, <15% of the trauma patients seen in the Accident and Emergency Center of the Lagos University Teaching Hospital are critical emergencies. This suggests that the severely injured die at the scene of the accident.

South Africa has a population of 47 million, and although it has a relatively sophisticated medical system, it is currently being overwhelmed by trauma because of violence and increasing road traffic accidents. A recent study looked at the annual trauma case loads by provinces, and this is shown in Table 5.[50] Minimum case load per facility is >2,300, and the maximum is 11,000. This type of case load could clearly overwhelm prehospital, hospital, and any rehabilitation services available.

China and India are the two most populous nations in the world, yet trauma systems and trauma care are confined to very few communities, essentially the highly populated cities.[51–53] The farther one gets from a large city, the more sparse prehospital services are, as well as hospitals that specialize in trauma care. The same can be said for Asia, including Indonesia and Southwest Asia. In many instances, it is the university hospitals in these countries that provide trauma care for the severely injured. Many of the patients in the rural areas simply do not make it to these centers.

Japan is a densely populated series of islands with a fairly advanced and sophisticated health care system.[54–56] Again, the universities and large metropolitan hospitals serve as resources of care for the trauma patient. Prehospital care is excellent in most areas, and rehabilitation is an important component of care for the injured patient.

In Australia also a countrywide trauma system is emerging. They have now designated and verified 12 trauma centers (Level I and Level II) and have in the past had a unique way of approaching some of the rural prehospital

TABLE 4
AIRWAY MANAGEMENT

	Facility Level[a]			
	Basic	**GP**	**Specialist**	**Tertiary**
Airway: Knowledge and Skills				
Assessment of airway compromise	E[b]	E	E	E
Manual manoeuvres (chin lift, jaw thrust, recovery position, etc.)	E	E	E	E
Insertion of oral or nasal airway	D	E	E	E
Use of suction	D	E	E	E
Assisted ventilation using bag—valve—mask	D	E	E	E
Endotracheal intubation	D	D	E	E
Cricothyroidotomy (with or without tracheostomy)	D	D	E	E
Airway: Equipment and Supplies				
Oral or nasal airway	D	E	E	E
Suction device: at least manual (bulb) or foot pump	D	E	E	E
Suction device: powered: electric/pneumatic	D	D	D	D
Suction tubing	D	E	E	E
Yankauer or other stiff suction tip	D	E	E	E
Laryngoscope	D	D	E	E
Endotracheal tube	D	D	E	E
Oesophageal detector device	D	D	E	E
Bag—valve—mask	D	E	E	E
Basic trauma pack	D	E	E	E
Magill forceps	D	D	E	E
Capnography	I	D	D	D
Other advanced airway equipment	I	D	D	D

[a]In this and subsequent resource matrices, the following key is used to indicate different levels of facilities; Basic: outpatient clinics, often staffed by non-doctors; GP: hospitals staffed by general practitioners; Specialist: hospitals staffed by specialists, usually including a general surgeon; Tertiary: tertiary care hospitals, often university hospitals, with a wide range of specialists.
[b]Items in the resource matrices are designated as follows:
E: essential; D: desirable PR: possibly required; I: irrelevant (not usually to be considered at the level in question, even with full resource availability).
From Guidelines for essential trauma case, Courtesy or World Health Organsiation, 2004.

TABLE 5
ANNUAL TRAUMA CASELOADS IN SOUTH AFRICA BY PROVINCE

	No. of Facilities Supplying Caseloads	**No. of Reported Cases**	**Mean No. of Cases per Facility (Standard Error)**
	(1)	(2)	(3)
Eastern Cape	33	150,705	4,567 (1,321)
Free state	21	79,626	3,619 (1,181)
Gauteng	18	198,406	11,023 (2,386)
KwaZulu-Natal	38	200,144	5,267 (1,106)
Mpuma langa	18	41,759	2,320 (376)
Northern Cape	15	50,414	3,361 (996)
Northern province	22	52,112	2,369 (1,058)
North West Province	14	36,954	2,640 (1,091)
Western Cape	30	236,032	7,868 (1,065)
All provinces		1,046,152	4,742 (284)

Modified from Matzopoulos RG, Prinsloo MR, Bopape JL, et al. *Estimating the South African trauma caseload as a basis for injury surveillance.* South African Medical Research Council; 1999.

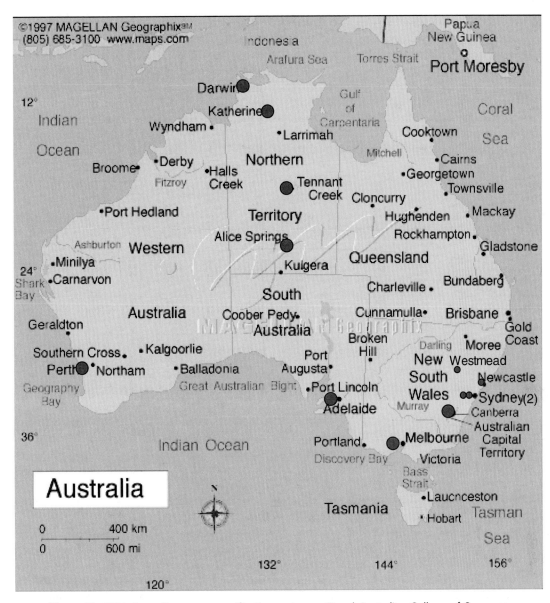

Figure 7 2006 Australian trauma verification system – (Royal Australian College of Surgeons, *Personal communication*, 2007.)

care. The flying doctor and flying surgeon programs were extremely innovative. New Zealand consists of two long narrow islands with four population centers and two medical schools (see Fig. 7). There is no country-wide trauma system; however, the two universities provide excellent trauma care, as do Wellington and Christchurch.

As pointed out in the first section of this chapter, trauma care and war are inextricably linked. It would be inappropriate not to review the current issues facing the US military with regard to providing care for US military troops in current "military actions" around the world.[57] These include Afghanistan (Operation Enduring Freedom) and Iraq (Operation Iraqi Freedom). Special Forces and troops are also involved in the Philippines and sub-Saharan Africa. Approximately 30 years ago, the

Department of Defense (DOD) adopted a "total force" policy, which occurred at a time when there was a transition to an all-volunteer active duty military force.[58] As part of this planning process, there were a number of force structure plans that looked at manpower and the needs to simultaneously engage in two major regional conflicts (MRCs). The Army has its input through total army analysis (TAA), and the penultimate TAA has been criticized by the General Accounting Office (GAO) in that there are not enough active duty and reserve components to meet a first MRC in a timely way. This is certainly highlighted by the current problems in Iraq and President Bush's decision to surge new forces into theater. This will overextend the active duty forces such that it is now doubtful if we should even consider a second MRC. Forces needed for an MRC would arrive late, and insufficient reserve components cannot make this up in a timely way. This is a particular problem in supplying medical support for two MRC scenarios.

Since Operation Desert Storm, more problems have been identified in military medicine. There were several reports from the GAO that documented problems with medical shortage and medical capability.[59-63] The four general categories outlined by the GAO report were mobilization and deployment of medical personnel, problems with medical supplies, doctrinal employment of hospitals, and problems with patient evaluations and regulations. The GAO reports documented that many personnel were either incompletely trained or untrained for wartime missions. The GAO found that air evacuation support during Operation Desert Storm was neither adequate nor responsive, particularly at night. This difficulty with the evacuation system extended into evacuation from theater. There appeared to be contention between services regarding roles, responsibility, and equipment. The end result was a poorly responsive system. Finally, there were two other problems that occurred during Operation Desert Storm that ran contrary to previous conflicts. The first is that there was no in-theater research. The second was that there were no civilian surgeons appointed as consultants to monitor health care in theater.

After September 11, 2001, even more demands and challenges were placed on the military in providing support for medical planning, disaster medical planning, and curbing terrorism. This led the Army, in 2002, to come up with TAA09, which now has the army force structure requirement, including Homeland Security, deterrence of aggressor, major combat operations, and small scale contingency. Using all volunteer active duty medical resources and reserves makes it almost impossible to provide medical support for all of these requirements and still try to maintain the two MRC requirements.

After the adverse reports on Operation Desert Storm from the GAO, the DOD did make some changes to address combat care capability.[64] Military attending surgeons and residents can now train in several civilian trauma centers. In addition, a few military academic centers are caring for civilian trauma injuries. Problems have been identified. We do not have an evaluation of the effectiveness of civilian trauma training for military personnel. The experience is not continuous, and we do not know whether exposure on an *ad hoc* basis is consistent with maintaining skills and experiences. In those few military academic health centers that care for injured patients, there has been one failure to meet ACS verification standards.

In theory, reserve units are a major resource for medical and nursing personnel in combat or conflict. Reserve unit trauma training is essentially nonexistent. An additional demand for medical personnel, particularly surgeons, is the disaster medical assistance teams (DMATs) currently under the Department of Health and Human Services. They are supposed to respond to civilian disaster, either secondary to natural events or terrorism. Surgeons, anesthesiologists, and nurses may or may not have continuous trauma experience in their civilian jobs. How do we maintain trauma experience and skills in active duty reserve and DMATs? An option is to support the concept that all military academic health centers should be actively involved in caring for civilian trauma injuries. This would maintain the skills of those surgeons, anesthesiologists, and nursing personnel that treat trauma patients on a continuous basis. DOD has had an opportunity to implement such a program, but it has failed to do so.

DOD has not addressed training of reserve personnel in trauma care. We do not even have requirements or normative standards that define what our expectations are for a nurse or surgeon in a reserve unit who may be activated to treat a trauma patient.

THE FUTURE

In order to anticipate what is needed for the future management of trauma care and development of trauma systems, we must return to the Burden of Disease Study by Murray and Lopez. They have projected that in 2020 on a world-wide basis, road traffic accidents will be the number three cause of DALYs. War injuries will be the number eight cause of DALYs. In developed regions, road traffic accidents will be number five, and self-inflicted injuries will be the number 10 cause of DALYs. In developing regions of the world, such as sub-Saharan Africa, road traffic accidents will be the number two cause of DALYs, and war injuries will be the number eight cause of DALYs. If one examines the 10 leading causes of death in 2020 worldwide, road traffic accidents will be the number five cause, and self-inflicted injuries will be number nine cause. In the developed regions of the world, self-inflicted injuries will be the number eight cause of death, and road traffic accidents number nine. In the developing regions of the world, road traffic accidents will be the number four cause of death (see Tables 6, 7, 8, 9, 10).

In discussing this section entitled "Future," I will continue to use the model developed by Murray and Lopez and breakdown the world into two parts: the developed and the developing. I believe it is fair to say, with few exceptions, that the developed world has an imperfect system of trauma care. It has been reported in the United States that 44% of patients in most states do not have access to a trauma system or trauma care (Level I or Level II).[65] In the United States, many states are not willing to provide the resources necessary to have a system or to complete it. I have previously commented that our national health care system in the United States is dysfunctional and contributes problematically to a cohesive and complete development of a nation-wide trauma system.[66] There are other fundamental problems, including work force shortages and even lack of some health resources. In 2002,

TABLE 6
LEADING CAUSES OF DEATH, WORLD, DEVELOPED AND DEVELOPING REGIONS, BY SEX, 1990

	Both Sexes			Males			Females		
Rank	Cause	Deaths (thousands)	Cumulative %	Cause	Deaths (thousands)	Cumulative %	Cause	Deaths (thousands)	Cumulative %
World									
	All Causes	50,467		All Causes	26,692		All Causes	23,775	
1	Ischaemic heart disease	6,260	12.4	Ischaemic heart disease	3,126	11.7	Ischaemic heart disease	3,134	13.2
2	Cerebrovascular disease	4,381	21.1	Lower respiratory infections	2,196	19.9	Cerebrovascular disease	2,359	23.1
3	Lower respiratory infections	4,299	29.6	Cerebrovascular disease	2,022	27.5	Lower respiratory infections	2,103	32.0
4	Diarrhoeal diseases	2,946	35.4	Diarrhoeal diseases	1,533	33.3	Diarrhoeal diseases	1,414	37.9
5	Conditions arising during the perinatal period	2,443	39.8	Conditions arising during the perinatal period	1,266	37.8	Conditions arising during the perinatal period	1,177	42.1
6	Chronic obstructive pulmonary disease	2,211	43.7	Chronic obstructive pulmonary disease	1,214	42.2	Chronic obstructive pulmonary disease	997	45.4
7	Tuberculosis	1,960	45.8	Tuberculosis	1,166	44.9	Tuberculosis	794	47.6
8	Measles	1,058	47.9	Road traffic accidents	730	47.6	Measles	512	49.7
9	Road traffic accidents	999	49.8	Trachea, bronchus and lung cancers	708	49.6	Malaria	400	51.6
10	Trachea, bronchus and lung cancers	945	51.7	Measles	547	51.6	Self-inflicted injuries	330	53.3
Developed Regions									
	All Causes	10,912		All Causes	5,567		All Causes	5,345	
1	Ischaemic heart disease	2,659	24.7	Ischaemic heart disease	1,297	23.3	Ischaemic heart disease	1,398	26.1
2	Cerebrovascular disease	1,427	37.8	Cerebrovascular disease	561	33.4	Cerebrovascular disease	867	42.4
3	Trachea, bronchus and lung cancers	523	42.6	Trachea, bronchus and lung cancers	399	40.5	Lower respiratory infections	205	46.2
4	Lower respiratory infections	385	46.1	Chronic obstructive pulmonary disease	205	44.2	Breast cancer	174	49.4
5	Chronic obstructive pulmonary disease	324	49.1	Lower respiratory infections	180	47.5	Colon and rectum cancers	142	52.1

(continued)

TABLE 6 (CONTINUED)

		Both Sexes			Males			Females		
Rank		Cause	Deaths (thousands)	Cumulative %	Cause	Deaths (thousands)	Cumulative %	Cause	Deaths (thousands)	Cumulative %
6		Colon and rectum cancers	277	51.6	Road traffic accidents	165	50.4	Trachea, bronchus and lung cancers	124	54.4
7		Stomach cancer	241	53.8	Self-Inflicted injuries	143	53.0	Chronic obstructive pulmonary disease	119	56.6
8		Road traffic accidents	222	55.8	Stomach cancer	142	55.5	Diabetes mellitus	107	58.6
9		Self-Inflicted injuries	193	57.6	Colon and rectum cancers	135	58.0	Stomach cancer	99	60.5
10		Diabetes mellicus	176	59.2	Cirrhosis of the liver	110	59.9	Dementia and other degenerative and hereditary CNS disorders	70	61.8
Developing Regions										
		All Causes	39,554		All Causes	21,124		All Causes	18,430	
1		Lower respiratory infections	3,915	9.9	Lower respiratory infections	2,016	9.5	Lower respiratory infections	1,899	10.3
2		Ischaemic heart disease	3,565	18.9	Ischaemic heart disease	1,829	18.2	Ischaemic heart disease	1,736	19.7
3		Cerebrovascular disease	2,954	26.4	Diarrhoeal diseases	1,529	25.4	Cerebrovascular disease	1,492	27.8
4		Diarrhoeal diseases	2,940	33.8	Cerebrovascular disease	1,461	32.4	Diarrhoeal diseases	1,410	35.5
5		Conditions arising during the perinatal period	2,361	38.7	Conditions arising during the perinatal period	1,217	37.7	Conditions arising during the perinatal period	1,144	40.2
6		Tuberculosis	1,922	43.4	Tuberculosis	1,137	42.5	Chronic obstructive pulmonary disease	878	44.5
7		Chronic obstructive pulmonary disease	1,887	46.1	Chronic obstructive pulmonary disease	1,009	45.2	Tuberculosis	785	47.3
8		Measles	1,058	48.7	Road traffic accidents	565	47.8	Measles	512	50.0
9		Malaria	856	50.9	Measles	546	50.3	Malaria	399	52.4
10		Road traffic accidents	777	52.8	Malaria	457	52.4	Self-Inflicted injuries	280	54.6

From Murray CJL, Lopez AD. *The global burden of disease.* Harvard University Press for the World Health Organization; 1996.

TABLE 7
TEN LEADING CAUSES OF DALYS IN 2020

	Both Sexes			Males			Females		
Rank	Disease or Injury	DALYs (thousands)	Cumulative %	Disease or Injury	DALYs (thousands)	Cumulative %	Disease or Injury	DALYs (thousands)	Cumulative %
World									
	All causes	1,388,836		All causes	796,144		All causes	592,692	
1	Ischaemic heart disease	82,325	5.9	Ischaemic heart disease	53,238	6.7	Unipolar major depression	51,075	8.6
2	Unipolar major depression	78,662	11.6	Road traffic accidents	49,719	12.9	Ischaemic heart disease	29,087	13.5
3	Road traffic accidents	71,240	16.7	Cerebrovascular disease	36,819	17.6	Cerebrovascular disease	24,573	17.7
4	Cerebrovascular disease	61,392	21.1	Chronic obstructive pulmonary disease	33,023	21.7	Chronic obstructive pulmonary disease	24,563	21.8
5	Chronic obstructive pulmonary disease	57,587	25.3	Unipolar major depression	27,587	25.2	Road traffic accidents	21,520	25.4
6	Lower respiratory infections	42,692	28.4	Violence	25,274	28.3	Lower respiratory infections	19,508	28.7
7	Tuberculosis	42,515	31.4	War	23,934	31.4	Tuberculosis	19,414	32.0
8	War	41,315	34.4	Lower respiratory infections	23,184	34.3	War	17,381	34.9
9	Diarrhoeal diseases	37,097	37.1	Tuberculosis	23,101	37.2	Diarrhoeal diseases	16,445	37.7
10	HIV	36,317	39.7	Diarrhoeal diseases	20,652	39.8	Conditions arising during the perinatal period	16,070	40.4
Developed Regions									
	All causes	1,60,534		All causes	95,126		All causes	65,408	
1	Ischaemic heart disease	17,997	11.2	Ischaemic heart disease	12,316	12.9	Unipolar major depression	6,423	9.8
2	Cerebrovascular disease	9,875	17.4	Cerebrovascular disease	5,568	18.8	Ischaemic heart disease	5,681	18.5
3	Unipolar major depression	9,825	23.5	Trachea, bronchus and lung cancers	5,508	24.6	Cerebrovascular disease	4,307	25.1
4	Trachea, bronchus and lung cancers	7,253	28.0	alcohol use	5,211	30.1	Osteoarthritis	3,416	30.3
5	Road traffic accidents	6,852	32.3	Road traffic accidents	4,812	35.2	Dementia and other degenerative and	3,414	35.5

(continued)

TABLE 7 (CONTINUED)

Rank	Both Sexes Disease or Injury	DALYs (thousands)	Cumulative %	Males Disease or Injury	DALYs (thousands)	Cumulative %	Females Disease or Injury	DALYs (thousands)	Cumulative %
6	Alcohol use	6,088	36.1	Unipolar major depression	3,401	38.7	Road traffic accidents	2,039	38.7
7	Osteoarthritis	5,580	39.5	Chronic obstructive pulmonary disease	3,164	42.0	Chronic obstructive pulmonary disease	1,746	41.3
8	Dementia and other degenerative and hereditary CNS disorders	5,506	43.0	Self-inflicted injuries	2,935	45.1	Trachea, bronchus and lung cancers	1,746	44.0
9	Chronic obstructive pulmonary disease	4,910	46.0	Osteoarthritis	2,164	47.4	Breast cancer	1,733	46.6
10	Self-inflicted injuries	3,879	48.4	Dementia and other degenerative and hereditary CNS disorders	2,092	49.6	Diabetes mellitus	1,360	48.7
Developing Regions									
	All causes	1,228,302		All causes	7,01,018		All causes	5,27,284	
1	Unipolar major depression	68,837	5.6	Road traffic accidents	44,907	6.4	Unipolar major depression	44,652	8.5
2	Road traffic accidents	64,388	10.8	Ischaemic heart disease	40,922	12.2	Ischaemic heart disease	23,406	12.9
3	Ischaemic heart disease	64,328	16.1	Cerebrovascular disease	31,252	16.7	Chronic obstructive pulmonary disease	22,817	17.2
4	Chronic obstructive pulmonary disease	52,677	20.4	Chronic obstructive pulmonary disease	29,859	21.0	Cerebrovascular disease	20,266	21.1
5	Cerebrovascular disease	51,518	24.6	Unipolar major depression	24,185	24.4	Road traffic accidents	19,481	24.8
6	Tuberculosis	42,364	28.0	Violence	23,911	27.8	Tuberculosis	19,382	28.4
7	Lower respiratory infections	41,107	31.4	War	23,285	31.1	Lower respiratory infections	18,766	32.0
8	War	40,190	34.6	Tuberculosis	22,982	34.4	War	16,905	35.2
9	Diarrhoeal disease	36,960	37.6	Lower respiratory infections	22,341	37.6	diarrhoeal diseases	16,379	38.3
10	HIV	33,962	40.4	Diarrhoeal diseases	20,581	40.5	HIV	15,605	41.3

DALYs, Disability Adjusted Life Years
From Murray CJL, Lopez AD. *The global burden of disease.* Harvard University Press for the World Health Organization; 1996.

TABLE 8

TEN LEADING CAUSES OF DEATH IN 2020

		Both Sexes			Males			Females	
Rank	Disease or Injury	Deaths (thousands)	Cumulative %	Disease or Injury	Deaths (thousands)	Cumulative %	Disease or Injury	Deaths (thousands)	Cumulative %
World									
	All Causes	68,337		All Causes	38,788		All Causes	29,549	
1	Ischaemic heart disease	11,107	16.3	Ischaemic heart disease	6,077	15.7	Ischaemic heart disease	5,030	17.0
2	Cerebrovascular disease	7,698	27.5	Cerebrovascular disease	3,977	25.9	Cerebrovascular disease	3,721	29.6
3	Chronic obsgtructive pulmonary disease	4,726	34.4	Chronic obstructive pulmonary disease	2,620	32.7	Chronic obstructive pulmonary disease	2,107	36.7
4	Lower respiratory infections	2,472	38.1	Trachea, bronchus and lung cancers	1,809	37.3	Lower respiratory infections	1,197	40.8
5	Trachea, bronchus and lung cancers	2,415	41.6	Road traffic accidents	1,623	41.5	Tuberculosis	986	44.1
6	Road traffic accidents	2,338	45.0	Tuberculosis	1,310	44.9	Road traffic accidents	715	46.5
7	Tuberculosis	2,296	48.4	Lower respiratory infections	1,275	48.2	Trachea, bronchus and lung cancers	606	48.6
8	Stomach cancer	1,588	50.7	Stomach cancer	1,069	50.9	Diarrhoeal diseases	550	50.5
9	HIV	1,250	52.5	Liver cancer	885	53.2	HIV	522	52.2
10	Self-inflicted injuries	1,229	54.3	Violence	841	55.4	Stomach cancer	519	54.0
Developed Regions									
	All causes	13,505		All causes	7,345		All causes	6,160	
1	Ischaemic heart disease	3,259	24.1	Ischaemic heart disease	1,730	23.6	Ischaemic heart disease	1,529	24.8
2	Cerebrovascular disease	1,705	36.8	Cerebrovascular disease	760	33.9	Cerebrovascular disease	945	40.1
3	Trachea, bronchus and lung cancers	804	42.7	Trachea, bronchus and lung cancers	577	41.8	Trachea, bronchus and lung cancers	227	43.8
4	Chronic obstructive pulmonary disease	551	46.8	Chronic obstructive pulmonary disease	345	46.5	Lower respiratory infections	219	47.4

(continued)

TABLE 8 (CONTINUED)

	Both Sexes			Males			Females		
Rank	Disease or Injury	Deaths (thousands)	Cumulative %	Disease or Injury	Deaths (thousands)	Cumulative %	Disease or Injury	Deaths (thousands)	Cumulative %
5	Lower respiratory infections	429	50.0	Stomach cancer	217	49.4	Chronic obstructive pulmonary disease	206	50.7
6	Colon and rectum cancers	364	52.7	Lower respiratory infections	210	52.3	Breast cancer	183	53.7
7	Stomach cancer	332	55.1	Colon and rectum cancers	198	55.0	Colon and rectum cancers	167	56.4
8	Self-inflicted injuries	234	56.9	self-inflicted injuries	171	57.3	Diabetes mellitus	149	58.8
9	Diabetes mellitus	228	58.5	Prostate cancer	163	59.5	Stomach cancer	115	60.7
10	Road traffic accidents	221	60.2	Cirrhosis of the liver	155	61.6	Dementia and other degenerative and hereditary CNS disorders	109	62.5
Developing Regions									
	All causes	54,832		All causes	31,443		All causes	23,390	
1	Ischaemic heart disease	7,848	14.3	Ischaemic heart disease	4,347	13.8	Ischaemic heart disease	3,501	15.0
2	Cerebrovascular disease	5,993	25.2	Cerebrovascular disease	3,217	24.1	Cerebrovascular disease	2,776	26.8
3	Chronic obstructive pulmonary disease	4,175	32.9	Chronic obstructive pulmonary disease	2,275	31.3	Chronic obstructive pulmonary disease	1,901	35.0
4	Tuberculosis	2,273	37.0	Road traffic accidents	1,475	36.0	Tuberculosis	979	39.1
5	Road traffic accidents	2,117	40.9	Tuberculosis	1,294	40.1	Lower respiratory infections	978	43.3
6	Lower respiratory infections	2,043	44.6	Trachea, bronchus and lung cancers	1,231	44.0	Road traffic accidents	642	46.1
7	Trachea, bronchus and lung cancers	1,611	47.5	Lower respiratory infections	1,065	47.4	Diarrhael diseases	548	48.4
8	Stomach cancer	1,256	49.8	Stomach cancer	853	50.1	HIV	509	50.6
9	Diarrhoeal diseases	1,208	52.0	Liver cancer	832	52.8	self-inflicted injuries	454	52.5
10	HIV	1,160	54.1	Violence	795	55.3	War	426	54.4

From Murray CJL, Lopez AD. *The global burden of disease.* Harvard University Press for the World Health Organization; 1996.

TABLE 9
CAUSES OF DALYS (PERCENTAGE OF TOTAL) IN DESCENDING ORDER, 1990

		World		Developed Regions			Developing Regions		
Rank	Disease or Injury	DALYs (thousands)	Cumulative %	Disease or Injury	DALYs (thousands)	Cumulative %	Disease or Injury	DALYs (thousands)	Cumulative %
	All Causes	1,379,238		All Causes	160,994		All Causes	1,218,244	
1	Lower respiratory infections	112,898	8.2	Ischaemic heart disease	15,950	9.9	Lower respiratory infections	110,506	9.1
2	Diarrhoeal diseases	99,633	7.2	Unipolar major depression	9,780	6.1	Diarrhoeal diseases	99,168	8.1
3	Conditions arising during the perinatal period	92,313	6.7	Cerebrovascular disease	9,425	5.9	Conditions arising during the perinatal period	89,193	7.3
4	Unipolar major depression	50,810	3.7	Road traffic accidents	7,064	4.4	Unipolar major depression	41,031	3.4
5	Ischaemic heart disease	46,699	3.4	Alcohol use	6,446	4.0	Tuberculosis	37,930	3.1
6	Cerebrovascular disease	38,523	2.8	Osteoarmritis	4,681	2.9	Measles	36,498	3.0
7	Tuberculosis	38,426	2.8	Trachea, bronchus and lung cancers	4,587	2.9	Malaria	31,705	2.6
8	Meales	36,520	2.7	Dementia and other degenerative and hereditary CNS disorders	3,816	2.4	Ischaemic heart disease	30,749	2.5
9	Road traffic accidents	34,317	2.5	Self-inflicted injuries	3,768	2.5	Congenital anomalies	29,441	2.4
10	Congenital anomalies	32,921	2.4	Congenital anomalies	3,480	2.4	Cerebrovascular disease	29,099	2.4
11	Malaria	31,706	2.3	Chronic obstructive pulmonary disease	3,365	2.3	Road traffic accidents	27,253	2.2
12	Chronic obstructive pulmonary disease	29,136	2.1	Conditions arising during the perinatal period	3,120	2.1	Chronic obstructive pulmonary disease	25,771	2.1
13	Falls	26,680	1.9	Schizophrenia	3,106	1.9	Falls	24,232	2.0
14	Iron-deficiency anaemia	24,613	1.8	Diabetes mellitus	3,022	1.9	Iron-deficiency anaemia	23,465	1.9
15	Protein-energy malnutrition	20,957	1.5	Bipolar disorder	2,543	1.6	Protein-energy malnutrition	20,758	1.7
16	War	20,019	1.5	Falls	2,448	1.5	War	18,868	1.6
17	Self-inflicted injuries	18,967	1.4	Lower respiratory infections	2,392	1.5	Tetanus	17,513	1.4
18	Tetanus	17,517	1.3	Cirrhosis of the liver	2,345	1.5	Violence	15,632	1.3
19	Violence	17,472	1.3	Colon and rectum cancers	2,298	1.4	Self-inflicted injuries	15,199	1.3
20	Alcohol use	16,661	1.2	Obsessive-compulsive disorder	2,098	1.3	Drownings	14,819	1.2

DALYs, Disability Adjusted Life Years
From Murray CJL, Lopez AD. *The global burden of disease.* Harvard University Press for the World Health Organization; 1996.

TABLE 10
TEN LEADING CAUSES OF DALYS AT AGES 15–44 YEARS, 1990

Rank	Both Sexes Disease or Injury	DALYs (thousands)	Cumulative %	Males Disease or Injury	DALYs (thousands)	Cumulative %	Females Disease or Injury	DALYs (thousands)	Cumulative %
World									
	All Causes	419,144		All Causes	217,153		All Causes	201,991	
1	Unipolar major depression	42,972	10.3	Road traffic accidents	15,554	7.2	Unipolar major depression	27,651	13.7
2	Tuberculosis	19,673	14.9	Unipolar major depression	15,321	14.2	Tuberculosis	8,736	18.0
3	Road traffic accidents	19,625	19.6	Alcohol use	13,096	20.2	Iron-deficiency anaemia	7,508	21.7
4	Alcohol use	14,848	23.2	Violence	11,040	25.3	Self-inflicted injuries	7,095	25.2
5	Self-inflicted injuries	14,645	26.7	Tuberculosis	10,937	30.4	Bipolar disorder	6,453	28.4
6	Bipolar disorder	13,189	29.8	War	7,899	34.0	Obstructed labour	6,419	31.6
7	War	13,134	32.9	Self-inflicted injuries	7,550	37.5	Chlamydia	5,964	34.6
8	Violence	12,955	36.0	Bipolar disorder	6,736	40.6	Schizophrenia	5,896	37.5
9	Schizophrenia	12,542	39.0	Schizophrenia	6,646	43.6	Maternal sepsis	5,367	40.1
10	Iron-deficiency anaemia	12,511	42.0	Falls	5,098	46.0	War	5,235	42.7
Developed Regions									
	All Causes	61,707		All Causes	36,943		All Causes	24,764	
1	Unipolar major depression	7,574	12.3	Alcohol use	4,677	12.7	Unipolar major depression	4,910	19.8
2	Alcohol use	5,477	21.2	Road traffic accidents	4,167	23.9	Schizophrenia	1,450	25.7
3	Road traffic accidents	5,304	29.7	Unipolar major depression	2,664	31.1	Road traffic accidents	1,137	30.3
4	Schizophrenia	3,028	34.7	Self-inflicted injuries	2,072	36.8	Bipolar disorder	1,106	34.7

		DALYs	%		DALYs	%		DALYs	%
5	Self-inflicted injuries	2,641	38.9	Schizophrenia	1,578	41.0	Obsessive-compulsive disorders	933	38.5
6	Bipolar disorder	2,241	42.6	Drug use	1,404	44.8	Alcohol use	801	41.7
7	Drug use	1,829	45.5	Violence	1,196	48.1	Osteoarthritis	783	44.9
8	Obsessive-compulsive disorders	1,652	48.2	Ischaemic heart disease	1,160	51.2	Chlamydia	599	47.3
9	Osteoarthritis	1,634	50.9	Bipolar disorder	1,135	54.3	Self-inflicted injuries	569	49.6
10	Violence	1,507	53.3	HIV	911	56.7	Rheumatoid arthritis	549	51.8
Developing Regions									
	All Causes	357,437		All Causes	180,211		All Causes	177,227	
1	Unipolar major depression	35,398	9.9	Unipolar major depression	12,658	7.0	Unipolar major depression	22,740	12.8
2	Tuberculosis	19,451	15.3	Road traffic accidents	11,387	13.3	Tuberculosis	8,703	17.7
3	Road traffic accidents	14,321	19.4	Tuberculosis	10,747	19.3	Iron-deficiency anaemia	7,135	21.8
4	War	12,382	22.8	Violence	9,844	24.8	Self-inflicted injuries	6,526	25.5
5	Iron-deficiency anemia	12,033	26.2	Alcohol use	8,420	29.4	Obstructed labour	6,033	28.9
6	Self-inflicted injuries	12,004	29.5	War	7,448	33.6	Chlamydia	5,364	31.9
7	Violence	11,448	32.7	Bipolar disorder	5,601	36.7	Bipolar disorder	5,347	34.9
8	Bipolar disorder	10,948	35.8	Self-inflicted injuries	5,478	39.7	Maternal sepsis	5,226	37.8
9	Schizophrenia	9,514	38.5	Schizophrenia	5,068	42.5	War	4,934	40.6
10	Alcohol use	9,371	41.1	Iron-deficiency anaemia	4,898	45.3	Abortion	4,856	43.4

DALYs, Disability Adjusted Life Years

From Murray CJL, Lopez AD. *The global burden of disease.* Harvard University Press for the World Health Organization; 1996.

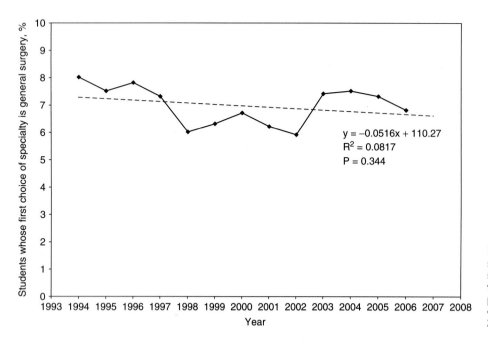

Figure 8 Trend in medical school student applications to general surgery residency programs (Modified from Bland KI, Isaacs G. Contemporary trends in student selection of medical specialties. *Arch Surg.* 2002;137:259–267).

Cooper published an article on physician supply.[67] He predicted that there would be a shortage of physicians that would not be relieved by physician extenders, including nurse practitioners and physicians' assistants. A follow-up paper in 2004 stated that by 2020, the deficit would be as great as 200,000 physicians, primarily specialists, particularly in the surgical fields, but also gastroenterology and cardiology.[68] This shortage will have a profound negative effect in several areas—including rural surgery, military surgery, and care for the elderly—and as noted in the ACS' White Paper, it is already a major problem in trauma and emergency surgery.[66] Cooper's work does not take into consideration that one fourth of all physicians in the United States are currently international medical graduates.

The shortage of trauma surgeons exists now and will be worse in 2010 when the Baby Boomers begin to reach age 65. The average age of a general surgeon in the United States is 52 years. There has been a recent decline in applicants to general surgery programs, and this is further influenced by gender[69] (see Figs. 8 and 9). Graduating medical students are at least 50% women and rightly so, but very few apply to general surgery (7% or a little >500 applicants). Part of this disinterest in general surgery seems to be the hours required, part of it is lifestyle, and part of it is a desire to combine a professional career with a traditional role as a parent, and it also reflects that the general surgery programs have not provided a structure whereby surgical residents can do both.

In addition, general surgery continues to become more fragmented and specialized, but the general surgery specialists have one commonality: they do not want to take trauma calls. In a 1990 study, Esposito polled all surgeons in Washington State about treating trauma patients (response rate of 50%).[70] The top four factors influencing the decision not to treat trauma patients were time commitment, compensation, dissimilar reimbursement, and a perceived increased medical/legal risk.

In the ACS' White Paper, similar findings were found.[66] The report indicated that surgeons are taking calls 5 to 10 times a month; they may do this at two or more hospitals, and the hospital bylaws, which typically require surgeons to participate in on-call panels, may allow surgeons to opt out. There was a perception by surgeons that they were being sued by patients who were first seen in the Emergency Department.

It is important to emphasize that the growing crisis in patient access to emergency surgical care exists now. In 2002, the Lewin Group of the American Hospital Association showed there is a nonavailability of neurosurgeons, orthopaedic surgeons, general surgeons, and plastic surgeons to cover emergency department on-call panels.[66] This was further emphasized by the Schumacher Group and two similar surveys carried out by the American College of Emergency Physicians in 2005. In that particular study, they showed that approximately three fourths of emergency department medical directors believe that they have inadequate on-call specialist coverage, which was an increase over 2004 data. The surgeons involved include orthopaedics, plastic surgeons, neurosurgeons, otolaryngologists, and hand surgeons. This is compounded by the flat or decreasing rate of general surgeons who are completing training, as well as neurosurgeons. Orthopaedic surgeons have increased the number of residents admitted to their programs.

A problem that is not mentioned in the White Paper is that specialty surgeons and general surgeons are increasingly asking for exorbitant on-call pay. These monetary requests range anywhere from $1,000 per night to >$7,000 in some of the subspecialties such as neurosurgery.

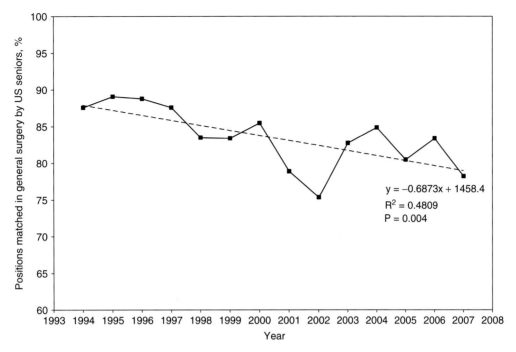

Figure 9   Positions matched in general surgery residency programs (Modified from Bland KI, Isaacs G. Contemporary trends in student selection of medical specialties. *Arch Surg.* 2002;137: 259–267).

A major problem by 2010 will be the 30% increase in the elderly population. It used to be that the peak in death rate from injury was in the age range of 16 to 24 years. We are now seeing a bimodal distribution, with an increased death rate in the elderly (see Fig. 10). They are more active, and unfortunately the mortality rate for an Injury Severity Score >15 is 3.5 times higher than the rate for their younger counterparts. They spend more time in the intensive care unit and do not have a good return to independent living status or quality of life after acute trauma care.[71]

The lack of general surgeons also negatively affects the DOD and its need for surgeons. Approximately 20% of DOD surgeons are active duty surgeons; 80% must come from the reserves. Unfortunately, young surgeons do not

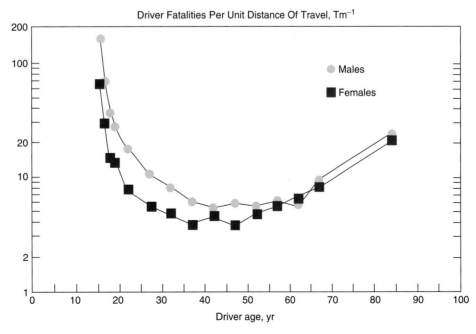

Figure 10   Driver fatalities per unit distance of travel.

join the reserves. Studies conducted by the US GAO after Operation Desert Storm show that surgeons were not being trained properly for trauma, particularly active duty surgeons; however, the DOD, as mentioned earlier, has recently improved this over the last 4 years.

One solution is for DOD and Health and Human Services, working with Homeland Security, to increase by one third the surgical, anesthesia, and nursing personnel in ACS–verified Level I and Level II trauma centers. These individuals would then belong to a reserve unit and serve as a reserve manpower pool. They would be subject to instant call-ups for DOD, DMAT, or Homeland Security needs. This would be similar to pilots who fly commercial jets and belong to reserve units and can be called to active duty. Holland has been doing this for approximately 10 years, and it works well for them. Another solution would be to encourage surgeons, anesthesiologists, and nurses to join military reserve units. Cancellation of medical school debts might be an incentive. Conscription is highly unlikely, secondary to current attitude in Congress; however, renewal of a "Berry-Plan" program might be possible. Somehow, we have to convince surgeons, anesthesiologists, and nurses that if our government commits to a war, a small scale contingency operation, or anti-terrorism activities, and our soldiers are placed in harm's way, they deserve the very best combat care possible. Objection to these governmental actions on a political basis should not be a consideration for medical and nursing personnel.

Another negative impact on trauma care is that many trauma centers are closing or downgrading their level of care. Since 2003, "dumping" has become an increasing problem for Level I and Level II trauma centers. Emergency medical treatment and active labor act (EMTALA), which was originally designed to prevent "dumping," now actually contributes to "dumping." This phenomenon is characterized by a community hospital ER physician calling the trauma centers and speaking to an emergency physician or surgeon because they have a trauma case that they "cannot provide care for" either because of lack of personnel or because the patient's case is too complex. Many of these patients reach the trauma center; they are observed and then discharged the following morning.

Another major problem in trauma care is that rehabilitation beds are not available after a severe injury. The GAO did a study showing that only one in eight patients with traumatic brain injury received appropriate rehabilitation following their acute care.[72] Rehabilitation is particularly a problem in patients who have no insurance.

A particularly vexing problem is the importation of physicians and nurses to the United States. In many ways, this confirms Friedman's book, *The World is Flat*.[73] He points out that the United States is already outsourcing pharmaceuticals, and we even outsource some surgical procedures. We have been importing health care professionals for many years — primarily nurses, but more recently physicians and surgeons. In order to fill general surgery slots,

18% to 23% are being filled by foreign medical graduates. There are many disadvantages to a "world is flat" model. Most importantly, this involves a "brain drain" from the developing countries that need these physicians most.

Another problem exists with regard to importing surgeons from these countries. The only test they must pass is the US Licensing Medical Examination. This examination does not include knowledge or psychomotor skills related directly to surgery. Knowledge tests could be developed that would be similar to the ones that the American Board of Surgery administers, and with virtual simulators, psychomotor skills could be tested. These virtual simulators, however, are quite costly. Many of these imported surgeons can go to rural hospitals and be credentialed by hospital medical staff. This not only reflects the shortage of general surgeons in rural areas but also highlights the need for competency testing. Probably the biggest disadvantage of "The world is flat" approach is that it is a short-term solution. It does not ensure a steady output of nurses, physicians, and/or specialists in the United States. For example, by 2020, the United States will be short of 800,000 nurses. At present, 140,000 applicants to US nursing schools are turned down each year because there are not enough positions due to lack of nursing instructors. Importing nurses is *not* the answer.

Another vexing issue is one of gender. At the present time, female medical students mostly have not been attracted to the field of surgery. This is potentially the largest pool of talented individuals that could help solve the shortage of general surgeons. In order to attract them into the specialty, we will have to solve lifestyle issues, such as protected time, both during training and during their practice. At the University of Melbourne in Australia, women residents are given extra time to finish their surgical training. Emergency Medicine has increasingly become an attractive career choice for women because they can do shift work. The concept of the emergency general surgeon who would do trauma and emergency surgery is most likely going to be accomplished by full-time surgeons who do shift work in acute care hospitals. On the basis of a 40-hour work week, full-time surgeons work approximately 160 hours a month. To assign 12 or 13 shifts of 12 hours each would come close to this, which means that within a 2-week period, a surgeon could fulfill his or her workload and have the next 2 weeks off. (There are obviously many variations of this model.) This is precisely what occurs in Emergency Medicine. Hospitals could participate by providing 24-hour childcare for physicians and nurses. There are probably few perks that would be more attractive from the standpoint of maintaining a professional career and a traditional role as a parent.

Canada is rich with resources. It is difficult to understand why they have not moved toward a nationwide trauma system. The central plains and mountainous west coast do have a problem with remote frontier and rural prehospital care. I think that most economists would consider Mexico being a middle-income developing country. It is quite probable that over the next 10 to 15 years, as their economy improves, so will the trauma system across the country. Costa Rica, with its excellent commitment to health care for all citizens, could easily have a nationwide trauma system. Other countries within Central America and South America will have a mixed solution to state-wide trauma systems. This will partly depend on natural resources and the economy, but the need is extreme in some areas with increased violence, such as Colombia and Brazil. It will also depend on how stable the government is and the degree of corruption. The Pan American Trauma Association could apply the "Essentials" of the WHO to the various countries and determine what optimal criteria each country could reach most easily. These essentials would be updated on a regular basis, and as the economies improve, trauma should be a high priority and reflect the additional resources.

The solutions in Europe will be somewhat problematic. I believe it is safe to say that there are no overall standards agreed upon in the EU to address what constitutes optimal prehospital care. The Royal College of Surgeons of Edinburgh has a faculty of prehospital care, which is setting the standards and verifying it by a peer review process. These could easily be applied across the EU, but at this time there is not a concerted effort to do so. I think it is also safe to say that medical education, and specifically surgical training, varies markedly from country to country. The same could be said for those who are involved in critical care and the standards adopted by them. The current approach to training a trauma surgeon in the EU is variable, and different specialists tend to provide this training. This is not necessarily bad, but there should be some standards which constitute the bare minimum in order for surgeons to go across the various borders and practice within this standard of care. Within Europe, rehabilitation is also variable, and yet, one of the best examples of an excellent trauma rehabilitation program exists in Israel. This might represent a model for the EU. The best place to start would be for the EU to develop a document similar to the ACS' Optimal Criteria that would apply to all countries. It cannot be overemphasized that all three components of a trauma system (prehospital, acute care, and rehabilitation) must have some type of review and verification.

Eastern Europe represents a challenge in development of trauma care and trauma systems. Western Turkey is well on its way to having an excellent trauma system; however, Eastern Turkey has yet to benefit from such planning and resources. As the economies in the Balkan states improve, it is inevitable that trauma systems will develop, but not necessarily at the same rate in the various countries. With the collapse of the former Soviet Union, the European portion of Russia has more resources, but there is no state-wide system of trauma care or trauma systems.[74] The Asian portion of the former Soviet Union is quite problematic because of the huge distances and sparse resources. Again, it would be worthwhile to implement the *Pre-hospital Trauma Care Systems* and *Guidelines for Essential Trauma Care* that have been developed by the WHO.

Japan evaluated in 2002 whether they had preventable deaths. It was shown to be approximately 40% of expired trauma patients. This led to the development of Japan Pre-hospital Evaluation and Care Program and the Japan Advanced Trauma Evaluation and Care Program for Physicians. A trauma registry has been started, and the process of designation of a trauma care hospital is well on its way nationwide.

China is not only in an economic growth countrywide but also in addressing health care. They have four military hospitals in Shanghai, Beijing, Guangzhou, and Chongqing that serve a fairly large military need and also the families of individuals who belong to the military. What is lacking is a system of trauma care for a population of more than one billion people. The boom in the economy is leading to increased automobile use and the predictable increase in road traffic crashes. Industrial accidents are also increasing. Fortunately, the boom in the economy has led to a significant surplus in government funds. Hopefully, some of this money will be spent on development of prehospital, hospital, and rehabilitation facilities that will serve a very large land mass. They have already developed a "120" EMS system, but it covers less than half of the population.

In addition to the four cities mentioned in the preceding text, Hong Kong has a more developed system of trauma care.[75] This is a city of 6.4 million in a total area of 1,100 km². They have a fairly sophisticated prehospital system, and initially, the ambulance attendants were trained to the first aid standard of the *St. John First Aid Manual* of the United Kingdom. More recently, they have advanced this training to an EMA-II modeled after British Columbia, Canada. Trauma management is essentially Basic Trauma Life Support. They have 33 ambulances and 173 ambulance men. In addition to prehospital care, they have a hospital authority with 14 accident and emergency departments. There are 11 major acute care hospitals, but only 8 have neurosurgeons in attendance. The two large university hospitals, Queen Mary Hospital (The University of Hong Kong) and Chinese University Hospital are Level I facilities. In addition, there is an ACS Hong Kong Chapter that provides ATLS courses. More than 180 doctors have attended this course. Rehabilitation exists in a number of centers.

Unfortunately, India lacks an organized trauma care system, and has been characterized as being in a "nascent stage."[76] It is agreed that approximately 10.1% of all deaths in India are due to accidents and injuries. Prehospital care is described as "virtually nonexistent in most rural and semi-urban areas." There is no minimal education and training standards for paramedics. Acute trauma care is offered by some government hospitals, corporate hospitals, and small clinics. University hospitals provide a reasonable level of care, but this is not universal. Of the 205 medical schools, 20 are private, and 60% of the state-run medical schools have deficiencies in infrastructure, facilities, and faculty.[77] On the positive side, India is in a major economic growth, and by using the WHO Guidelines, could easily establish the essentials for both prehospital and acute care facilities.

In Thailand, the number of trauma-related deaths has dramatically increased, and is second only to heart diseases. An effort is being made to improve care within the various provinces and to provide high-quality EMS and trauma care, but this is not consistent across the country.[78]

Malaysia, a country of 20 million people, is also addressing trauma care and trauma systems.[79] Prehospital care lacks cohesiveness, and in many instances, tow car operators often transport the injured to hospital, but not necessarily one with trauma care resources. This is particularly true in rural areas. Trauma care in the large university hospitals in the heavily populated areas such as Kuala Lumpur is quite good, but the farther one gets from a large metropolitan area, the more problematic it becomes. Rehabilitation centers are few, and patients with traumatic brain injury and spinal cord injury suffer as a consequence. Most of the resources are in Peninsula Malaysia.

Indonesia has a significant problem with trauma system development because of the multiple islands (>18,000). Indonesia is on a very active tectonic plate, and they have a number of natural disasters. In addition, they have a number of terrorist activities. The Asian Surgeons' Association is active in trying to establish a "118" Emergency Ambulance Service, and to also develop prehospital EMS. These are embryonic. Trauma care, even in the large urban areas, can also be problematic because of lack of ambulances and resources to care for road traffic accidents and to deal with the ongoing violence, particularly terrorism. The WHO Essentials of Pre-hospital Care and Pre-hospital Systems would be a reasonable guideline to use in prehospital and trauma care facilities.

Australia is well on its way to having a country-wide trauma system (Fig. 7). New Zealand has yet to systematize its prehospital and acute trauma care. New Zealand has two large university hospitals that provide Level I care. There are also a number of institutions that could provide either Level I community care, or more probably, Level II care. Rehabilitation units do exist. Prehospital care is only problematic from the standpoint of very remote areas and very long islands with a long coastline and mountains.

The last area to be discussed is Africa. The Northern Crescent of Africa is somewhat problematic from the standpoint of getting the various countries to cooperate and come up with a system of trauma care that transcends the various state borders. Many of these countries serve as attractions for tourists, and some have natural resources that provide more resources for their economy. Violence and terrorism are a problem. As noted earlier, the university hospitals serve as a focus for trauma care, but once into the rural area, problems exist with prehospital transport and transfer to higher centers of care. Rehabilitation is disjointed, and in many instances, inadequate. South Africa has a trauma system; however, it borders on being overwhelmed.[80]

Between this Northern Crescent and South Africa is sub-Saharan Africa. Almost all of these countries would qualify as low income developing countries. There is no area on earth that exemplifies the problems with health care, and in particular, the concept that Friedman extols in his book, *The World is Flat*. Billions of dollars have been put into sub-Saharan Africa over the last few years. For example, the Bill and Melinda Gates Foundation has given away $6.6 billion for global health programs; the great majority of which is going to Africa. The United States has increased its overseas development assistance to $27.5 billion in 2005. One would think that this would lead to better health care, but this has been challenged. Laurie Garrett, writing in *Foreign Affairs*, makes a very persuasive argument that this may actually be harmful.[81] She argues that this money is paying for largely uncoordinated efforts and is directed mostly at specific, high profile diseases rather than at public health in general. She also argues that aid is tied to short-term numerical targets and is not being used to develop a sustained health care system. She points out that there are no built-in methods of assessing efficacy or sustained ability of many of these programs. It is compounded further by corrupt governments that siphon away up to 80% of the dollars intended for health care projects. A typical example is Ghana. In 2006, the World Bank reported that approximately half of all funds donated for health efforts in sub-Saharan Africa never reached the clinics and hospitals at the end of the line. Yet another problem, which is called "stove-piping," is where money is put down through narrow channels relating to a particular program or disease. Most of these are infectious diseases, and very little money is going for problems such as trauma.

Another problem is that the nongovernment organizations that are involved in some of these health care programs in sub-Saharan Africa are actually contributing to making the problems worse. They often try to recruit doctors and nurses to come back to developed countries. In Ghana, out of 871 medical officers, 604 have left the country and now practice overseas. Similarly, in Zimbabwe, 1,200 doctors were trained in the 1990s, but only 360 remain in the country today. In Zambia, only 50 of the 600 doctors trained over the last 40 years remain. Kenya has lost 1,670 physicians and 3,900 nurses to emigration. Garrett argues that preventing the "brain drain" by bolstering the salaries of local officials would be enormously expensive, and even that might not work.

The answer to the above problem seems somewhat straightforward. At present, global health improvement is being funded at $20 billion annually. This money cannot go just for pet projects, such as human immunodeficiency virus (HIV), tuberculosis, and malaria. Some, if not most, of this money should go to build the infrastructure for a public health system, including ambulances, clinics, and hospitals. Obviously, I would push for a system of trauma care. Such a solution would probably not cost that much more in dollars on an annual basis, particularly if one could control the corruption and waste. Using the WHO Guidelines, sub-Saharan Africa could very well solve its trauma problems. In addition, communication would have to be addressed. Although there is a designated 999 number for emergencies, rural areas have almost no access to phone communication or even radio communication. Similar to Europe, there should be an organization within the various African states that could establish triage criteria that would transcend national borders. All physicians should be encouraged to be trained in ATLS. Professional organizations could be an impetus for the various national governments to make training a priority and to establish criteria based on the WHO's essentials that all countries should meet. Finally, working with the WHO and the United Nations, the brain drain of physicians and nurses must be halted. Developed countries must agree not to recruit health care professionals, and instead, should cooperate with the developing countries to provide education and training.

SUMMARY

It is clear from this review and history that trauma care and trauma systems are in their infancy worldwide. Some countries are ahead of others, but very few countries, if any, can state that they have a perfect system. I think it can also be appreciated that in a global economy, the medical world is flat too. Professional resources, such as doctors and nurses, can be recruited, but this is not in the best interest of the countries recruiting, and certainly not for the countries that these professionals come from.

SUGGESTED READINGS

Breasted JH. *The Edwin Smith surgical papyrus.* Chicago: University of Chicago Press; 1930.

Cannon WB. *Traumatic shock.* New York: Appleton & Company; 1923.

Churchill ED. *Surgeon to soldiers. Wound shock and blood transfusion.* Philadelphia: JB Lippincott Co; 1972:51.

Cunningham HH. *Doctors in gray: The confederate medical service.* Louisiana State University Press; 1958.

Diamond J. *Guns, germs and steel: The fates of human societies.* New York: WW Norton and Co; 1999.

Fraser J. The evolution of abdominal surgery of war. In: Bailey H, ed. *Surgery of modern warfare.* Baltimore: Williams & Wilkins; 1944.

Harvey W. *Exercitatio anatomica de motu cordis et sanguinis in animalibus (The Keynes english translation of 1928). Classics of Medicine Library.* Birmingham: LB Adams; 1978.

Hunter J. *A treatise on the blood, inflammation, and gunshot wounds. Classics of Medicine Library.* Birmingham: LB Adams; 1982.

Larrey DF. *Memoirs of military surgery and campaigns of the french armies,* Vol 1. Classics of Surgery Library. Birmingham: Gryphon Editions; 1985.

Leonardo RA. *History of surgery. American surgery.* New York: Froben Press; 1943:297–330.

Loria FL. *Historical aspects of abdominal injury.* Springfield: Charles C. Thomas; 1968.

Majno G. *The healing hand: Man and wound in the ancient world.* Cambridge: Harvard University Press; 1975.

The medical and surgical history of the war of the rebellion, 6 Vol. 2nd Issue. Washington, DC: Government Printing Office; 1875.

Nuland SB. *The origins of anesthesia. Classics of Medicine Library.* Birmingham: LB Adams; 1983.

Packard FR. *Life and times of ambroise paré.* New York: Paul B. Hoeber; 1921.

Rutkow IM. *Bleeding blue and gray: Civil war surgery and the evolution of American medicine.* New York: Random House; 2005.

Wangensteen OH, Wangensteen SD. *The rise of surgery from emperic craft o scientific discipline.* Minneapolis: University of Minnesota Press; 1978.

REFERENCES

1. Shires T, Brown FT, Canizaro P, et al. Distributional changes in extracellular fluid during acute hemorrhagic shock. *Surg Forum.* 1960;11:15.
2. Shires T, Coln D, Carrico J, et al. Fluid therapy in hemorrhagic shock. *Arch Surg.* 1964;88:688.
3. Murray CJL, Lopez AD. *The global burden of disease.* Harvard University Press for the World Health Organization; 1996.
4. Trunkey DD. History and development of trauma care in the United States. *Clin Ortho Relat Res.* 2000;374:36–46.
5. Trunkey DD. Trauma. *Sci Am.* 1983;249:29–35.
6. Cales RH, Trunkey DD. Preventable trauma deaths: A review of trauma care system development. *JAMA.* 1985;254:1059–1063.
7. Smith RF, Frateschi L, Sloan EP, et al. The impact of volume on outcome in seriously injured trauma patients: Two years experience of the Chicago trauma system. *J Trauma.* 1990;30:1066–1076.
8. Mullins RJ, Veum-Stone J, Hedges J, et al. Influence of a state-wide trauma system on location of hospitalization and outcome of injured patients after institution of trauma system in an urban area. *JAMA.* 1994;271:1919–1924.
9. West JG, Williams MJ, Trunkey DD, et al. Trauma systems: Current status – future challenges. *JAMA.* 1988;259:3597–3600.
10. Bazzoli GJ, Madura KJ, Cooper GF, et al. Progress in the development of trauma systems in the United States. *JAMA.* 1995;273: 395–401.
11. Bazzoli GJ. Community-based trauma system development: Key barriers and facilitating factors. *J Trauma.* 1999;47(Suppl 3):S22–S24.
12. MacKenzie EJ. Review of evidence regarding trauma system effectiveness resulting from panel studies. *J Trauma.* 1999;47(Suppl 3):S34–S41.
13. MacKenzie EJ, Rivara FP, Jurkovich GJ, et al. A national evaluation of the effect of trauma center care on mortality. *N Engl J Med.* 2006;354(4):366–378.
14. Papa L, Langland-Orban B, Flint L, et al. Assessing effectiveness of a mature trauma system: Association of trauma center presence with lower injury mortality rate. *J Trauma.* 2006;61(2):261–266; discussion 266–267.
15. Liberman M, Mulder D, Sampalis JS, et al. Multicenter Canadian study of prehospital trauma care. *Ann Surg.* 2003;237(2):161–162.
16. Liberman M, Mulder DS, Jurkovich GJ, et al. The association between trauma system and trauma center components and outcome in a mature regionalized trauma system. *Surgery.* 2005;137(6):647–658.
17. Arreola-risa C, Mock CN, Jurkovich GJ, et al. *Trauma care systems in urban Latin America: The priorities should be prehospital and emergency room management. J Trauma.* 1995;39:457–462.
18. Arreola-Risa C, Speare JOR. Trauma in Mexico. *Trauma Q.* 1999; 14(3):211–220.
19. Arreola-Risa C, Mock C, de Boer M, et al. Evaluating trauma care capabilities in Mexico with the World Health Organization Guidelines for Essential Trauma Care publication. *Pan Am J Pub Health.* 2006;19(2):94–103.
20. World Health Organization. *Prehospital trauma care systems.* World Health Organization; 2005.
21. World Health Organization. *Guidelines for essential trauma care.* World Health Organization; 2004.
22. Feoli E, Badilla V, Bermudez M, et al. Surgery in Costa Rica. *Arch Surg.* 2002;137:1435–1440.
23. Scarpelini S, de Andrade JI, Passos ADC. The TRISS method applied to the victims of traffic accidents attended at a tertiary

level emergency hospital in a developing country. *Sci Direct.* 2006;37(1):72–77.

24. Yates DW, Woodford M, Hollis S. Preliminary analysis of the care of injured patients in 33 British hospitals: First report of the United Kingdom major trauma outcome study. *Br Med J.* 1992;305:237–240.
25. Nicholl J, Turner J. Effectiveness of a regional trauma system in reducing mortality from major trauma: Before and after study. *Br Med J.* 1997;315:1349–1354.
26. Oakley PA, Kirby RM, Redmond AD, et al. Improvements have occurred since study. (Letter on effectiveness of a regional trauma system in reducing mortality from major trauma: Before and after study). *Br Med J.* 1998;316:1382.
27. Parr MJA, Nolan JP. Wrong comparisons were made. (Letter on effectiveness of a regional trauma system in reducing mortality from major trauma: Before and after study). *Br Med J.* 1998;316:1383.
28. Wright J. Data do not support conclusions. (Letter on effectiveness of a regional trauma system in reducing mortality from major trauma: Before and after study). *Br Med J.* 1998;316:1383.
29. Nicholl J, Turner J. Authors' reply. (Letter on effectiveness of a regional trauma system in reducing mortality from major trauma: Before and after study). *Br Med J.* 1998;316:1383.
30. Edinburgh Orthopaedic Trauma Unit. http://www.trauma.co.uk/history.htm. Accessed 2005.
31. Schmidt U. The German trauma system: Infrastructure and organization. *Trauma Q.* 1999;14(3):227–231.
32. Pape H, Oestern HJ, Leenen L, et al. Documentation of blunt trauma in Europe. *Eur J Trauma.* 2000;5:233–247.
33. Westhoff J, Hildebrand F, Grotz M, et al. Trauma care in Germany. *Injury, Int J Care Injured.* 2003;34:674–683.
34. ten Duis HJ, van der Werken C. Trauma care systems in The Netherlands. *Injury, Int J Care Injured.* 2003;34:722–727.
35. Leppäniemi A. Trauma systems in Europe. *Curr Opin Crit Care.* 2005;11:576–579.
36. Trunkey DD. Trauma in modern society: Major challenges and solutions. *Surgeon.* 2005;3(3):165–170.
37. Leppaniemi A. Trauma systems in Europe. *Curr Opin Crit Care.* 2005;11(6):576–579.
38. Nijs SJB, Broos PLO. Trauma care systems in Belgium. *Injury, Int J Care Injured.* 2003;34:652–657.
39. Guenther S, Waydhas C, Ose C, et al. Quality of multiple trauma care in 33 German and Swiss trauma centers during a 5-year period: Regular versus on-call service. *J Trauma Inj, Infect, Crit Care.* 2003;54(5):973–978.
40. Uranüs S, Lennquist S. Trauma management and education in Europe: A survey of twelve geographically and socioeconomically diverse European countries. *Eur J Surg.* 2002;168:730–735.
41. Hamam AM, El-Sayed HF. Injury in Egypt: The hidden epidemic. *Trauma Q.* 1999;14(3):261–267.
42. Mock C. Traumatic injury as a health problem worldwide. *Trauma Q.* 1999;14(3):191–196.
43. Mock C, Quansah R, Krishnan R, et al. Strengthening the prevention and care of injuries worldwide. *Lancet.* 2004;363:2172–2179.
44. Mock C, Quansah R, Addae-Mensah L, et al. The development of continuing education for trauma care in an African nation. *Injury, Int J Care Injured.* 2005;36:725–732.
45. Mock C, Adjei S, Acheampong F, et al. Occupational injuries in Ghana. *Int J Occup Environ Health.* 2005;11(3):238–245.
46. Mock CN, Forjuoh SN, Rivara FP. Epidemiology of transport related injuries in Ghana. *Accid Anal Prev.* 1999;31:359–370.
47. Forjuoh SN, Mock CN, Freidman DI, et al. Transport of the injured to hospitals in Ghana. *Accid Anal Prev.* 1999;3:66–70.
48. Adeyemi-Doro HO, Sowemimo GOA. Optimal care for trauma victims in Nigeria. *Trauma Q.* 1999;14(3):295–300.
49. Solagberu BA, Kuranga SA, Adekanye AO, et al. Preventable trauma deaths in a country without emergency medical services. *Afr J Trauma.* 2004;2:3–4.
50. Matzopoulos RG, Prinsloo MR, Bopape JL, et al. *Estimating the South African trauma caseload as a basis for injury surveillance.* South African Medical Research Council; 1999.
51. Wang Z, Jiang J. Current status of trauma care in China. *Trauma Q.* 1999;14(3):233–240.

52. Joshipura MK, Shah HS, Patel PR, et al. Trauma care systems in India – an overview. *Indian J Crit Care Med.* 2004;8:93–97.
53. Sethi AK, Tyagi A. Trauma untamed –as yet. *Trauma Care.* 2001;11(5):89–90.
54. Mashiko K. Trauma systems in Japan: History, present status and future perspectives. *J Nippon Med Sch.* 2005;72(4):194–202.
55. Kobayashi K. Trauma care in Japan. *Trauma Q.* 1999;14(3):249–252.
56. Matsumoto H, Mashiko K, Hara Y, et al. Effectiveness of a "doctor-helicopter" system in Japan. *Isr Med Assoc J.* 2006;8:8–11.
57. Henman P. War surgery – the temporary expatriate surgeon in a conflict zone. *Trauma Q.* 1999;14(3):311–322.
58. Trunkey DD. In search of solutions. *J Trauma.* 2002;53:1189–1191.
59. *Operation desert storm: Full army medical capability not achieved.* Washington, DC: U.S. General Accounting Office; 1992. GAO/NSIAD-92-175.
60. *Operation desert storm: Full army medical capability not achieved.* Washington, DC: U.S. General Accounting Office; 1993. GAO/NSIAD-93-189.
61. *Operation desert storm: Problems with Air Force medical readiness.* Washington, DC: U.S. General Accounting Office; 1993. GAO/NSIAD-94-58.
62. *War time medical care: DOD is addressing capability shortfalls, but challenges remain.* Washington, DC: U.S. General Accounting Office; 1996. GAO/NSIAD-96-224.
63. *War time medical care: Personnel requirements still not resolved.* Washington, DC: U.S. General Accounting Office; 1996. GAO/NSIAD-96-173.
64. Holcomb JB. The 2004 fitts lecture: Current perspective on combat casualty care. *J Trauma.* 2005;59(4):990–1002.
65. Vassar MJ, Holcroft JJ, Knudson MM, et al. Fractures in access to and assessment of trauma systems. *J Am Coll Surg.* 2003;197:717–725.
66. Trunkey DD. A growing crisis in patient access to emergency surgical care: A different interpretation and alternative solutions. *ACS Bull.* 2006;91:2–22.
67. Cooper RA, Getzen TE, McKee HF, et al. Economic and demographic trends signal an impending physician shortage. *Health Aff.* 2002;21:140–154.
68. Cooper RA. Weighing the evidence for expanding physician supply. *Ann Intern Med.* 2004;141:705–714.
69. Bland KI, Isaacs G. Contemporary trends in student selection of medical specialties. *Arch Surg.* 2002;137:259–267.
70. Esposito TJ, Maier RV, Rivara FP, et al. Why surgeons prefer not to care for trauma patients. *Arch Surg.* 1991;126:292–297.
71. Trunkey DD, Cahn RM, Lenfesty B, et al. Management of the geriatric trauma patient at risk of death. *Arch Surg.* 2000;135:34–38.
72. *Traumatic brain injury: Programs supporting long-term services in selected states.* Washington, DC: General Accounting Office; 1998. GAO/HEHS-98-55.
73. Friedman TL. *The world is flat: A brief history of the twenty-first century.* New York: Farrar, Straus & Giroux; 2006.
74. Gavrilova NNS, Semyonova VG, Evdokushkina G, et al. *Problems with mortality data in Russia. PAA Annual Meeting,* Moscow. 2005.
75. Yuen WK, Chung CH. Trauma care in Hong Kong. *Trauma Q.* 1999;14(3):241–247.
76. Joshipura M, Mock C, Goosen J, et al. Essential trauma care: Strengthening trauma systems around the world. *Injury.* 2004;35(9):841–845.
77. Kumar S. Report highlights shortcomings in private medical schools in India. *Br Med J.* 2004;328:70.
78. *Project for development of the trauma center complex.* Japan International Cooperation Agency; www.jica.go.jp/english/evaluation/project/term/as/2004/tha_02.htm. 2004.
79. Yeoh E. Trauma care in Malaysia. *Trauma Q.* 1999;14(3):253–260.
80. Brooks A, Mcnab C, Boffard K. South Africa. *Trauma Q.* 1999;14(3):301–310.
81. Garrett L. Do no harm: The global health challenge. *Foreign Aff.* 2007;86:14–38.

Disaster Management

2

Eric R. Frykberg

Health care providers and facilities have been confronted with an increasing number and frequency of catastrophic events in recent years, which result in large numbers of injured casualties and substantial property damage. The defining characteristics of such *mass casualty disasters* include a sudden and unpredictable occurrence, a disruption of societal infrastructure that gives rise to *chaos*, and an *overwhelming* of medical resources by the urgent medical needs and sudden presentation of large numbers of casualties.[1-3] The medical management of mass casualties requires an entirely different approach from the routine care of emergency patients who usually present one at a time. A true disaster is more than just a large emergency. Simply doing more of the same will not work, and yet this is what is often done, as most medical personnel do not understand the unique demands of mass casualty management. This is not taught in medical or nursing schools, and is not generally a requirement of residency training. Consequently, medical preparedness for mass casualty events is woefully lacking across the United States.[4,5]

Approximately 80% of all disasters have resulted in physical trauma to casualties. This emphasizes how important it is that surgeons, and other acute health care providers who provide surgical capability (i.e., emergency physicians, emergency department [ED], operating room [OR], trauma and intensive care unit [ICU] nurses, prehospital professionals), play prominent roles in disaster planning and management. It is surgeons who will be on the front lines of mass casualty management as the most likely *first receivers* of casualties. Surgeons regularly confront the challenges of trauma care and rapid decision making in their everyday practices. Likewise, trauma centers should serve as the foundation of any disaster response system, as they have the experience, personnel, resources, and linkages most essential to a successful disaster response, even in disasters that do not involve physical trauma.[6-10]

This chapter will review the basic concepts of disaster preparedness and response, emphasizing the critical contributions that surgeons must make to these processes within the context of the many nonmedical elements that a disaster response also entails. These concepts will be presented in the framework of the six Ps of disaster management: preparedness, planning, prehospital considerations, procedures for hospital care, and pathophysiology and patterns of injury, with the pitfalls of each of these elements incorporated into the discussion of each of these issues.

PREPARATION

This component of disaster management refers to the acquisition of a basic level of knowledge and skills that are necessary for a successful medical response. The medical aspects of mass casualty care are so different from the routine approaches to medical care of emergency patients that substantial education and training of medical personnel must be provided. Many principles of a disaster medical response are counterintuitive, and even morally antithetical to the precepts and ethics of patient care that are enshrined in standard medical education. Since disasters occur suddenly and unexpectedly, physicians must be trained in advance for this necessary paradigm shift in casualty care in order to optimize casualty outcomes. The longer the learning curve, the more lives lost.

There are many classification schemes for disasters that should be understood (see Table 1). The most useful of these is based on the level of resources needed to manage the property damage and casualties, which correlates closely with the overall magnitude of the event. This classification best reflects the essential characteristic of disasters, being the mismatch between the needs of a community and its victims, and the resources available to meet these needs.

TABLE 1

DISASTER CLASSIFICATION SCHEMES

Mechanism
   Natural
      Weather-related (hurricane, tornado)
      Geophysical (earthquake, tsunami)
   Man-made
      Intentional (terrorist attack)
      Unintentional (industrial accident)
Number of casualties
Nature of injuries
Geographic extent
   Closed
   Open
Duration
   Finite
   Ongoing
Level of response
   Level I: Local resources
   Level II: Regional resources
   Level III: State or national resources

An extensive literature on the experiences with past disasters serves as a valuable learning tool to understand those patterns that typically follow disasters. A massive influx of casualties, most commonly into the hospital nearest to the event, should be anticipated. Generally, 50% of all disaster casualties that will present to a hospital will do so within the first hour of the event, and 75% will arrive within 2 hours. The first wave of casualties will not be critically injured and largely not even require hospital care. However, this wave jeopardizes the hospital's ability to care for that minority (10% to 20%) who will be critically injured and in need of immediate life-saving care, and who will arrive in later waves, unless established mechanisms are in place to *lock down* the hospital and screen out those casualties, bystanders, curious onlookers, and volunteers who do not belong there. A major challenge facing physicians in this setting is the need for an orderly but expeditious process to rapidly identify those who need urgent care from among the majority who do not, as treatment delays for the latter could be fatal. Another challenge is to provide appropriate treatment to all with limited and overwhelmed resources. This may require a *rationing of care* according to how salvageable a casualty may be and the extent of resources needed, so as not to squander the scarce resources on one casualty that could better be applied to save many other more salvageable lives. Our standard approach to medical care of providing the greatest good for each individual, must change in a mass casualty event to the *greatest good for the greatest number*, requiring the focus of care to change from the individual to the casualty population as a whole. It must be recognized that optimal care for all casualties is impossible in this setting. The *altered standards* of medical care described in the preceding text must apply in order to maximize casualty salvage.[11,12] This basic principle of disaster management has been documented in the extensive experience in Israel with terrorist events, in which the hospital management of mass casualties has evolved to *minimal acceptable care* of all but the most severely injured, so as to be able to concentrate the limited resources where they are most needed.[3] These major changes in the goals of medical care are difficult and uncomfortable for health care providers to accept, and therefore difficult to learn. Physicians in the United States are generally not familiar with these principles of disaster preparedness and response; this includes surgeons, who are the most likely medical specialists to be among the frontline providers for disaster victims.[13]

There are many challenges and barriers to disaster education in the civilian medical sector (see Table 2). The rarity of true disasters tends to dampen the urgency of learning, as most physicians may never see one in their entire careers. The new approaches to medical care that disasters entail require time-consuming study and an unlearning of some habits and practices. The command structure of a major disaster response is also new to physicians, involving much more than medical care, placing medical providers in a subservient role, and requiring new levels of cooperation and teamwork with unfamiliar entities, all of which may cause discomfort and angst among physicians who do not understand the purpose of command structure.[14] The complexity of the injuries resulting from many disasters are a magnitude beyond that normally encountered by emergency care providers, and are made more difficult by the rapid decisions and treatment that are necessary to accommodate the large casualty influx.[3] There are major disconnects between the military and civilian medical sectors that prevent the latter from learning the effective procedures used by the military for disaster planning and response. Similar disconnects exist between the US health care sector and the many government and nongovernmental organizations that comprise the disaster response infrastructure of this country, effectively preventing medical personnel from

TABLE 2

CHALLENGES IN DISASTER EDUCATION FOR US HEALTH CARE PROVIDERS

Rarity of events
Different approaches to medical care
Incident Command structure and role
Complexity of injury patterns and decision making
Civilian vs. military disconnect
Health care sector vs. government/nongovernment agencies
   disconnect
Apathy and complacence
Failure to learn lessons from past disasters
Multiple disaster courses

engaging in the existing disaster system and becoming an integral and necessary component of a disaster response. There is a striking failure of the medical sector to learn the lessons from the mistakes of past disasters, which results in the same problems arising in every successive disaster response, with no progress being made to improve this response. Finally, there are so many educational efforts in disaster management being propagated in a disjointed manner by multiple groups, all with very different goals and target audiences, with no attempt made to coordinate and consolidate these efforts, that health care providers can easily be confused and discouraged from pursuing this necessary education. A standard curriculum in this discipline should be established in medical and nursing schools, and residency training, in order to provide all health care personnel with a basic core of knowledge and skills in disaster planning and management. All of these educational barriers must be overcome, as *preparation*—education and training—must be the most basic and essential component of a successful medical response to disasters, which in turn allows us to achieve the ultimate goal of any medical effort, that of saving lives.

PLANNING

The Challenge

There is a misguided tendency to think that there can be no effective planning in advance to deal with major disasters, given their sudden, unpredictable, random, and rare occurrence. The word *"disaster"* is derived from the Latin roots for "evil star," promoting the idea that they are acts of God or Fate, uncontrollable, and cannot be anticipated. This perception is largely untrue, but it discourages any form of preparedness, and leads to prolonged chaos when disasters strike, because people only then begin thinking about what to do.

The fact that disasters will always occur lends urgency to planning and preparation for them. There are several aspects of the modern world that increase the risk and frequency of disruptive and catastrophic events, including growing population density, an aging population, increased settlement in high-risk areas (i.e., flood plains, ocean fronts, earthquake-prone fault zones, unstable cliffs), increasing transport of hazardous materials through populated areas, increased technologic hazards (i.e., nuclear reactors, toxic chemical storage sites), the emergence of new and resistant strains of microorganisms, and the increased threat of terrorism.[15]

In fact, there are numerous opportunities to prepare for the unique contingencies of disasters. Many geographic areas are vulnerable to natural disasters that have occurred in the past, such as tornadoes in the American Midwest, hurricanes along the southern US coast, floods in major river valleys, and earthquakes in California. The patterns of property damage and injuries that occur in these events are well documented and easily anticipated. Many areas have known risks from industrial and environmental hazards. A Hazards Vulnerability Analysis (HVA) should be the first step in a disaster planning process by any hospital or community, analyzing all local threats, collating past experiences with these hazards, and developing a plan for responding to these potential problems that may threaten the population.[16] The identified risks should be prioritized according to their probability so as to most fully prepare and allocate resources for the most likely threats.

Planning must also anticipate the need for local assets to be on their own without outside help for several days. This has been confirmed time and again in most disasters, and when ignored has led to major ongoing losses of property and life, and prolonging of recovery, as occurred in New Orleans following Hurricane Katrina in 2005.

An appropriate medical response is greatly facilitated by analyzing the documented results of past disasters to identify common patterns of injury, and casualty and responder behaviors. For instance, abundant evidence from major terrorist bombings consistently shows that most surviving casualties are not seriously injured (see Fig. 1), a pattern that in fact characterizes most forms of mass casualty disasters. This allows hospitals to anticipate the need to keep most arriving casualties out with a restrictive screening

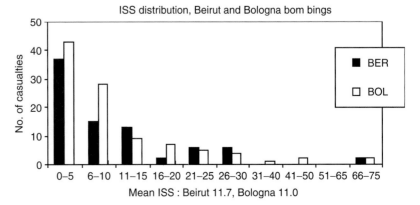

Figure 1 Graphic comparison of injury severity among survivors of the terrorist bombings of the Bologna, Italy train terminal in 1980 (*BOL*) and the US Marine barracks in Beirut, Lebanon in 1983 (*BER*), showing the consistently similar pattern of only a small minority of surviving casualties being critically injured (Injury Severity Score [ISS] >15). (From Frykberg ER, Disaster and mass casualty management. In: Britt LD, Trunkey DD, Feliciano DV, eds. *Acute care surgery: Principles and practice.* New York: Springer Science + Business; 2007;229–262, reprinted with permission.)

process, so as to apply the limited hospital resources most efficiently to only those who need urgent care.[3,17,18]

An *all-hazards approach* to disaster planning recognizes that all disasters have many patterns of injury, infrastructure damage, human behaviors, and resource requirements in common, which permits a basic plan template to be developed that can apply to virtually any disaster. Then, using such tools as an HVA to identify likely disaster mechanisms, this broad plan can be adapted to the specific and unique aspects of each individual disaster once it occurs. A single flexible and all-encompassing plan is far preferable and more workable than multiple plans to cover a multitude of specific events, as every possibility can never be covered, and responders will not be able to know the details of every plan.

The most effective disaster plans include the following elements[19]:

- Valid assumptions of injury patterns, threats, human behavior and needs
- Lessons learned from the results of past disasters
- Evidence-based principles of disaster response
- An integrated collaborative "systems" approach of many different entities working toward a common goal
- Inclusion in the planning process of those who will participate in the response
- Knowledge and agreement of the plan by the response participants
- Training and education of the participants in the elements of the plan
- Regular hospital drills and community exercises to test the plan's workability, and revision of the plan as necessary to address weaknesses and problems uncovered by the drills

A postevent debriefing and critique should follow all disaster drills and actual disasters, preferably within 24 hours. All key participants in the response should critically analyze its effectiveness and weaknesses, from which the lessons learned can be documented, disseminated, and used to revise the original plan.[20]

Planning Pitfalls

One of the most common pitfalls in disaster planning is the *paper plan syndrome*, which is the false sense of security that can be imparted by a written plan. This can be made worse by a failure to rehearse the plan to uncover its flaws. Realistic planning and rehearsal require a major effort that includes extensive research and collaboration of all elements and stakeholders in a disaster response (see Table 3). This is usually not done because of its substantial expense and time commitment. This is confirmed by accounts of most disasters, in which the original disaster plan was uniformly discarded early on when it was found unrealistic and unworkable for the actual circumstances.[20] In fact, the planning *process* should be considered more important

TABLE 3	
HOSPITAL AND COMMUNITY STAKEHOLDERS IN DISASTER PLANNING	
Hospital Participants	**Community Participants**
Medical and nursing staffs	Emergency Operations Center
Administration	Public health department
Security	Prehospital emergency medical services (EMS)
Food services	Law enforcement
Hospital Incident Command (HICS)	Fire department
Volunteer pool	Search and rescue
Blood bank/laboratory	Media
Pathologist/morgue	
Imaging services	Transportation/evacuation services
	Medical examiner/morgue
Operating room staff	Area blood banks/Red Cross
Intensive care unit staff	Area hospital representatives
Public information office	Mental health services
Chaplains	Local medical society
Rehabilitation assets	Structural engineers

than the written plan, to the extent that it involves a serious multidisciplinary effort to anticipate the problems and understand everyone's proper role in the response. This tends to encourage initiative and creativity in solving problems as they arise.[16]

Deviating from the all-hazards approach is another pitfall of planning. It is common for planners to concentrate on the last disaster (e.g., terrorist attacks in Washington, DC), or the most "popular" disasters regardless of their likelihood (e.g., bioterrorism), or worst-case but low-probability scenarios (e.g., global thermonuclear war), which tend to neglect the most basic principles and on the most likely threats that all disaster plans should encompass.[1]

Another planning pitfall is the application of faulty assumptions and stereotypes about human behavior in disasters to the structure of the plan, which usually arise more from the imagination of inexperienced planners than from a critical analysis of how people actually behave in this setting. There is a tendency to assume that behaviors will conform to the plan, rather than developing the plan according to likely behaviors that consistently occur. The belief that disasters result in widespread panic, or that casualties will go where directed in an orderly manner, are examples of common misperceptions that in fact rarely happen. Casualties and many uninjured people, most of whom do not need hospital care, consistently flock to the nearest hospital, and many times are sent there by first responders (i.e., the *geographic effect*), overwhelming the ability of these facilities to render effective care. Rather than resisting this inevitable casualty flow, plans should anticipate this, and direct that these inundated hospitals be converted to *triage hospitals*, otherwise termed *ground zero*, or *evacuation* hospitals, that do not treat casualties but take over the function, which should have occurred from the scene, of distributing casualties systematically to all other hospitals in the area.[3]

Failure to engage trauma centers and acute care medical personnel, who regularly manage trauma, in the planning process and in the established disaster infrastructure, is among the most common pitfalls of disaster planning. Trauma systems are already established throughout the United States, which should serve as the template for local, regional, statewide, and national disaster systems, because their resources, experience, and linkages are all important assets necessary for a successful medical response to disasters.[10,16,17]

PREHOSPITAL CONSIDERATIONS

The initial focus of a disaster response is at the scene of the event, where the nature and extent of the damage must be assessed, further damage minimized, and plans for dealing with the destruction and injured casualties formulated and implemented. Some forms of disasters do not have a specific "scene" or prehospital phase, such as disease pandemics or bioterrorist attacks, which evolve over long periods of time without a clear beginning or end. However, most disasters do have a readily identifiable scene, although it can vary quite extensively in size. The many challenges and complexities of the prehospital component of a disaster response may best be understood in the context of the classic phases through which most responses evolve[3] (see Table 4).

Phases of Response

All major disasters are characterized by an initial phase of *chaos*, with people dazed, frightened, and confused, running for shelter, and confronting the horrors of dead bodies and property destruction. There is no leadership or authority, and no organization of efforts. This is the period in which the geographic effect occurs, with the nearest hospital rapidly being inundated by arriving casualties, worried well, and volunteers trying to help, all usually without warning. In urban areas this chaos lasts only 30 to 60 minutes, but in more isolated locales where resources are fewer and further away, it may last several hours. The longer this phase lasts, the harder it becomes to achieve order, emphasizing the importance of a rapid prehospital response.[21] Critically injured casualties are most vulnerable in this phase, and the longer it lasts, the more lives may be lost. The ultimate goal at this time is to establish order, for the primary purposes of maximizing casualty survival and minimizing further damage and injury.

Initial response and reorganization represents the start of the *crisis management* phase of a disaster response, and

TABLE 4
PHASES OF PREHOSPITAL/HOSPITAL DISASTER RESPONSE

Chaos
Initial response/reorganization
    Establish command post
    Needs assessment
    Security and safety procedures
    Casualty evacuation to casualty collection areas (CCAs)
Site clearing
    Search and rescue/recovery
    Casualty distribution from CCAs to hospitals
    Clearing debris
    Initial hospital medical care
Late/recovery
    Rebuilding infrastructure
    Definitive hospital medical care/secondary casualty distribution
    Provider and casualty mental health follow-up
    Postevent critique and analysis of disaster response
    Community recovery

From Stein M, Hirshberg A. Medical consequences of terrorism: The conventional weapons threat. *Surg Clin North Am.* 1999;79: 1537–1552.

begins with the arrival at the scene of first responders, such as emergency medical services (EMS), law enforcement, and fire department assets, who assume responsibility for securing the disaster scene and establishing *command and control*. Generally, the first responders to arrive at the scene assume command and establish communications with the central command authority that is located in an Emergency Operations Center (EOC). A command post is established in an area near the scene, but located far enough to assure safety. Protection of first responders must be the first priority of prehospital efforts, to prevent them from becoming *secondary casualties*, and thereby depriving the disaster casualties and response of their necessary skills. Protection of casualties from further harm must be the next priority. The designated *incident commander* (IC) of the scene assumes authority from the interim commander upon arrival, with the responsibility to survey the damage and develop a *needs assessment*, which allows the EOC to mobilize the required resources. Any contamination of the scene with toxic materials must be determined at this time, and if present a decontamination process is established. A mechanism for transporting casualties must be developed. Security of the scene must also be established to restrict access to its potential dangers to all except those trained to be there with a defined role, to handle the predictable influx of onlookers and volunteers, to maintain order in the assessment and clearing process, to preserve forensic evidence if a crime is involved, and to keep traffic lanes open to ensure the flow of casualties and resources to their proper destinations.[2,22]

The *site-clearing phase* involves the work of casualty rescue and evacuation, and addressing ongoing dangers to provide a safe environment for the rescue and clearing operations. Active fires, downed power lines, gas leaks, and toxic chemical spills are usually addressed by the fire department. Structural engineers inspect damaged buildings for stability. Specialized response teams may be required to detect and neutralize hazardous materials, and contain flow of blood and bodily fluids from casualties, as decontamination procedures are begun. Heavy equipment is brought in to clear debris. A major danger that must be addressed is the possibility of delayed *second-hit* events that could jeopardize first responders. Unstable buildings may collapse during rescue efforts, aftershocks may continue following earthquakes, gas leaks could explode, and terrorist bombings are often followed by a second explosion after a short period of time to allow first responders, onlookers, and volunteers to arrive and also to be killed.[3,17]

Search and rescue operations are carried out in the site-clearing phase. Unlike routine emergencies, casualties following major disasters may be buried beneath debris or fallen buildings, or widely scattered, and search is required to find them. This calls for highly trained and specialized personnel, including hazardous materials specialists, structural engineers, heavy equipment operators for extrication, and those who understand search and rescue principles and methodology. Caring for casualties who are entrapped in locations that are difficult to reach, and in confined spaces, also requires special training that most hospital-based providers do not have, such as treating airway and breathing problems in poorly accessible locations, hypothermia, dehydration, and crush injuries. Extrication may be prolonged and require persistence with several shifts of rescue workers. Pressure is on the rescue personnel to find casualties as quickly as possible, as survivors are rarely found after 24 hours. After this time, rescue efforts are supplanted by efforts to recover the dead, which poses another set of emotional burdens on workers.[3]

Human casualties are first assessed and transported for eventual care during the site-clearing phase. There should be no attempt to render care to casualties who do not require extrication. The goal must be only to determine who is alive and who is dead, and move survivors away from the dangers of the scene to safer, more distant *casualty collection areas* (CCAs). It is best not to send large numbers of casualties directly to hospitals before determining their need for care and decontamination. The dead should be segregated in different areas from the living to allow eventual identification and forensic analysis, and to avoid wasting resources on their evaluation. At the CCAs, prehospital personnel should quickly assess injuries and the need for hospitalization, rendering no care beyond emergent life-saving interventions that are deemed appropriate according to the available resources (i.e., pressure on active bleeding).[2,22] Triage, or the sorting of casualties according to priority of treatment needs,

should be simple and minimal at these sites, limited to determining only who needs hospital care and who does not. Ideally, those requiring hospitalization should be distributed among all available hospitals in a systematic manner from the scene that avoids any one facility from being overloaded, termed *leap-frogging*, preferably matching the needs of each casualty to each hospital's resources.[17,23] Moving casualties through multiple sequential CCAs for repeat evaluation will tend to improve the accuracy of these triage decisions, and the efficiency of casualty care, by assuring that only those needing the limited hospital resources will finally be admitted. This further prevents hospitals from being unnecessarily overwhelmed by the geographic effect, and assures that the limited resources are applied where they are most needed. The initial phase of acute hospital care usually occurs simultaneously with these prehospital operations.

Those casualties not requiring immediate hospital care should be transported to other areas and monitored by medical personnel for any deterioration that may require an alteration of the original triage decision, and possibly sending for immediate care. This is one of the ways to mitigate the adverse consequences of initial triage errors, to ensure an *error-tolerant* system.

Personal protective equipment must be worn by all scene workers, and safety procedures for search, rescue, and extrication must be strictly followed. Experience from many disasters has shown that 70% of fatalities in confined-space rescue operations are the rescuers themselves, who become secondary casualties. Furthermore, 35% of these secondary casualties were the most experienced rescue supervisors. Occasionally, extrication of a casualty may require the emergent amputation of a limb, as happened following the bombing of the Murrah building in Oklahoma City in 1995, and following an expressway collapse after the 1989 San Francisco earthquake. This is only one of the indications for physicians to be at a disaster scene, yet even these medical personnel should be trained in the hazards of disaster management. It is the responsibility of a safety officer at the scene to oversee all rescue and site-clearing operations, to assure provider and casualty protection, and to report directly to the central command authority at the EOC.

The *late phase* of disaster response, otherwise known as the *consequence management* phase, involves the long-term clearing of all debris and damaged property, and the rebuilding of infrastructure in the community. It also includes the later phases of definitive hospital care after the acute casualty influx subsides, and secondary casualty distribution between hospitals to expedite care, which may involve evacuation of casualties over long distances. A post-disaster critique and analysis of the entire response should be carried out within 24 to 48 hours of its completion, to identify weaknesses and the lessons that should be learned to improve future responses. Confidential personal debriefings should be carried out among all active response participants to address emotional issues as a means of recognizing and preventing long-term problems such as post-traumatic stress disorder (PTSD). There should be a mechanism for addressing the short- and long-term mental health needs of responders, casualties, and the community as a whole, as a part of their long-term recovery to pre-event levels.

Incident Command

The many disparate jurisdictions, agencies, organizations, and personnel who must suddenly work together in a seamless coordinated effort to achieve the common goals of management and recovery following major disasters can succeed only with a strong and organized command structure. The Incident Command System (ICS) was developed for this purpose during wildfires in California in the 1970s, and has proved effective in all forms of major emergencies and disasters because of its modular and adaptable structure around the essential functional elements of command, planning, logistics, operations, and finance/administration. The ICS encompasses the concepts of *unity of command*, in which all personnel have specific assigned roles contributing to the ultimate goals; *chain of command*, in which all personnel have specific positions in the overall command structure and know who they report to and who reports to them, with limited *spans of control* in which no more than five to seven people report to any one position; and *unified command*, in which multiple independent entities with differing experience, training, and functions are all brought together to submit to one central authority for the purpose of achieving common goals. The Incident Commander (IC) is located in the EOC to direct the entire disaster response through the other four section chiefs. The IC staff is comprised of safety, public information, and liaison officers to facilitate this function. Planning, logistics, and finance/administration sections serve to support the operations section in its management of the disaster response with search and rescue, casualty transport, scene clearance, and other such nuts and bolts functions. The operations section is the only one that interacts directly with the public. It is critical that all participants in a disaster response understand this structure and their role in it, which requires education and training, as well as involvement in the planning process.[2,24]

Prehospital Pitfalls

Accounts of most mass casualty disasters document common and predictable patterns of mistakes and failures in prehospital management (see Table 5), from which we have the opportunity to learn and improve future responses.[20] Unfortunately, the very consistency and predictability of these established pitfalls demonstrate how little has been learned, as they continue to occur.

Communication between all elements of a disaster response typically fails very early, preventing the very *interoperability* of these elements that is essential for their

TABLE 5
PITFALLS IN DISASTER RESPONSE

Communications/interoperability
Authority and responsibility
Security
Medical care strategy
Original disaster plan

coordinated functioning, and for the overall success of a disaster response. Standard telephone lines and cellular phones routinely fail within minutes due to overload and, in many cases, due to destruction of their infrastructure in the disaster event. Redundancy must be built into the system in the planning process to anticipate this certainty, with the specification of several backup methods to have in reserve, such as satellite phones, dedicated land lines only used in disasters, dedicated radio frequencies (e.g., 800 MHz radios), walkie-talkies, HAM radio operators, web-based systems, and even the broadcast media to help get messages disseminated. In many disasters the final common denominator of communications is the human messenger who personally travels between various elements to obtain and receive information. Contingencies must be made for power outages, with supplies of batteries to allow all these methods to work.

Who is in charge is an extremely important factor that must be designated in advance and known by all participants. Otherwise, everyone thinks they should be in charge, and therefore nobody will be in charge, which will prolong the period of chaos through a failure to provide command and control. A failure to establish a command authority in a timely manner also leads to a failure of security, permitting unrestricted access to the scene by well-meaning volunteers and untrained providers, who then become potential secondary casualties.

Failure to adhere to the necessary altered standards of medical care for casualty management in the prehospital setting of a disaster response is a pitfall that jeopardizes maximal casualty salvage. In the absence of this knowledge, providers will default to standard medical care, which will cause major delays in casualty evacuation and traffic flow. Triage must be minimal in the prehospital sectors. Complex and outdated schemes that typically involve many categories of color-coding tags must be avoided, and efficiency of care should be optimized by applying the principle of minimal acceptable care, with casualty evacuation away from the scene and no medical treatment established as the primary goal.[3,11,12] Failure of prehospital personnel to rapidly establish a systematic leap-frog casualty distribution among all available hospitals tends to result in the geographic effect of overloading one hospital, preventing those casualties in most need of life-saving care from receiving it.[3,17,23]

PROCEDURES FOR HOSPITAL CARE

Surge and Casualty Handling

Hospitals in the area of any major disaster event must be prepared for the sudden and unannounced influx of mass casualties. In view of the typical failure of communications between the disaster scene and the hospital, there may be no warning of this influx. In fact, arriving casualties may be the first indication to hospital personnel that an event has happened. News reports on broadcast media are also common first warnings to hospitals. If advance warning does reach the hospital, there is only approximately 10 minutes to prepare for the casualty influx as the disaster response plan is activated. This time is best spent clearing all the spaces possible to accommodate a large number of casualties far beyond normal hospital capacity, to develop what is termed *surge capacity*. The ED, ICUs, and inpatient wards should move out or discharge existing patients, and the OR should cease all elective surgery, as these are the hospital resources that are in most demand following disasters.[25] Provisions must also be made for the ongoing care of those everyday emergencies that will continue to arrive (e.g., acute chest or abdominal pain, urgent obstetric deliveries, strokes, uncontrolled hypertension), but which are easily forgotten in this setting. Extra personnel must be called in, and equipment stores must be made available. Simultaneously a *hospital lockdown* must be rapidly accomplished by security personnel in anticipation of the geographic effect of casualty inundation, closing most hospital entrances to restrict access to all except those personnel with assigned and necessary functions, and only to those casualties who require urgent care and have been triaged and decontaminated.

Surge capacity is more than simple beds or space. It must be linked with *surge capability* if the medical response is to be at all effective. This refers to the ability to care for casualties in those beds, including physicians and nurses, as well as specialized skills and resources to handle special needs populations, such as dialysis; OR availability for specialty surgery; pediatric, geriatric, and burn care; and mental health resources.[26] Hirshberg et al. have combined these concepts to most appropriately define surge capacity as the *arrival rate* of critically injured casualties that can be treated optimally without any degradation in the quality of care.[27] Their computer modeling study, utilizing data from suicide bombings in Israel, showed this rate to be only 4.6 critical casualties per hour in a major American trauma center, beyond which the casualty load overwhelmed medical resources with a logical reduction in the quality of care that could be delivered (see Fig. 2). Maximizing the salvage of the most critical casualties is the essential mission of

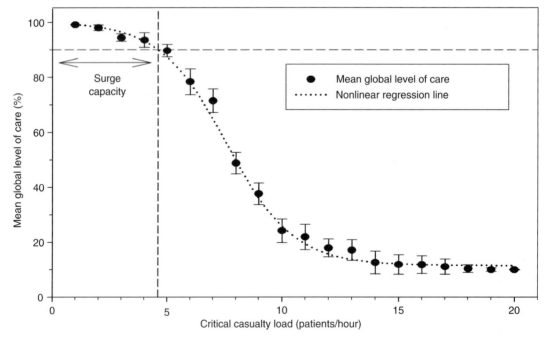

Figure 2 Graphic relationship between the arrival rate of disaster mass casualties into a hospital and the quality of care able to be provided, using data from suicide bombing victims in Israel as applied to how they would be cared for in an American trauma center, derived from a computer modeling program. Surge capacity is defined as the maximal arrival rate of critically injured casualties that permits at least 90% of the optimal level of care to be applied (4.6 critical casualties/hour in this model), after which the level of care degrades as resources are overwhelmed. (From Hirshberg A, Scott BG, Granchi T, et al. How does casualty load affect trauma care in urban bombing incidents? A quantitative analysis. *J Trauma*. 2005;58:686–695. Reprinted with permission, Lippincott Williams & Wilkins.)

a hospital's disaster response, and those factors that can expand this capability should be identified and optimized, while avoiding those factors that impair this capability. An effective development of surge capacity and capability has been related to reducing mortality among disaster mass casualties.[28]

Studies of the impact of mass casualties and their injury patterns on hospital resource utilization provide several predictable factors to be anticipated in the planning and execution of a hospital's disaster medical response.[25,29-32] A computer simulation of a hospital response to mass casualties from an urban suicide bombing shows that the number of ED beds for casualty evaluation, and the extent to which radiographic imaging and laboratory testing are applied, are typically underestimated in disaster plans. Conversely, the number of physicians and OR beds that are actually needed are typically overestimated.[29] Analysis of more than 1,000 casualties from more than 60 terrorist–related mass casualty events in Israel[25,31,32] shows that the ED, OR, and ICU pose the greatest resource demands during the initial period of casualty influx; that these demands are simultaneous and overlapping; that most early operations require multidisciplinary surgical teams of anesthesiologists and general, thoracic, and vascular surgeons; and that orthopaedic surgeons, plastic surgeons, and anesthesiologists are needed for more prolonged periods of time exceeding 24 hours because they do less urgent delayed procedures. Most operations are performed in the first 4 to 6 hours. Most casualties with Injury Severity Score (ISS) <25 are transferred to the ICU directly from the ED without surgery, whereas the most severely injured with ISS >25 require urgent surgery before ICU admission. Only 4.7% of all casualties were admitted to the ICU, but 73% of these required mechanical ventilation, and 77% had evidence of serious blast injuries to the lung and abdominal viscera. These studies confirm that noncritical casualties are always the first to arrive at a hospital following a mass casualty event.

This information permits accurate disaster planning for optimal resource use, especially in view how consistent these patterns are in most disasters, regardless of mechanism. Relatively few physicians and nurses are needed in the ED with a system in place that moves casualties rapidly to successive echelons of care, allowing the ED to have providers in reserve to take over after several hours. The use of imaging and laboratory testing is clearly a major impediment to overall casualty flow, and must be kept to a minimum initially to prevent backlogs and delays in care.[3,29,31] A common strategy for evaluating incoming casualties in the ED is to assign small teams of medical personnel to each stretcher to assess each casualty, record findings and triage decisions, and rapidly send them to the next appropriate care level with minimal to no treatment, thereby freeing up the stretcher team for the next casualty.[20,33,34] An accurate and reliable method of record keeping is essential for this to work, as the rapid casualty flow creates a potential for loss of continuity and casualty tracking. Records are best attached to each casualty, and if possible a central log is also kept in each care area. This also allows an overall assessment of the response to be analyzed in the future.[17]

Surprisingly few ORs and surgeons are needed in this setting, as most casualties do not need immediate surgery, and the surgery that is done must be abbreviated according to *damage control* principles, allowing rapid OR room turnover. In fact, these studies advocate *surgical conservatism*, meaning that surgery should be delayed as long as possible during the acute casualty influx so as not to deplete the OR resources too early before the most critical casualties arrive, who may need the most urgent interventions.[25] Those surgical specialists most required during the casualty influx should be available.

Of all hospital resources, ICU beds tend to be in greatest demand following a mass casualty event. ICU beds must be anticipated for only a minority of casualties, but they will require extensive resource use owing to the severity of their injuries. One idea to expand ICU capacity and capability is to use the recovery room (postanesthesia care unit [PACU]) as the ICU for postoperative casualties needing this level of care, thereby sparing beds in the actual ICU.[31] The inability to apply ICU resources to critically injured casualties has been shown to increase mortality, not surprisingly,[35] although a rationing of this scarce resource may be necessary to maximize casualty salvage.[36]

It is important that "controllers" be designated for the ED, OR, and ICU in mass casualty events to enforce the procedures for streamlining and abbreviating care in these spaces as outlined in the preceding text. Prolonged casualty evaluation, extensive imaging and other diagnostic procedures, and prolonged operations must be avoided to keep spaces cleared and accommodate continuing casualty influx. Controllers not involved in the actual care of casualties can best do this by maintaining the "big picture," or *situational awareness*, of the broader aspects of casualty flow and resource utilization, and of what is needed to accommodate incoming casualties to assure that all are seen, requiring that only the appropriate casualties are sent to the OR and ICU, and that minimal time is spent by surgeons in the OR. Generally, senior ED physicians, surgeons, and intensivists are the best controllers.[3,31]

Triage and Error Tolerance

The sorting of casualties according to urgency of need and severity of injury is *triage*, and is one of the most critical elements impacting casualty outcome in the medical response to disasters. This is the process whereby decisions are made as to the best use of limited medical resources in a mass casualty setting. Triage decisions are made on a relatively small scale in the routine management of emergency and trauma patients in developed countries, where resources are essentially unlimited, and optimal care for every patient is the guiding principle. However, disaster triage decisions must consider the additional factor of salvageability, and the extent of time, resources, and personnel that a specific casualty may require, which would have to be taken away from many other casualties with a better chance of survival. In disasters, the most severely injured, who would normally be the first priority for care, may have to be denied care in order to fulfill the new principle of the *greatest good for the greatest number*. The focus of medical care must change from the individual to the population. This *expectant* category of triage is difficult for health care providers, and society as a whole, to accept because it is morally antithetical to our training and philosophy, which is why education is so necessary to break through the barrier imposed by standard care to maximize the salvage of mass casualties.[2,17,36-39]

The unique challenge of mass casualty triage lies in the need to *rapidly* identify that consistent minority of 10% to 20% of survivors who are in need of immediate care from among the great majority who are not critically injured. Unfortunately, many critical injuries are not clearly evident on a quick examination. However, there are several high-risk injury patterns that have been correlated with the need for urgent care or close observation, such as traumatic amputation, blast lung injury (BLI), tympanic membrane rupture, penetrating torso injuries, and multiple system injuries. Furthermore, casualties with little or no signs of life and extensive burns, open fractures, or head trauma have such a high probability of death or extensive resource use that they should be considered expectant, and care should be denied.[36,39] This emphasizes the important role of the *triage officer*, who must have knowledge and experience in the injuries to be expected following any mass casualty event, must understand the unique requirements of making these decisions in the context of mass casualty principles, must exert authority and leadership in making these decisions that should not be second-guessed, and must have the quality of *situational awareness* of all elements of the ongoing disaster response.

Triage errors consist of *undertriage*, or the assignment of critical casualties to a delayed category, and *overtriage*, or the assignment of noncritical casualties to immediate care. The triage officer must minimize both in a mass casualty setting, as both have been shown to increase the mortality rate of critically injured casualties (*critical mortality rate*) who are most at risk of death.[12,17,38,40] Overtriage impairs the ability to care for casualties by reducing the rate of critical casualties arriving every hour, who can be cared for optimally (see Table 6), which effectively moves the casualty care curve in Fig. 2 to the left.[27]

Triage errors can be minimized in the prehospital areas by keeping the triage scheme simple, determining only who is alive and who is dead, and who among the living needs hospitalization and who does not. Once in the hospital, the decision should involve only who needs immediate OR or ICU care and who may be directed away from these limited

TABLE 6

EFFECT OF OVERTRIAGE ON SURGE CAPACITY (CRITICAL CASUALTY ARRIVAL RATE)

Overtriage Rate (%)[a]	Surge Capacity (cc/hour)[b]	Overtriage (Non-cc/hour)[c]
0	4.7	0
25	4.6	1.6
50	3.8	3.8
75	2.7	8.1

[a]No. of casualties not requiring urgent care as percentage of total casualties triaged to urgent care in hospital.
[b]No. of critical casualties arriving per hour into hospital.
[c]No. of noncritical (overtriaged) casualties arriving per hour into hospital.
cc, critical casualties.
From Hirshberg A, Scott BG, Granchi T, et al. How does casualty load affect trauma care in urban bombing incidents? A quantitative analysis. *J Trauma*. 2005;58:686–695. With permission from Lippincott Williams & Wilkins.

resources. Once the acute casualty influx subsides, triage categories may be expanded and decisions reconsidered in the light of the remaining resources.

However, in the chaos and rapid decision making during mass casualty events, it must be anticipated that triage errors will always occur even with the best triage officers.[41] Rather than strive for the impossible goal of eliminating all errors, a flexible system of care must be built into the disaster response that will mitigate the adverse consequences of triage errors. Examples of such an *error-tolerant system*[3] include the assignment of medical providers to delayed and nonurgent casualties, to identify any deterioration that may require reassignment to urgent care, and thereby minimize the effects of the initial undertriage error; and having multiple triage stations in both the prehospital and hospital areas to allow those who do not need hospital care to be successively screened out, so that only those who truly need hospitalization, or OR or ICU care, arrive at these places, thereby minimizing the consequences of overtriage. This process recognizes that triage must evolve with the response and be repeated frequently, precisely because injury is a dynamic process.[41]

Command Structure, Evacuation, Response Assessment

An effective unified command structure is as necessary in the hospital as it is in the prehospital sector of disaster response, to assure the proper flow and distribution of casualties and the logistic support for their care. The Hospital Incident Command System (HICS) is the most common and effective organization of this authority, representing the same structure and functional elements as ICS, as adapted to hospital functions. The modular nature of HICS allows it to expand or contract as required for the size of the disaster, and each hospital's command structure functions within the operations section of the community ICS, which in turn functions within the operations section of the regional or state ICS.

An evacuation mechanism must be in place if a disaster medical response is to be effective, as, by definition, no single hospital is able to fully care for a mass casualty burden. The role of the hospital is to provide the minimal care necessary to keep casualties alive until they reach definitive care. If the geographic effect overwhelms hospitals nearest to the disaster scene, these hospitals should plan to become *triage hospitals*, otherwise known as *evacuation*, or *ground zero* hospitals, which only triage and distribute their casualty load among all remaining available hospitals to more evenly distribute the burden and facilitate care for all, because they cannot treat them adequately. Triage hospitals may be able to keep those casualties they are best able to treat once the casualty influx dissipates and resources become available. All hospitals should consider a *secondary casualty distribution* to other hospitals at this time to expedite definitive care when space and specialty resources may be available elsewhere.[3,42]

One mechanism for expanding available hospital space to accommodate disaster victims is to create *alternate site surge capacity* outside of the hospital, mainly for those not in urgent need of hospital resources, and thereby conserving them. Using tent-covered open parking lots or parking decks in the area of a hospital is an easily implemented option, where triage and decontamination facilities are often set up to prevent the hospital from being overcrowded with these functions. Sports stadiums are very suitable for this purpose, such as the Superdome in New Orleans and the Astrodome in Houston used for this purpose following Hurricane Katrina in 2005.[43] These alternate sites are of most value for the long-term medical care of displaced and special needs populations during the late recovery consequence management phase of open and ongoing disasters that evolve over a long period of time, such as Hurricane Katrina in 2005, Hurricane Andrew in 1992, and Hurricane Hugo in 1989. They are not feasible for acute medical care in the crisis management phase of short-term closed and finite disasters, such as an urban terrorist bombing, because they cannot provide such short-term critical needs as ORs and ICUs.

A postevent critique and analysis is an essential element of any disaster response that should occur within 24 hours of the deactivation of the response, and includes the leading participants. An objective assessment of the strengths and weaknesses of the effort and of the original disaster plan should lead to appropriate revisions of the plan that should improve future responses. Errors of triage and medical treatment must be assessed. The lessons learned should then be organized and disseminated as an important educational tool. Of course, without an effective method of recordkeeping and casualty tracking such an analysis is impossible, and lessons will be lost, leading to the same mistakes being made in the future.[20]

Pitfalls of Hospital Response

The major barriers to an effective hospital disaster response are similar to those that occur during the prehospital phase (Table 5). All of these pitfalls are best avoided by education and training in the principles of disaster planning and management.

The disaster plan is typically found to be unworkable early on, usually because it is not based on realistic assumptions and has never been adequately tested in drills or exercises. This prolongs the initial chaos in the hospital as the response must develop *de novo*. Medical providers do not know their responsibilities, and do not understand the changes they must make in their approach to medical care. The command structure is uncertain in terms of who is in charge overall and of which hospital unit, which leads to poor coordination between hospital units and between the hospital and EMS, public health, the EOC, and the many other prehospital and community response elements.

Security is often inadequate due to small numbers of personnel and inadequate training, delaying hospital lockdown and restriction of access to care spaces, and providing little or no protection to the facility and medical personnel. Security breakdowns also result in failures of mechanisms for handling the onslaught of casualties as well as providers, volunteers, media, and families who wish to help or seek information, which can rapidly overwhelm any capability for providing medical care.

The system of medical care delivery is often inadequate owing to a failure to accommodate and rapidly assess casualties and move them through the system efficiently with constant forward flow and without traffic gridlock. ED, OR, and ICU controllers are often not designated to enforce the appropriate casualty care and traffic flow. Without adequate education and training, medical providers will often default to doing things as they normally do, which will not work. Altered standards of care, such as minimally acceptable care and recognition of expectant casualties, must be applied to allow all casualties to be seen and those who need urgent care to receive it expeditiously, while not diverting scarce resources to those with little chance of survival. Expenses and procurement related to medical care are often not properly recorded and tracked, leading to major financial losses and prolonging long-term recovery.

Failure of communications remains the most common and predictable pitfall in the hospital response to a disaster, which indicates how little is learned from past disasters. Redundant backup systems are not planned in advance. There can be no effective situational awareness without communications, and therefore the hospital cannot prepare for what will be arriving from the scene or know the status of other hospitals. Resources are thereby poorly utilized, and misinformation and delayed information prevails.[20,44]

PATHOPHYSIOLOGY AND PATTERNS OF INJURY

Although all disasters are unique in their mechanism, location, timing, and extent of damage, they all tend to have many features in common. Bodily injury is the most common affliction of disaster casualties, allowing a reliable anticipation of the medical personnel and resources needed during the crisis management phase of the medical response. There is also a very consistent pattern of injury following disasters, in which most survivors are not severely injured and do not require urgent medical treatment (Fig. 1).[17,21] Disaster planning should therefore always involve acute care medical personnel who provide surgical capability (i.e., anesthesiologists, surgeons, emergency physicians, surgical and ED nurses), as they will be the most likely first receivers of disaster casualties. Surge capability requires the availability of specialists in trauma, burns, orthopaedics, neurosurgery, and critical care. Trauma centers should be the foundation of disaster preparedness. However, mass casualty disasters frequently result in unusual forms of injury, and levels of severity and complexity of injuries, that are rarely a part of surgical education and practice, such as blast trauma and biological, chemical, and radiologic injuries. All medical providers should be familiar with the pathophysiology and treatment of these conditions, the distinct approaches to their care in the context of mass casualties, and the many consistent patterns of casualty injuries and disaster response evolution that will form the environment in which medical care will be rendered.

Unconventional Weapons of Mass Destruction

Modern terrorism poses the threat of several forms of mass casualty disasters, in fulfillment of its goal of maximizing casualty generation and lethality.[45] Although the "weapons of mass destruction" of biological, chemical, and radiologic agents have been rarely if ever used for the deliberate infliction of widespread injury and death, they certainly have that potential. These agents are also subject to accidental release and dissemination, risking large segments of the surrounding population. Therefore, it is important that all health care providers who are likely to participate in the medical response to disasters be familiar with the medical implications of these agents.

Biological Agents

Bioterrorism or biological disasters involve the deliberate or accidental dissemination of microorganisms, or their toxins, to inflict widespread disease and death. The Centers for Disease Control and Prevention (CDC) classifies biological agents according to their likelihood of being used for terrorist purposes. Category A agents are those considered to have the greatest potential for effective dissemination and widespread lethality. They include

anthrax, plague, tularemia, smallpox, and botulin toxins, all of which can be readily transmitted in aerosolized forms and have a proved capability to afflict large populations. The feature that most distinguishes biological mass casualty events from other causes is the slower time course of evolution of disease manifestation over days to weeks, which leads to a more prolonged disaster response. This allows more time for organization of resources, but on the other hand may result in a large number of deaths before the nature and magnitude of the event is known. Early detection is essential to minimize disease spread, and this requires a system of recognition of patterns of illness over wide areas, known as *syndromic surveillance*. Widespread vaccination programs and stockpiling of antibiotics and antitoxins are important preventive measures that can mitigate the consequences of biological disasters. Personal protection measures and isolation procedures must be followed by health care providers to prevent them from becoming secondary casualties. Public health officials and infectious disease specialists should be integrally involved in the medical response to biological disasters.[46]

Chemical Agents

Toxic substances exert their deadly effects through inhalation of aerosolized or gaseous forms, ingestion of poisoned foods, and absorption through direct contact with the skin, eyes, or mucous membranes. These agents have a long history of causing widespread injury and death among large populations through their deliberate or accidental dissemination. As many as one million casualties in World War I were attributed to the use of chemical warfare with poison gases. The worst industrial accident in history occurred in Bhopal, India in 1984, where the accidental release of gaseous methyl isocyanate resulted in more than 6,000 deaths and 400,000 injuries in the surrounding population. In 1995, the first example of chemical terrorism involved the release of the nerve agent Sarin in the Tokyo subway system, resulting in 12 deaths and 5,000 injuries, which included hundreds of poorly prepared health care providers. Explosives are a possible means to disseminate toxic chemicals. In the 1993 World Trade Center bombing in New York City, enough cyanide was contained in the bomb to contaminate the entire building, but fortunately was destroyed in the blast. There remains great potential for chemical poisoning on a large scale, with large amounts of toxic substances being regularly stored and transported through major urban areas.

Early detection of a chemical mass casualty disaster is essential to minimize injury and death, and is best accomplished by a heightened awareness on the part of emergency room personnel for patterns of similar symptoms among large numbers of patients (see Table 7). This provides the opportunity to lock down the hospital before it is overwhelmed and rendered ineffective by contamination, and to institute triage and decontamination procedures outside of the hospital before allowing any

TABLE 7

SYMPTOMS OF ORGANOPHOSPHATE POISONING

Diarrhea
Urination
Miosis
Bronchorrhea
Bronchospasm
Emesis
Lacrimation
Salivation

TABLE 8

CATEGORIES OF CHEMICAL TOXINS POSING MASS CASUALTY THREATS

Category	Agents	Treatment/Antidote
Nerve agents (organophos-phates)	Tabun, sarin, soman, VX	Decontamination atropine, pralidoxime (2-PAM), diazepam, airway control
Incapacitating agents (anticholinergics)	BZ	IV hydration, physostigmine
Vesicants (blistering agents)	Mustard, lewisite, phosgene oxime	Decontamination, hypochlorite, dimercaprol
Pulmonary irritants	Phosgene, chlorine	Decontamination, oxygen, water cleansing, bronchodilators, mechanical ventilation
Blood agents	Cyanide	Decontamination, hyperbaric oxygen, amyl nitrite
Irritants (riot control agent)	Tear gas, mace, pepper spray	Oxygen, saline eyewash, water irrigation, decontamination

casualties in.[47] Any casualty with wet clothing should be assumed as contaminated, especially if there are obvious noxious fumes detectable, and decontamination should then be instituted. *Gross decontamination* is the first step in management, which involves removing all clothing and quickly washing down the casualties with water. This removes approximately 90% of all contamination. Technical decontamination then follows, with thorough soap-and-water scrubbing, the use of detergents and bleach for specific agents, washing and shaving of hair, and careful collection of all clothing and runoff fluids for controlled disposal. All medical personnel should wear personal protection equipment (PPE), and have a working knowledge of the clinical manifestations and treatment of the most common chemical agents that may cause mass casualty events (see Table 8). Toxicologists, pharmacologists, and poison control centers should be an integral part of the planning and response to chemical disasters.

Radiologic Agents

Ionizing radiation damages body tissues through direct energy, and indirect effects from the production of toxic hyperoxide molecules in living cells. The two major forms of ionizing radiation are *particle radiation* (i.e., low energy α and β particles, high-energy neutrons), and *wave, or electromagnetic radiation* (i.e., high-energy γ rays and x-rays). Although α and β particles have low penetrance into body tissues, they are highly destructive and lethal if ingested. The most commonly used unit of measurement of the absorbed dose of radiation into body tissues following exposure is the rad, or its International Unit counterpart the Gray (Gy), with 1 Gy = 100 rads.

The two major means of deliberate or accidental dissemination of radiation over wide areas to afflict large populations are through conventional explosives, or *dirty bombs*, which contain and disperse commonly available radioisotopes (cobalt Co 60, cesium Cs 137, iridium Ir 192), and through the atmospheric release of large doses of intense ionizing radiation from sabotage or leaks from nuclear reactors, or from the detonation of nuclear

weapons. Dirty bombs are relatively easy and inexpensive to construct, and are unlikely to create much property damage or personal injury beyond the blast effects alone, with little danger from the low levels of radiation dispersed. Fear and panic in the surrounding population due to the radiation threat probably pose more danger than the actual injuries and damage, which is why dirty bombs are frequently labeled *weapons of mass disruption*. Nuclear leaks or detonations pose a substantial threat of widespread property damage and death, but are highly unlikely and therefore considered a low risk.

Detection of radiation following any mass casualty disaster must occur as early as possible at the scene during the prehospital response phase, and requires the use of radiation dosimeters to assess the magnitude of contamination. This should lead to gross and technical decontamination procedures before allowing casualties into the hospital unless medical needs dictate otherwise. Experts in radiation physics and radiobiology should be integrally involved in scene assessment, decontamination, and hospital triage and treatment.

The major determinants of radiation injury among casualties are *time* of exposure, *distance* from the source, and degree of *shielding*. All medical personnel should be familiar with the clinical manifestations of *acute radiation syndrome*, consisting primarily of gastrointestinal (nausea, vomiting, hematemesis, diarrhea) and hematopoietic (bone marrow suppression, pancytopenia) symptoms. The close correlation between the timing of these symptoms and

TABLE 9
MAJOR GLOBAL TERRORIST BOMBINGS

Event	Year	Explosive Force (TNT Equivalent)	No. of Casualties (Deaths)
Bologna train terminal	1980	20 kg TNT	291 (85)
US Marines barracks, Beirut[a]	1983	6–10 tons ($NHNO_3$)	346 (241)
World Trade Center, NY	1993	600 kg TNT/cyanide	1,042 (6)
AIMA building, Buenos Aires[a]	1994	660 lb ($NHNO_3$)	286 (85)
Oklahoma City[a]	1995	2 tons ($NHNO_3$)	759 (168)
Atlanta Olympics	1996	2 kg TNT	111 (2)
Khobar Towers, Saudi Arabia	1996	2.5 tons C-4	574 (20)
US embassies, Africa[a]	1998	600 lb Semtex	~5,000 (274)
USS Cole, Yemen	2000	600 lb C-4	52 (17)
U.N. headquarters, Baghdad[a]	2003	600 lb ($NHNO_3$)	100 (17)
Madrid train terminals	2004	100 kg TNT	2,092 (191)
London subways and bus	2005	18 kg acetone peroxide	~700 (55)

[a]Involved building collapse.

the degree of exposure facilitates triage and treatment decisions, and the determination of expectant casualties who are destined to die and should receive only comfort care. Absorbed doses of more than 10 Gy (1,000 rads) in casualties result in the rapid appearance of symptoms within minutes, and are generally not survivable even with maximal medical therapy. Treatment of radiation injury is largely supportive, using antibiotics, isolation, and volume repletion. Open wounds should be cleansed and closed as early as possible to prevent them from becoming lethal portals of entry into the body, and wound excision should be considered in cases of contamination with long-lived radionuclides (e.g., α emitters). Radiation exposure and contamination of casualties pose very little risk to medical personnel or hospital facilities that adhere to no more than standard universal precautions. Therefore, triage decisions need not be altered by the possibility of radiologic contamination, as treatment needs have priority over decontamination in this setting for those casualties requiring urgent life-saving hospital care. No casualty should be denied any intervention, or admission to the hospital, solely because of radiation concerns, although gross decontamination can be carried out quickly and should suffice for most casualties requiring immediate care. Technical decontamination can follow in less urgent casualties.[48,49] Provisions must be made for psychoemotional issues in radiologic disasters, as the mystique of radiation among the public, and even among health care providers, has led to many misperceptions and hysterical reactions that are far out of proportion to the actual dangers. Education is the best tool to combat this.

Explosions and Blast Injury

Explosives are generally considered conventional weapons. However, the great blast magnitudes and casualty numbers that can be achieved with high-energy explosives that are easily accessible and inexpensive, and require little education and training to create and detonate, clearly make this the "fourth weapon of mass destruction." The increasing frequency of deliberate and accidental explosive disasters over the past several decades (see Table 9), which is far out of proportion to any other weapon of mass destruction, emphasizes that this mechanism is the most common and therefore the most likely threat for which we must prepare. This requires a thorough knowledge of the physics and pathophysiology of a blast.[17,45,50–52]

High-energy explosives are those most likely to produce mass casualty incidents. These result in a sudden large magnitude increase in the ambient pressure of the surrounding medium (*peak overpressure*) that forms a *blast wave* which travels radially out from the source at supersonic speeds of 3,000 to 8,000 m per second. The leading edge of this wave is the *blast front*, which has a shattering ability known as *brissance*. This wave rapidly dissipates in air according to the cube of the distance from the blast, so that moving three times further away reduces the blast force by 27-fold. This dissipation of pressure actually continues into a negative pressure phase before returning to ambient pressure, resulting in some implosive effects in high-energy explosions, and even tidal waves along coastal areas as the water is sucked into this temporary vacuum. *Blast wind* refers to the large air movements resulting from these effects. In confined spaces, the blast wave is magnified, rather than dissipated, by reflecting off floors, walls, and ceilings, and with a large enough blast this can lead to building collapse. This explains why indoor or confined-space blasts cause higher levels of damage, and higher rates of injury and death among victims, than open air blasts, especially if accompanied by building collapse[33,40,53] (Table 9). Underwater blasts are more powerful than air blasts, as the increased density of water propagates the blast wave three times faster and more distant.

There are four categories of blast injury. *Primary blast injury* is caused by the passage of the blast wave through the body, leaving no external signs of trauma. Air-containing organs such as the lungs, bowels, and ears are severely disrupted by this wave through turbulence at air–liquid interfaces, called *spalling*. The lung is most severely injured in air blasts, whereas hollow viscera of the abdomen are injured in underwater blasts. Blast Lung Injury (BLI) is characterized by progressive pulmonary insufficiency and air emboli, with a radiologic and pathologic picture similar to pulmonary contusions. It is highly lethal, with most afflicted casualties being killed immediately from cerebral and coronary air emboli. Less than 1% of bombing survivors in the past have manifested BLI,[40] although this has been more common among survivors of recent urban bombings due to rapid transport to hospital care.[28,54] Tympanic membrane rupture is a relatively benign injury, but serves as a marker for exposure to the blast wave. Although this finding does not correlate reliably with the presence of severe BLI, it should at least mandate careful observation of these casualties for delayed pulmonary effects.

Secondary blast injury is caused by the impact of objects and debris displaced by the blast into the body, and *tertiary blast injury* results from the body itself being thrown into other objects. These result in typical blunt and penetrating trauma and are the predominant injury among survivors of major explosive disasters. However, this high-energy trauma tends to be more severe than that encountered in routine surgical practice, with a level of complexity that is further magnified by the need for rapid evaluation and treatment of large numbers of casualties. Terrorist bombings are also increasingly characterized by destructive metal fragments placed in the bombs, as well as occasional attempts to disseminate toxic chemicals with bombs, to further enhance injury and lethality. The term *multidimensional injuries* has been used to describe these challenging aspects of the medical management of mass casualties and the difficult decision making as to their disposition, especially following explosive events.[12,18]

Quaternary blast injury refers to miscellaneous forms of injury only indirectly related to the blast. These include burns from the initial fireball of major explosions, inhalation injuries from dust and toxic materials, crush injuries from structural collapse, and biological, chemical, or radiologic contamination from the dissemination of these agents in dirty bombs.

An understanding of the well documented injury patterns following explosive events allows accurate triage and treatment of the casualties who survive the initial blast. Primary BLI, trauma to the head, chest, and abdomen, and traumatic amputation are all markers of severity that are associated with substantial mortality, and should prompt triage decisions for immediate care.[12,39,40] Furthermore, a thorough knowledge of all elements of explosive disasters

TABLE 10

EXPLOSIVE DISASTERS: FACTORS THAT IMPACT CASUALTY OUTCOMES

Physical factors
　Magnitude of blast force
　Distance from blast
　Occurrence of building collapse
Environmental factors
　Medium: Air vs. water
　Confined space vs. open air
　Proximity of resources: Urban vs. isolated locale
Casualty management factors
　Interval to treatment
　Rapidity of casualty flow
　Forward traffic flow
　Surge capacity/capability
　Triage accuracy
　Surgical capability
Anatomic injury factors
　Primary blast injury
　Traumatic amputation
　Blunt and penetrating torso injuries
　Multidimensional injuries
　Severe head injury
　Early symptoms of chemical or radiation exposure

that impact casualty outcome[40,52] facilitates effective planning and achievement of a successful medical response to these disasters (see Table 10).

Pitfalls

The major problems that occur in this area relate to a failure to understand the biology, pathology, clinical manifestations, and patterns of occurrence, of those injuries that typically follow disasters. This results in poor planning and implementation of an effective medical response. Another pitfall is the failure to engage acute medical care providers, and trauma centers, in the planning process and the infrastructure of disaster management and response. These are the clinical assets that are best able to care for the most likely forms of injury documented to occur following disasters. Education of medical providers in the pathophysiology and treatment of those relatively unusual injuries that some disasters may produce, in the levels of severity and complexity of otherwise common injuries that may follow disasters, and in the unique requirements of the evaluation and treatment of all injuries in the setting of a mass casualty event, is the most important tool for assuring successful outcomes.

SUMMARY

Disaster planning and management should be an essential component of surgical practice and expertise. Most disasters and mass casualty events are characterized by large numbers of casualties with bodily injury, who require the skills and experience of surgeons to evaluate and treat. All acute medical care personnel who comprise the team that routinely manages trauma, and provides surgical capability, must be leaders in this field if the medical response to disasters is to succeed. Preparation and planning for disaster response requires a thorough knowledge of the unique aspects of mass casualty management, including the principles of disaster triage, prehospital and in-hospital casualty management, the structure and function of a unified command and the role of medical care within that command, the concepts of surge capacity and surge capability, the appropriate casualty flow and distribution, and the pathophysiology and patterns of injury most likely to occur following disasters. The lessons from past disasters must be learned and assimilated in order to maximize casualty outcomes in future events.

REFERENCES

1. Auf der Heide E. *Disaster response: Principles of preparation and coordination*. St. Louis: CV Mosby; 1989.
2. Waeckerle JF. Disaster planning and response. *N Engl J Med.* 1991;324:815–821.
3. Stein M, Hirshberg A. Medical consequences of terrorism: The conventional weapons threat. *Surg Clin North Am.* 1999;79:1537–1552.
4. Treat KN, Williams JM, Furbee PM, et al. Hospital preparedness for weapons of mass destruction incidents: An initial assessment. *Ann Emerg Med.* 2001;38:562–565.
5. Mann NC, MacKenzie E, Anderson C. Public health preparedness for mass casualty events: A 2002 state-by-state assessment. *Prehospital Disaster Med.* 2004;19:245–255.
6. Frykberg ER. Disaster and mass casualty management: A commentary on the American College of Surgeons position statement. *J Am Coll Surg.* 2003;197:857–859.
7. Jacobs LM, Burns KJ, Gross RI. Terrorism: A public health threat with a trauma system response. *J Trauma.* 2003;55:1014–1021.
8. Torkki M, Koljonen V, Sillanpaa K, et al. Triage in a bomb disaster with 166 casualties. *Eur J Trauma.* 2006;32:374–380.
9. Ciraulo DL, Barie PS, Briggs SM, et al. An update on the surgeon's scope and depth of practice to all hazards emergency response. *J Trauma.* 2006;60:1267–1274.
10. Rivara FP, Nathens AB, Jurkovich GJ, et al. Do trauma centers have the capacity to respond to disasters? *J Trauma.* 2006;61:949–953.
11. Phillips SJ, Knebel A, eds. *Mass medical care with scarce resources: A community planning guide*. Prepared by Health Systems Research, Inc., an Altarum company, under contract No. 290-04-0010. AHRQ Publication No. 07-0001, Rockville: Agency for Healthcare Research and Quality; 2007.
12. Kluger Y. Bomb explosions in acts of terrorism – detonation, wound ballistics, triage and medical concerns. *Isr Med J.* 2003;5:235–240.
13. Ciraulo DL, Frykberg ER, Feliciano DV, et al. A survey assessment of preparedness for domestic terrorism and mass casualty incidents among Eastern Association for the Surgery of Trauma members. *J Trauma.* 2004;56:1033–1041.
14. O'Neill PA. The ABC's of a disaster response. *Scand J Surg.* 2005;94:259–266.
15. Arnold JL. Disaster medicine in the 21st century: Future hazards, vulnerabilities, and risk. *Prehospital Disaster Med.* 2002;17:3–11.
16. Hammond JS. Mass casualty incidents: Planning implications for trauma care. *Scand J Surg.* 2005;94:267–271.
17. Frykberg ER. Medical management of disasters and mass casualties from terrorist bombings: How can we cope? *J Trauma.* 2002;53:201–212.
18. Kluger Y, Peleg K, Daniel-Aharonson L, et al. The special injury pattern in terrorist bombings. *J Am Coll Surg.* 2004;199:875–879.
19. Auf der Heide E. The importance of evidence-based disaster planning. *Ann Emerg Med.* 2006;47:34–49.
20. Klein JS, Weigelt JA. Disaster management: Lessons learned. *Surg Clin North Am.* 1991;71:257–266.
21. Berry FB. The medical management of mass casualties: The scudder oration on trauma. *Bull Am Coll Surg.* 1956;41:60–66.
22. Barrier G. Emergency medical services for treatment of mass casualties. *Crit Care Med.* 1989;17:1062–1067.
23. Jacobs LM, Goody MM, Sinclair A. The role of a trauma center in disaster management. *J Trauma.* 1983;23:697–701.
24. Irwin RL. The incident command system (ICS). In: Auf Der Heide E, ed. *Disaster response: Principles of preparation and coordination*. St. Louis: Mosby; 1989:133–163.
25. Einav S, Aharonson-Daniel L, Weissman C, et al. In-hospital resource utilization during multiple casualty incidents. *Ann Surg.* 2006;243:533–540.
26. National Center for Injury Prevention and Control. *A moment's notice: Surge capacity for terrorist bombings*. Atlanta: Centers for Disease Control and Prevention; 2007.
27. Hirshberg A, Scott BG, Granchi T, et al. How does casualty load affect trauma care in urban bombing incidents? A quantitative analysis. *J Trauma.* 2005;58:686–695.
28. Aylwin CJ, Konig TC, Brennan NW, et al. Reduction in critical mortality in urban mass casualty incidents: Analysis of triage, surge, and resource use after the London bombings on July 7, 2005. *Lancet.* 2006;368:2219–2225.
29. Hirshberg A, Stein M, Walden R. Surgical resource utilization in urban terrorist bombing: A computer simulation. *J Trauma.* 1999;47:545–550.
30. Shamir MY, Weiss YG, Willner D, et al. Multiple casualty terror events: The anesthesiologist's perspective. *Anesth Analg.* 2004;98:1746–1752.
31. Avidan V, Hersch M, Spira RM, et al. Civilian hospital response to a mass casualty event: The role of the intensive unit. *J Trauma.* 2007;62:1234–1239.
32. Roccaforte JD, Cushman JG. Disaster preparation for the intensive care unit. *Curr Opin Crit Care.* 2002;8:607–615.
33. Frykberg ER, Tepas JJ, Alexander RH. The 1983 Beirut airport terrorist bombing: Injury patterns and implications for disaster management. *Am Surg.* 1989;55:134–141.
34. Mahoney EJ, Harrington DT, Biffl WL, et al. Lessons learned from a nightclub fire: Institutional disaster preparedness. *J Trauma.* 2005;58:487–491.
35. Simchen E, Sprung CL, Galai N, et al. Survival of critically ill patients hospitalized in and out of intensive care units under paucity of intensive care unit beds. *Crit Care Med.* 2004;32:1654–1661.
36. Shapira SC, Adatto-Levi R, Avitzour M, et al. Mortality in terrorist attacks: A unique modal of temporal death distribution. *World J Surg.* 2006;30:2071–2079.
37. Almogy G, Belzberg H, Rivkind AI. Suicide bombing attacks: Updates and modifications to the protocol. *Ann Surg.* 2004;239:295–303.
38. Frykberg ER. Triage: Principles and practice. *Scand J Surg.* 2005; 94:272–278.
39. Almogy G, Luria T, Richter E, et al. Can external signs of trauma guide management? Lessons learned from suicide bombing attacks in Israel. *Arch Surg.* 2005;140:390–393.
40. Frykberg ER, Tepas JJ. Terrorist bombings: Lessons learned from Belfast to Beirut. *Ann Surg.* 1988;208:569–576.
41. Ashkenazi I, Kessel B, Khashan T, et al. Precision of in-hospital triage in mass-casualty incidents after terror attacks. *Prehospital Disaster Med.* 2006;21:20–23.
42. Einav S, Feigenberg Z, Weissman C, et al. Evacuation priorities in mass casualty terror-related events – implications for contingency planning. *Ann Surg.* 2004;239:304–310.

43. Gavagan TF, Hamilton D, Palacio H, et al. Hurricane katrina: Medical response at the Houston Astrodome/Reliant Center complex. *South Med J.* 2006;99:1–7.

44. Rubin JN. Recurring pitfalls in hospital preparedness and response. *HSI J Homeland Secur.* http://www.homelandsecurity.org/newjournal/Articles/displayArticle2.asp?article=101, Accessed June 20, 2007.

45. Slater MS, Trunkey DD. Terrorism in America: An evolving threat. *Arch Surg.* 1997;132:1059–1066.

46. Eachempati SR, Flomenbaum N, Barie PS. Biological warfare: Current concerns for the health care provider. *J Trauma.* 2002; 52:179–186.

47. Schecter WP, Fry DE. The surgeon and acts of civilian terrorism: Chemical agents. *J Am Coll Surg.* 2005;200:128–135.

48. National Council on Radiation Protection and Measurement. *Management of terrorist events involving radioactive material.* NCRP report no. 138. Bethesda: National Council on Radiation Protection and Measurement; 2001.

49. Mettler FA, Voelz GL. Major radiation exposure – what to expect and how to respond. *N Engl J Med.* 2002;346:1554–1560.

50. Born CT. Blast trauma: The fourth weapon of mass destruction. *Scand J Surg.* 2005;94:279–285.

51. DePalma RG, Burris DG, Champion HR, et al. Blast injuries. *N Engl J Med.* 2005;352:1235–1242.

52. Ciraulo DL, Frykberg ER. The surgeon and acts of civilian terrorism: Blast injuries. *J Am Coll Surg.* 2006;203:942–950.

53. Mallonee S, Shariat S, Stennies G, et al. Physical injuries and fatalities resulting from the Oklahoma City bombing. *JAMA.* 1996;276:382–387.

54. Guiterrez de Ceballos JP, Turegano-Fuentes F, Perez-Diaz D, et al. 11 March 2004: The terrorist bomb explosions in Madrid, Spain – an analysis of the logistics, injuries sustained and clinical management of casualties treated at the closest hospital. *Crit Care.* 2005;9:104–111.

Trauma System Management and Financing

Paul A. Taheri

Trauma centers and systems should be financed in a manner consistent with an integrated public health–trauma care plan. Individually, trauma centers function as the critical linkages leading to achieving a truly viable trauma system. Although seemingly straightforward, realizing this funding goal has been elusive for several reasons; these include lack of understanding of the basic business model of health care, poor understanding of what costs should be included in a trauma system, who should pay for these costs, and how they should be paid. This chapter will provide insights into these issues.

BASIC BUSINESS MODEL OF HEALTH CARE AND TRAUMA CENTERS

Clinically, health care delivery is a complex and interdependent series of processes that must function in a coordinated manner to deliver efficacious care. Understanding the basic business model of a hospital requires an understanding of the three basic costs associated with the delivery of care. These costs—variable, fixed, and indirect—are not unique to health care; rather they are present in virtually all businesses.

Variable Costs

These are the costs that are directly attributable to an individual patient and vary with each care episode.

Examples of these are the costs associated with the delivery of an antibiotic; usage of durable medical equipment; obtaining a radiograph, laboratory tests, and the like. Typically, variable costs are those costs that are controllable by clinicians. Because more of these resources are consumed during a patient care encounter, the higher the medical bill will be. The corollary to this observation is that the sicker the patient the higher the resource consumption, and the greater the variable costs that will be incurred.

Fixed Costs

These are the costs associated with the physical plant, real property, and equipment required to deliver care. Specifically, the fixed costs can be seen as the cost of the "brick and mortar" associated with a given care unit (e.g., intensive care unit [ICU], operating room [OR], emergency department [ED]). Fixed costs can also be human resources such as the salary associated with the unit clerk, charge nurse, or trauma nurse coordinator. These costs are easy to allocate to a single unit, but not simple to allocate to a specific patient. To best understand the fixed costs associated with a trauma ICU, think of how much it costs to keep the ICU open regardless of patient volume. In other words, the institution bears these fixed costs even if there are no patients in the unit. Cost accountants typically allocate these costs by applying a fixed tax rate to every patient encounter based on the variable costs associated with thespecific clinical encounter. For patients with high variable costs, a tax rate is applied which is typically high (i.e., 50%) and this is then added to the patients' variable costs. Therefore for a patient who accumulates $5,000 in variable costs, the fixed costs allocated to the unit would be an incremental $2,500 in addition to the aforementioned variable costs. The total charge for the patient would then be $7,500.

Indirect Costs

These are the costs that cannot be directly allocated to a specific patient because the cost cannot be readily attributed to a geographically distinct area within the hospital. These include chief executive officer (CEO) salary; cost of maintaining a parking garage, the cafeteria, admissions office, marketing; and the like. Trauma care is emblematic of a system in which substantial investments are required in advance of the patient's episode of care. Trauma centers must invest in both the physical plant and most importantly the human capital to accept the critically ill. These investments include capacity within the nursing, radiology, and technician staff to be immediately available upon the arrival of an injured patient. Moreover, other forms of capacity such as OR, interventional radiology suites, and ED space must be available. These resources, like all other investments, are expensive and the investment in capacity must be made long in advance of the first patient arrival. Such investments are termed *sunk* in hospital financial management terminology. Scheduling and prioritizing trauma care are extremely difficult to achieve and never a clinically viable option. The financial management challenges to trauma centers are, therefore, significant.

For trauma centers, a large proportion of the indirect cost is consumed in supplying medical specialist coverage, nursing and other specialized medical personnel, equipment, and space. These costs are experienced from the moment the institution decides to become a trauma center and the costs cannot be easily allocated or recovered from patient billings. These costs are termed the *cost of readiness*. A study of Florida trauma centers completed in 2002 showed that

the "cost of readiness" averaged $2.7 million annually for each of the 20 trauma centers.[1] The cost of readiness is a main determinant of the financial health of a trauma system. Despite the fact that a trauma center hospital may have a positive "bottom line," the cost of readiness is an important factor which may limit the flexibility of the institution in financial markets. This cost may alter the manner in which trauma centers invest in construction to increase capacity. Downstream revenues realized from trauma patients who return to the hospital for treatment rendered after the patient receives funding for health care costs serve to reduce the impact of these outlays.[2] Understanding the relationship between cost and reimbursement method for each patient category may also allow for strategic decisions that maximize trauma patient revenue.[3] Finally, the cost of readiness is the main reason trauma systems seek durable funding from government sources through local and state taxation schemes, surcharges on fees such as automobile license tags and health insurance costs, as well as "sin taxes" on alcohol and traffic violations.

Although all of the components of hospital indirect costs are important to the operational success of the organization, identifying and allocating a specific portion of these costs to a specific patient is remarkably difficult. For example, how much of the CEO's salary should be allocated to an ICU patient or an ambulatory care patient? The answer to this question is difficult, yet the cost accountants must cover the costs associated with these important functions. In aggregate, hospital fixed costs plus indirect costs are termed *overhead*.

The Mythology of Health Care Cost Reduction Strategies

For decades, physicians have been asked to reduce the cost of care by rationing resources. This rationing includes reducing the patients' lengths of hospital stay. To illustrate why this does not work as intended, consider the data in Table 1 on the cost of one hypothetical patient's stay

TABLE 1

COST DETAILS FOR A HYPOTHETICAL INPATIENT STAY, AUGUST 5–7

Date of Service	Department Group Name	Variable Direct Cost ($)	Allocated Overhead ($)	Total Cost ($)
08/05/99	Emergency services	471	480	951
08/05/99	Laboratory	7	18	25
08/05/99	Nursing-routine	437	725	1,161
08/05/99	Radiology	235	658	893
08/05/99	Laboratory	26	80	107
08/06/99	Nursing-routine	199	310	508
08/06/99	Pharmacy	8	11	19
08/06/99	Radiology	28	97	125
08/07/99	Nursing-routine	134	222	356
		1,544	2,600	4,145

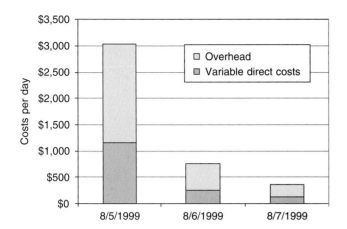

Figure 1 Costs per day, August 5–7, 1999.

in August 1999. This table provides little data on the patient's diagnosis or care, but it documents the resources consumed. For example, the patient had spent $25 for laboratory tests on August 5, and $18 of this amount was allocated as overhead. The test involved only $7 in variable direct costs. Similarly, the patient incurred $8 in variable direct pharmacy costs on August 6, and the hospital's accountants added $11 in overhead to help recover other (indirect) costs. The total 3-day cost was $4,145, of which $2,600 was overhead and $770 was the variable direct cost of routine nursing. Variable direct costs on the final day of the patient's stay were a mere $134.

Figure 1 shows the total daily costs. It is easy to see that resource consumption is front-loaded, with the majority expenses being incurred on the first day of the patient's stay.[4] If the caregivers responsible for this patient had somehow succeeded in discharging the patient on the evening of August 6 rather than on August 7, costs would have fallen by only $356, and the true resource savings would have been a mere $134, or just 3.4% of the $4,145 total! Lopping off a full day of this patient's stay would

have saved little. Indeed, from Table 1 it is clear that at most a few hundred dollars could be saved even if this encounter could have been done on an outpatient basis. What is true for this patient is true generally—resource consumption tends to be composed largely of overhead and front-loaded variable costs.

There are few savings attainable from rationing the variable resources needed to treat individual patients. To illustrate, suppose a hospital invests $500,000 in fixed costs for a new clinical service, including space, durable equipment, a salaried administrator, and other capital and human resources. These are the service's fixed costs, and the hospital incurs them whether it treats 1 patient or 100. This $500,000 investment constitutes "overhead," and Fig. 2 shows how the overhead cost per case varies with the number of patients treated. If there are only 20 patients, then $25,000 of overhead is allocated to each patient; if there are 50 patients, then overhead falls to $10,000 per patient; and if the hospital can somehow treat 100 patients, the overhead is a mere $5,000 per case. In other words, Fig. 2 shows how fixed cost per case falls as a result of treating more patients. This is the simple logic of "amortizing" fixed costs by spreading the cost over a larger group of patient encounters by increasing "throughput." This fact of business life is no more or less compelling in health care than in other high fixed-cost industries. The benefits are readily apparent in industries ranging from manufacturing to transportation to publishing to software. It is worth noting that amortization does not depend upon achieving "economies of scale." Economy of scale refers to producing products in large volumes to reduce unit costs, whereas amortization focuses on making full use of all available fixed resources. A pediatrician has high fixed costs but enjoys few economies of scale. Even operating on a relatively small scale the pediatrician must schedule as many patients as possible during the course of a working day.

If a hospital functions at high capacity utilization, then inpatient length of stay is important, not because

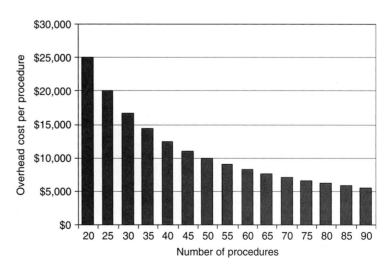

Figure 2 Fixed costs/case with $500,000 in overhead.

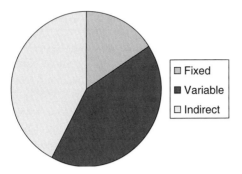

Figure 3   Hospital/health system cost structure displayed graphically.

discharging a patient early saves resources. But because reducing length of stay frees up capacity, thereby creating opportunities to admit more patients, improvement of throughput leads to more efficient capacity utilization, and a healthier financial status for the institution. The goal is not to discharge patients early from hospital or to rush them from beginning to end. Basic operations management techniques expedite care, thereby improving service and outcomes while raising patient satisfaction. Understanding the distribution of these costs is relevant to understanding how hospitals and health systems make investment decisions. In general, the distribution is as follows (see Fig. 3): The fixed cost accounts for approximately 15% to 20% of the total cost of care. The indirect and variable costs account for approximately 40% to 45% and 35% to 40%, respectively, of the care. In aggregate, these overhead costs account for approximately 60% to 65% of all the costs associated with the delivery of patient care. An alternative way of thinking of these "overhead costs" is how much it would cost to have the hospital functioning if no patients were admitted. From an economist's point of view, a hospital and health system is a high fixed cost and relatively low variable cost business. This economic model applies to programs within the institution such as trauma, transplant, and others. Understanding this fundamental economic tenet regarding the business of health care is critical to understanding trauma center financing. Once it is understood that most costs are fixed, this business model requires high volumes of patients to be financially viable. The goal is to optimize the system by high throughput volume (putting more patients through the system, center, or service) in order to amortize the large fixed costs over

as many patients as possible. This model is common in industries such as education, automobile manufacturing, oil and gas exploration, and pipeline construction.

Understanding these costs allows for enhanced insight into the management perspectives of health systems and trauma centers. From a management perspective, health systems must invest large amounts of capital in both the physical plant and in training and maintaining the requisite specialized human capital. The plant investments are easily seen and quantified, such as a new computed tomography (CT) scanner, new ORs, or new space in the ED. In addition, a portion of the human capital such as nursing and various therapists can be assigned or allocated to a specific region within the hospital (OR, ED, radiology). In the case of trauma, much of this expense comes in the form of trauma center readiness. Trauma centers by their very nature require a high level of on-demand support staff including physicians, specialists, and others to function properly. Several observations are important in understanding how these costs impact care. First, most costs are in "overhead" (fixed and indirect costs), not variable costs. For more than a decade, clinicians and administrators have focused their cost reduction efforts on the variable costs (per diem charges, laboratory costs, medications, and supplies), yet the bulk of the costs are in "overhead." Second, hospitals and health systems are by fiscal necessity, required to treat increasing volumes of patients to remain viable. Moreover, how these costs are specifically allocated at the patient level can then create some unfortunate consequences related to the financial interpretation of a given patient care episode. For example, legal and fiscal restraints prevent hospitals from discounting the billings for patients who are "self-pay" or who have no funding. This fact leads to the appearance of differential billing favoring patients who are more affluent at the expense of indigent patients.

How is Care Financed?

Health care is financed through multiple links and various financial intermediaries. Figure 4 depicts some but not all of the contractual relationships, with employees "up" stream as ultimate purchasers of care and providers all the way "down" stream as ultimate sellers. It describes three contractual interfaces—between employer and employee, between employer and third-party payer, and between third-party payer and health care provider. Each interface

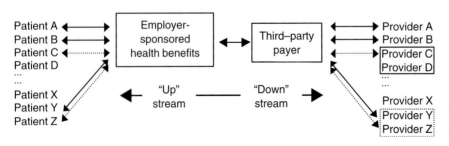

Figure 4   Diagrammatic representation of the complex relationships between payers, providers, and consumers of health care.

is complex and made more difficult by their many interactions. Therefore, for example, employees' covered benefits depend on the contractual relationships that third-party payers negotiate with providers downstream, while downstream contracts are negotiated with upstream relationships in mind.

THIRD-PARTY PAYERS

One way to parse these contracts is to identify third-party payers as the nexus through which contracting occurs. As an empirical matter, this makes sense, because the two largest payers, Medicare and Medicaid, are huge government agencies that set their contractual terms unilaterally. The terms they dictate *anchor* health care financing, even if other third-party payers cannot (or choose not to) follow Medicare and Medicaid. The approach, therefore, is to describe these third-party payers; then explain how they contract with other parties upstream and downstream.

Figure 5 shows the percentage of the US population covered by health insurance in 2005.[5] Medicare and Medicaid together cover 29% of Americans; various Blue Cross Blue Shield (BCBS) plans cover 19%; other private payers have a 32% share; and 15% of the population is uninsured. This section briefly summarizes each payer category.

Government Payers: Medicare, Medicaid, TRICARE, and Others

Medicare and *Medicaid* are the largest and most influential third-party payers. Medicare is the federal government's health insurance for elderly Americans. It also covers some disabled patients and patients with end-stage renal disease. Medicare is financed through a payroll tax (currently 2.9%) on all workers. When workers retire, they are then entitled to Medicare coverage at a nominal fee. Medicare "Part A" is available at no charge and covers hospital and skilled nursing facility care; Medicare "Part B" is Supplementary Medical Insurance (SMI) that reimburses

physicians' professional fees, diagnostic tests, radiology, pathology, and various other services. Part B is optional, but nearly everyone who is eligible pays the modest premium. In 2003, Congress added prescription drug coverage which began in 2006.

Medicaid provides health coverage for the poor. Eligibility is narrow, however, with an emphasis on families with children. (According to Harvard's Health Care Insurance Report[5] of 31 million Americans living in poverty in 2003, only 12 million were covered by Medicaid.) Medicaid also covers nursing home care for the elderly, if they have exhausted their Medicare coverage as well as their personal savings. Finally, Medicaid also provides benefits to the disabled. Medicaid is financed out of the general revenues of the federal government and the individual states, which together share the financial burden. Medicaid is administered by individual states. There are other government payers. *TRICARE* insures active duty military and uniformed retirees, along with their families. The *Federal Health Benefits Program* (FEHB) covers approximately 9 million federal employees and their dependents through 350 health plans nationwide. The *State Children's Health Insurance Program* (SCHIP) provides insurance to children in families that earn more than Medicaid allows but too little to afford other coverage. To cover the health care costs of their workers' job-related injuries, employers pay into a state fund called *Workers Compensation*.

"The Blues"

BCBS plans are collectively the nation's oldest and largest health insurers. Historically, they have been state-based not-for-profit firms (e.g., BCBS of Michigan). "The Blues" began consolidating in the 1980s, and of 110 plans in 1987, only 39 remained in 2003. Wellpoint is the largest BCBS plan, formed by the merger of many state plans, and it has converted from not-for-profit to a for-profit publicly traded company. Other BCBS plans have also converted to for-profit. In 2003, not-for-profit BCBS plans provided coverage to 88 million Americans.

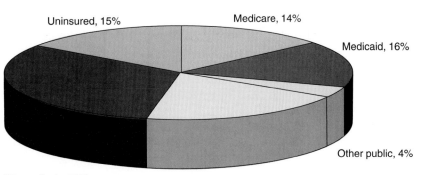

Figure 5 Proportions of US health care financing by payer source.

Other Private "Commercial" Payers

Compared to other industries, private health insurance is "fractured," meaning that many firms have small market shares. In recent years, the industry has consolidated, and even now payers in the second decile are, combined, not as large as the Blues. The largest of these "commercial payers" are Wellpoint (33 million enrollees), Health Group (23 million), Aetna (14 million), and United and CIGNA (10 million). Another tier includes Kaiser Permanente (8 million) and Humana (7 million). These commercial payers are consolidating, with more mergers likely. Many health systems also have system-owned or affiliated health insurance companies. As described in the subsequent text, each of these insurers offers multiple health plans, which they typically market to employers.

Employers' Self-Funded Plans

Many employers are partially or fully self-insured, or "self-funded," meaning that they bear the financial risk directly from providing for their employees' health care needs. They pay with their own cash. Employers often procure "stop-loss" insurance to guard against very high individual claims or group claims beyond a high threshold amount. Self-funded plans are attractive to large corporations that are well-positioned to bear the attendant financial risk, as well as smaller employers that for various reasons have difficulty procuring fully funded insurance from the health plans in their area. Employers rarely administer self-funded plans themselves. Instead they hire third-party administrators (TPAs) or administrative service organizations (ASOs).

Health Savings Accounts

In 2003, Congressional legislation created *health savings accounts* (HSAs), which enable individuals to set money aside to pay for health care services over their lifetimes. Money that remains unspent at the end of each year is "rolled over" and invested tax-free in the next. HSAs are also portable, meaning that employees may take their HSAs from one employer to another. HSAs must be coupled with a high-deductible health plan as a contingency against very large claims. Some Blue Cross plans and other commercial insurers, in turn, are marketing high-deductible plans that also provide the buyer with access to the plans' provider networks, so that patients can enjoy the contractual discounts and provider access that those plans have negotiated.

The Uninsured

In 2004, a total of 46 million Americans lacked health insurance for at least part of the year. This group is diverse—55% of the uninsured are working adults, 20% are children, and roughly one third earn more than $50,000 per year. As such, it is difficult to generalize about how the uninsured access and pay for health care. More details appear in the subsequent text, and in many of the modules that follow.

REIMBURSEMENT OF PROFESSIONAL FEES

Traditional Indemnity Insurance

Through the early 1990s physicians typically set their own reimbursements, provided only that their fees were "customary, prevailing, and reasonable." As long as a physician was not charging more than his or her peers, health insurers paid up. This arrangement is often referred to as *traditional indemnity insurance* because insurers made no attempt to regulate or negotiate prices, or otherwise manage the care that patients and physicians arrange on their own.

The Resource-Based Relative Value Scale

In 1992, Medicare began using a *Resource-Based Relative Value Scale* (RBRVS) to describe and measure physician services. Other payers followed. The RBRVS offers a common scale to meter physicians' work and resource costs. As illustrated in Table 2 it has three key elements:

TABLE 2
RESOURCE-BASED RELATIVE VALUE SCALE

Service	CPT Code	Physician Work	Practice Expense	Malpractice	Total RVU	Conversion Factor	Physician Reimbursement ($)
Office visit, detailed, established patient	99213	0.67	0.69	0.03	1.39	37.8975	53
Office visit, complex, established patient	99215	1.77	1.32	0.08	3.17	37.8975	120
Transplantation of kidney	50360	31.48	15.47	3.78	50.73	37.8975	1,923
Across all CPTs, percentage of total RVUs		55	41	4	100	—	—

CPT, current procedural terminology; RVU, relative value scale.

Current Procedural Terminology (CPT) Codes identify the particular services that physicians perform, including new patient office visits and specific procedures. CPT codes serve as a common language for describing and reporting services and getting paid for them

Relative Value Units (RVUs) quantify the relative work and resource costs associated with each CPT code and assign a numeric value. Each RVU is the sum of three components: (i) a *physician work RVU*, which measures the amount of physician time and effort required to provide the service; (ii) a *practice expense RVU*, which captures overhead and other nonphysician expenses required to provide the service; and (iii) a *malpractice cost RVU*, which is intended to compensate physicians for the cost of procuring professional liability ("malpractice") insurance. Across all physician services, physician work RVUs add up to approximately 55% of total RVUs, whereas practice expense and malpractice cost RVUs amount to 41% and 4%, respectively.

Finally, the total of these three RVUs are translated into reimbursement through a *conversion factor* and various *adjustment factors*. In 2005, the conversion factor was $37.90 per RVU. There are also geographic adjustment factors, for example, that reflect local and regional differences in costs. Medicare updates all elements of this reimbursement methodology annually.

Private Payers and Percent of Medicare

Many other third-party payers reimburse physicians with this same RBRVS methodology. Often they do not pay exactly what Medicare offers, but rather a percentage of Medicare. They may pay 115% of Medicare, for example, or just 85%, depending on local conditions and the relative bargaining power of specific physician groups and third-party payers.

Capitation

Some third-party payers contract with a physician group practice to take clinical and financial responsibility for *all* of a patient's medical care. Under such a *capitation* arrangement, a member of the payer's health plan chooses a primary care physician (PCP), and the payer reimburses the PCP's physician group a set amount per member per month (PMPM). The group then commits to meet clinical needs of all members and to assume all of the attendant financial risk.

Balance Billing

If a physician bills a patient $100 for an office visit but the patient's insurance only pays $75, what happens to the balance? If the physician holds the patient accountable and insists that he or she pay the remaining $25, then that physician has engaged in "balance billing." Most health plans insist that physicians agree not to balance bill their patients as a condition of payment.

Emergency and Trauma Call Stipends

Traditionally, nearly all hospitals required medical staff members to take ED call as a *quid pro quo* for admitting privileges. This obligation usually extended until the medical staff member reached a certain age, usually 50 to 60 years. Night and weekend ED call can be disruptive, and reimbursement for inpatient care of patients admitted from the ED is no longer adequate in many cases to cross-subsidize low professional fees in the ED. Because care migrates from inpatient to outpatient settings, and from outpatient to off-site venues, some physicians have decided to narrow or give up their admitting privileges. Others have negotiated "on-call stipends" from their hospitals for standing "ready and willing" to provide emergent care, and are paid in addition to the physicians' professional fees.

Viewed from the perspective of amortization, the logic of providing on-call compensation to trauma surgeons and other medical specialists is clarified. The on-call specialist's total compensation depends on throughput just as hospital revenue does. If the specialist is forced to defer or cancel a revenue-producing patient care encounter because of on-call obligations, the consequences extend beyond an economic loss to alienation of the patient from the specialist and the hospital, the specialist from the hospital, and ill feelings among all parties. The downstream effect on hospital throughput may be significantly negative. Moreover, the presence of the specialist has economic advantages for the hospital. During the on-call interval, the presence of the specialist improves hospital throughput by ensuring efficient medical decision making and optimum patient care processes leading to improved outcomes.[6] Increased patient satisfaction ensures that patients and their families will utilize the institution in the future. From an economic perspective, on-call stipends can be easily justified.

PAYING HOSPITALS FOR INPATIENT CARE

Fee-for-Service and "Full Billed Charges"

Health systems bill for their "facility services" separately from physicians' professional services. Like physicians, health systems could historically set their own charges and be assured of full reimbursement so long as their charges were "customary, prevailing, and reasonable." Although this is no longer generally the case, there are instances where third-party payers continue to pay "full billed charges" for inpatient care. If a patient travels to Chicago, for example, from Nashville and is admitted to a Chicago-area trauma center after a motor vehicle crash, it is possible that the patient's health insurer has no contract with the local trauma center already in place. In this case, the hospital can bill the third-party payer and insist upon payment in full.

Discounted Charges (Fee-for-Service) and Inpatient Per Diems

The prospect of paying full billed charges provides an incentive for third-party payers to negotiate with health systems for negotiated discounts. Hospitals often extend these discounts to third-party payers willing to include their health system in the payer's provider network, thereby making it easier for patients to access the health system. The discounts often take the form of *percentage of charges* or *inpatient per diems*. The percentage of charges methodology is also known as *fee-for-service*. The Health Care Advisory Board estimates that 37% of inpatient care nationwide was reimbursed through discounted fee-for-service, whereas 25% was reimbursed using a lump sum reimbursement per day.

Diagnostic-Related Groups and the Prospective Payment System

In 1983, Medicare adopted a *Prospective Payment System* (PPS). At discharge, each patient is grouped by principal and secondary diagnoses, and in some cases by age (e.g., 0 to 17 years) and treatment strategy (e.g., surgical vs. nonsurgical) into one of 25 *major diagnostic categories* (MDCs). Within these MDCs, patients are identified with one of 516 *diagnostic-related groups* (DRGs), which determine how much the hospital is paid. For each DRG, Medicare reimburses a lump sum base payment that is adjusted according to several factors, such as local costs of providing care, and whether the hospital has resident training programs or a disproportionate share of low-income patients. The lump sum payment for each DRG is designed to cover the costs of providing high-quality, cost-effective care. The payment does not vary with the actual costs that a hospital incurs for caring for individual patients, except in a small fraction of cases that reach "outlier status," meaning that they have exceptionally high costs. Once a patient reaches "outlier status," the payer provides added reimbursement as a percentage of incremental charges.

Because DRG-based payments take the form of a lump sum, hospitals are rewarded for controlling their costs. Medicare, Medicaid, and some other government health plans use this methodology to reimburse inpatient care nationwide, as do "the Blues." Table 2 lists the 25 MDCs, and for each MDC it provides an example of one DRG. Therefore, for example, the most common DRG nationwide is 391, "Normal Newborn," which is MDC 15, "Normal Newborns and Other Neonates."

The implications of prospective payment on trauma centers are far reaching. A number of studies have shown that the DRG reimbursement system is relatively insensitive to variations in cost for patient care depending on the severity of illness and the frequency with which the hospital treats a certain condition.[3,7] Trauma center reimbursement falls short of trauma center cost under prospective payment methodologies and this shortfall is not compensated for by alterations in case-mix severity or DRG outlier status.[8] Hospitals must respond by engaging in "portfolio management," a strategy that balances patient resource consumption, payer characteristics, reimbursement methods, and the revenue cycle to maximize revenue per patient encounter and provides flexibility for investment and acquisition of new technology.[9]

HOW MEDICARE REIMBURSES HOSPITALS FOR OUTPATIENT SERVICES

In 2000, Medicare began using a PPS to reimburse facility costs for hospitals' outpatient care. The individual outpatient services that hospitals provide are classified by reported CPT codes into groups that are clinically and financially similar. These groups are called *Ambulatory Payment Classifications* (APCs). The APC methodology sets a fixed prospective amount for each APC regardless of the actual cost to the hospital. The result is an outpatient facility fee schedule that operates much like the physician fee schedule, with CPT codes determining both the facility and professional reimbursement.

The cost of the facility itself and most other required resources (e.g., pharmaceuticals, supplies and equipment, and nursing services) are bundled into this outpatient service and are not paid separately. Patients with Medicare coverage share in the cost of this outpatient care through a mechanism known as *coinsurance*, which is described in the subsequent text. Other third-party payers may or may not follow Medicare's lead, though many third-party payers have already adopted this payment methodology and more are likely to do so.

OTHER OUTPATIENT REIMBURSEMENT

Third-party payers also reimburse other outpatient care, including skilled nursing facilities, durable medical equipment used in patients' homes, home health care services, hospice care, outpatient dialysis, outpatient laboratory services, surgeries performed in freestanding facilities, long-term hospital care, and psychiatric services. While it is important that residents are aware that these services are reimbursed, the methodologies vary across payers and types of outpatient care. As such, further details are beyond the scope of this brief overview.

PROVIDER NETWORKS AND THE MARKETING OF HEALTH PLANS TO EMPLOYERS

The term *managed care* can be applied narrowly or broadly to have different meanings. In its broadest interpretation, it includes any effort by third-party payers to negotiate the terms on which providers offer care. Some third-party payers negotiate strict contracts and maintain tight control over their providers, in the extreme, for example, by hiring salaried physicians who are devoted to a single health plan. For various reasons, other insurers may opt for much looser contractual arrangements.

Health Maintenance Organizations, Preferred Provider Organizations, and Point of Service Plans

Health maintenance organizations (HMOs) offer patients restricted access to a tightly controlled provider network. Patients must use "in-network" physicians who are under contract with the HMO, and they may access specialty care only after obtaining a referral from their PCP. Often the providers enlisted to deliver care to patients enrolled in HMOs have capitated contracts, which present these providers with keen incentives to reduce costs. In return for these tight controls and cost reduction measures, the members of HMOs enjoy lower monthly premiums, reduced out-of-pocket costs, and in some cases broader coverage (e.g., for preventive medicine).

Preferred provider organizations (PPOs) are less tightly controlled. Patients may choose their own providers, but they pay a premium for using services that are not "in-network." PPOs do not have gatekeepers, but patients must get prior approval for services such as hospitalizations.

Point of service (POS) plans combine HMO and PPO features. "In-network" care is tightly controlled, much like an HMO, with gatekeepers and other cost reduction measures. Yet patients may choose to go out-of-network if they are willing to pay a premium.

Both PPOs and POS plans require more cost sharing, which typically takes one of three forms: (i) *deductibles*, which refer to a specific dollar amount that a patient must pay before insurance provides any coverage; (ii) *co-payments*, which refer to a fixed dollar amount that a patient must pay for a specific service; and (iii) *coinsurance*, which requires the patient to pay a percentage of the amount owed to a provider. Recently, PPOs and POS plans have gained market share at the expense of HMOs, as part of a larger "backlash" against the strict controls that HMOs impose on their members. However, HMOs still command the largest share of the market.

HEALTH CARE COVERAGE AS AN EMPLOYEE BENEFIT

Employers are not required by law to provide health insurance to their employees, but the federal tax code gives them very strong incentives to do so. Most companies do offer significant health benefits, at least to their full-time employees. This coverage typically extends to the employee and his or her dependents. It often includes various choices for medical and wellness, dental, and vision care, and in many cases pharmacy and behavioral health. Employees in larger companies often choose from a menu of choices, with the employer paying the bulk of the cost of baseline coverage and employees paying most or all of the incremental cost of more expensive options.

Employees typically enroll in a health plan at the time they are hired, and they may change plans annually but only during an "open enrollment period." Their premiums do not depend on their own history of resource use; eligibility is not dependent on medical examination, nor is it restricted by age; and an employee's own coverage cannot be canceled by the third-party payer. Employee premiums are usually administered through a simple payroll deduction.

Finally, if workers leave their jobs, they may still purchase health coverage through their former employer for up to 18 months by paying the full premium plus a modest administrative fee. Employers are required by law to provide former employees and their families with this option under "*COBRA (Consolidated Omnibus Budget Reconciliation Act),*" which is the acronym for the legislation that created it. This COBRA coverage provides an important bridge for those who find themselves temporarily unemployed.

How Do Those Without Formal Employment Relationships Procure Health Care?

The previous discussion explains that two types of insurance coverage account for the bulk of all US health care financing: (i) government plans such as Medicare, Medicaid, and TRICARE, along with (ii) employer-based private plans offered by Blue Cross and commercial insurers such as Aetna and CIGNA. Individuals and families that cannot secure insurance through one of these two channels are in jeopardy on at least three key levels. First, even if they can pay for routine care, they face the financial risk of catastrophic claims if a family member becomes seriously ill. Second, employer-based insurance enjoys very generous tax breaks. Third, those who lack access to payers' in-network discounts are often faced with paying full billed charges for their care. In short, those without conventional forms of health coverage pay the entirety of their own bills, no matter how large, with neither the tax breaks nor negotiated discounts that are available to others. Not surprisingly, families that find themselves without health coverage often go without care.

Steps have been taken to reduce some of the more glaring inequities. COBRA coverage, for example, enables families to maintain their existing coverage during bouts of unemployment, and recent legislative enhancements to HSAs provide them with the same tax benefits as employer-provided insurance. HSAs are also coupled with stop-loss insurance from large third-party payers that provides access to those payers' in-network discounts and insures against catastrophic claims. There are disadvantages to HSAs, which are beyond the scope of this brief, but HSAs are a timely and important innovation.

Finally, health care for those who are uninsured or underinsured is underwritten by health care providers who bill for services rendered but then cannot collect. Providers, in other words, bear some of the cost of providing an imperfect safety net. Hospitals that provide a disproportionate share of nonreimbursed care are funded through Medicare and by other means, as well, so that they can better handle the financial burden.

TRAUMA CENTER FINANCING

Financing for individual trauma centers should take into consideration the broader trauma system and the public health perspective. The community wants trauma centers to be there when they need it regardless of the time of day or day of the week. Trauma systems, centers, and services have a requirement to be available 365/7/24. This capability to be "ready" 24/7 has a substantial cost, which is typically not recouped in the traditional health care reimbursement models.

Traditional fee-for-service reimbursement models reflect reimbursement based on the services rendered (transaction by transaction). In this model, trauma centers are only paid for the clinical activity that is delivered at that specific patient care episode. While this is appropriate, this model of reimbursement does not capture the underlying costs associated with readiness.

The goal of trauma center and system financing is to provide the public with a consistent, reliable, and readily available health care safety net for injured patients. Currently, the typical funding mechanisms do not provide optimal financial support for trauma centers because they are designed to fund incremental patient activity rather than support the larger fixed costs associated with maintaining a trauma center.

HOW SURGEONS CAN APPLY BASIC MANAGEMENT PRINCIPALS AND LEAD INSTITUTIONAL CHANGE

Conventional wisdom among health care workers and experts is that the principles that guide nearly every other business do not apply to health care, unless, of course, those principles are modified, qualified, adapted, or otherwise altered to take into consideration all of the idiosyncrasies the industry entails. This chapter rejects this conventional wisdom while providing concrete examples of how trauma centers can look critically at their service line.

Indeed, the first axiom sets out the position that "basic business principles are as applicable to health care delivery as they are to any other industry." Health care is not the only industry where reimbursement methodologies blunt incentives, or where quality is hard to measure. The problems that trouble the health care industry may be somewhat worse than they are elsewhere, but the differences are only a matter of degree. Many businesses suffer from conflicting regulations, constant technology innovation, and workforce shortages.

Physicians are not only educators but also excellent learners who can readily acquire the necessary business principles and apply them to the clinical delivery system. Moreover, physicians have an obligation to be good stewards of clinical resources and provide a platform for change. The three critical axioms imply that physicians are up to the task of transforming health care delivery, and only they can do it.

What business principles should guide physicians? First, they should proceed with the view that good medicine and fiscally responsible behavior need not be at odds. Indeed, economics is nothing more or less than the study of scarce resource allocation, so the scarcer the health care resources are, the more relevant familiarity with economic reasoning should become. More generally, business principles bring to physicians a toolkit for handling difficult choices. These principles are *not* constraints that foreclose, complicate, or distort those choices. If clinicians have suffered historically from adversarial relationships with administrators, third-party payers, and other business entities, it is because business principles have been misapplied; it is not because the principles themselves are flawed or inappropriate. Therefore, the first guiding principle introduced in this chapter is that well-conceived and designed initiatives allow good medical processes and fiscally responsible behavior to go hand-in-hand.

The second guiding principle, this chapter argues, is that physicians must have timely, accurate, and credible data. Data acquisition and information management are at the very core of management activity. Physicians and trauma directors are no different than other managers in their need for meaningful timely data.

The third guiding principle is that comprehensive health care reform must come one project at a time. There is no magic cure for what ails the industry. There are only incremental steps that advance health care delivery and trauma care forward. From an operational perspective, there is only continuous process improvement. Lessons learned in one clinical domain must be applicable to many others, so that a good idea that is well executed in a small corner of the enterprise can spread quickly. We can learn from others' successes; you do not need to "reinvent the wheel." Scalability is critical to reaping maximum rewards for both invested capital and physician time. Physicians should always be asking, "How might this project scale?"

Axiom 1: Basic Business Principles Apply to the Health Care Industry and Trauma Centers

The ORs are delayed again. The ICU is full. Patients are stacked up in the emergency room. Clinics are booked for months. Patients' laboratory tests are late or missing. The list goes on and on. How can we spend so much money on health care delivery and yet have such poor service? How is it that caregivers and patients put up with ineptness and inefficiency that they would not tolerate anywhere outside of health care?

To illustrate, no one would put up with a bank asking for personal information each and every time he/she walked into a branch office. No bank could get away with asking a customer when he/she made the last deposit, or which bank employee handled the transaction. No hotel could remain in business for long if it consistently failed to generate an itemized bill at the time its patrons checked out, or to discuss and remedy charges on the spot that these patrons deem incorrect or unfair. No airline could survive for long if its pilots submitted "professional fees" separate and distinct from what the parent company charged for the ticket. Yet, these activities are all considered acceptable in health care.

Physicians typically assert that health care delivery is complex; that health care delivery involves matters of life and death; that health care delivery suffers from obligations and burdens that other industries do not face, such as caring for the uninsured; and that in every sense the industry is special. As such, they conclude, the health care industry must have its own rules and its own laws of physics. Although the health care industry has some differences when compared to other industries, this is only partially true. Automobiles, to give just one example, are also complex; their manufacture and maintenance involves consideration of life-and-death safety issues; manufacturers are obliged to invest billions into the design and production of vehicles (electric, hydrogen, ultra low-emissions, etc.) that they have no reasonable prospect of ever selling; they face the same tort liabilities as physicians (even when vehicle owners do not exercise appropriate care); and they are heavily regulated.

Moreover, even if the health care industry was unique, it is not clear what any of the industry's differences have to do with long queues in ORs and clinics, missing or late laboratory results, poor medical records, arbitrary and incontestable charges, and the like. One might think, for instance, that in a life-or-death environment, laboratory tests would *less often* show up late or missing, and that capacity would be *more readily available*. The pretext that "we're different" or "this is a hospital problem" is, therefore, inexcusable.

Axiom 2: Physicians Can Learn and Apply Fundamental Business Principles

The basics of economics, cost accounting, finance, operations management, and marketing are not inherently difficult to understand. Costs are relatively straightforward to parse into all of their many different components; net present value (NPV) or return on investment (ROI) is a straightforward idea; throughput is intuitive; and targeting market niches is not complex.

A modest understanding of business principles and open lines of communication can provide enormous opportunities to clarify the miscommunication and misunderstandings between physicians and administrators. Simply understanding the basic lexicon of business allows physicians to more clearly communicate to the hospital leadership. Moreover, it is easier for physicians to understand the fundamentals of business, than for the administrative core to understand the clinical delivery and the complexity associated with care.

Axiom 3: Physicians Can Lead Fundamental Health System Change

Historically, physicians have been handicapped by a lack of access to financial data, strategic institutional planning, and other high-level executive suite functions, which administrators monopolized more out of necessity than by choice. As recently as 5 to 10 years ago, data were difficult to gather, authenticate, and distribute, and physicians were rarely asked to be in the loop. Now physicians must be provided with timely and credible data because clinical directors are being held accountable for the financial consequences of their clinical decisions. With data, physicians are health systems' natural leaders; without data, they are uninformed and therefore incapable of thoughtful change.

Trauma directors and faculty are uniquely positioned to leverage business principles into their daily practice. Trauma care touches virtually all areas of the hospital, and coordinated delivery is the hallmark of a well-organized trauma center. Because physicians are ultimately accountable for the processes by which their patients receive care, physicians are patient advocates and system navigators while being clinical providers. Physicians have clear incentives to optimize care because they are not compensated for the time patients spend awaiting test results or accessing the system. Not only are these delays expensive but they are also stressful for clinicians.

Perhaps even more important, process deficiencies translate into significant opportunity costs and frustration. Surgeons earn more in the OR than in their clinics or by making rounds. Interventional radiologists receive more for performing catheterizations than reading chest x-rays. Gastroenterologists generate more revenue from colonoscopies than inpatient consults. Delays are costly. Because delays are often unanticipated (they are *not* unpredictable), they can be all the more disruptive. Physicians are held accountable by patients and their families not only for ultimate clinical outcomes but also for the quality of services rendered.

To be successful managers, physicians must have good, reliable data to inform their decisions. Peter Drucker's[10] famous truism, "You cannot manage what you do not measure," is ingrained in our culture. Yet we are often attempting to manage our services with little timely or meaningful data. Trauma directors should insist on having the same information hospital administrators have, in the same level of detail, and with the same timeliness.[11] The information between the hospital leadership and the clinical leadership should be symmetrical. Conversely, physicians must also work with health systems to help design their own operations management and reporting tools. Physicians have a responsibility to engage their systems to build better reporting mechanisms and meaningful reporting structures.

One avenue for physicians to demonstrate their management skills is to take a project approach. Utilizing individual projects allows for a demonstration of the clinicians management skills and an opportunity to measure the outcome of the project. What follows are a few examples of "projects" that have provided valuable learning opportunities to both the participants and the institution.

CASE 1

"FLEXING" AN ICU

The demand for trauma and burn care is highly variable and nearly impossible to predict. Admissions are entirely random, and two or more critically injured or burned patients may arrive simultaneously. A ten-bed ICU may have seven patients a day, ten the next, and only five a few days later. It is virtually impossible to predict exactly how many patients and what their acuity is going to be on a given day. This uncertainty is very costly and complicates many aspects of trauma care.

In early 2000, our ten-bed trauma-burn ICU set out to better manage this variability. Leveraging our limited understanding of basic business principles, we determined that an ICU bed is assigned higher *fixed* costs

than a floor bed. Essentially, this means that the cost associated with an ICU bed is greater than the costs associated with a floor bed independent of the level of nursing care required. The goal of this project was to attempt to amortize the higher fixed costs associated with the ICU, by driving more admissions into the unit. To achieve this increased throughput, we continue admitting all trauma and burn patients directly to the ICU (i.e., patients in need of intensive care). If beds are available, we also admit patients requiring any aspect of monitoring that is consistent with a "step-down" status. This change ensured that going forward the trauma-burn ICU is always full or nearly full. Once patients are admitted, their care is managed according to three simple rules:

- *Rule 1*: Retain all ICU patients in the unit until they are discharged from the hospital, or until the ICU reaches capacity. If the ICU is oversubscribed, transfer as many low-acuity patients to the floor as necessary to accommodate arrivals.
- *Rule 2*: Continue to update patients' billing from ICU to "step-down" to floor status at the same point in their care.
- *Rule 3*: Adjust ICU staffing downward to reflect the care that patients would receive in the step-down unit or on the floor.

This arrangement is administered using colored refrigerator door magnets fixed to the outside of each patient's room: red for "ICU status," yellow for "step-down," and green for "floor status." Magnet color is determined each morning on physician-charge nurse rounds, also at that time physicians and nursing coordinate staffing associated with procedures to be undertaken that day (e.g., central line placement, bronchoscopy, and wound dressing changes). After rounds, the ICU clerk checks the magnets and adjusts room charges based on acuity (magnet color); and the charge nurse arranges the ICU nursing staff with a full understanding of the clinical requirements for each ICU patient.

The most immediate benefits are improved nurse staffing and better coordinated care. Yet the hospital reaps other benefits that include the following:

- Better ICU yield management, meaning higher capacity utilization and allocated revenue
- Better yield management in the step-down unit and floor as well because arrivals to these areas is smoother and more predictable
- Frees floor beds for nontrauma patients
- Better amortization of ICU fixed costs
- Lower nursing costs, that is, less overtime *and* less frequent over-staffing—decreasing the wide variability associated with nurse staffing
- Much-improved nurse morale, greater nurse productivity, and a reduction in nurse turnover

- In addition, patients have the opportunity to be discharged directly home from the ICU (if no admissions have "bumped" them, so they also benefit in the following ways:
  - Greater familiarity with their environment and less disruption
  - Ongoing relationships with their original nurses and residents
  - Closer proximity to caregivers even when they no longer require intensive care

Under this arrangement payers are relatively unaffected because the administration of the colored magnets results in a list of charges that is identical to what it would be under the model of care that prevailed before flexing the ICU.

CASE 2

THE SURVIVAL FLIGHT AEROMEDICAL SERVICE

At many hospitals, some patients arrive by aeromedical transport. These patients tend to comprise a very small fraction of total admissions, and yet they are much, much sicker on average than other patients. As such, they consume resources out of all proportion to their numbers. Moreover, these patients gravitate toward specific clinical domains such as trauma and burns, transplantation, and neonatal intensive care, which as a result rely very heavily on this form of transport to generate patient activity. In short, it is easy to underestimate the importance of these services, especially for specific areas of a hospital.

Governance of these aeromedical services is often poor. Individual clinical domains may account for only a small fraction of the business of an aeromedical service, and individual physicians are typically ignorant of helicopters and their operations. No physician, in other words, has either the incentive or the expertise to take ownership. And because the number of patients is so small, hospital leaders often overlook them too. In many cases, aeromedical services tend to operate quasi-independently of the hospital, without much oversight or control.

There are other complicating factors. The communities that benefit most from a hospital's aeromedical service are located far away, and the service, although quite valuable, is also exceedingly expensive. Many health plans do not automatically cover aeromedical transportation, and few employees take the time to compare aeromedical coverage when choosing between competing insurers. It is not a service that anyone expects to use. There is only a small peer-reviewed literature on aeromedical services,

and the relatively little evidence available is undecided on the overall clinical benefits. The operation of an aeromedical service entails very high costs, the bulk of them fixed, and so a small decline in business can be extremely damaging to the bottom line. Finally, in a health care world dominated by prospective payment schemes and capitation, it is difficult to justify a service that attracts resource-intensive patients who are reimbursed on the same terms as patients coming from nearby.

Our own aeromedical service, Survival Flight, fits this pattern. Survival Flight is large with three helicopters and a fixed wing jet. It is well regarded nationally. It operates with only clinical oversight from the ED, and historically it is a service perceived to lose money. In early 2001, our hospital's CEO broached the possibility of selling one helicopter to save money. In response, some of the leading stakeholders in Survival Flight formed a team that included the chairman of the ED, Survival Flight's medical director, the trauma director, representatives from among the pilots and nurses that staff Survival Flight, and personnel from finance, billing, and contracting. The specific goal was to determine the clinical, financial, and educational impact of selling one helicopter for the hospital at large and for the affected clinical domains.

We embarked on a comprehensive data analysis and a schedule of stakeholder interviews. The final result was a recommendation that the hospital keep all three helicopters, and a written document that detailed the importance of Survival Flight and included more than a dozen significant changes in the service. The importance of Survival Flight is illustrated by the following findings:

- Hospital-wide, in 1997, Survival Flight patients contributed 3% of all admissions, 7% of inpatient days, 22% of ICU days, 11% of *all* clinical revenues, and 15% of inpatient revenues.
- The ten largest admitting services for Survival Flight derived 11% of their patients and 22% of their revenues from admissions generated by Survival Flight.
- Measured downstream clinical activity generated incremental revenues for the University of Michigan Health System accounting for 43% of the initial inpatient revenue.
- Survival Flight accounts for a very large portion of the complex cases for the Medical School's educational mission.

There were many other interesting discoveries during our analysis. First, Survival Flight's helicopters were state of the art, and staffed with two critical care nurses (many other services have only one critical care nurse and a paramedic), and yet our charges were among the lowest in the entire Midwest, and far below other academic health systems. Second, Survival Flight had hired an outside company to supply pilots but was not enforcing key provisions of the contract.

There had been no negligence of Survival Flight responsibilities on the part of any individual or group, but there was also no comprehensive input or oversight. Billing had performed its function competently; the ED was supervising clinical care; the aircraft were properly maintained; and so forth. But there was no one in charge, and no one overseeing or coordinating the entire enterprise, and important tasks fell between functions.

Because Survival Flight is a fixed cost business, there are many avenues for increasing activity and improving the clinical and financial returns without significant new investments. In summary, physician leadership of the Survival Flight analysis has led to a better understanding of the aeromedical service's clinical value, financial intricacies, and a richer understanding of how this critical service dovetails with the health system's research, education, and patient care missions.

These projects highlight an important aspect that is fundamental to clinical redesign; physicians must lead these initiatives. They are ideally positioned to implement initiatives as they have the clinical credibility. Projects may have closure, but the underlying clinical franchise continues, and it is clinicians and their patients who then deal with the consequences (good or bad) of these initiatives. To ensure the best long-term outcomes, clinicians must lead.

The projects outlined in this section are "scalable," meaning that both the specific process improvements and the more general insights can be applied to many other settings. Yield management techniques are not unique to the health care industry—they have been applied with great success in myriad other settings—but once they are unleashed in one health care venue, the value becomes immediately apparent in others. There is no reason that flexing cannot occur in other areas of the hospital, and in other hospitals. More aeromedical flights mean better amortization of helicopters, but the incremental admissions also help spread fixed costs in the transplant service, the trauma-burn and neoneonatal ICUs, and for that matter, all of the other expensive fixed resources in the health system that these admissions draw upon. The knowledge gained from the aeromedical initiative can provide a platform for project initiation and implementation in other areas of the hospital such as magnetic resonance imaging (MRI), CT scanners, dialysis units, catheterization laboratories, primary care clinics, private offices indeed, virtually anywhere within the system. As capacity tightens going forward, more focus on sound yield management techniques is as important as any other operational initiative that health systems can undertake, and is likely to drive success or failure of both health systems and individual clinical services.

Physician leaders must keep "scalability" in mind as they conceive of new initiatives and design and push them forward. Scalability is a means to leverage ROI, to manage risk, and to maximize clinical and financial impact. A CEO may be unwilling to take the chance on a $100,000 investment if the best-case payoff is a one-time $120,000 payday; the same CEO may jump at the opportunity to invest $100,000 in a risky pilot project that, if successful, yields a $20,000 profit many times over.

Moving a project forward that is scalable also provides a huge opportunity for a physician to demonstrate a willingness to participate at a high organizational level. From a cultural and political standpoint, executive officers within a system are keen to adopt physician-led initiatives that are scalable because these benefit the entire organization, not just a single physician.

Finally, physicians and their administrative liaisons must look at their service line as "franchises." Physician leaders need to understand how the franchises function within their larger health systems. They can no longer manage care for individual patients or optimize individual functions (e.g., patient referrals) without considering how functions complement one another throughout the entire franchise, and across the organization.

REFERENCES

1. Taheri PA, Butz DA, Lottenberg L, et al. The cost of trauma center readiness. *Am J Surg.* 2004;187(1):7–13.
2. Taheri PA, Maggio PM, Dougherty J, et al. Trauma center downstream revenue: The impact of incremental patients within a health system. *J Trauma.* 2007;62(3):615–619; Discussion 619–621.
3. Taheri PA, Butz DA, Greenfield LJ. Paying a premium: How patient complexity affects costs and profit margins. *Ann Surg.* 1999;229(6):807–811; Discussion 811–804.
4. Taheri PA, Butz DA, Greenfield LJ. Length of stay has minimal impact on the cost of hospital admission. *J Am Coll Surg.* 2000;191(2):123–130.
5. Government M-RCfBa. *Health care delivery customers by market segment: summary of findings.* Boston: John F. Kennedy School of Government; 2005.
6. Luchette F, Kelly B, Davis K, et al. Impact of the in-house trauma surgeon on initial patient care, outcome, and cost. *J Trauma.* 1997;42(3):490–495. Mar discussion 495–497.
7. Taheri PA, Butz DA, Dechert R, et al. How DRGs hurt academic health systems *J Am Coll Surg.* 2001;193(1):1–8; Discussion 8–11.
8. MacKenzie EJ, Steinwachs DM, Ramzy AI, et al. Trauma case mix and hospital payment: The potential for refining DRGs. *Health Serv Res.* 1991;26(1):5–26.
9. Gapenski LC, Langland-Orban B. Predicting financial risk under capitation. *Healthc Financ Manage.* 1995;49(11):38–40, 42–33.
10. Drucker PF. *Managing for the future: the 1990s and beyond.* New York: Tuman Talley Books/Dutton; 1992.
11. Taheri PA, Wahl WL, Butz DA, et al. Trauma service cost: The real story. *Ann Surg.* 1998;227(5):720–724; Discussion 724–725.

Identifying Trauma System Components

4

Paul M. Maggio

In the United States, injuries are the leading cause of death for ages 1 to 44 and are the fourth leading cause of death for all ages.[1] The magnitude of traumatic injury as a public health problem is enormous. As an epidemic affecting all ages, the cost of caring for injured patients is approximately $260 billion each year and the resulting loss of productive life years is greater than any other single cause.[2] Yet, the importance of injuries as a public health problem fails to be fully appreciated by the community.

Efforts to develop an organized response to injuries have been made through government initiatives such as the U.S. Department of Health and Human Services (HRSA) and legislation, as well as through organizations such as the American College of Surgeons Committee on Trauma (ACSCOT). Their most recent recommendations have focused on the development of an inclusive system that incorporates all acute care facilities as opposed to a system that focuses solely on designated trauma centers. As a result, guidelines for trauma system development in the United States have evolved from single centers to more coordinated and integrated networks of trauma care delivery, capable of delivering better care in both urban and rural environments, as well as in the event of mass casualties.

DEVELOPMENT OF TRAUMA SYSTEMS IN THE UNITED STATES

A trauma system is an integrated multidisciplinary organization to care for the injured patient. Ideally, it should provide timely, appropriate, and standardized care for a defined geographic region. In conjunction with a means of monitoring system performance, it must also incorporate a system for process improvement.

The first proposal by ACSCOT to provide formal guidelines for the structure of a trauma system was published in 1976 in the document titled, *Optimal Hospital Resources for Care of the Seriously Injured*.[3] These initial guidelines were institutionally based and resulted in a relatively *exclusive* system that concentrated largely on the acute care of the injured patient, as well as defining the structure, staffing, and necessary equipment required for development of a trauma center. It has served as the basis for trauma center verification and designation. The ACSCOT guidelines were remarkable in standardizing the provision of health care to the injured patient, and subsequent studies have demonstrated that in contrast to centers without such expertise, designated trauma centers achieve better outcomes.[4-8]

The first model for the development of trauma systems to emphasize the importance of an *inclusive* system was initiated over a decade later by HRSA. Directed by the Trauma Systems Planning and Development Act of 1990, HRSA created the *Model Trauma Care System Plan* in 1992.[9] Never officially published by the federal government, it serves as a "living" document that continues to be revised and guides trauma system development in the United States. In contrast to an *exclusive* system, this model incorporates all acute care facilities and services at a state or regional level in a system designed to care for all injured patients by matching them with the appropriate facilities and available resources.[10] Integrating all facilities into a single state or regional system will limit the number of duplicative services and directs the most severely injured patients to a few high-volume institutions. This design is expected to reduce the overall injury-related mortality through a more efficient and cost-effective process in which the needs of all injured patients can be met by the most appropriate institutions.[11-13] In addition, as an integrated system capable of providing a continuum of services from injury prevention to prehospital care, acute care, and subsequent patient rehabilitation, it is better prepared to address traumatic injury as a public health problem. Traumatic injury is no longer viewed as an "accident," but in the context of a public health model it is viewed as a disease that can be predicted and prevented. The outcome, therefore, can be improved through a multidisciplinary and coordinated approach that not only improves the delivery of acute and subsequent care but also reduces its incidence and severity.

TRAUMATIC INJURIES AS A PUBLIC HEALTH PROBLEM

Public health is defined as "what we as a society do collectively to assure the conditions in which people can be healthy."[14] Recognition of traumatic injuries as a public health problem was highlighted by a 1966 publication from the National Academy of Sciences and the National Research Council, *Accidental Death and Disability: The Neglected Disease of Modern Society*.[15] This document identified trauma as a major public health problem, made specific recommendations to reduce the associated death and disability, and provided the impetus for trauma system development over the next 30 years. Further emphasis of traumatic injuries as a public health problem was spurred by the events of September 11, 2001, and natural disasters such as Hurricane Katrina that devastated the north-central Gulf Coast of the United States in 2005. Shortly after the September 11 attacks, an assessment of state and regional responses to emergency medical events was performed by HRSA and the resulting publication—*A 2002 National Assessment of State Trauma System Development, Emergency Medical Services Resources, and Disaster Readiness for Mass Casualty Events*—found that although trauma system development continued to progress on a local level, funding and personnel were inadequate and communication and coordination on a state and regional level were too limited.[16] Organizations such as the Institute of Medicine (IOM) and American College of Surgeons (ACS) have echoed these findings,[17,18] and in response, ACSCOT and HRSA have recently provided recommendations for the most comprehensive and inclusive model for trauma systems to date.

COMPONENTS OF AN INCLUSIVE TRAUMA SYSTEM

To fulfill its role in coordinating a multidisciplinary response to prevent injuries and care for the injured patient, a comprehensive and integrated trauma system must seamlessly provide a wide spectrum of care. This care ranges from public education and preventive intervention to prehospital care, triage and transportation, emergency department care, operative intervention, general and intensive care, rehabilitative services, social services, and medical follow-up (see Fig. 1). Importantly, it must perform these functions in both a rural or urban setting and maintain the capability to provide all-hazard care in the event of mass casualties. ACSCOT in its latest version of Resources for the Optimal Care of the Injured Patient 2006 has defined the necessary administrative and clinical components (see Table 1).[19] The administrative components address the requisite leadership to implement a trauma system including cooperative efforts with governmental agencies and the creation of new legislation. The clinical and operational components form the infrastructure for a coordinated, multidisciplinary, and multi-institutional approach to caring for the injured patient. On the basis of a facility's capabilities and available resources, patients are triaged to receive standardized and evidence-based care that is performed in conjunction with a system of data collection, research, and process improvement.

Injury Prevention

The epidemiology of traumatic injuries provides an opportunity to identify high-risk groups, assess individual risk factors, and develop evidence-based preventive interventions. Injury prevention programs are required for all trauma systems and can be categorized as primary, secondary, or tertiary preventions.[19] Primary injury prevention is the avoidance of the injury itself, for example, restricting the sale of alcohol to minors in order to decrease the incidence of alcohol-related motor vehicle collisions.[20] Secondary prevention efforts are intended to limit the severity of injury, such as legislation enforcing the use of seat belts. Tertiary prevention activities are designed to limit the effects of the injury or improve patient outcome after the injury has already occurred. Improving access to definitive care facilities and following evidence-based treatment guidelines are examples of tertiary preventive measures.

Preventive interventions raise the public awareness of traumatic injuries as a public health problem, modify public behavior through legislation and education, and familiarize the public with the function and capabilities of a trauma system. Since one third to one half of trauma deaths occur in the field before receiving treatment, investing in injury prevention programs that decrease the incidence and severity of injuries may improve public health and reduce health care costs more so than focusing primarily on postinjury care.[7,21]

Patient Triage

Patient triage depends on a reliable communication network that matches a patient's needs with the most appropriate available resources. The challenge of field triage, faced by emergency medical services (EMS), is timely

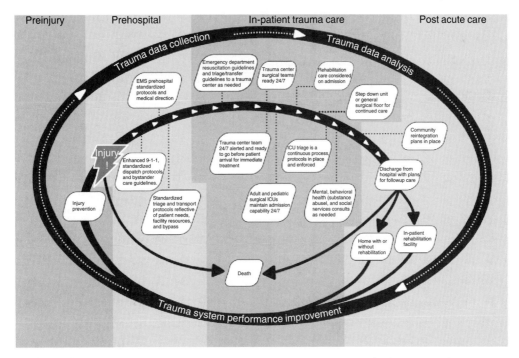

Figure 1 Preplanned trauma care continuum. EMS, emergency medical services, ICU, intensive care unit. (Source: U.S. Department of Health and Human Services, Health Resources and Services Administration. *Model trauma systems planning and evaluation.* Available at www.hrsa.gov/trauma/model.htm. February, 2006.)

transfer to an appropriate definitive center despite limited diagnostic capabilities. Decreased duration of prehospital care is vital in optimizing patient outcomes.[22-26] To efficiently evaluate a patient's needs, a number of triage scoring systems based on physiologic and anatomic data as well as the mechanism of injury have been developed. Examples include the Revised Trauma Score (RTS), Prehospital index (PHI), circulation, respiration, abdominal, thoracic, motor, and speech (CRAMS) scale, and the ACS Field Triage Scheme. These scoring systems have all been shown to correlate with outcome, but no single system has been proved to be significantly better than the others.[27-29] Regardless of the scoring system used, it must include a process of monitoring and evaluation of system performance coupled with a plan for process improvement. Monitored parameters must include the number of undertriaged and overtriaged patients. Undertriaging patients to lower level acute care facilities when they actually would be better served in a trauma center may adversely affect patient outcome, whereas overtriaging patients to trauma centers when they would be managed equally as well in a nontertiary care setting may overburden the system and impair access to care. Therefore, measures to improve the performance of a triage system should be guided by the goals of lowering undertriage and overtriage rates in order to more closely match a patient's needs with the appropriate resources. A field triage system must therefore be standardized, easy to

use, reproducible, and its assessment score should correlate with patient outcome.

Transportation

Choice of transportation should be based on patient safety and the expeditious transport to a definitive treatment center. Although ground transportation meets the needs of most patients, air transportation plays an increasingly important role in trauma patient evacuation.[30-32] On the basis of experience from helicopter evacuations in the Korean and Vietnam Wars, air medical dispatch units have been used for the civilian population to improve the speed of transportation and are now a well-established part of many EMS systems. Although guidelines for air medical dispatch have been published by the National Association of EMS physicians, appropriate use of air transportation remains somewhat controversial.[33-35] Additional studies are needed to determine the clinical benefits and cost-effectiveness of air transportation compared to other modes.

Air transportation may be particularly important in rural trauma systems where geographic variability of trauma centers leaves a large portion of the population without timely access to trauma care. One third of the US population resides in rural areas where the injury-related mortality rates are disproportionately high. Motor vehicle collisions and unintentional injuries are 50% higher in rural than in urban areas.[36,37] Low population density correlates with worse outcomes and more than half of motor vehicle-related

---

TABLE 1

BASIC COMPONENTS OF A TRAUMA SYSTEM

Administrative Components

Leadership	■ Lead agency providing oversight and administration to activities of the trauma system ■ Trauma system advisory committee to guide planning and review system performance ■ Trauma medical leadership
System Development	■ Formal trauma plan for the state or region ■ System guidelines and standards ■ Process to build collaborative constituency for trauma care
Legislation	■ Agency authority to develop and/or approve regional trauma plans ■ Authority to implement regional or state trauma plan, establish or adopt guidelines for care, and designate specialized definitive care facilities ■ To provide a sustainable source of funding for the trauma system and to support trauma care
Finances	■ Established process for trauma system financial analysis and reporting

Clinical Components

Injury Prevention	■ Overall system plan to promote injury control ■ System-wide injury control coalition
Human Resources	■ Sufficient workforce resources to allow coordinated operation of the trauma system ■ Process for evaluating adequacy of human resources ■ Educational programs sufficient to ensure adequate and ongoing trauma-related education
Prehospital Care	■ Identified agency responsible for prehospital care, continuing education, quality improvement, and so forth ■ Standardized certification ■ Ambulance and nontransporting medical unit guidelines ■ Communication systems integrated with emergency medical services (EMS) and disaster preparedness
Definitive Care Facilities	■ Specifically designated acute care facilities to provide acute trauma care ■ Designation process using established standards for acute trauma facilities ■ Established transfer agreements facilitating access to specialized trauma centers ■ Acute care facilities integrated by the trauma plan into an inclusive system of care ■ Rehabilitation facilities to provide post-acute care
Information Systems	■ System-wide information system allowing the timely collection and analysis of patient-related data
Evaluation	■ System-wide structures that allow monitoring of system performance, including compliance with standards and improvement opportunities
All Hazards Preparedness	■ Disaster preparedness capability that integrates prehospital and hospital response with the EMS ■ Involvement of private and public sectors in planned response ■ Inclusion of a performance improvement component
Research	■ Active research programs ideally linked to specific problems identified by prevention, quality improvement, or clinical efforts within the system

Source: American College of Surgeons Committee on Trauma. *Resources for optimal care of the injured patient.* 2006.

---

deaths occur in rural areas.[38,39] As of 2005, approximately 47 million Americans living in rural areas were more than an hour's drive from the nearest Level I or Level II trauma center, and more than 81 million relied on helicopters as their sole means of accessing a trauma center (see Fig. 2).[31,40] Although there have been efforts to designate trauma centers on the basis of needs, more than 90% of Level I trauma centers are located in metropolitan areas.[12] Expanding access to trauma systems through new flight programs may be more practical in some cases than increasing the number of trauma centers in rural areas. An additional benefit to limiting the number of trauma centers is higher patient volumes leading to greater trauma care experience and improved outcomes.

Inpatient Trauma Care

Similar to field triage, inpatient triage (secondary triage) should be a coordinated effort between the prehospital and hospital personnel to optimally care for the injured patient. It must be coordinated with activation of a trauma team and match a patient's needs upon admission with the appropriate hospital resources. This may result in initial care being provided in an urgent care area to resuscitation in a trauma bay or operating room. Similar to primary

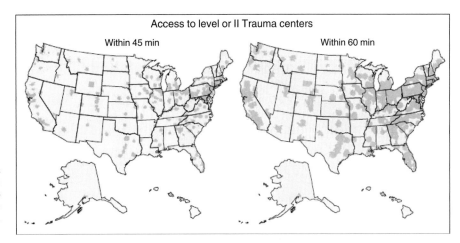

Figure 2   Areas in the United States with access to Level I and Level II trauma centers. (Branas CC, MacKenzie EJ, Williams JC, et al. Access to trauma centers in the United States. *JAMA.* 2005;293(21):2626–2633.)

triage, the design of inpatient triage must incorporate a system for process improvement, monitoring and reducing the number of over- and undertriaged patients.

Subsequent inpatient care must be protocol-driven and evidence-based to ensure that the right care is delivered in a timely manner. ACSCOT has greatly advanced the practice of trauma care by developing the advanced trauma life support (ATLS) course. ATLS provides an organized, standardized, and evidence-based approach to evaluating and managing injured patients. Although most injured patients can be adequately managed in nontertiary care centers, some patients require more comprehensive care. Ensuring the timely transfer to a more comprehensive trauma center requires well-established networks of communication among all acute care facilities in a trauma system in conjunction with preestablished transfer agreements and protocols. Interhospital transfer should occur only after the patient has been resuscitated and stabilized, and as with initial patient transportation in the field, should be based on the safest and swiftest method available.

Designation and verification of trauma centers occur through an external review process that categorizes hospitals on the basis of level of available resources. Verification can be accomplished by state and regional authorities or by verification from ACSCOT. An outline of the necessary resources for verification and designation are published in the Resources of Optimal Care of the Injured Patient, and classifies hospitals into four levels of verification[19]:

- *Level I*: Usually serves as the lead institution in a trauma system; manages a large number of severely injured patients with 24-hour availability of in-house surgeon; provides community leadership in trauma research, education, and prevention; admits >1,200 patients or 240 severely injured patients annually.
- *Level II*: Supplements the function of a Level I center in population-dense areas; serves as the lead trauma facility in less population-dense areas; provides full range of trauma care with 24-hour availability of in-house

surgeon; coordinates outreach programs to incorporate smaller regional institutions.

- *Level III*: Capable of initial patient management; surgeons must respond promptly and transfer agreements should be in place to facilitate transfers to Level I or Level II centers; provides injury prevention, outreach activities, and education programs for nurses, physicians, and allied health care workers.
- *Level IV*: Located in a rural environment; supplements care within a larger trauma system; requires 24-hour coverage by a physician; most patients require transfer to a higher level trauma center.

Categorization of all hospitals in an inclusive system is designed to improve the quality of trauma care. All participating hospitals must meet the necessary requirements for their level of verification as part of a trauma system. These requirements include the immediate availability of essential resources, a commitment to continuing medical education, use of quality improvement processes, and the adoption of evidence-based practice guidelines recommended by the ACS.

In a rural environment, patient discovery and transportation times are invariably longer and access to Level I and Level II trauma centers is limited. Furthermore, due to lower rural patient volumes EMS providers and physicians have less experience in managing trauma patients. Given that trauma-verified receiving hospitals are better prepared to provide initial care and preestablished transfer agreements and protocols facilitate patient transfer, an inclusive trauma system would be expected to improve the quality of trauma care in rural settings.[19] Although the benefits of an inclusive system have been demonstrated in an urban environment, they remain less apparent and unproven in rural areas.[41–43] Implementation of an inclusive trauma system in Oregon failed to show a significant improvement in overall survival.[44] Among other factors, the benefits of a designation process are lesser than expected because many rural trauma deaths are nonpreventative and would not survive under any circumstances.[38]

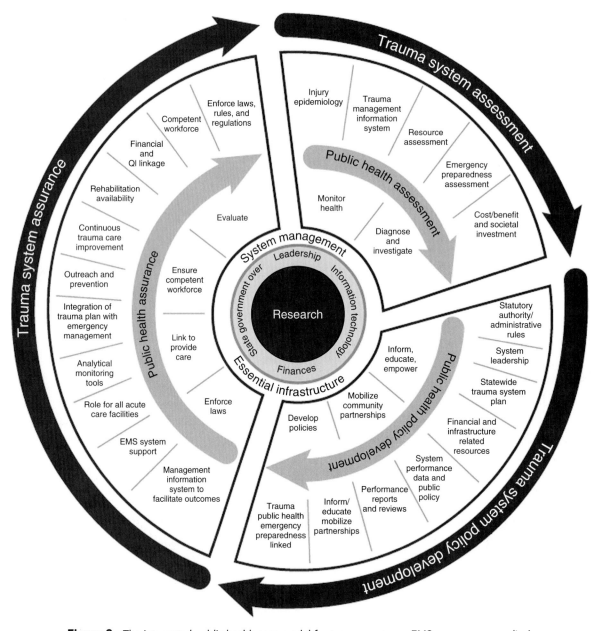

Figure 3 The integrated public health care model for trauma systems. EMS, emergency medical services, QI, quality indicators. (Source: U.S. Department of Health and Human Services, Health Resources and Services Administration. *Model trauma systems planning and evaluation.* Available at www.hrsa.gov/trauma/model.htm. February, 2006.)

Rehabilitation and Reintegration (Post-Acute Care)

Social services and rehabilitation are essential components of comprehensive care for the injured patient. Provided through an inpatient rehabilitation unit or a free-standing rehabilitation hospital, postacute care is critical to return a patient to regular activities of daily life and for successful reintegration into the community.[45] Future research incorporating a system-wide database is necessary to evaluate the long-term benefits and to develop evidence-based guidelines for rehabilitation and reintegration.

System Evaluation and Process Improvement

System evaluation and process improvement ensure the delivery of standardized, efficient, cost-effective, and quality health care. By monitoring how all the individual components of a trauma system function and interact, from prehospital care to rehabilitation, deficiencies and problems are identified and solutions are created. HRSA, in its recently revised *Model Trauma Care Systems Plan*, incorporates a public health approach for this purpose.[46] The public health system serves as a logical conceptual framework because it has extensive expertise in disease prevention, an integrated network with government agencies at all levels, and a well-established performance improvement process. The public health model is centered around the three core functions of assessment, policy development, and assurance (see Fig. 3):

- *Assessment*: The systematic collection and analysis of injury-related data to understand the status of a problem and identify potential opportunities for intervention.
- *Policy Development*: Establishment of comprehensive policies derived from assessment and goals of the organization.
- *Assurance*: Ensuring the provision of agreed-on services through surveillance of system components and performance and by adherence to policies and regulations.

In this model problems are identified as part of assessment, policies are then developed in response to the assessment, and the provision of services is ensured through monitoring and adherence to necessary standards.

The three core functions result in continuous process improvement as the process repeatedly loops from assurance back to assessment. Within the three core functions are ten essential services, which provide the foundation of the public health strategy. Research serves all the core functions driving system development and process improvement. System-wide registries and population-based data are essential and provide the means to study system performance, current practice methodologies, and outcomes. This information shapes future trauma care delivery through the creation of evidence-based policies and protocols. Government oversight, leadership, information technology, and finances ensure necessary support and continued function of these components. In the outer ring of this model are 24 functional benchmarks defining specific system attributes and how they relate to the three core functions. Each benchmark is accompanied by several indicators or performance measures (not present in Fig. 3) that are assessed and scored on a predetermined scale. There are currently a total of 113 indicators, and each one is related to a specific functional benchmark. Together, they serve as a means to evaluate the state of an inclusive trauma system. Demonstrating areas of strength and weakness, this model directs future system development to overcome its insufficiencies. Adopting the iterative system evaluation and process improvement of the public health model will ensure the delivery of standardized quality health care for patients with traumatic injuries.

SUMMARY

Inclusive trauma systems must provide comprehensive care that incorporates processes for continued system improvement. ACSCOT has provided guidelines for the necessary infrastructure including classification of trauma centers based on their available resources. This is essential for matching patients' needs with the appropriate acute care facility. In addition, ACSCOT has developed evidence-based guidelines for providing patient care, a well-established patient outcome database, and essential resources for all-hazard care. These components are applicable to both rural and urban settings, and well-coordinated networks of trauma care are capable of delivering better care in both environments. Furthermore, adoption of a public health framework can augment the function of current trauma systems. Viewing trauma as a disease, it offers expertise in population-based data analysis and epidemiology, which will improve current injury prevention programs. It also offers a model for system assessment, planning, and implementation, which will advance system-wide performance and development through dynamic and iterative organizational processes. Further collaboration and integration of trauma and public health systems will help implement a more comprehensive and inclusive health care delivery system for all injured patients.

REFERENCES

1. National Vital Statistics System, National Center for Health Statistics. Retrieved May 25, 2007, from http://www.cdc.gov/nchs/data/nvsr/nvsr55/nvsr55_10.pdf. 2003.
2. National Center for Injury Prevention and Control. *CDC injury fact book*. Atlanta: Centers for Disease Control and Prevention; 2006:2–8.
3. American College of Surgeons Committee on Trauma. *Optimal hospital resources for care of the seriously injured*. Chicago: American College of Surgeons; 1976.
4. Mullins RJ, Veum-Stone J, Helfand M, et al. Outcome of hospitalized injured patients after institution of a trauma system in an urban area. *JAMA*. 1994;271(24):1919–1924.
5. MacKenzie EJ. Review of evidence regarding trauma system effectiveness resulting from panel studies. *J Trauma*. 1999;47(Suppl 3):S34–S41.
6. Cayten CG, Quervalu I, Agarwal N. Fatality analysis reporting system demonstrates association between trauma system initiatives and decreasing death rates. *J Trauma*. 1999;46(5):751–755; discussion 755–756.
7. Trunkey DD. Trauma. Accidental and intentional injuries account for more years of life lost in the U.S. than cancer and heart disease. Among the prescribed remedies are improved preventive efforts, speedier surgery and further research. *Sci Am*. 1983;249(2):28–35.
8. MacKenzie EJ, Rivara FP, Jurkovich GJ, et al. A national evaluation of the effect of trauma-center care on mortality. *N Engl J Med*. 2006;354(4):366–378.
9. U.S. Department of Health and Human Services: Public Health Service Health Resources and Services Administration. *Model trauma care system plan*. Washington, DC: U.S. Department of Health and Human Services; 1992.
10. Utter GH, Maier RV, Rivara FP, et al. Inclusive trauma systems: Do they improve triage or outcomes of the severely injured? *J Trauma*. 2006;60(3):529–535; discussion 535–537.
11. Eastman AB. Blood in our streets. The status and evolution of trauma care systems. *Arch Surg*. 1992;127(6):677–681.
12. MacKenzie EJ, Hoyt DB, Sacra JC, et al. National inventory of hospital trauma centers. *JAMA*. 2003;289(12):1515–1522.
13. Nathens AB, Jurkovich GJ, Maier RV, et al. Relationship between trauma center volume and outcomes. *JAMA*. 2001;285(9):1164–1171.
14. Institute of Medicine. *The future of the public's health in the 21st century*. Washington, DC: National Academy Press; 2003:28.

15. National Academy of Sciences. *Accidental death and disability: the neglected disease of modern society.* Washington, DC: National Academy of Sciences; 1996.
16. U.S. Department of Health and Human Services. *A 2002 national assessment of state trauma system development, emergency medical services resources, and disaster readiness for mass casualty events.* Washington, DC: U.S. Department of Health and Human Services; 2002.
17. American College of Surgeons Division of Advocacy and Health Policy. *A growing crisis in patient access to emergency surgical care.* Chicago: American College of Surgeons; 2006.
18. Institute of Medicine. *Hospital-based emergency care at the breaking point.* Washington, DC: National Academy Press; 2006.
19. American College of Surgeons Committee on Trauma. *Resources for optimal care of the injured patient 2006.* Chicago: American College of Surgeons; 2006.
20. Schermer CR. Alcohol and injury prevention. *J Trauma.* 2006; 60(2):447–451.
21. Sauaia A, Moore FA, Moore EE, et al. Epidemiology of trauma deaths: A reassessment. *J Trauma.* 1995;38(2):185–193.
22. MacLeod JB, Cohn SM, Johnson EW, et al. Trauma deaths in the first hour: Are they all unsalvageable injuries? *Am J Surg.* 2007;193(2):195–199.
23. Sampalis JS, Lavoie A, Williams JI, et al. Impact of on-site care, prehospital time, and level of in-hospital care on survival in severely injured patients. *J Trauma.* 1993;34(2):252–261.
24. Carr BG, Caplan JM, Pryor JP, et al. A meta-analysis of prehospital care times for trauma. *Prehosp Emerg Care.* 2006;10(2):198–206.
25. Grossman DC, Kim A, Macdonald SC, et al. Urban-rural differences in prehospital care of major trauma. *J Trauma.* 1997;42(4):723–729.
26. Demetriades D, Martin M, Salim A, et al. The effect of trauma center designation and trauma volume on outcome in specific severe injuries. *Ann Surg.* 2005;242(4):512–517; discussion 517–519.
27. Lerner EB. Studies evaluating current field triage: 1966–2005. *Prehosp Emerg Care.* 2006;10(3):303–306.
28. Bulger EM, Maier RV. Prehospital care of the injured: What's new. *Surg Clin North Am.* 2007;87(1):37–53, vi.
29. Tamim H, Joseph L, Mulder D, et al. Field triage of trauma patients: Improving on the prehospital index. *Am J Emerg Med.* 2002;20(3):170–176.
30. Bledsoe BE, Wesley AK, Eckstein M, et al. Helicopter scene transport of trauma patients with non–life-threatening injuries: A meta-analysis. *J Trauma.* 2006;60(6):1257–1265; discussion 1265–1256.
31. Petrie DA, Tallon JM, Crowell W, et al. Medically appropriate use of helicopter EMS: The mission acceptance/triage process. *Air Med J.* 2007;26(1):50–54.
32. Shatney CH, Homan SJ, Sherck JP, et al. The utility of helicopter transport of trauma patients from the injury scene in an urban trauma system. *J Trauma.* 2002;53(5):817–822.
33. Thomson DP, Thomas SH. Guidelines for air medical dispatch. *Prehosp Emerg Care.* 2003;7(2):265–271.
34. Diaz MA, Hendey GW, Bivins HG. When is the helicopter faster? A comparison of helicopter and ground ambulance transport times. *J Trauma.* 2005;58(1):148–153.
35. Karanicolas PJ, Bhatia P, Williamson J, et al. The fastest route between two points is not always a straight line: An analysis of air and land transfer of nonpenetrating trauma patients. *J Trauma.* 2006;61(2):396–403.
36. Baker SP, Whitfield RA, O'Neill B. County mapping of injury mortality. *J Trauma.* 1988;28(6):741–745.
37. Peek-Asa C, Zwerling C, Stallones L. Acute traumatic injuries in rural populations. *Am J Public Health.* 2004;94(10):1689–1693.
38. Rogers FB, Shackford SR, Osler TM, et al. Rural trauma: The challenge for the next decade. *J Trauma.* 1999;47(4):802–821.
39. Baker SP, Whitfield RA, O'Neill B. Geographic variations in mortality from motor vehicle crashes. *N Engl J Med.* 1987; 316(22):1384–1387.
40. Branas CC, MacKenzie EJ, Williams JC, et al. Access to trauma centers in the United States. *JAMA.* 2005;293(21):2626–2633.
41. Nathens AB, Jurkovich GJ, Rivara FP, et al. Effectiveness of state trauma systems in reducing injury-related mortality: A national evaluation. *J Trauma.* 2000;48(1):25–30; discussion 30–21.
42. Mullins RJ, Mann NC, Hedges JR, et al. Preferential benefit of implementation of a state-wide trauma system in one of two adjacent states. *J Trauma.* 1998;44(4):609–616; discussion 617.
43. Nathens AB, Jurkovich GJ, Cummings P, et al. The effect of organized systems of trauma care on motor vehicle crash mortality. *JAMA.* 2000;283(15):1990–1994.
44. Mullins RJ, Hedges JR, Rowland DJ, et al. Survival of seriously injured patients first treated in rural hospitals. *J Trauma.* 2002;52(6):1019–1029.
45. Liberman M, Mulder DS, Jurkovich GJ, et al. The association between trauma system and trauma center components and outcome in a mature regionalized trauma system. *Surgery.* 2005;137(6):647–658.
46. U.S. Department of Health and Human Services: Public Health Service Health Resources and Services Administration. *Model trauma system planning and evaluation.* Washington, DC: U.S. Department of Health and Human Services; 2006.

Quantifying Trauma System Effectiveness

5

Gerald McGwin, Jr.

The objective of this chapter is to provide an overview of issues related to quantifying trauma system effectiveness. In order to offer a contextual perspective, the chapter begins with an overview of the injury problem in the United States. Following this is a brief description of the history of trauma systems and their development including a summary of the current status of trauma systems in the United States and globally. The chapter discusses measures used to evaluate the effectiveness of trauma systems. The reader should be aware that the following information is not meant to be a systematic and detailed review of published research regarding trauma system effectiveness as such information is abundant. Rather, an overview of our current state of knowledge regarding trauma system effectiveness will be provided with a specific emphasis on the merits of various approaches to assessing it as well as the nature of selected outcomes.

THE MAGNITUDE OF THE INJURY PROBLEM

Injuries represent a significant cause of mortality in the United States. In 2004, unintentional injuries alone were the fifth leading cause of death. Although intentional injuries (including homicide and suicide) have a lower mortality rate, they are among the top ten leading causes of death.[1] It is important to note that although fewer overall deaths are attributed to injuries than to chronic diseases such as heart disease and cancer, injuries are the leading cause of death for those aged 1 to 44 years. In fact, injuries represent half of all deaths among children aged 1 to 14 and 73% of all deaths among those aged 15 to 24 years; this is compared to approximately 6% of deaths overall.

Therefore, when measured using metrics that account for the unequal age distribution such as years of potential life lost, relative to other causes of death, injuries represent a much larger problem.

Although unintentional injury mortality rates have declined continuously since the late 1970s and early 1980s, recent data suggests that the rate may be increasing.[2] A similar pattern has been reported for suicide.[3] On the other hand, homicides have experienced a significant increase from the mid-1960s to the mid-1970s and then remained high until the mid-1990s when it declined sharply and has remained stable in recent years.[4]

Although death represents an important barometer for measuring the public health importance of disease, it is rare, relatively easy to measure, and inexpensive—that is, fatal injuries are associated with less medical care costs compared to severe yet nonfatal injuries. The overall incidence of medically treated injuries in the United States is approximately 18,135 per 100,000 (i.e., ~18%); this is compared to a mortality rate of approximately 53 per 100,000. Since the 1980s, injury-related hospital discharge rates have declined continuously, although in more recent years a plateau appears to have been reached.[5]

Although the vast majority of medically treated injuries that occur annually are considered minor and do not require hospitalization, the acute and chronic repercussions from these injuries are not insignificant. According to one study, minor injuries account for 80% of the morbidity during the first 6 months after injury and approximately 75% of the estimated lifetime morbidity.[6] It has also been estimated that nonfatal medically treated injuries are associated with an average of 11 days of temporary work loss.[7] Moreover, most of the estimated $400 billion in total injury costs in 2000 is attributed to productivity losses.[8] For most of those injured there is likely to be little long-term impact; however, for those who sustain serious injuries long-term sequelae will be frequent. Research suggests that return to preinjury function is protracted and that reductions in quality of life are significant.[9,10]

The information presented in the preceding text is useful in two regards; first, it places the injury problem in the proper context, and second, it provides an overview regarding the most commonly used metrics to measure the burden of injury. The latter point is important because this will be the same metrics used to evaluate the effectiveness of trauma systems.

TRAUMA SYSTEMS: DEFINITION AND HISTORY

Trauma System Defined

According to Hoyt and Coimbra, "A trauma system is an organized approach to patients who are acutely injured. It should occur in a defined geographic area and provide optimal care, which is integrated with the local or regional emergency medical services (EMS) system."[11] They further state that, "The major goal of a trauma system is to enhance community health." These authors also remind us that trauma systems must be viewed as part of a larger public health approach toward reducing injury-related mortality, morbidity, and years of potential life lost. As such it does not exist to provide only optimal care during the acute and late phases of injury, rather it must exist within a multidisciplinary environment and work collaboratively toward reducing injury incidence as well.

Trauma Systems History

Mullins and Nathens et al. describe the development of trauma systems and suggest that their history parallels that of major military conflicts dating back to the late 1700s with the development of the "flying ambulance" that, during the Napoleonic Wars, ferried wounded soldiers from the battlefield to definitive care.[12,13] Perhaps the most significant developments in military medicine that have impacted modern trauma systems occurred during 20th century conflicts. During World War I, the injured were evacuated from the battlefield through echelons of treatment facilities, each with greater resources than the prior one; approximately 2 decades later the same protocol was employed during World War II. However, as compared to World War I when the average time from injury to treatment was 12 to 18 hours, during World War II this time interval had decreased to 4 hours, attributable to the increased availability of motorized transportation.[12,13] Other changes involved the routine use of blood transfusion during a novel phase

of trauma care—resuscitation. Additionally, new surgical techniques for head, extremity, thoracic, and abdominal injuries required that systems for patient triage be developed and implemented. Between World War I and II, the mortality rate from battlefield injuries decreased from 8.5% to 5.8%.[14]

While a system of progressive levels of care remained in place during the Korean and Vietnam Wars, several changes in resources and the process of care led to a further reduction in the mortality rate to 2.4% in Korea and 1.7% in Vietnam.[14] First, the availability of definitive care was moved closer to the battlefield with the use of Mobile Army Surgical Hospitals. Second, the use of helicopters to transport the injured to such facilities resulted in a decrease in the time to definitive care to 2 to 4 hours in Korea and <1 hour in Vietnam. Third, the availability of organized care in the battlefield provided by specially trained medics meant that the process of resuscitation and triage could begin almost immediately following injury.

At the time of the Vietnam War, the collective military experience in treating injured soldiers over the prior 6 decades resulted in an organization of medical resources such that no soldier was more than 35 minutes away from definitive, live-saving treatment.[15] Moreover, this experience produced a continuum of care beginning as soon as possible following injury and served as a model for the development of civilian trauma care systems.

The application of the military system of trauma care to the civilian environment was fostered in 1966 with the publication of a National Academy of Sciences report, which highlighted trauma as a public health problem.[16] This report called for organized systems of trauma care such that civilian populations might enjoy the same benefits observed among soldiers in combat. It specifically recommended standards for prehospital care, ambulances, and emergency rooms, reflecting the manual on emergency care for the sick and injured of American College of Surgeons Committee on Trauma.[17] Following legislation by Congress in 1966, the states of Maryland, Illinois, and Florida developed and implemented organized emergency medical systems, trauma centers, and systems. In the 1970s, standards for categorizing hospitals with respect to their ability to provide trauma care were proposed and debated.[18,19] This process culminated with the publication of the first edition of the American College of Surgeons Committee on Trauma *Optimal Hospital Resources for Care of the Seriously Injured* in 1976.[20] This document described a categorization scheme for trauma centers and outlined the necessary resources associated with each level in this scheme. The organization of trauma systems, including a description of their specific elements and operation and the resources that define and differentiate the different levels of trauma centers, are beyond the scope of this chapter and such information is readily available elsewhere.[11,13,14,21] However, the essential characteristics of a trauma system have been described and they provide a brief yet comprehensive summary (see Table 1).

TABLE 1
ESSENTIAL ELEMENTS OF TRAUMA SYSTEMS

- Presence of a lead agency with legal authority to designate trauma centers
- Use of a formal process for designation of trauma centers
- Use of American College of Surgeons (or similar) standards for verification of trauma centers
- Use of an out-of-state survey team for designation of trauma centers
- Mechanism to limit the number of designated trauma centers in a community on the basis of community need
- Written triage criteria that form the basis for bypassing nondesignated centers
- Presence of continuous monitoring systems for quality assurance
- Statewide availability of trauma centers

Nathens AB, Brunet FP, Maier RV. Development of trauma systems and effect on outcome after injury. *Lancet.* 2004;422:17–22.

These elements underscore principles published in the American College of Surgeons' document that make it clear that in order for trauma centers to be effective they must exist within a larger system of trauma care. In fact, when viewed from a public health perspective, the components of a trauma system extend far beyond the process of providing care to critically injured patients (see Fig. 1). This perspective highlights not only the integration of trauma centers with familiar entities such as prehospital care providers but also less familiar individuals such as politicians, health policy specialists, and epidemiologists. Subsequent editions of the American College of Surgeons Committee on Trauma's document have been published, each reflecting lessons learned regarding the optimal structure and function of trauma centers and systems. This reflects the fact that although the basic elements of trauma systems have not changed over the last several decades, our understanding of their successful implementation is ongoing. The use of technology to more seamlessly link trauma centers within a trauma system represents an important evolution[22] as does the integration of automotive technology to further reduce the time to definitive care.[23] Finally, it should be noted that contemporary military conflicts represent novel opportunities to further evaluate and refine the provision of trauma care.[24]

TRAUMA SYSTEMS: EARLY DEVELOPMENTS TO CURRENT STATUS

As described earlier, by the early 1970s there was ample momentum for trauma center and system development and implementation. While this momentum was fueled by political will (and financial resources) and by organizations such as the American College of Surgeons and the American Medical Association, the successful implementation of the early systems likely had a significant impact as well. But perhaps more importantly, that these early efforts produced measurable outcomes provided even more support for trauma system development elsewhere. Following the implementation of trauma systems, Cowley et al. reported a reduction in the mortality rate for seriously injured patients in Maryland;[25] a similar reduction was reported by Mullner and Goldberg in Illinois, although this was limited to rural areas only.[26] In Jacksonville, Florida, the implementation of an emergency medical care system was associated with a reduction in motor vehicle collision–related mortality.[27]

These early successes were followed by other important developments. In the late 1970s in Orange County, California a study documented the inadequate care available to seriously injured patients.[28,29] Such patients were treated at a large number of hospitals, none of which were presumably dedicated to the care of such patients. Approximately three quarters of trauma-related deaths were judged to be preventable, this is compared to 1% of such deaths in San Francisco, California, where seriously injured were treated at a single institution. As a result, a trauma system was developed and implemented in Orange County, California and the care of critically injured patients was limited to just five trauma centers; subsequent studies reported significant reductions in injury-related mortality.[30,31] The experience of Orange County, California is important not only as an example of early trauma system implementation but perhaps more importantly as an example of the role of data for future trauma center and system development. That is, the Orange County experience underscores the importance of quantifying the injury problem in a community as an integral part of assessing the need for a trauma system. Although routinely quantifying trauma system effectiveness is vital, evaluating outcomes before system implementation is crucial for planning purposes and such information serves as a baseline against which postsystem outcomes can be compared. In fact, in the late 1970s and mid-1980s trauma systems developed in San Diego, California and Portland, Oregon took a similar approach to that used by Orange County, California.[32–36] Trauma system development and implementation in these two areas were viewed as a public policy issue and, as such, quantifying the injury problem served to highlight a need as well as demonstrate success following implementation.

By the late 1980s, only 2 states had all the essential components of a trauma system (Table 1) and 20 others had some of the components; 29 states had not begun the process of developing trauma systems.[37] Approximately 10 years later a report indicated that the number of states that possessed all of the essential components of a trauma system had risen to 5; however, only 14 had developed and implemented some of the components, a decrease since 1988.[38] By 1998, the picture had become more encouraging. Although the number of states with all essential trauma system components remained at 5,

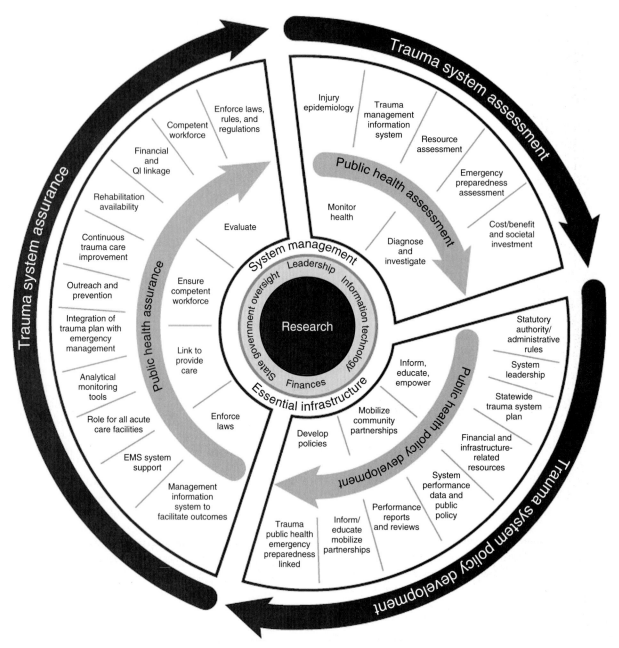

Figure 1   A public health perspective on trauma system planning and evaluation. QI, quality indicators; EMS, emergency medical services. (From the United States Department of Health and Human Services Health Resources and Services Administration. Model trauma system planning and evaluation. Available at: ftp://ftp.hrsa.gov/hrsa/trauma/Self-Assessment_Tool.pdf. Accessed July 15, 2007.)

the number with some components had increased to 38.[39] In 2005, Mann et al. reported that 8 states met all trauma system criteria, 27 had some criteria, and 14 had none.[40] Focusing on trauma center versus trauma system resources, MacKenzie et al. reported that in 2003 there were 1,154 trauma centers (190 Level I and 263 Level II) in the United States.[41] (It is perhaps important to note that the definition of a trauma center varied widely.) This represents a more than twofold increase since 1991 when there were a reported 471 trauma centers.[42] During this

time, the largest increase has been in Level III and Level IV/V centers, although Level I and II centers increased by 21%. Geographically the expansion of trauma center resources has not been uniform, with the south experiencing a greater increase than other areas.

Underlying the improvement in the availability of trauma care resources in the United States is the question, how much is enough? It has been suggested that one to two Level I or II trauma centers per million population is adequate.[43] This same study indicated that in the

35 states with formal trauma systems most meet this criterion, whereas in those without formal trauma systems, approximately 50% do. Therefore, despite the fact that trauma care resources are more abundant and better organized than at any time in the past, Nathens et al. calculated that more than one third of major trauma cases in the United States is received at institutions not formally designated for trauma care.[43] Branas et al. reported similar findings and additionally noted that this problem is greater in rural compared to urban areas.[44] It is perhaps important to note that the availability of trauma care resources in the United States is discordant with the public's perception and expectation of the availability of these same resources.[45]

Finally, although much of the material presented herein is in reference to the United States, trauma center and system implementation and development is active elsewhere in the world. A recent issue of the journal *Injury* provides an overview of trauma care systems in many other countries including Australia, China, Germany, and South Africa, among others.[46] There are opportunities to learn from the experiences of these countries, particularly those that have faced many of the challenges currently facing future trauma system development in this country.

MEASURING TRAUMA SYSTEM EFFECTIVENESS

General Considerations

It is important to place trauma system effectiveness within a larger context of the injury problem and the natural history of approaches to address it. This context helps provide perspective regarding what is meant by the word "effectiveness" when evaluating trauma centers and systems. It has been demonstrated that trauma systems are part of a larger approach to reducing the burden of injury that include injury prevention initiatives among others. Despite this, the success of trauma system, at least as described thus far, has been measured on the basis of mortality. Although mortality is clearly the most significant outcome that one might experience, there are many nonfatal outcomes and several non–health-related outcomes (e.g., quality of life, financial) that are important. These nonfatal and non–health-related outcomes will be discussed in turn.

Reflecting upon the definition of a trauma system provided by Hoyt and Coimbra, one should recall that, "The major goal of a trauma system is to enhance community health."[11] With respect to mortality, "community health" can be taken to mean the number of injury-related deaths per population. As will be discussed subsequently, many studies have used this very measure to quantify trauma center and/or system performance. Yet, a population-based injury mortality rate comprises two separate entities:[1] injury incidence (injury episodes per population) and[2]

injury case fatality (deaths per injury episode). A public health approach suggests that primary prevention (i.e., injury prevention) initiatives, valid components of a trauma system, seek to impact the incidence of injury, whereas tertiary prevention initiatives (i.e., the provision of organized and appropriate trauma care) seek to impact injury fatality rates. However, although primary prevention is viewed as an important element of a trauma system *per se*, the reality is that most systems function with the goal of tertiary prevention. This is important to keep in mind when evaluating studies reporting population-based injury mortality rates; the reality is that trauma centers are likely impacting but one component of these rates.

It is also important to note that trauma centers and systems cannot prevent all trauma-related deaths. The trimodal distribution of trauma deaths was first described in 1983.[47,48] As a function of elapsed time after injury, deaths from traumatic injury were classified as generally falling into one of three categories: immediate, early, and late. Immediate deaths were those that occurred <1 hour following injury, making up approximately 50% of the total; early deaths occurred within the first few hours of injury and accounted for 30%; and late deaths occurred days to weeks following injury and were 20% of all trauma deaths. Immediate deaths were largely due to neurologic injury (brain, brain stem, and spinal cord) or laceration of the heart or major vessels and classified as not preventable. Early deaths were largely due to severe blood loss from the head, respiratory system, and abdominal organs. These deaths were largely treatable and therefore possibly preventable. Finally, most late deaths were due to infection and multiorgan failure. Reducing the number of injury-related deaths during each period largely relies on expedient and optimal medical care, although less so for some periods than others. For example, injury prevention efforts are likely to be important for reducing immediate deaths, whereas trauma systems should have the greatest impact for early and late deaths.

And finally returning to nonfatal and non–health-related outcomes, although rarely evaluated in the literature, such measures are important when considering trauma system effectiveness. They are, however, more difficult to measure than deaths and in some instances they make suggest worse performance following trauma center/system implementation. For example, patients with major injuries who receive appropriate and timely care at a trauma center have improved chances of survival compared to similar patients treated at nontrauma facilities. However, care may be protracted for such patients and, related to this and their extensive injuries, their risk of complications is increased. Therefore, attempts to quantify trauma center/system effectiveness in terms of complications may find such rates elevated following implementation or compared to nontrauma facilities. A similar illustration could be made for length of stay and cost of care. Although appropriate study designs and statistical tools can help account for such changes or differences in patient characteristics within and between facilities, recognition of the potential for such seemingly unexpected is important.

The following sections will provide an overview of research regarding trauma system effectiveness according to various metrics (e.g., deaths, complications).

Mortality

A comprehensive review of trauma system effectiveness was published in 1999 in a supplement to the *Journal of Trauma* that served as the proceedings for a meeting, commonly known as the *Skamania Conference*, on the current state of trauma systems. Mann et al. summarized the literature on trauma system effectiveness published as of May 1998 and separated this work into three categories: panel studies, registry comparisons, and population-based studies.[49]

Panel Studies—Design and Interpretation

MacKenzie has reviewed the strengths and limitations of the panel study approach to trauma system assessment as well as provided a review of the literature as it existed at the time (i.e., 1998).[50] Generally described, these studies utilize a group of experts, that is the panel, to judge whether a group of deaths were potentially preventable and the role of specific errors that led to such deaths. Panel studies were among the first approaches used to demonstrate the need for trauma systems and to demonstrate their effectiveness. Early panel studies utilized subjective implicit criteria to determine whether deaths were potentially preventable and relied upon panels that were small in number. Inconsistent results across studies can be attributed to the less than rigorous conduct of these early studies. Indeed a lack of clear definitions regarding preventability and heterogeneous patient populations have been shown to result in low inter-rater reliability of judgments regarding preventability.[51] However, when designed and executed correctly panel studies can provide strong evidence regarding trauma system effectiveness. Therefore, how does one accomplish this task?

First, an understanding of the definition of a potentially preventable death must be uniformly understood. According to MacKenzie a potentially preventable death is, "any death that might have been prevented if optimal care had been delivered."[50] Implicit in this definition are three important criteria that must be met in order for preventability to be assessed—the injury or its sequelae must be survivable; the care provided is judged to be suboptimal; and care-related errors must be implicated, directly or indirectly, in the patient's death.[50] Only after a given death meets each of these criteria can an assessment of preventability be made. A related consideration is whether to view preventability as a binary choice or to provide a larger number of options. More recently, studies have utilized three categories: not preventable, possibly preventable, and definitely preventable. Perhaps the most important element of panel studies is the use of a consistent set of criteria against which to judge preventability. This increases validity and allows for uniform comparisons across studies. Fortunately, such criteria for judging preventability have been published along with guidelines for this application.[51]

A second consideration when conducting or evaluating panel studies is the study population; this is particularly important when comparing across studies or potentially across time within a single geographic region. The primary concern regarding case mix is which deaths are included in the preventability assessment and the group of deaths frequently omitted is prehospital deaths. These deaths are often excluded due to limited clinical information on which to base an assessment of preventability. As will be discussed in the subsequent text, information quantity and quantity are critical issues in panel studies. This is a legitimate reason for excluding such deaths and enhances the internal validity of the study; however, this also changes the nature of the question being answered. By excluding prehospital deaths while inferences to hospital trauma care can be readily made, those to trauma system performance are more tenuous. For studies that only include hospital deaths, the choice of which patients to include and exclude is similarly important. This is because preventable deaths are not uniformly distributed across injury types and mechanisms.

The quality and quantity of information on which to base assessments of preventability is a topic of debate. Although research has indicated that the use of prehospital, clinical, and autopsy information enhances the reliability of preventable death judgment, the availability and quality of both prehospital and autopsy information is often questionable. When multiple data sources have been used, these studies rarely provide sufficient detail regarding the extent to which each source was available and complete for all patients and the adequacy of this information for preventability assessment. For any given patient the more quality data that is available, the greater the likelihood of a reliable and valid judgment; however, in the aggregate heterogeneity may introduce bias and thereby reduce internal and external validity.

The size and composition of the review panel is another important consideration when evaluating and conducting panel studies; MacKensize's review of panel studies published as of 1998 suggests wide variability.[50] While there are statistical considerations regarding panel size there is little consensus regarding optimal size. Rather, that the panel be multidisciplinary in nature appears to be of greater importance.

Finally, the actual process of making preventable death judgments is crucial for establishing the reliability and validity of a panel study. Although most studies to date involve an independent review of each case by panel members some go further to include subsequent panel discussion; in either case final judgments are based on majority opinion. Other approaches include panel discussions for only those cases wherein independent reviews did not produce either a majority or unanimous judgment.

Panel Studies—Assessment of the Evidence

The literature regarding trauma system effectiveness as measured by panel studies has been reviewed by MacKenzie and Chiara et al.[50,52] The former review included ten preventable death studies published as of 1998; the paper includes details regarding each of these studies and their results and will not be recapitulated herein. Of these ten studies, only two provided a valid comparison of preventable deaths pre- and posttrauma system implementation and despite their limitations both provide evidence in support of the effectiveness of trauma systems. The remaining studies provide evidence of varying degrees and quality in support of the fact that the implementation of trauma centers and systems are associated with less inappropriate care and fewer preventable deaths. However, as noted earlier, because prehospital deaths are excluded from many of these studies, inferences with respect to trauma *system* effectiveness are less appropriate than trauma *center* effectiveness. Chiara et al. reviewed panel studies published as late as 2003 and came to the same general conclusions as MacKenzie, that is, panel studies are an important component of trauma center and system assessment.[50,52] They are particularly important when planning for such resources in a community; moreover, they serve as an important tool for continuous quality improvement. Therefore, although panel studies do not provide the highest level of evidence regarding trauma system effectiveness, they serve an important role and should be encouraged for both emerging and existing trauma centers and systems.

Registry-Based Studies: Design and Interpretation

Generally, trauma registries are a systematic accounting of all patients treated at a trauma center. The patients captured by any one institution's trauma registry may differ from another. For example, some institutions include deaths in the emergency room whereas others may not; some institutions only include patients admitted for at least 48 hours. Trauma registries also differ with respect to the information they collect. Few attempt to capture every aspect of a patient's hospital stay. The abundance of laboratory results and other diagnostic testing results makes such an endeavor time consuming and unwieldy. However, because hospitals increasingly manage patient information in electronic database rather than paper medical records, the exploitation of these electronic resources may make such comprehensive trauma registries more common. Currently, the most common approach is to collect data representing a cumulative picture of each patient's experience, including demographic, diagnosis, and outcome-related information. Trauma registry data is useful in many respects; it commonly serves administrative, quality improvement, and research needs. With respect to quantifying trauma center and system effectiveness, trauma registry data can be used to compare the experience of any given trauma center with[1] itself during a period when the institution was not participating in an organized system of trauma care,[2] another trauma or nontrauma center, or [3] national norms.

Jurkovich and Mock have summarized the relevant issues surrounding registry-based comparisons as well as the evidence for trauma system effectiveness derived from studies of this type.[53] Celso et al. have also reviewed this literature, although with a more circumscribed group of studies than discussed by Jurkovich and Mock.[54] Collectively, these authors raise several important issues that must be considered when evaluating and conducting effectiveness studies based on trauma registry data. Whether the comparison involves a single institution or multiple institutions, studies that compare the mortality experience before and after trauma system implementation are intuitively attractive. And, in fact, just like crossover studies wherein each patient serves as his/her own control thereby reducing between patient confounding, this attraction is validated methodologically because comparing institutions to themselves should also reduce between institution confounding. However, this design is not without limitations, the first of which is the availability of data. That is, is there a preexisting trauma registry or another source of historical information regarding trauma patients at a given institution against which to compare postsystem outcomes? Another issue is the comparability of any data, in terms of quality and quantity, which is available over time. Have there been changes in what data is being collected on what patients? Systematic (and nonsystematic) changes in inclusion and exclusion or variable definitions can result in biased results when conducting such comparisons. Despite stable variable definitions and data collection procedures, the role of temporal trends in patient composition or trauma care resources (beyond those attributed to trauma center/system implementation) is also a potential concern because this can also yield biased results. For example, nationally there has been a decrease in penetrating trauma over the last decade or more, and such injuries are associated with higher mortality than blunt trauma. Therefore, should an individual institution experience a decline in mortality coincident with the implementation of a trauma system as well as a change in patient mix, it may not be clear whether the observed change is attributable to the trauma system or a decrease in penetrating trauma. Similar changes in institutional resources or improvements in technology could produce the same, potentially misleading result. Finally, changes in mortality may not be immediately apparent. For example, a study from Oregon reported that a measurable reduction in trauma-related mortality was not apparent until several years after implementation of the trauma system.[55] Similarly, a nationwide study on the impact of regionalized trauma care on motor vehicle–related mortality reported that the observed 8% reduction took more than 10 years to manifest.[56] These delays in positive outcomes reflect the fact that system implementation is a gradual process and not as well demarcated as might be inferred from before and after study designs.

Many of these same concerns described in the preceding text can be leveled against comparisons between individual trauma centers and between trauma and nontrauma centers. By their very nature, trauma registry–based studies do not routinely include prehospital deaths. Therefore, even for studies wherein data from all trauma centers participating in given trauma system is being evaluated, the exclusion of prehospital deaths makes inferences regarding trauma system (vs. center) effectiveness difficult. Fortunately, many, though not all, of these concerns can be alleviated by proper study design and rigorous statistical analysis.

In addition to comparing patient outcome pre- and postsystem implementation, another frequently employed technique for measuring trauma system effectiveness based on trauma registry data is comparing outcomes for a given trauma center or set of trauma centers with national norms. These national norms are most commonly derived from the Major Trauma Outcome Study (MTOS).[57] Between 1982 and 1989, data from approximately 160,000 trauma patients from multiple hospitals throughout the United States and Canada were pooled to establish the MTOS. Data from the MTOS was used to calculate survival probabilities based on selected patient demographic, clinical, and injury severity characteristics, commonly referred to as the *Trauma and Injury Severity Score (TRISS) coefficients*.[58,59] Associated with these probabilities is an equation complete with regression coefficients. Provided that one has the necessary data to input into this equation, it is possible to calculate the expected probability of survival given a fixed set of characteristics. Therefore, by collecting these same characteristics from trauma center or system patients and applying them to this equation, it is possible to determine whether survival is different from this national norm. Associated statistical tests can be easily employed to quantify whether such differences are statistically significant. Using this same approach it is also possible to calculate the *expected* number of deaths that would have occurred had those patients experienced the same care received at the institutions included in the MTOS. These *expected* deaths can then be compared to the *observed* deaths and associated statistical tests performed to quantify whether any observed difference is statistically significant. This latter approach has the additional benefit of quantifying not only the presence of a difference but also its magnitude. Although the MTOS is the most widely used resource in studies of this type, other resources exist. For example, Wald et al. sought to determine whether the absence of a trauma system adversely affected outcome in patients with severe head trauma using the National Trauma Coma Data Bank as a reference population.[60] Cooper et al. compared pediatric trauma patients in a state lacking a trauma system (i.e., New York) to national norms using the National Pediatric Trauma Registry.[61]

This approach to quantifying trauma center or system effectiveness is appealing in that one need not devote resources to collecting a reference or comparison population. This is particularly attractive for trauma centers or systems that do not have data from a preimplementation time period readily available. Another advantage of this approach is that it is better suited to quantifying trauma system effectiveness than registry-based studies; however, the failure to include prehospital deaths means that a comprehensive assessment of system effectiveness is not possible. Additionally, the large number of studies that have used the MTOS allows for a uniform comparison with other published work.

Not unexpectedly, the advantages of using national norms to evaluate trauma center or system effectiveness have several important limitations, many of which have been previously discussed by Pollock.[62] Because most studies to date have used the MTOS database and associated TRISS methodology, many of these limitations are associated with this resource. One of the greatest concerns regarding the MTOS is whether it truly represents a national norm for trauma care outcomes. The participating hospitals did so on a voluntary basis and therefore the MTOS should not be viewed as a population-based resource, which it does not purport to be. Another limitation of the MTOS is that approximately 11% of the data submitted was incomplete and had to be excluded from the study. These two factors raise concerns regarding the external validity of this resource in that the participants may represent a biased pool of trauma patients who do not adequately reflect the national experience. There is also considerable concern regarding the measurement of injury severity. The TRISS calculations utilize the Injury Severity Score (ISS), which has been shown to have its own limitations in terms of adequately capturing probability of survival. Although the TRISS methodology attempted to keep pace with these issues, the last revision was in 1990 and subsequent developments in the characterization and quantification of injury severity have been made since that time.[63] Questions have also been raised regarding the statistical approach that was utilized to derive the TRISS coefficients. The simple pooling of data fails to reflect the likely heterogeneity inherent across multiple institutions. Moreover, the simple application of data from a single institution to the TRISS coefficients fails to acknowledge the complicated statistical issues that arise when conducting such analyses. Clark has proposed some techniques that make more effective use of the MTOS or any reference database.[64] An important, and frequently ignored, underlying assumption is that the statistical associations originally reported by the MTOS are universal. Although the MTOS is a large study, it may not be large enough to compensate for such concerns. Jurkovich and Mock also mention the problems of data quality and heterogeneous variable definitions.[65] Assuming that these problems occur randomly, they should result in nondifferential bias in the MTOS and in studies that utilize it for comparison purposes; however, differential bias is conceivable. They also point out that the MTOS last enrolled patients in 1989 and therefore comparing current trauma center or system outcomes to data that is approximately 20 years old would nearly always show improvement.

Finally, with respect to trauma registry comparisons, there is also a hybrid approach that, although rarely used, warrants mention. This approach uses a pre- and postdesign to compare the trauma system effectiveness. However, instead of using an internal comparison and directly comparing the same trauma center or system with itself, the MTOS is used as the comparison for both time periods. Studies reported by Norwood et al. and Stewart et al. serve as good examples of how to utilize this approach and to interpret the results.[65,66]

Registry-Based Studies: Assessment of the Evidence

In a 1999 publication, Jurkovich and Mock reported the results of a systematic review of trauma system effectiveness based on registry comparisons.[53] Most studies included in this review were based on comparison to the MTOS. More recently, Celso et al. reported the results of their systematic review of outcomes of severely injured patients treated in trauma centers following the establishment of trauma systems.[54] These authors specifically excluded panel studies and those using comparisons to national norms. Additionally, they conducted a meta-analysis quantifying results across various studies. As with the results from panel studies described earlier, these two reviews of the published literature depict a literature that overwhelmingly supports the notion that trauma centers and systems are effective in reducing mortality. They also arrive at a consistent estimate as to the magnitude of this effectiveness. Using a random effects model to combine the results of 14 individual studies, Celso et al. reported an overall quality-weighted odds ratio of 0.85. That is, according to the authors, a 15% reduction in mortality in favor of the presence of a trauma system. Similarly, of the 11 studies reviewed by Jurkovich and Mock those with relative risk estimates each report risk reductions of approximately 15%.

Although the consistency observed in registry-based studies is at first encouraging, one cannot help but wonder if there are explanations beyond reality underlying this pattern, the most obvious of which is publication bias. That is, studies reporting null or negative (i.e., trauma systems produce worse outcomes) associations never percolate their way into the literature. Assuming that the consistent results from published studies truly reflect reality, one must also be concerned regarding the quality of this research. The quality-weighted association reported by Celso et al. forestalls this concern somewhat. However, the widespread and persistent use of the MTOS will mean that many of its well-described limitations[67] will hamper the quality of

research in the future. Therefore, the future of registry-based trauma system effectiveness requires a contemporary national reference norm that is truly population-based. Such a resource should include critically injured patients who require advanced trauma care, yet succumb to their injuries before having the opportunity to receive it. The use of standardized inclusion criteria and variable definitions would greatly enhance the interval validity of this resource as would the inclusion of measures known to impact mortality following trauma such as comorbid medical conditions. And finally, in order to increase its utility, nonfatal outcomes including functional status and quality of life should be measured.

Population-Based Studies: Design and Interpretation

Population-based studies compare injury outcomes (usually mortality) in a given geographic area either to another, often similar, area or to the same area over time. For example, in 1985 the state of Oregon mandated that over a 5-year period a statewide trauma system be implemented and subsequent research compared the injury mortality rate for the entire state before and after this implementation.[35,36,68] As the name suggests, population-based studies take a more comprehensive perspective on trauma system effectiveness than either panel or registry-based studies. The important distinction between population-based studies and registry-based studies that compare outcomes pre- and postsystem implementation is that the former includes all injured patients, regardless of whether or where they received care. Therefore, frequently mentioned weakness of excluding prehospital deaths common in panel and registry-based studies is overcome when using this design. And, as a by-product, population-based designs are better able to truly evaluate trauma *system* effectiveness because they capture deaths that occurred during all phases of prehospital, hospital, and postdischarge care. This broader assessment of effectiveness comes at a price, that is, less detailed information regarding individuals. The most common source of information utilized in population-based studies is death certificates that provide basic demographic and cause of death information, yet do not contain information on injury severity and other characteristics of interest. In certain instances, it is possible to link death certificate data with hospital discharge data in order to increase the amount and detail of information available.[69,70] An additional advantage of death certificate data is that it is geographically comprehensive, readily available and, with the proper expertise, relatively easy to manipulate.

Another source of information for population-based studies is hospital discharge data sets, which contain summary information regarding individual patient's hospitalization such as diagnosis, procedure codes, and discharge status. Standard demographic information is also available. Like death certificate data it can be easy to work with. Although the availability of hospital discharge data sets varies, in some areas it may be possible to obtain them from individual hospitals in a given geographic region of interest. Also, some states maintain statewide hospital discharge data sets. Similar in principle to trauma registry data, hospital discharge data is significantly less detailed and contains information from both trauma and non-trauma centers. Although the present discussion is focused on mortality, by including data from all hospitals within a geographic region, hospital discharge data can be used to evaluate changes in the distribution of injured patients.

Regardless of the data source, population-based studies are attractive because they can often be conducted using existing data resources and, as mentioned, provide a more inclusive picture of trauma system effectiveness. However, this breadth of data is offset by the lack of depth. These designs have a number of other limitations to consider. Population-based studies that attempt to quantify whether trauma system implementation alters the trajectory of outcomes cannot easily rule out the impact of temporal trends. That is, external factors occurring coincident with trauma system implementation might also be responsible for any observed changes. For example, temporal trends as an explanation for the decline in injury-related mortality rates in Oregon before and after the implementation of a statewide trauma system cannot be ruled out. To counter this concern, additional research compared injury mortality in Oregon and Washington during similar periods of time.[30,71] That is, during a time when neither state had a trauma system and during a time when the Oregon system was in place and the Washington system was in the planning phase. While the former comparison demonstrated similar rates, the latter indicated better survival in Oregon.

In summary, population-based studies are more readily able to truly quantify trauma *system* effectiveness than the previously discussed study designs. Although overcoming certain limitations associated with this design is straightforward (e.g., temporal trends), others are more difficult to overcome (e.g., lack of detail in death certificate date).

Population-Based Studies: Assessment of the Evidence

Mullins and Mann reviewed the published evidence regarding the effectiveness of trauma systems on the basis of population-based studies.[72] These authors identified 14 such studies although several of them were repeated assessments of the same trauma system; all told, nine trauma systems were evaluated. Overwhelmingly, this evidence points to the fact that organized systems of trauma care improve survival. On average, these studies suggest that the implementation of trauma systems results in a 15% to 20% reduction in the risk of death. Only one study reported no difference;[73] however, a number of limitations including small sample size and the short duration of time between the time periods compared could explain the lack of an association. However, outcomes were

significantly improved for patients who sustained multiple serious injuries secondary to motor vehicle collisions. A more recent study not included in the Mullins and Man review compared motor vehicle collision death rates in states with and without trauma systems.[74] Although this study demonstrated that states with trauma systems had significantly lower death rates, the authors suggested that this could not be solely attributed to the presence of trauma systems. They also suggest that future work should focus on identifying which components of trauma systems are most beneficial. In their review several years earlier, Mullins and Mann pointed out that this evidence regarding trauma system efficacy could be mostly attributed to improvements in prehospital care.[72] They also indicated that the observed benefits were largely limited to seriously injured patients. Although research has long surmised that the availability and quality of prehospital resources can explain variations in injury-related mortality,[75,76] few studies have simultaneously evaluated the role of trauma system resources and their impact on outcomes. Studies that have evaluated the impact of prehospital resources solely have been criticized for failing to consider in-hospital resources as well.[77] Melton et al., in an ecologic study, reported that in-hospital resources were associated with lower injury-related mortality rates whereas no impact of prehospital resources was observed.[78] Other studies that have attempted to address this same issue have faced methodological challenges, underscoring the complexity of such studies.[79]

Summary

Most research to date supports the role of trauma centers and systems in reducing mortality following injury. However, inferences from this body of research regarding trauma system effectiveness must be made with caution. Despite the abundance of literature regarding this topic, few studies have evaluated injury and mortality at the community level and those that have done so face methodological limitations inherent to the study designs employed. This is not to suggest that current and future trauma system development be curtailed in anticipation of better evidence regarding effectiveness. Rather, this is a cautionary note to those developing, implementing, and evaluating trauma systems that they are fully aware as to what trauma systems can deliver in terms of mortality-related outcomes. Such awareness comes from an understanding as to what specific questions the study designs discussed in the preceding text are able to address and those they cannot and do not. The *definitive* study on trauma system effectiveness will never be conducted. However, despite its limitations, in aggregate the published evidence to date can only lead to one conclusion and that is that trauma systems are effective in reducing injury-related mortality. Therefore, the greatest illumination regarding trauma system effectiveness is derived when a combination of well-designed and focused approaches are utilized.

Nonmortality Outcomes

Morbidity-Related Outcomes

Mortality is the standard metric for quantifying trauma system effectiveness; however, other outcomes are also relevant yet rarely addressed in the literature. With respect to patient clinical outcomes (e.g., complications), one can hypothesize that providing timely and appropriate care to critically injured patients would decrease the incidence of such events. However, as extensively discussed in the preceding text such care improves patient survival, particularly for those with the most serious injuries. Such critically injured patients are at increased risk of complications both due to the nature of their injuries and their protracted length of stay. Therefore, had these patients died, and done so relatively early in their hospital course, then their trauma system-related survival may be associated with, on average, an increase in complications. Despite this, it is also possible that no change in complications is observed. This may be due to the increase in complications being offset by a decrease among those patients with a low-to-moderate mortality risk who experience less morbidity due to improved prehospital and trauma care resources. Scenarios wherein outcomes improve for all patients are also possible. Finally, morbidity is heterogeneous and it is possible that some complications are more responsive to trauma system resources than others. Unfortunately, there is little data against which to evaluate these hypothesized patterns of results. DiRusso et al. compared patient outcome and hospital performance before and after preparation for American College of Surgeons' Level I trauma center verification.[80] Among the complications evaluated, only the incidence of urinary tract infections decreased. However, the duration of time between these time periods was short and therefore the absence in complications rates cannot be easily interpreted. Over a 9-year period, Peitzman et al. reported a decline in the incidence of several types of complications following trauma center designation.[81] Yet the authors provided no data regarding the predesignation complication rates; this is important because the observed decline may have already been occurring.

The absence of research on morbidity-related patient outcomes likely reflects the fact that, compared to mortality, measuring such outcomes in a uniform and valid manner is difficult, thereby hampering comparisons between institutions. Within an institution, before and/or after, comparisons are also hampered by a number of issues including the lack of national norms for these outcomes as well as changes in diagnostic technology and the development of novel therapies. However, these are not insurmountable problems and although they increase study design complexity, this should not preclude investigations into morbidity-related outcomes regarding trauma system effectiveness.

Functional Status and Quality of Life

In addition to morbidity, nonclinical patient outcomes also have relevance when addressing the question of trauma system effectiveness. Functional status and quality of life are frequently used metrics when assessing trauma patient outcomes. Cameron et al. provide a very good review of issues surrounding the importance of these measures as an outcome measure in trauma systems research.[82] Despite the fact that numerous studies have quantified the magnitude of and risk factors for these outcomes, they have not been used to evaluate trauma system effectiveness. The importance of these outcomes is reflected by the fact that a panel of experts in trauma care, in developing research recommendations to facilitate trauma system implementation and evaluation, ranked functional outcome and quality of life as most important.[83] However, this document was published in 1999 and to date studies incorporating such outcomes have not appeared in the literature. This is not unexpected because conducting such research is complicated by many factors. First, there are numerous measures of functional status and quality of life available for use in clinical research, some with better provenances than others. Elvik evaluated several "health state indices" with reference to motor vehicle–related injury and reported different results depending on which measure was used.[84] More recently, Holbrook et al. has demonstrated the utility of the Quality of Well-being scale in trauma patients.[85] There are, of course, measures such as the Medical Outcomes Study Short Form 36 (SF-36) that have been widely used in outcomes research, including trauma, and whose validity has been established. An additional benefit of measures such as the SF-36 is the existence of national norms. Despite attempting to quantify some aspect of quality of life, personal well-being, or functional status, there is great heterogeneity among these tools in terms of what they ultimately measure. For example, some were developed for specific conditions whereas others were principally designed for specific demographic groups. Therefore, despite the wealth of resources in this area, the choice of which measure to use is not always immediately clear. It is beyond the scope of this chapter to provide guidance regarding this process. That being said, two important considerations are the knowledge of what constructs (e.g., function vs. psychological impairment) one is interested in measuring and the marriage of those constructs with valid and reliable instruments.

A second issue regarding the use of functional status and quality of life measures is patient follow-up. While morbidity outcomes are mostly limited to the inpatient phase of care and therefore easy to capture, functional and quality of life outcomes are more long term in nature and therefore require contact with the patient following discharge. Measuring these outcomes during the hospital course is important and not unexpectedly they are likely to be significantly impaired at the time of hospital discharge. However, improvements may not be apparent for 12 months or more. Therefore, there must be adequate resources to maintain contact with discharged patients; this is often a time-consuming endeavor. An additional consideration is that heterogeneity in patient follow-up can result in a biased depiction of these outcome measures if those who are assessed routinely and systematically differ from those who are not.

A third issue that has likely hampered the use of these measures in quantifying trauma system effectiveness is lack of information on preinjury status. That is, a patient's level of functional status and quality of life before being injured. An important consideration in evaluating whether organized trauma care returns improve these outcomes in trauma patients by returning them to preinjury functional status is knowing what that status is. It may not be reasonable to expect that trauma centers or systems will return patients to the highest level of functional status or quality of life, particularly if they were not at this level before their injury. As opposed to morbidities, which can be expected to be nonexistent preinjury, there is no expectation regarding preinjury functional status and quality of life. This means that preinjury status assessment must occur retrospectively, which may be hampered by a patient's inability to communicate; the opportunity for bias in collecting such information retrospectively must also be considered.

Finally, functional status and quality of life measures are not routinely captured as part of a patient's medical care; therefore in order for them to be used for quantifying trauma system effectiveness, resources must be available to collect this information. Although some instruments can be self-administered, some patients may be unable to do so. Regardless of the manner of administration, there must be resources to ensure that these assessments produce high-quality information. Moreover, in addition to ensuring that this data is collected uniformly between patients and over time at a given institution, when multiple institutions are involved additional effort is required to ensure homogeneity between them.

The barriers to quantifying trauma system effectiveness using functional status and quality of life measures are significant. However, the success of the Trauma Recovery Project in conjunction with the San Diego Regionalized Trauma System demonstrates that many of these limitations can be overcome and high-quality work produced.[9,10,85] Unfortunately, for existing trauma systems, it is not possible to retrospectively evaluate the impact of system implementation outcomes. However, in regions wherein trauma systems are currently being planned or discussed, the early integration of functional status and quality of life measures into the process of patient care and follow-up is imperative. This is not to suggest that such measures have no utility in existing trauma centers and systems. Data from such institutions is vital for providing a more comprehensive perspective regarding

patient outcomes that are not truncated at the time of hospital discharge.

Institutional Outcomes

Although patient-oriented outcomes are of primary importance when evaluating the question of trauma system effectiveness, the impact of such systems on the institutions themselves is also relevant. In fact, a number of studies have measured the impact of trauma system development and implementation on length of stay and financial outcomes. Harbrecht et al. observed a decline in the lengths of hospital stay for patients with splenic injury over a 15-year period following trauma center designation, despite no change in injury severity.[86] Over a 9-year period following trauma center designation, Peitzman et al. observed a similar decline for all trauma patients.[81] Neither of these studies presented data presystem implementation; therefore, one cannot be certain that the observed trends were not already in place. However, DiRusso et al. did compare hospital and intensive care unit length of stay before and after trauma center verification.[80] These authors reported declines in both measures, although only length of hospital stay was significant. Abernathy et al. reported a decreased length of stay for the most severely injured patients following the implementation of the regional trauma system.[22] Despite these findings, changes in length of stay following trauma system implementation may not always decrease, at least not immediately. As trauma systems shift the distribution of trauma patients to the proper facilities, changes in patient mix may cause certain institutions to see more seriously injured patients and fewer with less serious injuries. This, in conjunction with the survival of patients previously expected to die, may cause an increase in lengths of hospital stay. This may or may not offset shorter lengths of stay for patients who benefit from the system by receiving more timely and appropriate care.

Associated with length of stay are financial outcomes. Research evaluating the impact of trauma system development and implementation on the cost of care has generally yielded positive results. Abernathy et al. reported a lower cost of care following trauma system implementation. Durham et al., in a detailed economic analysis, reported that the cost per life saved compares favorably with other major public health expenditures.[87] With an eye toward productivity and return to work, these authors concluded that trauma systems provide significant returns on investment. Other studies have reported significant increases in the cost of care.[88] It is important to note that any observed cost savings must be viewed with respect to the additional costs incurred by operating a trauma center, although it has been demonstrated that cost savings still exist despite these expenditures.[22,80] What must also be considered is trauma care reimbursement and how changes in payer mix can impact the bottom line despite improvements in the cost of care.[89] Quantifying trauma system effectiveness in financial terms is complex yet vital because it often serves as a barometer for institutional support for such endeavors.

Trauma systems, by their nature, result in changes in the process of care both in the prehospital and in-hospital setting. There have been few studies evaluating process of care outcomes, although those that have report improvements following trauma system implementation.[90,91] Monitoring process of care outcomes is vital to ensuring that trauma systems not only get the right patient to the right place but also provide timely and appropriate care once the patient arrives.

Terrorism and Mass Casualty Events

The question of trauma system effectiveness has been addressed on the basis of long-term perspective. As mentioned previously, a nationwide study on the impact of regionalized trauma care on motor vehicle–related mortality reported that the observed 8% reduction took more than 10 years to manifest.[56] However, terrorism and natural disasters will produce a large number of critically injured patients in a very short period of time. Trauma systems have an important role in delivering timely, appropriate, and high-quality care and producing beneficial outcomes in response to acute events. Fortunately such events are rare, thereby producing few opportunities for evaluating performance and effectiveness. However, when such events occur, in addition to having adequate resources to provide appropriate care, trauma systems should also have the necessary resources to perform quantitative assessments of performance following the events. Several excellent examples of such assessments have been published.[92-94] The role of these assessments is clear—the identification of strengths and weakness throughout the system. This is not to suggest that such assessments can only occur in the face of an actual terrorist event or disaster. The development of disaster preparedness plans and participation in mock events represent important components of ongoing trauma system quality improvement.[92] The American College of Surgeons Ad Hoc Committee on Disaster and Mass Casualty Management is a useful source of information regarding the role of the trauma center in these types of events.

CONCLUSION

In medicine, quantifying effectiveness is frequently the by-product of applying specific interventions in individual patients. Great care is taken to eliminate all but the role of that specific intervention from the evaluation process. Quantifying trauma system effectiveness is a much more complex process owing to the fact that the intervention in question is an approach to care and the role of external factors cannot easily be manipulated. Despite this, there exists an ample body of research that only

leads to one conclusion—trauma systems improve survival following injury. Although the results of individual studies must be tempered with their limitations, the consistent finding of a survival benefit across geography, time, and study designs supports this conclusion. Whether trauma systems improve nonmortality outcomes remains an open question in desperate need of an answer. While assessments of mortality are vital for evaluating the performance of novel trauma systems and the maintenance of existing ones, there must be a greater emphasis on morbidity outcomes, functional status and quality of life institutionally, and process of care measures in future trauma system effectiveness research.

REFERENCES

1. Minino AM, Heron MP, Smith BL. Deaths: Preliminary Data for 2004. *National Vital Statistics Reports*, Vol. 54, No. 15. Hyattsville: National Center for Health Statistics; 2006.
2. Paulozzi LJ, Ballesteros MF, Stevens JA. Recent trends in mortality from unintentional injury in the United States. *J Safety Res*. 2006; 37:277–283.
3. Centers for Disease Control and Prevention. *Wed-based injury statistics query and reporting system (WISQARS)*. Available at: http://www.cdc.gov/ncipc/wisqars/. Accessed 2007.
4. Fox JA, Zawitz MW. *Homicide trends in the United States*. Bureau of Justice Statistics. United States Department of Justice. Available at: http://www.ojp.usdoj.gov/bjs/homicide/homtrnd.htm. Accessed 2007.
5. Heinen M, Hall MJ, Boudrealt MA, et al. *National trends in injury hospitalizations, 1979–2001*. Hyattsville: National Center for Health Statistics; March 2005.
6. McClure RJ, Douglas RM. The public health impact of minor injury. *Accid Anal Prev*. 1996;28:443–451.
7. Lawrence B, Miller T, Jensen A, et al. Estimating the costs of non-fatal consumer product injuries in the United States. *Inj Control Saf Promot*. 2000;7:97–113.
8. Corso P, Finkelstein E, Miller T, et al. Incidence and lifetime costs of injuries in the United States. *Inj Prev*. 2006;12:212–218.
9. Holbrook TL, Anderson JP, Sieber WJ, et al. Outcome after major trauma: Discharge and 6-month follow-up results from the Trauma Recovery Project. *J Trauma*. 1998;45:315–323.
10. Holbrook TL, Anderson JP, Sieber WJ, et al. Outcome after major trauma: 12-month and 18-month follow-up results from the Trauma Recovery Project. *J Trauma*. 1999;46:765–771.
11. Hoyt DB, Coimbra R. Trauma systems. *Surg Clin North Am*. 2007; 87:21–35.
12. Mullins RJ. A historical perspective on trauma system development in the United States. *J Trauma*. 1999;47:S8–14.
13. Nathens AB, Brunet FP, Maier RV. Development of trauma systems and effect on outcome after injury. *Lancet*. 2004;363:1794–1801.
14. Hoff WS, Schwab CW. Trauma system development in North America. *Clin Orthop Relat Res*. 2004;422:17–22.
15. Neel S. Army aeromedical evacuation procedures in Vietnam: Implications for rural America. *JAMA*. 1968;204:99–103.
16. National Committee of Trauma and Committee on Shock. In: *Accidental death and disability: a neglected disease of modern society*. Washington, DC: National Academy of Sciences/National Research Council; 1966.
17. American College of Surgeons Committee on Trauma. In: Kennedy RH, ed. *Emergency care of the sick and injured: a manual for law-enforcement officers, fire-fighters, ambulance personnel, rescue squads and nurses*. Philadelphia: WB Saunders; 1966.
18. American Medical Association Commission on Emergency Medical Services. *Categorization of hospital emergency capabilities*. Chicago: American Medical Association; 1971.
19. Detmer DE, Moylan JA, Rose J, et al. Regional categorization and quality of care in major trauma. *J Trauma*. 1977;17:592–599.

20. Committee on Trauma, American College of Surgeons. Optimal hospital resources for care of the seriously injured. *Bull Am Coll Surg.* 1976;61:15–22.

21. Committee on Trauma, American College of Surgeons. *Resources for optimal care of the injured patients: 2006.* ChicagoIL: American College of Surgeons; 2006.

22. Abernathy JH, McGwin G, Acker JE, et al. Impact of a voluntary trauma system on mortality, length of stay, and cost at a level I trauma center. *Am Surg.* 2002;68:182–192.

23. Hunt RC. Emerging communication technologies in emergency medical services. *Prehosp Emerg Care.* 2002;6:131–136.

24. Eastridge BJ, Jenkins D, Flaherty S, et al. Trauma system development in a theater of war: Experiences from operation iraqi freedom and operation enduring freedom. *J Trauma.* 2006; 61:1366–1373.

25. Cowley RA, Hudson F, Scanlan E, et al. An economical and proved helicopter program for transporting the emergency critically ill and injured patient in Maryland. *J Trauma.* 1973;13:1029–1038.

26. Mullner R, Goldberg J. Toward an outcome-oriented medical geography: An evaluation of the Illinois trauma/emergency medical services system. *Soc Sci Med.* 1978;12:103–110.

27. Waters JM, Wells CH. The effects of a modern emergency medical care system in reducing automobile crash deaths. *J Trauma.* 1973;13:645–647.

28. West JG, Trunkey DD, Lim RC. Systems of trauma care: A study of two counties. *Arch Surg.* 1979;114:455–460.

29. West JG. Validation of autopsy method for evaluating trauma care. *Arch Surg.* 1982;117:1033–1035.

30. West JG, Cales RH, Gazzangia AB. Impact of regionalization: the Orange County experience. *Arch Surg.* 1983;118:740–744.

31. Cales RH. Trauma mortality in Orange County: The effect of implementation of a regional trauma system. *Ann Emerg Med.* 1984;13:1–10.

32. Lowe DK, Gately HL, Goss JR, et al. Patterns of death, complications, and error in the management of motor vehicle accident victims: Implications for a regional system of trauma care. *J Trauma.* 1983;23:503–509.

33. Neuman TS, Bockman MA, Moody P, et al. An autopsy study of traumatic deaths; San Diego County, 1979. *Am J Surg.* 1982; 144:722–777.

34. Shackford S, Mackersie RC, Hoyt DB, et al. Impact of a trauma system on outcome of severely injured patients. *Arch Surg.* 1987;122:523–527.

35. Mullins RJ, Veum-Stone J, Hedges JR, et al. Influence of a statewide trauma system on location of hospitalization and outcome of injured patients. *J Trauma.* 1996;40:536–545.

36. Mullins RJ, Veum-Stone J, Helfand M, et al. Outcome of hospitalized injured patients after institution of a trauma system in an urban area. *JAMA.* 1994;271:1919–1924.

37. West JG, Williams MJ, Trunkey DD, et al. Trauma systems: Current status-future challengers. *JAMA.* 1988;259:3597–3600.

38. Bazzoli GJ, Madura KJ, Cooper GF, et al. Progress in the development of trauma systems in the United States: Results of a national survey. *JAMA.* 1995;273:395–401.

39. Bass RR, Gainer PS, Carlini AR. Update on trauma system development in the United States. *J Trauma.* 1999;47:S15–S21.

40. Mann NC, MacKenzie EJ, Teitelbaum SD, et al. Trauma system structure and viability in the current healthcare environmenv: A state-by-state assessment. *J Trauma.* 2005;58:136–147.

41. MacKenzie EJ, Hoyt DB, Sacra JC, et al. National inventory of hospital trauma centers. *JAMA.* 2003;289:1515–1522.

42. Bazzoli GJ, MacKenzie EJ. Trauma centers in the United States: Identification and examination of key characteristics. *J Trauma.* 1995;38:103–110.

43. Nathens AB, Jurkovich GJ, MacKenzie EJ, et al. A resource-based assessment of trauma care in the United States. *J Trauma.* 2004;56:173–178.

44. Branas CC, MacKenzie EJ, Williams JC, et al. Access to trauma centers in the United States. *JAMA.* 2005;293:2626–2633.

45. Champion HR, Mabee MS, Meredith JW. The state of US trauma systems: Public perceptions versus reality – implications for US response to terrorism and mass casualty events. *J Am Coll Surg.* 2006;203:951–961.

46. Colton CL. World trauma care systems. *Injury.* 2003;34:643.

47. Baker CC, Oppenheimer L, Stephens B, et al. Epidemiology of trauma deaths. *Am J Surg.* 1980;140:144–150.

48. Trunkey DD. Trauma. *Sci Am.* 1983;249:28–35.

49. Mann NC, Mullins RJ, MacKenzie EJ, et al. Systematic review of published evidence regarding trauma system effectiveness. *J Trauma.* 1999;47:S25–S33.

50. MacKenzie EJ. Review of evidence regarding trauma system effectiveness resulting from panel studies. *J Trauma.* 1999;47: S34–S41.

51. Shackford SR, Hollingsworth-Fridlund P, McArdle M, et al. Assuring quality in a trauma system – the Medical Audit Committee: Composition, cost, and results. *J Trauma.* 1987;27:866–875.

52. Chiara O, Cimbanassi S, Pitidis A, et al. Presentable trauma deaths: From panel review to population based studies. *World J Emerg Surg.* 2006;1:12.

53. Jurkovich GJ, Mock C. Systematic review of trauma system effectiveness based on registry comparisons. *J Trauma.* 1999;47: S46–S55.

54. Celso B, Tepas J, Langland B, et al. A systematic review and meta-analysis comparing outcome of severely injured patients treated in trauma centers following the establishment of trauma systems. *J Trauma.* 2006;60:371–378.

55. Mullins RJ, Mann NC, Hedges JR, et al. Preferential benefit of implementation of a statewide trauma system in one of two adjacent states. *J Trauma.* 1998;44:609–617.

56. Nathens AB, Jurkovich GJ, Cummings P, et al. The effect of organized systems of trauma care on motor vehicle crash mortality. *JAMA.* 2000;283:1990–1994.

57. Champion H, Copes W, Sacco W, et al. The Major Trauma Outcome Study: Establishing national norms for trauma care. *J Trauma.* 1990;30:1356–1365.

58. Champion H, Sacco W, Copes W. Injury severity scoring again. *J Trauma.* 1995;35:94–95.

59. Boyd C, Tolson M, Copes W. Evaluating trauma care: The TRISS method. *J Trauma.* 1987;27:370–337.

60. Wald S, Shackford S, Fenwick J. The effect of secondary insults on mortality and long-term disability after severe head injury in a rural region without a trauma system. *J Trauma.* 1993;34: 377–381.

61. Cooper A, Barlow B, String D, et al. Efficacy of pediatric trauma care: Results of a population-based study. *J Pediatr Surg.* 1993;28:299–305.

62. Pollock DA. Summary of the discussion: Trauma registry data and TRISS evidence. *J Trauma.* 1999;47:S56–S58.

63. Meredith JW, Evans G, Kilgo PD, et al. A comparison of the abilities of nine scoring algorithms in predicting mortality. *J Trauma.* 2002;53:621–628.

64. Clark DE. Comparing institutional trauma survival to a standard: Current limitations and suggested alternatives. *J Trauma.* 1999;47:S92–S98.

65. Norwood S, Myers M. Outcomes following injury in a predominantly rural-population-based trauma center. *Arch Surg.* 1994;129:800–805.

66. Stewart T, Lane P, Stefanits T. An evaluation of patient outcomes before and after trauma center designation using trauma and injury severity score analysis. *J Trauma.* 1995;39:1036–1040.

67. Glance LG, Osler T. Beyond the Major Trauma Outcome Study: Benchmarking performance using a national contemporary, population-based trauma registry. *J Trauma.* 2001;51:725–727.

68. Hedges JR, Mullins RJ, Zimmer-Gemback M, et al. Oregon trauma system: Change in initial admission site and post-admission transfer of injured patients. *Acad Emerg Med.* 1994;1:218–226.

69. Clark DE, Anderson KL, Hahn DR. Evaluating an inclusive trauma system using linked population-based data. *J Trauma.* 2004;57:501–509.

70. Clark DE, Hahn DR. Hospital trauma registries linked with population-based data. *J Trauma.* 1999;47:448–454.

71. Hulka F, Mullins RJ, Mann NC, et al. Influence of a statewide trauma system on pediatric hospitalization and outcome. *J Trauma.* 1997;42:514–519.

72. Mullins RJ, Mann NC. Population-based research assessing the effectiveness of trauma systems. *J Trauma.* 1999;47:S59–S66.

73. Kane G, Wheeler NC, Cook S, et al. Impact of the Los Angeles county trauma system on the survival of seriously injured patients. *J Trauma.* 1992;32:576–583.

74. Shafi S, Nathens AB, Elliott AC, et al. Effect of trauma systems on motor vehicle occupant mortality: A comparison between states with and without a formal system. *J Trauma.* 2006;61:1374–1378.

75. Baker SP, Waller A, Langlois J. Motor vehicle deaths in children: Geographic variations. *Accid Anal Prev.* 1991;23:19–28.

76. Clark DE. Effect of population density on mortality after motor vehicle collisions. *Accid Anal Prev.* 2003;35:965–971.

77. Marson AC, Thomson JC. The influence of prehospital trauma care on motor vehicle crash mortality. *J Trauma.* 2001;50:917–920.

78. Melton SM, McGwin G, Abernathy JH, et al. Motor vehicle crash-related mortality is associated with prehospital and hospital-based resource availability. *J Trauma.* 2003;54:273–279.

79. Maio RF, Green PE, Becker MP, et al. Rural motor vehicle crash mortality: The role of crash severity and medical resources. *Accid Anal Prev.* 1992;24:631–642.

80. DiRusso S, Holly C, Kamath R, et al. Preparation and achievement of American College of Surgeons level I trauma verification raises hospital performance and improves patient outcome. *J Trauma.* 2001;51:294–300.

81. Peitzman AB, Courcoulas AP, Stinson C, et al. Trauma center maturation. *Ann Surg.* 1999;230:87–94.

82. Cameron PA, Gabbe BJ, McNeil JJ. The importance of quality of survival as an outcome measure for an integrated trauma system. *Injury.* 2006;37:1178–1184.

83. Mann NC, Mullins RJ. Research recommendations and proposed action items to facilitate trauma system implementation and evaluation. *J Trauma.* 1999;47:S75–S78.

84. Elvik R. The validity of using health state indexes in measuring the consequences of traffic injury for public health. *Soc Sci Med.* 1995;40:1385–1398.

85. Holbrook T, Hoyt DB, Anderson JP, et al. Functional limitation after major trauma: A more sensitive assessment using the Quality of Well-being scale – the trauma recovery pilot project. *J Trauma.* 1994;36:74–78.

86. Harbrecht BG, Zenati MS, Ochoa JB, et al. Evaluation of a 15-year experience with splenic injuries in a state trauma system. *Surgery.* 2007;141:229–238.

87. Durham R, Pracht E, Orban B, et al. Evaluation of a mature trauma system. *Ann Surg.* 2006;243:775–785.

88. Cohen MM, Fath JA, Chung RS, et al. Impact of a dedicated trauma service on the quality and cost of care provided to injured patients at an urban teaching hospital. *J Trauma.* 1999;46:1114–1119.

89. Rutledge R, Shaffer VD, Ridky J. Trauma care in rural hospitals: Implications for triage and trauma system design. *J Trauma.* 1996;40:1002–1008.

90. Hedges JR, Mann NC, Mullins RJ, et al. OHSU Rural Research Group. Impact of a statewide trauma system on rural emergency department patient assessment documentation. *Acad Emerg Med.* 1997;4:268–276.

91. Olson CJ, Arthur M, Mullins RJ, et al. Influence of trauma system implementation on process of care delivered to seriously injured patients in rural trauma centers. *Surgery.* 2001;130:273–279.

92. Jacobs LM, Burns KJ, Gross RI. Terrorism: A public health threat with a trauma system response. *J Trauma.* 2003;55:1014–1021.

93. Feeney JM, Goldberg R, Blumenthal JA, et al. September 11, 2001, revisited. A review of the data. *Arch Surg.* 2005;140:1068–1073.

94. May AK, McGwin G, Lancaster LJ, et al. The April 8, 1998 tornado: Assessment of the trauma system response and the resulting injuries. *J Trauma.* 2000;48:666–672.

Injury Prevention and Control

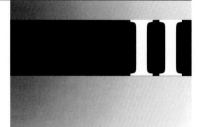

Injury Prevention

6

Charles C. Branas

Although tragic, the 1997 Paris car crash death of Diana, Princess of Wales, is an excellent opportunity to reflect on the basics of injury prevention. Five fundamental opportunities for prevention were overlooked and very likely resulted in the crash itself and its three deaths, including the princess'. First, the princess, in the rear right passenger seat, was not wearing a seat belt, along with two other occupants. The one occupant who did survive the crash was in the front passenger seat and was wearing a seat belt. Second, the princess' car was being pursued by photographers and was traveling at high speed, far beyond typical urban speed limits. Third, the chauffeur of the princess' car had been drinking alcohol before getting behind the wheel and was above the proscribed level of intoxication. Fourth, the princess' car drove into a tunnel where it hit a pillar that was very close to the road and then crashed into a wall. The aging urban roadway they had been driving on had not been updated with modifications such as guardrails or flared barriers. Fifth, a medically trained bystander who arrived minutes after the crash reported that the princess was conscious. Although emergency medical services quickly responded to the scene of the crash, it took as much as 90 minutes to then transport the princess to a hospital, which was only a few miles away. This tragic event is a helpful case study for new injury prevention strategists and will serve to reinforce an understanding of the topics discussed in this chapter—injury as disease, the history of injury prevention, the magnitude of the injury problem, and injury prevention strategies.

THE BIOMEDICAL DISEASE OF INJURY

Injury, or trauma, occurs when at-risk people, unsafe environments, and hazardous objects converge. As such, injuries are often thought of as simply unavoidable social accidents, not worthy of systematic study and, by extension, thoughtful prevention efforts. But injury clearly deserves

attention as a leading cause of death and disability in the United States and around the world. Injury also deserves attention because it occurs as part of a unique disease process: violence, suicide, falls, and automobile crashes are all disease-generating events that can very suddenly kill or disable otherwise healthy people. This is in contrast to other leading diseases, which generally become noticeable only after months or years of risk exposure. Therefore, injury develops in a fraction of a second, often after a similarly sudden exposure to one or more risk factors, making its prevention especially challenging.

Injury is a biomedical disease process brought about by a fast-acting, external force. The external force in question is created by the transfer of thermal, mechanical, electrical, or chemical energy onto the human body. This transfer of energy often occurs very rapidly and the pathologic damage that results is quickly recognizable. More recent definitions of injury have also included a damaging transfer of psychological energy (for instance, as with post-traumatic stress disorder).[1] The risk factors that precede this transfer of energy can occur almost simultaneously to the event itself or accumulate in the near or far past. The repercussions of this energy transfer also occur almost simultaneously to the event itself but with both immediate and long-term consequences. Given this fundamental disease paradigm, injury reduction strategists typically eschew the notion of injuries as unavoidable social accidents and instead rely on rational, scientific approaches to prevention.

HISTORY OF INJURY PREVENTION

The pluralism of injury prevention, as evidenced by its close ties to at least three different cabinet-level agencies in the United States—Health and Human Services, Justice, and Transportation—has made it one of three areas cited by the Institute of Medicine as highly suitable for interdisciplinary study.[2] In this way, the 20th century has been rife with

TABLE 1
A SELECT CHRONOLOGY OF TWENTIETH CENTURY INJURY PREVENTION ACCOMPLISHMENTS

1924—Cadillac offers the first car with safety windshield glass standard
1933—Congress charters the National Safety Council
1934—National Firearms Act passed as the first major federal gun legislation
1942—Hugh de Haven, a World War I pilot and crash survivor-turned-physiologist, publishes landmark article on importance of injury biomechanics
1949—Seat belts introduced by Nash Motors
1949—John Gordon suggests that injuries behave like classic infectious diseases and can be studied using epidemiologic methods
1951—First medical evacuation by helicopter during Korean War
1956—United States Public Health Service establishes an Accident Prevention Program
1965—Ralph Nader publishes *Unsafe at Any Speed* documenting the resistance of car companies to seat belts and the three Es of road safety: engineering, enforcement, and education
1966—National Research Council report, *Accidental Death and Disability*, is released
1972—First live product demonstration of Dupont Kevlar bulletproof vest that was invented by Richard Davis after he was shot at in an attempted robbery
1973—Congress passes the Emergency Medical Services Act
1974—General Motors produces first air bags
1986—Injury Prevention Act signed into law paving the way for the National Center for Injury Prevention and Control at the CDC

CDC, Centers for Disease Control and Prevention.

landmarks in injury prevention. Some of these events are accomplishments at singular points in time although many formed the basis of activities that continue today. The traffic safety movement of the 1920s and the home safety movement of the 1950s are two such examples[3-5] (see Table 1).

Given its landmark achievements in injury prevention thinking and study, the 20th century has also witnessed some noteworthy reductions in injury. In fact, motor vehicle safety has been cited as one of the top ten public health achievements in the United States over the last century. This is largely based on reductions in traffic deaths due to safer vehicles and highways, increased use of safety belts, child safety seats, and motorcycle helmets, as well as decreased drinking and driving.[6]

However, it is worth noting that in the last century mortality reductions from injuries of all causes (not simply motor vehicle crashes) have been far less than those of other diseases, such as influenza, tuberculosis, and gastroenteritis[7] (see Fig. 1). This relatively low level of success may be related to the fact that the federal research investment in injury prevention has been, and continues to be, very low proportional to the public health burden posed by the disease of injury[8] (see Fig. 2). Certain mechanisms of injury have been limited or even proscribed in terms of receiving resource support from certain federal agencies. For instance, since 1997 the Centers for Disease Control and Prevention (CDC) have not been legally permitted to fund "activities designed to affect the passage of specific Federal, State, or local legislation intended to restrict or control the purchase or use of firearms."[9] Correspondingly, the National Institutes of Health (NIH), the largest public health research agency in the United States, has only

granted one major research award per million firearm injury cases per decade in the last 30 years[10] (see Table 2). Therefore, federal public health support of firearm injury research has been in short supply relative to the magnitude of the problem.[11]

MAGNITUDE OF THE INJURY PROBLEM

Around the world, injury is the leading cause of death for the first half of the human life span and a regular source

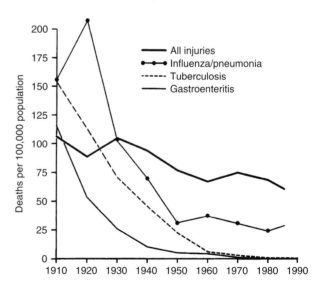

Figure 1 Twentieth century mortality reductions from injuries of all causes have been far less than those of other diseases. (Taken from Baker SP, Ginsburg MJ, O'Neill B. *The injury fact book*, 2nd ed. New York: Oxford Publishing; 1992.)

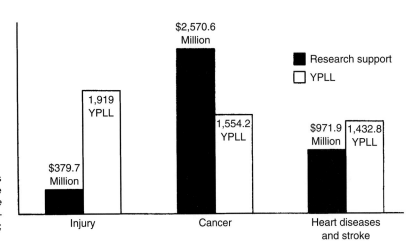

Figure 2 Years of potential life lost (YPLL) versus federal research investment. (Taken from Bonnie RJ, Fulco CE, Liverman CT, eds. *Reducing the burden of injury: advancing prevention and treatment*. Washington, DC: National Academy Press; 1999:19.)

of disability and disfigurement.[12-18] As a leading cause of death, injury is fourth behind heart disease, cancer, and stroke (see Fig. 3). As an actual cause of death injury also ranks quite high; this is especially true for certain mechanisms of injury such as motor vehicles and firearms[19] (see Table 3).

Injury and its repercussions have a significant impact on health and well-being. Each day in the United States more than 320,000 men, women, and children are injured severely enough to seek medical care. Approximately 200 of these people will sustain a long-term disability due to their injuries and an additional 400 will die.[20-23] Globally, approximately 16,000 people die from injuries each day and this incidence is growing.[24]

Annually, more than 5 million people die from injuries worldwide.[25] In the United States, injury touches as many as one in three people[26]—approximately 150,000 Americans will die due to injuries each year (the population of Center City Philadelphia), approximately 2.5 million Americans will be hospitalized due to injuries each year (half the entire Philadelphia metro area), and approximately 70 million Americans will require medical attention due to injuries each year (one quarter of the US population) (see Fig. 4).

Injury generates significant death, irreversible disability, and copious health care utilization. More than one third of all US emergency department visits, an estimated 39 million, are related to injury.[27] The most common injuries, accounting for approximately 40% of injury-related emergency department visits, are from falls and motor vehicle crashes. Each year an estimated 80,000 Americans experience the onset of long-term or lifetime disability from traumatic brain injury.[28,29] An estimated 10,000 new cases of spinal cord injury occur annually, with more than 240,000 persons currently living with paraplegia, tetraplegia, or related limitations.[30]

The consequences of injury also go well beyond these examples of physical disability. For both individuals and families, repercussions of injury are profound, including loss of independence,[31-34] loss of work,[35] loss of sexual function,[36] and fatigue.[32,37] The lifetime cost of injuries occurring in a single year in the United States totals an estimated $406 billion[38] in medical expenses and productivity losses (including lost wages, fringe benefits, and ability to perform normal household responsibilities).

INJURY PREVENTION STRATEGIES

Beginning in 1962, William Haddon developed and refined a list of ten general strategies for injury prevention[39] (see Table 4). From the standpoint of prevention, these ten injury countermeasures incorporated three basic themes: (i) when to intervene, (ii) on what to intervene, and (iii) how to intervene. These countermeasures were not supposed to be a formula for prevention as much as they were intended to be of assistance in thinking about prevention logically and systematically.[3]

TABLE 2

MAJOR NATIONAL INSTITUTES OF HEALTH (NIH) RESEARCH AWARDS AND CUMULATIVE MORBIDITY FOR SELECT CONDITIONS IN THE UNITED STATES, 1973 TO 2002

Condition	Total Cases	NIH Research Awards
Cholera	373	101
Diphtheria	1,337	54
Polio	266	106
Rabies	55	59
Total of four diseases	2,031	320
Firearm injuries	>3,000,000	3

(Taken from Branas CC, Wiebe DJ, Schwab CW, et al. Getting past the "F" word in federally funded public health research. *Inj Prev.* 2005;11(3):191.)

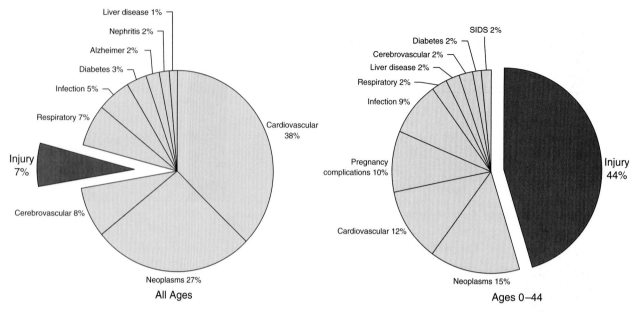

Figure 3 Leading causes of death in the United States, 1999 to 2000. SIDS, sudden infant death syndrome.

Injury occurs across a timeline or continuum, from early precursors to the defining disease event to immediate and long-term consequences. Consideration of when to intervene over the course of the pathophysiologic process is of great importance as pathologic changes may become fixed or irreversible. The time sequence in injury prevention is based on a traditional epidemiologic approach to disease prevention in which three levels exist. Opportunities to prevent or ameliorate injury correspondingly change across these three levels on the injury continuum: primary

prevention, applied during the stage of susceptibility, seeks to completely avert injuries by altering vulnerability or reducing exposure; secondary prevention, applied during early disease, employs early detection and immediate treatment of injuries once they occur; and tertiary prevention, applied during advanced disease or disability, focuses on limiting disability and restoring function for injured individuals.[40]

Primary prevention of injuries is considered to be in the pre-event category of countermeasures. Examples of pre-event/primary injury prevention activities include driver education campaigns and loaded chamber indicators on firearms. Secondary prevention of injuries is considered to be part of the in-the-event category of countermeasures. Because injury pathophysiology progresses so rapidly

TABLE 3

ACTUAL CAUSES OF DEATH IN THE UNITED STATES, 1990 AND 2000

Actual Cause	No. in 1990[a] No. (%)[b]	No. in 2000 No. (%)[b]
Tobacco	400,000 (19)	435,000 (18.1)
Poor diet and physical inactivity	300,000 (14)	400,000 (16.6)
Alcohol consumption	100,000 (5)	85,000 (3.5)
Microbial agents	90,000 (4)	75,000 (3.1)
Toxic agents	60,000 (3)	55,000 (2.3)
Motor vehicle	25,000 (1)	43,000 (1.8)
Firearms	35,000 (2)	29,000 (1.2)
Sexual behavior	30,000 (1)	20,000 (0.8)
Illicit drug use	20,000 (<1)	17,000 (0.7)
Total	1,060,000 (50)	1,159,000 (48.2)

[a]Data are from McGinnis and Foege.
[b]The percentages are for all deaths.
(Taken from Mokdad AH, Marks JS, Stroup DF, et al. Actual causes of death in the UNITED STATES, 2000. *JAMA*. 2004;291(10):1238–1245.)

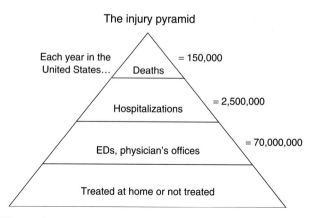

Figure 4 Annual burden of injury in the United States. EDs, emergency departments.

TABLE 4

TEN BASIC INJURY PREVENTION COUNTERMEASURES PROPOSED BY HADDON

1. Prevent the creation of the hazard in the first place
2. Reduce the amount of the hazard brought into being
3. Prevent the release of the hazard that already exists
4. Modify the release of the hazard that already exists
5. Separate, in time and space, the hazard and that which is to be protected
6. Separate, by material barrier, the hazard and that which is to be protected
7. Modify the relevant basic qualities of the hazard
8. Make that to be protected more resistant to damage from the hazard
9. Counter damage already done by the hazard
10. Stabilize, repair, and rehabilitate the object of the hazard

once it begins, secondary/in-the-event countermeasures are often immediate and/or automated. Examples include football helmets, automobile air bags, and bulletproof vests. Finally, tertiary prevention of injuries is considered to be in the postevent category of countermeasures. Examples include rapid response by emergency medical services systems, improved surgical and damage control techniques, and access to appropriate rehabilitation services. Injury prevention strategists often focus first on preventing the disease from occurring and then applying ameliorative or curative strategies, if necessary. However, because so many injury phenomena cannot realistically be eradicated, a strong emphasis on primary prevention should not completely overshadow the need to also develop and sustain secondary and tertiary prevention programs.

A second epidemiologic paradigm of disease can also be applied to prevent injury. This provides the prevention strategist a way to consider on what they are to intervene.

The "what" here is the basic epidemiologic triangle—host, agent-vector, and environment—and although its most common application has been infectious diseases, injury as a disease also benefits from the application of this epidemiologic triad. Understanding these basic modifiable factors can guide the selection of injury prevention strategies.

Injury occurs when an external agent capable of causing the disease meets a host that is vulnerable to the agent. The agent can then transmit the disease-causing vector, assuming that the environment permits the agent, vector, and host to interact. If we were to apply this paradigm to a disease such as malaria, prevention efforts might be directed at a human host or human populations (for instance, restricting people's entry into low-lying areas), the agent containing the disease vector (for instance, spraying of pesticides to kill mosquitoes), the disease vector itself (for instance, administering mefloquine against the *Plasmodium falciparum* parasite), or the environment within which agent, vector, and host interact (for instance, draining swampy areas of stagnant water). This paradigm can be extended to injury as a disease. For example, if we were to apply this to firearm injury, prevention efforts might be directed at a human host or human populations (for instance, restricting criminal access to firearms), the agent containing the disease vector (for instance, modifying firearms so that they can only be discharged by authorized users), the disease vector itself (for instance, restricting civilian access to armor piercing bullets), or the environment within which agent, vector, and host interact (for instance, disbanding illicit drug markets that encourage young men to arm themselves) (see Fig. 5). Together with the temporal sequence of injury pathology, this host-agent-vector-environment triad forms the traditional "Haddon matrix." It is also useful to note that Haddon distinguished between physical and social environments.

A third dimension that is worth adding to the traditional Haddon matrix is the distinction between active and passive injury prevention strategies. These are the routes of

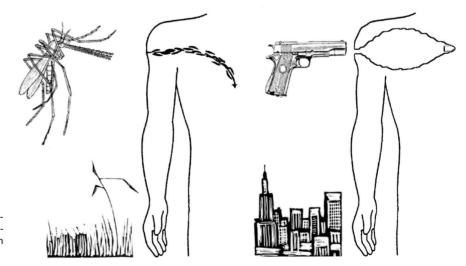

Figure 5 Comparison of the epidemiologic triangle (host-agent-vector-environment) for malaria and firearm injury.

administration that guide the injury prevention strategist on how best to intervene. Active strategies are those that require action on the part of people or their guardians to prevent injury. Many active prevention strategies involve education campaigns or behavior modifications. Classic examples of active prevention strategies include driver education programs or public service campaigns to get automobile occupants to use seat belts. Passive injury prevention strategies require no action for the intervention to be successful. Classic examples of passive prevention strategies include automobile air bags or clothing with cushioned protectors sewn into it. Although many injury prevention strategists favor passive, or automated, prevention strategies because they may have higher probabilities of success, it should be recognized that mixed strategies with both active and passive components are likely the best choice.

Taken together, the dimensions of when, on what, and how to intervene constitute a three-dimensional representation of options that the injury prevention strategist has at their disposal (see Fig. 6). As with Haddon's ten countermeasures, the use of this matrix is not intended to somehow be a recipe for injury prevention but a guide in logically and systematically thinking about prevention. Prevention strategists are encouraged to fill in every cell in the matrix as they consider the best ways to address a given injury problem. It is inevitable that they will be unable to implement every possible strategy in the matrix but thinking through all the possibilities, and their relative benefits and challenges, insures that the best one or two strategies will be identified and efficiently implemented.

The former Director of the CDC, Dr. William Foege, has stated that "injury is the principal public health problem in America."[26] A better understanding of injury as a biomedical disease, the history of injury prevention, and the magnitude of the injury problem, can inform the selection and implementation of successful injury prevention strategies. From Princess Diana to the average American, injuries have enormously tragic repercussions on people, their families, and society at large. They are, however, very preventable with some thoughtful effort.

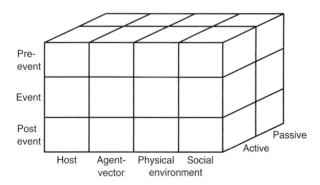

Figure 6 Three-dimensional representation of injury prevention options.

REFERENCES

1. Brewin BR, Holmes EA. Psychological theories of post traumatic stress disorders. *J Clin Psychol Rev*. 2003;23:339–376.
2. Pellmar TC, Eisenberg L, eds. *Bridging disciplines in the brain, behavioral and clinical sciences*. Washington, DC: National Academy Press; 2000:30.
3. National Committee for Injury Prevention and Control. *Injury prevention: meeting the challenge*. New York: Oxford University Press; 1989.
4. De Haven H. Mechanical analysis of survival in falls from heights of fifty to one hundred and fifty feet. *War Med*. 1942;2:586–596.
5. Gordon JE. The epidemiology of accidents. *Am J Public Health*. 1949;39:504–515.
6. Centers for Disease Control and Prevention. Ten great public health achievements – United States, 1900–1999. *Morb Mortal Wkly Rep*. 1999;48(12):241–243.
7. Baker SP, Ginsburg MJ, O'Neill B. *The injury fact book*, 2nd ed. New York: Oxford Publishing; 1992.
8. Bonnie RJ, Fulco CE, Liverman CT, eds. *Reducing the burden of injury: advancing prevention and treatment*. Washington, DC: National Academy Press; 1999:19.
9. Binder S, Manning SR. *Letter to grantees: restriction of funding*. National Center for Injury Prevention and Control, Centers for DiseaseControl and Prevention. Available at http://www.cdc.gov/ncipc/res-opps/restrictions.htm, accessed 4 January 2005.
10. Branas CC, Wiebe DJ, Schwab CW, et al. Getting past the "F" word in federally funded public health research. *Inj Prev*. 2005;11(3):191.
11. Kassirer JP. A partisan assault on science—the threat to the CDC. *N Engl J Med*. 1995;333:793–794.
12. Richmond TS, Kauder DK, Hinkle J, et al. Early predictors of long-term disability after injury. *Am J Crit Care*. 2003;12:197–205.
13. Richmond TS, Kauder DK, Strumpf N, et al. Characteristics and outcomes of serious traumatic injury in older adults. *J Am Geriatr Soc*. 2002;50:215–222.
14. Richmond TS, Thompson H, Deatrick J, et al. The journey towards recovery following physical trauma. *J Adv Nurs*. 2000; 32:1341–1347.
15. Richmond TS, Kauder DK. Predictors of psychological distress following serious injury. *J Trauma Stress*. 2000;13:681–692.
16. Richmond TS, Kauder DK, Schwab CW. A prospective study of predictors of disability at 3 months following non-central nervous system trauma. *J Trauma*. 1988;44:635–643.
17. Richmond TS. An explanatory model of variables influencing post-injury disability. *Nurs Res*. 1997;46:262–269.
18. National Research Council and the Institute of Medicine. *Injury in America: a continuing public health problem*. Washington, DC: National Academy Press; 1985:2.
19. Mokdad AH, Marks JS, Stroup DF, et al. Actual causes of death in the United States, 2000. *JAMA*. 2004;291(10):1238–1245.
20. Barss P, Smith GS, Baker SP, et al. *Injury prevention: an international perspective. epidemiology, surveillance, and policy*. New York: Oxford University Press; 1998:1–11.
21. Baker SP, O'Neill B, Ginsburg MJ, et al. *The injury fact book*. New York: Oxford University Press; 1992:14–15.
22. National Research Council Committee on Trauma Research. *Injury in America: a continuing public health problem*. Washington, DC: National Academy Press; 1985:1–19.
23. Rice DP, MacKenzie EJ. *Cost of injury in the United States: a report to congress, 1989*. San Francisco: Institute for Health and Aging, University of California and Johns Hopkins University; 1989.
24. World Health Organization. *Injury: a leading cause of the global burden of disease*. www.who.int/violence_injury_prevention/injruy/gbi. Accessed 11/18/2003, 2003.
25. Murray JL, Lopez AD. Global burden of mortality, disability and the contribution of risk factors: Global burden of disease study. *Lancet*. 1997;349:1436.
26. Foege WH, Baker SP, Davis JH, et al. *Committee on trauma research. Injury in America. A continuing public health problem*.Washington, DC: National Academy Press; 1985.
27. McCraig LF, Burt CW. National hospital ambulatory medical care survey: 2001 Emergency department summary. *Adv Data Vital Health Stat, CDC*. 2003;7:1.

28. Centers for Disease Control and Prevention. *Spinal cord fact sheet*. http://www.cdc.gov/ncipc/factsheets/scifacts.htm. Accessed 11/19/03. 2003

29. Centers for Disease Control and Prevention. *Traumatic brain injury fact sheet*. http://www.cdc.gov/ncipc/factsheets/tbi.htm. Accessed 11/19/03. 2003.

30. National Spinal Cord Injury Statistical Center. *Facts and figures at a glance december 2003*. http://www.spinalcord.uab.edu/show.asp?durki=21446. Accessed 1/29/04. 2004.

31. Brenneman FD, Katyal D, Boulanger BR, et al. Long-term outcomes in open pelvic fractures. *J Trauma*. 1997;42:773–777.

32. Haukeland JV. Welfare consequences of injuries due to traffic accidents. *Accid Anal Prev*. 1996;28:63–72.

33. Jurkovich G, Mock C, MacKenzie E, et al. The sickness impact profile as a tool to evaluate functional outcome in trauma patients. *J Trauma*. 1995;39:625–631.

34. Morris JA, Sanchez AA, Bass SM, et al. Trauma patients return to productivity. *J Trauma*. 1991;31:827–834.

35. Anke AG, Stanghelle JK, Finset A, et al. Long-term prevalence of impairments and disabilities after multiple trauma. *J Trauma*. 1997;42:54–61.

36. McCarthy ML, MacKenzie EJ, Bosse MJ, et al. Functional status following orthopedic trauma in young women. *J Trauma*. 1995;39:828–837.

37. Thiagarajan J, Taylor P, Hogbin E, et al. Quality of life after multiple trauma requiring intensive care. *Anesthesia*. 1994;49:211–218.

38. Finkelstein EA, Corso PS, Miller TR. *Incidence and economic burden of injuries in the United States*. New York: Oxford University Press; 2006.

39. Haddon W. The basic strategies for reducing hazards of all kinds. *Hazard Prev*. 1980;10:8–12.

40. Mauser JS, Kramer S. Epidemiologic orientation to health and disease. In: *Epidemiology: an introductory text*. Philadelphia: WB Saunders; 1985:9–13.

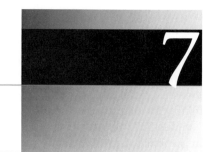

Firearm Injury Prevention

Douglas J. Wiebe   *Edmund M. Weisberg*

Reducing the overall level of violent acts committed in our society is a necessary goal. Violence committed with firearms specifically is a priority issue because gunshot wounds are more lethal than trauma inflicted using other weapons. In addition to being highly lethal, firearm violence has devastating effects on victims' families and communities, places heavy demands on trauma centers and health care systems, and creates serious physical and mental challenges for survivors.

The surgical management of gunshot trauma is of paramount importance, making the difference between life and death for those who have been shot. However, the trauma community does not bear the burden of firearm injury prevention itself. Far from it, in fact. Trauma surgery represents only one of the multiple points at which elements of the shooting event and its aftermath can be intervened upon in an attempt to achieve firearm injury prevention. Firearm injury prevention is a comprehensive concept, and is defined here as the public health goal of preventing shootings from occurring, as well as minimizing the likelihood that negative outcomes will result when shootings occur. These outcomes include mortality; physical, mental, and emotional morbidity; and costs to the medical system, as well as the impact on families, communities, and society.

This chapter describes a framework for firearm injury prevention. The framework follows the public health approach, which is interdisciplinary and science based.[1] This approach draws upon knowledge from many disciplines including medicine, epidemiology, sociology, psychology, criminology, education, engineering, and economics. The combined contributions of each discipline have allowed the field of public health to be innovative and responsive

to a wide range of diseases, illnesses, and injuries. As one example, the ability of the field to build knowledge of risk and subsequently reduce motor vehicle crash–related fatalities despite an increase in miles driven is cited by the Centers for Disease Control and Prevention (CDC) as one of the injury prevention successes of the 20th century.[2] With the focus here being on firearm injury prevention, this chapter provides a conceptual model for the shooting event, its precursors, and its aftermath, and presents a tool for identifying opportunities for prevention.

MAGNITUDE OF THE PROBLEM

Gunshot wound injury is the second most common trauma mechanism treated at United States trauma centers, surpassed only by motor vehicle crash–related injuries, and is the second leading cause of death in the United States in the 15- to 34-year-old age-group.[3] Moreover, it is the leading cause of violence-related injury deaths in all age-groups up to the age of 34. According to the National Trauma Data Bank (NTDB) 2006 annual report (on data from 2000 to 2005), 15% of cases of gunshot wound injury result in death after arrival at the hospital or trauma center, which is the highest percentage for any type of penetrating injury. During that period, 60,377 gunshot wound patients were treated at trauma centers and for survivors the average length of hospital stay was 6.5 days.

The average medical cost of gunshot injuries in 1998 was an estimated $16,500 per case, with average costs of $22,400 for unintentional gunshot injuries, $18,400 for assault-related injuries, and $5,400 for self-directed shootings.[4] Significantly, a substantial portion of the costs of treating gunshot victims is shouldered by government programs and less so by private insurers; in both cases, though, higher costs are transferred to the general public in terms of higher taxes and higher insurance premiums.[4]

Opportunity costs in terms of disability and lost productivity also create a significant impact. For Americans, firearm injuries in 2000 accounted for an estimated $35.2 billion in total lifetime productivity losses.[5] Considered in terms of life expectancy, firearm violence shortens the life of an average American by 104 days (151 days for white males, 362 days for black males).[6] Using a more expansive definition that also considers societal burdens such as security systems in schools and subsidizing urban trauma centers, Cook and Ludwig estimated that $100 billion is a more accurate assessment of the annual cost of gun violence in the United States.[4] Regardless of how narrowly or broadly we may define or identify the costs of gun violence, such violence exerts a considerable burden on individual victims, their families, and society at large. This public health problem is not confined to the United States, we should note, and in fact is identified as a global health priority by the World Health Organization.[4,7] For many reasons, then, it is a priority to consider how firearm violence can be prevented.

THE SHOOTING EVENT: INJURY PRECURSORS, INJURY EVENT, AND INJURY CONSEQUENCES

The gunshot injury event—the moment the firearm is discharged—provides us with a focal point from which to consider the event more broadly, including the circumstances that led up to the shooting, and the aftermath of the shooting. This notion of the shooting event has been diagramed by Cheney et al. (see Fig. 1)[8] and used to promote interdisciplinary collaboration for the study and prevention of firearm injury. It has been used successfully in broader applications to all injury categories (see Chapter 11).

The star in the center of the diagram, the focal point, represents the gunshot injury event. The issue that is key to appreciate here is that the gunshot injury event represents only one distinct moment, whereas the chronologic trajectory of events in the life of the gunshot injury victim includes the sequence of precursors as well as consequences. The firearm injury event can be thought to have occurred as a result of the culmination of preceding events that converged at the focal point. The routine activities theory of criminology, for example, conveys this notion well, and explains that for a gunshot injury to occur, there must be a convergence in time and space of three factors: a motivated perpetrator, a suitable target, and the lack of a capable guardian.[9,10] Also depicted in Fig. 1 is the fact that the firearm injury event is followed by ramifications for the victim and for others as well, including the victim's family, the community, the health care system, and society.

Having framed gunshot injury as a public health problem that consists of these three periods—the injury precursors, the injury event, and the injury consequences—we can overlay this model with the concepts of primary, secondary, and tertiary prevention, respectively. As we shall see more concretely in the subsequent text, each stage refers to a way of identifying strategies to address the problem of firearm injury toward the goal of prevention. Primary prevention activities are those that are designed to *prevent* instances of an illness, disease, or injury in a population and thereby to reduce, as much as possible, the risk of new cases arising. Therefore, primary prevention activities apply to the injury precursor phase. Secondary prevention activities are those designed to reduce the progress of a disease or injury and occur during the natural history of the disease or injury. Therefore, secondary prevention activities apply to the injury event phase itself—the moment of firearm discharge and the moment of penetrating trauma. Tertiary prevention activities are those designed to limit death and disability from disease and injury, and therefore apply to the injury consequences phase of Fig. 1. In considering that the realm of options available for our work toward the goal of firearm

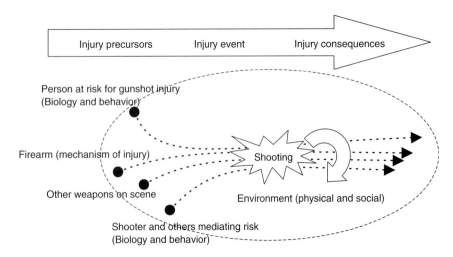

Figure 1 A conceptual model for interpersonal assault, unintentional, and self-directed gunshot injury.

injury prevention includes strategies of primary, secondary, and tertiary prevention, we start to frame this problem as one that can be approached in a deliberate and methodical manner. As a result, we can start to view firearm violence as a public health problem that is not intractable, but rather as one with aspects that can be targeted for prevention. The ways in which firearm violence can be targeted become even more concrete by proceeding one step further and considering the Haddon matrix.

PREVENTION

The goal of firearm injury prevention can be approached through the conceptual model that William Haddon, Jr. developed more than 3 decades ago during his work on motor vehicle crash injuries.[11,12] His influential model, known as the *Haddon matrix* (see Table 1), has since been used to conceptualize and develop approaches to prevent injuries of various types.

The Haddon Matrix

Haddon's model assists in suggesting which linkage points in a causal chain offer the most promise for a specific intervention. An excellent example exists in Runyan's application of the Haddon matrix to the problem of school-based firearm violence.[13] As mentioned in the preceding text, by breaking the problem of gunshot injury into its constituent parts, the goal most generally is to take what might be seen at first as an overwhelming problem and frame it, and in the process render it a problem that is tractable. We see this principle applied by Runyan insofar as her example does not address gunshot injury in its totality. Instead, Runyan's example specifically addresses firearm violence in schools, as a way to ensure that nuances of the problem are appreciated and opportunities for prevention can be detected and therefore targeted with precision.

Composed of four columns and three rows, the Haddon matrix unites the public health concepts of host-agent-environment as targets of intervention with the concepts of primary, secondary, and tertiary prevention.[14,15] For our purposes here in applying the matrix to firearm injury, the factors identified as the columns in the matrix denote the interdependent or interacting factors involved or essential in the shooting event. The first column, labeled as "host," pertains to the individual at risk of injury by shooting. Although in most areas of health, increased knowledge is believed to be a necessary but not sufficient ingredient for change, increased knowledge in the injury realm has not been shown to be associated with behavioral change. Nevertheless, some intervention options include teaching children to steer clear of guns, discouraging adults/parents from purchasing guns, demonstrating safe storage methods to gun owners, and providing gun owners with trigger locks to promote safe storage. The agent or vehicle in our application of the matrix is the firearm.

The physical environment entails all aspects of the setting in which the shooting occurs, including the home, streets, schools, and other public venues in which such violence takes place. The social environment comprises the legal and cultural or community norms, standards, and practices in the geographic region in which the shooting occurs. This category is also the most appropriate setting for traditional public health interventions, so we would include the hospital in this column. In Haddon's original design, the rows in the matrix referred to phases or time periods in which change would exert its effect. In our adaptation, the corresponding phases refer to the preshooting period, the shooting event (up to initial

	Host	Agent/Vehicle	Physical Environment	Social Environment
TABLE 1				
THE HADDON MATRIX				
Pre-event				
Event				
Postevent				

treatment), and the postshooting period (i.e., pre-event, event, and postevent). Identifying interventions that are apropos to each cell in the matrix facilitates the process of devising suitable strategies for reducing or preventing firearm injury. The table presented in the subsequent text is an adaptation by Runyan of the Haddon matrix to firearm violence in schools and serves as the model for our conception of the Haddon matrix as applied to general firearm injury (see Table 2).[13]

Significantly, Runyan emphasizes the need to carefully define the rows and columns (or dimensions) in the matrix, because the range of possibilities can be a function of one's perspective. Clarity in this definition helps to facilitate the process of considering the antecedent and subsequent events, which, in turn, contributes to the identification of potential prevention interventions. In Runyan's example of school violence by firearms, the event could be defined as the moment the shooter displays the weapon, the moment when she/he first points the firearm at another person, the moment the gun is first discharged, or the precise moment when an individual is shot.

Runyan's selection of the event as the moment the gun is exposed to be fired yields the period of time before the student uses the firearm as the pre-event phase. This

period is fertile ground for intervention at all sources. At the host level, parents can be educated regarding the risks of permitting their children to have access to guns. Children can be enlightened about the dangers of bringing a gun to school; they can also be taught to identify peer behavior that may indicate a predilection toward violence. In terms of the agent or vehicle, a pre-event intervention would be represented by the modification of firearms so that only the licensed owner can use them. The physical environment can be the scene of pre-event phase intervention through the installation of metal detectors and elimination/renovation of potential storage areas where students might consider hiding guns. In the social environment, several policies or laws could be enacted to reduce the likelihood of shooting events occurring at schools (e.g., a school policy to alert school leadership and the police if a student is suspected of possessing a gun on the premises; prohibiting gun possession on school grounds; and enforcing laws banning or restricting gun ownership by minors).

As the event unfolds, the most appropriate host intervention as suggested by Runyan is teaching students how best to avoid the line of fire. The event and agent/vehicle converge in terms of measures to diminish the capacity of firearms to discharge multiple rounds quickly

TABLE 2
HADDON MATRIX APPLIED TO THE PROBLEM OF SCHOOL VIOLENCE BY FIREARMS

Time of Violence	Host (Students at School)	Agent/Vehicle (Firearm and Bullets)	Physical Environment (School)	Social Environment (School and Community Norms, Policies, Rules)
Pre-event (before teen uses weapon)	Educate teens about the dangers of carrying guns to school Educate parents about dangers of allowing teens access to guns Teach students to recognize and report student behaviors indicative of possible violent behavior	Modify guns so that they are only operable by the owner	Install metal detectors at entrances to schools Eliminate storage places in schools (e.g., lockers) where guns might be kept	Adopt school procedures/policies to notify authorities if a student is suspected of having a gun at school Prohibit gun carrying on school grounds Enforce restrictions on the sale or transfer of handguns to teenagers
Event (when gun is taken out to be fired)	'Teach students to take cover when they see guns or hear gunfire'	Reduce capacity of weapons to fire multiple rounds quickly Modify bullets to be less lethal	Install alarm systems to call law enforcement as soon as weapons are visible	Have law enforcement officers on duty at school to intervene during fights Develop safety plans to help students move to safety in the event of violent episode
Postevent (after students are shot)	'Teach students first aid skill'	Reduce the capacity of the gun to continue firing	Make school grounds readily accessible to ambulances	Ensure well-trained emergency medical personnel and access to trauma facilities Provide postevent counseling to students, staff, and families

Reproduced with permission from the BMJ Publishing Group, Ltd., publishers of *Injury Prevention* (Inj Prev. 1998 Dec;4(4):302–307), to whom we are grateful.

without requiring reloading as well as altering bullets to render them less deleterious. The physical environment at the event phase can be intervened upon through the use of alarm systems that alert the police upon the first visible signs of a weapon. In the social environment, a contingent of police officers might be kept on duty, or the school might at least be included on the list of areas to routinely patrol, so that law enforcement officials can readily intercede upon the potentially harmful display of hostilities. Plans and procedures might also be devised in the social environment for implementation in the event phase, such as helping students find a safe haven during a shooting episode. Further, legislation to re-enact the ban on assault weapons could reduce the likelihood of such firearms being used during a shooting event.

Teaching first aid to students is a possible host postevent intervention. It also meets the definition of an *active intervention*, which is a term used in public health to indicate that action is required on the part of an individual for the intervention to have its impact. The flip side of this coin is the passive intervention, which requires no action on the part of the host to be effective. An example of a passive intervention in the agent/vehicle phase, as suggested by Runyan, might be reducing the capacity of firearms to continue firing, which again addresses bullet and gun technology, particularly gun magazines. An appropriate physical environment intervention for the postevent period is ensuring that school grounds and facilities are readily accessible by emergency medical teams and ambulances. The social environment is ripe for intervention in the postevent phase, and it is in this cell of the matrix where the surgical management of trauma is appropriately featured. Also in this cell, potential interventions could include emergency medical personnel being well trained and convenient access to trauma facilities being ensured. Counseling of students, staff, and families can be made available through the school system. In addition, counseling of traumatized witnesses and surviving victims, as well as their families, can be conducted at the hospitals. Counseling perpetrators who may wind up in the hospital may also serve as a significant postevent intervention. Indeed, the trauma center can also serve as a site from which to launch efforts to prevent recidivism.[16] While this would serve as a postevent intervention, it can also be considered as occurring in the pre-event phase in the context of preventing recidivism, in other words, a future event. Importantly, the clear delineation of the dimensions of the Haddon matrix sets the stage for brainstorming the most suitable and potentially effective interventions to prevent additional firearm injury.

ADDITIONAL CONSIDERATIONS

We hope that what has emerged in the preceding text is evidence that opportunities to prevent firearm injury can abound, and that the many constituencies that comprise and support the field of public health share the responsibility for identifying, creating, and implementing firearm injury prevention strategies. In a recent effort by this community, the National Research Collaborative on Firearm Violence set forth a research agenda dedicated toward the goal of the prevention of firearm injury.[17] The agenda identified the following five overarching research needs to reduce firearm violence: (i) central data collection, quality and control; (ii) qualitative research; (iii) partnerships between university-based researchers and community-based law enforcement, criminal justice, and public health professionals; (iv) formative research and pilot studies; and (v) increased research funding, particularly from the federal government. The Collaborative called for research to be conducted in these areas to identify strategies for reducing firearm violence and to evaluate the efficacy of those strategies.

Briefly, to accomplish this research, data on gun ownership, storage, use, and markets are desperately needed, along with data on gun-tracing as well as the protective, defensive, and deterrent effects of firearms. Research on firearms, according to the Collaborative, should be subject to the same effective standards as those employed in other research fields involving sensitive information.

Qualitative methods, such as ethnographic study of select populations, yield data transcending statistical analyses and would be best evaluated in conjunction with quantitative techniques to illuminate the complex etiology of firearm violence.

Partnerships between researchers and "practitioners," including trauma surgeons, would facilitate brainstorming, resource sharing, creating evidence-based interventions, and arriving at appropriate policy recommendations.

Calling for formative research and pilot studies is equivalent to recommending that researchers and practitioners improve their efforts to develop interventions that take into account the attitudes, beliefs, motivations, knowledge, and behaviors of their target audiences, with the results likely manifesting in better designed and more effective firearm violence interventions.

The research agenda of the Collaborative will require significant increases in federal funding, along with support from foundations, because federal funding for firearm injury prevention research has been scant.[18] To enact this ambitious agenda, the Collaborative acknowledges that it will also be necessary for the United States to reframe the issue of firearm violence as an issue of public health, which it notes the World Health Organization and several countries have already done.

The work, not to mention the name, of the Collaborative reinforces the notion that efforts to reduce the incidence and severity of firearm violence should indeed be an interdisciplinary endeavor involving the many fields that play some role in monitoring and improving public health. Researchers, physicians, nurses, law enforcement officials, criminologists, lawyers, social workers, emergency medical personnel, politicians, school administrators, members of the media, parents, and children all have important roles to play in this vital effort. The field of public health is best positioned to marshal such forces so that more effective approaches to developing and implementing firearm injury prevention can be achieved.

REFERENCES

1. Mercy JA, Rosenberg ML, Powell KE, et al. Public health policy for preventing violence. *Health Aff (Millwood)*. 1993;12(4):7–29.
2. Centers for Disease Control and Prevention. Ten great public health achievements–United States, 1900-1999. *MMWR Morb Mortal Wkly Rep*. 1999;48(12):241–243.
3. Centers for Disease Control and Prevention. *WISQARS leading cause of death reports, 2004. Vol. 2007 Office of Statistics and Programming*. National Center for Injury Prevention and Control, CDC; available at http://www.cdc.gov/nciplc/wisqars. Date accessed: April, 2007.
4. Cook PJ, Ludwig J. *Gun violence: the real costs*. New York: Oxford University Press; 2000.
5. Finkelstein EA, Corso PS, Miller TR, and associates. *Incidence and economic burden of injuries in the United States*. New York: Oxford University Press; 2006.
6. Lemaire J. The cost of firearm deaths in the United States: Reduced life expectancies and increased insurance costs. *J Risk Insur*. 2005;72(3):359–374.
7. Krug EG, Mercy JA, Dahlberg LL, et al. The world report on violence and health. *Lancet*. 2002;360(9339):1083–1088.
8. Cheney RA, Weiner NA, Seide MH, et al. A measurement framework for firearm research, intervention, and evaluation. *Conference Proceedings: National Meeting of the American Public Health Association*. Philadelphia: 2002.
9. Felson M. *Crime and everyday life: insights and implications for society*. Thousand Oaks: Pine Forge Press; 1994.
10. Felson M. Routine activities, social controls, rational decisions and criminal outcomes. In: Cornish D, Clarke RV, eds. *The reasoning criminal*. New York: Springer-Verlag New York; 1986;119–128.
11. Haddon W. On the escape of tigers: An ecologic note. *Am J Pub Health*. 1970;60:2229–2234.
12. Haddon W Jr. Options for the prevention of motor vehicle crash injury. *Isr J Med Sci*. 1980;16(1):45–65.
13. Runyan CW. Using the Haddon matrix: Introducing the third dimension. *Inj Prev*. 1998;4(4):302–307.
14. Susser M. *Causal thinking in the health sciences – concepts and strategies of epidemiology*. New York: Oxford University Press; 1973.
15. Kleinbaum DG, Kupper LL, Morgenstern H. *Epidemiologic research: principles and quantitative methods*. New York: Van Nostrand Reinhold; 1982.
16. Ford K. A hospital based violence prevention intervention reduced hospital recidivism for violent injury and arrests for violent crimes. *Evid Based Nurs*. 2007;10(2):50.
17. Weiner J, Wiebe DJ, Richmond TS, et al. Reducing firearm violence: A research agenda. *Inj Prev*. 2007;13(2):80–84.
18. Branas CC, Wiebe DJ, Schwab CW, et al. Getting past the "f" word in federally funded public health research. *Inj Prev*. 2005;11(3):191.

Gunshot Injury: Overview of Ballistics, Wounding, and Clinical Management Principles

8

Mark L. Gestring   *Brian James Gestring*

No injury is associated more strongly with the field of trauma surgery than the gunshot wound. Despite the fact that blunt trauma occurs more commonly than penetrating trauma, firearms represent a significant injury mechanism and remain a fact of life in the United States. More Americans have lost their lives to firearms since 1933 than the combined total of all American soldiers killed in every war they fought.[1] Despite this, firearm injury and fatality rates in the United States continue to increase.[2,3] According to recent Federal Bureau of Investigation (FBI) statistics, almost 30% of all violent crimes and close to 70% of all homicides in the United States involve firearms.[4] In addition, firearm injury is becoming a significant health problem for the nation's youth. A 75% increase in firearm deaths has been reported in the 15- to 19-year-old population over the last 2 decades,[5] and death by firearm has become the fifth leading cause of mortality in children younger than 14 years.[6] Furthermore, an increase in the overall severity of firearm injury has also been noted. In one study, the proportion of patients with two or more gunshot wounds increased from 26% in 1987 to 43% by 1990.[7] The widespread availability of firearms combined with improvements in weapon design and capacity have conspired in the development of this public health crisis.

Gunshot wounds are no longer unusual and their management is no longer restricted to the inner city, urban emergency room. A basic understanding of how firearms work, how tissue is injured, and how medical care is influenced by these principals is required to provide proper care for these patients. This chapter will provide an overview of the technical aspects of gunshot injury including basic ballistic theory, a review of factors contributing to firearm wound creation and, lastly, a review of proper legal procedure and evidence management.

BASIC BALLISTICS

Classically described, ballistics is the study of projectile motion. Currently, however, this term applies to both the study of projectile behavior as well as the physics of firearm design and function.[8] While there are many types of projectiles and firearms, the basic principles that govern their relationship remain remarkably constant. When treating patients with gunshot wounds, an understanding of the factors that determine and maintain this relationship can be very helpful.

The study of ballistics is best divided into three distinct components—internal, external, and terminal or wound ballistics. Internal ballistics is the study of projectile behavior within the firearm. Although this includes all aspects of projectile construction and design, the primary focus is on the internal workings of the firearm and the conversion of chemical energy in the form of propellant to kinetic energy (KE) in the form of projectile motion. External ballistics refers to the forces that act on a projectile during its flight to the target. Lastly, terminal or wound ballistics describes the interaction of target tissue with the projectile and the factors involved with wound creation. A complex topic can be simplified somewhat when each of these is discussed individually.

Internal Ballistics

Internal ballistics refers to the study of projectile motion and behavior within the weapon itself. The projectile, or bullet, is initially contained within a cartridge, which is inserted into the weapon for firing. Virtually all cartridges are similar in design, consisting of a shell casing that contains the other components necessary to fire the bullet. At the base of the cartridge, there is a very reactive chemical known as the *primer*. The firing pin from the weapon strikes the primer causing an explosion. This explosion ignites the less reactive propellant powder, which is housed in the shell casing and causes it to expand to fit the diameter of the barrel. The gases produced by the burning powder can only escape by forcing the bullet down the barrel (see Fig. 1). As the bullet accelerates through the barrel, it acquires spin from rifling, or spiral grooves, cut into the inner core of the barrel. Rifling increases the accuracy and velocity of the projectile in flight and imparts certain markings on the bullet that can later be used to identify the specific barrel that fired the bullet. Generally, a bullet will continue to increase its velocity as long as it remains within the barrel because of the contained gases propelling it in the closed space. Once the bullet leaves the barrel, the propulsive gases are quickly dissipated and the projectile is moving at its highest speed, referred to as its *muzzle velocity*. In addition to the bullet, hot gases and propellant powder in different states of thermal decomposition exit the barrel as a result of the process described in the preceding text (see Fig. 2). This is clinically relevant because these gases can cause burns to tissue known as *powder stippling*, which can be used to estimate firing distance. A burn found in conjunction with

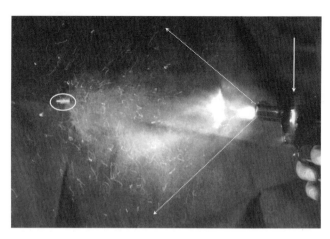

Figure 2   High-speed photograph of a revolver being fired. This picture illustrates the projectile in flight (circle), the inverted cone of residue propelled from the barrel toward the target, and the residue escaping from the space between the barrel and the cylinder (arrow). (Photo courtesy of Peter A. Pizzola, Ph.D, Kirby Matir, M.S., and Peter De Forest, D.Crim.)

a gunshot wound suggests close-range injury. Despite the intense heat associated with this process, bullets are not sterile and can be the source of clinical infection.[9,10]

Because the muzzle velocity of a projectile is ultimately determined by the amount of gunpowder propelling it, the weight of the projectile, and the length of the barrel through which it accelerates, velocity is an important characteristic used to classify firearm groups. Most handguns currently encountered are considered low-velocity weapons with muzzle velocities <2,000 ft per second. The classic high-velocity weapon, by comparison, is the rifle which has a longer barrel, a large propellant-rich cartridge, and muzzle velocities frequently in excess of the 2,000 ft per second range. Firearms can be further classified by caliber, which refers to the diameter of the bullet and can be designated in metric (mm) and standard (inches) units. This classification can be used to differentiate specific types of guns, but should not be used to predict injury patterns because there are many variables for each type of weapon.

Bullets can be composed solely of soft lead or lead covered by another, harder metal. This design modification is known as *jacketing* and is used for bullets fired from semiautomatic weapons to prevent the soft lead of un-jacketed rounds from jamming autoloading mechanisms. Jacketing also helps maintain the shape of the bullet and limits fragmentation when it reaches its target. It is possible for the jacketing to separate from its lead core on impact. The presence or absence of jacketing, as well as the extra missile that is created if the jacket separates, has significant implications on wound creation, which is discussed later in this chapter.

Once the bullet leaves the barrel, the spent cartridge must be removed to fire the next round. Depending on the type of firearm, the cartridge case is either retained in a cylinder for later removal or automatically ejected by the weapon

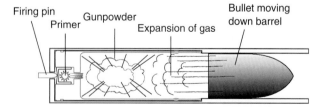

Figure 1   Diagrammatic representation of a cartridge being fired. (Illustration by Mark Schoemann, MD.)

Firing pin
Primer
Gunpowder
Expansion of gas
Bullet moving down barrel

as the next round is fired. Both the sides and the base of the shell casing may be used to associate it with a specific weapon, and fingerprints can sometimes be obtained from the shell casing itself.[11] For this reason, ejected cartridges are important forensic evidence and should be handled appropriately if they are encountered in the clinical setting.

External Ballistics

External ballistics refers to the study of projectile behavior while in flight. It includes those factors which impact forward motion and flight stability of the bullet. The concept of external ballistics, however, starts with an understanding of how the ballistic coefficient, or the ability of a bullet to overcome air resistance, affects its flight characteristics. This is based largely on the sectional density and shape of the projectile where pointed bullets encounter less air resistance than round ones. Most modern bullets have a pointed shape with the notable exception of shotgun pellets, which exhibit poor flight characteristics over longer distances.

The study of external ballistics is, in fact, the study of total KE transfer from the weapon to the target. Firearm designers have employed numerous modifications and enhancements to both weapons and bullets to increase the efficiency of this process and maximize transmission of KE to the final target. The main contributors to the final KE are velocity (V) and mass (M) of the projectile. This relationship is expressed by the formula KE $= \frac{1}{2}$ MV^2. Velocity is believed to be one of the major determining factors in predicting the effectiveness of a bullet; however, it is easier in practice to increase the mass of a projectile than to increase its velocity without major structural changes to the weapon. Because KE is measured in ft-lb and bullets are measured in grains of weight (7,000 grains in 1 lb), a conversion to mass must be performed using the formula M $=$ W/7,000 g. The resulting KE value provides an indication of the potential of the bullet for tissue destruction. The actual wounding potential, however, depends on additional factors, which will be discussed in further detail later in this chapter.

As described in the preceding text, rifling within the barrel of the firearm imparts a stabilizing spin on the bullet in its flight from the weapon. Without this spin, the path of the bullet would be far less predictable and tumbling as well as other aberrations may interfere with the motion of a bullet. A similar effect is observed when bullets are destabilized by striking intermediate targets. This often accounts for unusual trajectories and nontraditional entry wounds.

Terminal or Wound Ballistics

This aspect of ballistic study deals with wound creation and the interaction of the moving projectile with the target tissue. As described in the preceding text, potential tissue destruction is predicted by the relationship between velocity and mass. Actual tissue destruction, however, is dictated by projectile shape, projectile construction, and target tissue type.[12,13]

In general, an impact velocity of only 125 to 230 ft per second is required for a bullet or fragment to penetrate the skin.[14,15] A bullet causes tissue injury in three main ways. First, it directly crushes the tissue as it penetrates leading to what is referred to as the *permanent cavity*. The size of the permanent cavity is largely dependent on bullet size and design. Many modifications have been applied to bullets to allow deformation on impact with resultant larger permanent cavity formation in target tissue. Second, the bullet forces surrounding tissue outward away from the missile path as it penetrates. This tissue stretch is responsible for the temporary cavity,[16] which is a transient displacement of tissue, or a localized blunt trauma, caused by the cavitation of the passing projectile and is usually directly related to velocity. Elastic tissues such as bowel, lung, and muscle are relatively resistant to damage by stretch, whereas solid organs such as liver and brain are not.[17] The actual wound produced by a particular penetrating projectile is characterized by the amount and location of tissue crush and the degree of stretch. Although all bullets cause a permanent cavity when they penetrate tissue, the creation of a temporary cavity is usually limited to high-velocity weapons such as rifles. Stretch from temporary cavity tissue displacement can disrupt blood vessels or break bones at some distance from the projectile path; however, this phenomenon is also limited to wounds caused by high-velocity weapons. Fortunately, most wounds are created by handguns that usually cause injury by damaging tissue in the path of the permanent cavity. Cavitation and temporary cavity formation are generally not significant factors in wounds created by handguns.[18]

The third major factor in wound creation is fragmentation. This happens when the bullet separates or splits apart into smaller pieces on impact with the target tissue or, on occasion, before tissue penetration. This is common with soft lead bullets and can result in major tissue disruption. Each individual fragment of the bullet is capable of creating its own wound tract and increasing the overall destruction within the target tissue, resulting in a larger permanent channel. Fragmentation can be recognized on x-ray as debris, which is distributed widely along the bullet tract.[19] (see Fig. 3) A bullet striking bone may cause fragmentation of the bone as well as the bullet with subsequent formation of numerous secondary missiles, which are often more destructive than the primary missile and often take erratic and unpredictable courses (see Fig. 4).

Bullet wounds can be classified as low- or high-velocity wounds based on the criteria described in the preceding text. Low-velocity projectile wounds are generally considered to be less severe, more common in the civilian population, and typically attributed to projectiles with muzzle velocities <2,000 ft per second. While significant injuries and death can occur in this group, they are usually

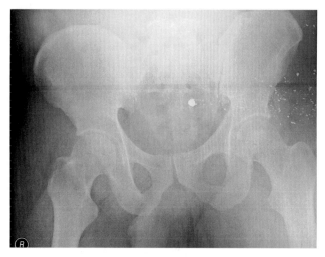

Figure 3 Pelvic radiograph of a high-velocity AR-15 wound to pelvis. Note the significant fragmentation, which delineates the bullet path on x-ray.

the result of direct bullet penetration and permanent cavity formation through specific tissues or vital structures. In an attempt to increase tissue destruction, however, various projectile modifications have been developed. The most common of these is the hollow-point, soft-tip, deforming bullet. This bullet is designed to flatten out on impact in order to create a larger wound tract and to transfer as much KE to the target as possible. Although there are many theoretic advantages to such a design, many factors interfere with the reliable expansion of these bullets.

Overall, tissue damage is usually more severe with high-velocity (>2,000 ft per second) military and hunting

weapons, where the effects of the temporary cavity described in the preceding text may be seen.[20,21] It is misleading, however, to assume that the severity of a gunshot wound is solely due to velocity.[22,23] As described earlier, many factors including bullet deformation, bullet fragmentation, and biologic characteristics of target tissues are responsible for the ultimate wounding capability of a weapon.

WEAPON TYPE

Most available firearms can be divided into three main groups—rifles, handguns, and shotguns. Rifles and handguns function similarly and share many behavioral properties, whereas shotguns vary in design and performance features and warrant separate discussion. All these weapon groups are commonly available and are capable of producing clinically significant wounds. Although not usually as severe, air gun injuries have been noted to be on the increase. Design modifications and enhancements have increased the ability of the air gun to cause injury, and it has become a weapon worthy of mention.

The Rifle

Rifles are consistently the most powerful of the three main weapon groups. To remain effective over long ranges, rifles have been designed to accommodate the increased chamber pressures that are associated with explosion of increased amounts of gunpowder contained in larger cartridges. In addition, the longer barrel allows increased acceleration of the bullet and accounts for the high velocities and increased amounts of KE that most rifles are capable of generating. A

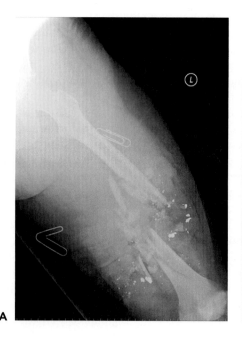

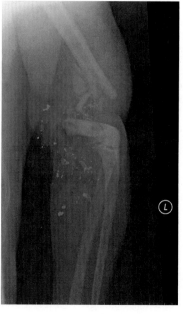

A   B

Figure 4 Radiograph of low-velocity gunshot wound with fracture and bullet fragmentation of lower extremity (**A**) and upper extremity (**B**). Note the significant debris field consisting of shattered bone and bullet fragments in each image. Paper clips may be used to mark skin wounds.

wide variety of rifles in many different calibers are currently available and in use.[24]

Rifles are usually divided into those used for military purposes and those used by civilians. One main difference is that military rifles may have a fully automatic mode that allows the operator to fire in three round bursts, continuously, or as long as the trigger is depressed. This feature is not available on civilian rifles. By convention, military weapons usually utilize full metal-jacketed bullets. The presence of a jacket permits greater velocity because unjacketed lead bullets cannot travel faster than 2,000 ft per second and ensures continued mechanical operation of the weapon.[25] This minimizes deformation and fragmentation of the bullet on impact and minimizes resultant tissue damage. Because this convention does not apply to civilian weapons, wounds inflicted using conventional ammunition may be more severe and more threatening than those sustained in military combat from bullets of comparable size and velocity.

With higher muzzle velocities, larger projectile masses, and greater total energy ratings, rifles are capable of causing massive injury. The most common cause of these injuries is related to hunting and recreational accidents. The overall size of most rifles makes them difficult weapons to conceal, and for this reason rifle injuries are not commonly seen as the result of criminal activity.

The Handgun

Although handguns are typically considered to be low-velocity weapons with most muzzle velocities <1,400 ft per second, they are the most frequently used firearms in fatal[26] and nonfatal[27] gunshot injuries. Handguns are the least powerful of the three main groups of weapons. They are difficult to aim effectively and tend to be harder to master than other types of weapons, with an average effective range of 25 yards or less for most shooters. Police and FBI department statistics show that most handgun shootings occur within 7 yards, and even at this close range, most shots miss. In a study of police shootouts, only 11% of assailant's bullets and 25% of bullets fired by police officers hit their intended target.[28]

Most handguns currently in use have barrels ranging in length from 1.5 to 6 in. Shorter barrel length translates to lower velocity, lower total KE, and decreased accuracy. Despite this, handguns are more commonly used in crimes because they are cheaper, lighter, easier to handle and, most importantly, easier to conceal.

Handguns can be classified into two main categories based on whether the weapon is considered to be a semi–automatic or a revolver. Revolvers have a cylinder which usually holds five or six cartridges. The bullets are fired by individual pulls on the trigger, and cartridge removal and reload are required to continue firing. Semi-automatic pistols, in contrast, utilize a replaceable magazine, which contains preloaded cartridges aligned along a mechanism that feeds them into the weapon automatically each time the gun is fired. Once the weapon is loaded it can be fired over and over until the magazine is empty. Older model weapons held five to seven cartridges in the magazine but newer models can hold significantly more rounds of ammunition. In addition, the process of switching magazines allows reloading to be completed very quickly.

Historically, most handgun injuries treated in urban emergency settings were of the small-caliber, low-velocity type.[29] As weapon technology improved, however, more powerful handguns with increased firing capacity were found to be responsible for an increase in on-scene shooting deaths[30] as well as an increase in complex wounds seen in urban trauma centers.[31] An analysis done in Washington DC showed that almost 60% of confiscated weapons in 1999 were semiautomatic handguns. This represented a significant change when compared to the 1970s and 1980s when smaller-caliber, revolver-style handguns represented most weapons confiscated.[32] This trend was also recognized in the midwest, where handguns accounted for 89% of firearm homicides and 71% of firearm suicides. Notably, a shift toward the use of larger-caliber, semiautomatic handguns during the study period was recognized.[33] Yet another analysis reported a steady increase in the size of bullets removed at surgery or autopsy over a 16-year period ending in 1997.[34]

The Shotgun

Shotguns are powerful weapons at close range, and they are commonly available because of their widespread appeal to the recreational user. Shotguns are smooth bore, long-barreled weapons that differ significantly from rifles or handguns in terms of ballistic performance and wounding potential.[35] Shotgun terminology also differs from conventional weapons. Instead of using caliber to indicate the barrel diameter, shotguns use the term *gauge*. Smaller gauge designations indicate larger barrels.[36] Instead of the single projectiles commonly fired by rifles and handguns, shotguns fire cartridges, or shells, loaded with pellets of varying size and number. The type of load varies widely and can range from many small pellets to a single, large shotgun slug.[37] Usually, the total weight of lead pellets in a shotgun shell remains the same regardless of pellet size. A shell with double 00 buckshot, for instance, would hold nine pellets for a total weight of 1 oz, whereas a shell with number 8 birdshot would hold 410 pellets for a total weight of 1 oz. The shotgun shell differs in its design and construction from the previously described conventional cartridge. The standard shotgun shell consists of a plastic body atop a brass head, containing primer, wadding, powder charge, and shot charge (see Fig. 5). The wadding acts to keep the pellets of the shot load together and allows all the pellets to move down the barrel together when fired. At ranges of <6 m, the wadding or shot charge components may be propelled into the

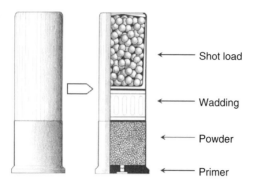

Figure 5 Cross-sectional representation of a conventional shotgun shell. The shot load varies from many small pellets to a single large slug, depending on shell type. The area of the shell that contains the shot, however, remains constant so that the number of pellets decreases as their size increases. (Illustration by Ludovit Gondkovsky.)

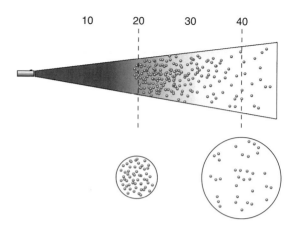

Figure 6 Diagrammatic representation of the effect of distance on shotgun pellet spread. At close distances, the pellet concentration is high and the spread is narrow. Significant injury is possible at close range. At further distances, pellet concentration is less dense and the spread is significantly wider. The pellets contain less energy and cause less injury as the distance from the weapon increases. (Illustration by Mark Schoemann, MD.)

wound.[38] The presence of wadding material in a wound provides strong presumptive evidence that the range was <2 m.[39] These components are frequently not apparent radiographically and may be overlooked if a high index of suspicion is not maintained when treating shotgun injuries. For this reason, an aggressive search for these components should be undertaken in the operating room (OR) at the time of exploration. A high degree of wound contamination has been reported when the wadding is found to penetrate tissue.[40,41] As the firing distance increases, the wadding may also produce another injury in a different location than the original wound. This injury may only be superficial when compared to the main injury, but should be documented if observed. This information is important in the determination of firing distance and may be overlooked because it is rarely as impressive as the principal wound.

Range is critical to the understanding of shotgun ballistics. At close range, all the pellets essentially act as one mass, and a typical shell would give the mass of pellets a muzzle velocity of approximately 1,300 ft per second and a KE of 2,100 ft-lb.[42] If the energy is divided between the pellets, it becomes apparent that fewer, larger pellets can carry more KE, but the spread may carry them away from the target. Pellets, in general, are poor projectiles due to their spherical shape and most small pellets are unable to penetrate skin at increased distances. For this reason, close-range wounds are usually severe, but wounding is decreased with distance as pellets scatter and slow in flight (see Fig. 6). The ability of the shotgun to disperse its pellets accounts for its unique wounding characteristics. At close range, the pellets stay together and act as one mass delivering significant KE to the target tissue resulting in massive wounds. When firing 00 buckshot with nine pellets in the load, for example, the total energy of 2,000 ft-lb is divided among the pellets for an individual KE of approximately 200 ft-lb per pellet. With 280 pellets in a load of number 6 birdshot, however, the energy averages

out to 7.21 ft-lb per pellet.[43] As the individual pellets spread out and travel through the air, they continually lose KE. After traveling approximately 80 yards, most pellets will not penetrate skin. Most pellets will lose all their energy and hit the ground within 200 yards. By comparison, many rifle bullets can travel 3,000 to 5,000 yards before losing their energy.[44] The same design that gives shotgun pellets a very poor ballistic coefficient and large retardation effect insures their ability to destroy huge quantities of tissue at close range. Because human tissue is 800 times denser than air, these pellets will decelerate even quicker in the body releasing all their energy to the target. Even point blank shots rarely form exit wounds.

One important exception to the ballistic pattern described in the preceding text, however, is the shotgun slug. This is a large, single projectile that is used by hunters predominantly for larger animals. They are more accurate over longer distances than pellet-style loads and produce very high KE values due to their large size and high muzzle velocities. These are formidable weapons capable of creating devastating injuries at ranges further than the conventional shotgun load.[45]

The Air Gun

Air guns can fire either small round balls known as *ball bearings* (BBs) or formed lead pellets. These pellets can range in size from the most popular .177 to .25 calibers. Either projectile can achieve muzzle velocities between 200 and 900 ft per second. Although usually considered low energy and relatively safe for children to use, they are capable of causing severe injury. The projectiles have been reported to penetrate to a depth of 25 mm at a range of 1 m and up to 15 mm at a range of 5 m.[46] Newer designs allow the user to increase the air pressure within the weapon with external pumping mechanisms, thereby increasing the velocity of the projectile. Because air guns are not considered firearms in the traditional sense, they are not usually included in gun regulations. Despite this, both homicides and suicides have been reported with this weapon and airguns should not be underestimated.[47,48]

Technical Considerations in Gunshot Wound Management

Certain aspects of clinical management are unique to those patients who have sustained gunshot trauma. Although the overall care of specific injuries is discussed in great detail throughout this text, some general principles regarding practical considerations deserve special attention.

Trajectory Determination

The clinical approach to the patient with a gunshot injury should include an attempt to elicit the trajectory of the bullet or bullets whenever possible. Trajectory refers to the actual path taken by the bullet through tissue. In a practical sense, this can be affected by many factors including a patient's position at the time of being shot, as well as involvement of intermediate targets such as windows, doors, or belt buckles which are all capable of altering the path of a missile.

The actual determination of trajectory can be accomplished quickly in most cases and begins with a complete and accurate physical inspection supplemented by selected radiographs as indicated. It is imperative that every portion of the patient be examined to avoid missing an injury. This includes underarms, between buttocks, and between skin folds. A complete inventory of wounds is required before an attempt at trajectory determination can be effectively undertaken. Once identified, all external wounds should be marked with metal before performing radiographs to allow for identification of the wounds on x-ray. Paper clips with tape make cheap and easily available markers, but any radiopaque marker will suffice. Care must be taken to include the entire area of interest on the radiograph to avoid missing a projectile. In larger patients, it may be necessary to make several attempts to complete the series. The goal is to identify all external wounds and internal projectiles. The number of wounds plus the number of bullets should equal an even number. If this is not the case, examination should be repeated to be sure no external injury was missed. Once the projectiles are located on anterior-posterior (AP) views, a directed lateral view can be helpful in pinpointing the location of the bullet (see Fig. 7). Ultimately, injuries will be anticipated on the basis of the suspected trajectory and a preliminary therapeutic plan will be based on this early information. Although most cases lend themselves well to such an analysis, trajectory determination may be very challenging in some instances. It will sometimes be necessary to reevaluate wounds or redirect radiographs to obtain the desired information. The determination of trajectory, however, should not delay the care of the unstable patient and indicated surgical intervention should never be delayed in these cases.

Documentation of Gunshot Wounds

Typical entrance wounds are generally round in shape with a circumferential margin of abrasion surrounding

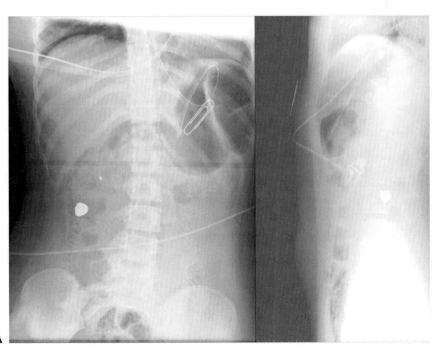

Figure 7 Anterior-posterior (AP) **(A)** and lateral **(B)** radiographs of a patient with single, low-velocity gunshot wound to left upper quadrant. The entrance is marked with a paperclip, which is visible on both images. It is evident from these two simple studies that this bullet crossed the midline and traveled from front to back. It is also apparent that the chest is likely not involved. These studies are performed quickly on patient arrival and do not delay transport of this patient to the operating room. The information obtained is useful in predicting potential injuries based on the bullet trajectory. **A**

B

the defect produced by the bullet. This abrasion ring is a scraping or scuffing of the skin caused by the bullet as it pushes inward. This abrasion ring may be concentric or eccentric based on many factors present at the time of injury. Atypical entrance wounds are commonly seen and generally result from ricochets or the passage of a bullet through an intermediate target such as a window or a door. Exit wounds, by comparison, can assume many shapes and sizes. In general, the main difference between entrance and exit wounds is the absence of the abrasion ring from the exit wounds.[49]

More important, however, is the realization that most clinicians *lack* the proper training and experience to differentiate entrance from exit wounds and should refrain from doing so to avoid confusion and potential conflict during later legal proceedings. Previous reports have documented that clinical charts routinely lack adequate descriptions of gunshot wounds[50,51] and that clinicians were shown to mistake entrance and exit wounds in up to 50% of cases.[52] In cases of gunshot injury, clinicians would be well advised to refrain from identifying any wound as an entrance or an exit and instead simply record the location, size, and shape of the wound in the medical record. Similarly, it is usually not possible to determine the caliber of the bullet from the size of the wound.

Evidence Management and Medicolegal Considerations

Bullets recovered at surgery or during nonoperative patient care represent important evidence and should be treated as such. If potential evidence is mishandled, whether by the surgeon, the nurse, the OR technician, or the investigators assigned to the case, it diminishes the likelihood of that material being of value during any subsequent trial. Most institutions have a formal protocol in place to handle evidence recovered during patient care. Whatever the procedure, it is imperative that the chain of custody be maintained and that each person with access to the evidence is accounted for.

Any bullet or fragment extracted from the body should be handled carefully and without the use of instruments that may scratch or otherwise alter the markings found on the projectile. Each bullet or fragment recovered should be placed directly in a clear plastic container and sealed with tape or a patient-identity sticker. This container should then be placed in a plastic bag with the patient's name, time, and date of recovery and the name of the person who recovered the evidence clearly noted. It is important not to mark the actual bullet in any way to avoid altering potentially important markings. Once the evidence is sealed and labeled, it should be secured until it can be turned over to law enforcement. It is important that the record reflect the name of each person who had custody of the material and the date and time that it was turned over to the investigating authority.

It is not always possible for clinicians to identify a specific bullet type with accuracy; therefore, it is best to refrain from speculating on bullet type and, instead, document general size, shape, color, and any unusual or distinguishing characteristic on the recovery record. In addition, there will be occasions where other foreign debris will be found within the wound. This could provide additional important evidence and should be treated in the manner described earlier. These precautions will ensure that there will be no dispute regarding admissibility of evidence when the matter comes to trial.

In addition to bullets, clothing worn at the time of injury and personal property such as cell phones and pagers should be treated as evidence and a chain of custody should be established and preserved as previously described. Whenever possible, care should be taken to avoid cutting through suspected bullet holes when clothing is removed. Blood-soaked clothing should be allowed to dry before packaging and should never be packaged in plastic. Clothing items should be packaged individually and should be handled minimally to preserve potential gunshot residue and other trace evidence. If a weapon is encountered, extreme care should be taken until the weapon is secured by law enforcement. All such weapons should be considered fully loaded. In addition to the risks inherent to such a discovery, care should be taken to avoid touching the weapon in an effort to avoid disruption of important forensic data such as fingerprints or evidence of recent use.

CONCLUSION

The appropriate care of gunshot injury requires expertise beyond the conventional boundaries of standard medical training. An appreciation for the many aspects of management must include a rudimentary understanding of firearm function and the factors that are responsible for wound creation. In addition, an appreciation of the medicolegal issues which frequently surround these injuries is necessary to avoid making or documenting statements that may prove to be incorrect.

It is important to recognize that the proper management of potential evidence often begins at the gunshot victim's bedside. Although evidence processing is not the clinical team's first priority, the importance of proper evidence collection and preservation procedures cannot be overstated. The successful prosecution of those who would use firearms for criminal purposes is a worthwhile objective for clinicians committed to breaking the cycle of violence and preventing future, similar injuries.

REFERENCES

1. Schwab CW, Frykberg ER, Bloom T, et al. Violence in America: A public health crisis – the role of Firearms. *J Trauma*. 1995;38: 163–168.

2. Centers for Disease Control and Prevention. Deaths resulting from firearm and motor vehicle-related injuries. United States 1968–1991. *MMWR Morb Mortal Wkly Rep*. 1994;43:37.

3. Fingerhut LA, Jones C, Makuo D. Firearm and motor vehicle injury mortality – variation by state and race and ethnicity: United States, 1990–1991. *Vital and Health Statistics*, No. 242, National Center for Health Statistics; 1994.

4. Department of Justice- Federal Bureau of Investigation. *Crime in the United States 2005*, September 2006.

5. Christoffel KK. Pediatric firearm injuries: Time to target a growing population. *Pediatr Ann*. 1992;21:430.

6. Schetky DH. Children and handguns: A public health concern. *Am J Dis Child*. 1985;139:229.

7. Zawitz MW. *Firearm injury from crime and criminal justice*. United States Department of Justice Programs, Bureau of Justice Statistics; NCJ-160093, 1996.

8. Barach E, Tomlanovich M, Nowak R. Ballistics: A pathophysiologic examination of the wounding mechanisms of firearms: Part 1. *J Trauma*. 1986;26:225–235.

9. Tzeng S, Swan KG, Rush BF. Bullets: A source of infection? *Am Surg*. 1982;48:239–240.

10. Wolf AW, Benson DR, Shoji H, et al. Autosterilization in low-velocity bullets. *J Trauma*. 1978;18:63.

11. Given BW. Latent fingerprints on cartridges and expended cartridge casings. *J Forensic Sci*. 1976;21:587–594.

12. Fackler ML. Gunshot wound review. *Ann Emerg Med*. 1996;28:194–203.

13. Santucci RA, Chang Y. Ballistics for physicians: Myths about wound ballistics and gunshot injuries. *J Urol*. 2004;171:1408–1414.

14. DiMaio VJ, Copeland AR, Besant-Matthews PE, et al. Minimal velocities necessary for perforation of skin by air guns and bullets. *J Forensic Sci*. 1982;27:894–898.

15. Hopkinson DW, Marshall TK. Firearm injuries. *Br J Surg*. 1967;54:344–353.

16. Fackler ML. Wound Ballistics: A review of common misconceptions. *JAMA*. 1988;259:2730–2736.

17. Fackler ML, Surinchak JS, Malinowski JA, et al. Wounding potential of the Russian AK-74 assault rifle. *J Trauma*. 1984;24:263–256.

18. Ragsdale BD. Gunshot wounds: A historical perspective. *Mil Med*. 1984;149:301–315.

19. Fackler ML, Surinchak MA, Malinowski JA, et al. Bullet Fragmentation: A major cause of tissue disruption. *J Trauma*. 1984;24:35–39.

20. Brettler D, Sedlin ED, Mendes DG. Conservative treatment of low velocity gunshot wounds. *Clin Orthop*. 1979;140:26–31.

21. Mendelson JA. The relationship between mechanisms of wounding and principles of treatment of missile wounds. *J Trauma*. 1991;31:1181–1202.

22. Fackler ML. Ballistic injury. *Ann Emerg Med*. 1986;15:1451–1455.

23. Fackler ML. Wound ballistics and soft-tissue wound treatment. *Tech Orthop*. 1995;10:163–170.

24. Barach E, Tomlanovich M, Nowak R. Ballistics: A pathophysiologic examination of the wounding mechanisms of firearms: Part II. *J Trauma*. 1986;26:374–383.

25. Hollermann JJ, Fackler ML, Coldwell DM, et al. Gunshot wounds: Bullets, ballistics and mechanisms of injury. *AJR Am J Roentgenol*. 1990;155:685–690.

26. Zawitz MW. *Guns used in crime: Firearms, crime and criminal justice*. United States Department of Justice Programs, Bureau of Justice Statistics; NCJ-148201, 1995.

27. Gotsch KE, Annest JL, Mercy JA, et al. Surveillance for fatal and non-fatal firearm related injuries: United States, 1993–1998. *MMWR Morb Mortal Wkly Rep*. 2001;50:1–31.

28. Lesce T. Gunfighting tactics. *Survival Guide*. 1984;6:28–31.

29. Marcus NA, Blair WF, Shuck JM, et al. Low-velocity gunshot wounds to the extremities. *J Trauma*. 1980;20:1061–1064.

30. McGonigal MD, Cole J, Schwab CW, et al. Urban firearm deaths: A 5-year perspective. *J Trauma*. 1993;35:532–537.

31. Wintemute GJ. The relationship between firearm design and firearm violence: Handguns in the 1990's. *JAMA*. 1996;275:1749–1753.

32. Simpson BM, Grant RE. A synopsis of urban firearm ballistics: Washington, DC Model. *Clin Orthop Related Res*. 2003;408:12–16.

33. Hargarten SW, Karlson TA, O'Brien M, et al. Characteristics of firearms involved in fatalities. *JAMA*. 1996;275:42–45.

34. Caruso RP, Jara DI, Swan KG. Gunshot wounds: Bullet caliber is increasing. *J Trauma*. 1999;46:462–465.

35. Rybeck B, Janzon B. Absorption of missile energy in soft tissue. *Acta Chir Scand*. 1976;142:201–207.

36. Demuth WE. The mechanism of shotgun wounds. *J Trauma*. 1971;11:219–229.

37. Amato JJ, Billy LJ, Lawson NS, et al. High velocity missile injury. An experimental study of the retentive forces of tissue. *Am J Surg*. 1974;127:454–459.

38. Ordog GJ, Wasserberger J, Balasubramanian S. Shotgun wound ballistics. *J Trauma*. 1988;28:624.

39. Shepard GH. High-energy, low-velocity close-range shotgun wounds. *J Trauma*. 1980;20:1065.

40. Hoekstra SM, Bender JS, Levinson MA. The management of large soft tissue defects following close range shotgun injury. *J Trauma*. 1990;30:1489–1493.

41. Patzakis MJ, Harvey JP, Ivler D. The role of antibiotics in the management of open fractures. *J Bone Joint Surg*. 1974;56A:532–541.

42. Demuth WE, Nicholas GG, Munger BL. Buckshot Wounds. *J Trauma*. 1976;18:53–57.

43. Wilson J. Shotgun injuries and shotgun ballistics. *West J Med*. 1978;129:149–155.

44. Sights WP. Ballistic analysis of shotgun injuries to the central nervous system. *J Neurosurg*. 1969;31:25–33.

45. Gestring ML, Geller ER, Akkad N, et al. Shotgun slug injuries: Case report and literature review. *J Trauma*. 1996;40:650–653.

46. Grocock C, McCarthy R, Williams DJ. Ball Bearing (BB) guns, ease of purchase and potential for significant injury. *Ann R Coll Surg Engl*. 2006;88:402–404.

47. Cohle SD, Pickelman J, Connolly JT, et al. Suicide by air rifle and shotgun. *J Forensic Sci*. 1987;32:1113–1117.

48. DiMaio VJ. Homocidal death by air rifle. *J Trauma*. 1975;15:1034.

49. Denton JS, Segovia A, Filkins JA. Practical pathology of gunshot wounds. *Arch Pathol Lab Med*. 2006;130:1283–1289.

50. Fackler ML, Riddick L. Clinician's inadequate descriptions of gunshot wounds obstruct justice. *Wound Ballistics Rev*. 1996;2:40–43.

51. Shuman M, Wright RK. Evaluation of accuracy in describing gunshot wound injuries. *Proc Am Acad Forens Sci*. 1998;4:159–160.

52. Collins KA, Lantz PE. Interpretation of fatal, multiple and exiting gunshot wounds by trauma specialists. *J Forensic Sci*. 1994;34:94–99.

Drugs, Alcohol, and Injury Prevention

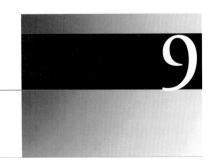

Jeffrey D. Kerby *Andrea T. Underhill* *Phillip Jeffrey Froster, Jr.*

In the United States currently, motor vehicle crashes involving alcohol result in a nonfatal injury requiring medical intervention every 2 minutes and in a death every 31 minutes.[1] As recently as 2005, a total of 16,885 people died in alcohol-related motor vehicle crashes. This figure accounts for approximately 40% of all traffic-related deaths for that year. An additional 254,000 people sustained varying nonfatal injuries, many of which resulted in catastrophic, life-long disabilities. Other drugs, generally in combination with alcohol, are involved in approximately 20% of all motor vehicle driver deaths.[2] In addition, 30% of those killed in motorcycle crashes have a blood alcohol content (BAC) over the legal limit.[1] Clearly, alcohol plays a major role in contributing to the number and severity of injuries seen in trauma centers each year.

For the purposes of this chapter, we use the commonly referred to definition of problem drinkers as persons at risk for developing alcohol-related problems, particularly being injured, as a result of their drinking. This chapter also provides a historic perspective of Screening and Brief Interventions (SBI), some information about its theoretical underpinnings, evidence supporting its effectiveness and guidance for its practical application in trauma centers, including potential obstacles to its effective implementation. Although the focus will be on those who are defined as problem drinkers, the information can be generalized to virtually all substance abusers.

RELEVANCE TO TRAUMA CENTERS

Injuries are the single greatest killer of Americans between 1 and 44 years of age and the fifth overall leading killer for all age-groups combined.[4] As described by Gentilello "alcohol and other drug (AOD) use disorders are the leading risk factors for injury."[5] Therefore, it is the importance of the cause–effect relationship between alcohol and injury that has stimulated interest in developing mechanisms to promote a change in behavior to prevent further injury.

Alcohol is a drug. Unlike many other abused drugs, its naturally occurring state is that of a liquid. It is unique because it requires no digestion, is quickly absorbed unchanged into circulation, is water and lipid soluble, and is therefore rapidly transported to and concentrated in the brain and central nervous system (CNS). It has the capacity to shorten the attention span, slow reaction time, interfere with performance of motor tasks and impair reasoning ability. Inebriated drivers often develop impaired perceptions that can lead to speeding, reckless driving, and failure to wear safety belts. This constellation of potentially lethal motor and cognitive consequences has resulted in a public health problem of monumental proportions.[6]

Recent studies have shown that 40% of patients admitted to trauma centers are BAC positive on admission.[7] In 2005, 85% of those with a positive BAC met the legal definition for intoxication or impairment[1] and studies have shown a mean BAC in those patients as nearly twice the legal limit.[8-11] Forty percent of motor vehicle passenger crash deaths involve alcohol and the same 40% figure is reported among pedestrians who die after being struck by a vehicle. Alcohol is also commonly associated with intentional violent injuries.[5] These alarming statistics illustrate, albeit rather simplistically, the public health importance of this problem.

Excessive alcohol consumption is the third leading cause of preventable death in the United States.[12] In the United States each year, more than half of the estimated 80,000 alcohol attributable deaths are due to intentional and unintentional injuries.[6] Moreover, in addition to the direct lethal effects, alcohol contributes significantly to trauma-related morbidity, years of productive life lost, and breathtaking costs.[6,13]

In the United States in the year 2000, the annual economic burden attributed to alcohol-related crashes was $51 billion.[14] Alcohol intoxication increases treatment costs by complicating the clinical examination and even obscuring signs of injury, which often results in the need for unnecessary additional diagnostic testing. Additionally, intensive resources are sometimes required for alcohol-positive patients who are uncooperative or who have severely altered mental status due to their level of intoxication. Alcohol-positive patients tend to have more severe injuries that require longer lengths of stay.[15] Further, patients with chronic alcohol use who develop alcohol withdrawal syndromes (AWS) during their hospitalizations have been shown to have more prolonged and costly hospitalizations.[16]

TRAUMA RECIDIVISM

There is a known high incidence of recurrent injuries in patients who screen positive for alcohol following trauma.[17–19] One frequently cited study shows that patients who are injured while intoxicated are two-and-a-half times more likely to be readmitted for an injury over a 2-year period than patients who were not intoxicated when injured.[18] The frequency of recidivism in this population has led to the suggestion that it causes an additional fourth peak of mortality beyond the established trimodal distribution of mortality after trauma.[20,21]

Although several studies note the incidence of patients returning again to their centers with traumatic injuries, this underestimates the problem. There are other patients who die from subsequent injuries without being treated. One large study from Baltimore followed up all trauma patients discharged alive for subsequent mortality. Of the 29,354 patients followed up, those who were toxicology positive during their initial trauma center admission were nearly twice as likely to die as a consequence of injury compared to the toxicology-negative group (1.9% vs. 1.0%). Of those who died in the period of follow-up, toxicology-positive patients were more than twice as likely to have died from injury (34.7% vs. 15.4%).[19]

Clearly, recidivism is a costly cycle affecting the injured party, the hospital, and society as a whole. The patient's self-destructive behavior frequently results in the injury or death of themselves and/or others. Therefore, reducing this costly cycle of alcohol-driven injury recidivism will save trauma care facilities and society millions of dollars while helping

to reduce alcohol-related morbidity and mortality. Given the high incidence of alcohol-related injuries requiring admission to trauma centers and the high rate of recidivism among problem drinkers, it is imperative that health care providers take advantage of the teachable moment provided by the treatment of a problem drinker following injury.

RECOMMENDED ACTION AND EVIDENCE SUPPORTING IT

In January 2006, the American College of Surgeons Committee on Trauma (ACS-COT) added requirements for trauma center verification to include the need for a focused program to identify and provide an intervention for problem alcohol users as part of routine trauma care.[15] Level I centers are now required to establish a program to both screen and provide an intervention, whereas Level II centers will be required to screen patients. The addition of this requirement has evolved over time as leaders in the trauma community have elevated the issue of alcohol and trauma and painstakingly detailed its impact on the incidence, outcome, and cost to trauma centers and to society as a whole.

A large portion of patients who are harmed secondary to alcohol use are not, by standard definition, true alcoholics.[11] While dependent use may provide for more potential exposure to traumatic situations over time, the largest segment of the population and the great majority of patients sustaining alcohol-related injuries drink excessively only on occasion and would not be classified as truly dependent drinkers. This is largely the rationale behind a 1990 Institute of Medicine (IOM) report titled *Broadening the Base of Treatment for Alcohol Problems.*[22] This report recommended expansion of the existing focus on patients with severe dependence to include patients with less severe problems who put themselves and others at risk by the nature of their drinking patterns. The report also called on medical specialties outside of those focused on drug addiction to share the responsibility of addressing those with alcohol problems. Given the large number of patients with alcohol problems that the trauma community cares for every day, it seems intuitive that we should become a cornerstone of that base identified in the IOM report. The report also recommended that those with nondependent alcohol problems receive brief on-site counseling, whereas those with true alcohol dependence should be referred for more intensive treatment.

A great deal of experimental effort has been put forth by those in the trauma community to validate SBI as a simple, yet effective approach to the problem. Given that SBI is now a mandated requirement for Level 1 trauma center verification,[15] early workers such as Gentilello and a number of his contemporaries are, at long-last, being acknowledged for their vision and efforts to validate its theoretic underpinnings and encourage its nationwide implementation based on a substantial body of supportive evidence.[23-43]

For example, in 1993 Bien et al. reviewed 32 international brief intervention (BI) trials and concluded that BI was more effective than no counseling and often just as effective as more extensive interventions.[44] In 1997, Wilk et al. described a dozen randomly controlled BI trials and determined that they were nearly twice as effective as no intervention, demonstrating an odds ratio of 1.9.[45] In 1999, Gentilello reported that BIs with injured patients reduced the risk of future injuries by 47%.[27]

In 2001, the Centers for Disease Control and Prevention (CDC) convened a conference focusing on the identification and intervention of alcohol-related problems in patients in the emergency department (ED). Participant contributors included scientists, practitioners, and a variety of additional stakeholders from around the country. They evaluated and assessed the current knowledge about alcohol problems among patients in the ED and the effectiveness of ED-based screening and intervention methods. Eventually, conference organizers produced a list of recommendations to enhance research and clinical practice in hospital EDs and provided impetus and direction for attacking the problem.[46]

One year later, D'Onofrio and Degutis[47] published their findings from a systematic meta-analysis launched to evaluate the strength of the recommendations for SBI for alcohol-related problems in the ED setting. Their methodology consisted of multiple Medline searches coupled with a comprehensive review of the Cochrane Collaboration Library. They identified and reviewed 27 new articles in addition to 14 primary articles appearing in an earlier *US Preventive Services Task Force Report*.[48] Their final SBI meta-analysis consisted of 39 reports. These included 30 randomized controlled and 9 cohort studies, of which 32 demonstrated a positive SBI effect. This led to their published recommendation that SBI be incorporated into clinical practice for alcohol-related problems in hospital EDs. In 2003, Burke et al. confirmed earlier reports by other workers that BIs were effective in reducing alcohol consumption and alcohol-related problems in various settings including hospital EDs.[49]

In 2004, Dinh-Zarr et al. reported another systematic review of the alcohol intervention effectiveness literature focused on problem drinkers.[50] Their effort represented an important departure because prior SBI evaluations had attempted to measure the effects of the intervention on alcohol consumption, maintenance of abstinence and reduction of ED recidivism. Still other trials attempted to evaluate the effects of interventions on a variety of negative consequences linked directly or indirectly to drinking such as hospitalizations, rehospitalizations, and social or occupational maladjustment. This exhaustive study yielded the following conclusions: (i) interventions for problem drinking are likely to reduce the incidence of injuries and their antecedents, but current data are insufficient

to draw firm conclusions, particularly in terms of effects on violent injuries; and, (ii) interventions for problem drinking appear to have beneficial effects on injury risk, but this benefit does not necessarily correlate with the effect of the intervention on abstinence, alcohol consumption, or drinking-related hazardous behavior. Therefore, one may reasonably conclude that a key finding of the Dinh-Zarr et al. review was that the trials they studied reported imprecise effect estimates, and often had methodological weaknesses, underscoring the requirement for further research.

The CDC organized a second conference in May 2003, which focused on trauma surgery and trauma centers titled *Alcohol Problems Among Hospitalized Trauma Patients: Controlling Complications, Mortality, and Trauma Recidivism*.[51] Participants in this conference included clinicians and researchers from emergency medicine and trauma surgery, psychiatrists, psychologists, alcohol researchers, epidemiologists, policy advocates, and representatives from federal and state agencies focused on alcohol research and substance treatment efforts.[52] The result of this two-and-a-half day conference was a list of seven recommendations.[52] The most immediate impact on trauma centers from this conference was the eventual change in the ACS-COT's *Resources for Optimal Care of the Injured Patient* as noted in the preceding text. The Steering Committee for the conference endorsed recommendations to disseminate the evidence in support of SBI to the trauma community, to fund implementation research involving the trauma community, to change insurance regulations to prevent denial of medical expense coverage for those patients found to be intoxicated, and to reimburse trauma center staff for SBI for substance abuse disorders.

THEORETIC BASIS FOR SCREENING AND BRIEF INTERVENTIONS

Although operating in friendly waters it is warranted to identify and review behavioral theories supporting the BI concept. Doing so is important for a variety of reasons, not the least of which is that BIs have been viewed with a measure of skepticism by some rather highly regarded behavioralists.[53] Because we are aware of legitimate skeptics, failure to acknowledge them and their reasons for their skepticism would be intellectually dishonest.

For example, Roche and Freeman[54] wrote a compelling article examining characteristics of brief interventions and the personnel responsible for conducting them. In it, they explored reasons for the apparent failure of BIs to move from efficacy to effectiveness. In fairness, Roche and Freeman demonstrated quite clearly that they were well acquainted with a substantial body of evidence supporting the efficacy of BIs, most notably for alcohol and tobacco. Nonetheless, they describe how, in their opinion, much of this evidence has been used to encourage a variety of physicians to use BIs, especially in hospital EDs. Therefore, it was to them (and to us) of more than casual interest that they found that internationally, SBI or similar secondary prevention efforts have largely failed. Yet, because they are objective scientists operating without a preconceived notion regarding the efficacy of SBI, they do not dismiss BIs as being without promise. In fact, they speak to the *possible effectiveness of BIs*, qualifying their conclusions by underscoring the *"prevention potential* that rests with brief interventions." But they add the caveat that there are crucial questions remaining unasked such as "why frontline workers have failed to embrace these proven interventions?" Another question is whether BI advocates have identified "the right vehicle but the wrong driver" which really asks whether BIs might prove more effective if they were conducted by trauma center personnel other than physicians. Elsewhere in this chapter we address obstacles and barriers to successfully implementing SBI practices resulting from professional skepticism, apathy, and institutional inertia. Briefly, a common obstacle to screening is a widely held perception that attempts at intervention are ineffective.[26] Furthermore, research has found that only 55% of 2,500 randomly selected ED physicians reported believing that psychologists and psychiatrists were even capable of addressing alcohol problems effectively. As if this was not discouraging enough, their reported perception of alcohol treatment efficacy provided by other staff physicians and surgeons was only 23%.[55]

Although not abundant, other critics of BIs were readily identified as we sought to assure that information presented herein was objective and unbiased. We concluded that although they appear to be in the minority among behavioral scientists and practitioners who specialize in substance abuse, the positions of BI critics must be thoughtfully considered. Our assessment of their research is that it was generally well done; that their conclusions and explanations for reaching them were entirely reasonable and the critiques, options, and alternatives they offered were invariably constructive.

These few but compelling examples from the literature reflect a measure of entrenched skepticism coupled with a lack of current awareness regarding progress that has been made in alcohol treatment. In fact, based on the literature we reviewed and Gentilello's own conclusions, pervasive skepticism appears closer to "the rule rather than the exception" among large numbers of ED physicians, surgeons, and allied health personnel.[26,55,56]

The *coefficient of skepticism* is not as robust among all clinical observers. For example, as reported by Blow et al., the efficacy of SBIs as an alcohol intervention strategy has been tested in a number of clinical trials.[57] These approaches have been reported to be effective in reducing alcohol consumption among patients in primary care[44,45,58–60] and hospital settings[27,61] with effects varying somewhat by study population, setting,

and intervention intensity (length of session, number of sessions, etc.).[49,62–64] By way of a specific example, in their study referred to earlier, Gentilello et al. screened more than 2,500 patients (70%) from a larger trauma center population of just under 3,600. They randomized approximately 30% (762 patients) into a control group ($n = 366$) and an intervention group ($n = 366$), of which 300 (82%) actually completed the intervention. According to their report, subsequent follow-up showed that 47% had a reduction in return to the ED within the first year; and, 48% had a reduction in inpatient readmissions over the next 3 years. They reported that other outcomes such as traffic violations, driving under influence (DUI) arrests, and so on, "occurred statistically much less in the intervention group" although further inspection revealed that the differences did not attain actual statistical significance.[27] Further, several ED-based studies using brief alcohol interventions have been conducted with evidence of modest positive impact on either alcohol consequences[65,66] or consumption,[27] but not both.

Perhaps, the most important and promising findings reported by Blow et al. is that before their work was published there had been few studies of tailored messaging for alcohol problems in any setting. By comparison, they found that generic and tailored ED-based interventions, with and without advice, could reduce quantity, frequency, and some consequences of alcohol use and did not require a post-ED visit booster session to be effective.[65] Additionally, theirs was the first study to examine the potential benefits of tailored versus generic written messages for at-risk alcohol use. Their work sought to determine the impact of brief advice along with detailed written feedback. They concluded that determining the efficacy of tailored messages and advice versus no-advice conditions is a critical step in disentangling the crucial elements in BIs used in ED settings. They maintained that such questions are particularly relevant to a busy ED where, given current health care costs and restrictions, staff advice sessions must be very brief.[67]

Our earlier published assessment of prevention research[68] suggests two mandatory requisites: first, successful prevention strategies must incorporate theory-based interventions and methods and second, prevention strategies can be improved upon, in virtually all instances, by adopting and implementing underlying theory. Moreover, the use of theory in prevention programs will provide an improved understanding of the nature of targeted health behaviors and can explain the dynamics of behavior, processes for changing behavior, and the effects of external influences on behavior. Whereas theory alone does not and cannot produce effective prevention programs, theory-based planning, implementation, and monitoring can and does. Theory is essential in determining what to look for (research strategy), what to achieve (preventive intervention goals), and in helping to explain intervention outcome.

Theory enables us to consider ideas and strategies that we might otherwise never have envisioned. Experience has demonstrated *that no single theory is dominant in prevention programs*. In fact, one of the major problems facing public health workers is the challenge of adapting a particular theory so that it works with a particular issue. To meet this sort of challenge, the fit must be logical and consistent with everyday observations. Also, the theoretic strategy should be similar to those used successfully in other programs, and, for reproducibility and validity, the theory should be supported by rigorous research.

It goes without saying that if one reviews the annals of behavioral research, two impressions emerge and are left lingering. First, there is an abundance of theories, each with proponents and critics and each characterized by underlying research of varying quality. Second, behavioral theories not unlike new drug therapies are often greeted with great enthusiasm, attain measurable peak acceptance within a comparatively short period of time (i.e., become fashionable and in vogue) and then, invariably, decline in their popularity, adaptation, and use. They seldom bottom out completely or are summarily dismissed as invalid, although this is not always the case. Nevertheless, it seems fair to conclude that almost all eventually decline in popularity among practitioners. This is not meant to imply they are without validity or usefulness. Rather, it acknowledges that much as a lake turns over to refresh itself, scientists continually strive to identify the Holy Grail of interventions. In other words, as long as there is good science there will be research activities that seek to build upon and expand existing bodies of knowledge. Therefore, it seems to be a given that behavioral theories come in and out of vogue, some disappearing from sight, some becoming less frequently applied, and some serving as logical building blocks for the next generation of behavioral research and clinical applications.

Table 1 provides an easily referenced summary of those theories linked most closely to SBI. The four principal theories are identified by title, rationale for use, underlying concepts, and the scientists most commonly credited for the advancement of each theory in the realm of SBI.

IMPLEMENTATION OF SCREENING AND BRIEF INTERVENTIONS IN TRAUMA CENTERS

In 2007, the Substance Abuse and Mental Health Administration (SAMHA) published *Alcohol Screening and Brief Interventions (SBI) for Trauma Patients—Committee on Trauma Quick Guide*.[69] This resource was sponsored by the American College of Surgeons, United States Department of Health and Human Services, and The Department of Transportation and written by leaders and innovators in the field of alcohol and trauma. It posits "because excessive drinking is a significant risk factor for injury, it is vital for trauma centers to have protocols in place to identify and help patients." Although it is too soon to know whether

the COT *Quick Guide* will become the seminal reference for trauma centers and those who plan for and staff them, there are many reasons it should. The *Quick Guide* is a well-written, appropriately brief synopsis of how and why the SBI practice should and can be adopted. In our opinion, the usefulness of the *Quick Guide* to those involved in trauma center planning, certification, operation and patient care cannot be overstated. At the same time, the value of the procedural blueprint it provides might well be underestimated because of its physical brevity and overall simplicity, which was of course by design. The *Quick Guide* provides keys to the proverbial kingdom for those implementing SBI programs.

In toto, the *Quick Guide* provides the novitiate as well as the experienced trauma professional with a readily understood, thumbnail sketch of *The Problem* and the rationale behind *The Response* (to *The Problem*):

> "Trauma centers can use the **teachable moment** generated by the injury to implement an effective prevention strategy, for example, alcohol counseling for problem drinking. Alcohol is such a significant associated factor and contributor to injury that it is vital that trauma centers have a mechanism to identify patients who are problem drinkers. Such mechanisms are essential in Level I and II trauma centers. In addition, Level I centers must have the capability to provide an intervention for patients identified as problem drinkers..."

It goes on to describe that which is, in our opinion, the *sine quo non*—the indispensable condition underpinning the entire SBI concept:

> "... Although this guide is intended to help Level I and II trauma centers implement SBI, the Committee on Trauma recommends that **all trauma centers** incorporate alcohol screening and brief intervention as part of routine trauma care."

In sum, the COT's *Quick Guide* clearly defines a constellation of essential trauma center criteria. These include, but are not limited to, protocols capable of identifying, distinguishing between, and intervening effectively with trauma patients who abuse alcohol (and other substances). Once again, it is important to underscore the *Quick Guide* targets patients who are most likely to benefit from this interventional approach. Such individuals are not "problem, hard core drinkers." Rather, they are persons who have experienced episodes of drinking, including periodic binge drinking or recreational drug use and who have, as a consequence, found themselves in hospital EDs requiring care.

OVERVIEW OF THE COMMITTEE ON TRAUMA *QUICK GUIDE*

Alcohol SBI in trauma centers has been reduced to a straightforward, three-step process: (i) screening, (ii) BI and (iii) follow-up. While not "rocket science" by any stretch

TABLE 1
BEHAVIORAL THEORIES LINKED MOST CLOSELY WITH BRIEF INTERVENTIONS (BIs)[a]

Theory	Rationale for Use	Underlying Concept	Origin
Health belief model	Addresses why trauma center hospitalization is a good time to intervene	One must feel personally **susceptible** (at risk) for an illness or bad event that is **severe** (injury) and one must believe that the benefits of taking action (quitting or cutting down) outweigh the costs and the barriers	**Rosenstock IM, Strecher VJ, Becker MH.** Social learning theory and the Health Belief Model. Health Educ Q. 1988;15(2):175-83.
Social cognitive theory	Addresses why the BI focuses on importance of changing and confidence in ability to change	One must believe that performing a new behavior (quitting or cutting down) is **important** because it makes something very bad go away or something very good come to you and one must believe that one has the necessary skills and abilities to perform the new behavior, which is **confidence or self-efficacy**	**Bandura A**. Social cognitive theory: an agentic perspective. Annu Rev Psychol. 2001;52:1-26.
Trans-theoretic model of change	Addresses various readiness profiles encountered when conducting BIs	People go through common stages when changing a behavior: **precontemplation** (not seeing a problem as status quo); **contemplation** (seeing a problem but stuck); **preparation** (deciding to change); **action** (early, experimental change in behavior); **maintenance** (having sustained the new behavior for many months to have become a habit) *NOTE: The motivational tasks for people in different stages of readiness vary, requiring different interventions for each stage to facilitate movement to the next stage*	**Prochaska JO, DiClemente CC, Norcross JC.** In search of how people change. Applications to addictive behaviors. Am Psychol. 1992;47(9):1102-14.
Theory of reasoned action	Addresses why some patients are given normative feedback on their drinking during BI and encourages patients to think about significant others in their lives who would expect them to change	One's strong intention to perform a behavior is the best predictor and immediate precursor of action; BUT, intention to act depends on one's perceived ability to do it, the expected outcomes of the behavior and **one's subjective norms** e.g., what one perceives to be normal drinking behavior and what one perceives their significant others to expect in terms of one's own drinking	**Ajzen, I., & Fishbein, M.** (1980). *Understanding attitudes and predicting social behavior.* Upper Saddle River, NJ: Prentice-Hall.

[a]Courtesy of Dr. Chris Dunn. Dr. Dunn is an internationally acknowledged behavioral scientist specializing in SBI research. Along with his colleague and coworker Dr. Craig Field, they are also at the forefront of SBI training activities sponsored by the ACS-COT. Therefore, when compiling information for this chapter, the authors concluded that eventual readers would be served best by identifying a constellation of behavioral theories underlying current SBI practices and then seeking Dunn's expert guidance in selecting and briefly describing those theories considered to be of greatest relevance and importance (Fine's Personal Communication with Dunn).

of the imagination, to be effective the SBI must be well planned before being implemented. To this end a generic performance axiom is applicable: "If you are going to do it, do it well." Therefore, planning must address identifying program staff, defining the target population of patients who will be screened, developing or adapting one or more screening protocols, developing a record-keeping protocol, establishing one or more mechanisms to assure patient privacy protection and confidentiality, and developing a reimbursement strategy ... because no matter how well intended or altruistic the motive, to become perpetual, SBI needs to demonstrate efficacy AND show that it can pay its way or at least, be able to offset some of its associated expense.

Moreover, subjective judgment is an unreliable means of identifying at-risk drinking.[69] Therefore, it is incumbent upon the hospital provider to select an evidence-based screening instrument and process and to employ it for as many trauma admissions as possible.

Several validated screening instruments, each with their unique characteristics and advantages, are available. These include the **Alcohol Use Disorder Identification Test** known by the acronym **AUDIT**;[70] the **Consumption + CAGE** (feeling the need to Cut down, Annoyed by criticism, Guilty about drinking, and need for an Eye-opener in the morning) Questionnaire[69,71] (see Fig. 1); **CRAFFT** (riding in Car with someone who was drinking, using alcohol to Relax, using alcohol while Alone, Forgetfulness, criticism from Friends and family, Trouble—CRAFFT, a mnemonic that cues six items covering a "part year" time frame), which was specifically designed to screen for alcohol and drug problems in adolescents;[72] **BAC** a quick, simple laboratory measure that requires no additional personnel or functions other than acting on the results; or, a single "**Binge Drinking**" question that can be piggy-backed on a routine intake questionnaire.[73]

As described in detail sufficient enough to warrant acquisition, the *Quick Guide* explains, "The overall aim of a BI is to help patients decide to lower their risk for alcohol-related problems." To this end, the *Quick Guide* elaborates on the three key components of BIs: (i) giving information and acquiring feedback, (ii) understanding patients' views of drinking and enhancing motivation, and (iii) giving advice and negotiating. There is also an array of thoughtfully suggested and selected Frequently Asked Questions and Answers that address most, if not all, of the issues and concerns those considering an SBI program might raise.

Of particular utility is a sample SBI narrative that illustrates the ease and simplicity with which this unobtrusive intervention process can be accomplished. In fact, the attempt:success ratio of the SBI may be markedly increased if the screening process becomes a transparent component of the trauma center's normal routine. This will increase the likelihood that the patient will not conclude that they have been singled out or labeled, *a priori*, as a person with a drinking problem.

TRAUMA CENTER CHALLENGES TO SCREENING AND BRIEF INTERVENTIONS IMPLEMENTATION

Evidence shows that there is widespread support for the concept of implementation of an SBI program for problem drinking in trauma programs. In a recent survey

---

CAGE

1. Have you ever tried to cut down on your drinking?

2. Have you ever been annoyed by someone criticizing your drinking?

3. Have you ever felt guilty about your drinking?

4. Have you ever had an eye-opener in the morning?

Consumption

1. On average, how many days per week do you have a drink containing alcohol?

2. On a typical day when you drink alcohol, how many drinks do you have?

3. How many times in the past year have you had x (x=5 for men; x=4 for women) or more drinks in a day?

(A drink is equal to one beer, or one 5 ounce glass of wine, or one standard mixed drink containing 1.5 ounces of 80 proof spirits)

Any of the following situations are indicative of a need for further screening and counseling:

- *Two or more positive answers on the **CAGE***

- *The product of responses to items one and two of **Consumption** is greater than 7 for women and anyone over age 65, or greater than 14 for men under 66*

- *The response to item 3 of **Consumption** is greater than 0*

Figure 1   The Consumption + CAGE Questionnaire (69, 72).

of surgeons, 83% of the respondents agreed that the trauma center was an appropriate place for intervention with problem drinking but only 55% were screening their patients while 37% were currently performing BIs at their centers.[33] This suggests that attention still needs to be paid to making the transition from support of the concept in principle to actual commitment of resources and time to the practical development of an SBI program. The requirement by the ACS-COT for SBI programs for trauma center verification has stimulated necessary interest in the need for these programs beyond the compelling data proving their efficacy. However, several obstacles remain at individual centers committed to initiation of an SBI program.

Although lack of knowledge and skepticism of the effectiveness of SBI is the primary obstacle to implementation of SBI programs,[37] its impact is decreasing as the body of evidence supporting it continues to grow and as more clinicians are educated on its potential impact. Additional secondary concerns do exist, however, that could cause some to continue to hesitate.[21]

The potential impact of alcohol screening on reimbursements for trauma centers has to be considered and needs to be discussed. The Uniform Accident and Sickness Policy Provision Law (UPPL) still exists in many states and allows insurance carriers to deny payment to patients based on whether they were alcohol or drug positive. This has led many trauma centers to stop testing for BAC on admission. Because it still appears that most trauma centers are using BAC as their main method for alcohol screening, <100% use of this tool to identify patients with the potential for problem drinking behavior will mean that some patients will be missed with no BI rendered. Although the National Association of Insurance Commissioners (NAIC), the same

organization that drafted the model law in 1947, amended the UPPL in 2001 to prohibit its application to medical expense policies, states are under no obligation to do so. As of January 1, 2006, in fact, 34 states still had these laws in effect (see Fig. 2). A recent survey has shown that the majority of legislators are not familiar with the UPPL but support the concept of elimination of laws allowing denial of medical insurance payments based on intoxication.[39] However, getting individual states to prohibit denial of medical claims based on this exclusion will require additional effort. Partnering with advocacy groups such as Mothers Against Drunk Driving (MADD) is one approach trauma centers can take in an effort to repeal these laws. In the meantime, trauma centers that do not routinely measure BAC on admission to the hospital are encouraged to use other screening methods (see the preceding text) to identify patients who may be at risk.

The cost of initiation and maintenance of an SBI service is another area of concern for trauma centers. Although the cost benefit of these programs has been established,[36] it is still up to the trauma centers to bear the initial investment in the SBI program. However, it appears that the resources required to run these programs may be much less than currently perceived. A feasibility study on alcohol screening and intervention performed at four trauma centers showed that it requires the addition of only one half-time employee to provide the service.[74] Currently, trauma surgeons and social workers cannot bill directly for these services, but there are others in the medical care community with alcohol counseling credentials who can bill for these services. Given the relative small contribution of resources necessary and the potential for reimbursement on some level, establishment of a service aimed at intervention is likely, at the minimum, to be self-supporting.

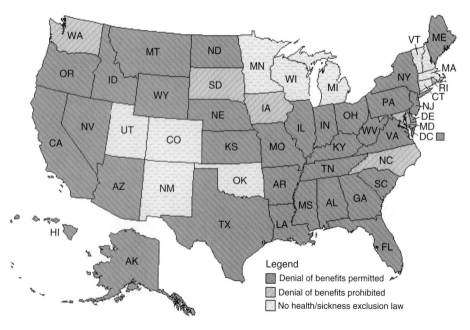

Figure 2   Insurers' Liability for Health/Sickness Losses Due to Intoxication ("UPPL") as of January 1, 2006. Picture taken from http://www.alcoholpolicy.niaaa.nih.gov

Legend
- Denial of benefits permitted
- Denial of benefits prohibited
- No health/sickness exclusion law

Finally, there exist concerns over patient privacy and confidentiality that must be taken into account.[40] Trauma surgeons must understand that asking patients about their alcohol and drug use is well accepted by the patients and not viewed as an invasion of their privacy.[27] However, given the stigma associated with alcohol and drug use and those seeking treatment for these disorders, one must be aware of the laws governing this information. Federal regulations ensuring patient confidentiality (42 Federal Confidentiality Rules [CFR] Part 2) were designed to encourage individuals to seek alcohol and drug treatment. These regulations apply specifically to hospitals that have specialized alcohol treatment programs. In 1990, the regulation was amended to exclude the medical record from emergency and trauma center visits (52 Fed. Reg. 21796, 21797, 1990). This allows an exemption to trauma surgeons who obtain BAC for the primary purpose of making clinical management decisions. However, if the BAC becomes part of the screening process or if a screening questionnaire is administered for the purposes of identifying and referring a patient for treatment, this information should be kept confidential under the provisions of the regulation. To insure the highest degree of confidentiality for the patient, records related to SBI should be kept separate from the main medical record.

PRIMARY PREVENTION EFFORTS

While the establishment of effective SBI programs in trauma centers will provide a public health benefit beyond the direct impact on trauma care, they are primarily aimed at prevention of trauma recidivism and therefore do not encompass preventive efforts aimed at the entirety of the problem of alcohol and trauma. Therefore, it is imperative that primary prevention efforts continue to be supported and established to address this problem. Strong legislative efforts to control drunk driving as well as effective health promotion activities need to continue to limit the impact of alcohol on the generation of traumatic injury.

SUMMARY AND CONCLUSIONS

There is a large body of evidence that supports the efficacy of SBI in trauma centers and this is now a requirement for Level I trauma center verification. Although Level II centers are only required to screen patients, it would be desirable for trauma care providers in any situation where the teachable moment exists to provide, requirement or not, BIs that have been shown to minimize the chance of a trauma center reunion between staff and patient. The optimal outcome from the multitude of research and education in this field is to establish the importance of these efforts in trauma centers so that effective screening and intervention services can be established. In other words, we need to move beyond merely checking the box to fulfill

a COT requirement and make these services a top priority with the necessary resources and focus they need to be successful. In addition, by partnering with local colleagues and advocacy groups focused on the negative effects of alcohol consumption, a complete program of both primary and secondary prevention efforts can be established to limit the impact that alcohol has on both the volume and severity of traumatic injury.

REFERENCES

1. Department of Transportation (US), National Highway Traffic Safety Administration (NHTSA). *Traffic safety facts 2005: alcohol.* Report No.: DOT HS 810616. Washington, DC; 2006.
2. Jones RK, Shinar RK, Walsh JM. *State of knowledge of drug-impaired driving.* Report No.: DOT HS 809642. Washington, DC: Dept of Transportation (US), National Highway Traffic Safety Administration (NHTSA); 2003.
3. Zonies DH, Jenkins DH. Substance abuse and withdrawal in the intensive care unit. In: Flint L, Meredith W, Taheri P, et al. eds. *Trauma: contemporary principles and therapy,* 1st ed. Philadelphia: Lippincott Williams & Wilkins; 2007.
4. Heron MP, Smith BL. Deaths: leading causes for 2003. *National vital statistics reports,* Vol. 55. No 10. Hyattsville: National Center for Health Statistics; 2007.
5. Gentilello LM. Alcohol and drugs. In: Moore EE, Feliciano DV, Mattox KL, eds. *Trauma,* 5th ed. McGraw-Hill; 2004:1007–1020.
6. Midanik LT, Chaloupka FJ, Saitz R, et al. Alcohol-attributable deaths and years of potential life lost. *MMWR Morb Mortal Wkly Rep.* 2004;53(37):866–870.
7. Soderstrom CA, Dischinger PC, Smith GS, et al. Psychoactive substance dependence among trauma center patients. *JAMA.* 1992;267(20):2756–2759.
8. Rivara FP, Jurkovich GJ, Gurney JG, et al. The magnitude of acute and chronic alcohol abuse in trauma patients. *Arch Surg.* 1993;128(8):907–912.
9. McLellan BA, Vingilis E, Liban CB, et al. Blood alcohol testing of motor vehicle crash admissions at a regional trauma unit. *J Trauma.* 1990;30(4):418–421.
10. Schermer CR, Apodaca TR, Albrecht RM, et al. Intoxicated motor vehicle passengers warrant screening and treatment similar to intoxicated drivers. *J Trauma.* 2001; 51(6):1083–1086.
11. Schermer CR. Alcohol and injury prevention. *J Trauma.* 2006; 60(2):447–451.
12. Mokdad AH, Marks JS, Stroup DF, et al. Actual causes of death in the United States, 2000. *JAMA.* 2004;291(10):1238–1245.
13. Maier RV. Controlling alcohol problems among hospitalized trauma patients. *J Trauma.* 2005;59(Suppl 3):S1–S2.
14. Blincoe L, Seay A, Zaloshnja E, et al. *The economic impact of motor vehicle crashes, 2000.* Report No.: DOT HS 809446. Department of Transportation (US); National Highway Traffic Safety Administration (NHTSA); 5-2-2002; 2002.
15. Committee on Trauma. *Resources for optimal care of the injured patient.* Chicago: American College of Surgeons; 2006.
16. Bard MR, Goettler CE, Toschlog EA, et al. Alcohol withdrawal syndrome: Turning minor injuries into a major problem. *J Trauma.* 2006;61(6):1441–1445.
17. Schermer CR, Qualls CR, Brown CL, et al. Intoxicated motor vehicle passengers: An overlooked at-risk population. *Arch Surg.* 2001;136(11):1244–1248.
18. Rivara FP, Koepsell TD, Jurkovich GJ, et al. The effects of alcohol abuse on readmission for trauma. *JAMA.* 1993;270(16):1962–1964.
19. Dischinger PC, Mitchell KA, Kufera JA, et al. A longitudinal study of former trauma center patients: The association between toxicology status and subsequent injury mortality. *J Trauma.* 2001;51(5):877–884.
20. Trunkey DD. Trauma. *Sci Am* 1983;249(2):28–35.

21. Gentilello LM. Alcohol and injury: American college of surgeons committee on trauma requirements for trauma center intervention. *J Trauma*. 2007;62:S44–S45.

22. Institute of Medicine, National Academy of Sciences. *Broadening the base of treatment for alcohol problems*. Washington, DC: National Academy Press; 1990.

23. Gentilello LM, Duggan P, Drummond D, et al. Major injury as a unique opportunity to initiate treatment in the alcoholic. *Am J Surg*. 1988;156(6):558–561.

24. Gentilello LM, Donovan DM, Dunn CW, et al. Alcohol interventions in trauma centers. Current practice and future directions. *JAMA*. 1995;274(13):1043–1048.

25. Dunn CW, Donovan DM, Gentilello LM. Practical guidelines for performing alcohol interventions in trauma centers. *J Trauma*. 1997;42(2):299–304.

26. Danielsson PE, Rivara FP, Gentilello LM, et al. Reasons why trauma surgeons fail to screen for alcohol problems. *Arch Surg*. 1999;134(5):564–568.

27. Gentilello LM, Rivara FP, Donovan DM, et al. Alcohol interventions in a trauma center as a means of reducing the risk of injury recurrence. *Ann Surg*. 1999;230(4):473–480.

28. Gentilello LM, Villaveces A, Ries RR, et al. Detection of acute alcohol intoxication and chronic alcohol dependence by trauma center staff. *J Trauma*. 1999;47(6):1131–1135.

29. Gentilello LM, Rivara FP, Donovan DM, et al. Alcohol problems in women admitted to a level I trauma center: A gender-based comparison. *J Trauma*. 2000;48(1):108–114.

30. Rivara FP, Tollefson S, Tesh E, et al. Screening trauma patients for alcohol problems: Are insurance companies barriers? *J Trauma*. 2000;48(1):115–118.

31. Zatzick DF, Jurkovich GJ, Gentilello L, et al. Posttraumatic stress, problem drinking, and functional outcomes after injury. *Arch Surg*. 2002;137(2):200–205.

32. Dunn C, Zatzick D, Russo J, et al. Hazardous drinking by trauma patients during the year after injury. *J Trauma*. 2003;54(4):707–712.

33. Schermer CR, Gentilello LM, Hoyt DB, et al. National survey of trauma surgeons' use of alcohol screening and brief intervention. *J Trauma*. 2003;55(5):849–856.

34. Donovan DM, Dunn CW, Rivara FP, et al. Comparison of trauma center patient self-reports and proxy reports on the Alcohol Use Identification Test (AUDIT). *J Trauma*. 2004;56(4):873–882.

35. Neumann T, Neuner B, Gentilello LM, et al. Gender differences in the performance of a computerized version of the Alcohol Use Disorders Identification Test in subcritically injured patients who are admitted to the emergency department. *Alcohol Clin Exp Res*. 2004;28(11):1693–1701.

36. Gentilello LM, Ebel BE, Wickizer TM, et al. Alcohol interventions for trauma patients treated in emergency departments and hospitals: A cost benefit analysis. *Ann surg*. 2005;241(4):541–550.

37. Gentilello LM. Confronting the obstacles to screening and interventions for alcohol problems in trauma centers. *J Trauma*. 2005;59(Suppl 3):S137–S143.

38. Gentilello LM. Alcohol interventions in trauma centers: The opportunity and the challenge. *J Trauma*. 2005;59(Suppl 3):S18–S20.

39. Gentilello LM, Donato A, Nolan S, et al. Effect of the uniform accident and sickness policy provision law on alcohol screening and intervention in trauma centers. *J Trauma*. 2005;59(3):624–631.

40. Gentilello LM, Samuels PN, Henningfield JE, et al. Alcohol screening and intervention in trauma centers: Confidentiality concerns and legal considerations. *J Trauma*. 2005;59(5):1250–1254.

41. Worrell SS, Koepsell TD, Sabath DR, et al. The risk of reinjury in relation to time since first injury: A retrospective population-based study. *J Trauma*. 2006;60(2):379–384.

42. Gentilello LM. Let's diagnose alcohol problems in the emergency department and successfully intervene. *MedGenMed*. 2006;8(1):1.

43. Neumann T, Neuner B, Weiss-Gerlach E, et al. The effect of computerized tailored brief advice on at-risk drinking in subcritically injured trauma patients. *J Trauma*. 2006;61(4):805–814.

44. Bien TH, Miller WR, Tonigan JS. Brief interventions for alcohol problems: A review. *Addiction*. 1993;88(3):315–335.

45. Wilk AI, Jensen NM, Havighurst TC. Meta-analysis of randomized control trials addressing brief interventions in heavy alcohol drinkers. *J Gen Intern Med*. 1997;12(5):274–283.

46. Hungerford DW, Pollock DA, eds. *Alcohol problems among emergency department patients: proceedings of a research conference on identification and intervention*. Atlanta: National Center for Injury Prevention and Control, Centers for Disease Control and Prevention; 2002.

47. D'Onofrio G, Degutis LC. Preventive care in the emergency department: Screening and brief intervention for alcohol problems in the emergency department: A systematic review. *Acad Emerg Med*. 2002;9(6):627–638.

48. US Preventive Services Task Force. *Guide to preventive clinical services*, 2nd ed. Baltimore: Williams & Wilkins; 1996.

49. Burke BL, Arkowitz H, Menchola M. The efficacy of motivational interviewing: Meta-analysis of controlled clinical trials. *J Consult Clin Psychol*. 2003;71(5):843–861.

50. Dinh-Zarr T, Goss C, Heitman E, et al. Interventions for preventing injuries in problem drinkers. *Cochrane Database Syst Rev*. 2004;3: CD001857.

51. *J Trauma*. 2005;59(Suppl).

52. Hungerford DW. Recommendations for trauma centers to improve screening, brief intervention, and referral to treatment for substance use disorders. *J Trauma*. 2005;59(Suppl 3):S37–S42.

53. Welfel ER. Ethical challenges of brief therapy. In: Charman DP, ed. *Core processes in brief psychodynamic psychotherapy advancing effective practice*. Mahwah: Lawrence Erlbaum; 2004:343–360.

54. Roche AM, Freeman T. Brief interventions: Good in theory but weak in practice. *Drug Alcohol Rev*. 2004;23:11–18.

55. Chang G, Astrachan B, Weil U, et al. Reporting alcohol-impaired drivers: Results from a national survey of emergency physicians. *Ann Emerg Med*. 1992;21:284–290.

56. Soderstrom CA, Dailey JT, Kerns TJ. Alcohol and other drugs: An assessment of testing and clinical practices in US trauma centers. *J Trauma*. 1994;36:68–73.

57. Blow FC, Barry KL, Walton MA, et al. The efficacy of two brief intervention strategies among injured, at-risk drinkers in the emergency department: Impact of tailored messaging and brief advice. *J Stud Alcohol*. 2006;67(4):568–578.

58. Fleming MF, Barry KL, Manwell LB, et al. Brief physician advice for problem alcohol drinkers. A randomized controlled trial in community-based primary care practices. *JAMA*. 1997;277(13): 1039–1045.

59. Fleming MF, Manwell LB, Barry KL, et al. Brief physician advice for alcohol problems in older adults: A randomized community-based trial. *J Fam Pract*. 1999;48(5):378–384.

60. Babor TF, Grant M, Acuda W, et al. A randomized clinical trial of brief interventions in primary care: Summary of a WHO project. *Addiction*. 1994;89(6):657–660.

61. Welte JW, Perry P, Longabaugh R, et al. An outcome evaluation of a hospital-based early intervention program. *Addiction*. 1998;93(4):573–581.

62. Poikolainen K. Effectiveness of brief interventions to reduce alcohol intake in primary health care populations: A meta-analysis. *Prev Med*. 1999;28(5):503–509.

63. Dunn C, Deroo L, Rivara FP. The use of brief interventions adapted from motivational interviewing across behavioral domains: A systematic review. *Addiction*. 2001;96(12):1725–1742.

64. Barry KL. *Brief interventions and brief therapies for substance abuse: Treatment Improvement Protocol (TIP) series 34*. Rockville: U.S. Department of Health and Human Services, Public Health Service, Substance Abuse and Mental Health Services Administration, Center for Substance Abuse Treatment; 1999.

65. Longabaugh R, Woolard RE, Nirenberg TD, et al. Evaluating the Effects of a brief motivational intervention for injured drinkers in the emergency department. *J Stud Alcohol*. 2001;62(6):806–816.

66. Monti PM, Colby SM, Barnett NP, et al. Brief intervention for harm reduction with alcohol-positive older adolescents in a hospital emergency department. *J Consult Clin Psychol*. 1999;67(6):989–994.

67. Hungerford DW, Pollock DA. Emergency department services for patients with alcohol problems: Research directions. *Acad Emerg Med*. 2003;10(1):79–84.

68. Fine PR, Foster J, Underhill AT, Harper KT. The prevention of spinal cord injury. In: Lin VW, ed. *Spinal cord medicine: principles and practice*. New York: Demos Medical Publishing, Inc; In press.

69. US Department of Health and Human Services, Substance Abuse and Mental Health Services Administration, Center for Substance Abuse Treatment. *Alcohol screening and brief intervention (SBI) for trauma patients: committee on trauma quick guide*. Report No.: SMA 07-4266; 2007.

70. Babor T, Ramon de la Fuent J, Saunders J, et al. *The alcohol use disorders identification test: guidelines for use in primary health care*. Geneva: World Health Organization; 1989.WHO Publication No. 89.4.

71. Ewing JA. Detecting alcoholism. The CAGE questionnaire. *JAMA*. 1984;252:1905–1907.

72. Knight JR, Shier LA, Bravender TD, et al. A new brief screen for adolescent substance abuse. *Arch Pediatr Adolesc Med*. 1999;153: 591–596.

73. Cook RL, Chung T, Kelly TM, et al. Alcohol screening in young persons attending a sexually transmitted disease clinic. Comparison of AUDIT, CRAFFT, and CAGE instruments. *J Gen Intern Med*. 2005;20(1):1–6.

74. Schermer CR, Bloomfield LA, Lu SW, et al. Trauma patient willingness to participate in alcohol screening and intervention. *J Trauma*. 2003;54(4):701–706.

Burn Prevention

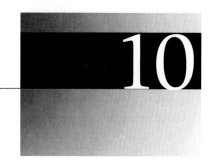

10

James H. Holmes

Burns are the sixth or seventh most common cause of injury, depending on the classification scheme of injury definition used. The most recent year for which accurate, composite burn incidence and cost data are available is 2000.[1] In that year, approximately 4,000 people died from burns or in fires (~1 per 100,000) and approximately 775,000 sustained burns requiring treatment of some sort (~280 per 100,000). These burn injuries consumed close to $7.5 billion in lifetime costs. However, compared to 1985, the incidence decreased by more than 50% from 616 to 280 per 100,000.

For the approximately 40,000 burn injuries requiring hospitalization, approximately 25,000 are admitted to dedicated burn centers.[2] On the basis of this data from the National Burn Repository, the overall survival rate now approaches 95%. For patients treated at burn centers, approximately 50% are <10% total burned surface area (TBSA), 40% are 10% to 29% TBSA, and only 10% are >30% TBSA in size. The vast majority are white males, and most injuries occur in the home. Flame and scald injuries account for 80% of all burns.

Although relatively uncommon, burn injuries are nonetheless associated with significant morbidity and costs, and most importantly, virtually all burn injuries are preventable.

HISTORICAL PERSPECTIVE

In the United States, large-scale burn prevention measures really did not begin until the 1940s and 1950s. These initial efforts were in response to a catastrophic Boston nightclub fire and to injuries sustained by children wearing costume clothing. The Cocoanut Grove Nightclub fire in 1942 remains one of the single most important events in the development of burn prevention in the 20th century.[3,4] A flame from a lit match caused the fire, and the resulting 491 deaths and hundreds of casualties were mainly due

to the violation of several fundamental principles of fire safety and burn prevention. This led to extensive changes in fire safety regulations that remain in effect currently, such as laws prohibiting the use of revolving doors as principal exits, doors to all public buildings being required to open outward, and emergency lighting systems and nonflammable decorations being made mandatory for public buildings. Further, this disaster resulted in many advances in burn care and stimulated the formal organization of burn centers, public safety legislation, and burn prevention. Also in the 1940s, publicity stemming from children sustaining burns to the legs while wearing "Roy Rogers chaps" made of highly flammable brushed rayon focused attention on the dangers of flammable clothing.[5] Thereafter, a rash of burns sustained by young girls wearing "torch sweaters" reinforced this. These incidents resulted in federal legislation (Flammable Fabrics Act of 1953) that subsequently led to extensive research into fabric flammability and measures to reduce it.

BURN PREVENTION EFFORTS AND INITIATIVES

Hot Water Burns

First and foremost, *all* tap water scald burns are preventable. Full-thickness scald burns occur in adult skin in 2 seconds on exposure to water temperatures of 150°F (66°C), in 4 seconds at 140°F (60°C), in 30 seconds at 130°F (55°C), and in 5 minutes at 120°F (49°C).[6] These times are variably reduced in children who have a much thinner dermis than adults. To date, tap water scald burn prevention initiatives have involved legislation and manufacturers' voluntary standards.

The states of Florida and Washington enacted laws in the 1980s mandating preset water heater temperatures at 125°F (52°C) and 120°F (49°C), respectively. An epidemiologic follow-up study in Washington, done 5 years after the legislation, demonstrated a 50% reduction in the average number of scald burns per year requiring admission to the hospital—5.5 per year in the 1970s to 2.4 per year in the 1980s.[7] Further, the severity of the burns decreased following the legislation as manifest by reduced TBSA involved, lower mortality, fewer number of operations required, reduced scarring, and decreased hospital length of stay. In addition, the state of Connecticut requires the installation of tempering valves in all new domestic dwellings that prevent the passage of water through showerheads or bathtub inlets if the water temperature exceeds 115°F (46°C).[8]

The manufacturers of water heaters have agreed upon voluntary standards for factory preset temperatures. Gas units are set at 120°F (49°C), whereas electric units are set at 125°F (52°C).[9] Unfortunately, there is neither any formal monitoring of compliance nor published analysis of the effects of the standards.

Residential Fires

Flame burns sustained in the home are the most common type of thermal injury. The National Fire Protection Association (NFPA) data indicate that house fires result in approximately 3,000 deaths per year and annually account for $5 to $6 billion in direct property losses.[10] Effective strategies to reduce residential fire-related injuries include the installation of smoke detectors and the use of automatic sprinkler systems.

Smoke detectors have been commercially available in the United States since the late 1960s, and their use has been widely accepted. Ongoing data from the Centers for Disease Control indicate that almost 95% of US residences have at least one smoke detector. Studies have demonstrated that both voluntary educational efforts and legislative measures are effective in increasing smoke detector use and subsequent residential fire-related injuries. In Pittsburgh, pediatricians tried to increase smoke detector installation by counseling parents about the importance of smoke detectors and then offering them low-priced ones for purchase in the office. Approximately half of the experimental families purchased smoke detectors, and of those, approximately 75% installed them compared to none in the control families.[11] After experiencing an increase in fire-related deaths in 1982, the City of Baltimore initiated a citywide smoke detector giveaway program. In a follow-up study 8 to 10 months after the giveaway, 92% of the homes had installed the detectors with 88% of them functional.[12] In Oklahoma City, a smoke detector giveaway program in an area with a high rate of residential fire-related injuries produced an 80% reduction in the injury rates during the 4 years following the intervention.[13] Similarly, in St. Louis, the project "Alarms for Life" that was designed by a group of burn survivors resulted in a 50% reduction in residential fire-related deaths in the target

population compared to the year before the project. The success of the project precipitated passage of an ordinance mandating smoke detectors in all city residences.[14] Finally, legislative efforts in Montgomery County, MD in 1978 required smoke detectors in all homes. A follow-up study 5 years later demonstrated that Montgomery County had significantly fewer homes with no functioning detectors or no detectors compared to a control county.[15] Of note, the NFPA estimates that homes with smoke detectors have approximately 50% fewer fire-related deaths than homes without detectors. To promote the maintenance of existing smoke detectors, "Change Your Clock, Change Your Battery" is a biannual campaign at daylight savings time organized by Energizer Batteries and the International Association of Fire Chiefs.

Automatic sprinklers are designed to control or extinguish a developing fire and are complementary to smoke detectors. Residential sprinkler systems have been available in the United States since the late 1970s, and it is estimated that installation increases the total costs of a new home by approximately 2%. As noted in the preceding text, the presence of smoke detectors reduces the risk of residential fire mortality by approximately 50%, and this mortality risk is further reduced to 3% by adding sprinklers according to the NFPA. There have been no multiple loss of life scenarios due to fire or smoke in fully sprinkler-covered buildings, and property loss has been reduced 80% compared to buildings without sprinklers.[16–18] More than 200 cities and towns in the United States have existing residential sprinkler laws. The first to enact such legislation was San Clemente, CA in 1978 followed by Scottsdale, AZ in 1985. Common to these, and typical of other communities' sprinkler ordinances, is that they only apply to new residential construction; retrofitting ordinances for homes have yet to be implemented.

Clothing Ignition and Flammability

Untreated fabric flammability is quite variable.[19,20] Wool tends to burn very slowly and does not ignite; it melts with a red glow, retracts, and extinguishes itself. Conversely, cotton burns intensely and is rapidly destroyed. A combination of cotton and wool burns less than either alone. Rayon and polyester ignite easily but do not burn as intensely as cotton. Nylon melts but then sticks to the underlying surface. Silk produces a red glow but rapidly extinguishes. Raised cut materials are quite flammable, whereas tight weaves are more flame retardant than loose weave fabrics. Overall, loose-fitting clothing burns more intensely, because air currents have access to both sides of the material, than tight-fitting clothing.

As noted earlier, pediatric burns associated with particular garments led to landmark burn prevention efforts. The Flammable Fabrics Act of 1953 resulted in burn units collecting epidemiologic data about burns from clothing ignition, research into fabric flammability and testing standards, and the development of flame-retardant fabrics. Initially, the Act only covered clothing materials and excluded industrial fabrics. Then, in 1967, the Act was amended to cover industrial fabrics and interior furnishings such as paper, rubber, plastic, synthetic films, and foam, as well as clothing materials. Flammability standards were also formalized for children's sleepwear during the early 1970s. "Tris" (2,3-dibromopropyl phosphate) was the common agent used to create flame-retardant clothing in the United States. Although inexpensive and highly effective as a flame retardant, "tris" was banned by the Consumer Product Safety Commission (CPSC) in 1977 based on mutagenic/carcinogenic potential in rodent models. At the same time, data from the Boston Shriners Burn Center revealed a decrease in sleepwear-related burns during the first half of 1970.[21] Unfortunately, accurate national statistics to support its individual center's experience were lacking; therefore, other explanations in addition to the flame-retardant sleepwear standards were proposed to account for the observed decrease in sleepwear-related burns. Collection of national statistics continued to be a problem, and in 1996, the CPSC relaxed the children's sleepwear standards. A current effort under way, between the CPSC, American Burn Association, and the Shriners—the National Burn Center Reporting System (NBCRS), is attempting to capture data on all clothing-related burns for children younger than 15 years. It has been effective since July 2003, and data analysis is pending further collection at this time.[22] Nonetheless, the safest sleepwear, and for that matter clothing in general, is a snug-fitting, flame-resistant (i.e., synthetic) garment.

Fire-Safe Cigarettes

Smoking-related fires are the leading cause of fire/burn deaths in the United States. According to the NFPA, in 2003, there were 25,600 structure fires, 760 deaths, 1,520 injuries, and $481,000,000 in direct costs resulting from smoking-related fires.[23] Approximately 25% of the fatalities were not the smoker whose cigarette started the fire. A cigarette, when left unattended, can burn for up to 40 minutes. When combined with alcohol consumption, there is an even greater risk of fire/burn injury and death; however, smoking appears to be the greater risk factor.[24]

The concept of a fire-safe cigarette dates back to 1929, when, following a cigarette-ignited fire, Massachusetts Congresswoman Edith Nourse Rogers called for the National Bureau of Standards to develop technology for "self-snubbing" cigarettes. After 3 years of research and testing, the Bureau was successful in developing a "self-snubbing" cigarette; however, no subsequent federal or state legislation or efforts followed until 1974. In that year, a bill was introduced in the US Senate mandating the manufacture of only "self-extinguishing" cigarettes, but the bill stalled in the Congress.[25] In the 1980s, multiple states introduced fire-safe cigarette proposals with no success.

In 1984, the federal Cigarette Safety Act created a study group for analyzing the technical and economic feasibility of producing a fire-safe cigarette. Their report, in 1987, confirmed both economic and technical feasibility with multiple cigarette redesign options to decrease fire ignition propensities: reducing cigarette circumference, lowering tobacco density, using less porous paper, and reducing the citrate content in the paper.[26] To date, no federal legislation has resulted. However, since 2000, nine states (New York, Vermont, California, Illinois, New Hampshire, Massachusetts, Utah, Kentucky, and Oregon) have passed fire-safe cigarette legislation.

New York was the first state to enact fire-safe cigarette legislation and has been the model for the subsequent states' legislation. The fire-safe cigarette technology being used in current state legislation is based on a design change developed by the Philip Morris tobacco company. This involves a simple manufacturing alteration whereby two to three bands of less porous paper are incorporated in the paper binder of the cigarette. These bands effectively act as "speed bumps," thereby slowing the burning process and causing the cigarette to extinguish if not puffed. Since enactment of the New York state fire-safe cigarette law in June 2004, smoking-related fire/burn deaths have decreased.[25]

EVALUATING BURN PREVENTION EFFORTS AND INITIATIVES

In this day and age of evidence-based medicine and increasing cost containment, burn prevention strategies have to be demonstrably effective or they cannot/will not be funded. Many apparently effective burn prevention programs have been developed and implemented on the local level utilizing the locally generated data for efficacy analysis. Unfortunately, this typically leaves the study underpowered. To perform a study sufficient to demonstrate a burn injury decrease of 50% ($\alpha = 0.05$ and $\beta = 0.80$) requires a population of 9,330, whereas demonstrating a 10% reduction requires 295,082. To demonstrate the same reductions in burn mortality requires populations of 4,672,000 and 148,175,000, respectively.[27] It is quite apparent that no single burn center or even community will have a large enough patient population to perform meaningful studies. Therefore, burn prevention efforts truly need to be coordinated and conducted on the regional or national level.

REFERENCES

1. Corso P, Finkelstein E, Miller T, et al. Incidence and lifetime costs of injuries in the United States. *Inj Prev.* 2006;12:212–218.
2. American Burn Association. website: http://www.ameriburn.org/resources_factsheet.php?PHPSESSID=bc78be8572b1dba75cddd7638f39cb77 (accessed 4/20/2007).
3. Moulton RS. *The Cocoanut Grove Nightclub fire, Boston, 28 November 1942.* Boston: National Fire Protection Association; 1943:1–19.

4. Saffle JR. The 1942 fire at Boston's Cocoanut Grove Nightclub. *Am J Surg* 1993;166:581–591.

5. Burnett WE, Caswell HT. Severe burns from inflammable cowboy pants. *JAMA*. 1946;130:935–936.

6. Moritz AR, Henriques FC. Studies of thermal injury: The relative importance of time and surface temperature in the causation of cutaneous burns. *Am J Pathol*. 1947;23:695–720.

7. Erdmann TC, Feldman KW, Rivara FP, et al. Tap water burn prevention: The effect of legislation. *Pediatrics*. 1991;88:572–577.

8. Stephen FR, Murray JP. Prevention of hot tap water burns – a comparative study of three types of automatic mixing valves. *Burns*. 1993;19:56–62.

9. Schieber RA, Gilchrist J, Sleet DA. Legislative and regulatory strategies to reduce childhood unintentional injuries. *Uninten Injuries Child*. 2000;10(1):111–136.

10. National Fire Protection Association. website: http://www.nfpa .org/itemDetail.asp?categoryID=953&itemID=23071&URL= Research%20&%20Reports/Fire%20statistics/ The%20U.S.%20fire%20problem (accessed 4/20/2007).

11. Miller RE, Reisinger KS, Blatler MM, et al. Pediatric counselling and subsequent use of smoke detectors. *Am J Public Health*. 1982;72:492.

12. Gorman RL, Charney E, Holtzman NA, et al. A successful citywide smoke detector giveaway program. *Pediatrics*. 1985;75:14–18.

13. Mallonee S, Istre GR, Rosenberg M, et al. Surveillance and prevention of residential fire injuries. *N Engl J Med*. 1996;335:27–31.

14. Schmeer S, Stern N, Monafo WW. An effective burn prevention program initiated by a recovered burn patient group. *J Burn Care Rehabil*. 1986;7:535–536.

15. McLoughlin E, Marchone M, Hanger SL, et al. Smoke detector legislation: Its effect on owner-occupied homes. *Am J Public Health*. 1985;75:858–862.

16. Cote AE. Field test and evaluation of residential sprinkler system: Part I. *Fire Technol*. 1983;19:221–232.

17. Cote AE. Field test and evaluation of residential sprinkler system: Part II. *Fire Technol*. 1984;20:48–58.

18. Cote AE. Field test and evaluation of residential sprinkler system: Part III. *Fire Technol*. 1983;20:41–46.

19. Crikelair GF. Flame-retardant clothing. *J Trauma*. 1966;6:422–427.

20. Crikelair GF, Agate F, Bowe A. Gasoline and flammable and nonflammable clothing studies. *Pediatrics*. 1976;58:585–594.

21. McLoughlin E, Clarke N, Stahl K, et al. One pediatric burn unit's experience with sleepwear-related injuries. *Pediatrics*. 1977;60:405–409.

22. American Burn Association. website: http://www.ameriburn.org/ advocacy_safechildrenssleepwear.php (accessed 4/20/2007).

23. National Fire Protection Association. website: http://www.nfpa .org/itemDetail.asp?categoryID=294&itemID=19303&URL= Research%20&%20Reports/Fact%20sheets/ Safety%20in%20the%20home/ Smoking%20material-related%20fires (accessed 4/20/2007).

24. Ballard JE, Koepsell TD, Rivara F. Association of smoking and alcohol drinking with residential fire injuries. *Am J Epidemiol*. 1990;135:26–34.

25. *Coalition for fire-safe cigarettes*. website: http://firesafecigarettes.org/ categoryList.asp?categoryID=10&URL= About%20fire-safe%20cigarettes (accessed 4/20/2007).

26. Brigham PA, McGuire A. Progress towards a fire-safe cigarette. *J Public Health Policy*. 1996;16:433–439.

27. Peck MD, Maley MP. Population requirements for statistical analysis of efficacy of burn prevention programs. *J Burn Care Rehabil*. 1991;12:282–284.

Injury Control Research

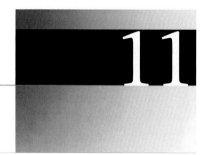

11

Rose A. Cheney   *Therese S. Richmond*

INJURY

Injury and its repercussions have a significant impact on health and well-being. Each year, more than 150,000 people die from injuries in the United States and more than 5 million people die from injuries worldwide.[1] It is the leading cause of death for Americans younger than 45 years and the burden of injury is not limited to deaths. Injury is a significant source of morbidity, disability, and disfigurement, generating substantial health care costs and lost productivity.[2-11]

More than one third of all US emergency department visits, an estimated 39 million, are related to injury.[12] Each year, approximately one of every six Americans will require medical treatment for injuries and more than 2 million Americans will be hospitalized for injuries.[8,13-15] In 2000, the total medical costs attributable to injury were estimated to be $117 billion, or approximately 10% of all medical costs in the United States.[16]

The estimated lifetime costs of injury for the >50 million Americans who experienced a medically treated injury in 2000 was $406 billion (inclusive of medical care and lost productivity).[17] Disabling injury can have lasting impact. Each year an estimated 80,000 Americans experience the onset of long-term or lifetime disability from traumatic brain injury.[18] And 11,000 new cases of spinal cord injury are estimated to occur annually, with more than 250,000 persons currently living with paraplegia, tetraplegia, or related disability.[19,20] The consequences of injury extend well beyond these physical disabilities. The repercussions of injury for individuals and families are profound, including decline in physical ability,[21-24] loss of work,[25,26] loss of sexual function,[27] fatigue,[22,28] and emotional health.[29]

The circumstances of injury are often classified across two dimensions—intent (unintentional and intentional) and mechanism (e.g., motor vehicle, firearm, submersion, and fall).[30] Data on injury mortality and morbidity, classified by external cause of injury codes[31] (formerly known as *E codes*[32]), are categorized across these two dimensions. In the United States, motor vehicle traffic injuries (27%) are the leading cause of injury deaths, followed by poisoning (18%), firearm (18%), falls (12%), and suffocation (8%).[9,33] The five leading causes of injury deaths in those younger than 15 years are motor vehicle, fire and burns, drowning, suffocation, and firearm-related deaths. For youth and young adults, aged between 15 and 24, and older adults, aged between 65 and 74, traffic- and firearm-related injuries are the leading cause of injury death. Among adults older than 85 years, falls become the most important injury mechanism.

CURRENT ISSUES IN INJURY CONTROL RESEARCH

Injury differs from many other leading diseases, making injury control and its study particularly challenging: violence, falls, and automobile crashes all are events that can suddenly kill or disable otherwise healthy people. For the most part, injury happens in a fraction of a second, often after sudden exposure to immediate risk factors. In the past, injury has often been thought of as the result of unavoidable accidents—neither preventable nor likely to yield to systematic study. A closer look at the possible causal paths for many injuries suggests that this does not need to be the case. While an injury event is quite rapid and some risks may be almost simultaneous to the event, many injuries are likely to follow from a series of accumulating and converging risks for people, mechanisms, and environments, some of which span decades.[34] The multiple factors and risks involved in different injuries suggest areas of systematic study and multiple points for intervention. Finally, although there are immediate repercussions of an injury, there is also the potential for long-term consequences.[35]

The nature of emergency care for serious injury, occurring under less than optimal conditions, presents unique challenges for research. A narrow time window for intervention coupled with limited patient information and the inability of patients to give their own consent can raise ethical complications for resuscitation research.[36–38] Emergency research studies that seek exception from, or waiver of, informed consent require consultation with the community and public notification to that community.[39] In the case of trauma care, geographic designations of community may not capture the population at risk.[36] Clinical injury research needs to be thoughtful in the development of pragmatic and ethically appropriate approaches to study design.

Successful response to injury, once it has occurred, is highly time dependent.[40] Serious injury is usually followed by an extremely limited window of time for preventing disability or death. In some instances the damage caused by injury can be mediated for the event itself, by a restraint system or helmet, for example. Medical care systems must quickly be mobilized. Successful responses require a working knowledge of the many body systems that are activated in response to an injury (biochemical, cellular, connective, organ, and psychological systems). The wide range of interconnected physiologic responses involved in the injury event, coupled with the need for extremely rapid medical care, is a research and methodological challenge to injury science. Published research on clinical practice guidelines reveals that retrospective studies and case reports dominate clinical trauma research, with only 4% of studies based on more methodologically rigorous randomized prospective designs.[41]

The complexity of elements relevant to an injury event, its risks, and its repercussions encompasses many spheres of knowledge, making injury science an important yet developing field of interdisciplinary research.[42] Research is often conducted within a single discipline, without crossing boundaries of traditional knowledge domains. An analysis of systematic reviews of injury research from the Cochrane Collaboration and the Campbell Collaborative illustrates this point.[43–47] In these reviews, only 10 out of 48 (21%) involved more than one knowledge domain (e.g., biology and behavior or mechanism and environment). As a complex and uniquely challenging disease process, injury research has not yet leveraged the full potential of systematic, integrated, interdisciplinary research.

Injury as a field of public health has grown in size, scope, cohesion, and sophistication; there are now a wide variety of disciplines, specialties, and practitioners participating in the field of injury prevention and treatment.[48] Also important for the advancement of the field of injury control has been a growing connection between prevention and treatment.[48] Although debate continues on the boundaries of the field, the application of appropriate methods, and the degree of scientific rigor, there has been much progress.[9]

Is the prevention of intentional injuries a valid area of injury control research?[48] Some in the injury field see the inclusion of violence as a deviation from the field's core mission, diverting resources needed for the study and prevention of unintentional injury. However, violence is increasingly being seen as a public health problem.[49] Indeed, there are calls to integrate injury research across intentional and unintentional causes to improve injury prevention and health.[50] This increasing interest by medical and public health professionals should not imply that injury control research should supplant criminology or mental health research, but rather it should complement the approaches of these and other fields.

Another tension in the field has been between active and passive approaches to injury prevention. Although the field initially focused on attempts to change individual behaviors, there was increasing skepticism about the effectiveness of individually focused behavioral interventions.[48] This skepticism, coupled with injury control advances in the 1960s, led to a shift toward passive interventions that focused on changing mechanisms and environment. In recent years, however, the field has begun to integrate both as complementary rather than competing approaches. In addition, scientists have also broadened the focus from individual behavior to societal behaviors that might mitigate risks.[51]

The field also suffers from tensions over tradeoffs with other important societal values—the relative costs of interventions and curtailment of freedom and policies perceived as paternalistic. Increasing research on cost-effectiveness and cost benefits is important to addressing these concerns, and the restriction of personal freedom should be considered as one of the potential costs of any intervention.[48]

The approaches, resources, and tools of public health provide a scientific foundation for injury control science. To be fully effective, injury control needs coordinated efforts that build interdisciplinary studies in prevention and treatment.[9] The advancement of injury science would benefit from a more systematic and methodologically rigorous approach across a range of inquiry, including genes, cells, organ systems, body, mind, individuals, social groups, and the environment. This integration across biology, environment and behavior can illuminate new ways to consider risk for injury.[52] Research on the precursors of injury, the injury event, and the consequences of injury has tended toward descriptive studies or less methodologically rigorous designs.[53] Further, injury research generally focuses on behavioral approaches for the precursors of injury, bio-engineering approaches for the injury event, and clinical approaches for the consequences of injury. Injury research has not harnessed the full potential of the biomedical sciences. This limits our ability to significantly reduce the overall impact of injury, both in terms of prevention, mortality, and long-term repercussions.

PROGRESS FOR INJURY CONTROL RESEARCH

Despite these many challenges, the field of injury control has made great strides toward redefining injury as preventable. With the advent of industrialization, work-related injuries came under increasing scrutiny leading to developments in industrial safety. Modern injury science evolved as a distinct field of public health in the mid-1960s using epidemiologic tools and incorporating interactions between human and environmental factors.[48]

The field has contributed one of the 20th century's public health success stories—the systematic and multidisciplinary approach of reducing the rate of death attributable to motor vehicle crashes in the United States.[54] Annual death rates declined dramatically, from 18 per 100 million vehicle miles traveled in 1925 to 1.7 in 1997. In 1966, with the passage of the Highway Safety Act and the establishment of the National Highway Safety Bureau (NHSB), a systematic approach to motor vehicle–related injury prevention was begun. The federal government was authorized to set and regulate standards for motor vehicles and highways. Behavioral changes for drivers and passengers were addressed through public education and the enactment of traffic safety laws.

The first director of the NHSB, Dr. William Haddon changed the approach to injury control in traffic safety, suggesting a framework that is now used to organize factors affecting injury risks and fatalities as pre-event, event, and postevent, and around host (person), agents (vehicle), and environment.[55] This framework, known as the *Haddon matrix*, and its variants, have been successfully employed not only in the field of traffic safety but also expanded to forms of intentional and unintentional injury. The NHSB used this matrix to initiate an injury control campaign that systematically identified, collected data, and conducted research to address these factors (human, vehicle, and environmental) during each phase of a motor vehicle crash. Further, the NHSB had regulatory power to enact changes to reduce risks for motor vehicle crash.

Other injury control policies and initiatives during this era included the creation of a federal program on emergency medical services in the 1970s, the establishment of poison control centers, funding of state injury control programs, and the founding of the American Trauma Society in 1968.[48] The National Highway Traffic Safety Administration (NHTSA) established the Crash Injury Research

and Engineering Network (CIREN) in 1996. This system links trauma center clinicians and crash investigators to a national computerized network, serving as a valuable resource for both clinical care and engineering safety designs.[48] NHTSA also oversees the Fatality Analysis Reporting System, an important surveillance system that makes data available to researchers for studies focused on motor vehicle crashes.[56] Recently, more comprehensive injury approaches, either locally or nationally, are being developed in countries around the world.[57] The World Health Organization (WHO) has provided recommendations and guidance to policymakers in both high-income and less-developed countries.[58]

Injury data are collected through numerous national, state, and local surveillance systems. These data have been used to (i) establish injury control priorities, (ii) monitor trends, (iii) identify new injury problems, and (iv) evaluate prevention and intervention efforts.[9] National data systems were an important component of the comprehensive progress in reducing motor vehicle injuries in the United States. Surveillance data were used in the enactment and assessment of legislation.[9] As surveillance data have improved, they have played an increasingly important role in injury prevention and treatment. The international resources of the WHO have promoted surveillance for both higher-income and less-developed countries, providing guidelines for collecting, coding, processing, and using injury data.[58] Despite these accomplishments, further progress for all causes will require long-term commitments to funding, supporting, expanding, and linking surveillance data.

The National Academy of Sciences has sought to unify and strengthen a scientific approach to injury control, with committees developed through the National Research Council and later through the Institute of Medicine (IOM) crafting recommendations for mobilizing resources to reduce injury and its repercussions: *Accidental Death and Disability: The Neglected Disease of Modern Society* in 1966;[59] *Injury in America: A Continuing Public Health Problem* in 1985;[8] and *Reducing the Burden of Injury: Advancing Prevention and Treatment* in 1999.[9] The work of each of these committees has resulted in recommendations for strengthening the field of injury control and its scientific infrastructure, and improving policy and practice.

INJURY CONTROL RESEARCH AND EVALUATION METHODOLOGIES

Given limited resources for the prevention and treatment of injury, the field of injury control needs a strong scientific foundation built on evidence of effectiveness. The public health approach provides a systematic process to (i) define the injury problem, (ii) identify risk and protective factors, (iii) develop and test prevention interventions and strategies, and (iv) ensure adoption of effective interventions and strategies.[60] To do this, injury control research needs to address etiologic research, followed by intervention research and evaluation.[61]

Surveillance systems or linked databases are important tools for identifying injuries and understanding their causes. However, care must be taken to understand and address selection biases, representativeness, and data quality. Qualitative methods are important in the early design and planning stage. Foundational and developmental research are important at this stage, creating explanatory models and pilot research on how interventions could affect key variables in the causal chain of an injury. Appropriate measures of exposure and denominator are also important in understanding risk. Quantifying the role of risk and protective factors should rely on the strongest possible methods available, whether randomized controlled trials, cohort studies, case–control studies, or other rigorous statistical approaches.[61]

Understanding the etiology of injury and physical impact within the context of a body of intervention theory can inform the development of interventions. Systematic reviews provide the best source for evidence of intervention effectiveness, from prevention to treatment and rehabilitation. Systematic reviews critically examine evidence of effectiveness, using carefully structured protocols to weigh the scientific rigor of research findings. These include the Cochrane and Campbell Collaboratives,[62,63] the Centers for Disease Control (CDC) Community Guide,[64] and Harborview Injury Prevention Research Center Best Practices.[65] Information from systematic reviews of effectiveness can also be found in peer review articles, and through professional society reviews, recommendations, and evidence-based protocols. Recommendations for conducting and presenting reviews using meta-analytic techniques should be followed to improve the systematic approach to synthesizing findings.[66]

In addition to identifying effective or promising practices, systematic reviews have been successful in identifying types of interventions with potential for unintended consequences.[67] For example, the systematic review of Scared Straight programs, which was designed to deter youth from criminal activity by organizing visits to prisons, found that not only did this intervention fail to deter crime but it also led to more offending behaviors.[62] Unfortunately, there are many issues in injury with insufficient research for evidence of effectiveness. A large number of injury interventions have not been evaluated. Even if they do not cause harm to vulnerable populations, programs with no proven effectiveness may have an overall negative impact through lost opportunity costs for economic and human resources. In the face of limited information on effectiveness, injury researchers need to (i) work to contribute to a body of evidence, (ii) use the best possible evidence and theory in designing interventions, and (iii) include

as rigorous an evaluation as possible, when fielding an intervention.

The field of injury control research and prevention has moved away from earlier simpler approaches.[68] The complexity of injury problems requires researchers to look for complementary prevention strategies that build on both active and passive strategies of injury control. This requires integrating knowledge from the behavioral sciences into mainstream injury prevention. Although a significant knowledge base does exist for promoting individual and community health in general, this is underrepresented in injury control research. The limited success of behavior-change efforts in the field of injury control has been attributed to (i) the complexity of the issues involved, (ii) a failure to understand the determinants of behavior, and (iii) failure to properly apply health behavior theory.[68] Fortunately, there is now movement in the field to address this by building more connections between these two areas of knowledge.

The complexity of issues involved in injury control suggests that researchers should look at a more complex model to coordinate multiple intervention opportunities. Injury occurs across a timeline or continuum from early precursors to the defining disease event to immediate and long-term consequences. Opportunities to intervene in order to prevent or ameliorate injury correspondingly differ across this continuum: *primary prevention* seeks to completely avert injuries by altering susceptibility or reducing exposure; *secondary prevention* employs early detection and prompt treatment of injuries once they occur; and *tertiary prevention* focuses on limiting disability and restoring function for injured individuals,[69] and reducing recurrent injuries.[70] In this way, the continuum provides a comprehensive and logical framework for considering scientific approaches to interventions.

The model in Fig. 1, in the subsequent text, was initially developed and used to foster interdisciplinary collaboration for one type of injury—intentional injury.[71] Its success in communicating and translating across a wide range of disciplines makes it useful for broader adaptation to all injuries. This model provides a focal point for thinking about injury, anchoring areas of knowledge that can then lead to better interdisciplinary approaches. The focal point is the injury event (shown as a star in the center of Fig. 1). This is where the precursors of injury converge and the consequences of injury begin and continue forward, potentially throughout the lifetime of injured individuals. Other persons or mechanisms also may mediate a risk, either by raising it (for instance, a drunk driver or an illegal firearm) or helping protect against it (for instance, a cautious parent or a highway barrier). These trajectories are relevant to prevent injury, improve short-term outcomes, maximize healthy function, and avoid reinjury or other consequences.

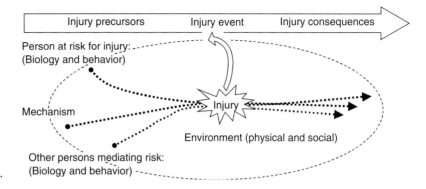

Figure 1   A conceptual model for injury science.

DATA AND METHODS

Once injury-related risks are identified and targeted and interventions designed, plans for evaluation should be developed as an integral part of any implementation. Evaluations can be designed to answer questions on the processes, the outcomes or the cost-effectiveness of injury prevention or treatment interventions. Evaluation research can provide generalizable knowledge about the effectiveness of an injury intervention (intervention research) or specific information relevant to decisions to continue, improve or expand a specific intervention program (program evaluation). Individual outcomes can range from more immediate measures of reported knowledge, attitudes, and behaviors to observed behavior, injury, functional impairment, or death. Program outcomes can include operations, costs, and impact measures. Overall evaluation goals, information gaps, stakeholders and audiences (funders, providers, and policymakers), and resources (time, financial, and program size) will influence decisions on evaluation design.[72]

In response to the complexity of injury control prevention and treatment, the CDC brought together an impressive array of internal and external prevention professionals to develop guidelines for evaluation.[73] The findings of this group are useful for guiding injury control evaluation in a systematic way to improve prevention and treatment and provide accountability for interventions. The report seeks to integrate evaluation with routine program operations, complementing program management and providing explicit formal evaluation procedures. It raises important questions regarding potential values of program activities, including merit, worth or cost-effectiveness, and significance. The framework identifies six steps that must be taken for a successful evaluation—engaging stakeholders, specifying the intervention, focusing the evaluation design, gathering credible evidence, justifying conclusions, and ensuring the use and sharing of lessons learned.

Engaging stakeholders is central to identifying the injury problems worthy of study, in designing culturally sensitive and community-specific interventions, and creating sustainable programs.[74] Stakeholders include community residents, nonprofit organizations, local businesses, faith-based institutions, and government organizations. Although there are different models informing community involvement in research, these commonalities have community stakeholders involved in each step of the project design from identifying the problems to be addressed through evaluation and dissemination of findings.[75,76]

Focusing the evaluation design and gathering credible evidence are central to injury science. To gather credible evidence on intervention effectiveness, injury control researchers will need to identify the best level and types of evidence to determine effectiveness. Randomized designs are considered a gold standard for evidence-based interventions, but may not be appropriate or feasible for many important unanswered questions in injury control.[72] Quasi-experimental techniques have been developed in response to logistic or ethical limitations to randomized techniques. Qualitative methods can be important for informing interventions or interpreting results. Limited resources, along with complex issues of causality, confounding factors, and secular trends challenge existing approaches and methods. Injury control researchers need to conduct the most rigorous evaluations possible, using the best design, measurements, and statistical tools available.

To justify conclusions, injury researchers must carefully evaluate outcomes and work with engaged stakeholders to interpret the findings. It is also critical to distinguish between findings that are generalizable across populations or geographic locations versus findings that may require testing in new and different populations. Given that injury is one of the leading causes of death in children and younger adults in almost every country in the world, injury researchers have a wealth of opportunities to adapt effective strategies or develop new approaches to injury control for populations in less-developed countries, as well as for those in high-income countries.[77]

Researchers should publish and disseminate their results, positive, null or negative, to inform practitioners and provide the data necessary for later systematic reviews. Circling back to engaging stakeholders, it is essential that injury researchers disseminate their results to the communities of interest. Lessons learned, both positive and negative, are essential to include in dissemination of results to all parties because these lessons have an impact on the sustainability of prevention programs.

RESEARCH FUNDING

Injury control research has been consistently underfunded, relative to its overall public health importance. Funding for research in injury has been approximately 1% of the total budget of the National Institutes of Health (NIH), which traditionally funds biomedical and health research.[78] In 1966, the National Research Council recommended the establishment of a National Institute of Trauma at the NIH.[9] Although this was not implemented, subsequent reports by the National Research Council and the IOM have called for the strengthening and coordination of injury control research.[9] Injury prevention research occurs through numerous federal agencies: NHTSA; National Center for Injury Prevention and Control (NCIPC) and the National Institute for Occupational Safety and Health (NIOSH) at the CDC; the Occupational Safety and Health Administration (OSHA) in the US Department of Labor; Consumer Product Safety Commission (CPSC); National Institute of Justice (NIJ); the Department of Defense; and various institutes within the NIH; Other funding sources include industry, nonprofit foundations, and state and local injury control efforts.

The CDC's NCIPC is interested in a comprehensive injury control research agenda.[60] It recently convened a panel of internal and external researchers, practitioners, and policy makers to establish a research agenda for the prevention of unintentional and intentional injury.[79] This agenda represents research priorities for foundational, developmental, effectiveness, and dissemination research. The specific injury topics and cross-cutting issues identified in this agenda suggest priority areas for future injury control research funding opportunities. A similar agenda of priority areas has been identified by NIOSH.

The field of motor vehicle injury has demonstrated the success of long-term, stable funding and focus in injury control research, although important opportunities for continued research remain. Inadequate funding has hampered the field for many other areas of injury. The IOM report found that *"abundant opportunities for scientific advancement in all aspect of the field"* justified substantially higher funding for injury control research and that trauma research should receive a higher allocation in the NIH budgets.

ADVOCACY, POLICY, AND SCIENCE

The field of injury control has made impressive gains in the last few decades in communication, advocacy, and building national interest in promoting injury prevention. These gains, while including higher visibility in government at all levels, have been influenced by strong private sector engagement. Public–private partnerships in injury control need to continue to advocate for a strong foundation in injury control research.

The IOM report recommends national investment to promote informed policymaking. This includes improved information systems, and setting priorities for injury control research and interventions.[9] Additionally, researchers need to better communicate findings—interventions known to be successful should be more widely disseminated and implemented. The dissemination of public health practices relies on advocacy for prevention policies and efforts. Injury researchers can and should be evidence-based advocates, taking positions that are grounded in the evidence.[80] It is important, however, that injury control scientists balance the demands of science and those of injury control advocacy, taking care not to become so invested in a particular policy decision to the detriment of public perceptions and confidence in their science. On the other hand, researchers should craft research questions and the dissemination of their results in a way that is useful and accessible to policy makers. Examining feasibility and cost-effectiveness, in terms of financial, social, and individual costs and benefits, also helps support evidence-based policy decisions.

REFERENCES

1. Murray JL, Lopez AD. Global burden of mortality, disability and the contribution of risk factors: Global Burden of Disease Study. *Lancet.* 1997;349:1436.
2. Richmond TS, Kauder DK, Hinkle J, et al. Early predictors of long-term disability after injury. *Am J Crit Care.* 2003;12:197–205.
3. Richmond TS, Kauder DK, Strumpf N, et al. Characteristics and outcomes of serious traumatic injury in older adults. *J Am Geriatr Soc.* 2002;50:215–222.
4. Richmond TS, Thompson H, Deatrick J, et al. The journey towards recovery following physical trauma. *J Adv Nurs.* 2000; 32:1341–1347.
5. Richmond TS, Kauder DK. Predictors of psychological distress following serious injury. *J Trauma Stress.* 2000;13:681–692.
6. Richmond TS, Kauder DK, Schwab CW. A prospective study of predictors of disability at 3 months following non-central nervous system trauma. *J Trauma.* 1988;44:635–643.
7. Richmond TS. An explanatory model of variables influencing post-injury disability. *Nurs Res.* 1997;46:262–269.
8. National Research Council Committee on Trauma Research. *Injury in America: a continuing public health problem.* Washington DC: National Academy Press; 1985.
9. Institute of Medicine. In: Bonnie R, Fulco R, Liverman, C, eds. *Reducing the burden of injury: advancing prevention and treatment.* Washington DC: National Academy Press; 1999.
10. Manwell LB, Mindock S, Mundt M. Patient reaction to traumatic injury and inpatient AODA consult: Six-month follow-up. *J Subst Abuse Treat.* 2005;28:41–47.
11. Pagulayan KF, Temkin NR, Machamer J, et al. A longitudinal study of health-related quality of life after traumatic brain injury. *Arch Phys Med Rehabil.* 2006;87:611–618.
12. McCraig LF, Burt CW. Center for Disease Control. National Hospital Ambulatory Medical Care Survey: 2001 emergency department summary. *Adv Data Vital Health Stat.* 2003;1.
13. Barss P, Smith GS, Baker SP, et al. Injury prevention: an international perspective. *Epidemiology, surveillance, and policy.* New York: Oxford University Press; 1998:1–11.

14. Baker SP, O'Neill B, Ginsburg MJ, et al. *The injury fact book*. New York: Oxford University Press; 1992:14–15.

15. Rice DP, MacKenzie EJ. *Cost of injury in the United States: a report to congress*. xv. 1989.

16. Finkelstein EA, Fiebelkorn IC. Medical expenditures attributable to injuries – United States, 2000. *Morb Mortal Wkly Rep*. 2004; 53(1):1–4.

17. Corso P, Finkelstein E, Miller T, et al. Incidence and lifetime costs of injuries in the United States. *Inj Prev*. 2006;12:212–218.

18. Center for Disease Control. *Traumatic brain injury fact sheet*. http://www.cdc.gov/ncipc/factsheets/tbi.htm. Accessed 11/19/2003.

19. Center for Disease Control. *Spinal cord fact sheet*. http://www.cdc.gov/ncipc/factsheets/scifacts.htm Accessed 12/19/2006.

20. National Spinal Cord Injury Statistical Center. *Facts and figures at a glance December 2003*. http://www.spinalcord.uab.edu/show.asp?durki=21446. Accessed 12/20/2006.

21. Brenneman FD, Katyal D, Boulanger BR, et al. Long-term outcomes in open pelvic fractures. *J Trauma*. 1997;42:773–777.

22. Haukeland JV. Welfare consequences of injuries due to traffic accidents. *Accid Anal Prev*. 1996;28:63–72.

23. Jurkovich G, Mock C, MacKenzie E, et al. The sickness impact profile as a tool to evaluate functional outcome in trauma patients. *J Trauma*. 1995;39:625–631.

24. Morris JA, Sanchez AA, Bass SM, et al. Trauma patients return to productivity. *J Trauma*. 1991;31:827–834.

25. Anke AG, Stanghelle JK, Finset A, et al. Long-term prevalence of impairments and disabilities after multiple trauma. *J Trauma*. 1997;42:54–61.

26. Read KM, Kufera JA, Dischinger PC, et al. Life-altering outcomes after lower extremity injury sustained in motor vehicle crashes. *J Trauma*. 2004;57:815–823.

27. McCarthy ML, MacKenzie EJ, Bosse MJ, et al. Functional status following orthopedic trauma in young women. *J Trauma*. 1995; 39:828–837.

28. Thiagarajan J, Taylor P, Hogbin E, et al. Quality of life after multiple trauma requiring intensive care. *Anesthesia*. 1994;49:211–218.

29. Rapoport MJ, Kiss A, Feinstein A. The impact of major depression on outcome following mild-to-moderate traumatic brain injury in older adults. *J Affect Disord*. 2006;92:273–276.

30. Centers for Disease Control and Prevention. Recommended framework for presenting injury mortality data. *Morb Mortal Wkly Rep*. 1997;47:RR–14.

31. Centers for Disease Control and Prevention, National Center for Injury Prevention and Control. *ICD-10 each cause list*. Available from: ftp://ftp.cdc.gov/pub/Health_Statistics/NCHS/publications/ICD10/. [Accessed 12/20/2006].

32. U.S. Department of Health & Human Services, Public Health Service, Health Care Financing Administration. *International classification of diseases, 9th revision, clinical modification, sixth revision*. October 1, 1996.

33. Centers for Disease Control and Prevention, National Center for Injury Prevention and Control. *Web-based injury statistics query and reporting system (WISQARS)*. [online]. (2005). Available from: www.cdc.gov/ncipc/wisqars. [Accessed 12/06/2006].

34. Berk RA, Soenson SB, Wiebe RJ, et al. The legalization of abortion and subsequent youth homicide: A time series analysis. *Anal Soc Issues Public Policy*. 2003;3:45–64.

35. Gillies ML, Barton J, DiGallo A. Follow-up of young road traffic accident victims. *J Trauma Stress*. 2003;16:523–526.

36. McGee G, McErlean M, Triner W, et al. Keynote address: Toward a pragmatic model for community consultation in emergency research. *Acad Emerg Med*. 2005;12(11):1019–1021.

37. Vanpee D, Gillet JB, Dupuis M. Clinical trials in an emergency setting: Implications from the fifth version of the declaration of Helsinki. *J Accid Emerg Med*. 2004;26(1):127–131.

38. Silverman H, Lemaire F. Ethics and research in critical care. *Intensive Care Med*. 2006;32:1697–1705.

39. Kerner T, Ahlers O, Veit S, et al. The European DCLHb Trauma Study Group. DCL-Hb for trauma patients with severe hemorrhagic shock: The European on-scene multicenter study. *Intensive Care Med*. 2003;29:378–385.

40. American College of Surgeons Committee on Trauma. *Resources for optimal care of the injured patient:1999*. 1998:19.

41. Malcynski JT, Hoff WS, Reilly PM, et al. Practice management guidelines for trauma patients: Where's the evidence? *Internet J Emerg Med Intensive Care Med*. 2001;5:2.

42. Institute of Medicine. In: Pellmar T, Einsenber L eds. *Bridging disciplines in the brain, behavioral and clinical sciences*. Washington, DC: National Academy Press; 2000.

43. Cochrane Injury Review Group. *Injury review*. http://www.cochrane-injuries.lshtm.ac.uk/. Accessed 1/05/2004.

44. The Campbell Collaboration. http://www.campbellcollaboration.org/Fralibrary.html. Accessed 1/05/2004.

45. Guide to Community Preventive Services. http://www.thecommunityguide.org/. Accessed 1/05/2004.

46. *Youthsafe*. http://www.youthsafe.org. Accessed 1/05/2004.

47. Harborview Injury Prevention and Research Center. http://depts.washington.edu/hiprc. Accessed 1/05/2004.

48. Bonnie R, Guyer B. Injury as a field of public health: Achievements and Controversies. *J Law Med Ethics*, 2002;30:267–280.

49. Krug EG, Dahlberg LL, Mercy JA, et al. *World report on violence and health*. Geneva: World Health Organization; 2002.

50. Cohen L, Miller T, Sheppard MA, et al. Bridging the gap: Bringing together intentional and unintentional injury prevention efforts to improve health and well being. *J Safety Res*. 2003;34:4773–4483.

51. Guth AA, O'Neill A, Pachter HL, et al. Public health lessons learned from analysis of New York City subway injuries. *Am J Public Health*. 2006;96:631–633.

52. George DT, Phillips MJ, Doty L, et al. A model linking biology, behavior and psychiatric diagnoses in perpetrators of domestic violence. *Med Hypotheses*. 2006;67:345–353.

53. Rivara FP. Prevention of injuries to children and adolescents. *Inj Prev*. 2002;8:iv8.

54. Centers for Disease Control and Prevention. Achievements in public health, 1900–1999. Motor vehicle safety: A 20th century public health achievement. *Morb Mortal Wkly Rep*. 1999;48(18):369–374.

55. Haddon W. The changing approach to the epidemiology, prevention, and amelioration of trauma: The transition to approaches etiologically rather than descriptively based. *Am J Public Health*. 1968;58:1431–1438.

56. Marmor M, Marmor NE. Slipper road conditions and fatal motor vehicle crashes in the Northeastern United States, 1998–2002. *Am J Public Health*. 2006;96:914–920.

57. Linqvist K, Timpka T, Schelp L, et al. The WHO safe community program for injury prevention: Evaluation of the impact on injury severity. *Public Health*. 1998;112:385–391.

58. World Health Organization. *National policies to prevention violence and injury*. Available from: www.who.int/violence_injury_prevention/policy.[Accessed 12/20/2006].

59. National Research Council. *Accidental death and disability: the neglected disease of modern society*. Washington DC: National Academy Press; 1966.

60. Centers for Disease Control and Prevention, National Center for Injury Prevention and Control. *CDC injury research agenda*. Atlanta: Centers for Disease Control and Prevention; 2002.

61. Rivara F. Introduction: The scientific basis for injury control. *Epidemiol Rev*. 2003;25:20–23.

62. Cochrane Injury Review Group. *Injury topics, index*. Available from: http://www.cochrane.org/reviews/en/topics/74.html. [Accessed December 11, 2006].

63. The Campbell Collaboration. Available from: http://www.campbellcollaboration.org/Fralibrary.html. [Accessed 1/05/2004].

64. Guide to Community Preventive Services. Available from: http://www.thecommunityguide.org/. [Accessed 1/05/2004].

65. Harborview Injury Prevention and Research Center. Available from: http://depts.washington.edu/hiprc/index.htm. [Accessed 1/05/2004].

66. Stroup DF, Berlin JA, Morton SC, et al. The MOOSE Group. Meta-analysis of observational studies in epidemiology. *JAMA*. 2000;283:2008–2012.

67. Binder S. Injuries among older adults: The challenge of optimizing safety and minimizing unintended consequences. *Inj Prev*. 2002;8:iv2–iv4.

68. Geilen A, Sleet D. Application of behavior change theories and methods to injury prevention. *Epidemiol Rev.* 2003;25:65–76.

69. Mauser JS, Kramer S. Epidemiologic orientation to health and disease. *Epidemiology: an introductory text.* Philadelphia:WB Saunders; 1985:9–13.

70. McGwin G, May AK, Melton SM, et al. Recurrent trauma in elderly patients. *Arch Surg.* 2001;136:197–203.

71. Cheney RA, Weiner NA, Seide MH, et al. A measurement framework for firearm research, intervention, and evaluation (abstract). *Presented at the National Meeting of the American Public Health Association,* Philadelphia, PA (130th Meeting). 2002.

72. Doll L, Bartenfeld T, Binder S. Evaluation of interventions designed to prevent and control injuries. *Epidemiol Rev.* 2003;25:51–59.

73. Centers for Disease Control and Prevention. CDC framework for program evaluation in public health. *Morb Mortal Wkly Rep.* 1999;48(RR111):1–40.

74. Reed MS, Fraser EDG, Dougill AJ. An adaptive learning process for developing and applying sustainability indicators with local communities. *Ecol Econ.* 2005;59:406–418.

75. Lavery SH, Smith ML, Esparza AA, et al. The community action model: A community-driven model designed to address disparities in health. *Am J Public Health.* 2005;95:611–616.

76. Richmond TS, Schwab CW, Riely J, et al. Effective trauma center partnerships to address firearm injury: A new paradigm. *J Trauma.* 2004;56:1197–1205.

77. Mock C, Quansah R, Krishnan R, et al. Strengthening the prevention and care of injuries worldwide. *Lancet.* 2004;363:2172–2179.

78. Pruitt B. Centennial changes in surgical care and research. *Ann Surg.* 2000;3:287–301.

79. Centers for Disease Control and Prevention. *CDC injury research agenda fact Sheets.* Available from: http://www.cdc.gov/ncipc/anniversary/media/fact.htm. [Accessed 12/15/2006].

80. Friedlaender E, Winston F. Evidence based advocacy. *Inj Prev.* 2005;10:324–326.

The Trauma Center

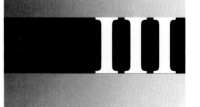

Design of the Trauma Resuscitation Area

12

William Scott Hoff

The resuscitative phase of trauma is the specific period of time when events that have transpired during the prehospital phase are linked to the care which will be provided in the hospital. Clinically, this phase represents a time when a rapid primary survey is performed to exclude immediately life-threatening injuries and a coordinated effort is initiated to maintain or restore normal perfusion.[1] Subsequently, an organized physical assessment is performed to catalog injuries and prioritize treatment. Successful resuscitation is time dependent. As such, a systematic, organized approach to evaluation and resuscitation is of vital importance in the resuscitative phase of care.

This chapter will outline the necessary elements to optimize trauma resuscitation with regard to physical plant and equipment. Important ergonomic considerations in the design of a trauma resuscitation area will be emphasized.[2] A limited list of medications required in the acute phase of trauma care will be reviewed. Finally, large-scale natural disasters and threats of terrorist-initiated catastrophes are pervasive considerations in modern emergency medicine (EM). Accordingly, there are important elements of design that must be considered for the contemporary trauma resuscitation area.

PHYSICAL SPACE—THE TRAUMA RESUSCITATION AREA

All emergency departments (EDs) should be prepared in some capacity to receive injured patients. In general, the national or state-based designation/accreditation standards for trauma centers require some dedicated space in the ED for receiving trauma patients. The American College of Surgeons Committee on Trauma classifies trauma centers as follows:

Level I: An in-house trauma team is available 24 hours a day. The facility can provide full resuscitation and definitive surgical care for all injured patients. Level I trauma centers are typically located in population-dense regions. In addition to providing the highest level of clinical care, these centers have a commitment to training, research, and community outreach.

Level II: The level of clinical care available is very similar to that available at a Level I trauma center. An in-house trauma surgeon is not required, but must be immediately available. Level II centers usually provide trauma care in regions where the population is less dense (e.g., suburban, rural).

Level III: These centers are often the initial contact for injured patients in rural areas. An in-house general surgeon is not required, but must be available in a timely manner. In addition, higher-level sub-specialists (e.g., neurosurgeons) are not required. Formalized transfer agreements with Level I/II trauma centers are central to providing optimum patient care in this environment.

Level IV: Physicians skilled in trauma management at the advanced trauma life support (ATLS)–level are available to begin resuscitation and evaluation of injured patients. Surgical resources may be limited and are not mandatory. Level IV trauma centers are designed to stabilize injured patients in remote areas; most patients will require transfer.

For trauma centers and EDs that receive a significant volume of trauma patients or where the luxury of prehospital notification is not existent, a dedicated space

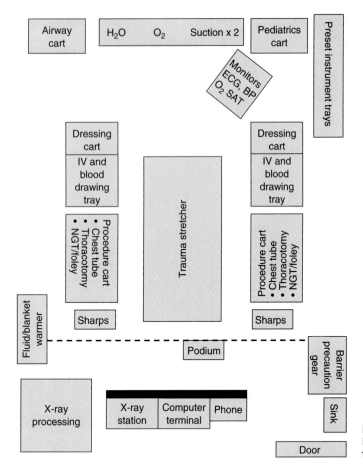

Figure 1 Trauma resuscitation area ECG, electrocardiogram; BP, blood pressure; SAT, oxygen saturation; NGT, nasogastric tube.

for trauma resuscitation is recommended. The size of the trauma resuscitation area largely depends on the volume and acuity of trauma managed by the institution. Figure 1 illustrates a potential layout for a dedicated trauma resuscitation area, including equipment, specialty carts and clerical components (see the following text). At the very least, the space must comfortably accommodate the full trauma team, necessary equipment, and allow for the performance of the following emergency procedures:

- Endotracheal intubation
- Cricothyroidotomy/surgical airway
- Insertion of central venous catheters
- Thoracostomy
- Placement of urinary catheters
- Resuscitative thoracotomy
- Diagnostic peritoneal lavage (DPL)
- Splinting of fractures

Whenever possible, the trauma resuscitation area should be adjacent but physically separate from the general ED. Distinct entrances and exits for the trauma patient from the remainder of the ED are considered ideal. Maintaining separate access and a dedicated area facilitates security and minimizes disruption to the main ED while focusing the trauma team to trauma resuscitation and care only. Access to nonmedical and any nonessential personnel should be limited. At the same time, convenient access to the radiology suite, operating room, and intensive care unit should be considered. If possible, a radiologic suite with access to plain radiography and computed tomography should be contiguous to or located within the ED.

Preventing hypothermia, an important component of the resuscitative phase, is facilitated by independent temperature control and radiant heaters in the trauma resuscitation area. Sufficient room lighting and an overhead operating room light for each trauma stretcher are imperative and fixtures should not impede movement around the patient. To permit unimpeded circumferential access to the patient, monitoring equipment, suction, and gases should be mounted above the patient on fixed columns or movable overhead booms; the floors should be free of fixed hardware to avoid tripping! The ceiling mounts should be higher than the height of tall members.

LEVEL OF RESPONSE

Regardless of the type of institution (i.e., designated trauma center, community hospital, etc.), a preestablished response to injured patients is essential for organized care of injured patients. In designated trauma centers, trauma teams consisting of attending physicians, residents, nurses and ancillary personnel routinely respond. In nondesignated hospitals, where a full trauma team is not available, an established procedure (e.g., personnel, tasks) will facilitate the resuscitation/evaluation process. Many institutions have established levels of response to efficiently mobilize personnel. Response levels are determined ideally by field triage criteria or following initial evaluation by an emergency physician:

> *Full Response ("Level One Response," "Trauma Code," etc.):* A level designed for patients who are physiologically unstable or who present with life- or limb-threatening injuries. Full response generally mobilized higher-level personnel (e.g., anesthesiologist, trauma surgeon) to the ED.
>
> *Modified Response ("Level Two Response," "Trauma Alert," etc.):* This level is intended for patients with normal prehospital physiology, but with potentially serious injury based on mechanism of injury. In some institutions, EM physicians are the primary physicians for this level of response.
>
> *Trauma Consult:* These patients have typically sustained a "low-energy" mechanism of injury and present with normal physiologic parameters. Their evaluation is usually completed by the emergency physician with no formalized team mobilization required. After the initial workup is complete, a referral is made to the trauma surgeon or the appropriate surgical subspecialist for further evaluation.

UNIVERSAL PRECAUTIONS

Exposure to various bodily fluids, which are potential sources of transmissible disease, is both highly likely and nonpredictable. Therefore, barrier precautions should be mandatory for all health care providers during the resuscitation/evaluation of an injured patient. Barrier precautions include (i) gown, (ii) cap, (iii) nonsterile gloves, (iv) surgical mask, (v) protective eyewear, and (vi) shoe covers.[3] These items are ideally located in a designated, fully visible area adjacent to the trauma resuscitation area. In this way, all providers may easily locate and wear protective gear before entering the trauma workspace.

EQUIPMENT

Resuscitation stretchers should be located in the central portion of the resuscitation space. The number of stretchers is dependent on trauma room, size, and the potential for arrival of multiple patients at a single time or frequent arrival of patients (without prenotification). A modicum of equipment, sufficient to temporarily begin trauma resuscitation for all clinical situations and transfer, should be stored under the stretcher:

- Patient gowns
- Blankets
- Small oxygen tank
- Nasogastric/orogastric tubes
- Urinary catheter sets
- Irrigation tray
- Automatic blood pressure cuff
- Electrocardiogram (ECG) leads
- Pulse oximeter leads

A comprehensive list of equipment and materials required for the resuscitative phase of trauma care is outlined in Table 1. Equipment necessary for management of the most life-threatening injuries (e.g., airway cart, intubation drugs, and thoracotomy trays) should be stored close to the patient. Other equipment (e.g., mechanical ventilators) may be stored along the walls but should be visible and readily available. In addition, key equipment for procedures should be stored closest to the person performing the procedure (i.e., functional arrangement) or near the region of the body where it will be used (i.e., anatomic arrangement).[4] For example, equipment for airway management is best stored near the head of the

---

TABLE 1

TRAUMA RESUSCITATION AREA EQUIPMENT

1. Airway control/ventilation
   (a) Laryngoscopes
   (b) Endotracheal tubes
   (c) Bag-valve masks
   (d) Oxygen source/oxygen tubing
   (e) Mechanical ventilator
2. Pulse oximetry
3. End-tidal capnography
4. Suction devices (minimal two)
5. Electrocardiogram machine
6. Defibrillator
   (a) External paddles
   (b) Internal paddles
7. CVP monitoring
8. Standard IV fluids/administration devices/IV catheters
9. Rapid infuser/fluid warmer
10. Sterile procedure trays
    (a) Thoracostomy (chest tube)
    (b) Thoracotomy
    (c) Cricothyroidotomy/tracheostomy
    (d) Laceration repair
    (e) Central venous catheterization
    (f) Arterial catheterization
11. Temperature control/warming devices
    (a) Patient/radiant heater, convection, etc.
    (b) Blood/IV fluids
    (c) Room
12. Skeletal immobilization devices
13. Ultrasound
14. X-ray equipment

CVP, central venous pressure.

stretcher; thoracostomy trays should be located on both sides of the stretcher.[5]

Inventory in the trauma resuscitation area should be carefully managed to avoid overstocking; quickly locating a specific item is difficult in an overstocked storage area.[4] In general, two of each item should be stocked in the immediate resuscitation area; additional inventory to replenish supplies utilized should be located nearby in a separate locked storage area. Materials and equipment trays should be accurately labeled and openly displayed on shelves or mobile carts. In the trauma resuscitation area, cabinets and drawers are not recommended. Equipment and disposal containers (e.g., sharps containers) should be positioned such that wasted effort is minimized during resuscitation. Procedure trays should include only those instruments that are necessary and should be arranged on the tray in a standard manner that allows easy access. Scalpels should be preassembled with protective covers and any necessary suture packs should be included in the tray. The type of trays, instruments, sutures, and so on must be standardized by protocol and change should occur only with full interdisciplinary trauma team agreement and communication.

Equipment appropriate for resuscitation of pediatric patients should be stored on a dedicated cart or in a preassigned pediatric resuscitation area. The pediatric cart or pediatric resuscitation area should be equipped with a Broselow tape for calculation of medication doses and a selection of appropriate-sized equipment based on a rapid estimation of the patient's size and weight.

MEDICATIONS

A modest inventory of medications should be stocked in a secure but easily accessible location in the trauma resuscitation area (see Table 2).[5] Instantly available drugs include those used for rapid sequence induction/endotracheal intubation. Other drugs, such as sedatives and opioids, should be promptly and readily available based on the time sensitivity of their administration. Commonly used antibiotics,

antiseizure drugs, vasoactive drugs, and so on should also be stored in the trauma resuscitation area to facilitate ease of access and timely administration.

COMMUNICATION

Effective communication is a vital component of trauma care. Communication with prehospital providers enables the resuscitation team to be better prepared for arrival of the patient. A dedicated phone line for the prehospital medical command provides effective two-way communication between prehospital and EM personnel. Once the resuscitation team is assembled, the prehospital medical command physician or emergency medical services (EMS) provider should provide a verbal report, ideally in the trauma resuscitation area. Although this verbal report is the most efficient means of communication, installation of a "listen-only" line in the trauma resuscitation area offers the resuscitation team the luxury of a real-time report during transport of the patient.

Efficient methods of communication must continue in the trauma resuscitation area such that essential information is recorded and repetition is minimized. A simple marker board can be used to record brief history, physical findings, and pertinent test results. A computer terminal, with access to laboratory results and medical records, and a dedicated and separate digital x-ray station in a "dark" area should be readily available.

A podium designated for documentation of the resuscitation should be centrally located. Dedicated telephone lines must be available to the operating room, blood bank, radiology department, and intensive care unit. Accurate daily call schedules with pager numbers should be prominently displayed in close proximity to the telephones. Trauma outcomes often depend on rapid access to the operating room. A standardized method for communicating potential surgical needs to the operating room facilitates access when necessary. The following classification system offers a standardized method for communication with the operating room:

TABLE 2

TRAUMA RESUSCITATION AREA MEDICATIONS

Immediately Available	Promptly Available	Readily Available
■ Succinlycholine	■ Lorazepam	■ Diphenylhydantoin
■ Sodium thiopental	■ Morphine sulfate	■ 50% Dextrose
■ Etomidate	■ Fentanyl	■ Methylprednisolone
■ Vecuronium	■ Naloxone	■ Mannitol
■ Midazolam	■ Tetnus toxoid	■ Thiamine
	■ Cefazolin	■ Magnesium
	■ Aminoglycoside	■ Dopamine ismalol
		■ Calcium

Class A: An unstable trauma patient has arrived who requires immediate surgical intervention. No further evaluation is planned in the ED. Immediate access to the operating room is necessary.

Class B: An unstable trauma patient has arrived who will likely require surgical intervention within 15 to 30 minutes. A limited diagnostic evaluation is in progress.

Class C: A stable trauma patient has arrived who may require surgical intervention in the next 2 hours. A thorough diagnostic evaluation is in progress.

Class D: A stable trauma patient has arrived with minor injuries and minimal probability of surgical intervention.

Using this system, the operating room can automatically hold surgical cases when notified of a Class A/B and plan for later modifications to the schedule (Class C) when necessary. In high-volume trauma centers, unless an operating room is maintained open at all times, a communication such as this is imperative.

THE TRAUMA TEAM

The "trauma team" is an organized group of providers who perform the initial assessment and resuscitation of injured patients. The composition of the trauma team will, of necessity, be institution specific. Predetermined guidelines for responsibilities of the trauma team members are important for efficient management of the trauma patient. Typical team members include the following:

Trauma Surgeon: An attending general surgeon who has demonstrated interest, skills, and training in trauma. Depending on the institution, the trauma surgeon may be available in-house. In Level I trauma centers, the trauma surgeon serves as the trauma team leader in "full response" trauma alerts.

Emergency Physician: EM physicians have typically completed ATLS and are skilled in trauma resuscitation. They serve as the trauma team leader in the absence of the trauma surgeon (e.g., Level II/III trauma centers) and, in many institutions, for the "modified response" trauma alert, multiple patient survivors. In more rural areas they may be the principal physician in early trauma diagnoses and management.

Airway Manager: One individual is available to perform endotracheal intubation when necessary. Depending on the institution, this role may be assigned to the emergency physician, an anesthesiologist, or a certified registered nurse anesthetist (CRNA).

Trauma Nurse(s): EM nurses with specialized interest and training in trauma function as the primary nurse for the patient. Additional nurses may be required to assist as needed.

Resident Physicians: In teaching hospitals, surgical and EM residents and trauma fellows assume active, graded roles in trauma resuscitation. Capable senior surgical residents (PGY-4/5) may serve as trauma team leaders in designated trauma centers.

Other Health Professionals: Other personnel who may assume active roles on the trauma team include respiratory therapists, radiology technicians, laboratory technicians, and EM technicians. Individual involvement will be determined by the individual institution.

MULTIPLE TRAUMA SCENARIOS

All hospitals, even Level I trauma centers, must have a plan for the arrival of multiple trauma patients. Obviously, the definition of "multiple patients" depends on the resources readily available and, as such, is institution specific. The key to optimal management of multiple patients is an effective and organized trauma team leader. Under these circumstances, the trauma team leader should assess the overall situation and assign the appropriate personnel to the appropriate patient. Patients should be assigned space based on their perceived needs. For example, more severely injured patients and those likely to survive should be placed in the trauma resuscitation areas. Less severely injured patients should occupy space in the ED but close to the trauma resuscitation area. A primary resuscitator is assigned to each patient with close oversight by the trauma team leader. Extraneous noise in the trauma resuscitation must be minimized because clear and concise verbal communication between primary resuscitator and trauma team leader is imperative. As the initial assessments are completed, patients may be moved out of the trauma resuscitation area and personnel and resources should be reallocated to each based on patient assessment, acuity, and injury severity. In scenarios where in-house capability *may be* excluded, "back ups" in surgery, EM, nursing, anesthesia, and so on should be called in early.

CONTEMPORARY ISSUES

The major issues in the design of contemporary EDs and trauma resuscitation areas are related to disaster preparedness. Four central themes in this regard are surge capacity, flexibility, information access, and security.[6]

Space does not permit a comprehensive discussion of disaster preparedness in the ED but some general statements are in order. Most EDs have developed simple plans for adapting to the common problem of overcrowding. However, the response necessary for a large-scale disaster is significantly more complex than managing a congested ED. Surge capacity must be incorporated into ED plans to handle a large number of injured patients arriving within a short period of time, all of whom need trauma evaluation and management. In this sense, flexibility is a key component of the contemporary trauma resuscitation area and trauma response.

General ED treatment areas must be rapidly converted into trauma resuscitation areas capable of providing the same level of patient care available in the trauma resuscitation area. Plans should be established to quickly convert space adjacent to the ED and trauma resuscitation area into triage space and patient treatment areas. Nonclinical space (e.g., waiting rooms), parking garages, and parking lots can be converted into expanded triage or treatment areas. Part of the expansion plan must include provisions for communication, materials management, and information technology. In addition, space and equipment for decontamination must be included in the surge capacity plan.

Surge capacity also applies to information systems; an adequate plan should be in place to make essential patient information available to providers in all of the areas that have been converted to clinical workspace. In addition, health care providers need ready access to important information relative to patient care ("just-in-time" training) such as patient decontamination and management of injuries from nonconventional weapons (e.g., biologic, chemical, nuclear).

Security, a prominent issue in many EDs, becomes a larger issue during a disaster response. To protect patients and health care providers, the ED must have the ability to enact a total lockdown. Access to the ED from inside and outside the hospital must be strictly controlled. Establishing a security perimeter, such that access to the hospital grounds is also limited is an additional consideration.

SUMMARY

The evaluation and resuscitation of a severely injured patient is best performed in a dedicated trauma resuscitation area. For designated trauma centers, a trauma resuscitation area is required and is essential. In all EDs, some space should be designated for trauma resuscitation. If trauma volume is sufficiently low, this space may be "flexed" for other major resuscitations. Regardless, the following principles to the designing of the resuscitation area are important:

■ The physical space allotted should be sufficiently large to accommodate the entire resuscitation team and permit safe completion of all necessary diagnostic testing and invasive procedures.
■ Equipment inventory in the resuscitation is best kept to a minimum and standardized by protocol. Additional stock is kept nearby.
■ Equipment and materials should be easily located in a logical position relative to the patient and provider and clearly labeled.
■ Dedicated communication must be available to the resuscitation team to facilitate patient flow, expedite care, and mobilize all in-house resources.
■ Provisions for rapid expansion of resuscitation space are an essential element of any trauma plan.

REFERENCES

1. American College of Surgeons Committee on Trauma. *Resources for optimal care of the trauma patient*. Chicago: American College of Surgeons; 1998.
2. Wears RL, Perry SJ. Human factors and ergonomics in the emergency department. *Ann Emerg Med*. 2002;40:206–212.
3. DiGiacomo JC, Hoff WS. Universal barrier precautions in the emergency department. *Hosp Physician*. 1997;33:11–16.
4. Yaron M, Ruiz E, Baretich MF. Equipment organization in the emergency department adult resuscitation area. *J Emerg Med*. 1994;12:845–848.
5. Hoff WS. Organization prior to trauma patient arrival. In: Peitzman AB, Rhodes M, Schwab CW, et al. eds. *The trauma manual*. Philadelphia: Lippincott Williams & Wilkins; 2002:69–77.
6. Woodland R, Lai M, Shapiro MJ, et al. Emergency department design after 9/11/2001. *Med Health R I*. 2003;86:204–206.

Design of the Trauma Operating Room

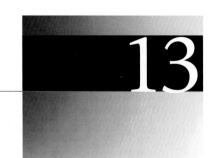

Richard Leslie George   *Arpan K. Limdi*

For many surgeons, getting involved in a major building project is a once-in-a-lifetime experience. Our focus throughout this chapter is to educate the reader about the core concepts and current trends in planning, design, and medical technology surrounding the operating room (OR) environment. In understanding the language, asking the correct questions, and providing the answers the consultants seek, the opportunity to build a durable and functional facility that embodies the visions of all members of the design team is realized. Furthermore, understanding the points along the project timeline beyond which the process cannot be revisited will set forth appropriate goals and expectations. In so doing, the reader will be a more effective leader in the design process.

The 2007 Construction Survey conducted by Health Facilities Management and the American Society of Healthcare Engineers (ASHE) indicates a significant and sustained surge in hospital construction activity.[1] Ongoing construction in excess of $40 billion is addressing aging facilities, accommodating new technology, providing larger private patient rooms, improving operating efficiency, and responding to population-based demand and competition.[1-5] In its 2006 survey, more than 20% of responding hospitals indicated ongoing construction projects in emergency departments (EDs) and surgery suites, with another 25% indicating plans within 3 years; areas of specific interest to this reader.[6] Flexibility, modularity, evidence-based design, and infrastructure for emergencies are the significant criteria driving the planning and design of new facilities.[1,2,7,8] With building costs in 2007 exceeding $300 per sq ft (and approximately twice as much in California to address new seismic requirements), the development of a new OR suite is a significant economic investment for a

health care institution.[1,9,10] Providing thoughtful and well-balanced input into this process will help the institution make optimal use of the usually limited capital funds.[3,11-13]

OVERVIEW OF THE PLANNING, DESIGN, AND CONSTRUCTION PROCESS

The planning, design, and construction process, shown in Fig. 1, may be broadly organized into six categories: strategic planning, master planning, predesign, design and award, construction, and occupancy.

Strategic Planning

On the basis of institution's vision and mission, strategic planning is the process through which the institution comprehends its situation in the context of its environment, defines key organizational objectives to achieve its vision, and develops broad strategies to achieve these objectives.[14,15] In simpler terms, the strategic plan establishes the criteria and parameters around which business decisions are made by the institution.

Master Planning

Before initiating a significant building program, it is necessary to assess whether the physical and functional design of the facility provides an appropriate, effective, and efficient environment to satisfy the mission and strategic plan of the institution.[3,16-18] The master planning process incorporates this assessment, identifies assets and constraints associated with the environment, and develops the actions

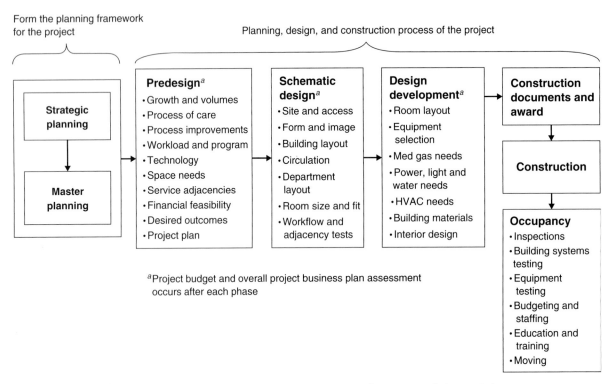

Figure 1   Planning, design, and construction process. HVAC, heating, ventilation, and air-conditioning.

necessary to address the constraints and implement the planned business initiatives.[3,16,19] Integrating the physical and functional evaluation with the future needs of the institution leads to a facility master plan that defines the overall planning criteria and articulates the highest and best use of available resources.[20] The facility master plan defines broad initiatives such as land acquisition, parking development, building replacement, and utility capacity development to accommodate projected future needs.[20,21] The master plan is reviewed and updated on a regular basis along with the strategic plan and the associated financial plan.[3,12]

Predesign

Planning for a specific project begins with the predesign process. In essence, this is the phase in which the specific needs and desired outcomes associated with the project are defined within the broader context of the strategic plan and facility master plan. Activities undertaken during predesign include more detailed facility and operational assessments, assessment of demand, development of growth projections, a financial feasibility study, and determination of project goals.[15,17,19,20] Once the financial and operational viability of the project is established, the team proceeds with development of the program.[15,20]

Program development involves determination of workload followed by preparation of the functional program, space program, and conceptual building plan.[17,22] The project implementation plan, preliminary project budget,

and project schedule are also developed at this time.[16,19,23] Medical and communication technology planning traditionally occurs during the design phase; however, it is important to identify transformational technologies (that have significant impact on care processes and outcomes) to be included in the project.

Determination of a design and construction delivery method is necessary to establish the project implementation plan. Design-award-build is the traditional method of project delivery based on a clear, formal, and standardized process.[16] Other options for project delivery focus on managing financial risk and accelerating implementation schedules. An increasingly common approach is for the owner to retain a construction manager (CM). The CM may work with the owner and architect to coordinate the design and then become the general contractor (often guaranteeing cost and schedule) or continue to manage the construction by coordinating with a builder on behalf of the owner.[16] The CM approach allows the team to benefit from the contractor's expertise in several areas such as building methods, prevailing costs, and early purchase of long-lead items.[16,19,24]

Design

Design is the process where the solution to address the needs specified during predesign is synthesized. Design activities are organized into two phases—schematic design and design development. The image, form, size, structural grid, and circulation plan of the building (project) are established during schematic design. The size, location, and arrangement of functional areas and building utility systems are also established at schematic design.[16,19] Each individual space in the building program is located within its assigned functional area using the size, dimensions, and desired adjacencies described in the functional program. However, not all desired adjacencies are achievable. A primary purpose of the schematic design review with the owner is to evaluate the developed plans against the desired functional program. Solutions for individual rooms or services that do not fit expectations are developed by reevaluating program, size, workflow, and prioritizing adjacencies.[19] A schematic level budget estimate is also prepared and titrated against the desired scope, proposed design, and the financial plan.

The design development phase takes the approved schematic design further to a level of detail necessary to describe the project for construction. The workflow within and between rooms is finalized, and medical equipment and associated utility systems required within each room are selected. The lighting, power, water, and medical gas requirements along with the heating, ventilation, and air-conditioning (HVAC) system requirements for each space are defined. Detailed design of the building interiors is undertaken, and building materials, interior finishes, and furnishings are selected and specified.[16,19] All this information is recorded on room data sheets prepared for each space within the building program.[16] Detailed drawings (floor plans, reflected ceiling plans, room elevations, and sections) and specifications are prepared from the gathered information showing the size, exact dimensions, exact location, and installation requirements for the items specified on the room data sheets.[16,19] The design team also prepares an updated project cost estimate to evaluate against the available project budget. With owner approval of the design development drawings and specifications, the team proceeds with preparation of construction documents. Any changes to the project scope and program after completion of design development will cause additional design expenses. In addition, if the changes are significant, it may also extend the project schedule and increase the cost of the project.

Construction Documents, Bidding, and Award

Construction documents or contract documents form the basis for a legally binding agreement between the owner and a builder to construct the specified project within a specified time and for a specified cost.[16,19,23] The documents consist of drawings, specifications, and general contract conditions. Contractors use the bid documents and issued addendums to determine the construction cost (and their profit), schedule, and means and methods of building the project. The owner and design team review bids or negotiate with interested builders to obtain the lowest responsible and fair cost and appropriate quality of construction for the project.[16,19,23] Changes in scope, program, or design after contract award will cause significant increases in the construction cost and delay the completion date of the project.

Construction and Occupancy

During the construction process, the owner's team is responsible for several issues. Construction progress is monitored against the schedule. The contractor's pay requests are reviewed against progress and approved for payment. Field inspections are performed to assure quality of construction and conformance to specifications. Changes to the design or specified materials, requested by the builder or end users, are evaluated and addressed. The specification, bidding, evaluation, award, and installation of owner-provided furnishings and equipment are also undertaken.

Another important set of activities for the owner's team is preparing the end users to take occupancy of the project at its completion. Occupancy planning involves orienting staff to the new facility, training to operate new systems, developing budgets, hiring staff, developing new procedures, and performing preoccupancy testing of clinical systems. The relocation plan for existing departments and the activation plan for the new facility is developed and communicated. Special attention should be placed on testing the environment for mold and spores, and if applicable, moving critically ill patients. For large building projects, a commissioning agent is hired to test, balance, and tune all electrical and mechanical (another term referring primarily to HVAC) systems; to prepare building systems documentation; and to provide enhanced training to facility maintenance staff.[25] Tuning building automation systems to produce energy efficient operations right from building start-up can avoid significant unnecessary expenses for an institution.[25]

GETTING ORGANIZED FOR THE PROJECT

Activities necessary to get organized for the project include selecting consultants, organizing the owner's project management team, and developing a project management and decision-making structure. With the team in place, the project delivery plan is developed and the predesign process can begin.[16,19,23,26]

Selecting Consultants

Selecting well-qualified and experienced professionals is essential to a successful building project. Key members of this team include the programmer or functional planner, the architect and associated engineers, and the contractor or CM. Additional criteria to evaluate include skill and experience, size of the firm and proposed team, knowledge of local conditions, commitment to the project, and their design fee. Consider the experience of not only the principals but also the staff that will be handling the bulk of the project development. Other consultants who may be necessary for the project include medical equipment planners, communication system planners, the developers or development consultant, financial consultants, and cost estimators.

The Owner's Team

The owner's team, at a minimum, is represented by three groups—the project management team, the end users, and administration. The project management team is responsible for all aspects of the administration of the project. It should be staffed by individuals with extensive experience in planning, design, and construction of facilities. Physicians, nurses, and allied health professionals are the end users who will utilize the facility. They should be heavily involved in the planning and design of the project. Administration is responsible for setting direction and making all final decisions on the project.

A comprehensive view of the clinical and functional requirements from a multidisciplinary perspective is necessary to develop an effective surgical suite design.[23] Therefore, be as inclusive as possible without making the team dysfunctional. In addition, tailor the structure of the team to the complexity of the project and to complement the social and operational dynamics of the organization. Being knowledgeable about workflow and paying attention to details are two important attributes necessary for members of the user team. To be effective, the teams need to develop trust and a sense of ownership in the process and design, eventually becoming strong advocates for the design.

Guiding Principles

At initiation, the executive team and key stakeholders should be clear about the objectives of the project. The strategic and financial plans, coupled with the facility master plan, provide the framework to define these objectives. A set of planning and design principles derived from the objectives should be used in evaluating options and making decisions throughout the course of the project.[23] Some of the common themes driving the current building boom are discussed in the subsequent text:

A predominant theme that will continue for several years is the need to address aging facilities while incorporating flexibility for the future.[1,16,17,27] For facilities built in the 1950s and 1960s, right-sizing and reorganizing core diagnostic and treatment space are essential to accommodate new technology, improve operational efficiency, address competition, and maintain marketshares.[1,2,8,28]

Patient care spaces built using a standards-based, modular design approach experience construction cost reductions, assure operational flexibility, bolster patient safety, and ease adaptation in the future.[29]

Medical technology has served as one of the major drivers of innovation in health care. These innovations are powering significant improvements in patient outcomes, productivity, and efficiency. However, due to rapid improvements, the useful life of major technologies (telecommunication systems, imaging, laboratory, pharmacy, and surgery) has shortened considerably. Therefore, planning for future flexibility in replacing technology has become a core guiding principle of building projects.[16]

There is a trend toward utilization of an evidence-based design approach reflecting an increasing level of maturity in the health care design process. Features such as larger private rooms with family space, introduction of natural light and nature into the care environment, improving ceiling design, introduction of art and color, and taking active measures to reduce noise levels are results of studies conducted, showing their beneficial effects on patients, family, staff, and revenues.[30,31]

Building project costs are rising at significant rates beyond inflation.[10] Health care institutions are caught between reduced reimbursement for services rendered and greater (and justifiable) demands for safety and efficiency (which require improved workflow and new technology).[3] Investment in the physical plant is essential, but the financial outlook is negative (reduced revenues from operations, deteriorating debt capacity, and lower bond ratings). Therefore, to extend the reach of available funds, executives are exploring functional flexibility through multiuse procedure spaces and acuity adaptable or universal patient rooms. In addition, heretofore unglamorous (but expensive) areas such as building structure, emergency generators, power plants, utility systems, and wiring conduit are also being planned with future expansion in mind.

THE PREDESIGN PROCESS

From the owner's perspective, most significant operational and financial decisions related to a project occur during the predesign or programming phase of the project.[11,17,23] The axiom "form follows function" is central to the planning of health care facilities, and the definition of function begins in the predesign process.[11] The tendency to begin drawing once the architect is selected should be curbed until the predesign process is completed. As reviewed in section II, the predesign process has several activities, which we will expand upon in this section.

Physical and Operational Assessment

For a renovation project, the assessment of existing physical, operational, and environmental conditions is an important task. As standards of care and technologies evolve, facilities accrue deficiencies requiring operational workarounds. Issues to evaluate in the existing OR include size; power, communication, and medical gas capacity; HVAC capacity and performance; and the ability to locate and power larger imaging equipment. Issues to evaluate in the existing surgery suite include preoperative holding and recovery capacity; equipment, instrument, and supply storage capacity; location and adjacency of key support services; and the workflow of patients, sterile supplies, and soiled goods. This evaluation, conducted by the architect, functional planner, or medical programmer, is best handled through tours, interviews, and a well-organized questionnaire system.[22]

Scope of Program

To develop the appropriate functional program, space program, and required adjacencies, the medical planner needs to develop an understanding of the scope and extent of the trauma program. Some of the key questions to address include the following:

- Is the trauma program a Level I or II service within the community?[32] Is there a full-time trauma surgical service at the institution?[33] Is the institution the only significant community resource for trauma care?
- Who are the other providers of trauma service in the local and regional geographic area? What level of service do the other providers support? Is this expected to change in the short- to medium-term future?
- How does the local or regional emergency management system operate?
- Are there any specific community social and behavioral trends that dictate specific arrival patterns to the trauma service?
- What are the demographics of the geographic area serviced by the institution? What are the long-term population trends? Are there seasonal and peak demand trends?
- What are the surge capacity requirements in the event of a mass casualty event?[32]
- What are the current and projected trauma patient volumes expected at the institution?

Answers to such questions (or a consensus, where clear data are not available) are used by the medical planner to understand future population trends, and develop volumes and capacity requirements for the functional and space programs.

Workload Projection

The number of ORs (or any other key room) is generally determined by the projected volumes for each type of procedure, the average length of each type of procedure (turnaround time) coupled with the hours of operation of the surgical suite, and a proposed utilization (or efficiency) factor.[22,32,34,35] A trauma surgery suite should be able to handle all emergency general surgery procedures. Institutions can elect to configure their ORs so that a trauma surgical procedure can be performed in any OR. However, for hospitals with a large trauma population, it would be advisable to have a block of rooms (on the basis of projected volumes) dedicated to trauma surgery. One OR should always be kept ready and available to handle emergency procedures. These arrangements not only assure availability of resources in critical situations, but also allow optimization of workflow, and improvements in efficiency and delivery of patient care for the entire surgical service.

Functional Program

The functional program is a detailed document that describes the planned future functions and operations of a service or department.[27] The program documents existing care processes, associated inefficiencies, future care processes, and associated improvements. A thorough understanding of workflows (patients, staff, and materials), operating metrics, shared resources, critical adjacencies, and special design concepts is assimilated and documented in the functional program.[22,27,36] Analyzing routine tasks, eliminating redundancies, and optimizing workflow can produce operating efficiency, additional capacity, and improved financial performance.[27,37–39]

The nature of the surgical disease of trauma mandates critical management. Rapid and timely access to resources is essential to successful management of a trauma service patient. In the development of efficient workflow, it is important to understand that the ED, the trauma bay, the OR, the postoperative care unit, the intensive care unit (ICU), and the surgery ward form an interdependent system through which the trauma patient will transit during their stay at the hospital.[40] Separating urgent surgical cases from the scheduled case workflow will significantly improve the throughput for both areas.[40]

There are several functional adjacencies to consider when planning a trauma program. Intake to the trauma surgical service generally occurs from the ED or a specified trauma unit within. Access to the ED and OR by helicopter and ambulance through dedicated circulation (including large elevators when required) facilitates timely and efficient patient flow. The adjacency of the principal care delivery spaces such as the ED, ICU, and OR is also an important functional planning consideration. Within the ED, the location of decontamination facilities;[32] location of the trauma pod and adjacency to dedicated imaging services; and adjacency to supply and medication rooms requires careful consideration. In the OR environment, location of ORs to large trauma elevators; quick access to the blood bank, pharmacy, anesthesia laboratory, and portable imaging equipment; and adjacency to the computed tomography (CT) service should be considered.

Associated adjacencies important to successful operation of the trauma suite include location of postanesthetic care unit (PACU) (recovery); location of sterile instrument trays and supplies; and location of central supply services where instruments may be washed, packed, sterilized, and transported to and from surgery.

Space Program

For large projects, space program development occurs at a conceptual level and is followed by a detailed, room-by-room development. The conceptual space program is a rapid method for the programmer to establish the total space need. The method is based on multiplying the total number of revenue generating spaces planned, also called key rooms (e.g., the OR), by a space assignment factor which incorporates the size of the key room as well as the size of all support spaces needed to make it functional. The factor most commonly used for this activity is the department gross square feet (DGSF) factor. Space needs for a surgery department are estimated using a factor ranging between 2,700 DGSF per OR and 3,500 DGSF per OR. The conceptual space program provides the design architect initial feedback regarding the total size of the project (building), and serves as a benchmark for the development of the detailed space program.

The detailed building or space program is a room-by-room space list organized by department, service, functional area, or building component. The program tabulation, prepared by the medical planner (or programmer), shows name, number, size, and purpose of all rooms, spaces, areas, and services to be included in the project and necessary to address the needs defined in the functional program.[22,34,35] A brief narrative describing the character of the key space and the criteria used to establish its size may be included in the tabulation.[16,19,22] The size of individual rooms in the space program is shown in net square feet (NSF). NSF represents the clear usable space within the walls of the room. Medical planners generally apply two factors to the total NSF of a department or functional unit. The first factor converts the NSF to the DGSF, which accounts for the space for walls, internal circulation, and interior building structure. A second factor is applied to the DGSF to account for common building areas such as lobbies and atria, primary building circulation, inter-departmental circulation, elevators, stairwells, mechanical and electrical shafts, and telecommunication risers.[16,22,41]

Size of Operating Rooms

OR size has tremendous impact on all aspects of the planning and design of the surgical suite. Minimum acceptable OR size standards are recommended by the American Institute of Architects (AIA) and adopted by most public health departments. In the 2006 Guidelines for Design and Construction of Health Care Facilities, AIA recommends a minimum 400 sq ft clear usable space with a minimum clear length of 20 ft for construction of a new general OR.[32] The size recommendation is increased to 600 sq ft for cardiovascular, orthopaedic, and neurosurgical ORs. It is important to note that these guidelines represent minimum acceptable standards. The information in the functional program is the key driver in establishing the size of the OR. A significant body of practical experiences indicates that for general OR design, a minimum of 600 sq ft OR is a desirable goal.[22,42–44] For environments with extensive use of minimally invasive surgery equipment, imaging equipment, and surgical instrumentation, a minimum size of 750 sq ft would be desirable.[22,42–45]

Physical and Functional Relationships

The physical and functional relationships identified in the functional program are blended with the detailed space program to produce relationship diagrams. The workflow (in terms of patients, staff, key services, and materials) within the department and between service entities, and the adjacencies necessary to satisfy the project requirements described in the functional program are pictorially depicted in these diagrams.[16,19,22] Relationship diagrams can take the form of simple bubble diagrams that depict the process and functional relationship or preschematic diagrams that show an optimal organization of physical spaces and circulation of patients, materials, and staff.[16,22] An example of a functional flow diagram is shown in Fig. 2.

Architectural Design Guidelines

During the predesign process, the owner and architect need to develop architectural and engineering design guidelines to direct and further define the character of the facility or project.[13] The design guidelines are derived from the guiding principles established at the inception of the planning process. The planning and design guidelines should be thoroughly explored and tuned during the interview process with clinicians, staff, and administrators. The resulting information is usually described in the scope of work and in the functional program. Design guidelines address issues such as the overall image and architectural character of the building, the aesthetic attributes of the interior spaces, the arrangement of services, flexibility within the building program, and circulation of public, patients, staff, supplies, and waste through the facility.[46–48] For projects involving renovation of existing space, consideration should be given to issues such as noise and vibration, coordination of utility shutdowns with patient care operations, daily construction schedule, and circulation routes for workers, supplies, and debris.

Patient and staff safety and infection control procedures during construction require special attention in the planning, design, and construction process.[49] Interim Life Safety Measures (ILSM) are actions required to compensate

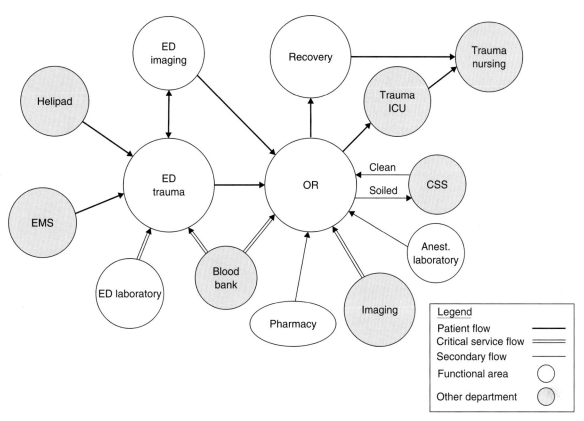

Figure 2 Functional flow diagram. CSS, central sterilizing service; ED, emergency department; ICU, intensive care unit; EMS, emergency medical services; OR, operating room.

for potential fire-related hazards that may be created during the process of construction. These actions are identified by the Joint Commission on Accreditation of Healthcare Organizations (JCAHO) and implemented by the builder and the institution's facility manager as applicable. During the planning process, the institution is required to conduct an Infection Control Risk Assessment (ICRA) and provide the results to the design team.[32,49] The ICRA identifies the potential risk of transmission of various air or waterborne biological contaminants in the facility. On the basis of this assessment, the owner provides design recommendations for inclusion in the program, and specific risk mitigation recommendations to avoid contamination during construction.[32,45,50] The final project construction documents and specifications should clearly delineate the physical and operational measures required to be undertaken by the contractor to implement ILSM and protect patients and staff from the risks identified in the ICRA.

Transformational Technologies

Another area of discussion during the predesign process is to identify transformational medical, information systems, and communication technologies that the institution is considering for the project. Transformational technologies refer to systems that will fundamentally change the care process, operational workflow, or clinical outcomes throughout the project. In surgery, significant transformations in care are being driven by technologies supporting a minimally invasive surgical (MIS) approach, sophisticated imaging systems for planning and guidance during surgery, the use of surgical robots, and expanded use of audio and visual communication systems coupled with digital control of the OR environment.[51-76]

The activities that constitute the predesign process are highly interdependent and iterative activities. Discovery of new information at each step of the predesign process may cause reevaluation of the assumptions, conclusions, and directions formed before that point in the process. Therefore, it is necessary (and more cost effective) to confirm the project goals, programs (volumes, functional program, space program, and desired adjacencies), and financial plans in an integrated manner before embarking into design development.

THE DESIGN OF THE OPERATING ROOM SUITE

The goal of the schematic design phase is to develop a clearly defined, feasible design plan along with the associated project budget and schedule. The output of the physical evaluation, functional program, space program, and relationship diagrams for each department in the project is integrated with the overall architectural configuration of the project (based on site, access, shape, image, structure, primary circulation, and building systems) to produce a relatively complete, dimensionally tested plan to realize the project. This is the point where the implications of desired functional spaces, their sizes, and adjacencies are understood and tested against the possibilities driven by available space and its architectural configuration. Several schematic designs are usually reviewed with the owner and end-user teams during the process of refinement of the plans.

Design of Building Foundation, Shell, and Core

The building foundation is the structure on which the building sits. The shell and core refers to the structure, mechanical spaces, the electrical, mechanical, plumbing and telecommunication risers and shafts, in addition to the elevators, stairwells, and primary circulation corridors of the building. Planning additional capacity in the underground utility systems (supplying water, power, and telecommunication capacity to the building) and planning additional load-bearing capacity within the foundation and structure can provide future flexibility to accommodate heavy imaging technology (e.g., intraoperative magnetic resonance imaging [MRI]) as well as future expansion capability. The planning of the building shell and core should also consider increased floor-to-floor heights to accommodate sophisticated mechanical and medical technologies, larger electrical and telecommunication risers, additional conduit, and larger mechanical rooms.

The structural columns, elevators, building infrastructure risers and shafts, and exit stairwells form the framework around which the functional space is arranged. In an ideal condition, maximum flexibility in the use of the clinical space can be achieved by aligning stairwells, risers, and shafts as close as possible to the immovable structural elements of the building (such as columns and shear walls).[16] The layout of the structural grid has important implications for the layout and design of clinical services. Practical experiences indicate that planning a structural column layout with a 30 ft distance between adjacent columns is generally the most efficient and cost-effective design direction in a multistory structure. This design grid offers the most optimal size and clear dimension options for laying out services such as the ED, ORs, imaging services, ICUs, and acute care beds. Although the 30 ft dimension may change in the future, the standardized design grid must work efficiently within the overall building envelope and be able to effectively accommodate the various key rooms (ED examination room, OR, imaging suite, and patient bed) effectively within the grid.[16,35,44,77]

While making provisions for future flexibility is important, the architect has to balance these considerations against other criteria such as construction cost, site constraints, connectivity to adjacent structures, impact on available functional space, and interior visibility.

Layout of the Surgery Suite

Key elements in the layout of the surgery suite include the location, size, and arrangement of the OR, adjacent substerile and storage space, the sterile supply and instrument holding area, and the patient and staff circulating corridor. Various planning topologies that address the movement of patients, staff, clean supplies and instruments, and soiled material have been developed and explored in the design of the surgical suite. In the single corridor design, patients, staff, clean supplies, and soiled materials travel to and from the OR through the same corridor. Although this plan does not separate flow of clean and soiled materials, it is an efficient plan and is adequate for a small surgical suite.[35] A more desirable arrangement for larger surgical suites involves the use of a clean core and a peripheral corridor system. In this plan, each OR has two entries on opposite walls with one corridor providing circulation for patients, staff, and soiled goods, while a separate corridor connects to the clean (or sterile supply) core that holds sterile supplies and instruments sent from the central sterile supply department.[35,36,78,79] This plan achieves the desired separation of clean and soiled material flow. It also provides the opportunity to bring natural light into the surgical suite. However, these benefits are achieved at the expense of additional space allocation and longer travel distances. Following placement of the core elements of the surgical suite and associated circulation within the envelope of the available space, important support services such as the blood bank, laboratory, and pharmacy can be located and evaluated. The floor plan of the surgery suite at University of Alabama Hospital at Birmingham (UAB) showing key elements associated with the trauma surgery service is shown in Fig. 3.

An additional level of flexibility can be planned in the OR environment by placement of "soft" space in appropriate locations within the suite. Soft space refers to support spaces such as storage and offices that can be relocated in the future without producing a serious detrimental effect on the function of the OR environment. Location of equipment storage space between adjacent ORs, which can be converted into future control rooms for intraoperative imaging equipment, is an example of planning flexibility for the future.

TRANSFORMATIONAL TECHNOLOGIES IN THE OPERATING ROOM

The emergence of MIS techniques, intraoperative imaging systems, robotic systems, and the digitization of the OR environment are technology trends with potentially

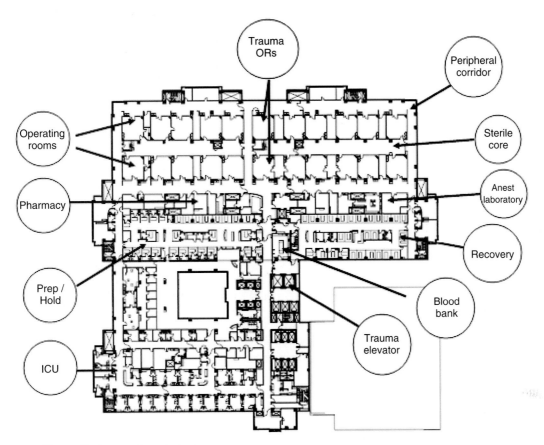

Figure 3 Layout of surgical suite.

significant impact on patient recovery, OR safety, and overall efficiency.[61] Some of these technologies are in various stages of early development, require significant capital investment, and have limited adoption in the mainstream OR environment. However, various trials and studies show tremendous growth in the future. With an eye toward flexible use of the OR and accommodating future technologies, the planning impact and design requirements to utilize these technologies must be explored.

MIS techniques are emerging into the mainstream of surgical practice primarily due to the perceived patient care benefits including smaller wounds, reduced postsurgical pain, shorter recovery periods, and reduced lengths of stay.[67,80,81] A concomitant development is the surgical video system (SVS), which integrates the components used to perform MIS and provides images of the procedure for all members of the surgical team to monitor.[52] These systems improve clinician visualization and comfort, provide enhanced documentation, and support educational and training activities.[52] SVSs are available as a part of an overall MIS system package from various endoscope system manufacturers. However, to maintain flexibility, the institution can work with a medical equipment planner to design an "open system," integrated digital OR (IOR) with SVS capability using "off-the-shelf" components.[53] This issue is explored further in the next section.

There are several design issues to consider when planning for MIS in the OR. Accommodating the equipment required for an MIS case requires more space and preparation, and can take significant additional time.[53,67,82] Considering the ergonomic configuration around the operating table (the position of the OR table, the height and position of the video displays, and the location of physiologic monitors) is important to provide relief from muscle fatigue and visual feedback to all members of the surgical team.[42,67,82,83] Owing to the extensive use of displays, the ability to manage lighting levels to reduce glare within the OR is another important design consideration.[42,43,53,67,82] The additional equipment involved in MIS and the SVS places greater energy demands on electrical systems and greater heat loads for HVAC systems to accommodate.[84] Room setup, access and circulation around the OR table, and maintaining a hazard free environment are also issues to address during design.[57,67] Ceiling-suspended articulating booms that hold MIS equipment and provide power, medical gases, and other connections can address some of these challenges. This issue is explored further later in this section.

Computer-aided surgery techniques using imaging systems are gradually emerging in the OR environment. These systems provide surgical planning information, guidance to various surgical instruments during procedures, and immediate feedback to the surgeon about the results of their intervention.[85–87] Radiography, fluoroscopy, CT, MRI, and ultrasonography are amongst the imaging modalities being utilized in these applications.[59,85,88] Digital angiography systems are being considered for use in combined interventional OR environments to handle cardiovascular surgical interventions.[74,89,90] Image-guided MIS procedures using intraoperative CT and MRI are being explored for use in spinal procedures.[71,91] Intraoperative MRI is being explored in neurosurgical tumor resection procedures to attain further precision in locating the tumor and obtaining immediate feedback on the results of surgical manipulation.[58,92] Virtual endoscopy, using three-dimensional (3D) reconstruction using thin-slice helical CT scans, has been shown to be as effective as traditional endoscopy and bronchoscopy procedures.[93] Studies are also exploring the use of image-guided MIS procedures using robotic arm technologies.[92]

The addition of fixed imaging equipment in the OR environment significantly increases the size and complexity of the space. Building structure, OR size, as well as floor and ceiling loading require careful consideration. The location and range of motion of the imaging system, medical utility booms, and surgical and procedure lighting require careful coordination with each other and with the workflow and positioning of the procedure table and staff.[94] Electrical, mechanical and plumbing system design, air flow, infection control, shielding, and safety are also important considerations in the planning of these spaces.[63]

Robotic systems in the OR environment provide direct assistance, extending and enhancing the abilities of the surgeon in a variety of ways.[51] "Third arm" robotic telescopic arm systems assist the surgeon during endoscopic procedures by holding (and positioning) the endoscope to provide steady images throughout the procedure. Robotic devices translate the surgeon's gross motor skills into microscopic motion while eliminating the impact of muscle tremor to enhance microsurgical procedures.[54,93,95,96] More sophisticated master-slave robotic systems perform MIS procedures by holding and manipulating several surgical instruments introduced through small incisions to the surgical site.[96,97] The motion of the instruments in the surgical field are controlled remotely from a console by the surgeon who is provided a stereoscopic view of the surgical site.[54,98]

In planning for the use of robotic systems, consideration must be given to the size, structure, and utility capacity (power, telecommunication) of the OR. In addition, the OR layout needs to consider location and workflow of people, supplies, instruments, and equipment, along with the robot and associated systems.

A significant portion of new hospital construction is incorporating planning for a digital information management and controls environment. In terms of patient flow and throughput management, institutions are investing in patient tracking systems. These systems post the location and status of patients, the ORs, and support services on displays at strategic locations within the surgical suite and associated services for staff to monitor.[43,99] Locations can include preoperative holding, OR control desk, PACU, and central sterile supply.[43,99] These systems can combine anesthesia status as well as video images from the OR to provide more precise information on the status of a particular surgical case.[99] Tracking of patients, devices, and instruments may be taken a level further through the integration of physical tracking technologies, such as radio frequency identification systems, with OR information and display systems.[100] Another area of innovation is the development of IOR, which makes it quicker and easier to set up and manage the OR environment. A single user interface connected to the MIS equipment, flat panel displays, OR lighting, HVAC, and medical equipment offers the circulating nurse the ability to rapidly set up and change the status of the OR environment.[101,102] For example, the circulating nurse can reroute images from the MIS system, physiologic monitor, in-room cameras, or portable imaging equipment to any display in the OR without reconnecting any video cables. The temperature and lighting levels within the OR can be changed from the same interface. Certain systems offer levels of integration allowing the circulating nurse to raise or lower the OR table and control robotic instruments from this interface. Additional capabilities allow consultation between the pathologist and the surgeon in the OR. The images from the microscope can be routed to displays in the OR along with audio and tele-illustrator capability to allow effective communication. Another significant improvement involves connectivity of the OR case management system with all sources of medical information (patient vital signs, anesthesia and drug levels, laboratory data, and images) to create a comprehensive electronic medical record. In addition to tracking patient status, such systems also offer significant benefits in the quality improvement and medicolegal arena.

Creating a digital information management and controls environment involves making significant infrastructure investments in the structured cabling system along with planning and integration of several elements such as the MIS, SVS, IOR, OR case management system, patient tracking system, medical devices with status information and control interfaces, and building automation system. Conduit and cable tray systems to accommodate all potential information sources and destinations, large telecommunication equipment management rooms, increased HVAC capacity to handle additional heat loads, and location of the circulating nurse are key areas of consideration in the design of OR.

Much of this technology can be accommodated into the existing OR environment by placing insufflators, light sources, and camera control units on one or more equipment carts. After the circulating nurse moves these carts into position, insufflation tubing, video cables, light cords, cautery lines, and foot controls can be positioned and connected. While this cart-based paradigm works for the occasional MIS procedure, for high volume surgery centers a cart-based paradigm creates significant deficiencies. The cart-based system requires additional time to set up, restricts ergonomically appropriate positioning of equipment,[53] and can be a source of hazard to the patient and the surgery staff.[57,67] In order to decrease clutter, reduce tripping hazards, improve setup times, reduce setup errors, ease staff movement, and provide better ergonomic positioning options, it is necessary to consider the use of alternate medical utility systems. Ceiling-suspended articulating booms can provide medical gases, power, low-voltage video connections, other utilities, hold the MIS equipment on shelves, and provide organized wire management support.[53,101–103] Flat panel displays suspended from ceiling-mounted articulating arms allow optimal ergonomic positioning for the surgeon and other members of the team.[53] The SVS can transmit the video information generated by the camera to the appropriate flat panel displays within the OR, to another OR for consultation with a colleague, and to a classroom setting for educational activity.

DESIGN OF THE OPERATING ROOM

A systematic approach to the design of the OR provides a structured method for developing and refining a design that is as standardized as possible, yet flexible enough to respond effectively to most procedural demands.

On the basis of functional program and the schematic design, the size of the OR and the layout of the surgical suite should already be established. An OR size between 600 and 750 sq ft can accommodate most surgical procedures that utilize MIS equipment, a robotic arm, or portable imaging equipment. If considering fixed imaging equipment in the OR, room sizing requires specific planning in the context of the modality and type of procedures to be performed. Again, during the predesign phase, such needs should be identified, programmed, and appropriately shown in the schematic design.

The design process involves development of concepts and plans during the schematic design phase of the project, and testing, further refinement, detailed development, and specification of these plans during design development. Design development usually involves the detailed design and refinement of individual rooms. At the end of design development, all significant components of the project should be identified, defined, described, sized, and located.[16,19]

The layout of the OR requires an understanding of the number of elements occupying space within the OR, their predominant location within the room, the range of motion of each element, interactions between elements, and the pathway for movement into and out of the OR.[94] Elements that occupy space within the OR are staff (e.g., surgeon, anesthesiologist, and circulating nurse), patient, supplies, surgical instruments, and equipment. These elements may occupy space only during the course of the procedure (e.g., the patient), may be brought in for a portion of the procedure (e.g., mobile C-arm), or be located permanently in the OR (e.g., booms). Once all the elements are identified, the travel path, desired (or predominant) location, and orientation of the significant clinical elements (patient, anesthesia system, circulating nurse station, key personnel, surgical instruments, and the sterile zone) should be visualized and documented for each type of surgical procedure. The layout of significant clinical elements for a trauma OR is shown in Fig. 4.

With knowledge of the reach and range of motion of the ceiling-mounted articulating booms, articulating surgical light, and display holders, the architect can propose appropriate locations for these devices in coordination with the significant clinical elements.[94] Through an interactive process of refinement with the end-user team, the architect can optimize these locations so that staff can set up the OR for a majority of procedures easily, while maintaining travel pathways and space for supplies, materials, and equipment.[102] With these elements established, the layout can be completed by locating HVAC diffusers, medical equipment, environmental controls, communication equipment, and computer systems. Figure 5 shows the results of this process on the layout of the trauma ORs at UAB.

It is highly advisable for the end users and the design team to carefully test and evaluate the results of the design by building a full-size mock-up of the proposed OR. The mock-up can also be used to evaluate the performance of booms, articulating arms, surgical lights, and other medical equipment being planned for use in the new OR.

PLANNING HEATING, VENTILATION, AND AIR-CONDITIONING, ELECTRICAL, MEDICAL GAS, LIGHTING AND SURGICAL BOOM SYSTEMS

Mechanical, electrical, plumbing, fire protection, and life safety systems account for 45% to 50% of the total construction cost of a new building. This percentage may be even higher for renovation projects.[104] A review of the detailed design of these systems is beyond the scope of this chapter. However, in this section we will review some of the significant issues of which the surgeon should be aware.

The HVAC system is the critical element providing environmental comfort, infection control, and patient recovery support within the OR and the surgery suite.[48] To develop the appropriate design, the engineer establishes the performance parameters with the end users, accommodates the current and projected heat load within the OR, satisfies the required (or desired) air exchange rate through the space, and makes accommodation for future flexibility.[104]

External circulation corridor

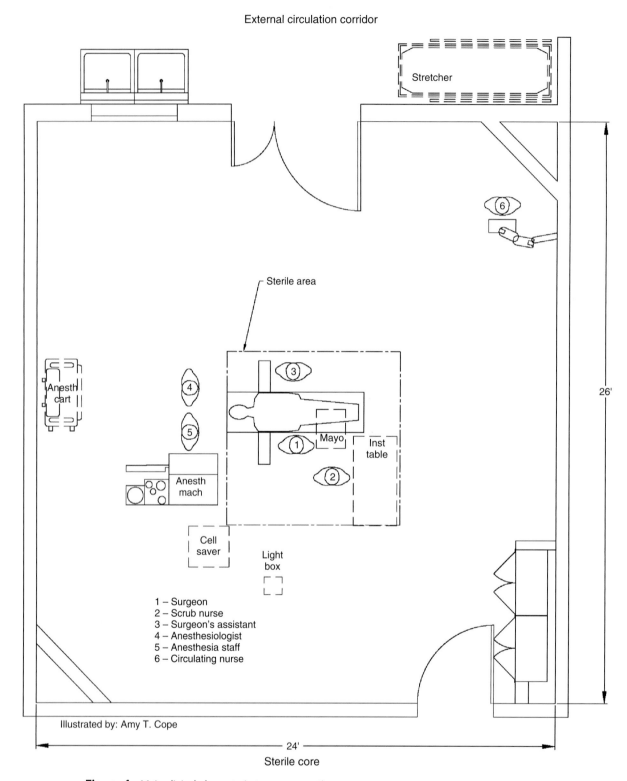

1 – Surgeon
2 – Scrub nurse
3 – Surgeon's assistant
4 – Anesthesiologist
5 – Anesthesia staff
6 – Circulating nurse

Illustrated by: Amy T. Cope

Sterile core

Figure 4 Main clinical elements in trauma operating room.

Air exchange rates establish a level of dilution of the particulate matter which, in turn, minimizes the risk of infection to the patient from bacterial counts within the environment. The acceptable rate of air changes per hour (ACH), the low temperature and high temperature desired, humidity levels, and the rate of change of temperature desired within the OR are the design specifications the engineer seeks from the end users.[48]

Ventilation requirements for areas affecting patient care are established by various agencies and societies

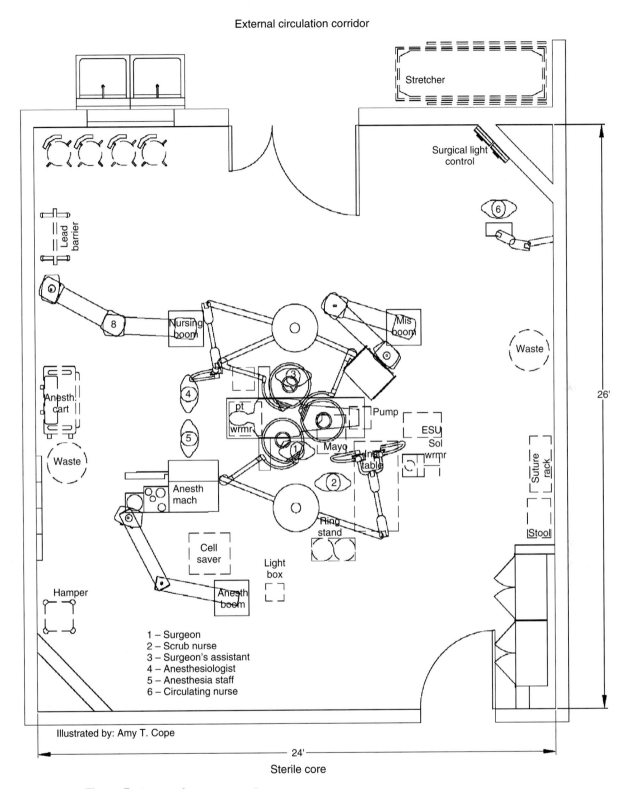

Figure 5 Layout of trauma operating room.

such as the Centers for Disease Control and Prevention (CDC), American Society of Heating, Refrigeration, and Air-Conditioning Engineers (ASHRAE), and the AIA. The AIA guidelines recommend a minimum of 15 ACH with a relative humidity range of 30% to 60% and a design temperature between 68°F and 73°F.[32,45] It is important to note that these are recommended minimum guidelines. Participation of the surgeons, anesthesiologists, and nursing staff is important in the determination of design conditions. With the plethora of equipment and personnel occupying the OR, a wider design temperature range (between 60°F and 85°F) should be considered.

From a reliability and flexibility perspective, engineers design the air handlers (that cool and push the air through the ducts) so that they deliver the required volume of air (at the necessary velocity) when running at 80% to 85% of their rated capacity. Another system level redundancy is to crossconnect supply ducts from the air handlers to provide some level of conditioning of the space in the event of failure of one of the devices.

For the OR environment, AIA and ASHRAE recommend a vertical downdraft air curtain system to reduce the opportunity for particulate matter to contaminate the surgical site and sterile field. Most airborne microorganisms are 0.5 to 5 μ in diameter.[48] To maintain an environment free of impurities, a design involving use of prefilters at the air handlers followed by high efficiency particulate air (HEPA) filters located above the diffusers through which the air enters the OR is recommended.[48] The prefilters may include charcoal filters to remove environmental contaminants. The efficiency of the HEPA filters (for 0.3 μ sized particle) may range between 90% and 99.97%. The diffuser panels in the ceiling should be located above the predominant position of the OR table (patient) to provide maximum benefit of the vertical downdraft air curtain effect.[48] Return air should be located near the floor level as far from each other as possible.

From the electrical system design perspective, the engineer works with the end users to identify all the potential devices requiring power within the OR, followed by a determination of the general location of each device and the associated power outlet.[104] The list of devices is usually extensive and includes items such as the OR table, surgical lights, anesthesia equipment, MIS equipment, portable imaging equipment, lasers, computer systems, light boxes, and general medical equipment. The engineer also accounts for items such as motorized booms and general room lighting. Provision of adequate power outlets (and capacity) from the ceiling-mounted articulating booms can provide significant flexibility in the arrangement and utilization of the OR. In addition to the specific equipment list, the design engineer will also give consideration to providing additional power outlets distributed around the OR (convenience outlets) and additional power capacity for future changes or additions.[104]

As an example, the new ORs at UAB are supported by two line isolation monitor (LIM) panels with 15 kVA capacity each. The electrical capacity is 20% to 33% greater than the maximum estimated load in the OR allowing for future additional load. A total of 80 electrical outlets are distributed around the OR including eight duplex power outlets and five emergency power outlets from each of the three booms. Power outlets also support the laser, circulating nurse station, portable imaging equipment, and other medical devices. Each isolation panel is powered from a separate set of electrical circuits tied to one of two parallel electrical bus systems. Each electrical bus is powered by normal power as well as two of the four emergency power generators. This design allows multiple levels of safety in the event of failure of general power, the electrical bus, or the emergency generators.

Medical gas requirements for the OR are determined in a manner similar to the electrical requirements. The engineer works with the end users to establish the type of medical gases required in the OR; the number, location, and connector type of the medical gas outlets, and determines whether the gases should be supplied from a central system or from local system supported by a tank room. To enhance the flexibility of the OR, consideration should be given to provide anesthetic gas and insufflation service from more than one boom. The arrangement of medical gas utility outlets on the booms in the ORs at UAB is shown in Table 1. The planned medical gas capacity is well in excess of the minimum recommended guidelines by the AIA.[32]

ORs are required to have general lighting as well as surgical lighting units located above the OR table. Surgical lights are preferably mounted on articulating arms, which provide a wide range of motion for positioning during various surgical procedures. General OR lighting and surgical lights are required to be on separate electrical circuits.[32] Owing to the extensive use of MIS techniques, glare-free visualization of the flat panel displays is very important.[43] Therefore, the ability to dim the general room lighting should be available at the circulating nurse station. To enhance viewing of flat panel displays, consideration

TABLE 1

MEDICAL GAS UTILITY ARRANGEMENTS IN OPERATING ROOMS AT UNIVERSITY OF ALABAMA HOSPITAL

Boom	Air	O_2	V	N_2	N_2O	CO_2	Other
Anesthesia	2	2	4	1	2	1	Waste anesthetic gas evacuation
MIS boom	2		4	2		2	Smoke evacuation system
Nursing	2	2	4	2	1	2	Waste anesthetic gas evacuation

MIS, minimally invasive surgery.

should be given to installation of a dimmable green down light.[105] Color temperature, color rendering index, shadowing, maneuverability, and integration with the OR environment control system are criteria to consider in the selection of surgical lights. Light sources available on the market include halogen, xenon, fluorescent, and light emitting diode (LED). Each light source has its advantages and issues. Conducting trials in a mock-up and in the OR environment is the best method of evaluating surgical lights.

Careful evaluation and selection of an appropriate surgical boom technology is an important activity for the end users and design team. Surgical boom technology promotes flexibility, assists in reducing clutter, facilitates accessibility, provides ease of connectivity to utilities, and improves visibility and organization within the OR.[103] There are several performance criteria to consider including boom placement, load capacity and installation requirements, number of articulating arms, reach and range of motion, degrees of rotation, vertical travel, braking system, equipment shelves, wire management, smoke evacuation capabilities and capacity to accommodate power, medical gas, and communication connections.[103] At UAB, three surgical booms are installed in each OR as shown in Fig. 5. Arrangements for installation of an additional boom in the future have also been made. Where possible, a unistrut grid should be considered to provide additional flexibility in location of booms, surgical lights, and displays.[42]

PLANNING COMMUNICATION INFRASTRUCTURE

High performance, IP-based Ethernet networks are becoming the standard in the health care industry. These networks enable rapid and accurate transmission of high volumes of information to and from all parts of the health care enterprise. The network provides an integrated connectivity platform for real-time collaboration, monitoring, and control, as well as a myriad of voice, data, video, and multimedia applications necessary for the quality, safe, and efficient delivery of patient care. Cabling infrastructure is the foundation for the development of an integrated, accessible, and flexible hospital information system.[106,107] A well-designed and installed structured cabling system provides the framework necessary for reliable and predictable performance, as well as the flexibility to grow and evolve over time without the need to make extensive changes in the cabling backbone.[69,106,107]

The structured cabling system provides the physical connections necessary to exchange information (data, voice, and images) between connected computers and other digital devices in real time. The primary elements of a structured cabling system are the routers that connect the network to the external world, network devices (hubs

and switches), which distribute information between the router and the internal network, patch panels through which the information is routed to the correct user or devices, the outlets in the walls, and the cables that connect these elements together. The ideal cabling infrastructure generally includes a mixture of copper and optical fiber based on a single standard. However, cost implications may force hospitals to mix Category 5, 5e, and 6 cabling components based on performance requirements in specific areas.[107] The category number refers to the material quality, winding, shielding, and other specifications of the cable in order to reliably produce the specified bandwidth. For example, Category 5–based networks, with the appropriate electronics, can produce manufacturer-certified bandwidths up to 100 Mbps, and Category 6–based networks can be certified for bandwidths up to 1 Gbps.

In the surgical suite, the integrated network generally connects and supports information exchange between a large number of medical devices, systems, and technologies referred to in earlier sections of this chapter. In addition, the structured cabling system and network also support systems such as telephone, nurse call, code 10, public addressing, intercom, dictation, energy management (building automation), building security, and access control.[108] Within the OR environment, additional conduit capacity, cable tray system, and large telecommunication equipment rooms (which could be 450 sq ft or more in size) are important elements to incorporate for future flexibility.[69] Consider placing equipment rooms between adjacent ORs. These spaces can hold computer servers, switches, and SVS routing gear that may clutter the OR and provide flexibility for future expansion. Institutions should also consider installing fiber optic cabling within the OR in order to support real-time image transmission from radiology systems in native resolution.

INTERIOR FINISHES

Interior finishes refer to the appropriate covering for the floors, walls, and ceilings. The primary design criteria are cost, comfort, aesthetics, durability, ease of cleaning, resistance to stains, and installation requirements.

AIA guidelines require the installation of a monolithic and joint-free (seamless) floor.[32] The floor should be nonporous, slip-resistant in wet and dry conditions, handle frequent hard cleaning, and capable of handling heavy rolling loads.[32,45] There are two major types of flooring materials to consider in the OR–terrazzo or broadcast epoxy and rolled goods (vinyl or rubber). Broadcast epoxy floors have superior durability but are hard underfoot (which is an important consideration for staff comfort and fatigue). Installation of this floor takes a longer time and is more labor intensive. When repairs are required, OR downtime is longer and repair costs are higher. Rolled goods such as rubber and vinyl are less durable compared to broadcast epoxy floors. However, their installation takes less time and is less labor intensive. Repairs and maintenance are quicker and easier to perform. In addition, rubber floors are more comfortable under foot and are a naturally green product. Regardless of floor type, careful preparation of the substrate is critical to successful, long lasting installations.

Wall finishes are required to be impermeable to fluids, free of fissures, open joints, or crevices that may retain dirt particles, and washable.[32,45] Use of high-impact resistant boards can protect walls from impact of equipment moving into and out of the OR. Tile is also an option for a wall covering; however, it is more labor intensive to install and can chip, crack, or break easily on impact. Epoxy paint is an acceptable wall finish, which seals the wall surface for infection control and is easy to clean; however, it does not offer impact wall protection.

Ceilings are required to be monolithic, scrubbable, and capable of withstanding chemicals.[32,45] Cracks or perforations are not allowed. Plaster or water-resistant, epoxy-coated, gypsum wall systems may be used to prepare the ceiling. All floor-, wall-, and ceiling-mounted fixtures and access panels are required to be sealed to prevent entry of dust and contaminants into the OR.

SUMMARY

Involving oneself in the design, construction, and occupancy of an OR can be a daunting task. Since the OR does not function in isolation, it positions the present chapter in the context of surgical suite and hospital design. Understanding the language used, the process outlined, and the goals desired allow the surgeon to come to the table as a team member, but with a skill set that affords the opportunity to be a team leader. Understanding the key design features for a fully functional and efficient system permits compromise on less critical issues, and knowing the point in the process beyond which changes are no longer practical or feasible defines a component of the timeline. However, as "form follows function," an exceedingly difficult task will be to convey in detail the subtle complexities of what is otherwise second nature to a surgical team such that the consultants understand the cumulative process. A successful project embodies a balance between an appropriate but expandable scope, necessary but adaptable quality, and judicious but feasible cost; the latter of which can be significantly controlled with a thoughtful, comprehensive planning and predesign process.[16] Of the comprehensive reference list, the selected readings provide a resource list to initiate supplemental reading.

SUGGESTED READINGS

Allison DJ. *Planning, design, and construction of health care environments.* The Joint Commission on Accreditation of Healthcare Organizations; 1997.

Hardy OB, Lammers LP. *Hospitals: the planning and design process,* 2nd ed. Aspen Publications; 1986.

Hayward C. Health care facility planning: Thinking strategically. In: *ACHE management series.* Health Administration Press; 2006.

Zuckerman AM. Health care strategic planning: Approaches for the 21st century. In: *ACHE management series.* Health Administration Press; 1998.

REFERENCES

1. Carpenter D, Hoppszallern S. Construction—still booming. *Hosp Health Netw.* 2007;81:44–46, 48, 2.
2. Carpenter D. The boom goes on. Technology and consumer demands keep driving construction and renovation. *Trustee.* 2006;59:6–10, 1.
3. Barker BT, Whelan CB. Maximizing ROI: Funding strategies for capital construction. *Trustee.* 2004;57(3):30–31.
4. Bazzoli GJ, Gerland A, May J. Construction activity in U.S. hospitals. *Health Aff (Millwood).* 2006;25:783–791.
5. Coile RC Jr. Competing by design. *Physician Exec.* 2002;28: 12–16.
6. Carpenter D. The boom goes on. *Hosp Health Netw.* 2006;48–54.
7. Moon S. Construction—and costs—going up. Even as expenses mount, pressured by rising commodity prices, health care building continues to boom, annual survey shows. *Mod Healthc.* 2005;35:30, 32–34, 36–38.
8. Carpenter D. Behind the boom. What's driving hospital construction? *Trustee.* 2004;57:6–11, 1.
9. Greene J. Climbing construction cost. *Hosp Health Netw.* 2006; 76–77.
10. Romano M. Through the roof. *Mod Healthc.* 2006;36:26–30.
11. Voyvodich ME, Pesce DS. Avoiding 'Builder's Remorse'—maximizing the value of your facilities investments. *Trustee.* 2005; 58:22–28.
12. Kauffman K. Best-practice capital allocation and financing. *Front Health Serv Manage.* 2004;21:33–36.
13. Goff DW. Planning and design health care facilities for maximum patient value. *J Acad Arch Health.* 2000;3.
14. Zuckerman AM. Health care strategic planning: Approaches for the 21st century. In: *ACHE management series.* Health Administration Press; 1998.
15. Grube ME. Strategic financial planning. What every trustee needs to know about facility replacement. *Trustee.* 2005;58:24–28, 30, 1.
16. Allison DJ. *Planning, design, and construction of health care environments.* The Joint Commission on Accreditation of Healthcare Organizations; 1997.
17. Hayward C. Health care facility planning: Thinking strategically. In: *ACHE management series.* Health Administration Press; 2006.
18. Capps DM. The impact of aging infrastructure and site on facility planning. *Healthc Facil Manag Ser.* 1993;1–9.
19. Hardy OB, Lammers LP. *Hospitals: the planning and design process,* 2nd ed. Aspen Publications; 1986.
20. Kabela R. Project /Pitfalls/: Nine common hospital planning mistakes. *Health Facil Manage.* 2006;19(7):39–44.
21. Kesler SP, Fagan D. Firm foundation. Successful facility expansion is built on robust MEP master planning. *Health Facil Manage.* 2005;18:31–33.
22. Woollard GW. *Functional and space programming.* 2006.
23. Axon DC. Medical facility planning 101: A primer for administrators and others. *J Acad Arch Health.* 2006;9.
24. Dubbs D. Taking charge: Keeping a tight rein on health facility construction costs. *Health Facil Manage.* 2002;15(2):16–19.
25. Stasiewicz PH. Basics of health facility commissioning. *Health Facil Manage Health Forum.* 2007.
26. Hill R. Hospital construction 101: Blueprints for success. *Nurs Manage.* 2005;36:46–51.
27. Chefurka T, Nesdoly F. Concepts in flexibility in health care facility planning. *J Acad Arch Health.* 2003.
28. Sadler BL. Designing with health in mind. Innovative design elements can make hospitals safer, more healing places. *Mod Healthc.* 2004;34:28.

29. Brown KK, Gallant D. Impacting patient outcomes through design: Acuity adaptable care/universal room design. *Crit Care Nurs Q*. 2006;29:326–341.

30. Ulrich RS Quan X, Zimring C, et al. The role of the physical environment in the hospital of the 21st century: A once-in-a-lifetime opportunity. In: *Designing the 21st century hospital project*. Princeton: Robert Wood Johnson Foundation; 2004.

31. Berry LL, Parker D, Coile RC Jr, et al. The business case for better buildings. *Front Health Serv Manage*. 2004;21:3–24.

32. American Institute Architects. AIA issues new guidelines for the design and construction of health care facilities. *Healthc Hazard Manage Monit*. 2006;20:1–6.

33. Cornwell EE III, Chang DC, Phillips J, et al. Enhanced trauma program commitment at a Level I trauma center: Effect on the process and outcome of care. *Arch Surg*. 2003;138:838–843.

34. Glasser BL. *Needs analysis and space programming. Health care planning and design for technology-driven "Super Departments": surgery, imaging and emergency*. 1999.

35. Coull A, Rostenberg B. *Planning concepts for surgical environments. Blurring the boundary: design and planning of imaging, interventional, and surgical environments*. 2003.

36. Friesen GA. Functional programming and planning for the operating suite: Location, traffic flow, supply lines. *Anesthesiology*. 1969;31:107–115.

37. Krupka DC, Sandberg WS. Operating room design and its impact on operating room economics. *Curr Opin Anaesthesiol*. 2006;19:185–191.

38. Cendan JC, Good M. Interdisciplinary work flow assessment and redesign decreases operating room turnover time and allows for additional caseload. *Arch Surg*. 2006;141:65–69, discussion 70.

39. Sandberg WS, Daily B, Egan M, et al. Deliberate perioperative systems design improves operating room throughput. *Anesthesiology*. 2005;103:406–418.

40. Haraden C, Resar R. Patient flow in hospitals: Understanding and controlling it better. *Front Health Serv Manage*. 2004;20:3–15.

41. Aliber J. Real numbers: Understanding square footages and building multipliers that work. *Health Facil Manage*. 2007;20:37–39.

42. Mathur NS. The next generation of operating rooms. *J Acad Arch Health*. 2005;8.

43. Gordon D. A state-of-the-future surgical platform at Memorial Sloan-Kettering Cancer Center. *J Acad Arch Health*. 2006.

44. Bardwell PL, Saba JL. Suite success: Applying 'universal' principles to surgical suites. *Health Facil Manage*. 2005;37–41.

45. Allo MD, Tedesco M. Operating room management: Operative suite considerations, infection control. *Surg Clin North Am*. 2005;85:1291–1297.

46. AORN Recommended Practices Subcommittee of the TPCC. Proposed recommended practices. Traffic patterns in the surgical suite. *Aorn J*. 1992;56:312–315.

47. Association of periOperative Registered Nurses. Recommended practices for traffic patterns in the peroperative practice setting. *Aorn J*. 2000;71:394–396.

48. Laufman H. Streamlining environmental safety in the operating room: A common bond between surgeons and hospital engineers. In: *Health care facilities management series*. American Society of Hospital Engineers of the American Hospital Association; 1994.

49. Sehulster L, Chinn RYW. *Guidelines for environmental infection control in health care facilities: recommendations of CDC and the Healthcare Infection Control Practices Advisory Committee (HICPAC)*. DoHaH Services; 2003.

50. Centers for Disease Control and Prevention. CDC report on environmental infection control. *Healthc Hazard Manage Monit*. 2003;17:1–8.

51. Pott PP, Scharf HP, Schwarz ML. Today's state of the art in surgical robotics*. *Comput Aided Surg*. 2005;10:101–132.

52. Surgical video systems. *Health Devices*. 2004;33:109–147.

53. Berci G, Phillips EH, Fujita F. The operating room of the future: What, when and why? *Surg Endosc*. 2004;18:1–5.

54. Camarillo DB, Krummel TM, Salisbury JK Jr. Robotic technology in surgery: Past, present, and future. *Am J Surg*. 2004; 188:2S–15S.

55. Coile RC Jr, Johnson T. Operating room of the future. *Russ Coiles Health Trends*. 2003;15:1, 4–6, 8.

56. Haugh R. The future is now for surgery suites. *Hosp Health Netw*. 2003;77:50–54, 2.

57. Herron DM, Gagner M, Kenyon TL, et al. The minimally invasive surgical suite enters the 21st century. A discussion of critical design elements. *Surg Endosc*. 2001;15:415–422.

58. Iseki H, Muragaki Y, Nakamura R, et al. Intelligent operating theater using intra-operative open-MRI. *Magn Reson Med Sci*. 2005;4:129–136.

59. Jolesz FA. Future perspectives for intra-operative MRI. *Neurosurg Clin N Am*. 2005;16:201–213.

60. Kavic MS. Robotics, technology, and the future of surgery. *JSLS*. 2000;4:277–279.

61. Kavic MS. Operating room design: "The devil is in the details". *JSLS*. 2001;5:297–298.

62. Rattner DW, Park A. Advanced devices for the operating room of the future. *Semin Laparosc Surg*. 2003;10:85–89.

63. Rostenberg B. 'Surgology' is coming! Designing for the convergence of surgery and interventional radiology. *Health Facil Manage*. 2005;18:49–52.

64. Satava RM. Future trends in the design and application of surgical robots. *Semin Laparosc Surg*. 2004;11:129–135.

65. Satava RM. The operating room of the future: Observations and commentary. *Semin Laparosc Surg*. 2003;10:99–105.

66. Satava RM. Emerging technologies for surgery in the 21st century. *Arch Surg*. 1999;134:1197–1202.

67. Reijnen MM, Zeebregts CJ, Meijerink WJ. Future of operating rooms. *Surg Technol Int*. 2005;14:21–27.

68. Goldman JM, Schrenker RA, Jackson JL, et al. Plug-and-play in the operating room of the future. *Biomed Instrum Technol*. 2005;39:194–199.

69. Miller T. Emerging from the twilight zone: Planning for future technology during renovation. *J Acad Arch Health*. 2004;7.

70. Ruskin KJ. Communication devices in the operating room. *Curr Opin Anaesthesiol*. 2006;19:655–659.

71. Cleary K, Clifford Mark, Stoianovici Dan, et al. Technology improvements for image-guided and minimally invasive spine procedures. *IEEE Trans Inf Technol Biomed*. 2002;6:249–261.

72. Holly LT, Foley KT. Intra-operative spinal navigation. *Spine*. 2003;28:S54–S61.

73. Merkle EM, Lewin JS, Liebenthal R, et al. The interventional MR imaging suite: Magnet designs and equipment requirements. *Magn Reson Imaging Clin N Am*. 2005;13:401–413.

74. ten Cate G, Fosse E, Hol PK, et al. Integrating surgery and radiology in one suite: A multicenter study. *J Vasc Surg*. 2004;40:494–499.

75. Vergnion M, Lambert JL. A protocol of trauma care in the emergency service including MDCT imaging. *Acta Anaesthesiol Belg*. 2006;57:249–252.

76. Merrell RC, Jarrell BE, Schenkman NS, et al. Telemedicine for the operating room of the future. *Semin Laparosc Surg*. 2003; 10:91–94.

77. Waldron M. *Planning for flexibility and efficiency. Health care planning and design for technology-driven "Super Departments": surgery, imaging and emergency*. 1999.

78. The peripheral corridor plan. *J Am Hosp Assoc*. 1969;43.

79. Jacobs RHJ. The surgical suite: Prototype designs reflect innovations in OR planning. *J Am Hosp Assoc*. 1969;43:124–130.

80. Rattner D. *The future of surgery: focus on minimally invasive technology. Health care planning and design for technology-driven "Super Departments": surgery, imaging and emergency*. 1999.

81. Bragg K, Vanbalen N, Cook N. Future trends in minimally invasive surgery. *Aorn J*. 2005;82:1006–1014, 1016–1018; quiz 1019–1022.

82. Gallagher AG, Smith CD. From the operating room of the present to the operating room of the future. Human-factors lessons learned from the minimally invasive surgery revolution. *Semin Laparosc Surg*. 2003;10:127–139.

83. Eckmann C, Olbrich G, Shekarriz H, et al. The empty OR-process analysis and a new concept for flexible and modular use in minimal invasive surgery. *Surg Technol Int*. 2003;11:45–49.

84. Kogut LE, Satko VA. Planning considerations for the minimally invasive surgical suite. *Healthcare Design*. 2006;57–60.

85. Holly LT. Image-guided spinal surgery. *Int J Med Robot.* 2006;2: 7–15.

86. Lipson AC, Gargollo PC, Black PM. Intra-operative magnetic resonance imaging: Considerations for the operating room of the future. *J Clin Neurosci.* 2001;8:305–310.

87. Liu H, Hall WA, Martin AJ, et al. MR-guided and MR-monitored neurosurgical procedures at 1.5 T. *J Comput Assist Tomogr.* 2000; 24:909–918.

88. Jolesz FA, Hynynen K. Magnetic resonance image-guided focused ultrasound surgery. *Cancer J.* 2002;8:S100–S112.

89. Murayama Y, Saguchi T, Ishibashi T, et al. Endovascular operating suite: Future directions for treating neurovascular disease. *J Neurosurg.* 2006;104:925–930.

90. Hastenteufel M, Yang S, Christoph C, et al. Image-based guidance for minimally invasive surgical atrial fibrillation ablation. *Int J Med Robot.* 2006;2:60–69.

91. Anderson DG. Image guidance in spinal surgery. *Instr Course Lect.* 2006;55:591–594.

92. Alexander E III. Optimizing brain tumor resection. Midfield interventional MR imaging. *Neuroimaging Clin N Am.* 2001;11: 659–672.

93. Maniscalco-Theberge ME, Elliott DC. Virtual reality, robotics, and other wizardry in 21st century trauma care. *Surg Clin North Am.* 1999;79:1241–1248.

94. Gehrki B. Key decisions in designing a new OR. *OR Manager.* 2002;18:15–18.

95. Ballantyne GH. Robotic surgery, telerobotic surgery, telepresence, and telementoring. Review of early clinical results. *Surg Endosc.* 2002;16:1389–1402.

96. McBeth PB, Louw DF, Rizun PR, et al. Robotics in neurosurgery. *Am J Surg.* 2004;188:68S–75S.

97. Mantwill F, Schulz AP, Faber A, et al. Robotic systems in total hip arthroplasty—is the time ripe for a new approach? *Int J Med Robot.* 2005;1:8–19.

98. Marescaux J, Rubino F. The ZEUS robotic system: Experimental and clinical applications. *Surg Clin North Am.* 2003;83: 1305–1315.

99. Hu PF, Xiao Y, Ho D, et al. Advanced visualization platform for surgical operating room coordination: Distributed video board system. *Surg Innov.* 2006;13:129–135.

100. Nagy P, George I, Bernstein W, et al. Radio frequency identification systems technology in the surgical setting. *Surg Innov.* 2006;13:61–67.

101. Brady JL. Inside the OR of the future. *Biomed Instrum Technol.* 2005;39:188–193.

102. Gehrki B. OR design and construction, Part 1. New Mayo ORs allow for rapid change. *OR Manager.* 2001;17:13–15, 19.

103. Pelczarski K. *Technology planning for surgical services in the 21st century. Health care planning and design for technology-driven "Super Departments": surgery, imaging and emergency.* 1999.

104. Caretsky W. *Engineering design for operating rooms. Blurring the boundary: design and planning of imaging, interventional, and surgical environments.* 2003.

105. Fischer AL. Medical lighting. *Biophotonics Int.* 2007;30–34.

106. Longo MC, Lockhart P. Structured cabling: Foundations for the future. *Healthc Inf Manage.* 1996;10:59–77.

107. Kish P. Structured cabling for health care networks. *Health Manag Technol.* 2006;27:76–77, 80–81.

108. Miller T. *Communications for the surgery department. Health care planning and design for technology-driven "Super Departments": surgery, imaging and emergency.* 1999.

Trauma Care, Medical-Legal Issues, and Risk Management

14

Sherry Morris   **Paul Kerr**

Medicine and law are two professions that frequently become necessarily intertwined. The practice of medicine is not only dictated by a strong understanding of science and the human body but also of the law. There are many issues that the trauma provider faces that can be simplified by involving a risk manager who is familiar with the state and federal laws that govern the practice of medicine. It is no longer good enough to just practice the best medicine you feel is applicable, you must also think about the standard of care set by your peers across the country and how the care you provide could carry you through a medical malpractice case.

There are many legal issues that will be part and parcel of relationships which physicians have with peers as well as with patients and their families. Knowledge of the applicable laws will assist in effective communication and help the physician feel more comfortable with practice decisions.

The information contained in this chapter is a sampling of some common legal issues you should be familiar with as a trauma physician. While it should be noted that laws vary from state to state, many of these issues are federal in nature and are applicable to all citizens of the United States. To familiarize yourself with state laws where you practice, contact your risk manager and ask for an informational session providing common areas specific to your geographic area.

THE ROLE OF THE RISK MANAGER

The successful risk manager must possess many of the same qualities as the successful trauma surgeon. Although the informational focus is dramatically different, the need for constant continuing education within the field and the overwhelming variety of areas of responsibility mandate that the risk manager stays updated on the happenings in the regulatory and legal community as it applies to medicine. The risk manager relies on the medical practitioner to paint an accurate medical picture and then relies on his or her own skill sets to perform legal analyses. The risk manager must be able to listen to and understand all of the information provided and use it to evaluate a situation and deliver a concise recommendation to the physician, administration, hospital staff, patient, or the health care decision maker. The risk manager must collaborate with the appropriate attorney to evaluate the situation and determine recommendation on the basis of past court decisions and legal evaluation. While the risk manager must know and be able to state the law for certain situations, an attorney may be necessary to determine how an unclear situation should be handled based on an analysis of relevant case law for the area.

As patients and their families take advantage of increased access to medical information through Internet searches, the questioning of physicians and the care they provide have become a daily part of medical diagnosis and treatment. Effective communication has long been a challenge for physicians and patients. The added element of scattered information gained from potentially unreliable Internet sources has made communication ever more complicated. In optimal situations, the informed patient is more aware of the options and able to better understand the treatment choices. Whatever the situation, communication with the patient is paramount to success as a physician. A patient who feels included in the decision-making process for his or her own health care and who feels informed throughout is generally a happier patient and one less likely to seek legal recourse in the event of an adverse outcome.

MEDICAL-LEGAL ISSUES THAT AFFECT TRAUMA CARE

Medical malpractice, related insurance costs, and tort reforms are factors that have entered into the trauma arena. Patients and their families are bombarded with advertisements from law firms promising money for medical wrongs. Many of these advertisements suggest that if a patient is injured or dies in a hospital, a medical provider must have done something wrong. Trauma facilities have certainly felt the impact of the litigious society the United States has become. Trauma providers, as well as many other medical specialists, have begun to practice defensive medicine and/or employ avoidance behavior. Avoidance behavior occurs when the medical specialist declines to provide trauma or emergency care because of the fear of litigation or fear of provoking an increase in the cost of malpractice insurance coverage. Defensive medicine occurs when diagnostic and therapeutic interventions go above and beyond what the practitioner feels is medically necessary for the treatment of a particular patient's complaints. In a research study performed by Harvard School of Public Health together with Columbia Law School and utilizing a professional survey organization, physicians who practice in Pennsylvania were asked to respond to a survey regarding defensive medicine. The survey found that 93% of the physicians surveyed reported that they sometimes practiced defensive medicine. The behaviors that defined defensive medicine for the purpose of this study included ordering more tests than medically indicated, prescribing more medications than medically indicated, referring patients to other specialists in unnecessary circumstances, suggesting invasive procedures to confirm diagnoses, and avoiding certain procedures or interventions.[1]

In each of these, and many other ways, the law has entered into the decision-making arena for health care providers. Even the most careful practitioner will face difficult legal dilemmas but armed with the proper knowledge, will handle the situation with confidence.

EMERGENCY MEDICAL TREATMENT AND ACTIVE LABOR ACT

Patient Scenario

A 31-year-old female presented to a small community hospital following an all terrain vehicle (ATV) accident. She was hypotensive and was complaining of abdominal pain. A computed tomography (CT) scan was performed and showed bleeding in her abdomen. The on-call surgeon for the emergency room (ER) was called. The surgeon for the community hospital did not come in to see the patient but told the staff to transfer her to a trauma center.

The ER physician at the community hospital phoned the trauma center's transfer center and reported the patient's condition to the trauma surgeon for transfer acceptance. The trauma surgeon said that he would be happy to take the patient as a transfer but that she needed to be hemodynamically stable before she could be transported. He expressed concern that she would die in transport with the reported vital signs. He said that the surgeon needed to come in to the community hospital, take her to the operating room (OR), and pack her abdomen with laparotomy sponges.

The surgeon at the community hospital called back to say that he wanted to transfer the patient and refused to take her to the OR. He stated that he did not have the proper equipment to perform the surgery because of not having a rapid infuser. The trauma surgeon had no choice but to send the trauma center flight team to transport the patient from the community hospital at that point and attempt to get her to the trauma center quickly enough to save her. The patient was brought to the trauma facility and expired before she could be taken to the OR.

What action was required by the small community hospital prior to transporting the patient? Did that facility violate Emergency Medical Treatment and Active Labor Act (EMTALA)?

The federal EMTALA was passed in 1986 in an effort to stop ERs from turning patients away based on their ability to pay. The materialization of the law was due to a public outcry rooted from the experiences of two distinct patients who were deemed victims of patient dumping.

The first, Eugene Barnes, was a 32-year-old unemployed mechanic who was stabbed in the head and suffered a gaping wound. He stumbled for a couple of blocks and then collapsed in front of a crowd and was taken by ambulance to Brookside Hospital in San Pablo, California. The emergency department at Brookside Hospital had an on-call neurosurgeon. He was called but he refused to assume care of the patient. The ER physician called a second neurosurgeon (this one was not on call) who also refused to take the patient. The ER physician then called another county hospital and asked the neurosurgeon there to take over care of the patient. That neurosurgeon said that he was too tired to appropriately care for this patient and could not accept him. Another hospital was contacted but it also refused to take Barnes as a patient. Finally, approximately 4 hours after his arrival, Barnes was transferred to San Francisco General Hospital. He immediately went to surgery but died 3 days later. News crews began investigating the story before he was even transferred and the series of events became national news.[2]

The second patient to have a serious impact on the creation of EMTALA was Sharon Ford, a young woman who was in active labor and reported to Brookside Hospital to deliver her baby. She arrived at the emergency department and gave her insurance information to a nurse. On the basis of her insurance information, she was transferred to Samuel Merritt Hospital because this institution had been identified as the indigent care facility which handled the bulk of the Medicaid births. Ms. Ford left Brookside Hospital and drove to Samuel Merritt Hospital. Unfortunately, due to a paperwork error, she was not on the list of insured for her Medicaid program. After an examination determining that she was indeed in active labor and consultation with the on-call obstetrician, she was again referred to another hospital. She was sent to Highlands General Hospital, Oakland's county hospital. Soon after arriving at Highlands General, she delivered a stillborn infant.[2]

During this time frame, the press seized upon the issue and touted stories of the many Americans who were injured or died as a result of this practice, dubbed "patient dumping." Emergency departments became newsworthy not for helping those in need of medical care but for neglecting the needs of the uninsured. The public cried out for change and the United States Congress heard their plea.[3]

The original legislation on this issue, as it was introduced to the Congress, was quite punitive and included criminal charges for a physician who caused harm to a patient as a consequence of a transfer. Upon its ultimate passing, it was less stringent but still forceful. "One of the most important pieces of health care legislation in the history of our country would be tucked away in the Consolidated Omnibus Budget Reconciliation Act of 1985 as Section 9121, "Examination and Treatment for Emergency Medical Conditions and Women in Active Labor Act." President Reagan signed the bill into law on April 7, 1986. Effective August 1, 1986, any person presenting to an acute care hospital with an emergency department would have a legal right to health care.[2]"

For the trauma surgeon, EMTALA plays a part almost exclusively with regard to patient transfers received at the trauma facility. The transferring physician or surgeon at the transferring facility has a legal obligation to stabilize the patient before sending them to another center for a higher level of care. According to the wording of the EMTALA, the emergency department staff must take "whatever medical measures are available and necessary to ensure that the individual's medical condition will not materially deteriorate during or as a result of transfer from the facility.[2]"

This fact adds to the complexity of the transfer process for injured patients because "stabilization" may mean a major procedure such as laparotomy or thoracotomy to achieve hemostasis if the patient is actively bleeding. The reluctance of specialty surgeons to take on the task of stabilizing an acutely injured patient is a major factor stimulating transfer of unstable patients. For the accepting trauma surgeon, it is imperative that the best interests of the patient remain in the forefront. It is appropriate to ask the transferring physician or surgeon to attempt hemostasis. On the other hand, if the expected elapsed time to achieve hemostasis exceeds the evacuation time to the trauma center, rapid evacuation with resuscitation in progress is indicated.

It is important to understand the obligations of the transferring facility when discussing patient care and transfer with the physicians involved at the outlying facility.

EMTALA applies to all hospitals with an emergency department that participate in a federal contract to provide Medicare services.[4] This, of course, means that almost all emergency departments are mandated to follow these directives. Emergency departments are required to screen all patients who request treatment (the request can come from the patient, another person for the patient, or by actions of the patient that would cause a lay person to recognize that the patient needed treatment) for an emergency medical condition. Emergency medical condition is defined as "when the absence of immediate medical attention may be expected to result in the patient's death or serious harm to either a major bodily function or body part.[2]

EMTALA mandates that a hospital that has an emergency department and determines that a patient has an emergency medical condition must treat that patient within the capacity of that facility. This includes any ancillary service that would routinely be available to a patient in that emergency department. The patient must either be stabilized in that emergency department or transferred to another facility according to the established guidelines. The appropriate transfer is described as follows:

Appropriate transfer—An appropriate transfer to a medical facility is a transfer—

(A) *in which the transferring hospital provides the medical treatment within its capacity, which minimizes the risks to the individual's health and, in the case of a woman in labor, the health of the unborn child;*
(B) *in which the receiving facility–*
   (i) *has available space and qualified personnel for the treatment of the individual, and*
   (ii) *has agreed to accept transfer of the individual and to provide appropriate medical treatment;*
(C) *in which the transferring hospital sends to the receiving facility all medical records (or copies thereof), related to the emergency condition for which the individual has presented, available at the time of the transfer, including records*

related to the individual's emergency medical condition, observations of signs or symptoms, preliminary diagnosis, treatment provided, results of any tests and the informed written consent or certification (or copy thereof) provided under paragraph (1)(A), and the name and address of any on-call physician who refused or failed to appear within a reasonable time to provide necessary stabilizing treatment;

(D) in which the transfer is effected through qualified personnel and transportation equipment, as required, including the use of necessary and medically appropriate life-support measures during transfer; and

(E) which meets such other requirements as the Secretary may find necessary in the interest of the health and safety of individuals transferred.[5]

The Department of Health and Human Services issued interpretive guidelines in 1998 that helped define some of the standards for EMTALA. They defined what a surveyor would look at while investigating if a patient transfer was appropriate by saying that the investigator would look in the medical record to find evidence that: "The receiving hospital had agreed in advance to accept transfers; the receiving hospital had received appropriate medical records; all transfers had been effected through qualified personnel, transportation equipment, and medically appropriate life support measures; and the receiving hospital had available space and qualified personnel to treat the patient.[6]"

Hospitals and physicians alike are responsible for following the mandates of EMTALA. Those who do not may find themselves facing a fine of up to $50,000. If the violation is extremely worrisome, the Centers for Medicare and Medicaid Services (CMS) may decide to terminate the participation of the provider or facility in Medicare. Of course, the patient injured by the EMTALA violation may also sue the physician and facility involved in their care.

HEALTHCARE INSURANCE PORTABILITY AND ACCOUNTABILITY ACT

A patient's right to privacy and confidentiality has long been understood by the medical profession. The Oath of Hippocrates states: "What I may see or hear in the course of the treatment or even outside of the treatment in regard to the life of men, which on no account must be spread abroad, I will keep to myself, holding such things shameful to be spoken approximately.[7]" A physician, by virtue of his or her role, must be given access to a patient's most personal information.

The patient–physician relationship relies upon the patient being honest and open with the physician so that the very best diagnosis can be attained. If there was not a promise of confidentiality when giving information to a physician, many people would not give the most personal

information nor would they report certain symptoms accurately. To have the best opportunity for complete medical care, patients must feel completely confident that the physician will hold their information confidentially.

The importance of confidentiality has never been more important nor more difficult to ensure than it is currently. In this electronic age where medical information is easily accessed through computer by health care providers, protecting the information from the public is quite a challenge. Physicians, working with many patients in limited time, also find themselves discussing patient information in public areas. This is one of the most common and least acceptable violations of a patient's confidentiality. Care must be taken when discussing or electronically transferring any information regarding patient care.

The federal government recognized the additional hazards of the information era and enacted the Healthcare Insurance Portability and Accountability Act (HIPAA) in 2003. HIPAA regulations bind all practitioners and health care facilities that practice in the United States and transmit health information electronically. HIPAA actually defines the protected health information (PHI) as "individually identifiable health information that is transmitted by or maintained in any other form or medium, and that relates to past, present, or future physical or mental health or conditions of an individual; the provision of health care to an individual; or the payment from the provision of health care.[8]"

Each facility has developed a means to follow HIPAA regulations and can most likely offer assistance to physicians in establishing their own HIPAA provisions.

Advance Directives

The Patient Self Determination Act of 1990 (which did not become effective until December 1991) mandated that a patient be informed of the treatments being offered as well as the risks, benefits, and alternatives available to them. The Patient Self Determination Act requires that facilities provide to patients information regarding their rights under applicable state law to make decisions concerning their medical care. Such care includes the right to accept or refuse medical or surgical treatment, and the right to formulate advance directives.[9]

Advance directives amount to written or verbal instructions that will become effective at the time when the patients can no longer speak for themselves. As long as these instructions are drafted according to the appropriate state law, they should be honored by health care providers without fear of legal action from the patients' family members.

A living will is one type of advance directive. It allows a patient to document the amount and types of care they want in particular medical conditions. A living will is defined as "an instrument, signed with the formalities necessary for a will, by which a person states the intention to refuse medical treatment and to release health care providers from all liability if the person becomes both terminally ill and unable to communicate such a refusal."[10] Living wills also allow a patient's family to follow wishes without second guessing that it is truly what the patient wanted. The use of a living will makes end-of-life decisions easier for everyone involved. Most importantly, the patient receives only the treatment he or she desired to have.

The durable power of attorney and naming of a health care surrogate are other types of advance directives. Each of these documents allows patients to name another person to substitute for them and make health care decisions in their stead. If patients are unable to decide for themselves, the named party has the duty, if they accept, to make the decision they feel the patient would have made in the same situation.

The absence of advance directives creates a situation in which the physicians must rely on someone to make the health care decisions for the patient. In many states, the law allows for the automatic appointment of a health care proxy from an ordered list of family members, some including personal friends at the end of the list.

A Patient's Right to Refuse

Patient Scenario

A patient presents to the ER via ambulance. He is a 35-year-old male who had just been ejected from a motor vehicle and thrown about 100 feet. His injuries include a C4-C5 fracture resulting quadriplegia, some left rib fractures, a left clavicle fracture, left humeral fracture, and a left hemothorax. After initial stabilization, the patient decides that he will not allow any nursing or medical care. He refuses to be turned or cleaned and, over time, develops large decubitus ulcers. He lies in stool for days at a time and even refuses vital signs most days. Upon examination by psychiatry he is deemed competent to make his own decisions.

He develops the beginnings of pneumonia and an infection in his sacral decubitus ulcer. Still, he refuses to allow care. What are the rights of the patient versus the obligations of the care providers?

A patient has the right to be informed of the risks and benefits of proposed medical care and then determine if they wish to have that particular treatment. Informed consent is a process that physicians participate in every day that they practice. Each time an intervention is chosen, it should be explained to the patient and the patient given an opportunity to accept or decline that treatment. It is when the patient decides against a treatment that will sustain their lives that we resist the process. These rights are guaranteed by the Patient Self Determination Act as well as past court cases.

In some instances, criminal charges could also be filed against a health care provider who performs a treatment against a patient's will. A patient has a right to tell another person not to touch his or her body. An unwanted touch could result in a criminal conviction for the provider.

In most situations, the decision to refuse care will not mimic the patient scenario given in the preceding text. Rather, the refusal will usually be in the form of withholding or withdrawing a life-sustaining treatment such as ventilator support, nutrition, or hydration. These issues have been hotly debated in the courts and have always ended up siding with the patient's, or their designee's, right to decide.

One of the most important cases in the patient's rights issue was that of Nancy Cruzan. This case was decided in 1990. Ms. Cruzan was in a persistent vegetative state after sustaining a brain injury from a motor vehicle crash. Her parents wanted to refuse treatment for her by having her nutrition and hydration withheld, thereby effectuating her death. The State and the family battled, and eventually the case wound up in front of the US Supreme Court. In the Cruzan versus the Director of the Missouri Department of Health case, the US Supreme Court said that competent adults have a common-law right to refuse medical treatment or to have unwanted treatment withdrawn. The Supreme Court Justices based this decision on a person's constitutional right to liberty.[11]

More recently, the case of Theresa Marie Schiavo[12] captured the attention of the medical and legal communities as well as the nation. Ms. Schiavo was also in a persistent vegetative state after a brain injury. Her husband's court battle to withdraw her life-sustaining treatment is one that made history in the legal system as the government stepped in and attempted to alter the law as an emotional response to the issue. This case also caused great confusion in the medical community when the court issued a ruling that a medical procedure be completed and then a different court ruling that the same procedure be withdrawn. The end result of that case was that the law remained as it had been. In general, patients and/or their decision makers have the right to decide what medical treatments they wish to have performed and how long they wish to have those treatments. Certainly, it is wise to involve risk management when there are potential conflicts regarding this issue.

There are exceptions to the rule for a patient's right to refuse care. The state's interest in a minor can preclude parents from deciding to withhold care for their child before the child can make decisions. An example of this situation is a Jehovah's Witness child who is severely injured and needs a blood transfusion but the parents refuse on the basis of their religious beliefs. If you encounter a situation in which your patient is a minor and the parents are refusing care that could result in the patient's death, you should involve the risk manager to help sort out the legal action that may become necessary to resolve the dilemma.

Another example of a situation in which the patient's wishes may not be followed would be a pregnant woman who elected to refuse treatment. The state could step in and protect the unborn child and force treatment upon the mother.[13] Again, this would require the assistance of risk management along with attorneys from the state.

Medical Futility

Patient Scenario

A patient presents to the ER via air transport. He is a 19-year-old male who had just been in a motor vehicle accident while involved in a police chase after stealing a car. He was the unrestrained driver and was ejected from the vehicle. He came to the ER with a Glasgow Coma Score of 15 and was initially hemodynamically stable. His workup is notable for a right talar fracture, right rib fractures, right pulmonary contusion, and an aortic transection picked up on CT angiogram.

He is stabilized and then taken to the OR for a thoracotomy and repair of the transected aorta including a femoral-femoral bypass. His orthopaedic injuries are also addressed at that time.

He is taken back to the OR several times over the next few days to address hypotension and cold legs. He has a reexploration of his left thoracotomy, right common femoral artery repair, axillofemoral bypass, right femoral thrombectomy, popliteal exploration, popliteal balloon thrombectomy, and facetectomies of the right lower extremity. Within a week of arrival, he has a right above-the-knee amputation performed due to vascular insufficiency in the area. After all of these surgeries, he developed acute renal failure. He is intubated and rarely able to follow any direction. His parents are jointly making his medical decisions.

His left lower extremity begins to show signs of ischemia and then necrosis, followed by wet gangrene. His parents are approached about amputation of his left leg and told that his prognosis is not good. They opt to decline the amputation even though the infection has now caused him to go into multiple organ failure. The line of demarcation from the infection is just below the umbilicus and pieces of his left leg are falling off during cleaning and examining. The patient is now on continuous venovenous hemodialysis (CVVHD) and multiple antibiotics for his infection. His parents are threatening the staff touting such statements as "If our son dies, I will make sure you die too."

There were no medical interventions that would change the condition of this young man. He was literally rotting in his hospital bed. His parents are demanding that no interventions be taken away and that he remain a full code. The patient now has gangrene in his left arm and has fingers falling off with examination.

The entire medical team believes that the only compassionate care for this patient would be to remove him from life support. His parents would not hear of it and involve an attorney to ensure that it is clear that there was to be no removal of life support and that the patient would remain a full code.

Everyone agrees that medical care is futile at this point except the patient's parents who are making his medical decisions. What are the appropriate actions for the trauma physician to take? Do the rights of the parents to make health care decisions for their son outweigh the medical opinion of the health care providers?

The right of patients to refuse care has been clearly delineated by the courts in the United States, but a patient's right to demand treatment when such treatment will be futile or ineffective is still unclear. The importance of open and honest communication between patient/family and medical providers is never more evident than when disagreements arise over end-of-life care. Patients and their families must have trust in their physician and the care provided in order to accept a message of futility and agree with the determination.

Futility is a term that medical scholars have struggled to define in a manner that can translate to the legal arena. Because futility is a concept that applies to particular situations differently, it cannot be adequately defined in such a way that it would not be the responsibility of the physician to make a unilateral declaration of the futility in the situation.

Professional associations began promoting futility policies in the 1990s. The American Medical Association recommended that facilities of all sizes should adopt a policy for medical futility.[14] Many facilities have followed this advice and adopted futility policies but they lack the backing of the courts at this point. The number of cases that have actually been heard by a court is small and none of the decisions have done much to help define what the duty of the physician will ultimately be.

Texas legislature adopted Section 166.046 of the Texas Advance Directives Act titled "Procedure if not effectuating a directive or treatment decision," in an attempt to answer many of the questions faced by medical providers and patients/families when futility comes into question. Under the directive of this statute, the facility must institute a series of steps when there is a disagreement between the treating physician and patient/family regarding futility of the patient's situation. The steps are outlined in the statute as follows:

§ *166.046. PROCEDURE IF NOT EFFECTUATING A DIRECTIVE OR TREATMENT DECISION.*

(a) *If an attending physician refuses to honor a patient's advance directive or a health care or treatment decision made by or on behalf of a patient, the physician's refusal shall be reviewed by an ethics or medical committee. The attending physician may not be a member of that committee. The patient shall be given life-sustaining treatment during the review.*

(b) *The patient or the person responsible for the health care decisions of the individual who has made the decision regarding the directive or treatment decision:*

    (1) *may be given a written description of the ethics or medical committee review process and any other policies and procedures related to this section adopted by the health care facility;*

    (2) *shall be informed of the committee review process not less than 48 hours before the meeting called to discuss the patient's directive, unless the time period is waived by mutual agreement;*

(3) at the time of being so informed, shall be provided:
  (A) a copy of the appropriate statement set forth in Section 166.052; and
  (B) a copy of the registry list of health care providers and referral groups that have volunteered their readiness to consider accepting transfer or to assist in locating a provider willing to accept transfer that is posted on the website maintained by the Texas Health Care Information Council under Section 166.053; and
(4) is entitled to:
  (A) attend the meeting; and
  (B) receive a written explanation of the decision reached during the review process.

(c) The written explanation required by Subsection (b)(2)(B) must be included in the patient's medical record.

(d) If the attending physician, the patient, or the person responsible for the health care decisions of the individual does not agree with the decision reached during the review process under Subsection (b), the physician shall make a reasonable effort to transfer the patient to a physician who is willing to comply with the directive. If the patient is a patient in a health care facility, the facility's personnel shall assist the physician in arranging the patient's transfer to:
  (1) another physician;
  (2) an alternative care setting within that facility; or
  (3) another facility.

(e) If the patient or the person responsible for the health care decisions of the patient is requesting life-sustaining treatment that the attending physician has decided and the review process has affirmed is inappropriate treatment, the patient shall be given available life-sustaining treatment pending transfer under Subsection (d). The patient is responsible for any costs incurred in transferring the patient to another facility. The physician and the health care facility are not obligated to provide life-sustaining treatment after the 10th day after the written decision required under Subsection (b) is provided to the patient or the person responsible for the health care decisions of the patient unless ordered to do so under Subsection (g).

(e-1) If during a previous admission to a facility a patient's attending physician and the review process under Subsection (b) have determined that life-sustaining treatment is inappropriate, and the patient is readmitted to the same facility within six months from the date of the decision reached during the review process conducted upon the previous admission, Subsections (b) through (e) need not be followed if the patient's attending physician and a consulting physician who is a member of the ethics or medical committee of the facility document on the patient's readmission that the patient's condition either has not improved or has deteriorated since the review process was conducted.

(f) Life-sustaining treatment under this section may not be entered in the patient's medical record as medically unnecessary treatment until the time period provided under Subsection (e) has expired.

(g) At the request of the patient or the person responsible for the health care decisions of the patient, the appropriate district or county court shall extend the time period provided under Subsection (e) only if the court finds, by a preponderance of the evidence, that there is a reasonable expectation that a physician or health care facility that will honor the patient's directive will be found if the time extension is granted.[15]

Since this piece of legislation was passed, it has been utilized by many hospitals throughout Texas. Although many situations made it to the ethics/medical committee stage, an agreement was usually reached between the families and health care providers at this stage. Therefore, the legality of the Act was not tested for some time. The first legal test came from Texas Medical Center in Houston in the winter of 2004–2005.[16]

The first case was regarding Sun Hudson, a child born with thanatophoric dysplasia, a rare and fatal form of neonatal dwarfism. The physicians established the diagnosis and then explained to the infant's mother that his condition was fatal and recommended that the life-sustaining treatments be withdrawn. The procedure for futility was started. The infant's mother sued the hospital and asked for an extension as allowed by the statute. The court declined her request reasoning that it was not an expectation that another provider would be willing to continue treatment on this child. The hospital was allowed to withdraw support and the infant died.[16]

The second case was regarding Spiro Nikolouzos, a 68-year-old man who had been an invalid since 2001, when he experienced bleeding related to a shunt in his brain. He was taken to the hospital in February 2005 with bleeding around his feeding tube. While in the hospital, his condition deteriorated and his physicians recommended that life-sustaining treatment be withdrawn. Mrs. Nikolouzos refused and the futility process began. Mrs. Nikolouzos asked the court to grant her an extension of the 10-day waiting period. The court refused saying that there was not sufficient evidence that the family would be able to effectuate the transfer if granted the extension. Mrs. Nikolouzos appealed and received the same outcome. She was able to have her husband transferred to a nursing home during the 10-day period and he lived there for another 3 months before dying.[16]

Although the Texas Advance Directives Act is a beginning to answering the medical futility issue, there is a long way to go before there is a nationally acceptable standard. Because this Act is challenged and modified, it will lead to a clearer path for physicians, facilities, and patients/families alike.

Disclosure of Errors

Communication with patients has long been an issue for medical practitioners. The trauma service, by nature, is the most difficult area to effectuate solid communication and trust of the patient. The trauma patient is usually seen by more than just the trauma service. It can be very confusing to the patient to see so many physicians and not know who to report what issues to. Open and honest communication with the patient and their family, as necessary, will help build trust in their providers. Especially during the unexpected and often catastrophic injury of a trauma admission, the patient and family need to have trust in their physician and the care being provided to them. This trust and open communication could mean a world of difference in the event of an adverse incident. Regularly scheduled meetings with the patient, the family, and/or representatives of the patient and family are an effective means of establishing consistent communication links.

When it comes to medical errors, hospitals and medical professionals have created an environment that is embedded with silence because of the fear of potential litigation, bad press, and reporting of the medical professionals to a state agency. Physicians have been taught not to discuss errors openly by their educational facilities, the hospitals in which they practice, their insurance companies, and their own legal counsel. These teachings will have to be overcome and physicians will ultimately have to learn the art of apology.

The public interest in medical errors came into the national spotlight in 1999 with the Institute of Medicine report "To Err is Human: Building a Safer Health System," which stated that approximately 48,000 to 98,000 patients die each year as a result of medical errors that occur in hospitals.[17] Those statistics outnumbered the fatalities for automobile accidents in the United States at that time. Those statistics also state that more people die from preventable medical errors in 6 months in the United States than the people lost in the entire Vietnam War.[18]

As a result of the public outcry, the Joint Commission for the Accreditation of Healthcare Organizations (JCAHO) passed a directive in 2001 (Standard RI 2:90) mandating that there will be disclosure to patients of unanticipated outcomes. "The JCAHO standards encourage clear, objective communication within the team of caregivers, as well as with the patient and family. This includes verbal notification of an unanticipated outcome, discussion of plan of care issues and changes, and documentation of the key points of those conversations.[19]"

Five states have now passed mandatory disclosure laws echoing the JCAHO mandate. Nevada enacted NRS §439.855 in 2004; Florida enacted F.S. §395.1051 in 2004, Pennsylvania enacted 40 P.S. §1303.308 (b) in 2004; New Jersey enacted N.J.S. §26:2H-12.25 in 2005, and Vermont enacted Vermont §310 in 2006. Each of these pieces of legislation involves mandatory notification of adverse events to patients.

The state of Illinois was the first to adopt a disclosure program to assist physicians and facilities alike in the difficult task of saying "I'm sorry." The program, titled "Sorry Works" was part of a medical liability reform bill (Illinois Senate Bill 472) and was passed in May 2005. This bill included a benefit for providers making a health care provider's apology nondiscoverable in court.[20] This law allows physicians to express their apology to a patient and/or their family members without worrying about their own words being used against them in court. This was the first step in creating a nonpunitive arena for open communication between a physician and their patient.

The Sorry Works! Coalition (http://www.sorryworks .net) believes that "apologies for medical errors, along with up-front compensation, reduce anger of patients and families, which leads to a reduction in medical malpractice lawsuits and associated defense litigation expenses.[21]"

How exactly does "sorry" work? The coalition advocates that after every bad outcome or adverse event, providers (in conjunction with their insurer and risk management team) should perform root cause analyses to determine if the standard of care was met. This process may take weeks to months and may involve the assistance of outside experts.

If the root cause analysis shows that the standard of care was not met through medical error or negligence, the providers (and their insurers) apologize to the patient or family, admit fault, provide an explanation of what happened and how the hospital will fix the procedures so the error is not repeated, and make a fair offer of up-front compensation (as determined by an actuary or qualified party). The attorney(s) representing the providers and plaintiffs' attorney usually negotiate the compensation, and the case is usually closed in a few months.

If, however, the standard of care was met—there was no medical error or negligence—the providers and their legal counsel still meet with the patient/family and their attorney(s) and explain what happened, apologize, and offer empathy but do not admit fault or provide up-front compensation. The providers open and explain medical charts, answer all questions, and basically prove their innocence. However, the providers do not settle or offer compensation for a nonmeritorious claim, and the hospital and insurer fight all charges when their doctors committed no error.[8]

Sorry Works! has been in existence since February 2005. Currently, 21 states have adopted some form of an apology law. It is unclear if the benefit of excluding these expressions of apology helps in jury trials or if there is greater benefit in showing the jury that the medical practitioner was concerned about the patient and was honest about the accident.

Since the inception of a full-disclosure program at the University of Michigan Hospital System in 2001, the number of lawsuits has dropped to half of what they were. They also claim a reduction in litigation costs "from an average of $65,000 per case to $35,000 per case, resulting in a total average annual savings of $2 million.[22]" Officials at the University of Michigan are careful to point out that the apology is only part of the process. The process must be carefully and thoughtfully set up and followed by all members of the health care team.

THE ANATOMY OF A TRAUMA LAWSUIT

A lawsuit is a process that one person (usually a patient for medical malpractice claims) uses to establish a legal obligation from another (the health care provider) to be compensated for a loss. The procedural systems used vary from state to state but all include the same basic components. Some states have adopted tort reform to cap the noneconomic damages that can be awarded for a single claim. Many other states are fighting for this reform because malpractice insurance rates are skyrocketing for many providers.

Negligence Theory

Pending litigation is not something physicians like to discuss with each other or anyone else for that matter. Being involved in a lawsuit makes anyone uncomfortable. For the most part, trauma surgeons will be involved in professional liability claims. This type of claim is also called *medical malpractice* or a *negligence claim*. The negligence claim usually involves allegations that the practitioner (known as the *defendant in the court system*) acted negligently in the care of the patient (known as the *plaintiff in the court system*) and that the negligence that caused physical harm. Negligence is generally known to be a departure from the standard of care by the health care provider. This departure can be either by an act or an omission of action. Negligence claims are filed in the civil court system and usually under the state law jurisdiction, although occasionally they can fall under federal law jurisdiction.

A negligence claim must meet a four-part criteria in order to successfully file with the court system. The four parts that constitute a negligence claim are duty, breach of the duty, injury, and damages.

Duty: One person must be under a duty to another person (or to society) before negligence becomes an issue. In the context of professional liability, duty usually attaches when the provider undertakes to care for the patient.

Breach of the duty: The person under the duty must breach the duty in some way (such as allowing a hazard to exist) to allow negligence to attach.

Injury: The plaintiff must suffer an injury as a result of the defendant's breach of duty. If the injury did not arise out of the breach of the duty, the plaintiff may not be able to prove causation, which is also a key element in negligence.

Damages: The plaintiff must be able to show legally cognizable damages as a result of the injury sustained. Damages typically include pain and suffering (sometimes capped by tort reform efforts), medical expenses, lost wages, emotional distress, loss of consortium or companionship, and so on.[23]

In the patient scenario given in the preceding text, it is easy to establish duty. This is usually the case with trauma cases as the trauma surgeon who is on duty at the time the patient enters the ER is usually the person who directs the patient's care and is clearly indicated in the medical record. The moment a patient–physician relationship is initiated, the physician owes a duty to the patient to treat them appropriately.

The second component, breach of the duty, is not as easy to allege. This area of the negligence theory is determined by the accepted standard of care. Standard of care is measured by "the degree of care and skill possessed by other physicians within the same or similar circumstances.[6]" There is no clear definition of the standard of care for each situation that comes before the court. The court relies on affidavits and testimony from expert witnesses to establish this aspect of the case.

The injury to the patient is usually ascertained from the medical record. Many times the plaintiff will have to undergo independent medical examinations to evaluate the permanency and/or accuracy of the injury as it is being alleged. Causation is also a part of this element. Causation is a hotly debated area in most cases. The plaintiff must prove that the alleged breach of duty by the defendant actually caused the injuries being claimed in the case. To prove causation, the plaintiff must hire an expert physician who is of the opinion that the breach of duty by the practitioner was, indeed, the cause of the injury.

Damages are quantified by the amount of money that the plaintiff seeks to compensate for their injury and the associated losses by the injured party or their family members. There are economic and noneconomic damage claims attached to most claims. Loss of consortium is defined as "A loss of the interests that one spouse is entitled to receive from the other, including companionship, cooperation, affection, and sexual relations." Loss of consortium can be recoverable as damages in a person injury or wrongful death action.[10]

The Legal Process

The legal process varies from state to state and the requirements for particular documents and time frames differ greatly. Generally, the plaintiff's attorney will evaluate the claim and have it reviewed by a physician to determine if there was a departure from the standard of care. If it is determined that the case has merit, the attorney will proceed with litigation. In some states, the plaintiff is required to give notification to the defendant of a potential lawsuit. This notification is called a *Notice of Intent* to file litigation. At this point in the case, there have been no documents filed with the court and there is no formal lawsuit. An investigative time frame is assigned to each side after the date of this filing to determine the validity of the claim and the manner in which to proceed.

The initiation of the actual lawsuit comes with the filing of the summons and complaint. This document is actually filed with the court and marks the time that the case becomes a formal litigation. The complaint document indicates the exact allegations from the plaintiff, the exact date of injury, and the circumstances surrounding it that the plaintiff feels indicate the failures on the part of the defendant(s). Upon receipt of the complaint, the defendant must seek legal counsel to have the complaint answered in the allotted time. As part of the answer to the complaint, the defendant is required to either admit or deny the claim. There are some circumstances in which the defendant's counsel will file a motion to have the case dismissed from the court process. One such situation would be a statute of limitation defense.

One of the most important factors in determining whether a lawsuit can be filed is the statute of limitation. This is the time period after the injury in which the court will allow legal action to be filed against the practitioner. This time period varies from state to state and some states offer a much longer time period for minors who suffer an injury. The general time frame is approximately 2 years from the date of injury. The first thing a defendant must check when a lawsuit is filed is whether the plaintiff has timely filed the claim with the court.

The next phase of the process is referred to as the *discovery phase*. During this phase, the plaintiff and defendant investigate the validity of the claim. Both sides use this time to gather facts and documents that are in the possession of the opposing side. Information is gathered by using interrogatories "lists of questions to be answered in writing and under oath,[2]" requesting the production of documents, and taking depositions. During this phase, there are usually settlement discussions and sometimes mediation. Mediation is a meeting between the plaintiff and defendant(s) and a neutral third party in which settlement is negotiated. Some states require that a case go through mediation before it can be placed on the trial docket.

Jury trial is the last phase of the litigation process and often occurs more than a year after the original filing of the case. A medical malpractice trial can last from a few days to a few weeks depending on the number of witnesses and depth of the expert testimony. A jury of lay people are gathered together to hear both the plaintiff and defendant present their version of the case. The jury is asked to evaluate the evidence presented to them and to decide a finding of liability or no liability. They also decide the amount of money awarded to the plaintiff, if any.

"Depending on the verdict, either the plaintiff or the defendant may allege errors that the trial that constitute grounds for appeal to a higher court.[2]" After the appeal is filed, an appellate court will read the appeal brief, which lays out the perceived error by the court and the trial court transcripts. There will generally be oral arguments also, but they are usually only attended by the attorneys from each side. The appellate court will review the information and determine if the trial judge committed a reversible error or not. Sometimes an entirely new trial at the trial court level is ordered.

Medical Liability and Litigation for Trauma Surgeons

Litigation is one of the most stressful experiences a medical provider will confront. Even the most careful and caring providers in the profession can be involved in malpractice litigation. The fear and misunderstanding of this situation as it pertains to trauma has driven some out of the service and forced some facilities to close or let go of their trauma designation. It is important to understand the realities of litigation in the United States as it pertains to trauma providers and to medicine in general.

Is there a higher medical malpractice risk for a trauma surgeon based simply on the nature of the patient population? This is a question posed by many in the trauma community and one that is not easily answered. Most hospitals and providers hold their liability claim information confidentially for fear of public reaction if the information was available. There have, however, been two studies specific to the reality of medical liability as it relates to trauma.

The first, from the University of Michigan, looked at general surgery/trauma specifically and determined the types of cases, the number of cases performed, and the outcome of these cases for their study results. They used existing data from the risk management database from 1992 through 2002. In part, their results were as follows:

> In general surgery, the most common diagnostic issues related to liability were problems associated with delay in diagnosis or misdiagnosis of cancer (27%), infections processes (27%), missed traumatic injury (18%), and compartment syndrome (9%). When examining the type of surgical error, the two most common errors were retained foreign body and neck dissection (27% each), followed by laparoscopic procedures (18%). Evaluation of nonsurgical procedural complications was approximately evenly distributed between retained foreign body, central line placement, missed intubation, and endoscopic complication.

The trauma service is typically thought to be a high-risk service for litigation. Yet our analysis revealed that the two largest payments (> $2 million each) to plaintiffs were related to elective surgery and a complication on another service in which the expense was allocated after discharge to the trauma service. A third claim, just under $1 million, was also related to the general surgical aspects of the case.

Excluding these three high-cost claims, no claim related to trauma exceeded $200,000 during the sample period.[24]

This study points out that trauma lawsuits made up approximately one half of the general surgery lawsuits and that the distribution of money spent was about even across the board for all services. It suggests that trauma may not be the high-risk litigation area it is perceived to be.[2]

The second study is a product of the University of Texas Health Science Center at San Antonio, the University Hospital, San Antonio, and the Audie L. Murphy Veterans Administration Hospital. This study looked at lawsuits filed against general surgeons from 1992 to 2004 at the three facilities and compared that number to the total number of surgeries performed during the same time period. The surgeries were broken down into three categories: elective, urgent, and trauma. A sampling of the study results follows:

> The ratio of lawsuits filed/operations performed and the incidence in the three groups is as follows: ELECTIVE 14/39,080 (3.0 lawsuits/100,000 procedures/year), URGENT 5/17,958 (2.3 lawsuits/100,000 procedures/year), TRAUMA 2/5,312 (3.1/100,000 procedures/year). There were no statistically significant differences between the groups. Considering trauma as a risk factor for increased malpractice, the relative risk for trauma was 1.1 (95% CI, 0.2632–4.8494). Considering emergent/urgent general surgery as a risk factor for malpractice suit, the relative risk was 0.77 (95% CI, 0.2830–2.1084). These relative risk calculations for all groups were based on the number of procedures performed.[25]

These studies suggest that the practice of trauma surgery is not a higher-risk area for litigation than general surgery alone. The perception of risk has potentially become a part of physician's choices to enter into specialty services. A greater understanding of these issues and the facts about litigation could open up the field of trauma surgery to the cautious group of physicians that would not have considered it in the past. Certainly, more research in this area could assist trauma facilities and physicians in arguing for malpractice tort reform and help to even out the rising costs insurance. Sorting out the actual versus perceived risks associated with trauma surgery is imperative for the future of this vital field of medicine.

CONCLUSION

This chapter has reviewed several aspects of the law and the legal process that relate to the care of injured patients. Circumstances of risk and risk management vary according to geographic area, the type of hospital (trauma center vs. nontrauma center), the medical circumstances of each individual patient care event, and the experience and approach of the trauma team members. The recurring theme that cannot be ignored is that frequent, open, honest, and compassionate communication is the single most important factor other than excellent patient care in determining the overall outcome from the risk manager's perspective. Of critical importance is the presentation of the trauma team as an integrated whole in which all team members have an active role. Involvement of nurses in team function and communication is important because of the extensive and intensive daily contact these professionals have with patients and families.

REFERENCES

1. Studdert D, Mello M, Sage W, et al. Defensive medicine among high-risk specialist physicians in a volatile malpractice environment. *JAMA.* 2005;293:21.
2. Bitterman R. *Providing emergency care under federal law: EMTALA.* American College of Emergency Physicians; 2000.
3. Hermer LD. The scapegoat: EMTALA and emergency department overcrowding. *J Law Policy.* 2006;14:695.
4. 42 U.S.C. §1395dd Examination and Treatment for Emergency Medical Conditions and Women in Labor.
5. Compilation of the Social Security Laws. *Examination and treatment for emergency medical conditions and women in labor.* http://www.ssa.gov/OP_Home/ssact/title18/1867.htm, 2006.
6. Lee T. An EMTALA primer: The impact of changes in the emergency medicine landscape on EMTALA compliance and enforcement. *Ann Health Law.* 2004;13:145.
7. Getachew T, Closson F. Emergency medical treatment and labor act: The basics and other medicolegal concerns. *Pediatr Clin North Am.* 2006;53:139–155.
8. 45 CFR Parts 160 and 164 December 28, 2000 as amended: May 31, 2002, August 14, 2002, February 20, 2003 and April 17, 2003. Healthcare Insurance Portability and Accountability Act.
9. 42 U.S.C. §1395cc (a) Advance Directive. Federal Patient Self Determination Act 1990.
10. Garner BA, ed. *A handbook of basic law terms from the Black's law dictionary series.* Minnesota: Est Group St. Paul; 1999.
11. Cruzan v. Director. Missouri Department of Health; 497 U.S. 261, 1990.
12. *A complete history of the Theresa Schiavo legal battle,* is available at http://www6.miami.edu/ethics/schiavo/timeline.htm, 2006.
13. Raleigh Fitkin Paul Morgan Memorial Hospital v. Anderson. 42 N.J. 421 cert. denied 377 U.S. 985, quoted in Macdonald, Health Care Law, 18–40, 1964.
14. 7 Marq. Elder's Advisor 313. *To be or not to be, should doctors decide? Ethical and legal aspects of medical futility policies.* 2006.
15. Texas Health and Safety Code Ann. § 166.046.
16. 43-JUN Hous. Law. 38. *The history, successes and controversies of the Texas "Futility" policy.* 2006.
17. Kohn L, Corrigan J, Donaldson M, eds. *Institute of medicine report on 1999, titled "To Err is Human".* Committee on Quality of Healthcare in America; 1999.
18. Hyman D, Silver C. The poor state of health care quality in the U.S.: Is malpractice liability a part of the problem or part of the solution? *Cornell Law Rev.* 2005;90:893–994.
19. Popp P. How will disclosure affect future litigation? *ASHRM J.* 2003;23:5–9.
20. Ill. Gen. Ass. Pub. Act 094-0677, 2005. An Act Concerning Insurance. Article 4. Sorry Works! Pilot Program Act. 2005.
21. Wojcieszak D, Banja J, Houk C. The sorry works! coalition: Making the case for full disclosure. *Jt Comm J Qual Patient Saf.* 2006;32(6):344–350.
22. Excited Actuaries at University of Michigan Hospital System. *Sorry works!.* Website. http://www.sorryworks.net/media22.phtml, accessed November 13, 2006.
23. Carroll R. *Risk management handbook for health care organizations,* 4th ed. J-B AHA Press; 2004.
24. Taheri P, Butz D, Anderson S, et al. Medical liability–the crisis, the reality, and the data: The University of Michigan Story. *J Am Coll Surg.* 2006;203(3):290–296.
25. Stewart R, Johnston J, Geoghegan K, et al. Trauma surgery malpractice risk perception versus reality. *Ann Surg.* 2005;241(6):969–975.

Regional Relationships and Transfer of Patient Care

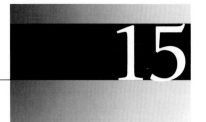

Jordan A. Weinberg   *Loring W. Rue, III*

Ideally, any patient sustaining a significant injury would be promptly transported to a hospital capable of providing immediate and comprehensive trauma care. In reality, however, patients are often taken to facilities that have neither the expertise nor resources to manage complex or life-threatening injuries. As an example, in the Birmingham, Alabama region (population 1.2 million), before the development of a regional trauma system, 60% of patients meeting physiologically unstable trauma triage criteria of the American College of Surgeons were being transported to hospitals that lacked any organized trauma response.[1] The development of regional trauma systems, both in Alabama and across the nation, has helped to improve field triage, whereby critically injured patients may be transported directly to designated trauma centers, possibly bypassing closer nontrauma hospitals. There are still circumstances, however, where patients will arrive at facilities incapable of providing definitive treatment. This may be intentional, owing to logistic concerns regarding weather or transport time (particularly in rural scenarios), or unintentional, as a result of field undertriage or arrival of the patient by private vehicle. Interhospital transfer of such patients to centers with the capability of rendering definitive care is therefore necessary, and the benefit of the efficient handling of such transfers is obvious. In this chapter, the process of interhospital transfer is reviewed, both within the context of well-developed trauma systems and outside of such systems. The impact of the US federal regulations as outlined in the Emergency Medical Treatment and Labor Act (EMTALA) on the interhospital transfer of trauma patients is also discussed.

REGIONAL RELATIONSHIPS

Before the development of trauma centers, victims of injury were generally transported to the closest hospital to the scene. Over time, specific hospitals (most commonly university hospitals) developed expertise and dedicated resources to trauma, realizing the development of the "trauma center." Formal designation of hospitals as trauma centers was spearheaded by the American College of Surgeons Committee on Trauma (ACSCOT), as outlined in the guideline, *Optimal Hospital Resources for the Care of the Seriously Injured*, published in 1976.[2] Despite the development of trauma centers, patients were still being transported to nondesignated hospitals, necessitating interhospital transfer to a trauma center when the patient's injuries overwhelmed the capabilities of the nondesignated hospital. Protocols for interhospital transfer, however, were uncommon, making for an onerous and inefficient process. This reflected the need for improved interhospital cooperation within a region to better deliver injured patients to appropriate facilities in a timely manner.

The concept of the regional trauma system then evolved, whereby the varying facilities within a defined geographic region would form a hospital network to provide care for patients injured within that region. Fundamental to this concept is the classification of hospitals within a region according to their level of expertise and available resources for the care of the injured patient. ACSCOT established well-defined trauma center designations, from Level I centers, which act as the region's lead hospital for the system, through Level IV centers, which can provide initial evaluation and resuscitation of injured patients, but will generally require transfer of most patients to higher level centers (see Table 1).

The evidence concerning the effectiveness of trauma systems is largely retrospective, but is becoming increasingly robust. Mann et al. performed a systematic review of the literature in 1999 and concluded that a 15% to 20% decrease in mortality is observed following the implementation of a regional trauma system.[3] Subsequently, Nathens et al. observed an 8% motor vehicle crash mortality reduction following trauma system implementation.[4] They also noted a lag effect; that is, the mortality reduction was not realized until 10 years following system implementation. Utter et al. recently analyzed survival according to the extent of

hospital participation within a trauma system and found that survival was greater in more "inclusive" systems although patients were no more likely to be hospitalized at a regional trauma center.[5]

Coordination of field triage is a fundamental aspect of a trauma system, and is typically centrally directed. An example of such a system is the Birmingham Regional Emergency Medical Services System, the trauma system for North Central Alabama. Its Trauma Communications Center (TCC) serves as the coordinating command center for prehospital personnel. The TCC tracks the trauma capacity of all participating hospitals in real time, using a computer-linked modem system, with the goal of avoiding situations where a particular facility may be overwhelmed with a surge of incoming patients. Prehospital personnel arrive at the scene and determine, with guidance from the TCC, whether the injured patient should be entered into the trauma system based on well-developed criteria (primary triage). These criteria are generally based on physiologic/clinical parameters, mechanism of injury, and anatomic factors (e.g., penetrating injury to torso). Secondary triage is then performed, in conjunction with the TCC, whereby the severity of injury, geographic concerns, and hospital capacities are taken into account. The secondary triage status then determines the hospital destination (i.e., closest Level III center vs. regional Level I center).

INTERHOSPITAL TRANSFER

Whether in the setting of a mature statewide trauma system, with well-developed field triage protocols, or in the setting where no system exists, it is inevitable that patients will be transported initially to centers incapable of providing definitive care, owing to lack of hospital resources and/or specialist expertise. Interhospital transfer to a facility with the required capabilities must then be initiated. Patient outcomes benefit when this process is efficient and well coordinated.

Determining the Need for Patient Transfer

It is fundamental that doctors caring for trauma patients be well aware of their own capabilities and limitations, as well as those of their institution. This allows for the early determination of those patients who may be cared for in the local hospital versus those who require transfer to a higher level of care. In general, patients who exhibit signs of shock or progressive neurologic deterioration require the highest level of care and should be considered for timely transfer. While stable patients with blunt abdominal trauma and documented solid organ injury may be candidates for nonoperative management, such management should be supervised by a surgeon in a facility with the capability for immediate operative intervention, should nonoperative

---

TABLE 1

DESCRIPTION OF AMERICAN COLLEGE OF SURGEONS TRAUMA CENTER LEVELS

Trauma Center Level	Description
I	■ Full range of specialists and equipment available 24 hr/d ■ Minimum annual volume of patients ■ Leader in trauma education and injury prevention ■ Conducts trauma-related research
II	■ May exist to supplement Level I center in population-dense area, or may serve as lead trauma center in relatively less population-dense region ■ 24 hr/d availability of all specialties and equipment
III	■ Capability to initially manage majority of injured patients ■ Continuous surgical coverage ■ Maintains transfer agreements with Level I and/or II centers for patients whose needs exceed resources of Level III facility
IV	■ 24 hr/d emergency department coverage ■ Specialty coverage may or may not be available ■ Provides initial evaluation and resuscitation, but most patients will require transfer to higher level center

Adapted from Committee on Trauma, American College of Surgeons. *Resources for optimal care of the injured patient 2006.* Chicago: American College of Surgeons; 2006.

TABLE 2

CRITERIA FOR CONSIDERATION FOR TRANSFER

A.   Critical Injuries to Level I or Highest Regional Trauma Center

1.   Carotid or vertebral arterial injury
2.   Torn thoracic aorta or great vessel
3.   Cardiac rupture
4.   Bilateral pulmonary contusion with PaO_2 to FIO_2 ratio <200
5.   Major abdominal vascular injury
6.   Grade IV or V liver injuries requiring >6 U RBC transfusion in 6 hr
7.   Unstable pelvic fracture requiring >6 U RBC transfusion in 6 hr
8.   Fracture or dislocation with loss of distal pulses

B.   Life-Threatening Injuries to Level I or Level II Trauma Center

1.   Penetrating injury or open fracture of the skull
2.   Glasgow Coma Scale score <14 or lateralizing neurologic signs
3.   Spinal fracture or spinal cord deficit
4.   More than two unilateral rib fractures or bilateral rib fractures with pulmonary contusion
5.   Open long bone fracture
6.   Significant torso injury with advanced comorbid disease (such as coronary artery disease, chronic obstructive pulmonary disease, type 1 diabetes mellitus, or immunosuppression)

RBC, red blood cells.
Adapted from Committee on Trauma. American College of Surgeons. *Resources for optimal care of the injured patient 2006.* Chicago: American College of Surgeons; 2006.

management fail. It is inappropriate for such patients to be treated expectantly at facilities that are not prepared for this scenario. Early transfer of such patients is optimal. Patients with certain specific injuries or combinations of injuries are also likely to benefit from early transfer to a higher level of care, as outlined in Table 2.

Once the decision for transfer has been made, it is the priority of the treating physician to perform evaluation and resuscitation measures within the capabilities of the facility as outlined by the Advanced Trauma Life Support Program.[6] Patients with airway instability from impaired cognitive status or otherwise should have the airway secured by intubation before transfer. Similarly, pneumothoraces should typically be managed with chest tube placement before transfer.

Control of hemorrhage before transfer is optimal but, in certain circumstances, may not be possible. External hemorrhage from wounds may be controlled with maintenance of pressure. Hemorrhage from an open book pelvic fracture may be contained by the application of a pelvic binder. Intra-abdominal hemorrhage, however,

requires surgical expertise and operating room resources often beyond the capability of the transferring facility. In such a scenario, the patient must be transported in a relatively unstable state, and the continuous administration of fluids and blood products during transfer is essential. When surgical expertise is available at the transferring hospital, it may be appropriate for the patient to undergo operative damage control of hemorrhage before transfer. Such procedures are warranted, particularly in the rural setting, when relatively long travel distances to definitive care put the patient at risk for exsanguination during transfer. Weinberg et al. reviewed a multicenter experience with 56 rural trauma patients who underwent emergency laparotomy before transfer to definitive care, and found that the 82% survival rate was similar to what would be expected for urban trauma patients after accounting for injury severity.[7] The decision to operate before transfer must take into account the injury severity, the capabilities of the transferring hospital (in particular blood bank resources), travel distance/times, and mode of transfer. Consultation between the transferring and receiving surgeon regarding this complex decision is beneficial.

Transfer Responsibilities

Both the referring and receiving physicians involved in the transfer of a trauma patient have specific responsibilities to ensure the appropriateness, timeliness, and safety of the transfer. It is the responsibility of the referring physician to initiate transfer by consulting with the receiving physician. Initiation of the transfer process should begin while resuscitative efforts are in progress to facilitate an expeditious transfer. As described in the preceding text, the referring doctor must stabilize the patient within the capabilities of his or her institution. Once the decision to transfer has been made, diagnostic imaging and laboratory tests should only be performed if they are necessary for the stabilization of the patient before transfer (e.g., chest x-ray to assess for pneumothorax). Such tests otherwise often result in unnecessary delays. Likewise, the performance of procedures such as wound care may be undertaken, but should not delay transfer. The emphasis should be on stabilization for transfer and not on definitive care.

It is the responsibility of the receiving physician to assess the appropriateness of the intent to transfer and to assure that his or her institution has the capacity to accept the patient. The receiving physician may also provide expertise regarding initial stabilization and ongoing resuscitation during transfer. If the receiving physician is unable to accept the patient due to lack of capacity, he or she should assist the referring physician by suggesting alternative facilities.

While it is ultimately the responsibility of the referring physician to select the mode of transportation and level of care required during transport, it is helpful for the receiving physician to assist in this decision. Consideration should

SAMPLE TRANSFER FORM
(Suggested information to send with the patient)

A. Patient Information
Name _____
Address _____
City _____ State ____ Zip_____
Age _____ Sex _____ Weight _____

Next of kin _____
Address _____
City _____ State ____ ZIP_____
Phone # (____)____ - _____

B. Date and Time
Date ___ / ____ / ____
Time of injury _____ am/pm
Time admitted to ED _____ am/pm
Time admitted to OR _____ am/pm
Time transferred _____ am/pm

C. AMPLE History:

D. Condition on Admission
HR_____ Rhythm_____
BP___ / _____ RR____ Temp_____

E. Probable Diagnoses:

F. Diagnostic Studies:
Lab data—Attach all results to form
Basic imaging studies—Send all
  films with patient
ECG
Send appropriate specimens, eg,
  DPL fluid

G. Treatment Rendered:
Medications given, amount and time

IV fluids, type and amount

Other

H. Status of Patient at Transfer:

I. Management During Transport:

J. Referral Information:
Doctor _____
Hospital _____
Phone # (___) ____ - _____

K. Receiving Information:
Doctor _____
Hospital _____
Phone # (___) ____ - _____

Figure 1 Sample transfer form. (Adapted from Committee on Trauma, American College of Surgeons. *Advanced trauma life support instructor course manual.* Chicago: American College of Surgeons; 1997.)

be given to both the mode of transport and the level of care available during transport (e.g., flight nurse with advanced training vs. basic life support–trained ambulance crew).

Pertinent patient data must precede or accompany the patient in transfer, including any laboratory or imaging results performed at the transferring institution. A conventional transfer form that documents the history, physical, and treatment administered facilitates the transfer of accurate information (see Fig. 1). Hard copies or digital files of imaging being performed should also accompany the patient, along with transcription of the interpretations of such imaging, if available.

Interhospital Transfer and Regional Trauma Systems

As emphasized by ACSCOT, the development of transfer agreements for the movement of patients between institutions is an essential part of a trauma system. The objective

of transfer agreements is to have in place a process for the expeditious movement of patients before the acute need for transfer. The transferring and receiving hospitals therefore benefit by having predetermined the needs and expectations of both institutions before the actual transfer process begins. Transfer agreements are mutually approved by participating hospitals and offer the opportunity for periodic review and possible revision.

The particulars of transfer agreements may vary from system to system, reflective of the particular needs of the region. In general, the transfer agreement outlines criteria for which patients should be transferred, and a process for initiating the transfer (see Fig. 2). Usually, transfer is initiated when the referring physician contacts the receiving physician, who then agrees to accept the patient, provided that the receiving facility has the capacity to take an additional patient. In the Birmingham, Alabama region, this process is expedited by relying upon the TCC. Because the system tracks trauma hospital resource availability

This agreement is made as of the (day) day of (month), (year) by and between (referring hospital) generally at (city, state), a nonprofit corporation, and (receiving hospital) at (city, state), a nonprofit corporation.

Whereas, both the (referring hospital) and the (receiving hospital) desire, by means of this Agreement, to assist doctors and the parties hereto in the treatment of trauma patients; and whereas the parties specifically wish to facilitate: (a) the timely transfer of such patients and medical and other information necessary or useful in the care and treatment of trauma patients transferred, (b) the determination as to whether such patients can be adequately cared for other than by either of the parties hereto, and (c) the continuity of the care and treatment appropriate to the needs of trauma patients, and (d) the utilization of knowledge and other resources of both facilities in a coordinated and cooperative manner to improve the professional health care of trauma patients.

Now, therefore, this agreement witnesseth: That in consideration of the potential advantages accruing to the patients of each of the parties and their doctors, the parties hereby covenant and agree with each other as follows:

1. In accordance with the policies and procedures of the (referring hospital) and upon the recommendation of the attending doctor, who is a member of the medical staff of the (referring hospital) that such transfer is medically appropriate, a trauma patient at the (referring hospital) shall be admitted to (receiving hospital) of (city, state) as promptly as possible under circumstances, provided that beds are available. In such cases, the (referring hospital) and (receiving hospital) agree to exercise their best efforts to provide for prompt admission of the patients.

2. The (referring hospital) agrees that it shall:
   a. Notify the (receiving hospital) as far in advance as possible of impending transfer of a trauma patient.
   b. Transfer to (receiving hospital) the personal effects, including money and valuables, and information relating to same.
   c. Effect the transfer to (receiving hospital) through qualified personnel and appropriate transportation equipment, including the use of necessary and medically appropriate life support measures. (Referring hospital) agrees to bear the responsibility for billing the patient for such services, except to the extent that the patient is billed directly for the services by a third party.

3. The (referring hospital) agrees to transmit with each patient at the time of transfer, or in the case of emergency, as promptly as possible thereafter, an abstract of pertinent medical and other records necessary in order to continue the patient's treatment without interruption and to provide identifying and other information.

4. Bills incurred with respect to services performed by either the (referring hospital) or the (receiving hospital) shall be collected by the party rendering such services directly from the patient, third party, and neither the (referring hospital) nor the (receiving hospital) shall have any liability to the other for such charges.

5. This Agreement shall be effective from the date of execution and shall continue in effect indefinitely, except that either party may withdraw by giving thirty (30) days notice in writing to the other party of its intention to withdraw from this Agreement. Withdrawal shall be effective at the expiration of the thirty (30)-day notice period. However, if either party shall have its license to operate revoked by the State, this Agreement shall terminate on the date such revocation becomes effective.

6. The Board of Directors of the (referring hospital) and the Governing Body of the (receiving hospital) shall have exclusive control of the policies, management, assets, and affairs of their respective facilities. Neither party assumes any liability, by virtue of this Agreement, for any debts or other obligations incurred by the other party to this Agreement.

7. Nothing in this Agreement shall be construed as limiting the right of either to affiliate or contract with any hospital or nursing home on either a limited or general basis while this Agreement is in effect.

8. Neither party shall use the name of the other in any promotional or advertising material unless review and approval of the intended use shall first be obtained from the party whose name is to be used.

9. The parties hereby agree to comply with all applicable laws and regulations concerning the treatment and care of patients designated for transfer from one health care institution to another, including but not limited to the Emergency Medical Treatment and Active Labor Act, 42 U.S.C 1395dd.

10. This agreement may be modified or amended from time to time by mutual agreement of the parties, and any such modification or amendment shall be attached to and become part of this Agreement.

In witness whereof, the parties hereto have executed this Agreement the day and year first above written.

_____   _____

By: _____   By: _____

Date: _____   Date: _____

Figure 2 Sample transfer agreement. (Adapted from Committee on Trauma, American College of Surgeons. *Advanced trauma life support instructor course manual*. Chicago: American College of Surgeons; 1997.)

in real time, interhospital transfer from a participating community hospital to the regional Level I center can be initiated without formal acceptance of the patient by the Level I center. Should the physician at the community hospital who first encounters the patient decide that immediate transfer to the Level I center would benefit the patient, the patient is routed through the trauma system and the transferring physician can then relay the patient's history and status to the receiving trauma center while transport is already under way.

Ideally, all injuries would occur within the boundaries of a regional trauma system, but in fact, trauma systems are in existence in only 50% of the states in the U.S.A.[8] However, many areas are served by geographically smaller regional systems, and *de facto* trauma systems may exist in the absence of formal systems. In Vermont, a state without a formal trauma system, the Level I center in Burlington serves the rural communities of both Vermont and upstate New York. Despite the lack of formal criteria for what determines a major trauma patient or any protocols governing patient transfers, the development of regional relationships over time has resulted in the community hospitals' awareness of the Level I facility as a resource for definitive care and trauma leadership in general. Analysis of patients stabilized at a community hospital before transfer to the Level I facility in Burlington demonstrated that survival was similar to those patients transported directly to Burlington.[9] Similarly, a population-based analysis of trauma care in Vermont demonstrated that overall trauma patient survival was no worse at community hospitals in the region than the Level I center.[10] The Level I center in Birmingham, Alabama, is the lead hospital for the regional trauma system, which serves six contiguous counties in North Central Alabama. This system is a voluntary system (i.e., not legislated by state or local government), whereby only 10 of the 24 hospitals in the region participate. Despite relatively marginal formal participation in the system, it is well appreciated by those nonparticipating hospitals and those outside of the immediate region that the Level I center is the closest resource for definitive trauma care. A significant decline in mortality was observed for the six-county region following the establishment of this voluntary trauma system.[11]

Interhospital transfer in such settings is facilitated by a centralized hospital transfer center. This duty may be performed by the communications center that coordinates prehospital care, or a separate entity dedicated to facilitating interhospital communication and transfer. The existence of such centralized communication centers allows for direct communication between both the transferring and receiving physicians, and the personnel at each facility who will ultimately coordinate the interhospital transport. In Southwest Texas, such a communications center was made operational in 1996. Retrospective review demonstrated a significant decrease in interhospital transport time with the communications center in place.[12]

INTERHOSPITAL TRANSFER AND UNITED STATES LAW

The EMTALA was signed into law in 1986 as part of the Consolidated Omnibus Budget Reconciliation Act (COBRA) of 1985. It was born of concern that hospital emergency rooms were refusing to accept or treat patients based on insurance status.[13] This legislation delineates the requirement that all hospitals must administer treatment to any individual with an emergency medical condition, regardless of the individual's ability to pay. It also addresses hospitals' responsibilities during the course of transferring and receiving patients in an emergency medical condition.

Essentially, the law requires any emergency department to provide a screening medical evaluation to determine whether an emergency medical condition exists or not. Should the presence of an emergency medical condition be determined, it is then the responsibility of the facility to either provide treatment or transfer the patient to another facility, should a higher level of care be required.

Elements of EMTALA relative to the initiation of transfer of a trauma patient include the following:

1. Identification of a higher level of care with the capacity and willingness to accept the patient
2. Not transporting hemodynamically unstable patients, except for medical necessity and only after providing treatment within the facility's capability and capacity
3. Providing appropriate transportation
4. Providing all pertinent medical records either with the patient, or as soon as possible, should providing it with the patient cause unnecessary delay
5. Completing a physician transfer certificate and obtaining consent for transfer

The receiving hospital also has specific obligations under the law. Hospitals that have "specialized capabilities" such as burn units, trauma units, or regional referral centers in general may not refuse to accept a patient in transfer if they have the capability and capacity to treat the individual. Capability refers to both the facility itself (i.e., equipment and supplies) and the staff (specialist coverage). Capacity refers to bed availability, but is not simply reflected by available beds; it includes whatever the hospital customarily does to accommodate patients in excess of occupancy limits (e.g., boarding patients on off-service floors, or calling in additional staff). When it is suspected by the receiving facility that the transferring facility has the capability to take definitive care of the patient's injuries, the patient must still be accepted in transfer in order to comply with the law (it is not up to the receiving hospital to determine capabilities of the transferring facility; complaint regarding transfer impropriety may be made to the Centers for Medicare and Medicaid Services).

The potential for the overburdening of trauma centers, particularly with a large proportion of uninsured patients, is clear given the implications of EMTALA. Nathens et al., in fact, demonstrated that insurance status was an independent predictor of transfer to a Level I trauma center; that is, patients without commercial insurance were 2.4 times more likely to be transferred to a Level I facility from a Level III or IV center than those with commercial insurance, after adjusting for differences in injury severity.[14] Recently, however, Spain et al. reviewed their experience with 692 transfer requests and found no significant difference in payer status compared with their primary catchment patients.[15] Further study of this issue on a national scale will be necessary to better quantify the impact of EMTALA, and ultimately determine how the burden of trauma care is best distributed.

SUMMARY

When a patient's acute injuries require resources and expertise beyond the capabilities of a hospital, expeditious interhospital transfer to a regional trauma center is necessary. A well-coordinated and orderly process facilitates the timely transport of such patients. Although the existence of a regional trauma system helps streamline the transfer process, efficient interhospital transfer may still be achieved outside of a formal trauma system. It is essential that both the transferring and receiving physician understand their respective roles and responsibilities to ensure both a safe and rapid transfer of the critically injured patient.

REFERENCES

1. Birmingham Regional Emergency Medical Services System. *Regional trauma system plan*. http://bremss.com/ Regional%20Trauma%20System%20Plan%206-01.pdf. 2001.
2. Committee on Trauma, American College of Surgeons. Optimal hospital resources for care of the seriously injured. *Bull Am Coll Surg*. 1976;61:15–22.
3. Mann NC, Mullins RJ, MacKenzie EJ, et al. Systematic review of published evidence regarding trauma system effectiveness. *J Trauma*. 1999;47(3 Suppl):S25–S33.
4. Nathens AB, Jurkovich GJ, Cummings P, et al. The effect of organized systems of trauma care on motor vehicle crash mortality. *JAMA*. 2000;283(15):1990–1994.
5. Utter GH, Maier RV, Rivara FP, et al. Inclusive trauma systems: Do they improve triage or outcomes of the severely injured? *J Trauma*. 2006;60(3):529–535; discussion 535–537.
6. Committee on Trauma, American College of Surgeons. *Advanced trauma life support course: faculty manual*. Chicago: American College of Surgeons; 2004.
7. Weinberg JA, McKinley K, Petersen SR, et al. Trauma laparotomy in a rural setting before transfer to a regional center: Does it save lives? *J Trauma*. 2003;54(5):823–826; discussion 826–828.
8. Hoyt DB, Coimbra R. Trauma systems. *Surg Clin North Am*. 2007;87(1):21–35, v–vi.
9. Rogers FB, Osler TM, Shackford SR, et al. Study of the outcome of patients transferred to a level I hospital after stabilization at an outlying hospital in a rural setting. *J Trauma*. 1999;46(2):328–333.
10. Rogers FB, Osler TM, Shackford SR, et al. Population-based study of hospital trauma care in a rural state without a formal trauma system. *J Trauma*. 2001;50(3):409–413; discussion 414.
11. Abernathy JH III, McGwin G Jr, Acker JE III, et al. Impact of a voluntary trauma system on mortality, length of stay, and cost at a Level I trauma center. *Am Surg*. 2002;68(2):182–192.
12. Epley EE, Stewart RM, Love P, et al. A regional medical operations center improves disaster response and interhospital trauma transfers. *Am J Surg*. 2006;192(6):853–859.
13. Teshome G, Closson FT. Emergency medical treatment and labor act: The basics and other medicolegal concerns. *Pediatr Clin North Am*. 2006;53(1):139–155, vii.
14. Nathens AB, Maier RV, Copass MK, et al. Payer status: The unspoken triage criterion. *J Trauma*. 2001;50(5):776–783.
15. Spain DA, Bellino M, Kopelman A, et al. Requests for 692 transfers to an academic Level I trauma center: Implications of the emergency medical treatment and active labor act. *J Trauma*. 2007;62(1):63–67; discussion 67–68.

Evaluating Trauma Center Performance

16

Turner Osler   *Laurent G. Glance*

The mission of trauma centers is to prevent death and optimize the recovery of injured patients. The performance of trauma centers is therefore of critical interest to patients and their families, and increasingly to those who pay for trauma care as well: insurers and the government.[1] But the evaluation of trauma center performance requires some measure or measures of performance, and such metrics have proved elusive. In part, this is because there are so many possible (and possibly conflicting) outcomes upon which a trauma center might be evaluated. The underlying heterogeneity of trauma patients further compounds the problem because we must always adjust our expectations for an individual patient predicated on his potential for a good outcome. Importantly, the required adjustment will depend on the outcome under consideration.

Perhaps because of these underlying difficulties the measurement of trauma center performance is still in its infancy. Tellingly, although the most basic and unequivocal outcome measure, survival, has been extensively examined over the last 25 years there is not yet agreement on the best model for this outcome: Injury Severity Score (ISS), International Classification of Disease Injury Severity Score (ICISS), Trauma and Injury Severity Score (TRISS), and A Severity Characterization Of Trauma (ASCOT) all have their advocates and still other survival models are likely to emerge. (See appendix for a brief discussion of these measures.) Early work suggests that the choice of outcome prediction model affects conclusions about trauma center performance,[2] and therefore the choice of scoring system is likely to be of considerable interest to all concerned, particularly if trauma center certification or reimbursement becomes contingent upon such measures.

If we consider outcomes for individual patients, we might think of survival as of primary interest, but the degree of residual disability that patients experience may be of even greater importance in the case of injuries that are rarely fatal. Many other outcomes are also of interest: the efficiency with which care is rendered (in terms of length of stay or cost), the effectiveness of care (complication rates, readmission rates, accuracy of medical decision making), satisfaction with care (patients, families, referring physicians), all are important. Developing risk-adjusted measures for any of these outcomes is likely to prove at least as challenging as finding a single risk-adjusted measure for survival to discharge has. Moreover, because the risk factors for different outcomes are likely to be different, every outcome of interest will require its own risk adjustment model. Some thoughtful authors have gone so far as to conclude that "outcome is neither a sensitive nor a specific marker for quality of care" and should be used only "...to help organizations detect trends and spot outliers...".[3] It is sobering to observe that to date we do not have a single risk-adjusted trauma outcome measure that is universally accepted.

Even if performance measures could be defined and measured, methodological difficulties remain. For these measures to be useful metrics of performance, they must be used to make comparisons, either within a single institution over time or between institutions. Deciding if two institutions with different patient mixes differ significantly on a given outcome measure is not trivial, however, as is evidenced by the number of statistical approaches that have been advocated. Although the simple "Z, W, and M statistics"[4,5] approach to comparing institutional mortality rates of 20 years ago never achieved mathematical respectability, subsequently many other methods have been explored: cumulative sum charts,[6] hierarchal models,[7] Bayesian methods,[8] propensity scoring,[9] and matching algorithms[10] have all been proposed, and other methods are likely to emerge.

Faced with the enormity of the task of "measuring performance" in terms of numbers of possible outcomes to be measured, the effort required to develop even a single such measure, and the statistical complexities of comparing institutions based on such measures, organizations such as the American College of Surgeons (ACS)[11] have wisely eschewed performance measures in favor of measures of structure and process. This approach, first outlined by Donabedian 25 years ago,[12] advocates the evaluation of structures that are believed necessary for excellent care (physical facilities, qualified practitioners, training programs, etc.) and processes that are believed conducive to excellent care (prompt availability of practitioners, expeditious operating room access, patients who underwent postsplenectomy receiving overwhelming postsplenectomy infection [OPSI] vaccines, etc.) Although outcome measures were also included in Donabedian's schema, he recognized that these would be the most difficult to develop and employ.

Although it might seem that measures of structure and process would be straightforward to posit and use, in practice difficulties immediately arise. The selection of structural characteristics requires that we know which aspects of a trauma center's design affect performance, and here intuition may mislead us. An instructive example of this was the suggestion of "case volume" as structural criteria for trauma centers. Although case volume has been shown to be associated with outcomes for some high-risk surgical procedures, when this criteria was examined for trauma centers it was unclear how "case volume" should be defined (all trauma admissions?, all "major" trauma cases?, "major" trauma cases per trauma surgeon?, etc.) or what actual volume of cases was adequate. Indeed, it is not even clear that there is an association between volume and outcome in trauma care.[13] Process measures are subject to these same difficulties with definition and implementation.

An entirely separate question is: "If accurate measures of trauma center performance were developed, how might such measures be employed?" One possible use would be to carefully examine centers with the best performance to determine which characteristics and practices lead to superior outcomes. This approach has been fruitfully employed by the Northern New England (NNE) Cardiovascular Disease Study, where a 24% reduction in hospital mortality rates was observed,[14] and by the National Surgical Quality Improvement Program[15] where a similar decrease in mortality in Veterans Administration Hospitals was described. Other approaches are possible, however. Insurers might simply require trauma centers to attain some benchmark before agreeing to pay for services. Government regulators might follow the "No Child Left Behind" model, and require that all trauma centers meet defined standards or face funding sanctions or perhaps state control. Although the experimental rigor of the NNE approach has been questioned and the unintended consequences of the latter two approaches are difficult to envision, it seems certain that, if predicated on inaccurate or unfair outcome measures, the result of performance evaluation is likely to be worse, not better, care of the injured. It is therefore imperative that any outcome measures be reliable before they are employed.

In this essay we will expand briefly on the philosophic and technical difficulties involved in measuring performance. We will find that measures of structure and process are much better developed at this time, but are not without serious problems in their application. We will then briefly describe how trauma centers are currently evaluated by the American College of Surgeons Trauma Center Verification process. In the end, we will conclude that the perceived need for measures of performance currently outstrips our ability to provide them. Indeed, it is uncertain if such measures can ever be developed.

PHILOSOPHIC CONSIDERATIONS

Any summary measure loses some of the information present in the data during the process of summarization, and this is true for measures of quality. Therefore, we must recognize that any single measure of quality is likely to hide as much as it reveals. For example, a hypothetical trauma center might be judged to have "satisfactory survival results," but the actual data may consist of poor results for patients with closed head injuries and excellent results for patients with penetrating trauma. To simply accept the judgment of "satisfactory" would be to miss an important opportunity to improve the care of patients with head injuries at that trauma center. Because care can vary over so many types of injuries, we are likely to need many measurements to gain a clear picture of quality of care. The problem is compounded because individual patients may have several types of injuries. Additionally, quality can vary in many dimensions. While it may be relatively easy to discern a difference in outcome between patients with blunt and penetrating trauma, care that varies from day to day, or care that is worse on weekends may be much more difficult to detect and will likely escape notice unless it is specifically sought.

Many different outcomes may be of interest, and some of these will inevitably be in conflict. Therefore, short length of stay may be regarded as a marker for good care, but high readmission rates would likely be regarded as a marker for poor care. It is a matter for considered judgment to decide what the appropriate balance for these two conflicting outcomes might be. Indeed different arbitrators (a patient's insurance company vs. the same patient's lawyer, for example) might have different perspectives of where the balance ought to be. As another example, although it is paramount for physicians to respect patients' wishes concerning medical treatment, such deference may lead to "unnecessary" deaths which might be held on superficial analysis to reflect "bad" care. It may be difficult to ferret out all such confounding circumstances.

Even after we decide on a dimension of care that we wish to evaluate, many different competing measures may be available. Problematically, different risk adjustment models may lead to different conclusions about the overall success of care,[16,17] and it is usually unclear which measure is the most valid. In the absence of a gold standard, it is likely that disagreements over the most appropriate measure will arise.

STATISTICAL CONSIDERATIONS

At its heart, statistical analysis is simply the mathematical procedure used to distinguish real differences from random variations. Although statisticians have developed powerful techniques to attack this fundamental problem over the last century, in practice comparisons between different trauma centers' performances present several challenges.

Because of the low incidence and binary nature of many measures that might be used in performance assessment, very little information is available per measurement. Therefore, large numbers of patients are usually required to reliably detect real differences between trauma centers. Consider the simple example of mortality rates. Suppose two trauma centers had identical patient populations and further, that trauma center A had a mortality rate of 3% whereas trauma center B had a mortality rate twice as great (6%). A simple calculation reveals that 1,000 patients from each trauma center would be required to have a 90% chance of declaring this difference significant. More subtle differences, say between mortality rates of 5% and 6%, would require more than 10,000 patients per trauma center, a number unlikely to be available in any reasonable time frame. Fortunately, binary outcomes with higher incidences (say complications) require fewer observations to establish significant differences, but to establish a difference between a 50% rate and a 60% rate still requires 500 patients per trauma center.

In reality it would be rare for two trauma centers to actually have identical patient populations, and therefore risk adjustment models are required. The science of risk adjustment is an evolving field, however, and as alluded to in the preceding text, many different statistical techniques for risk adjustment have been suggested.[18] It is still unsettled which approach is most reliable, but certain principles are clear. For example, risk adjustment models can be successful only if the patient populations of the centers being compared overlap significantly on predictors that affect the outcome of interest. Therefore, it would not be sensible to compare pediatric trauma centers to adult trauma centers unless the adult trauma center happened to also care for children, and further that such an analysis was limited only to outcomes for children. Although this example seems trivial, the same problem would complicate the comparison of a trauma center caring largely for patients with penetrating trauma to a center caring for patients with primarily blunt trauma.

A more technical issue associated with risk adjustment results from the correlation of outcomes for patients within any given center. Because the outcomes for a given center's patients are more similar to one another than to those of any other center, accurate modeling requires that we include this subtlety in our analysis. Unfortunately this sort of hierarchical modeling of "patients within trauma centers" is rarely a part of the analysis of trauma outcome data, although it has been a feature of analyzing school performance data ("pupils within schools") for many years, and has begun to appear in medical quality research.[19]

PRACTICAL CONSIDERATIONS

The practical problems involved in performance measurement are legion, and begin with settling on a definition for the outcome of interest. Although most clinicians feel that they understand the vocabulary of medical outcomes, even for as common place an outcome as mortality many different definitions are plausible: survival to hospital discharge, 30-day survival, survival excluding patients who request withdrawal of support; each of these definitions of "survival" might be appropriate in a particular context. Complication rates are another possible measure of performance, but are based on an arbitrary set of clinical events (Which events should be counted as complications?), each of which can itself be somewhat arbitrary (hyperkalemia might be defined as $K > 5$ or $K > 5.5$ or $K > 5.6$, or ...). In the absence of uniformity in the definitions employed, comparisons are impossible. It is unclear which organization should be responsible for establishing such definitions.

Data for the assessment of performance may come from many sources, but can be broadly classified as "administrative" (usually extracted from computer databases maintained by the hospital or clinic, often for billing purposes: e.g., international classification of disease-9 [ICD-9] codes) or "clinical" (usually extracted from the medical record). Administrative data is almost always easier and less expensive to acquire, but may lack detail necessary for robust risk adjustment models.[20] Clinical data, on the other hand, is expensive to acquire but is often a richer source of information. Although the detail available in clinical data may be desirable, such information often involves "self-reporting" by clinicians, and there is evidence that clinicians may not always be reliable reporters. When the medical record regarding deficiencies in airway management was compared to video recordings of airway management large discrepancies were found,[21] and this problem may undermine the reliability of clinical data. Finally, it is problematic that different sources of information have resulted in different conclusions about the performance of intensive care units.[22]

More generally, if achieving expected outcomes becomes associated with rewards or sanctions we may expect clinical data and even administrative data to be degraded by "upcoding" of patient risk factors used in modeling expected outcomes or even frank falsification of outcomes. The "No Child Left Behind" program has produced instances of teachers falsely improving their class performance by changing pupils' answers before submitting their standardized test forms,[23] as well as instances of principals falsifying students' dropout status.[24] Unfortunately, there is no reason to believe that the health care profession should be immune to the human weakness manifested in the teaching profession. Ensuring the reliability of clinical data used in benchmarking trauma center performance might require independent data collection, but such a step would likely be very expensive. Nevertheless, we must be aware that linking outcomes to rewards or sanctions may adversely affect the validity of the data upon which quality assessment rests. It is ironic that the greater the significance we attach to performance the more difficult it may become to measure, but this phenomenon is not unique to medicine. The corruption of indicators used to monitor important processes is so common that it has been given the name "Campbell's Law" by sociologists.[25]

PERFORMANCE MEASURES IN ACTUAL PRACTICE

The TRISS score is the oldest and most widely used survival prediction model in trauma registries in the United States currently. Because it predicts a likelihood of survival for individual patients it has often been used to designate patients as "unexpected survivors" and "unexpected deaths" to facilitate patient outcome review. However, in a recent review[26] of 270 patients from a single trauma center classified by TRISS as "unexpected survivors" only 11% were corroborated as unexpected survivors by a peer review process, prompting the authors to conclude that TRISS unexpected survivors were "a statistical phenomenon only." Other authors[27] have observed that when the TRISS methodology is applied to a cohort of trauma centers, most are "above average," a seeming statistical conundrum. Therefore, the most widely used outcome metric does not seem to provide plausible assessment of trauma center performance.

While survival is a metric of great interest, other measures of outcome have been proposed. "Good functional outcome" is also of obvious interest, but early work suggests that trauma centers with the best overall survival rates are not necessarily those with the highest rates of "good functional outcome."[28] It therefore seems that the assessment of trauma center performance may require many different metrics to capture the many dimensions of a "good outcome."

THE AMERICAN COLLEGE OF SURGEONS' VERIFICATION PROCESS

Approximately 20 years ago the ACS created a verification process by which structure, process, and outcome measures for individual trauma centers could be reviewed and this approach to trauma center evaluation has subsequently been carefully refined.[11] The process is a unique combination of facility inspection, outcome assessment, and "process improvement seminar" that serves to evaluate trauma center performance and suggest improvements. Interestingly, the ACS verification process does not rely upon statistical measures of performance but rather upon the judgment of seasoned, impartial trauma surgeons and nurses who review the medical records of individual trauma patients as well as the results of the trauma center's various quality improvement programs to assess a trauma center's performance. The ACS verification process is in practice far more useful than simply an isolated performance measure because it also suggests paths to improved outcomes, something that a simple performance measure cannot provide.

THE FUTURE

The measurement of trauma center performance is in its infancy. To date we do not have even a single agreed-upon risk-adjusted measure of performance and as a consequence we have no clear idea how much trauma centers actually differ in their performance. A few researchers have suggested that such differences do exist, but this work has been done using narrowly focused types of injuries[29] or small samples of trauma centers.[30] But the simple observation that the ACS verifies some trauma centers and not others suggests that differences in quality exist between trauma centers and may be substantial.

In the near term, administrative data sets (e.g., Health Care Cost and Utilization Project [HCUP][31]) and voluntary trauma databases (e.g., the National Trauma Data Bank [NTDB][32]) could be examined using existent (or perhaps improved) survival models to examine the variability of survival between trauma centers. Such an undertaking would give an idea of the variability of performance between trauma centers. If such an analysis disclosed significant differences in performance among trauma centers we would suspect that some centers' performance might be improved. More importantly, a careful evaluation of the most successful centers might provide valuable insights into which features of trauma centers are associated with outstanding performance. Unfortunately, "data sets of convenience" such as the NTDB and HCUP have substantial limitations: administrative data sets lack clinical information that can add substantially to the accuracy of any outcome model, whereas voluntary data from trauma registries may not be representative of trauma care generally. The most powerful tool to make inferences about trauma care would be a statistically valid sampling of clinical data from all hospitals providing trauma care, but such a data set does not now exist and would be expensive to develop and maintain.

In the longer term, larger and more widely available trauma data sets and better statistical tools will allow the development of better survival models, and these should be adopted whenever they show significantly better performance than our current models. Models to evaluate other endpoints of interest, such as complication rates or disability rates, will require clear, functional definition of these elusive terms. Questions such as "What is a complication?" and "What is a wound infection?" will require unambiguous, if somewhat arbitrary, answers. Moreover, such results will need to be consistently and reliably recorded for large numbers of patients if the promise of data to improve trauma care is to be realized.

CONCLUSIONS

To be assured that trauma centers perform well we require measures of trauma center performance. Unfortunately, such measures have proved elusive and those that are sufficiently robust and accurate to allow comparisons between trauma centers or track a given center's performance over time have not yet emerged. Nevertheless, government,[33] industry,[34] insurers, and patients feel a need to compare medical care among hospitals and providers. We should continue our search for such measures because we will learn much in the process. But we must resist the calls to employ such measures in the evaluation and comparison of trauma centers until they are robust enough to allow valid conclusions. If we succumb to the clamor for measures of performance and begin to make pronouncements on the quality of trauma centers based on inaccurate metrics we risk undermining the very quality we seek to ensure.

APPENDIX: CURRENTLY AVAILABLE MEASURES OF PERFORMANCE

Survival is a well-defined outcome following trauma, and risk adjustment for the same has been extensively studied over the last 35 years. Broadly, three factors can be thought of that might influence survival: the severity of anatomic injury, the severity of physiologic derangement, and the underlying resilience of the patient. To risk adjust, we must be able to measure each of these factors, and combine them into a single estimate of the likelihood of survival.

Currently the TRISS equation is the most widely used approach to generate risk-adjusted expected survivals:

$$P\ Survival_{Blunt} = 1/1 + e^{(-0.4499 + 0.8085 \times RTS - 0.0835 \times ISS - 1.7430 \times age)}$$

$$P\ Survival_{Penetrating} = 1/1 + e^{(-2.5355 + 0.9934 \times RTS - 0.0651 \times ISS - 1.1360 \times age)}$$

This equation allows a string of injuries (expressed in the lexicon of the Abbreviated Injury Scale [AIS] and summarized as an ISS, a measure of physiologic derangement (captured as Glasgow Coma Score, systolic blood pressure and respiratory rate and expressed as their weighted sum, the Revised Trauma Score [RTS]), a surrogate for resilience (age expressed as a binary variable: age >54 or age ≤54) and mechanism (blunt or penetrating) to be combined into a single prediction of survival.

Unfortunately, each of the subscores that contribute to TRISS was created before large data sets allowed the application of rigorous statistical methods, and none of these measures are therefore likely to be optimal. The ISS is a case in point. Created more than 30 years ago, the ISS was empirically defined as the sum of the squares of the AIS-defined severity of the worst injury sustained in each of the three worst-injured body regions. This score quickly became the standard measure of trauma severity and has proved remarkably durable. Although modifications of the ISS have been proposed, the formula used to calculate the ISS has remained unchanged over the last 30 years.

Despite its broad acceptance there are problematic features of the ISS approach to injury severity. By design the ISS allows a maximum of only three injuries to contribute to the final score, and in practice the actual number is often fewer. Moreover, because the ISS allows only one injury per body region to be scored, the scored injuries may not be the three most severe injuries that a patient has sustained. The idiosyncratic sum of squares formula used to compute ISS allows only 44 valid scores that are bounded between 0 and 75 but clustered below 26.

The performance of ISS in large data sets has been disappointing. Although scoring systems should be monotonic, there are several instances where higher ISS scores are correlated with lower mortality[35] (see Fig. 1). Curiously, a model based on the single worst injury a patient has sustained more accurately predicts survival than does ISS,[36] suggesting that the ISS fails to correctly extract the information present in a set of injuries. Finally, 11 ISS scores can be achieved as a result of more than one combination of three individual severities, and therefore occasionally different overall injury patterns are conflated into a single ISS scores. Unfortunately, these different patterns often have quite different observed mortality rates. The ISS may therefore be thought of as an algorithm that maps the 84 possible combinations of three or fewer AIS injuries into 44 possible scores that are distributed between 0 and 75 in a nonuniform way that roughly correspond to the likelihood of death. Although several alternatives to the

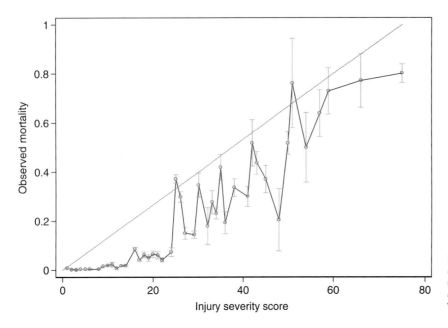

Figure 1   Observed mortality as a function of the 44 possible Injury Severity Scores (ISSs). (100,000 trauma cases selected randomly from the National Trauma Data Bank, V 6.1.)

ISS have been proposed (the ICISS[37], the Anatomic Profile [AP[38]], the New Injury Severity Score [NISS[39]]), none has achieved universal acceptance. Indeed, there is not even consensus regarding the data dictionary that should be used to describe injuries, because whereas the AIS provides more specific injury categories and severities, ICD-9 injury descriptors are more widely available.

Unfortunately, the other scores contributing to the TRISS equation are similarly flawed: the RTS, the Glasgow Coma Score, and even the dichotomization of age at 55 were all created using *ad hoc* methodologies. Because these subscores have been less studied, fewer alternatives have been advanced, but it is likely that these scores can be substantially improved upon.

Even if a method to reliably predict the survival of individual patients could be agreed upon, further statistical difficulties arise when we try to use these results to actually evaluate trauma center performance. An early statistical method that was developed specifically to address the evaluation of trauma centers was the "Z, W, and M statistics" approach. Using this technique, the W statistic provided an estimate of the number of patients who survived unexpectedly, the Z statistic was a measure of how likely such a difference was to have occurred by chance alone, and the M statistic represented an *ad hoc* measure of how likely this method was to provide reliable answers. Unfortunately, although logical in its approach, the Z, W, and M methodology has never been thoroughly evaluated, and its statistical properties and reliability are unknown.

It would be unwise to begin evaluating trauma center performance until the techniques used to produce performance estimates are known to be reliable. The premature general implementation of trauma center evaluation using inaccurate or unreliable methods risks discrediting the use of performance measures for many years to come.

REFERENCES

1. Iglehart JK. Linking compensation to quality—Medicare payments to physicians. *N Engl J Med.* 2005;353:870–872.
2. Glance LG, Osler TM, Dick AW. Evaluating trauma center quality: Does the choice of the severity-adjustment model make a difference? *J Trauma: Injury Infect Crit Care.* 2005;58:1265–1271.
3. Lifford R, Mohammed MA, Spiegelhalter D. Use and misuse of process and outcome data in managing performance of acute medical care: Avoiding institutional stigma. *Lancet.* 2004;363: 1147–1154.
4. Flora JK. A method for comparing survival of burn patients to a standard survival curve. *J Trauma.* 1978;18:701–705.
5. Boyd CR, Tolson MA, Copes WS. Evaluating trauma care: The TRISS method. *J Trauma.* 1987;27:370.
6. Steiner SH, Cook RJ, Farewell V, et al. Monitoring surgical performance using risk-adjusted cumulative sum charts. *Biostatistics.* 2000;1(4):441–452.
7. Leyland AH, Goldstein H. *Multilevel modeling of health statistics.* West Sussex, England: John Wiley and Sons; 2001.
8. Spiegelhalter DJ, Abrams KR, Myles JP. *Bayesian approaches to clinical trials and health-care evaluation.* West Sussex, England: John Wiley and Sons; 2004.
9. Huang I, Frangakis C, Dominici F, et al. Application of a propensity score approach for risk adjustment in profiling multiple physician groups on asthma care. *Health Serv Res.* 2005;40:253–278.
10. Trooskins SZ, Copes WS, Bain LW, et al. Case-matching methodology as an adjunct to trauma performance improvements for evaluating lengths of stay and complications. *J Trauma: Injury Infect Crit Care.* 1999;1018–1027.
11. http://www.facs.org/trauma/verificationhosp.html.
12. Donabedian A. *The definition of quality and approaches to its assessment.* Ann Arbor: Health Administration Press; 1980.
13. Glance LG, Osler TM, Dick AW Mukamel D. The relation between trauma center outcome and volume in the national trauma databank. *J Trauma: Injury Infect Crit Care.* 2004;56: 682–690.
14. O'Connor GT, Plume SK, Olmstead EM, et al. The Northern New England Cardiovascular Disease Study Group. A regional intervention to improve the hospital mortality associated with coronary artery bypass graft surgery. *JAMA.* 1996;275(11):841–846.
15. Khuri SF, Daley J, Henderson WG. The comparative assessment and improvement of quality of surgical care in the department of Veterans affairs. *Arch Surg.* 2002;137(1):20–27.
16. Glance LG, Osler T. Beyond the major trauma outcome study: Benchmarking performance using a national contemporary,

population-based trauma registry. *J Trauma: Injury Infect Crit Care.* 2001;51:725–727.

17. Glance LG, Osler T, Dick A. Rating the quality of ICUs—Is it a function of the ICU scoring system? *Crit Care Med.* 2002;30(9):1969–1975.

18. Iezzoni LI, ed. *Risk adjustment for measuring health care outcomes.* Chicago: Health Administration Press; 2003.

19. Glance LG, Dick AW, Osler TM, et al. Using hierarchical modeling to measure ICU quality. *Intensive Care Med.* 2003;29(12):2223–2229.

20. Hunt JP, Baker CC, Fakhry SM, et al. Accuracy of administrative data in trauma. *Surgery.* 1999;126(2):191–197.

21. MacKenzie CF, Jefferies JN, Hunter WA, et al. Comparison of self-reporting of deficiencies in airway management with video analysis of actual performance. *Hum Factors.* 1996;38:623–635.

22. Hartz AJ, Kuhn EM. Comparing hospitals that perform coronary artery bypass surgery: The effect of outcome measures and data sources. *Am J Public Health.* 1994;84(10):1609–1614.

23. http://pricetheory.uchicago.edu/levitt/Papers/JackobLevittToCatchACheat2004.pdf.

24. http://www.rethinkingschools.org/special_reports/bushplan/drop181.shtml.

25. Campbell DT. *Assessing the impact of planned social change.* Dartmouth College: Public Affairs Center; 1976.

26. Norris R, Woods R, Harbrecht B, et al. TRISS unexpected survivors: An outdated standard? *J Trauma: Injury Infect Crit Care.* 2002;52:229–234.

27. Glance LG, Osler TM, Dick AW. Evaluating trauma center quality: Does the choice of the severity-adjustment model make a difference? *J Trauma.* 2005;58(6):1265–1271.

28. Glance LG, Dick A, Osler T. Judging trauma center quality: Does it depend on the choice of outcomes? *J Trauma: Injury Infect Crit Care.* 2004;56:165–172.

29. Trooskin SZ, Copes WS, Bain LW, et al. Variability in trauma center outcomes for patients with moderate intracranial injury. *J Trauma: Injury Infect Crit Care.* 2004;57:998–1005.

30. Celso B, Tepas JJ, Flint LM, et al. *Effective comparison of trauma center performance is still an illusive goal.* American Association for the Surgery of Trauma Poster; 2003. www.aast.org/03abstracts/03absPoster_059.html.

31. http://www.hcup-us.ahrq.gov/overview.jsp.

32. http://www.facs.org/trauma/ntdb.html.

33. http://www.hospitalcompare.hhs.gov.

34. http://www.leapfroggroup.org.

35. Kilgo PD, Meredith JW, Hensberry R, et al. A Note on the disjointed nature of the injury severity score. *J Trauma: Injury Infect Crit Care.* 2004;57:479–487.

36. Kilgo PD, Osler T, Meredith W. The worst injury predicts mortality outcome the best: Rethinking the role of multiple injuries in trauma outcome scoring. *J Trauma: Injury Infect Crit Care.* 2004;56:928–934.

37. Osler T, Rutledge R, Deis J, et al. ICISS: An international classification of disease-9 based injury severity score. *J Trauma.* 1996;41:380–386.

38. Copes WS, Champion HR, Sacco WJ, et al. Progress in characterizing anatomic injury. *Proceedings of the 33rd Annual Meeting of the Association for the Advancement of Automotive Medicine.* Baltimore;1089.

39. Osler T, Baker SP, Long W. A modification of the injury severity score that both improves accuracy and simplifies scoring. *J Trauma.* 1997;43(6):922–925; Discussion 925–926.

The Trauma Team

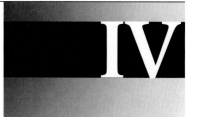

Overview—Making Music Out of Noise

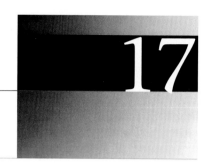

Janet McMaster *Mary Kate FitzPatrick* *Patrick Reilly*

To a newcomer, a trauma resuscitation can appear noisy, disorganized, and even chaotic. One sees and hears many health care providers, each performing unique tasks, each seemingly with a different purpose. Over time, with experience, one learns to appreciate the flow of resuscitation, the rhythm, and patterns, as the Airway, Breathing, Circulation (ABCs) are assessed and the primary and secondary surveys are performed. A well–run, well-organized trauma team functions as an orchestrated unit, with the trauma team leader as the director.

Similarly, the performance improvement (PI) process can appear chaotic and noisy, with unfamiliar acronyms and abbreviations, and seemingly random cases being discussed. A well-designed, well-structured PI program can eliminate the noise, and become an integral part of an efficient, harmonious trauma department.

PERFORMANCE IMPROVEMENT PLAN

The importance of a formal, written PI plan cannot be overemphasized. The PI plan should be a dynamic document, developed as the result of an integrated multidisciplinary effort, which should be reevaluated and updated periodically to encompass key changes within the hospital trauma system and trauma care standards. Recommended distribution of the plan might include hospital quality improvement staff, nursing leadership, physician leadership from medical divisions involved in trauma care, and trauma program staff. This plan could be used as part of the orientation process for new hospital leadership, which will be responsible for trauma patient care. The PI plan should include the following:

- Overview of the process (issue identification through resolution)
- Personnel involved and their roles
- PI forums/committees
- Link to hospital/system PI
- Problem identification and performance indicators
- Data management methods
- Guidelines for determining peer review judgment decisions (accountability)
- PI reports/provider profiles
- PI loop closure (reevaluation)
- Provision for protection of confidentiality

The PI plan should consider state, regional, and national standards related to trauma care. The American College of Surgeons document titled *Trauma Performance Improvement, A How to Handbook* provides practitioners with an operational manual for establishing and maintaining a trauma PI program.[1]

PERSONNEL

The trauma program's medical director sets the tone for the PI program, by leadership and active participation. Although tasks may be delegated to other personnel, the medical director is accountable for the PI activities.

Under various titles, the trauma nurse coordinator, program manager, or program administrator shares the responsibility for the PI program. In centers with high volumes of patients, the PI activities may be delegated to a PI coordinator, who is responsible for collecting and reporting data as well as for providing links with other hospital departments.

The attending physician staff should also have an active role in PI, which includes identifying problems, attendance at meetings, reviewing medical records, and participating in the peer review process. Ensuring physician attendance at PI meetings can be difficult. To facilitate attendance, a set calendar of meetings should be established on a routine day and time that are convenient for team members considering their clinical responsibilities. It may be helpful to incorporate trauma PI committees into existing hospital and departmental forums such as departmental morbidity and mortality conferences. There should be records of attendance to comply with the American College of Surgeons' (ACS) standard for participation in multidisciplinary peer review forums.

The roles and responsibilities of the personnel involved in the PI program should be part of the respective job descriptions, and these should be included in the PI plan.

PROCESS

The PI process can follow any one of a number of models, just one of which is outlined in the subsequent text.

FOCUS–PDCA, also called the *Shewhart cycle*

- Find a process improvement opportunity
- Organize a team that understands the process
- Clarify the current knowledge
- Uncover or understand the cause of variation
- Select a potential process improvement and start the "Plan-Do-Check-Act" cycle

Regardless of which model is utilized, the institution should have a systematic way to identify problems, analyze the issues, and take corrective action if indicated, and then reevaluate.

PROBLEM IDENTIFICATION—UTILIZING PERFORMANCE IMPROVEMENT INDICATORS: AUDIT FILTERS, OCCURRENCES, AND COMPLICATIONS

The trauma registry is a fundamental component of the center or trauma system, and there should be a strong interface between the registry and the PI program. Registry reports can provide information on audit filters; therefore, it is helpful to have the current registry data. This allows for real-time evaluation of care with impact to the patient at point of service. The utility of current audit filters has not been determined definitively. Research has been done on whether the audit filters have consistent links to improved outcomes.[2]

Literature suggests that although some have found existing audit filters to be useful, others have found them labor intensive and costly.[3]

Occurrences or complications can also be identified by registry reports, so an up-to-date registry is valuable. It is imperative that standard definitions for complications be adopted, so that occurrence rates can be compared or benchmarked with other institutions.

If the trauma center practices evidence-based medicine, in which high quality research leads to clinical guidelines, protocols, or algorithms, then variations in practice can be tracked and integrated into the PI process.

In addition to the registry, it is helpful to have a means for other health care providers to report issues on a concurrent basis, by way of a dedicated phone line, an electronic reporting system, or the use of issue identification forms, all of which should be set up to guarantee confidentiality. This encourages all members of the multidisciplinary trauma care team to participate in the PI program.

In addition to registry reports, other sources of information that can provide useful measures of outcome include patient satisfaction surveys, infection control reports, medical examiner reports and autopsies identifying missed injuries, utilization review data regarding readmissions, denied days, lengths of stay, and intensive care unit (ICU) lengths of stay.

MORTALITIES

Standard scoring systems provide a starting point for reviewing mortalities. In short, Trauma and Injury Severity Score (TRISS) tool methodology is based on the following:

- Physiologic parameters including respiratory rate (RR), Glasgow Coma Scale (GCS) score, and systolic blood pressure (SBP)
- Age (younger than 15 years, 15 to 55 years, and older than 55 years)
- Mechanism of injury (blunt or penetrating)
- Anatomic scoring of injuries by Injury Severity Score (ISS)

On the basis of these parameters, the probability of a patient's survival is calculated, and the outcome is expressed as expected death, unexpected death, or unexpected survivor. TRISS is useful in identifying unexpected outcomes, and it offers a standardized way to compare outcomes with those in other trauma centers, other states, and other populations. However, it has some limitations that reduce its usefulness in PI review. Because TRISS depends on physiologic parameters on admission, patients who arrive intubated, without a recorded respiratory rate, are excluded from analysis. Similarly, intubated patients lack the verbal component of the GCS, which excludes them from analysis.[4] While lack of verbal response and respiratory rate excludes a patient from TRISS, the intubation status is an independent predictor of mortality and should be included in future scoring systems.[5] Additionally, patients who arrive dead may have no injuries recorded; therefore, no ISS can be calculated. These patients are excluded from TRISS analysis until final anatomic diagnoses are determined from autopsy results. Another weakness of TRISS analysis is that it is based on the ISS, which was initially developed as a way to standardize severity of injuries for patients who were involved in motor vehicle crashes and had injuries to multiple body areas. The ISS is less accurate in classifying patients with multiple injuries to one body region, a disadvantage when calculating scores for patients with penetrating injuries.

Over the years, investigators have evaluated TRISS and tried to improve the method of evaluating trauma care objectively.[6-10] Some of the more recent innovations based on ICD-9-CM coding have the advantages of being more costefficient to calculate because they are based on injuries identified by medical record coders rather than specialized trauma registrars. In addition, they can be used to predict outcomes such as morbidity and lengths of stay, not just mortality. Another proposed method, the New Injury Severity Score (NISS), enhances ISS by including all the most serious injuries, not just the most serious in one body area.[11] These newer methods have been tested and compared to determine their validity and have the potential to enhance a trauma center's ability to predict mortality, if they become widely accepted.[12]

ANALYSIS

None of the scoring methods can replace a critical evaluation of patient care, in an interdisciplinary forum, using a framework for reaching peer review judgments. Participants at morbidity and mortality conferences should be prepared to come to a determination regarding the complication or death, whether it was nonpreventable, preventable, or potentially preventable. There are no clear-cut definitions for these terms because they are clinical judgments based on review of the available evidence from the medical records. Factors to be considered when reaching determinations should include the following:

- Was the outcome expected based on TRISS?
- Are the patient's injuries considered nonsurvivable (i.e., ISS = 75)?
- Were standard procedures, guidelines, and protocols followed?
- Was the care appropriate? Provider errors that could contribute to a death or complication include missed injuries, delayed diagnosis of injuries, technical errors, errors in judgment, and errors in management.
- Was system response optimal?
- Did the patient have preexisting medical conditions that contributed to the outcome?

Two useful techniques for analyzing unexpected outcomes are (i) FMECA (failure mode, effect, and criticality analysis), which is a systematic way to examine a process for possible ways in which failure can occur, usually initiated by a "near miss" incident and (ii) root cause analysis, which looks for the cause of variation after a sentinel event or an unexpected outcome has taken place.[13]

The purpose of determining preventability in the case of an unexpected outcome is not to place blame, but to provide an honest appraisal of what went wrong, to prevent future errors, and to enhance patient safety.[14,15]

ACTION PLAN—REEVALUATION

On determination that a provider- or system-related error has occurred corrective actions should be taken, which could include the following:

- Collection of data for a period of time to determine if the variation represents a trend or an isolated occurrence
- Change in or better enforcement of policy or procedure
- Development of clinical management guidelines
- Presentation of the issue as a topic in an educational setting
- Physician/provider counseling
- Mandatory continuing education
- Probation or suspension of staff members who have varied from accepted standards of care
- Notification of risk management

As mentioned previously, the PI process can be viewed as a cycle, as per the Joint Commission Accreditation of Healthcare Organizations (JCAHO) guidelines. One very important activity in closing a PI case is to ensure that the recommended actions are implemented and that the actions have the desired effect of improving patient care. This continuous reevaluation of the outcome guarantees that the PI process remains dynamic and responsive to the changing environment in medicine.

REFERENCES

1. American College of Surgeons, Committee on Trauma. *Trauma performance improvement, a how to handbook.* Chicago: American College of Surgeons; 2006.
2. Cryer HG, Hiatt JR, Fleming AW, et al. Continuous use of standard process audit filters has limited value in an established trauma system. *J Trauma.* 1996;41(3):389–395.
3. Rhodes M, Sacco W, Smith S. Cost effectiveness of trauma quality assurance audit filters. *J Trauma.* 1990;30:724–727.
4. Offner P, Jurkovich G, Gurney J, et al. Revision of TRISS for intubated patients. *J Trauma.* 1992;32:32–35.
5. Hannan EL, Farrell LS, Bessey PQ, et al. Accounting for intubation status in predicting mortality for victims of motor vehicle crashes. *J Trauma.* 2000;48(1):76–81.
6. Baker SP, O'Neill B, Haddon W, et al. The injury severity score: A method for describing patients with multiple injuries and evaluating emergency care. *J Trauma.* 1974;14:187–196.
7. Champion HR, Sacco WJ, Cornazzo AK, et al. A revision of the trauma score. *J Trauma.* 1989;29:623–676.
8. Sacco WJ, Copes W, Staz C, et al. Status of trauma patient management as measured by survival/death outcomes: Looking toward the 21st century. *J Trauma.* 1994;36:297–298.

9. Rutledge R, Osler T, Emery S, et al. The end of the Injury Severity Score (ISS) and the trauma and injury severity score tool (TRISS): ICISS, an international classification of diseases, the ninth revision-based prediction tool, out performs both ISS and TRISS as predictors of trauma patient survival, hospital charges, and length of stay. *J Trauma*. 1998;44:41–49.

10. Al West T, Rivara F, Cummings P, et al. Harborview assessment for risk of mortality: An improved measure of injury severity on the basis of ICD-9-CM. *J Trauma*. 2000;49(3):530–541.

11. Hoyt DB. Is it time for a new injury score (commentary)? *Lancet*. 1998;44:580–582.

12. Hannan EL, Waller CH, Farrell LS, et al. A comparison among the abilities of various injury severity measures to predict mortality with and without accompanying physiologic information. *J Trauma*. 2005;58(2):244–251.

13. http://www.jointcommission.org/SentinelEvents/se_glossary .htm, accessed November 1, 2006.

14. Gruen RL, Jurkovich GJ, McIntyre LK, et al. Patterns of errors contributing to trauma mortality: Lessons learned from 2,594 deaths. *Ann Surg*. 2006;244(3):371–380.

15. Pierluissi E, Fischer MA, Campbell AR, et al. Discussion of medical errors in morbidity and mortality conferences. *JAMA*. 2003;290(21):2838–2842.

Information Management to Improve Performance

18

Paul A. MacLennan   *E. Lanette Milligan*

Information management is a vast and important endeavor in the care of trauma patients. Their care often relies on a multitude of interrelated surgical and medical specialties, diagnostic tests, and therapeutic interventions that are time and resource intensive as well as costly. Health care delivery is inherently fragmented and poor documentation and miscommunication can lead to errors, duplicate testing, inappropriate care, increased costs, and reduced timeliness of care. Information management and health information technology have the potential to enhance timely care that is well organized and efficient through planning and communications while decreasing complications, lengths of stay, and adverse events. However, research shows that adoption of new technologies that contribute to quality and safety has not occurred as quickly as had been anticipated.[1]

A number of stakeholders, both inside and outside of medicine, are pushing for more integrated and sophisticated information management systems. This new emphasis is most always linked to the desires of health care facilities, providers, and third party payers to improve the overall quality of care and cost-effectiveness by streamlining bureaucracy, catching and correcting errors, assisting with decisions, and improving communications. A report in 2000 from the Institute of Medicine (IOM) dramatized the need for greater attention to quality. In their report, the IOM estimated that adverse events occurred in 2.9% to 3.7% of all hospitalizations and in light of approximately 34,000,000 hospital admissions per year, the number of deaths that resulted were between 44,000 and 98,000.[2]

Health care is an information intensive industry with an estimated annual 30 billion transactions.[3] Although it would seem important for health care to rely heavily on information management, the industry has historically underinvested in information systems, as compared to other industries.[3,4] Unlike other sectors of the economy, health care is very complex, making computerization of medical tasks very difficult. In addition, doctors have traditionally controlled decision making in health care and when lives are at stake, they are understandably conservative about changing the way they practice medicine.[5] Furthermore, introduction of information technology can produce stress among an entire organization because its integration often interferes with the existing workflow.[6] However, there is a serious need to overhaul the information system that has historically relied on paper, telephone, fax, and Electronic Data Interchange media to create a system that is often inefficient in communications within and between organizations.[7] The shift from paper-based processing and storage to electronic-based processing and storage has brought some disadvantages due to higher technologic complexity and advantages because of higher functionality and greater opportunities in using patient information and medical knowledge.[8]

Information is stored in many ways and in many locations with inherent fragmentation that often results in incomplete, inaccurate, and unclear communications based on which clinical decisions have to be made. The expected information technology overhaul is likely to be very expensive and many providers will need financial assistance for investments as well as a nudge from payers in how they pay for health care.[3] For example, Kaiser Permanente, an integrated managed care organization operating in nine US states, plans to spend approximately $3.2 billion on a paperless system over 10 years.[3] In the past, hospitals' boards of trustees have held medical staff responsible for developing and implementing activities and mechanisms for monitoring and evaluating patient care and to identify opportunities to improve patient care by recognizing and then resolving patient care problems; but with the impeding pay for performance standards the approach to information management may begin to be addressed strategically from the top levels of administration.[9,10]

Health care information is health care data that has been processed. Therefore, in order to have high quality health care information the data input must also be of high quality. Data is utilized for billing, research, decision making across professions, and for comparisons for health care issues. Poor data can result in diminished quality in patient care, poor communication among providers and patients, problems with documentation, reduced revenue generation due to problems with reimbursement, and a diminished capacity to effectively evaluate outcomes or participate in research activities.[3]

The Medical Records Institute identified five areas in which poor data can affect poor health care outcomes:

- Patient safety
- Public safety
- Continuity of patient care
- Health care economics
- Clinical research and outcomes analysis[3]

HISTORY OF HEALTH CARE INFORMATION SYSTEMS

The evolution of information systems in health care was primarily shaped by the needs of organizations to be reimbursed and external technologic developments.[3] Health care organizations began to seek out systems that could automate billing and process accurate cost reports in response to the payment systems established by Medicaid and Medicare in the 1960s. During this period, the Hill-Burton Act encouraged tremendous growth of new hospitals throughout the United States and provided access to capital for organizations to grow and expand. Driven by Medicare and Medicaid reimbursement practices that paid a little higher than the costs of services, known as *costs plus reimbursement*, and by demands to access capital through Hill-Burton, organizations needed a way to keep track of their accounting and finances, and patients. During the period of cost plus reimbursement practices, the larger the number of patients that organizations served, the more they grew, and the more money they

were reimbursed. Computers of this period were very large and needed a great deal of space for storage and maintenance. They were also quite expensive and typically only available to very large medical centers.[3] Centralized large mainframe computers were typically utilized for automating administrative functions such as accounting and financial services.[6]

The 1970s can be characterized by escalating costs in health care and the development of minicomputers and departmental information systems. It became necessary for departments (e.g., laboratory, radiology) to address efficiency of care and minicomputers were smaller and often more powerful than mainframe computers.[3] During this period turnkey systems were developed and marketed by vendors toward departments within health care facilities. Software systems could be put into functional operation in a department simply by being turned on, therefore the turnkey terminology.[3] The turnkey systems were limited in their inability to be adaptable to specific institutions.[3] However, the advent of the minicomputer allowed for technology to find its way into clinical applications rather than just administrative functions.

Health care costs continued to increase in the 1980s and Medicare transformed its reimbursement policies from the cost plus reimbursement to a prospective payment system based on diagnosis-related groups (DRGs). Health care organizations were now paid a specific amount for a specific diagnosis as opposed to being paid the costs determined by organizations to treat their patients. This new reimbursement system forced health care organizations to implement cost-reducing processes and policies and to strive for more efficiency in delivery of care. Also in response to increase costs, health insurance companies began to move from fee-for-service models toward managed care plans. The 1980s also saw privatization and integration of health care organizations and health care services were merged into one system to offer a range of services from ambulatory care to long-term care. The dramatic changes of this period welcomed the advent of the microcomputer, better known as the *personal computer* (PC).[3] The PC was powerful and small and could be utilized at workstations in departments. It was typical of this period for computers to be specific to departments, for example pharmacy or laboratories, and rarely were the systems integrated to enable different departments to communicate with one another. However local area networks (LAN) did allow for multiple computers to share pertinent information.[3] The microcomputer allowed for health care organizations other than large hospitals to acquire computer technology.

The 1990s were a dynamic era for health care and information technology. The success of DRGs ushered in similar changes of reimbursement policies for providers based on managed care models. The new system supported on resource-based relative value scale intended to put decisions into the more efficient and less costly primary care providers and therefore reimbursed them at better rates than specialist; however, the changes required good information management to administer these new reimbursement practices.[3] Other managed care components called for physicians to become better at disease management, and technology offered a mechanism to do so. In 1991 the IOM called for a gradual phase out of paper records, citing numerous problems and recommended the adoption of computer-based patient record (CPR).[3] In 1996 the Health Insurance Portability and Accountability Act (HIPAA) was signed into law and was designed to make insurance more affordable and accessible; however, the real impact of the law resides in its provision to protect the confidentiality of patient health records.[11] Up to this point, there was no federal legislation addressing the confidentiality of patient records. HIPAA ushered in the most sweeping change to the US health care system since Medicare and Medicaid.[10] During this time computers were becoming much more prevalent, with many households now owning PCs. The impact of the microcomputer in the 1980s parallels the introduction of the Internet in the 1990s as the *single greatest technologic achievement of this era.* The Internet impacted health care in a multitude of ways, from how health care professionals communicated, accessed information, and conducted business. Providers can access vast amounts of information quickly, patients and providers communicate through e-mail efficiently and in a timely manner, and organizations can share information internally and externally to improve business processes.[3]

In trauma care currently, hospital information systems are just one component of health information. The importance of information management begins at the time of injury in the prehospital setting and follows patients' continuum of care through the emergency department (ED), surgery, the intensive care unit (ICU), and hospital stay, until discharge and rehabilitation.

PREHOSPITAL INFORMATION

Enhanced information technology, information management, and communications are critical to trauma systems providing seamless transition between each stage of patient care. Efficient and rapid movement of patients through the system (prehospital assessment and treatment, transport, hospital resuscitation, evaluation, and care) results in maximum outcome potential and trauma survival.[12,13] Effective communication enables the systems to vary resource utilization and allow for maximum preparation from receiving trauma centers.[14]

To attain high performance and quality assurance, emergency medical service (EMS) systems must monitor the effectiveness of patient care delivery. Prehospital information is used to bridge the gap between education and competency. Reliable information can be used for educational reinforcement based on actual patient care

for the purpose of improving patient care. Current activities include the National Emergency Medical Services Information System (NEMSIS), a nationwide electronic EMS documentation system.[15] The NEMSIS will eventually be used for EMS education, to examine outcomes and evaluate trauma systems, and to generate research questions and evaluate cost-effectiveness.

AUTOMATIC COLLISION NOTIFICATION

Motor vehicle collisions (MVCs) are a significant cause of morbidity and mortality throughout the world. Trauma centers and systems have decreased mortality rates by providing MVC victims with appropriate and timely trauma care.[13] Currently available automotive technology represents an opportunity to further enhance patient survival in the prehospital setting. Automatic crash notification (ACN) systems utilize collision sensors and wireless technology to detect and transmit information regarding the occurrence of an MVC.[16-19] ACN systems provide an opportunity for decreasing the time between injury and EMS arrival, which may be especially important in rural areas where MVCs may go unobserved and therefore result in delayed notification of EMS. Moreover, the information available from newer systems (e.g., crash severity) can be used to estimate occupant injuries and aid in the delivery of prehospital care and thereby improve patient outcomes.[20] Currently, the two largest commercial providers of ACN services in the United States are OnStar and ATX Technologies.

ACN services utilize systems that are integrated with the vehicle electrical architecture. The systems are activated by in-vehicle crash sensors and the resultant crash messages are transmitted by cell phone call to the service provider call center that is operated by the ACN service. The crash location (i.e., vehicle latitude and longitude at the time of the crash) is determined using global positioning system (GPS) and reported as part of the crash message. All currently available ACN systems provide the time and location of the MVC; some of the newer systems can also provide information on the nature and severity of the crash. Potentially, future systems, utilizing available technology could also include information on the number and seating position of vehicle occupants, restraint and protection system use, and postcrash vehicle orientation (e.g., overturned, vehicle rollover, and occupant ejection). However, currently ACN systems are not integrated with EMS or public safety agencies (9-1-1 centers).

When an ACN-equipped vehicle is involved in an MVC, the vehicle automatically transmits a crash message to the national call center operated by the ACN telematics service provider (TSP) (e.g., OnStar). The TSP attempts to talk to occupants of the car and when necessary, calls the public safety dispatch organization (i.e., the 9-1-1 call center) serving the region in which the crash has occurred, and verbally provides them with crash information including crash location. Quantitative estimates of the potential benefit of ACN systems are dependent on the level of ACN market penetration (i.e., the number of vehicles on the road with ACN equipment). A recent estimate, assuming an ideal ACN system, suggested a 1.5% to 6% reduction in MVC deaths in the United States annually.[21]

HEALTH CARE AND MEDICAL INFORMATICS

Information management has many different components and plays a number of roles in health care; it is important to note that many of the terminologies are used interchangeably. At the basic level are health care data. Data are facts, images, or sounds that may or may not be useful.[6] For example a number, 13, is a datum that is not useful without context. Most often, not until the data has been formatted, filtered, and/or manipulated does it become useful and is now considered health information.[6] Health information is utilized to make comparisons and is shared across many professions.[3] "Transforming quality health care data into meaningful health care information is necessary to access the quality of patient care and to improve its effectiveness. The quality of health care depends upon the quality of health care information."[6] Clinical practice in health care relies on gathering, synthesizing, and acting on information. The relevance of a good hospital information system is obvious because without access to relevant data, no decisions on diagnostic, therapeutic, or other procedures can be made. Medical informatics is a scientific field concerned with improving health care through the management and use of medical information. The objective of medical informatics is to examine and optimally manage the flow of information in biomedicine and health care.

Health care information systems include all clinical and administrative applications and comprises interacting components such as people, work processes, data, and information technologies that have defined relationships that all work toward accomplishing a goal.[6] Health care organizations employ a multitude of information systems; for example, administrative, clinical, financial, and operational. Administrative information systems may include management information systems that enable decision making among managers. Clinical information systems include patient care and laboratory and radiology systems. Financial systems include billing, accounts receivable, and accounts payable systems. Operational information systems include admission, operating room scheduling, and inventory systems.[6]

The electronic medical record (EMR) has been defined as the set of databases (or repositories) that contains the health information for patients within a given institution or organization. Therefore, an EMR contains the aggregated data sets gathered from a variety of clinical service delivery processes, including laboratory data, pharmacy data, patient registration data, radiology data, surgical procedures, clinic and inpatient notes, preventive care delivery, ED visits, billing information, and so on. Research in the field of medical informatics has recently enabled the development of many applications relevant to clinical practice. These applications are also part of the EMR and include clinical information systems (e.g., EMR, laboratory information systems, picture archiving and communication systems (PACS) for radiographs), computerized provider order entry (CPOE), computerized patient care systems, computerized clinical decision support systems (CDSS), telemedicine, knowledge access and retrieval through online resources or those installed onto a PC or a personal digital assistant (PDA), and communication systems that utilize text messaging and automated patient alerts through PDAs. Applications that record information, for example, EMRs connected to medical devices and PACS, show that computerized data collection can be reliably captured in both computerized systems and noncomputerized systems.[22]

The IOM report in 2000 stated that a major cause of errors was due to providers not having access to complete patient data at the point of care because of decentralization and fragmentation of the health care system.[2] The concept of the electronic health record (EHR) extends EMRs to cross-institutional health information exchange (HIE) and would typically include subsets of a number of EMRs for each patient. The EHR includes a number of episodes of care rather than a single encounter and is only possible if EMRs from participating institutions are interoperable. In addition to its technical issues (e.g., lack of standards), EHR implication is complicated by legal issues regarding protected health information (PHI) privacy and data security. In the United States, there are currently 109 regional health information organizations in 45 states. An example is the Indiana Network for Patient Care, an HIE in Indianapolis that receives information from all local hospitals, physicians' offices, community health centers, health departments, laboratories and pharmacies; information is readily available to ED staff when a patient enters the ED. A potential benefit to future success of these organizations is today's more advanced and less expensive networking technologies, which rely on the Internet instead of stand-alone networks, enabling a decentralized approach to data sharing so that stakeholders can maintain their own information. In addition to their primary purpose of defragmenting patient health care information, the advancement of EHRs and regional health information organizations will eventually be used to support public health and epidemiologic research.[23]

The Agency for Health care Research and Quality (AHRQ) has defined the general framework (see Fig. 1) of health care information technology (HIT) as incorporating four levels: (i) application level, (ii) communication level, (iii) process level, and (iv) device level. The application

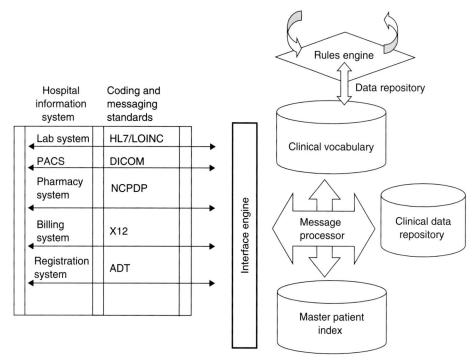

Figure 1 Health care data flow and inner relations of applications. (Adapted from AHRQ National Resource Center for Health Information Technology)

level includes CPOE, clinical decision support (CDS), electronic prescribing (e-prescribing), electronic medication administration records (eMAR), results reporting, electronic documentation, and interface engines; the communication level includes messaging standards (HL7, ADT, NCPDP, X12, DICOM, etc.) and coding standards (LOINC, ICD-9, CPT, NDC, RxNorm, SNOMED CT, etc.); the process level includes HIE, master patient index (MPI), HIPAA security/privacy, and so on; and the device level includes tablet PCs, application service provider (ASP) models, PDAs, and bar coding (see Table 1).[24]

Many Emergency Department Information Systems (EDIS) are stand-alone, proprietary products that can also be integrated into hospital information systems. Goals of an integrated EDIS include (i) minimizing redundant input by automating Admission Discharge and Transfer (ADT) software; automating laboratory,

electrocardiogram (ECG), radiology, and ancillary reports into the ED record; integrating discharge instructions and prescriptions into chart; and automating output for patients; (ii) improving tracking of patients, equipment, and staff through an automatic passive tracking system; (iii) providing cost-effective patient charting; and (iv) providing digital radiology (DR).[25] An effective EDIS can help streamline clinical workflow, reduce patient length of stay, decrease medication errors and duplication of tests, and enhance revenue by enabling coders to capture all performed procedures.

PATIENT INFORMATION FLOW

Understanding how technologies and work practices affect information flow in health care is becoming increasingly important. Information flow connects the units of a hospital with the health care providers within each unit. Specialized systems collect and store data within hospital information systems. For example, patients have blood drawn and analyzed by the hospital laboratory, then laboratory information systems collect all the data about processed specimens. Similar systems are in existence for radiology services, billing services, pharmacy services, and so on resulting in multiple silos of information.

All patient information is maintained in one place, the clinical data repository, which obtains data from the separate specialized hospital information systems so that information is more readily attainable. Because these hospital information systems may use different information to identify patients, the central data repository relies on an MPI to

TABLE 1		
APPLICATIONS AND DEVICES FOR PATIENT MANAGEMENT		
PDA/tablet	Results reporting	CPOE
Web/ASP	Clinical documentation	eMAR
Bar coding	Patient management	e-Prescribing

PDA, personal digital assistant; CPOE, computerized provider order entry; ASP, application service provider; eMAR, electronic medication administration records.

ensure that all the different identifying information about each patient can be resolved to a single patient identity.

Coding and messaging standards have been developed to pull data from these specialized systems into the clinical data repository. These standards (e.g., CPT, HL7) were developed so as to reach agreement on what each piece of data represents, and how to format each transmission of data. Because everyone does not use the same standards, health care organizations have developed interface engines that translate from one standard to another. However, the above-mentioned information is usually unknown to end users who are generally interested only in applications such as CPOE, CDS, and so on.

COMPUTERIZED PROVIDER ORDER ENTRY

CPOE systems are higher-level clinical applications in which providers write orders for tests, medications, services, or other clinical processes. Because most actions in health care follow an order, computerization allows for real-time decision support that implements guidelines and critical pathways. To enable clinicians to make an informed decision, ideally CPOE uses other clinical systems (e.g., clinical data repository of patient information, user interphase for data entry that might include CDS, and a clinical messaging system to communicate orders).

During the "ordering phase," CDS is concerned about the choices made by the provider. If, for example, a patient's prescribed medication conflicts with another medication then the ordering user is given an alert. An ideal CDS system will be able to access the patient's current clinical data and know the "best practices" within a given domain (expressed as electronic rules using Boolean or other logic). Given a new order within the CPOE, The CDS will apply these rules to the clinical data and provide appropriate guidance about potential problems.

Other Components of Computerized Provider Order Entry

E-Prescribing
Prescriptions that are generated and transmitted electronically can increase medication safety by checking drug doses, routes of administration, frequency of administration, patient allergies, and drug-to-drug interactions before a prescription is issued, and by alerting clinicians when patients are at risk because of a potential prescription. In addition, pharmacy bar coding of medications ensures that patients receive the ordered medication in the correct dose at the specified time.

Quality Improvement
CPOE systems can provide real-time quality of care through other forms of CDS such as evidence-based order sets given an indication or condition, and automated reminders and alerts embedded within the ordering process so that important interventions and actions are not omitted from the clinical service delivery.

Clinical Decision Support

AHRQ defines CDS as "...software that makes relevant information available for clinical decision making." CDS ranges from electronically available clinical data (e.g., information from a clinical laboratory system and information from a disease registry), to electronic full-text journal and textbook access, to evidence-based clinical guidelines, to systems that provide patient and situation-specific advice (e.g., ECG interpretation, and drug-to-drug interaction checking).[26] The functionality of CDS can be influenced by user-friendly presentation of data and the allowance of manipulation of data. Clinical effectiveness cannot be simply judged on the basis of whether patient outcomes are positively affected (e.g., health status and processes of care) but also by the acceptance of clinicians (e.g., adherence to CDS recommendations, satisfaction, efficiency).[22]

CDS has been shown to be effective in the trauma setting. McKinley et al. (2001) reported effective standardized mechanical ventilator support in trauma patients with acute respiratory distress syndrome.[27] Traditionally, this task had been performed by a respiratory therapist (RT) at bedside who reset mechanical ventilator controls based on physician orders. However, orders lack consistency and there is a lag between assessment-order and order-execution. The CDS system uses a computer at bedside that iteratively executes clinical logic and provides the bedside RT with data and instructions. The system not only standardizes care but also improves the quality of care by reducing errors.[28]

The key to increasing acceptance of CDS is in integrating it with other clinical systems and clinical workflow at the point of decision making. The development of the EMR will greatly enhance the prevalence of CDS functions such as reminders for appropriate care, drug-to-allergy alerting during order entry, and evidence-based order sets. CDS should also enable access to medical knowledge (full-text journals, trusted e-health portals, EMRs) at the point of care. Access requires trusted data sources and availability of these sources to those who need them.

IMPROVING SAFETY WITH INFORMATION TECHNOLOGY

Information technology can reduce the rates of errors in three ways: potentially preventing errors and adverse events, facilitating a rapid response after an adverse event has occurred, and by providing feedback about adverse events. Technology contributes to error prevention by improved communications, readily accessible knowledge, requiring key pieces of information (e.g., drug dosage); assisting in calculations, performing checks in real-time, assisting in monitoring, and providing decision support.[29] For example, in a study examining the utility of CDS in assisting adjustment of medication dosage among patients with renal insufficiency, Chertow et al. reported significantly improved rates of appropriate prescribing by dosage and frequency using this technology.[30]

IMPROVING COMMUNICATIONS

Discontinuity of care due to cross-coverage had been shown to increase the risk of an adverse event by as much as a factor of five[31]. Technology designed to improve the exchange of and access to clinical data, including computerized coverage systems for signing out, handheld PDAs, and wireless access to EMRs should have a significant impact in the reduction of these types of errors.

In addition, information systems can automatically identify and communicate laboratory abnormalities that require immediate attention to clinicians. One study reported that such systems had the potential to reduce response time by 11% and the duration of dangerous conditions by 29%.[32]

ACCESS TO INFORMATION

A number of reference materials, that is, Medline database and reference guides are available on desk-top and handheld computers. The portability that a PDA offers enables clinicians to access medical reference information to support decision making at the point of care with relative ease.[33,34]

RAPID RESPONSE AND TRACKING OF ADVERSE EVENTS

Computerized tools can be used in conjunction with the EMR to identify, intervene, and track the frequency of adverse events. The electronic ICU can use smart alarms to enhance efficiency, increase effectiveness, and standardize clinical and operating processes. In addition, performance can be improved through automated measure of outcomes and monitoring of resource utilization.

REQUIRING INFORMATION AND ASSISTING WITH CALCULATIONS

CPOE applications force prescriptions written on computers to be legible and complete. By having the capabilities to place limits on dosage and warn about potential adverse effects, these applications reduce error rates. Corollary orders

are dependent actions that are triggered by placing an order that may require other orders. Calculation errors, for example infusion rates, can be reduced using computers.

OTHER INFORMATION TECHNOLOGIES

Many hospitals are implementing PACS. Studies have shown that these systems work well when compared with conventional radiographs with the added benefit of saving time for the trauma team in the management of patients.[35,36] With DR, electronic transmitters capture radiographic images that can be transmitted for review within seconds. The process time is much faster than screen-film radiographic processing and has the added advantage that DR images can be transferred to a PACS with ease. Once the images are available in PACS, they can be reviewed and interpreted concurrently by a radiologist and the treating physician resulting in faster interpretation and time to treatment. A recent study compared the average time per image examination between a group of patients with mixed film and computed radiography (CR) to a group of patients with DR images only. The authors reported that although technicians had initial difficulty with learning DR, resulting in twice as many repeat images compared to the CR group, there was still a significant 23% decrease in time spent per image (2.51±1.16 minute compared to 3.27±1.50 minute).[37]

Telemedicine is the use of telecommunications to allow caregivers to interact with patients and/or other caregivers operating at remote locations. In the past, a number of telecommunications devices have been used including telephones, radios, facsimile, modem, and video. Rosenfeld et al. (2000) showed the utility of providing continuous patient management in a surgical ICU through remote 24-hour monitoring by an offsite intensivist using video conferencing and high bandwidth.[38] Computerized monitoring can examine large amounts of data for trends and relations before an adverse event occurs.[39]

Bar coding, long used in grocery stores, is now used to reduce pharmacy-dispensing errors. However, owing to its high start-up costs and maintenance it is estimated that currently only 5% of US hospitals use this technology.[40] Long-term studies suggest that it substantially decreases the incidence of adverse drug events (ADEs) and that over time, more than pays for itself by decreasing the costs associated with ADEs.[41,42] Another use of bar coding is for patient identification bracelets that are designed to reduce errors such as performing procedures on one patient that are intended for another.

Wireless alert pager systems serve as communication tools between staff members and as real-time clinical notification systems of critical laboratory results, medication problems, and critical patient trend information.[43] For the latter function, pagers linked to clinical information systems convey important clinical information to health care workers who are extremely mobile (e.g., within an ICU) and would otherwise be unaware of changes in critical values. Unlike one-way pagers, two-way pagers have the potential to send a message received confirmation, send a "message read" confirmation, and to send direct feedback to other caregivers. Pager systems can also allow for a hierarchical structure that resends the message to a supervisor if the message is unread or unanswered.

The Internet is a powerful tool that offers basic medical uses such as email and locating medical information online to more advanced uses such as access to patient information, wireless access, and critical events notification.[44] For remote access to patient information, the institution must maintain a "firewall" which requires a certificate server to authenticate who the user is. Information is further protected by encryption and through a secured and locked session. Access allows for real-time monitoring (e.g., ICU flow sheets) of the EMR. PACS may also be available online so that physicians can select from x-rays, magnetic resonance images, and computed tomography images; all of which can be manipulated (e.g., zoom, moved) by clicking a mouse.

PRIVACY AND CONFIDENTIALITY

The HIPAA was enacted by the US Congress in 1996 and defines PHI as "verbal or written information created or received by a healthcare provider, health plan, public health authority, employer, life insurer, school or university or healthcare clearing house that related to the physical or mental health of an individual, or payment for provision of health care."[11] Under HIPAA, PHI is protected from intentional or unintentional disclosure or misuse. A great deal of information is not PHI because it is not patient specific. The patient record generates most of the clinical information generated by a health care organization.[3]

The Joint Commission (formerly the *Joint Commission on Accreditation of Healthcare Organizations*), encourages health care organizations to take responsibility of health care information management just as they would their other resources, dividing health care information into the following:

- Patient-specific data and information
- Aggregate data and information
- Knowledge-based information
- Comparative data and information

The Joint Commission is a voluntary accrediting agency; however Medicare and Medicaid will not reimburse organizations that are not accredited. The Joint Commission has devoted a great deal to specifying information systems standards regardless of the technology used and expects information management systems "to support decision making to improve patient outcomes, improve health care documentation, assure patient safety, and improve

performance in patient care, treatment, and services, governance, management and support processes."[45] The Joint Commission states that organizations must "identify their information needs, design the structure of their information management system, capture, organize, store, retrieve, process and analyze data, and information, transmit, report display, integrate and use data and information and safeguard data and information," as well as maintain standards to ensure content and security of patient records.[3]

GUIDELINES, PATHWAYS, AND PROTOCOLS

Clinical guidelines are systematically developed statements designed to assist physician and physician extender decision making. They are generally specific to a disease, problem, or process and include recommendations, which are rated by the power of evidence. The AHRQ includes evidence-based guidelines that are accessible online through the National Guideline Clearinghouse (NGC), a public resource for evidence-based clinical practice guidelines.[46] Guidelines are derived from national organizations and societies (e.g., The Eastern Association for the Surgery of Trauma, The Society for Critical Care Medicine) and are intended at the appropriateness of care. Pathways and protocols are bedside tools for implementation of guidelines.[47] The former are designed to provide overviews of the care processes whereas clinical management protocols are derived from evidence-based national guideline but use institutional specific algorithms for patient care. For implementing these tools and accessing their effectiveness, it is necessary to integrate the hospital information system to enable decision support. The American College of Surgeons Committee on Trauma lists 26 evidence-based guidelines in its Trauma Performance Improvement Reference Manual.[48]

CONCLUSIONS

Health care delivery is perhaps the most complex of all human endeavors. Primarily for this reason, the transformation of health informatics from paper to electronic has often fallen short of its promise. Although there has been an explosion of informatics systems and applications, there are few assessments that have considered safety, functionality, technical performance, clinical effectiveness, economics, and organizational limitations.[22] There remains a large gap between the embedded logic of CPOE and CDS and how clinical work is actually performed. According to Wears and Berg (2007), the former are based on a different work model; one that is objective, rational, linear, localized, solitary, and single minded; whereas clinicians are interpretive, multitask, collaborate, distribute tasks, and are opportunistic and reactive.[49]

The potential benefits of CPOE are many: improved patient safety and efficiency of care, support of compliance efforts, and support of billing activities. For example, a study of a busy medical-surgical ICU reported significantly improved timeliness of diagnostic laboratory and imaging tests with CPOE.[50] However, there are pitfalls related mostly to disruptions in workflow when CPOE is introduced into an ICU, many due to the increased workload in coordination of activities because of improper workflow assumptions in the design of the CPOE.[51] In addition, one recent study found that a poorly designed CPOE system actually increased medication errors because of poor information display, concurrent use of a hybrid paper-electronic system that resulted in ignored notifications, separation of functions, and inflexible ordering formats that generated incorrect orders.[52] Although the technologic challenges of implementing these systems are great, it appears as if the sociocultural hurdles are even greater because system implementation dramatically alters the workflows of busy health care providers.

REFERENCES

1. Poon EG, Jha AK, Christino M, et al. Assessing the level of healthcare information technology adoption in the United States: A snapshot. *BMC Med Inform Decis Mak.* 2006;6:1.
2. Institute of Medicine Committee on Quality of Healthcare in America. *To err is human: Building a safer health system.* In: Kohn LT, Corrigan JM, Donaldson MS, eds. Washington, DC: National Academy Press, 2000.
3. Wager K, Lee FW, Glasser JP. *Managing health care information systems: a practical approach for health care executives.* San Fransico: Jossey-Bass; 2003.
4. Bottles K. Critical choices face healthcare in how to use information technology. *MedGenMed.* 1999;1:E24.
5. Gawande AA, Bates DW. The use of information technology in improving medical performance. Part I. Information systems for medical transactions. *MedGenMed.* 2000;2:E14.
6. Johns M. *Information management for health professionals.* Albany: Delmar; 1997.
7. Litvin CB. In the dark – the case for electronic health records. *N Engl J Med.* 2007;356:2454–2455.
8. Haux R. Health information systems – past, present, future. *Int J Med Inform.* 2006;75:268–281.
9. Kahn CN, Ault T, Isenstein H, et al. Snapshot of hospital quality reporting and pay-for-performance under Medicare. *Health Aff (Millwood).* 2006;25:148–162.
10. Skurka M, eds. *Health information management: principals and organization for health information services,* 5th ed. Chicago: Jossey-Bass; 2003.
11. *Health insurance portability and accountability act of 1996. Public law 104-191, 104th Congress.* Accessed June 30, 2007: http://www.cms.hhs.gov/HIPAAGenInfo/Downloads/HIPAALaw.pdf.
12. Sauaia A, Moore FA, Moore EE, et al. Epidemiology of trauma deaths: A reassessment. *J Trauma.* 1995;38:185–193.
13. Nathens AB, Jurkovich GJ, Cummings P, et al. The effect of organized systems of trauma care on motor vehicle crash mortality. *JAMA.* 2000;283:1990–1994.
14. BREMSS. *Overview of Birmingham Regional Emergency Medical Services System (BREMSS).* Accessed June 26, 2007. http://www.bremss.org/index_files/menu.htm.
15. NESIS. *History of NESIS.* Accessed June 30, 2007. http://www.NEMSIS.org.
16. Butler D, *Launching advanced automatic crash notification (AACN): A new generation of emergency response,* SAE Paper 2002–21–0066.
17. Berube J. Reducing the Extent Of Injury Using Telematics. *J Head Trauma Rehabil.* 2000;15:1186–1189.
18. Starosielec, EA, Funke, DJ, Blatt, AJ, *Automated Crash Notification: Preliminary Findings and Future Trends, Transportation Research News,* Transportation Research Board, No. 201, March 1999.
19. Akella MR, Bang C, Beutner R, et al. Evaluating the reliability of automated collision notification systems. *Accid Anal Prev.* 2003;35:349–360.
20. Champion HR, Augenstein J, Blatt AJ, et al. Automatic crash notification and the URGENCY algorithm: Its history, value, and use. *Top Emerg Med.* 2004;26:143–156.
21. Clark DE, Cushing BM. Predicted effect of automatic crash notification on traffic mortality. *Accid Anal Prev.* 2002;34:507–513.
22. Adhikari N, Lapinsky SE. Medical informatics in the intensive care unit: Overview of technology assessment. *J Crit Care.* 2003;18:41–47.
23. Shapiro JS, Kannry J, Lipton M, et al. Approaches to patient health information exchange and their impact on emergency medicine. *Ann Emerg Med.* 2006;48:426–432.
24. AHRQ. *Architecture of health IT.* Agency for Healthcare Research and Quality. http://healthit.ahrq.gov/portal/server.pt?open=514&objID=5554&mode=2&holderDisplayURL=http://prodportallb.ahrq.gov:7087/publishedcontent/publish/communities/k_o/knowledge_library/key_topics/health_briefing_03282006111834/architecture_of_health_it.html. Accessed June 30, 2007.
25. Taylor TB. Information management in the emergency department. *Emerg Med Clin North Am.* 2004;22:241–257.
26. AHRQ. *Clinical decision support.* Agency for Healthcare Research and Quality. http://healthit.ahrq.gov/portal/server.pt?open=514&objID=5554&mode=2&holderDisplayURL=http://prodportallb.ahrq.gov:7087/publishedcontent/publish/communities/k_o/knowledge_library/key_topics/health_briefing_01242006122700/clinical_decision_support.html. Accessed June 30, 2007.
27. McKinley BA, Moore FA, Sailors RM, et al. Computerized decision support for mechanical ventilation of trauma induced ARDS: Results of a randomized clinical trial. *J Trauma.* 2001;50: 415–424.
28. East TD, Heermann LK, Bradshaw RL, et al. Efficacy of computerized decision support for mechanical ventilation: Results of a prospective multi-center randomized trial. *Proc AMIA Symp.* 1999;251–255.
29. Bates DW, Gawande AA. Improving safety with information technology. *N Engl J Med.* 2003;348:2526–2534.
30. Chertow GM, Lee J, Kuperman GJ, et al. Guided medication dosing for inpatients with renal insufficiency. *JAMA.* 2001;286:2839–2844.
31. Petersen LA, Brennan TA, O'Neil AC, et al. Does housestaff discontinuity of care increase the risk for preventable adverse events? *Ann Droit Int Med.* 1994;121:866–872.
32. Kuperman GJ, Teich JM, Tanasijevic MJ, et al. Improving response to critical laboratory results with automation: results of a randomized controlled trial. *J Am Med Inform Assoc.* 1999;6:512–522.
33. Lapinsky SE, Wax R, Showalter R, et al. Prospective evaluation of an internet-linked handheld computer critical care knowledge access system. *Crit Care.* 2004;8:R414–R421.
34. Rothschild JM, Lee TH, Bae T, et al. Clinician use of a palmtop drug reference guide. *J Am Med Inform Assoc.* 2002;9:223–229.
35. Gouin S, Patel H, Bergeron S, et al. The effect of picture archiving and communications systems on the accuracy of diagnostic interpretation of pediatric emergency physicians. *Acad Emerg Med.* 2006;13:186–190.
36. Lucey BC, Stuhlfaut JW, Hochberg AR, et al. Evaluation of blunt abdominal trauma using PACS-based 2D and 3D MDCT reformations of the lumbar spine and pelvis. *AJR Am J Roentgenol.* 2005;185:1435–1440.
37. Lee B, Junewick J, Luttenton C. Effect of digital radiography on emergency department radiographic examinations. *Emerg Radiol.* 2006;12:158–159.
38. Rosenfeld BA, Dorman T, Breslow MJ, et al. Intensive care unit telemedicine: Alternate paradigm for providing continuous intensivist care. *Crit Care Med.* 2000;28:3925–3931.

39. Celi LA, Hassan E, Marquardt C, et al. The eICU: It's not just telemedicine. *Crit Care Med.* 2001;29:N183–N189.

40. Wright AA, Katz IT. Bar coding for patient safety. *N Engl J Med.* 2007;353:329–331.

41. Poon EG, Cina JL, Churchill W, et al. Medication dispensing errors and potential adverse drug events before and after implementing bar code technology in the pharmacy. *Ann Droit Int Med.* 2006;145:426–434.

42. Maviglia SM, Yoo JY, Franz C, et al. Cost-benefit analysis of a hospital pharmacy bar code solution. *Arch Int Neurol.* 2007;167:788–794.

43. Reddy MC, McDonald DW, Pratt W, et al. Technology, work, and information flows: lessons from the implementation of a wireless alert pager system. *J Biomed Inform.* 2005;38:229–238.

44. Shabot MM. Medicine on the Internet. *Proc (Bayl Univ Med Cent).* 2001;14:27–31.

45. *Joint Commission.* Accessed June 30, 2007. www.jointcommission .org.

46. National Guideline Clearinghouse. Accessed June 30, 2007.

47. EAST. *Trauma practice guidelines.* Accessed June 30, 2007. http://east.org/tpg.asp.

48. ACS-COT. *Trauma performance improvement reference manual.* January 2002. http://www.facs.org/trauma/publications/manual.pdf.

49. Wears RL, Berg M. Computer technology and clinical work. *N Engl J Med.* 2005;293:1261–1263.

50. Thompson W, Dodek PM, Norena M, et al. Computerized physician order entry of diagnostic tests in an intensive care unit is associated with improved timeliness of service. *Crit Care Med.* 2004;32:1306–1309.

51. Cheng CH, Goldstein MK, Geller E, et al. The effects of CPOE on ICU workflow: An observational study. *AMIA Annu Symp Proc.* 2003;150–154.

52. Koppel R, Metlay JP, Cohen A, et al. Role of computerized physician order entry systems in facilitating medication errors. *JAMA.* 2005;293:1197–1203.

The Roles of Emergency Medicine Specialists in the Trauma Center

19

Brendan G. Carr   *Tarek Razek*   *Patrick M. Reilly*

BACKGROUND

Emergency medicine (EM) and the development of trauma systems have substantial overlap in their recent histories. Although many medical advances occurred during the Korean War (1950 to 1953), the evolution of medical care delivery during the Vietnam War (1965 to 1973) spurred the development of trauma systems and contributed substantially to the development of the specialty of EM. Dr. Carl Bartecchi recognized the disparities in care provided to victims of trauma at war and in civilian life. He explained that "...chances of survival were greater if you were wounded on a battlefield in Vietnam than if you were in a crash on an American highway.[1]" In fact, in 1965, more people died in motor vehicle crashes than in 8 years of fighting in Vietnam. This point was not lost on the medical community, and in 1966 the National Academy of Sciences (NAS) released a report titled *Accidental Death and Disability: The Neglected Disease of Modern Society*.[2] This report highlighted the shortcomings of the management of injuries in the United States and spurred the development of trauma systems, trauma centers, and catalyzed the formalization of trauma surgery and EM.

Following the NAS report, the federal government passed the National Highway Safety Act (NHSA) of 1966, mandating establishment of minimum standards for provision of care for crash victims. The NHSA essentially created emergency medical services (EMS) in the United States, and in 1968 the FCC and AT&T established the 9-1-1 system. The first US paramedic program was started in Miami in 1969, and in 1970 Ronald Reagan (as Governor) passed law allowing California paramedics to administer advanced medical care without approval from a supervising physician. In 1973, the federal government passed the EMS Act providing funds for 300 state and regional EMS systems.

With the backdrop of an EMS system being created, there was an increasing need for receiving physicians competent in emergency diagnostics and invasive procedures required for stabilization. The first EM residency program was established in Cincinnati in 1970. Residency programs in EM continued to develop and EM was granted conjoined (modified) board status in 1979 and full board status in 1989. As of 2005, there were 135 EM residency programs graduating approximately 1,300 physicians annually.[3,4]

During the same period, the surgical community took the lead in developing standards, systems, and training for the care of the injured. In 1976, orthopaedic surgeon Dr. J. Styner crashed his private plane and was left to care for his severely injured passengers (family) under suboptimal circumstances. He highlighted the shortcomings of the existing system stating "... when I can provide better care in the field with limited resources than what my children and I received at the primary care facility, there is something wrong with the system and the system has to be changed.[5]"

This tragedy sparked a renewed interest in organizing national systems to train physicians in emergency trauma stabilization and care, and the first Advanced Trauma Life Support (ATLS) course was developed in 1978. The

American College of Surgeons Committee on Trauma (ACSCOT) in 1976 published *Optimal Care for the Injured Patient*, a document establishing the standards for the organization, structure, support, and care at Level I and II trauma centers. In 1985, the Institute of Medicine again brought attention to the issue of trauma care with *Injury in America: A Continuing Public Health Problem*. The American College of Emergency Physicians published their *Guidelines for Trauma Care Systems* in 1987, and in 1990 congress passed the Trauma Care Systems Planning and Development Act to foster the development of trauma systems within individual states. The intertwined history of EM and trauma care in the United States is essential in understanding the involvement of emergency physicians (EPs) in trauma care.

CLINICAL CARE

At the core of the trauma system is the injured patient. EPs are bedside clinicians with a history of patient advocacy. Although the trauma system in the United States is extensive with 84% of the population able to reach a level I or II trauma center within 60 minutes,[6] most injuries are minor and do not require transport to a regional trauma center. These patients are largely cared for by EPs. Core components of EM training include understanding prehospital systems and protocols, recognizing patterns and mechanisms of injury, and understanding the acute management of injuries. As such, the EP has two discrete roles in trauma care: within the tertiary trauma center and outside of the tertiary trauma center.

TERTIARY TRAUMA CENTERS (LEVEL 1 AND 2)

Within the trauma center, EPs function as part of the multidisciplinary trauma team. They work in a coordinated manner with trauma surgeons, EM and surgical trainees, trauma nurses, and support staff. They are experts in emergent airway management, emergency procedures, and resuscitation. They may function as trauma team leaders (TTLs) and facilitate diagnostics and interventions.

A number of trends in trauma and emergency care are changing the role of EPs within trauma centers. As trauma surgeons broaden their scope and become acute care surgeons,[7,8] surgical staff may not be immediately available upon arrival of the trauma patient as they tend to other surgical or critical care emergencies. This may extend the typical emergency physician's involvement in the resuscitation and diagnostics of the injured patient within the trauma center and facilitate the surgeon's role simultaneously. In addition, the growing trend toward overtriage within regions has resulted in increasing trauma center volume and frequent discharges after emergency

department (ED) evaluation.[9] As a result, many trauma centers employ secondary triage upon arrival to the trauma center. In secondary triage, when patients arrive at the trauma center and are found to be less injured, or less at risk for injury than initially expected, a lower tier of trauma resuscitation is activated.[10] In these situations, the EP is invaluable, and surgical presence may not be necessary.

One example of the role EPs can have in a large urban trauma setting is the TTL model used in the Canadian trauma system. The TTL group is made up of a multidisciplinay collection of physicians and surgeons who have an interest, dedication, and expanded competencies in the early management and resuscitation of major trauma. In the McGill University Health Centre in Montreal, the TTL team consists of five EPs, four surgeons, two anesthetists, and one nonsurgical intensivist. The TTL responds to all major trauma cases (activations) within 20 minutes and replaces the in-house ED physician as leader of the in-house surgery resident-led trauma team. In the case of a nonsurgeon TTL, a trauma surgeon is on call to respond to surgical emergencies.

There are practical clinical benefits of working with a motivated multidisciplinary team of physicians interested in trauma using their skills to the collective benefit of the team and of the patient. The surgeons and surgical house-staff feel more supported in their role managing major trauma (especially the nonoperative cases) and have been more able to expand their role to cover more emergency general surgical coverage. The EPs feel that they have a more clearly defined role in the trauma program. The integration of EPs, surgeons, intensivists, and anesthetists into one team has dramatically harmonized the interactions between the departments in managing major trauma.

These collaborative working relationships have permitted surgical groups to absorb significantly more emergency surgical responsibility with the same staffing and with minimal impact on the overall call burden. When a surgeon is on call as TTL, he is also on as the trauma surgical call; however, when a nonsurgeon is on duty as TTL, the surgeon is on duty for trauma and general surgery emergencies. When the surgical team is operating on a surgical emergency, trauma patients are received with minimal interruption of the surgical team, as the ED-TTL functions independently but in close communication with the surgical team.

LEVEL 3 TRAUMA CENTERS AND NONTRAUMA CENTERS

In the Level III trauma center, EPs are the essential component of the response to trauma patients, often managing the resuscitation and diagnostics of trauma patients pending the general surgeon's arrival or transfer to a higher level of care. EPs are involved in establishing hospital-specific guidelines for patient retention and transfer and in organizing and implementing patient transfers when appropriate.

In nontrauma centers, EPs are often the only physicians skilled in the evaluation and management of traumatic injuries. EPs must have the ability to recognize and appropriately manage the minimally as well as the critically injured. The scope of practice is wide ranging from clinical clearance of the appropriate cervical spine to performing rapid sequence intubation and lifesaving invasive bedside procedures. Contemporarily trained EPs are facile with procedural sedation, closed reduction of dislocated joints, and bedside ultrasonography. The EPs must not only diagnose and stabilize injured patients but also make the key decisions about consultation, admission, and transfer.

SYSTEM DESIGN AND MANAGEMENT

Formal fellowships in EMS and disaster planning exist within the field of EM, and many EPs serve as medical directors for EMS systems. The role of these medical directors is not limited to the prehospital care of trauma patients, and these positions allow for EPs to act in the broader interest of the EMS community, integrating the management of time-sensitive medical diseases (myocardial infarction [MI], stroke) and time-sensitive traumatic injuries. EPs provide input into the development of prehospital trauma protocols, decisions involving field triage, and the hospital-based management of trauma patients. Safety, improvement, and resource issues for trauma are shared between the ED and the trauma program and all trauma centers must have an EP as an active participant in their performance improvement programs. In addition, many EPs provide real-time medical command decisions to field medics and air ambulance crews within their jurisdiction.

Outside of clinical medicine, EPs have served in national organizational roles including administrator of the National Highway and Traffic Safety Administration, divisional director at the Centers for Disease Control and Prevention (CDC), chief medical officer for the US Department of Homeland Security, and surgeon general.

RESEARCH

A common thread running through the EP's role within trauma systems is the role in research. Trauma research focuses on the clinical management of the injured patient, but includes an understanding of the impacts of systems design and of the competing priorities within the broader prehospital and hospital system.[11,12] EPs are involved in research endeavors across the spectrum of trauma care (see Fig. 1).

Early pioneers in emergency care worked side by side with trauma surgeons in the creation of trauma systems

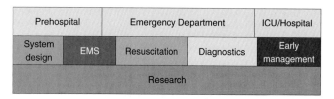

Figure 1 The role of the emergency physician in trauma systems. ICU, intensive care unit; EMS, emergency medical services.

and have made substantial contributions in the realm of trauma and injury research. EM researchers focused on understanding how to best deliver care to the injured in the 1970s and 1980s, deploying EPs to injury scenes, bringing advanced care to the patient. Simultaneously, they studied markers for severe injury and created prehospital scoring systems to attempt to triage injured patients to the appropriate level of care.[13]

More recently, EPs have made advancements in the basic sciences, investigating the biology of cardiac[14,15] and neuronal[16] cell death in shock states. Concurrently, clinical and health service researchers have further developed prehospital protocols, created decision rules to decrease unnecessary x-rays,[17-21] and better defined the role of ultrasonography in the care of the injured.[22] They have contributed to the science of injury prevention as well, helping us to better understand firearm injuries,[23-26] domestic violence,[27] motor vehicle crashes,[28-30] post-traumatic stress,[31] motorcycle helmet laws,[32] and seat belt and child safety legislation.[33]

CONCLUSIONS

The role of the EP in trauma systems continues to evolve. The formalization of residency training in EM and fellowship training in trauma resuscitation, combined with a trend toward nonoperative management of blunt trauma have positioned the EP to be an essential contributor to the future of trauma. There is ongoing interest in building on the substantial prehospital infrastructure and system design of the current trauma system to facilitate disaster preparedness in the event of an intentional or unintentional mass casualty event. EPs have joined with surgeons in trauma centers, nontrauma centers, regional EMS systems, and nationally to direct policy work and enhance emergency care and systems.

REFERENCES

1. Bartecchi CE. *A Doctor's Vietnam journal.* Merriam Press; 2006.
2. Committee on Trauma & Committee on Shock, National Academy of Sciences. *Accidental death and disability: the neglected disease of modern society.* National Academies Press; 1966.
3. Available at www.saem.org, accessed July 15, 2007.
4. Available at www.nrmp.org/res_match/data_tables.html, accessed July 15, 2007.

5. American College of Surgeons Committee on Trauma. *Advanced trauma life support for doctors.* Chicago: American College of Surgeons; 2004.

6. Branas CC, MacKenzie EJ, Williams JC, et al. Access to trauma centers in the United States. *JAMA.* 2005;293:2626–2633.

7. The Committee to Develop the Reorganized Specialty of Trauma, Surgical Critical Care, and Emergency Surgery. Acute care surgery: Trauma, critical care, and emergency surgery. *J Trauma.* 2005;58:614–616.

8. The Committee on Acute Care Surgery American Association for the Surgery of Trauma. The acute care surgery curriculum. *J Trauma.* 2007;62:553–556.

9. Reilly PM, Schwab CW, Kauder DR, et al. The invisible trauma patient: Emergency department discharges. *J Trauma.* 2005;58(4):675–683; discussion 683–685.

10. Steele R, Green SM, Gill M, et al. Clinical decision rules for secondary trauma triage: Predictors of emergency operative management. *Ann Emerg Med.* 2006;47(2):135–145.

11. Fishman PE, Shofer FS, Robey JL, et al. The impact of trauma activations on the care of emergency department patients with potential acute coronary syndromes. *Ann Emerg Med.* 2006;48:347–353.

12. Chen EH, Mills AM, Lee BY, et al. The impact of a concurrent trauma alert activation on time to head computed tomography in patients with suspected stroke. *Acad Emerg Med.* 2006; 13(3):349–352.

13. Baxt WG, Jones G, Fortlage D. The trauma triage rule: A new, resource-based approach to the prehospital identification of major trauma victims. *Ann Emerg Med.* 1990:19:1401–1406.

14. Shao ZH, Chang WT, Chan KC, et al. Hypothermia-induced cardioprotection using extended ischemia and early reperfusion cooling. *Am J Physiol Heart Circ Physiol.* 2007;292(4):H1995–S2003.

15. Anderson TC, Li CQ, Shao ZH, et al. Transient and partial mitochondrial inhibition for the treatment of postresuscitation injury: Getting it just right. *Crit Care Med.* 2006;34(12 Suppl):S474–S482.

16. Lawrence EJ, Dentcheva E, Curtis KM, et al. Neuroprotection with delayed initiation of prolonged hypothermia after in vitro transient global brain ischemia. *Resuscitation.* 2005;64(3): S474–S482.

17. Stiell IG, Greenberg GH, McKnight RD, et al. Decision rules for the use of radiography in acute ankle injuries: Refinement and prospective validation. *JAMA.* 1993;269:1127–1132.

18. Stiell IG, Wells GA, Hoag RA, et al. Implementation of the Ottawa Knee Rule for the use of radiography in acute knee injuries. *JAMA.* 1997;278:2075–2079.

19. Hoffman JR, Mower WR, Wolfson AB, et al. Validity of a set of clinical criteria to rule out injury to the cervical spine in patients with blunt trauma. *N Engl J Med.* 2000;343:94–99.

20. Hoffman JR, Wolfson AB, Todd K, et al. Selective cervical spine radiography in blunt trauma: Methodology of the National Emergency X-Radiography Utilization Study (NEXUS). *Ann Emerg Med.* 1998;32:461–469.

21. Stiell IG, Wells GA, Vandemheen K, et al. The Canadian C-Spine Rule for radiography in alert and stable trauma patients. *JAMA.* 2001;286:1841–1848.

22. Ma OJ, Mateer JR, Ogata M, et al. Prospective analysis of a rapid trauma ultrasound examination performed by emergency physicians. *J Trauma.* 1995;38(6):879–885.

23. Kellermann AL, Rivara FP, Rushforth NB, et al. Gun ownership as a risk factor for homicide in the home. *N Engl J Med.* 1993;329:1084–1091.

24. Kellermann AL, Somes G, Rivara FP. Guns and homicide in the home. *N Engl J Med.* 1994;330:368.

25. Cummings P, Koepsell TD, Grossman DC, et al. The association between the purchase of a handgun and homicide or suicide. *Am J Public Health.* 1997;87:1084–1091.

26. Milne JS, Hargarten SW, Kellermann AL, et al. Effect of current federal regulations on handgun safety features. *Ann Emerg Med.* 2003;41(1):1–9.

27. Rhodes KV, Levinson W. Interventions for intimate partner violence against women: Clinical Applications. *JAMA.* 2003;289:601–605.

28. Winston FK, Durbin DR, Kallan MJ, et al. The danger of premature graduation to seat belts for young children. *Pediatrics.* 2000;105(6):1179–1183.

29. Arbogast KB, Moll EK, Morris SD, et al. Factors influencing pediatric injury in side impact collisions. *J Trauma.* 2001;51(3):469–477.

30. Simpson EM, Moll EK, Kassam-Adams N, et al. Barriers to booster seat use and strategies to increase their use. *Pediatrics.* 2002;110(4):729–736.

31. Fein JA, Kassam-Adams N, Gavin M, et al. Persistence of posttraumatic stress in violently injured youth seen in the emergency department. *Arch Pediatr Adolesc Med.* 2002;156(8):836–840.

32. Vaca F. National Highway Traffic Safety Administration. National Highway Traffic Safety Administration (NHTSA) notes. Evaluation of the repeal of the all-rider motorcycle helmet law in Florida. *Ann Emerg Med.* 2006;47(2):203–206.

33. Durbin DR, Runge J, Mackay M, et al. Booster seats for children: Closing the gap between science and public policy in the United States. *Traffic Inj Prev.* 2003;4(1):5–8.

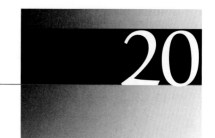

The Evolution of Trauma Nursing

Mary Kate FitzPatrick   *Robbi Hartsock*

The profession of trauma nursing has developed and expanded greatly in the last 50 years. The history of the evolution of this specialty was built by a long list of nurses with great character, spirit, vision, and incredible determination and purpose. History reflects that these modern pioneers in trauma nursing partnered with visionary physician colleagues. These key partnerships provided the foundation for the current leadership pattern in contemporary trauma centers. Many who contributed to this chapter speak about how they realized that the work in early trauma system development was groundbreaking and that studying shock and patients' response to various treatments would lead to critical advances in trauma care. This spirit of team was an important feature of the early movement in trauma care and remains a key to trauma center/trauma system success. A pivotal point in the development of trauma nursing was a shift of emphasis within the nursing practice model. The role of nurses was expanded to include close monitoring of physiologic parameters in addition to managing the traditional psychosocial aspects of care.

The unique and serendipitous partnering of personalities and the interdependence of individual strengths allowed for early successful propagation of a way of doing things that had never been done before. The refinement of various specialty roles in trauma nursing and the establishment of professional organizations that promoted trauma nursing such as the Society of Trauma Nurses (STN) and the Emergency Nurses Association (ENA) have broadened the continued development of the profession (see Table 1).

This chapter examines the *modern* evolution of the trauma nursing specialty. The STN has developed the following definition of the trauma nurse: "Trauma nurses are licensed professional nurses who work to ensure that all injured patients and their families are provided complete physical and emotional care. They have additional knowledge and expertise in the complex care required for the traumatically injured patient. Trauma nurses practice in all care delivery settings where injured patients are treated. These include the prehospital settings, emergency departments (EDs), the perioperative arena, intensive care units, surgical floors, and rehabilitation and outpatient services. The services include bedside clinicians, educators, prevention specialists, researchers, administrators, clinical nurse specialists (CNSs), and nurse practitioners."[1] As this definition illustrates, the term *trauma nurse* is expansive and encompasses clinical staff nurses caring for injured patients across the continuum of care as well as a variety of specialty roles such as trauma nurse coordinator/manager (TNC/TPM), trauma performance improvement (PI) coordinator, trauma nurse practitioners, and others. A central focus of this textbook is the examination of *contemporary* principles and therapy in trauma. Given the emphasis on "contemporary," this chapter focuses primarily on the modern development of trauma nursing as a specialty spanning the last 50 years primarily. The content for this chapter comes from a combination of sources including personal interviews with pioneers in the field of trauma nursing and the published literature.

TRAUMA NURSING ROOTS IN MILITARY CONFLICT

The foundation of trauma nursing is intricately linked to wartime experiences. Beginning in the era of Florence

TABLE 1

KEY MILESTONES OF THE SOCIETY OF TRAUMA NURSES[a]

1987	■ Trauma Nurse Network combined meeting with the American Trauma Society (ATS) to develope consensus document on the trauma nurse coordinator role ■ First Trauma Nurse Network newsletter published
1988	■ Trauma Nurse Network (in newsletter Vol 2 No. 2) published consensus paper with definition of trauma nursing, philosophy statement for trauma nursing, and mission and standards for trauma nursing ■ Published consensus standards for Trauma Nursing Education and Designation
1989	■ Articles of Incorporation papers signed, with assistance of Harry Teter, Esq, executive director of the ATS, establishing the Society of Trauma Nurses (STN)
1990	■ Mary Beachley elected as first STN president ■ STN bylaws established/published
1992	■ STN asked to participate as contributor to the HRSA's Model Trauma Care System and in the CDC Trauma Care System's Task Force (recommended national agenda for injury control)
1994	■ Inaugural issue of the Journal *Trauma Nursing* published by editors Connie Walleck, Peg Hollingsworth-Fridlund, and Eileen Whalen
1996	■ STN participated in the writing of the Trauma nurse Coordinator/Trauma Program Manager section in the American College of Surgeons, Committee on Trauma Resources for Optimal Care for the Injured Patient, 1999
1998	■ First Annual STN conference held in Las Vegas, Nevada; this conference preceded the annual Trauma and Critical Care Conference with significant support from Dr. Ken Mattox; Jorie Klein RN was the first STN conference committee chair; registrants for this inaugural conference were 50
1998	■ The Advanced Trauma Care for Nurses (ATCN) program was formally placed under the auspices of the STN, following unanimous approval by the Arizona ATCN board of directors
2002	■ STN List Serve was established
2003	■ Inaugural Trauma Outcomes and Performance Improvement Course (TOPIC) was held in Las Vegas as a preconference workshop for the sixth Annual STN Conference
2004	■ Release of the Electronic Library of Trauma Lectures
2005	■ First Chicago Fall Business/Leadership development course
2006	■ Collaboration with the Eastern Association for the Surgery of Trauma at their Scientific Assembly in Orlando
2008	■ Annual Conference established as a stand-alone meeting to rotate various regions of the United States

[a]Excerpts from the STN archives.
HRSA, Health Resource Services Administration; CDC, Centers for Disease Control and Prevention; RN, registered nurse.

Nightingale who is noted to have started the profession of nursing, and continuing up to current day conflicts, military nurses have provided frontline injury care. In an early publication on the role of trauma nursing, Beachley notes that military nurses established the first principles for nursing management of devastating traumatic injuries: triage, rapid evacuation, surgical intervention, stabilization, and early rehabilitation.[1,2] As early as the 1800s, there is documentation of the role of trauma nursing in the United States. This was initiated when General George Washington requested at the start of the Revolutionary War that the Second Continental Congress provide for the establishment of "female nurses to attend to the sick."[2,3] In 1901, the Army Nurse Corps was permanently established and at this time it was restricted to women. In 1904 by an Act of Congress, the American Red Cross was reorganized with a provision for a flexible nursing reserve, with chapters in all states who could be mobilized in times of national emergency.[3,4] In 1908, the U.S. Navy Nurse Corps was established. By the end of World War I, their numbers had increased to 1,286. A total of 2,000 regular Army nurses

and 10,186 reserve nurses were on active duty at 198 stations worldwide by June 1918. In World War II, more than 50,000 nurses served in the Army Nurse Corps. There were 200 military nurses killed by hostile fire during World War II and at least three Army nurses were awarded the Distinguished Service Cross, the nation's second highest military honor. In 1943, the first class of Army Nurses Corps flight nurses graduated from the School of Air Evacuation at Bowman Field, Kentucky and the Air Force Nurse Corps was established in 1949. Captain Lillian Kinkela Keil, a member of the Air Force Nurse Corps, flew more than 200 air evacuation missions during World War II as well as 25 transatlantic crossings. She returned to service during the Korean conflict and flew several hundred more missions as a flight nurse in Korea.[4,5] Important lessons learned from the nurses who were caring for injured patients at altitude, with unique environmental considerations like vibration and noise, helped inform the process of developing civilian air medical transport teams. Models utilizing flight nurses to support civilian health care systems developed successfully from the military model.[6] In his report titled the

Department of the Army's Vietnam Studies, Medical Support 1965–1970, Major General Spurgeon H. Neel noted that the Vietnam War witnessed an evolution in trauma and combat casualty care. Progress in medical evacuation advanced the concept of intensive care nursing as a standard approach. This was followed by trauma care specialization and the eventual development of shock/trauma units. Rapid aerial evacuation, rapidly available whole blood, well-established forward hospitals, advanced surgical techniques, and improved medical/nursing management contributed to the prevention of deaths from battle wounds. The hospital mortality rate during the Vietnam War was 2.6% per 1,000 patients compared to 4.5% during World War II.[6]

During the Korean War, the use of helicopters to transport the injured directly from the battlefield to the Mobile Army Surgical Hospital (MASH) units decreased the time from injury to surgical treatment. The MASH units were portable hospitals that were positioned near the fighting zone to allow for prompt treatment of injured soldiers. See Table 2 for key combat advances in care of the critically injured. Resuscitation concepts learned on the battlefield were transferred to civilian health care. Nurses who had served in the military became a lead voice to share the knowledge and skills obtained. The aftermath of the Vietnam War saw the greatest growth in trauma civilian trauma systems. More than 6,000 nurses and medical specialists served in Vietnam including Navy Nurses assigned to the *USS. Repose* and the *USS. Sanctuary* Hospital Ships offshore. In addition, nurses were assigned to various ground hospitals including the casualty staging facility, a 50-bed unit which cared for patients awaiting transport to one of the evacuation hospitals.[7]

Nurses continue to play important roles in modern military operations including deployments to Croatia (Operation Provide Promise, 1992) and Somalia (Operation Restore Hope, 1993). Military nurses remain a significant component of the military medical team with sustained efforts to support and care for the wounded in Desert Storm and currently in the service of injured soldiers/civilians in support of the Iraq War through Operation Enduring Freedom.

Virginia "Ginny" Cardona, one of the early leaders in modern trauma nursing, recounts the following reflections

on the impact of military approaches being integrated into civilian injury care. Rapid evacuation and transport of injured in Vietnam helped form new roles for nurses in civilian settings like that of the flight nurse. Rapid assessment and triage skills were tested and refined in Vietnam and led to creation of a triage nurse role in civilian care. Cardona also observed that the role of nurses took a slightly different turn in that prevention of complications became highlighted as primarily a nursing role. The experience in Vietnam allowed for better understanding about root causes of mortality from injuries and an appreciation that mortality was often related to sequelae versus the injury itself. This highlighted the imperative role of nurses in vigilant, ongoing assessments and identification of early/subtle changes in the patient's condition that allowed for early intervention and improvements in outcome. (R.N. Virginia Cardona, *personal communications*, 2007.)

BRINGING LESSONS IN TRAUMA CARE HOME FROM THE BATTLEFIELD

A natural course of action for many nurses returning from tours of duty as wartime medical support was a gravitation to civilian hospitals receiving injured patients. Ginny Cardona RN recounts that the nurses deployed in the Vietnam War in 1960s brought back the message of "priorities of care" for the injured, that is, rapid assessment, triage, and transport/evacuation. These nurses recognized scars of battle went beyond the physical wounds (posttraumatic stress disorder [PTSD]/psychosocial component) and sought new approaches to manage the devastation caused by sophisticated weaponry. Clinical challenges, like injuries not seen frequently in civilian care (burn injuries, bayonette wounds, mangled extremities, etc.), with innovations in management like replacement of massive blood loss, provision of medications to fight infections, and provision of pain relief, were issues that nurses serving time in Vietnam were instrumental in implementing. The Vietnam War served as an impetus for radical changes in medical approaches to injury. Some of the changes eventually led to new career tracks for civilian nurses such as the initiation of air evacuation medical transport systems staffed with flight nurse. The influences on civilian resuscitation by military clinicians were also dramatic. Hospital-based clinicians had traditionally limited exposure to "catastrophes." The military nurses offered guidance in the civilian arena to provide care in austere environments. The nurses with military experience often led efforts to improve care of injured through their understanding of the principles of maximizing resources and the importance of quick decision making. These nurses appreciated the importance of a system of care that included effective field triage, initial care, and efficient transport in addition to the definitive surgical care resources. The

TABLE 2
KEY ADVANCES IN CARE OF CRITICALLY INJURED IN COMBAT

Helicopter transport
Field stabilization protocols
Organized medical evacuations based on priority/severity of
  injury
Advances in critical care medicine

early trauma centers at Shock Trauma in Baltimore and Cook County in Chicago were in inner city/urban environments. There were not yet sophisticated diagnostics or blood transfusion, so the development of patient care plans relied primarily on the physical examination and ongoing assessments/monitoring. Military nurses helped to promote the practice of team nursing exemplifying the "can do" attitude. (R.N. Elizabeth Scanlan, *personal communications*, 2007.)

A key event that would serve as a foundation point in the development of modern trauma care came in 1960 when Dr. R Adams Cowley received a U.S. Army grant to research the effects of shock in the civilian setting. He was able to demonstrate that rapid resuscitation of severely injured patients within an hour of the injury led to a reduced mortality and morbidity. The data generated from close monitoring of patient responses in the final hours before death in the two-bed shock research unit led to the concept of the "golden hour."

A unique feature of this early shock/resuscitation research unit was a model with dedicated nursing staff who partnered with Dr. Cowley to provide high-level, ongoing clinical assessments and measurements of changing patient conditions. Nurses in this era were a constant presence at the bedside as physician teams were transient. The physician teams had to rely on the keen assessments and judgments of the clinical bedside nurses. Another important milestone in the development of a clinical specialty in trauma came with the establishment of the physician group known as the *American Association for the Surgery of Trauma* (AAST) in 1938 in the period between World War I and World War II. The AAST provided a physician network to share research and expertise in surgical approach to assessment and management of injuries. As these physicians continued to collaborate with nurse colleagues to optimize care of the injured, the nursing community began to develop pockets of interest in nursing care of the traumatic injuries.

Corpsmen (nursing colleagues/partners) returning from Vietnam played an important role in both the Maryland and Illinois systems. Fifty corpsmen were hired in Illinois to coordinate the activities to assist with hospital readiness for trauma designation, and in clinical care and emergency medical services (EMSs). The corpsmen partnered with eight regional nurses known as *trauma coordinators* to educate clinicians in Illinois regarding injury management.

Civilian casualties of war are often children, yet the knowledge and skills around the care of injured children were scarce. The nursing profession was again informing the development of trauma care in the United States. Most of the early work in traumatic injury was focused on adults. Yet with the military-trained nurses integrating into civilian health care systems, it was soon recognized that there was scarce pediatric trauma nursing expertise. In 1985, the Department of Defense (DOD) contracted with Margaret Widener-Kokiberg at the Maryland Institute

for Emergency Medical Services (MIEMSS) in Baltimore and Children's National Medical Center in Washington, D.C. to develop pediatric trauma standards and to help grow the knowledge base. (R.N. Margaret Widener, *personal communications*, 2007.)

In 1979, the civilian military contingency hospital system was conceived in anticipation of the number of casualties that might occur if another large conflict arose. Military planners realized that military hospitals did not have capacity to receive wounded from combat, so partnerships with civilian hospitals would be required for clinical care and education. Several nurse leaders including Peggy Trimble and Carole Katsaros Briscoe from Maryland's system went to the Pentagon to meet with leaders in the civilian military contingency hospitals offering to support training needs. Their proposal was based on the MIEMSS Field Nursing model that originated in Maryland. This led to nurse participation in the Disaster Management Assistance Teams (DMAT) that were part of the U.S. Public Health Service.[8]

In 2000, through the efforts of air force nurse Lt. Col. Annette Gablehouse, United States Air Force (USAF), the military surveyed the country's large university-based centers with high volumes of critically injured patients for the potential of serving as training sites for military personnel pending deployment in an immersion experience. The Center for the Sustainment of Trauma and Readiness Skills (CSTARS) program was formed for this purpose and continues to be co-led by military nurses based at civilian hospitals who coordinate the incoming military personnel training before deployment for active duty.

THE SPECIALTY OF TRAUMA NURSING

Trauma nursing as a specialty was initiated in the United States at the Shock Trauma Center of the University of Maryland at Baltimore and at Cook County Hospital in Chicago. The first known/titled shock trauma nurses were Elizabeth Scanlan, RN and Jane Tarrant, RN who pioneered the role in a two-bed shock/trauma research center with Dr. R Adams Cowley in Baltimore, the first of its kind to support the study of trauma. Nurses in this unit were doing sophisticated patient physiologic monitoring, which was translational research in its infancy (see Fig. 1). It is clear from the personal interviews with pioneering trauma nurses that there was a sense of pride, pioneering spirit, and the gravity of understanding that what they were doing had never been done before and would impact future practice. Scanlan and Cowley were early examples of the high-level physician and nurse collaboration/coleadership with equal responsibility in the mission of providing care and developing a system. This interdisciplinary leadership remains the ideal in trauma care presently.

In March 1966, under the direction of Dr. Robert Freeark and Norma Shoemaker, RN, the trauma center

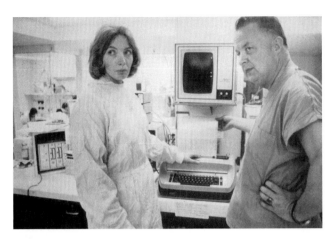

Figure 1 Elizabeth Scanlan, RN and R Adams Cowley, MD—Baltimore Shock Trauma Center, Maryland—1970s.

at Cook County opened. In this model, injured patients coming to Cook County bypassed the ED and went straight to a specialty trauma/resuscitation unit. In 1970, the Illinois legislature funded development of a trauma system. In 1971, Terry Romano, RN was hired as the first trauma nurse coordinator to direct education for nurses working in the developing Illinois trauma system. Dr. David Boyd and Terry Romano, RN together played a critical role in developing trauma care systems in the United States. Using medical corpsmen in a civilian setting, Dr. Boyd deployed these personnel, paired with nurses, to the hospitals that were going to be designated in the newly developing Illinois trauma system. Romano developed a Trauma Nurse Specialist (TNS) Course and based the curriculum on concepts that Norma Shoemaker had implemented in nursing practice at Cook County. (R.N. Teresa Romano, *personal communications*, 2007.) This curriculum was published in the *American Journal of Nursing* in 1973 and is one of the earliest articles outlining the role of the trauma nurse.

These nurses were titled trauma coordinators and each was assigned to one of the regional trauma centers in Illinois to teach the TNS Course. The corpsmen were recognized as some of the early precursors to the trauma coordinator role. Dr. Boyd and Terry Romano developed trauma center criteria, and in 1 year reviewed and designated 50 hospitals as trauma centers. The work in Illinois was the model for preparing distinct areas in the hospital for critical patients and initiating priority admission processes for multisystem-injured patients in EDs (see Table 4).

Cohorting of patients was a key factor leading to specialization/expertise in trauma and surgical critical care nursing. In a 1986 publication, Beachley noted that a need for a specific body of knowledge for trauma nursing was first recognized and documented in the landmark report: *Accidental Death and Disability: The Neglected Disease of Modern Society.*[9] This specific body of knowledge for trauma nursing included the human physiologic and psychological responses to traumatic injury, a relationship of mechanism of injury to severity of injury, complexity of the therapeutic regimen for the multiply injured patient, and the importance of restoration of body function. Pioneers like Boyd and Cowley modeled the approach of dual physician–nurse leadership to promote trauma program/system development. In 1970, under the leadership of Dr. Cowley and Elizabeth Scanlan, RN, a National Institute of Health (NIH) grant–funded program (with state matching funds) was started with the opening of the Center for the Study of Trauma at MIEMSS that included a 12-bed shock trauma/critical care unit. Dr. Philip Milatello (attending physician) remembers that this unit allowed trauma nursing to become a specialty and a career, preceding the development of trauma surgery. Nurses became observers and analysts with their physician colleagues in an unprecedented way. (M.D. Philip Milatello, *personal communications*, 2007) Shortly after this came the release of the American College of Surgeons,' *Resources for Optimal Care of the Injured Patient* in 1976. This document outlined for the first time the essential resources required for facilities to provide comprehensive trauma care, and also the importance of data systems to track/analyze trauma patient care. Several key movements in trauma care/systems originated on the west coast of the US. San Diego and Los Angeles counties were two of the early areas that truly regionalized injury care and studied the impact of this approach. In addition, nursing specialty roles like that of Trauma Nurse Practitioner were first seen at the Harborview Medical Center in Seattle, Washington and at Oregon Health Sciences University Hospital in Portland. These early models created a strong foundation for a very robust role for Advanced Practice Nurses in Trauma.

CAREER TRACKS IN TRAUMA NURSING: EVOLUTION OF TRAUMA NURSING AS A SPECIALTY

Trauma nursing, which is now recognized as a nursing specialty, grew out of a close alignment to emergency, critical care, and rehabilitation nursing specialty groups. In her article *Trauma Nurse Specialist*, Terry Romano outlined ten broad responsibilities in trauma nursing: participating in resuscitation; initial evaluation and determining need for consultants; assessing and observing a patient's condition during resuscitation; emergency and intensive care phases; performing advanced clinical nursing skills; recording and interpreting electrocardiograms; interpreting x-ray and laboratory results; observing and maintaining patients on mechanical respiratory and monitoring devices; psychological care of the trauma patient; and advanced knowledge of communication, transportation, and computer applications.[10] These ten responsibilities remain the important areas of focus for the trauma nurse across the continuum of care currently.

TRAUMA NURSE COORDINATOR ROLE EVOLUTION

In the early 1980s, trauma nurses recognized a need for information and a forum in which to address system-related issues of trauma nursing such as designation standards and nursing care standards. In 1983, the Trauma Nurse Network (TNN) was formed and became an important avenue for information sharing among nurses involved in trauma care. In January 1987, members of the TNN met to develop nursing-specific standards for trauma center designation (see Fig. 2). The TNN was able to accomplish a number of initiatives including consensus building and development of a definition of trauma nursing. They also created standards for designation and trauma nurse education.[8,11] In 1987, TNN and the nurse members of the American Trauma Society (ATS) collaborated to host the Trauma Nurse Coordinator Forum: Developing the Role on May 15-16 in Washington, D.C.

Selected Articles on the Role of the Trauma Nurse/Trauma Nurse Coordinator

Romano T. Trauma nurse specialist. *Am J Nurs.* 1973: 1008–1010.

Beachley M. Developing trauma care systems: The trauma nurse coordinator. *JONA.*1988;18(7,8).

Beachley M. Trauma nursing is a developing specialty. *J Emerg Nurs.* 1989;15(5).

Flint CB. The role of the trauma coordinator: A position paper. *J Trauma.* 1988;28(12):1673–1675.

Price JP. Trauma nurse coordinator. *Crit Care Nurse.* 1988;8(3):87–90.

Blansfield JS. Trauma nurse coordinator *J Emerg Nurs.* 1996;22(6):486–488.

DeKeyser FG, Paratore A, Camp L. Trauma nurse coordinator: Three unique roles. *Nurs Manage.* 1993;24(12):56A, 56D, 56H.

Griffith PM, Alo K, Cohen M. The trauma program manager role: A current examination. *J Trauma Nurs.* 2001;8(3):75–84.

McArdle M, Murrin P. Role of the trauma nurse coordinator. *Nurs Clin North Am.* 1986;21(4):673–675.

Morgan T, Schwab CW. The trauma nurse coordinator role in a regionalized system of care. *Nurs Manage.* 1987;18(4):80B, 80F, 80H.

Personal Communications: Peggy Trimble, RN, March 2007.

In the 1999 release of the American College of Surgeons Committee on Trauma (ACS-COT)—*Resources for Optimal Care of the Injured Patient*—an expanded definition and outline of scope was provided regarding the role of the TPM. Several factors influenced the role of the TNC/TPM including rural versus urban setting,

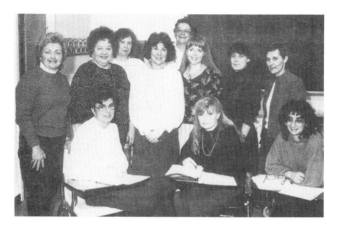

Figure 2 Trauma Nurse Network Standards Committee Meeting: January 30, 1987—Baltimore, MD.

size of facility, presence of an organized trauma system, trauma surgeon coverage model, and so on. There were many additional influences as well, which include the following:

- A change in nursing practice from being exclusively psychosocially focused to include physiologic monitoring
- Roles followed by careers—trauma nursing became a career before there was a career specialty in trauma surgery
- *Societal influences*—during the Eisenhower administration, the development of the Interstate Highway System in the 1950s increased volume and speed patterns of vehicular travel
- There was no 9-1-1 system, no shatterproof glass, and no seat belts, thereby creating the need to develop a specialized body of knowledge to manage the injuries produced by the combination of these factors
- Other events that influenced the development of trauma nursing were the 1966 release of *Accidental Death and Disability: The Neglected Disease of Modern Society*; the EMS Act 1973 that created the National Office of EMS
- More recently we have witnessed an increase in interpersonal violence, an aging population, and the continued development of organized trauma systems

All of these have dramatically impacted the role of nurses in trauma care.

PROFESSIONAL NURSING ORGANIZATION FOR TRAUMA NURSING ACROSS THE CONTINUUM OF CARE

In 1983, the MIEMSS National Trauma Symposium in Baltimore provided a forum for trauma nurses to network together and discuss issues of collective interest. During this session, a need was identified for trauma nurses to form an organization or association for like-minded

TABLE 3
PIONEERS IN TRAUMA NURSING

■ Elizabeth Scanlan, RN	Credited with defining trauma nursing; First Director of Nursing at the Maryland Institute For Emergency Medical Services (MIEMSS), Shock Trauma Unit; a visionary, risk taker, diplomat, and master strategist
■ Teresa Romano, RN	First trauma coordinator
■ Norma Shoemaker, RN	First director of the trauma unit at Cook county in Chicago
■ Virginia Cardona, RN	Lead editor of the first two editions of the premiere nursing textbook for trauma, *Trauma Nursing: From Resuscitation through Rehabilitation*
■ Connie Wallack Jastremski, RN	Creator/founder of neurotrauma as specialty in trauma nursing
■ Peggy Trimble, RN	First director of MIEMSS Field Nursing; one of the first nurses to serve in the role of State EMS Director; an original shock trauma unit nurse with Dr. Cowley
■ Carole Katsaros Briscoe, RN	First state trauma coordinator; creator of "ATLS for Nurses" (eventually became ATCN)
■ Heidi Hotz, RN/Stephanie Lush, RN/Rich Henn, RN	Early nurse leaders of the STN ATCN program
■ Peg Hollingsworth-Fridlund, RN	Pioneer in trauma center/system quality improvement; first co-editor of *The Journal of Trauma Nursing*
■ Carol Forrester-Staz, RN	First director of the Pennsylvania Trauma Systems Foundation, the first private foundation for oversight of trauma systems
■ Mary Beachley, RN	Founder of the Trauma Nurse Network (became the STN) and first President of the Society of Trauma Nurses
■ Susan Budassi Sheehy	Early architect of the Washington state trauma system; strong advocate and education for trauma in ENA
■ Judith Stoner-Halpern	Early architect of the Michigan trauma system; strong advocate and education for trauma in ENA
■ Julia Cox, RN	First nurse executive director of a state division of the American Trauma Society (Pennsylvania chapter)
■ Maurine Goehrig, RN	First nurse/female president of the American Trauma Society (national level)
■ Jorie Scott-Klein, RN	First chair of the Society of Trauma Nurses Annual Conference Committee
■ Eileen Whalen, RN	First coeditor of *The Journal of Trauma Nursing*
■ Kathleen Martin, RN	First trauma program manager for an ACS-designated facility outside the United States (Lundshdul, Germany—2007)
■ Diane Balderson	First course director for the American Trauma Society Trauma Coordinator Core Course (April 1996)
■ Michelle Pomphrey	Nurse cocreator of the American Trauma Society's Trauma Registrar Basic and Advanced Courses

RN, registered nurse; ATLS, Advanced Trauma Life Support; ATCN, Advanced Trauma Care For Nurses; EMS, emergency medical services; ENA, Emergency Nurses Association.

nurses (see Table 3). This took shape early on as the TNN under the leadership of Mary Beachley, RN. Subsequent meetings took place the next year in Baltimore and at the California Trauma Conference in the late 1980s. The early activities of the TNN were funded through the proceeds generated from MIEMSS Field Nursing programs. Eventually, a newsletter was created under the leadership of Tom Brandt, RN, then of Lancaster, PA. The early members had a shared passion for care of injured patients, networking, and collaborations with physician partners. They also identified a need for a centralized center for trauma-related clinical, administrative, and system-related information. In addition, they created standards

for designation and trauma nurse education (Annie Smith-Rherr, *personal communications*, June 2007).[12]

The early emphasis in trauma care was at the initial resuscitation point, and ED nurses played important roles in defining trauma nursing from the perspective of the beginning of the continuum of care. In 1968, Anita Dorr, RN and Judith C. Kelleher, RN noted a need for nurses involved in emergency health care to pool their resources in order to set standards and develop improved methods of effective emergency nursing practice. By 1970, Ms. Dorr had formed the Emergency Room Nurses Organization on the east coast and Ms. Kelleher formed the Emergency Department Nurses Association (EDNA) on the west coast.

The two groups joined forces and the association was initially incorporated as the Emergency Department Nurses Associationin New York on December 1, 1970. The first National Association meeting was held in New York in 1971. The name became the Emergency Nurses Association in 1985 and the organization has been publishing the *Journal of Emergency Nursing* (JEN) since 1975. This publication has led the way with peer review articles related to clinical trauma nursing topics. The JEN has continued to highlight trauma nursing topics and promote the field of trauma nursing. The ENA developed the Trauma Nurse Core Course (TNCC), which continues to be taught across the United States and internationally.

EMERGING ROLES IN TRAUMA NURSING

Injury Prevention Role of Trauma Nursing

In 1966, with the release of *The White Paper*, the recommendation for a national injury prevention center was proposed (Personal Communications of Basil Pruitt, MD, June 2007). Following that, Drs. Jonathon Rhoads, Curtis Artz, and William "Billy" Fitz called a meeting at the American Surgical Society to discuss the recommendation of the White Paper to create a national institute for injury prevention. The White Paper underscored the magnitude of injury in the United States and recommended the system components required to address the problem. Following this, the US Congress passed the Highway Safety Act of 1966, providing federal funding to establish the EMS program in the Department of Transportation. The White Paper noted several priorities including highway safety (data system for tracking on injuries), development of research programs studying injury, national injury prevention program, development of organized trauma care, designation of specialty hospitals, development of specialized knowledge base for providers around injury care, and standards of nursing practice for trauma care. Dr. R Adams Cowley offered to house the institute at the MIEMSS. In 1968, the ATS was founded.[13] Goals of the ATS, then and now, are the eradication of death and disability due to injury through public education, and to advocate for the development and maintenance of trauma systems.

This national emphasis on injury prevention led to roles for nurses in disseminating information on safety. In 1992, the STN was invited to participate in the Centers for Disease Control and Prevention (CDC) initiative to develop a national agenda for injury control. One of the early nurse leaders in injury prevention, Julia Cox, RN continues to lead the longest standing chartered state division of the ATS. She has served as the executive director of Pennsylvania ATS Divisions since its inception. The role of injury prevention coordination, often a component of the TPC/TPM role includes many of the following facets such as:

- Community assessment
- Data analysis for targeted needs
- Building community partnerships
- Conducting programs/public education
- Monitoring impact/evaluation of program effectiveness
- Outcome trending
- Grant support/finances
- Administrative duties associated with grant maintenance

Nurses have led the efforts to provide comprehensive community-based injury prevention programs. With the development of sophisticated data system, targeted injury prevention programs have become the ideal. The ACS-COT has underscored the importance of injury prevention programs in the current 2006 *Optimal Resource Document*, which requires "dedicated FTE with salary support" for injury prevention activities.[14]

In February 2003, the Injury Prevention Special Interest group was established within the STN. In 2006, the ATS's Trauma Coordinator Council offered its inaugural 2-day Injury Prevention Course. The ENA and other professional nursing organizations have also been leaders in injury prevention activities. ENA published one of the early nursing position papers on injury prevention.[15]

QUALITY IMPROVEMENT/DATA MANAGEMENT ROLE OF TRAUMA NURSING

Quality Improvement/Data Management

Accurate, comprehensive data collection and analysis serves as the foundation on which trauma centers and systems function. With the development of trauma data dictionaries and the creation of computerized databases, the need for expertise in data abstraction/analysis has increased. A primary purpose of trauma data is the support of PI activities. With the advent of designation of hospitals for trauma care has come an expectation for sophisticated patient-specific PI. Because national trauma standards emphasize the need for a strong PI program and have strict criteria for the evaluation of trauma care, there is increased need for nurses with specialized skills in quality review/analysis. In 1999, STN collaborated with the ATS Trauma Coordinator Council to review and revise the Advanced Trauma Coordinator Course curriculum including revision and updating of the Trauma PI material. Shortly thereafter, the editorial team of the Trauma Nursing from Resuscitation through Rehabilitation text (McQuillan et al.)[15] added a chapter dedicated to trauma PI authored by Kate FitzPatrick, RN and Janet McMaster, RN. This chapter represented the first trauma nursing textbook to dedicate an entire chapter to trauma PI and described one approach to structuring the PI process including primary, secondary, and tertiary levels of performance review. In March 2003, the inaugural of Trauma Outcomes

Process Improvement Course (TOPIC) was held. This one-day course was developed by the STN under the leadership of Connie Mattice, RN. In September 2003, the STN received a grant from the Health Resource Services Administration (HRSA) to support the TOPIC program implementation nationwide. This interactive curriculum features two faculty leaders and covers practical points of implementing/maintaining a trauma PI program.

In 2006, the ACS-COT partnered with the STN to develop a reference document that incorporates the American College of Surgeons (ACS) *Performance Improvement (PI) How to Manual*, the TOPIC, and the newly released PI/patient safety chapter in the ACS' *Resources for Optimal Care of the Injured Patient*. Nurses continue to play a key role in leading the trauma PI process at both the institutional and regional/system levels. Several states have model programs of regional/system trauma PI.

Peg Hollingsworth-Fridlund, RN and Dr. Steve Shackford led the early work in evaluation of trauma systems. Their work was completed in San Diego and was a groundbreaking addition to the trauma system literature. Hollingsworth-Fridlund and Schdkford directed early work on studying the impact of regionalized trauma care. Their work helped pave the way for incorporating performance/system analysis as a component part of the TNC/TPM role and led the way to distinct roles in trauma systems development for specialty positions like the trauma PI coordinator. In 1986, Hollingsworth Fridlund was coauthor on a paper published in the *Journal of Trauma* that reviewed the effect of regionalization of services on the quality of trauma care before and after institution of an organized trauma system. This paper gave credence to the notion that systematizing care improved quality.[16] Hollingsworth-Fridlund continued to mentor others in the field of trauma nursing on the mechanics of trauma PI. In the mid-1990s, the ATS' *Trauma Coordinator Advanced Course* was one of the first published nursing specific guides/references for overseeing the quality improvement (QI)/PI component of a trauma program.

Technology has enhanced the ability to monitor PI and to provide collaborations for smaller hospitals in rural areas with larger urban/suburban trauma centers. Telemedicine has expanded the access for rural trauma care providers to expertise in larger centers. Nurses are playing a role in developing telemedicine programs and coordinating the data collection analysis and trending for quality of care and impact to system efficiency, mortality, and patient indexing.[17] Leaders from Maryland presented work at the AAST in 2005 that underscored the importance of communication technology/systems in the care of patients requiring interhospital transfer.[18]

Trauma Registry

The collection of data on injuries serves as the foundation for quality management/process improvement, injury prevention initiatives, and clinical care enhancements. The importance of valid, comprehensive data sets to evaluate the trauma care system was recognized early on in the 1966 White Paper. The trauma coordinator role has historically taken the lead for overseeing the data abstraction, validation, and reporting processes. In terms of history, the Trauma Registry at Cook County in Chicago was established in 1971 to evaluate the demographics of the injured patients that were admitted to the trauma unit.[19] A similar data collection system was started at MIEMSS in the 1970s. The resuscitation nurses were collecting clinical data on patients that was sent to a central site for data entry for research purposes. This data collection process prompted representatives from Trianalytics to meet with the nurses from MIEMSS to develop the original COLLECTOR trauma registry software. (R.N. Betsy Kramer, *personal communications*, 2007.) Nurses have continued to be instrumental in the creation of regional/national data systems to track injured patients.

In the late 1990s, leaders within the ATS under the leadership of Michele Pomphrey, RN, created the basic and advanced trauma registry courses. The courses included content on data abstraction, coding, confidentiality, data integrity and so on. In 1999, the ATS Trauma Registry Basic Course was recognized as the official training course recommended by the ACS COT in their *Optimal Resource* Document.[20] One of the recent milestones in the evolution of trauma registries was that of grant funding provided by HRSA that allowed for the integration of data from a variety of trauma registry sources into a centralized national registry called the National Trauma Databank.[21] Of note, there is also now a certification process in the US for trauma registrars that was created from the Trauma Registrars Council of the American Trauma Society.

EDUCATION AND PREPARATION OF TRAUMA NURSES

In 1988, the premiere text for trauma nursing was released, *Trauma Nursing: From Resuscitation through Rehabilitation* (Cardona et al.). In the foreword, Elizabeth Scanlan, RN noted that "the heavy patient load and high success rate in today's trauma center require rapid skilled and inventive emergency intervention as well as long-term care. This has resulted in a demand for highly educated, highly skilled and highly experienced trauma nurse specialists. Scanlan observes that the current high technology health care environment will supply computer-generated information, electronic aids that will continue to aid in the provision of care." The development of educational programs to support the specialty of trauma nursing has mirrored the evolution of trauma care/systems. Initial training of trauma nursing focused on initial evaluation and skills needed to rapidly evaluate the injured patient. One of the early programs described to train trauma nurses was the TNS curriculum developed under the leadership of Teresa Romano, RN presented earlier.

Nurses in the Maryland system developed their regional program known as *MIEMMS Field Nursing*. This was implemented with a cadre of trained nurses working under a grant from the Department of Health Education and Welfare. The concept was to create a traveling curriculum for educating nurses in several emergency clinical areas including trauma, burns, and orthopaedics. The other curriculum areas included psychiatric and medicine/cardiac emergencies. Early faculty for the Field Nursing program included Sally Sohr, RN, Peggy Trimble, RN, Judy Bobb, RN, and Carol Katsaros Briscoe, RN. In the later years, a pediatric component was added with the expertise of Margaret Widener-Kolberg. The name for the program "Field Nursing" was designated by a retired military leader and was later renamed *EMS Nursing and Specialty Nursing Care*. At its peak, the programs numbered more than 100 per year held in 50 locations across Maryland and reaching 2,000 nurses per year. The goal was to provide training to nurses in community settings on how to care for patients in the first hours after injury and how to facilitate the transfers to trauma and specialty referral centers safely. It was during these early years that the inextricable links were made with the Maryland State Police (MSP) Aviation Division and the ground EMS providers.

Trauma Nurse Triad also grew out of Field Nursing. This was a 3-day program developed especially in response to requests from international visitors to observe care at MIEMSS. This later became a more formal international trauma seminar.

In 1982, another program was developed called *Advanced Trauma Life Support* (ATLS) for nurses. This course was considered a nursing tract in the physician ATLS program. Physician trauma leaders including Dr. Michael Rhodes taught in the nursing skill stations that were part of this program. The nursing and physician participants attended the didactic portion of the curriculum together, underscoring the teamwork that remains an important tenant in trauma care.

The nurse leadership for ATLS for nurses included Carol Katsaros Briscoe, RN, Judy Bobb, RN, and Peggy Trimble, RN. The ATLS for Nurses course (see Fig. 3) was quite successful. Sometime after it's initiation the name of the course (which is proprietary to the American College of Surgeons) was renamed. In response to this, a revised program was implemented for nurses with a similar format, under the new name of Trauma Nursing Course, and later changed again to Trauma Care for Nurses, which became a stand-alone traveling course. A team of trauma nurses from Arizona came to Baltimore to take the course and were impressed with its comprehensive content. Subsequently, they approached the Arizona Committee on Trauma regarding the idea to develop a companion course to ATLS that would be called *Advanced Trauma Care*

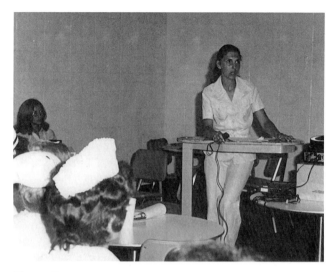

Figure 3   ATLS For Nurses Course—1970s Baltimore, Maryland, Instructor: Carole Katsaros Briscoe, RN. ATLS, Advanced Trauma Life Support.

for Nurses (ATCN). This was supported in Arizona and ATCN was born. After many successful years of partnership in Arizona, the course began expanding to other states. In 1998, ATCN was formally transitioned to the STN as a proprietary course. In 2000 the ACS unanimously approved the STN's proposal to deliver the concept of ATLS to nurses. This was a pivotal time for both organizations and opened the door to numerous other collaborations with the ACS-COT as this proposal served as a model for other proposals/programs. It continued to evolve and currently it is taught in numerous states in the United States and multiple other countries as well. To date, approximately 905 nurses have completed the program. This course is unique in that it not only continues to share the didactic content with the physician ATLS course participants but also includes interactive nursing skill stations that are relevant to nurses across the continuum of care.[22]

In 1986, ENA held the first Trauma Nurse Core Course. This popular curriculum is a free-standing program that includes both lecture and skills components and is geared primarily to the nurse providing care during the initial resuscitation phase of trauma. It is conducted throughout the United States and globally, and in some states/regions it is the entry level course for trauma nurse credentialing.

The ACS' *Resources for Optimal Care of the Injured Patient* originally outlined standards for hospitals wishing to function as trauma centers. Subsequent editions have defined leadership roles/responsibilities of key trauma center personnel along with current standard of care. The specific standards in the latest ACS document include recommendations for education/credentialing standards for physicians and nurses involved in acute trauma care.

As the role of trauma coordinator developed, courses that focused on developing skills in key areas of this role were created. For example, these courses included information on site survey preparation, prevention, quality/PI/data systems, and eventually business development/management of systems of care. The Core and Advanced Trauma Coordinator Courses of the ATS are two such curricula that offer this content.

The role of the trauma nurse specialty in hospitals was fueled by development of graduate nursing programs in critical care and trauma nursing. The early programs for masters level curriculum in trauma/critical care nursing were developed at the University of Washington in Seattle, the University of Maryland in Baltimore, and Widener University in Chester, PA. All of these programs offered a curriculum for preparing CNS; however, in many programs that exist currently a combined CNS and nurse practitioner curriculum is available.

ROLE OF NURSES IN TRAUMA SYSTEM DEVELOPMENT

The White Paper of 1966 initiated the early movement to develop comprehensive trauma systems. Later, in the early 1990s, the federal program through HRSA that established a competitive grant program continued the development of trauma systems and furthered the opportunities for nurses at the system level. Carol Katsaros Briscoe, RN (Maryland) and Terry Romano, RN (Illinois) were the first two trauma nurses with system level roles. They both had the title of trauma nurse coordinator training, education, legislative advocacy/advancement, QI/process improvement, data collection/analysis, networking/collaboration with the public health department, EMS, designation standards development/maintenance, writing/procurement grant acquisition, and public relations/community outreach were all part of their early roles. Although the scope has expanded, there has been little change in the core responsibilities of this role as it has evolved over 5 decades. The breadth of contributions to the field of trauma nursing is expansive. A summary of the major contributions to the profession by some of the key pioneers is detailed in Table 3.

TRAUMA NURSES AND PREHOSPITAL CARE

Both the trauma center and the system rely on competent and efficient prehospital care. There was early recognition that without trained prehospital providers, particularly in rural/remote areas, the patient outcomes were negatively impacted. Nurses have played an instrumental role in the growth of prehospital care and in linking the field to the hospital system, assuming pivotal roles as educators for EMS providers. Annie Smith Rehfeld, RN at MIEMSS, worked with R Adams Cowley to ensure that trained flight personnel were on the scene of injured patients. His initial strategy was to look at existing resources and adopt a cross-training approach. This led to collaboration with the MSP, who became the first law enforcement agency to provide aeromedical services. The early training was based on the then national paramedic curriculum and it was named the Aviation Trauma Technician (ATT) program.[11] Under Annie's leadership, resuscitation nurses developed the didactic and hands-on skills training that the ATT students (see Fig. 2) completed. Over the years, this group of troopers became well-trained prehospital providers and eventually became the MSP Aviation Division—the first model to successfully implement the threefold mission of Medevac—search, rescue, and law enforcement. Currently referred to as the Aviation Command with approximately 150 personnel, there are 54 trooper/flight paramedics providing care from 8 helicopter sections throughout Maryland.

Outreach and education for ground EMS providers were also accomplished in Maryland by utilizing a core group of trauma nurses from MIEMSS. Lou Jordan, a former military corpsmen, worked with Peggy Trimble, the director of MIEMSS Field Nursing, to take training and education to EMS providers statewide, similar to the model used for nursing.

In yet another example of nurses playing lead roles in the EMS system, Teresa Romano RN partnered with Dr. David Boyd and others to develop the 9-1-1 system in Illinois. This was one of the first of its kind in the country.

Prehospital care continues to be influenced by nurses in leadership roles. There are a number of state EMS directors in the United States who have been and are nurses. Nurses continue to provide direction and leadership for EMS systems. Evolution of the trauma nurse coordinator position has included links to EMS agencies in a liaison role. This role has been implemented in various ways. An early model saw the trauma nurse coordinator as link to EMS for patient feedback, QI, coordination of case reviews, traveling grand rounds for education, and improvement of care. Later models evolved to include a trauma PI trauma nurse that is the point of contact for EMS issues. There are also models where facilities have a formal EMS liaison nurse who works for the trauma program and provides QI reviews, regional education, skill development experiences at the facility, recertification/refresher courses, and individual patient follow-up.

Prehospital Trauma Life Support (PHTLS) was one of the early standardized courses for EMS trauma education. Will Chapleau, RN led the effort to develop PHTLS in collaboration with the National Association of Emergency Medical Technicians (EMTs). He worked hand in hand with Dr. Norman McSwain who was the lead from the ACS and Dr. Scott Frame on this initiative. Nurses continue to be integral to PHTLS and Basic Trauma Life Support (BTLS) EMS trauma training classes. Several serve as state directors for PHTLS training programs.

TRAUMA NURSING: WHERE ARE WE NOW?

Recent decades have seen tremendous advances in our ability to assess and manage critically injured patients. Development of comprehensive trauma systems has allowed for more appropriate routing of injured patients to centers best equipped to manage their clinical conditions. Changes in the demographics of injury have also impacted the profession of trauma nursing. In some areas of the country now, penetrating mechanisms from interpersonal violence is the leading cause of injury/death. In addition, there is an increase in incidents of mass injury from terrorism. As has always been the case, trauma nurses are caring for patients/families in crisis following devastating injuries. The impact on staff, including issues related to burnout and cumulative stress, continues to be a concern.

Changes in the medical training model resulting in the restriction of residency work hours have led to new opportunities for trauma nurses. One of the most notable changes is the expanded use of Advanced Practice Trauma Nurses. The utilization of trauma nurse practitioner has led to a number of improved outcomes and better continuity of care.[23,24]

Technology has greatly enhanced the ability of trauma care providers to network. E-mail, list serves, and telecasts have brought injury care providers from all over the globe closer together. The advent of telemedicine has led to real-time consultations that have improved trauma care in remote/rural areas and improved the efficiency of trauma systems.[23]

As of 2007, the Trauma Information Exchange Project (TIEP) reports more than 1,300 trauma centers (see Table 4) in the United States. Trauma nurses are coleading the trauma programs at these hospitals as a requirement of state and national standards.

The changing of nomenclature from "trauma nurse coordinator" to "trauma program manager" has changed this role's classification and compensation as well as its place on the organizational configuration, reporting structure, and scope of authority. Trauma nurses continue to be at the forefront of national initiatives involving trauma care. They have an important voice on issues with key partner organizations including the Eastern Association for the Surgery of Trauma, HRSA's Model Plan for Trauma Systems workgroup and Trauma/EMS Stakeholders, the ATS' Trauma Leadership Forums and TIEP, as well as the ACS Committee on Trauma Verification Review.

Changes in trauma nursing care are being driven by the evolution of trauma medical practice toward noninvasive surgery and nonoperative management. Therefore, the nursing care of patients has transitioned from preoperative resuscitation and postoperative care expertise to a more vigilant ongoing monitoring.

The Institute of Medicine released a report on Emergency Care in the United States in 2006. This document outlines a crisis in emergency care in terms of access and quality.

The threat of the loss of commitment of trauma centers and the liability insurance crisis has had a significant impact on trauma nursing. With the demise of local resources, patients and families are often transported out of their communities for injury care. They are forced to find support in an unfamiliar area for the duration of the hospitalization, and feel displaced, frustrated, scared, and often angry. Delays are also an issue with the lack of availability of specialty care beds needed for transfer to a higher level of care. Diversion hours, ED overcrowding, and higher nurse-to-patient ratios are all implications of these trends.

FUTURE

The metamhorphasis of the trauma program to include acute care surgery has implications for traditional nursing

---

TABLE 4

TRAUMA CENTER INVENTORY—2003

Level of Center	Designated or Certified by State or Region		ACS Verified Only	All Centers
	Not ACS Verified	ACS Verified		
I	102	60	32	194
II	143	65	38	246
III	246	12	20	278
IV/V/Unspecified	610	3	0	613
Pediatric Only	19	8	9	36
All	1,120	148	99	1,367

ACS, American College of Surgeons.
MacKenzie EJ, Hoyt DB, Sacra JC, et al. National Inventory of Hospital Trauma Centers2. *JAMA.*
2003;289(12):1517. ©2003 American Medical Association.

roles in trauma. The TPM of the future may become the acute care/emergency surgery manager with oversight of the program treating acute surgical illness. This shift will impact the data registry and PI components of the trauma program, along with educational requirements, budgetary planning, and personnel needs. The continued expansion of the TPM role has evolved in many areas to now be that of a trauma program nurse director with expanded scope and salary support in many cases.

It is becoming increasingly difficult to recruit and retain trauma nurses due to the nature of the patient profiles, acuity, and the reality that trauma occurs in predictable patterns during summer, weekends, nights, and holidays. Trauma volumes increase during these times when other hospital departments experience a converse decrease in volume. In addition, these are traditionally times when most nurses prefer to spend time outside of work.

It appears that there will be scarcity of next-generation trauma nursing leaders as there are other specialties in nursing that afford a more pleasant work-life balance. Technology will continue to advance creating new and faster diagnostic capabilities, which will continue to decrease patient lengths of stay and increase the need for more efficient discharge planning. The aging of America will require the evolution of an entirely new body of trauma nursing knowledge related to geriatric trauma care. More data to base decisions on physician shortage, trauma surgeon specialty, and loss of the federal program again. The American Trauma Society continues to develop a myriad of programs to support clinicians, patients and families. The Trauma Survivor's Network is a program in development that has several key components offering supports to patients and their families following during/after acute hospitalization for injury. The biggest challenges facing the future of trauma nursing include the continued threat (reality) of man-made and natural disasters and various forms of terrorism. In addition, the expanded utilization of technology offers great promise to improve the connectedness of trauma clinicians and improve care, particularly in rural or underserved areas. Telemedicine, the use of systems like VISICU (remote ICU monitoring system), incorporation of clinical decision support systems and electronic medical records have already changed the way patients are cared for and enhanced ability to perform quality reviews. The profession of trauma nursing while relatively young in its evolution has grown tremendously. New or enhanced roles for trauma clinical nurses and leaders continue to be developed. The future holds much promise for this rich and greatly important component of the nursing profession.

REFERENCES

1. Society of Trauma Nurses Website: www.traumanursesoc.org, accessed, July 2007.
2. Beachley M. Trauma nursing is a developing specialty *J Emerg Nurs.* 1989;15(5).
3. Army Nurse Corps History. Available at : http://history.amedd .army.mil/default index2.html.
4. Beachley M. The evolution of trauma nursing and the society of trauma nurses. *A Noble Hist.* 2005;12(4):105–115.
5. US Korean War Memorial. Available at: http://korea50.army.mil.
6. Vietnam Women Veterans Memorial Foundation - Available at: http://www.vietnamwomensmemorial.org/pages/framesets/ setvwmp.html.
7. 6 Gender Gap: Nurses on the Battlefieldhttp://www .vietnamwomensmemorial.org/pages/framesets/setvwmp.html.
8. Beachley M. Education standards/designation standards. *Trauma Nurse Newsl.* 1988;2(3):2–3.
9. Committee on Trauma and Committee on Shock, Division of Medical Sciences, National Academy of Sciences, National Research Council. *Accidental death and disability: the neglected disease of modern society.* Rockville Maryland: Department of Health, Education and Welfare; 1966.
10. Romano T. Trauma nurse specialist. *Am J Nurs.* 1973;73(6): 1008–1011.
11. Beachley M. Trauma nurse network standards. *Trauma Nurse Newsl.* 1988;2(2):2.
12. Emergency Nurses Association (ENA). Website www.ena.org accessed August, 2007.
13. American College of Surgeons, Committee On Trauma Resources for Optimal Care of the Injured Patient; 2006.
14. Shackford SR, Hollingsworth-Fridlund P, Cooper G, et al. The effect of regionalization upon the quality of trauma care as assessed by concurrent audit before and after institution of a trauma system: A preliminary report. *J Trauma.* 1986;26:812–820.
15. FitzPatrick MK, McMaster J. Trauma performance improvement. In: McQuillan K, Von Rueden K, Hartsock R, et al. eds. *Trauma nursing: from resuscitation through rehabilitation*, 3rd ed. WB Saunders; 2001.
16. Shackford SR, Hollingsworth-Fridlund P, Cooper GF, et al. The effect of regionalization upon the quality of trauma care as assessed by concurrent audit before and after institution of a trauma system: A preliminary report. *J Trauma.* 1986;26:812–820.
17. Rogers FB, Ricci M, Caputo M, et al. The use of telemedicine for real-time video consultation between trauma center and community hospital in a rural setting improves early trauma care: Preliminary results. *J Trauma.* 2001;51:1037–1041.
18. Hartsock RL, Leone SK, Dutton RP, et al. Statewide trauma system communication improves quality of care in interhospital transfer patients. Poster Presentation. American Association for the Surgery of Trauma, 64th Meeting, Atlanta, Georgia, September 2005.
19. *Ill Med J.* 1971:258–265.
20. American College of Surgeons. Resources for Optimal Care of the Injured Patient; 1993.
21. American College of Surgeons, National Trauma Data Bank (NTDB) http://www.facs.org/trauma/ntdb.html accessed June, 2007.
22. (REFERENCE Beachley article JTN page 112)
23. Cooper MA, Lindsay GM, Kim S, et al. Evaluating emergency nurse practitioner services: A randomized controlled trial. *J Adv Nurs.* 2002;40(6):722–730.
24. Christmas AB, Reynolds J, Hodges S, et al. Physician extenders impact trauma systems. *J Trauma.* 2005;58(5):917–920.

ACKNOWLEDGMENT

The authors would like to thank the following for their contributions to this chapter: John Ashworth, MHA; Diane Balderson, RN; Mary Beachley, RN; Sharan Bidle, RN; Judy Bobb, RN; David Boyd, MD; Jim Brown, MA; Ginny Cardona, RN; Jenny Delauter, RN; Carol Forrester-Staz, RN; Deana Holler, RN; Heidi Hotz, RN; Carole Katsaros Briscoe, RN; Paula Kelly, RN; Barbara Keyes, RN; Betsy Kramer, RN; Connie Mattice, RN; Philip Militello, MD; Michelle Pomphrey, RN; Basil Pruitt, MD; Teresa Romano, RN; Elizabeth Scanlan, RN; Brian Slack, BS; Annie Smith Rehfeld, RN; Johnese Spisso, RN; Harry Teter Esq.; Terese Trainum, RN; Peggy Trimble, RN; Connie Walleck Jastremski, RN; Margaret Widner Kolberg, RN.

Training and Development of Trauma Surgeons

Anthony A. Meyer   **Colin G. Thomas**

Surgical management of injured patients has been described as far back as we have written records. The type of injuries, methods of treatment, and skill and training of the "surgeons" who treated them is part of the continually changing process of human experience. This chapter will only examine the state of the training and development of trauma surgeons who will be providing care for the injured in the future.

Lack of exact knowledge of the change in injury patterns, health care expectations, and who will be the surgeons to deliver their care does not prevent a review of trauma surgeon's training and development. However, no matter how trauma care changes, what is known is that there will need to be surgeons leading the efforts to provide best care for injury victims.

This chapter will review the present state of surgical training and practice in trauma and the trainees available to pursue trauma careers. Approaches to train and develop future trauma surgeons will be presented. The considerations will be largely limited to the "general" trauma surgeon, rather than the subspecialties such as orthopaedics, neurosurgery, or plastic surgery. The care provided by these specialties will be considered, but the specifics of their training and development is not at the core of the looming problem of having enough trauma surgeons to cover the needs of the United States for injury management. Additionally, the focus of the discussion will be on US trauma systems, although there are even greater needs for surgeons involved in care of the injured in most of the world outside the United States.

TRAINING AND DEVELOPMENT OF TRAUMA SURGEONS

The evidence that the present organizational structure of trauma centers saves lives has most recently been presented by McKenzie et al.,[1] Durham et al. (June Annals of Surgery), and Demetriades et al.[2] The finding that survival from equivalent injury treated in Level I trauma centers is 25% better compared to patients treated in nontrauma facilities argues strongly for such a system, and the availability of surgeons trained in and committed to the care of the injured. The magnitude of this difference in outcome must be taken into context, in that there is at present no data to support a comparable difference in outcome in national comparisons of centers for managing cancer or heart disease. Those differences may exist but have not been demonstrated. Furthermore, when considering the impact of reduction in death and disability from injury, which is responsible for more years of productive life lost than cancer and heart disease combined,[3] the impact of trauma centers is further magnified. Finally, when considering the growing global importance of injury as a health problem, the adoption of organized trauma systems and the training of sufficient numbers of surgeons skilled and interested in care of the injured become more compelling.[4]

However, there is an increasing realization that the future availability of surgeons skilled and interested in management of the injured will be inadequate to meet the needs of the US health care delivery system.[5] Early indications of this problem were noted by Richardson, Esposito, and Trunkey[6–8] who found a lack of interest in trauma as a career choice for surgical residents. Several obvious perceptions contributed to this lack of interest, including time and call demands, unappealing patient population, and financial impact. Whether these perceptions are supported by evidence does not matter much because practice or subspecialty preference is more subjective than objective decision.

Review of surgical journals, web sites, and letters to program directors demonstrate a large number of open positions for trauma surgeons, or surgeons willing to cover trauma as part of their practice. Notably, many of these postings have been present for months or years. This suggests either that the position is not appealing, or that there are too few surgeons capable of or interested in filling that position. It is not feasible to accurately track the number of open trauma positions, or the number of surgeons taking such jobs. It is also difficult to determine how many trauma fellowship positions are filled because there is no official registry, although many are posted on several web sites. Surgical Critical Care (SCC) training is often associated with preparation for a career in trauma. Review of the number of SCC residencies and the number of residents in these positions over the last 6 years shows a 27% increase in the number of training programs and a 20% increase in the number of trainees from 2001 to 2006 (see Table 1). The actual number of SCC training positions is difficult to calculate, but usually only two thirds are filled.

Table 2 shows the number of surgeons who take the American Board of Surgery (ABS) examination in SCC for the years 2003 to 2005. Notably, fewer than half the first-time candidates finished their training the previous year. It appears that as many as a third of SCC trainees may never take the examination for certification. These findings

TABLE 1

NUMBER OF ACCREDITATION COUNCIL FOR GRADUATE MEDICAL EDUCATION (ACGME)-APPROVED SURGICAL CRITICAL CARE PROGRAMS AND TRAINEES

Year	No. of Programs	No. of Trainees
2000–2001	67	110
2002	71	93
2003	79	87
2004	82	111
2005	85	119
2006	85	132

TABLE 2

NUMBER OF SURGEONS TAKING AMERICAN BOARD OF SURGERY (ABS) EXAMINATION IN SURGICAL CRITICAL CARE

Year	No. of First-Time Examinees
2003	80
2004	99
2005	85

suggest that some, perhaps a significant proportion, of SCC training positions are occupied by trainees who may not be eligible for examination by the ABS. Most importantly, what is not known is how many of these SCC-trained and SCC-certified surgeons are in a clinical practice that includes trauma coverage.

The concern for the number of surgeons participating in trauma care now is compounded by the anticipated fundamental changes in the training of surgeons of all types, changes in the practice of trauma surgery, and the changes in the trainees themselves.

SURGICAL TRAINING IN TRAUMA

Significant decreases in the number of applicants to general surgery resulted in the failure to fill approximately 7% of general surgery residency positions in 2001. Although the numbers of US senior medical students matching into general surgery increased somewhat since then, probably in part due to the 80 hour per week work limit, subspecialties requiring general surgery training have continued to have problems filling their training positions. Thoracic surgery, vascular surgery, and pediatric surgery have all had reductions in the number of US-trained applicants.

This has led thoracic and vascular surgical program directors more to primary board certification, which does not require completion of general surgery training. The impact of these changes in established subspecialties is overshadowed by the anticipated restructuring of what has been "general surgery" into subspecialties. The proposed new subspecialties include surgical oncology, gastrointestinal (GI) surgery, transplantation, acute care surgery, and some formats of general surgery, possibly comprehensive general surgery and/or rural surgery. The exact divisions and training paradigms have not yet been determined, but the changes are in development. The reality of increasing knowledge and differing skills in each subspecialty, the pursuit of fellowship training in one of these areas by approximately 75% of all present graduating general surgery trainees, the cost in time and money for the present 5 years of general surgery before specialization, and the actual practice patterns of established surgeons continue to push toward this change, despite real concerns. These concerns include further fragmentation of patient care and major imbalances in workforce in the future.

The result of many of the proposed new paradigms will produce new surgeon subspecialists with only limited experience in trauma management whose certification will not include comprehensive trauma care, and who will not be able to be credentialed in trauma care at their hospitals.[9] In such a training structure, only surgeons trained and certified in either acute care surgery, or possibly comprehensive and/or rural general surgery, will be credentialed to comprehensively manage acutely injured patients. Given that training in comprehensive general surgery will be focused on preparing surgeons for practice in communities without large specialty hospitals, the number of trauma-capable surgeons to staff urban trauma centers will be significantly impacted. As the more broadly trained general surgeons who provide much of the trauma care leave practice, the care of injured patients in the United States will suffer greatly.

SURGICAL PRACTICE IN TRAUMA

The practice of trauma surgery has changed considerably in the last 25 years, and will continue to change. These changes are due to the frequency and types of injuries seen, as well as the methods of treatment.

Trauma has traditionally been perceived to be the management of penetrating trauma and motor vehicle crashes. Recent data has found that the incidence of penetrating trauma is down as much as 70% in some locales. Because most patients with major penetrating torso injuries require surgical interventions, this decrease in incidence has led to a decrease in operative procedures for trauma surgeons. At the same time, the surgical management of blunt truncal injuries has changed to more frequent nonoperative management. Hepatic, splenic, and renal injuries are most often managed nonoperatively.[10]

Although the drop in penetrating trauma and improved outcomes in some cases of blunt trauma managed nonoperatively has led to decreased trauma deaths, it has decreased the attractiveness of trauma surgery because of reduced operative activity.[11] The shift of trauma surgeons is out of the operating room (OR) and into the intensive care unit (ICU) to manage complex patients who require only orthopaedic and neurosurgical operations, or to meeting rooms to handle the increasing demand for policy changes, quality reviews, and process documentation. Although the critical care management role of the trauma surgeon has become more involved and comprehensive, it is difficult to interest enough young surgeons in a specialty with a low frequency of operative intervention, to meet the needs of trauma centers. Notably, as trauma surgeons bemoan their reduced operative activity, they continue to publish studies of nonoperative management of injuries in which the only outcome benefit is no surgery.

SURGICAL TRAINEE CHANGES

The demographics, and more importantly, the expectations, of surgical trainees continue to change. Graduating medical school classes have approximately the same number of men and women. General surgical training positions continue to attract more men than women, but the difference is decreasing. Studies have identified some impact of gender on the volume and type of practice activity. However, the differences are not large, and are mostly related to competing time demands for child rearing on women surgeons.[12]

A greater issue regarding surgical trainees than gender is the overall time commitment to career. The issues involved include income, time in training, time off clinical responsibility once in practice, changed standards for accomplishments, and many others. They are often lumped together as "lifestyle" issues, but reflect other factors as well.[13] This impacts not only how many surgeons enter careers in trauma surgery but also how long they continue to provide trauma care. Many surgeons drop out of trauma participation because of "lifestyle" interests.

A survey published by Esposito et al. lists the ideal practice characteristics from practicing trauma surgeons, as shown in Table 3.[14] Notably 8 of 10 are lifestyle related. Generational differences in goals and expectations are well described. It is not realistic to expect these to stop changing, or for them not to affect surgical trainees. It is likely that these differences in surgical trainees in the future will be further effected by additional influences such as the duty hour restrictions set by the Accreditation Council for Graduate Medical Education (ACGME).[15] The 80-hour average work week limits for residents has not been shown to adversely impact trauma care, or other specialty care management. The changes have documented some

---

TABLE 3

IDEAL PRACTICE CHARACTERISTICS

Ranking	Characteristic
1	Guaranteed appropriate salary
2	Guaranteed time away from work
3	Subsidized ancillary benefits
4	More general surgery
5	Less night call
6	Subsidized reliable coding and billing support
7	Addition of physician extenders
8	Less surgical critical care
9	Stipend for on-call services
10	Large group diversified practice
11	Addition of selected orthopaedic and neurosurgical procedures

Adapted from Esposito TJ, Leon L, Jurkovich GJ. The shape of things to come: Results from a National Survey of Trauma Surgeons on Issues Concerning Their Future. *J Trauma.* 2006;60:8–16.

decrease in fatigue in residents, but stress is unchanged or even worse.[16] Notably, there is no consistent evidence that patient safety is improved; possible gains in fatigue may be offset by problems with communication due to more frequent transfer of responsibility. Pressure for further reduction in resident duty hours is inevitable, especially given the European Union common goal of 40 hours.

There is no reason to support excessive duty hours for surgical residents or any other health professionals. However, progressive reduction in duty hour limits will have at least three serious impacts. First, it will decrease the educational experience. Residents will have seen fewer cases. Even if the resident spends time outside the duty hour limits in reading about surgery, the decrease in the actual time of clinical care, and its continuity, will result in surgeons less well prepared to care for the injured.

Second, their bedside participation will be more intermittent; this could lead to "shift mentality" toward patients and a lack of continuity of responsibility once the trainee enters practice. Van Eaton et al. have described how surgical practice is evolving from individual to team responsibility.[17] Surgical care has always been a team concept, with each team member taking individual responsibility for patients, not only their role, but for the total care of the patient. This leads to a redundancy that is important to reduce the risk of errors. If there is a qualitative decrease in "individual responsibility," given the psychological concept of a greater willingness to accept greater outcome risk when there is shared impact of adverse outcome, there may be greater risk to patient safety. There can be no increased tolerance for error in trauma or any other medical care just because the responsibility shifts to the "team."

Third, it is already apparent that residents training under duty hour limits usually expect to have no greater time demands once they finish training and begin practice than they did in residency. It is uncommon that surgeons in practice routinely spend more than 80 hours on one in four in-house night call. However, if training duty hour limits are significantly reduced, the change in resident experience will likely change what surgeons will be willing to do once in practice. This will not only impact the format and continuity of care of the injured but also the surgical workforce needed to provide trauma care. This would lead to an effective reduction in trauma surgeon workforce despite the same number of practitioners.

APPROACHES FOR TRAINING AND DEVELOPING TRAUMA SURGEONS FOR THE FUTURE

It is difficult to develop a strategy to provide trauma surgeons for the future when the training paradigm is undergoing major changes and the capabilities and number of trauma-capable surgeons is unknown. At the same time, the characteristics of a trauma surgeon's practice in the

future also remains unknown. Despite this difficulty, a strategy needs to be developed to help direct these evolving structures of training and practice to yield an educational system and workforce that will provide high-quality care to meet the needs of all injured patients for future generations.

Although the patterns of injury and the best approaches to treatment are changing, the fact that there will be injured patients who will be best served by an organized, quality-care focused health care team will not change. It is necessary to come up with educational and development programs that will produce trauma surgeons capable of leading these teams, and leading these changes, not just reacting to them.

TRAUMA SURGEON RECRUITMENT

The surgeons who provide trauma care in the future will come from among those surgeons who pursue training in acute care surgery (those trained in trauma, critical care, and emergency surgery) and those trained in the adapted forms of general surgery (comprehensive general surgery, rural surgery, or other variations of general surgery). The other evolving subspecialties of general surgery (oncology, transplant, and GI will not have comprehensive trauma care as one of their components of certification, and will likely not be able to get privileges at a hospital to do trauma except in the most extreme emergencies. General surgeons trained before the anticipated early subspecialization initiative (which will likely be finished between 2013 and 2018) will still be able to practice trauma surgery if they maintain continuing medical education (CME) and are active in trauma care. Having surgeons without sufficient training, experience, or commitment to trauma care provide a hospital's surgical trauma coverage would negatively impact outcomes and lead to loss of trauma center designation, and eventual breakdown of an organized trauma system.

It will be essential that active recruitment be done for medical students and preliminary surgical residents not yet matched into another subspecialty in order to bring enough quality trainees into acute care surgery or the general surgery specialties capable of meeting the needs of trauma systems. The essential elements of such recruitment are (i) role models with a passion for a career, which includes care of the injured, (ii) an understanding by the future surgeon about the value, both personal and professional, of a participation in trauma care, and (iii) overcoming the negatives of a career including trauma care. A list of these from the survey by Esposito et al. is seen in Table 4.[12]

Trauma surgery has had a history of great role models who helped recruit new surgeons into careers in which care of the injured is an integral part. These role models had or have a passion for what they do, and it is picked up by some of their trainees. This has become more difficult, possibly because fewer trauma surgeons have the

TABLE 4	
IMPEDIMENTS TO TRAUMA SURGERY AS A CAREER CHOICE	
Ranking	**Impediment**
1	Personal lifestyle issues
2	Length of training
3	Scope of practice
4	Income
5	Medicolegal risk
6	Malpractice premium cost
7	Professional respect
8	Disruptive nature of trauma care

Adapted from Esposito TJ, Leon L, Jurkovich GJ. The shape of things to come: Results from a National Survey of Trauma Surgeons on Issues Concerning Their Future. *J Trauma*. 2006;60:8–16.

charisma of Drs. Shires, Blaisdell, Walt, Trunkey, Carrico, or those too many to name, but more likely because the excitement of operating on trauma patients has been replaced by nonoperative management of patients, whereas other specialties do surgeries, and leave the complex care to the trauma team. There are still surgical leaders with the passion for care of the injured. It will be important for them to demonstrate to medical students and residents how they can get the satisfaction of providing excellent trauma care, while expanding their operative activity both in procedures not traditionally done by general surgeons in the United States (e.g., external fixation, intracranial pressure [ICP] monitoring, and catheter placement) and urgent and emergent general surgery procedures.

Medical students and preliminary residents will have to see this work for it to be effective. As the transition to acute care surgery occurs, attention to increasing operative activity and promotion of the care of the injured will be essential. Strategies to get students interested will be to involve trauma surgeons in the first year of medical school in anatomy and pathophysiology courses as well as in programs on prevention and epidemiology. These efforts will demonstrate the excitement of treating the injured based on physiologic principles and anatomic approaches to operative management of injuries. Participation in epidemiology and prevention programs raises the students' awareness of the societal and global impact of injury and the contributions they can make in a career which includes trauma care.

The exact number of surgeons necessary to provide trauma care in the United States is difficult to quantify. It includes surgeons at all levels of trauma centers, from rural to urban, Level IV to Level I. With the volume, patterns, and management of injury changing and the practice and capabilities of surgeon simultaneously changing, estimates at a surgeon workforce for trauma would be just a guess. Previous efforts by groups to predict specialty

workforce needs with fewer variables to consider have been very inaccurate. Rather than identify a number, these recommendations will focus on a strategy for producing surgeons capable of providing trauma care.

Medical students and preliminary surgical residents who demonstrate the capabilities and commitment necessary to be a good trauma surgeon should be encouraged to pursue careers in acute care surgery. Efforts should be made to reinforce their interests in the field, such as by bringing them to local, regional, or national trauma meetings. The American Association for the Surgery of Trauma has had a program to support medical students to do this since 1992. Residents as well as students should be encouraged to participate in scholarly activity in trauma care, clinical or basic science, or even useful case reports. The Committee on Trauma of the American College of Surgeons, the Eastern Association for the Surgery of Trauma, and the American Burn Association have had awards for the best papers presented by residents at their meetings. These efforts are effective in encouraging careers in trauma surgery.

No change in training development or practice structure will provide enough quality trauma surgeons if excellent students and residents are not recruited to the field. Recruitment will not be successful unless there is a genuine and concerted effort to reach out and bring these future surgeons into a specialty to which they see their role models genuinely committed.

TRAINING TRAUMA SURGEONS

As the training structure of surgery in the United States is changed, efforts are being made to make sure that the graduates of the new subspecialty of acute care surgery will have the skills necessary for comprehensive care of the injured.

Efforts are under way at the ABS, the Residency Review Committee for Surgery of the ACGME, and trauma surgery organizations including the American Association for the Surgery of Trauma and the Committee on Trauma of the American College of Surgeons to identify the necessary educational elements for training trauma surgeons.[9] It is not clear currently how this structure will look when implemented. Furthermore, each training program will have unique experiences and variations.

There are important discussions with leadership from Orthopaedic Surgery and Neurosurgery regarding the role of the acute care surgeon in the management of some injuries currently handled by these surgeons. These specialties have ongoing internal debates because many of their members have no interest in trauma care, whereas other members have career interests in trauma management. These issues will have to be resolved in order to have a trauma care system capable of providing excellent trauma care throughout the country, and not just represent local turf battles. In major trauma centers, it is likely to have enough orthopaedists and neurosurgeons committed to trauma care. The subspecialists who are an active part of the trauma team will provide the trauma care. In hospitals with insufficient orthopaedic or neurosurgery participation, acute care surgeons will likely need to expand their practice to include ventriculostomies and ICP management, and external fixation of unstable fractures and management of open fractures by debridement and wound coverage. Therefore, it will be important to have these elements as part of training programs for acute care surgery.

Since the practice of acute care surgery can be quite varied, its training has to include those subspecialty elements that may be necessary in a setting without much help. These acute care surgeons will need capability to manage many complex soft tissue wounds, vascular emergencies requiring open approach and management of basic emergent thoracic injury, and some of their sequelae. Involvement of other surgical specialists in the management of the injured patients will be dependent on the type of hospital, and the capabilities and interests of the other surgeons involved.

One subspecialty in acute care surgery that will require additional training will be burn surgery. Although acute care surgeons should be able to initiate care of burn victims, an acute care surgeon with additional training in burns will need to lead the team that provides comprehensive burn care.

The other elements of training of the acute care surgeon will include the traditional general surgery emergencies; intra-abdominal infection, obstruction or ischemia; and the management of other acute surgical problems such as necrotizing soft tissue infections.[11,18] This will require senior experience in GI surgery and plastic surgery in the acute care surgery training years. Similarly, senior residents in other specialties will need rotations on acute care surgery to see some of the problems they may treat depending on their practice situations.

The other specialty training that will provide surgeons with the certification and potential credentialing to manage trauma patients will be those that are most similar to what is now general surgery. There may be two tracks: comprehensive general surgery for practitioners who want to practice in locales that need only a few surgeons but ones who are capable of providing a wide spectrum of care including trauma and emergency surgery; and rural surgery, for practitioners in solo or small groups that provide not only traditional general surgery but some gynecology and other specialty support as well. Although elective general surgery will be a large part of the practice of these "general surgery" specialists, they will provide a good deal of trauma care, especially in rural areas.[19,20] These surgeons expand the pool of those capable of trauma management, as well as some career flexibility if they wish to pursue other practice options.

DEVELOPMENT OF TRAUMA SURGEONS

Once surgeons have been trained in a specialty that certifies them for patient care including trauma care, it is important to help them continue to provide high quality trauma care and meet the needs of their community for management of the injured. This means keeping them current in trauma management, and active in trauma care. Educational programs already exist to help trauma surgeons maintain their skills and acquire the new knowledge and techniques necessary to provide state-of-the-art care of the injured. It is not as easy to provide a structure to keep surgeons interested in providing trauma care. Attrition of surgeons from trauma care is a huge problem that can overwhelm any recruitment efforts. It is essential to limit this attrition because it will make any recruitment effort less effective.

Strategies to develop and retain trauma surgeons include those that help them attain their professional achievements, economic and lifestyle goals, and personal fulfillment. Meeting only one of these goals will be less effective in keeping a surgeon's or anyone's interest in trauma care or any profession. Helping trauma surgeons realize all three goals will be most successful in retaining them to provide care of the injured.

Professional achievement in trauma surgery or any profession is attained by capability, effort, and sponsorship. Capability is determined largely by training and effort, by behavior patterns established in childhood and focused by surgical role models. The sponsorship so important for professional achievement has been continually passed from one generation of trauma surgeons to the next. Senior trauma surgeons involve their more junior colleagues in local, state, and national organizations involved in the care of the injured. State emergency medical service (EMS) organizations and state chapters of the Committee on Trauma of the American College of Surgeons are some of the most effective groups involved in trauma care; and all are often in need of surgeon participation. Effective involvement in these efforts, as well as continued sponsorship by mentors, will lead to opportunities to participate in regional and national organizations committed to improved trauma care. These organizations have both academic and advocacy roles and include the American Association for the Surgery of Trauma, the Eastern Association for the Surgery of Trauma, the Western Trauma Association, and the National Committee on Trauma of the American College of Surgeons. There are many other organizations with more focused interest, such as the American Burn Association, or interests that overlap with injury, such as the Surgical Infection Society. Sponsorship for trauma surgeons to these organizations and their introduction to the organization's leadership will help cement a career interest in trauma care, as experienced by many present trauma surgeons.

These organizations are not an end in themselves, but vehicles to increase the quality of care for injured patients. It is participation in these efforts that helps surgeons realize professional achievement, not just membership or even leadership position in the organization. Again, it is the effort of their sponsors and role models that allows surgeons to see how this achievement is essential to patient care.

For surgeons in academic positions, scholarly accomplishments are part of their professional achievement. Some of this scholarship is achieved by scientific contributions, in basic or clinical science, or both. Many of our academic trauma centers have made major contributions to the care of the injured. These institutions are crucial in the recruitment, training, and development of trauma surgeons. They contribute notably by developing future role models for trauma surgeons who will populate trauma centers across the United States and the world, and help to keep governmental and health care systems reminded of the importance of injury on societies.

Economic and lifestyle issues dominated the list of ideal practice characteristics in Esposito et al.'s survey, reproduced in Table 3. Income and lifestyle concerns differ, but are inextricably involved because income and work effort are generally directly related, and lifestyle is inversely related to work effort.

The continued pressure on control of health care expenditures, increased competition for health care money, and a general lack of concern by the public for physician income will make it difficult to achieve gains in income for surgeons providing trauma care without an increase in the value of their efforts. This gain in value could potentially be achieved by the acute care surgeon and "general surgeon" specialists whose practices expand in the number and complexity of procedures. Hospitals which now pay large stipends to multiple subspecialists who cover trauma will be able to realign resources with effort and are likely to save money with the change.

It is important to note that trauma surgeons progressively see themselves as hospital or health care system employees, rather than as part of a professional group practice. This may be largely the result of local changes in the financial structure of health care systems, but it will accelerate the perception of the trauma surgeon as a "shift employee" rather than the leader of a team providing continuity of care to the injured. This may be consistent with the directions taken by duty hour limits for residents; however, great care will have to be taken to avoid a negative impact on trauma care. Efforts must be made to develop systems to avoid negative impact by a "shift work" approach,[13] but it will ultimately require a commitment to personal responsibility by all participants, not just team responsibility that will keep trauma care improving.

A final goal that needs to be met by trauma surgeons, and all professionals, is personal fulfillment. The particulars of this goal will vary between individuals and are different than professional achievement or economic and lifestyle success. Personal fulfillment, for a surgeon, can be most simply summarized as a feeling that the surgeon has made a positive difference to society, the profession, and family and friends. For many people, attainment of personal fulfillment is more important than professional achievement, economic status, and lifestyle gains. Again, role models of surgeons who acknowledge the personal fulfillment they get from a career including trauma surgery is important to help develop surgeons who look forward to the opportunity to care for the injured.

Despite changes in the patterns of injury, the approaches to trauma management and the training paradigm of surgery, care of the injured will be a crucial part of health care in the future. The evidence of surgeon-led trauma systems saving lives is clear, and emphasizes the need for surgeons skilled in and committed to care of the injured. It is necessary for us to meet this need by ensuring effective training and career development structure, and recruiting talented surgeons to this specialty.

REFERENCES

1. Mackenzie EJ, Rivara FP, Jurkovich GJ, et al. A national evaluation of the effect of trauma center care on mortality. *N Engl J Med.* 2006;354:366–378.
2. Demetriados D, Moartin M, Salim A, et al. Relationship between American College of Surgeons Trauma Center Designation and mortality in patients with severe trauma (injury severity score 715). *J Am Coll Surg.* 2006;202:212–215.
3. Trunkey DD. Trauma: Accidental and intentional injuries. *Sci Am.* 1983;249:28–35.
4. Meyer AA. Death and disability from injury: A global challenge. *J Trauma.* 1998;44:1–12.
5. Rodriguiez JL, Christmas AB, Franklin GA, et al. Trauma/critical care surgeon: A specialist gasping for air. *J Trauma.* 2005;59:1–7.
6. Richardson JD, Miller FB. Will future surgeons be interested in trauma care? Results of a resident survery. *J Trauma.* 1992;33:229–235.
7. Esposito TJ, Maier RV, Rivara FP, et al. Why surgeons prefer not to care for trauma patients. *Arch Surg.* 1991;126:292–297.
8. Trunkey DD. What's wrong with trauma care. *Bull Am Coll Surg.* 1990;733:11.
9. Committee to Develop the Reorganized Specialty of Trauma, Surgical Critical Care and Emergency Surgery. Acute care surgery: Trauma, critical care and emergency surgery. *J Trauma.* 2005;58:614–616.
10. Cryer GM III. The future of trauma care: At the crossroads. *J Trauma.* 2005;58:425–436.
11. Esposito TJ, Rotondo M, Barie PS, et al. Making the case for a paradigm shift in trauma surgery. *J Am Coll Surg.* 2006;202:655–667.
12. Schroen AT, Brownstein MR, Sheldon GF. Women in academic general surgery. *Acad Med.* 2004;79(4):310–318.
13. Meyer AA, Weiner TM. The generation gap. *Arch Surg.* 2002;137(3):268–270.
14. Esposito TJ, Leon L, Jurkovich GJ. The shape of things to come: Results from a National Survey of Trauma Surgeons on Issues Concerning Their Future. *J Trauma.* 2006;60:8–16.
15. Shackford S. How then shall we change. *J Trauma.* 2006;60:1–7.
16. Zare SM, Galanko J, Behrns KE, et al. Psychological well-being of surgery residents before the 80-hour work week:

A multiinstitutional study. *J Am Coll Surg*. 2004;198(4):633–640.

17. Van Eaton EG, Horvath KD, Pellegrini CA. Professionalism and the shift mentality. *Arch Surg*. 2005;140:230–235.

18. Scherer LA, Batistella FD. Trauma and emergency surgery: An evolutionary direction for trauma surgeons. *J Trauma*. 2004;56: 7–12.

19. Ruby BJ, Cagbill TH, Gardner RS. Role of the rural general surgeon in a statewide trauma system. *Bull Am Coll Surg*. 2006;91: 37–40.

20. Austin MT, Diaz JJ, Feurer ID. Creating an emergency general surgery service enhances the productivity of trauma surgeons, general surgeons, and the hospital. *J Trauma*. 2005;58:906–910.

Organizing the Continuum of Care for Injured Patients

22

Eddy H. Carrillo   Fahim Habib

Over the last decade, organizing the care of trauma has become increasingly more complicated. This is a multifactorial situation; however, the foremost reasons are: (i) the specialty of trauma has become less attractive; (ii) there is a perceived but not documented increase in litigation with skyrocketing malpractice premiums; (iii) the erroneous belief that there is an increased exposure to infectious diseases; and (iv) a significant decrease in reimbursement from traditional payers.[1] Trauma surgery is also seen by new general surgery graduates as a nonoperative specialty because most patients can be treated with nonsurgical management. Finally, trauma surgeons are seen as specialists who prepare patients for surgical procedures performed by other specialists.[2] Notwithstanding all these challenges, modern trauma systems and the surgeons who lead them have accomplished much in what is arguably the leading area of medical practice in terms of documentation of results and cost effectiveness. The purpose of this chapter is to highlight the efforts to create an efficient and effective continuum of care for injured patients, which integrates the contributions of multiple medical specialists and other professionals to produce high-quality effective patient care.

EVOLUTION IN TRAUMA CARE

The end of the 20th century witnessed a significant increased dependence in technology to care for trauma patients, a proliferation of systems of trauma care systems, and significant advances in prehospital and hospital care of trauma victims. The increasing number of patients treated by nonoperative means and advanced critical care support, as well as progress in imaging technology has dramatically changed our approach to trauma patients.[3] There is also an associated substantial decrease in the incidence of penetrating injuries. According to the Bureau of Justice Statistics of the Justice Department, violent crime in the United States is at its lowest level since the government began to survey victims in 1973. Unfortunately, these advances in trauma care have arrived at the expense of key changes in the way that trauma care is delivered in the United States.

EMERGENCY ROOM COVERAGE

Because of some, if not all of the changes in trauma surgery, the biggest change has been in the manner in which emergency room (ER) and trauma coverage is provided. On July 1, 2003, several regulations of working hours for residents were put forth by the Accreditation Council for Graduate Medical Education (ACGME). These measures restricted the number of hours and changed the quality of the training environment for residents. As a result of these measures, ER and overall service coverage has become more challenging. Numerous coverage alternatives have been proposed and we will describe some of the most common ones.

In-House Attending

The requirement for a surgical attending presence during initial resuscitation by the Committee on Trauma of the American College of Surgeons has been challenged lately and is the subject of intense debate at different levels. Most experts in the field postulate that there is a relationship between trauma center patient volume and mortality reduction.[4] Furthermore, it has been shown that outcomes are directly related to institutional commitment, and not just the individual surgeon's experience.[5] Prehospital hypotension has been questioned as an indicator of severity of injury or poor outcome.[6] It is the philosophy of most units, including ours, to have a trauma attending present or within an immediate response for those patients with the following physiologic findings: (i) a systolic blood pressure <90 mm Hg; (ii) a Glasgow Coma Score (GCS) <8, (iii) need for endotracheal intubations, and (iv) penetrating injuries to the neck and/or torso.[7] There is no data to support that in-house attending presence decreases mortality. However, patient disposition, coordination with other specialists, and perhaps increased reimbursement are associated with an in-house presence. Durham et al.,[8] recently examined outcomes of injured patients who met prehospital criteria for trauma team activation before and after instituting a system of in-house trauma surgeon attending presence. Preventable deaths, as defined by review of each death by a multidisciplinary panel, were reduced from 8% to 1% after provision of in-house attending coverage.

The Complexity of Emergency Room Coverage by Specialists

Tertiary hospitals must provide specialty coverage or risk a loss of substantial federal and state subsidies for their trauma centers. Furthermore, the lack of proper ER coverage can result in violation of the Emergency Medical Treatment and Labor Act (EMTALA). This has the potential to incur hefty fines or termination of agreements for Medicaid and Medicare reimbursement. The increase in the number of hospitals using hospitalists to relieve primary doctors of admissions, as well as alternative practice venues that have made outpatient surgeries common practice, has encouraged some surgical specialists to reduce or drop their clinical privileges including ER availability.

During the 2005 Spring Meeting of the American College of Surgeons in Washington, D.C., Dr. J. Wayne Meredith, Chairman of the Committee on Trauma, reported that the current yearly expenditure by hospitals to outsource ER call coverage is close to $1 billion annually. As a matter of fact, the difficulties with ER call coverage by specialists has been the number one complaint in a recent survey among physician executives.[9] This impact has been felt particularly in community-based trauma centers. Another significant contributing factor for the lack of a timely response to the

ER was a result of the 2003 decision by the Centers for Medicare and Medicaid Services to ease the 1985 EMTALA rules, permitting specialists to schedule elective surgeries while on-call provided the hospital is able to show that "their coverage was reasonable." Multiple efforts are under way to improve the ER coverage by specialists. However, most experts in the field believe that ER coverage by surgical specialists will remain a problem unless radical changes are made (see Table 1).

The American Medical Association states that physicians have a "moral responsibility" to provide emergency care to any patient regardless of their ability to pay. That principle is not currently followed, and it is not uncommon that physicians change their hospital privileges from "active" to "courtesy" to avoid ER coverage. An alternative to this dilemma is to secure locum tenens physicians. The *caveat* of this arrangement is the lack of continuity of care by the same physician, which is one of the fundamental goals of surgical care put forth by the American College of Surgeons since the time of its inception in 1912. The lack of consistent ER coverage is problematic for trauma centers for the specialties of neurosurgery, orthopaedic surgery, plastic surgery, and ophthalmology. Changes in the practice structure for these specialties have had the unintended consequence of

---

TABLE 1

POTENTIAL SOLUTIONS TO IMPROVE EMERGENCY ROOM (ER) COVERAGE BY SURGICAL SPECIALISTS

Outsource ER coverage to corporations or multispecialty groups

Pay ER availability stipend to specialists[a]

Collaboration at the local, state, and federal level to secure additional funding for uninsured or partly insured patients

Establish working networks within the jurisdiction of hospitals to minimize unnecessary transfers and prevent EMTALA violations

Increase awareness among community leaders of the crises of ER coverage to facilitate a designated tax increase dedicated for ER stipends coverage

Develop a fair distribution of the on-call schedule among the different specialists

Hospital recognition that the days of free ER coverage in order to maintain clinical privileges are over; most surgeons can be as productive in an office or alternative surgical centers as in a hospital

Negotiations of managed care contracts should include ER call coverage

Increase the number of nonsurgical or noncritical admissions to hospital-based practices (i.e., hospitalists)

Create additional sources of funding for trauma centers (i.e., red light violations, speeding tickets, and dedicated taxes)

---

[a]Stipends are unique to each hospital. Some of the criteria include type of specialty; need to be present while on-call; payer mix at the hospital; professional liability risks; and the number of physicians available in the specialty to take a call.

EMTALA, Emergency Medical Treatment and Labor Act.

worsening the problem of emergency specialist availability. Neurosurgical practice has moved away from intracranial surgery and neurocritical care toward spine surgery. Orthopaedic surgery is a highly compartmentalized specialty with narrow clinical focus for many specialists, which leads to a lack of confidence to manage acute musculoskeletal injuries. Plastic surgery and ophthalmology have moved increasingly to outpatient practice sites with many specialists practicing without active staff hospital privileges. Lack of proper specialist coverage causes delays in patient treatment and increases patient transfers between hospitals, with EMTALA violations. During the 2005 meeting of the Department of Health and Human Services, the EMTALA laws dominated the agenda. After extensive discussions, *no recommendations were issued at the meeting* other than the panel will try to meet at least twice a year.[10]

Clearly, the most common stated reason physicians drop ER coverage is because professional liability expenditures have risen. There is also a related increase of specialty consultation requests as defensive medicine practices increase. The scenario worsens as the number of ER patients continues to rise as the number of emergency department facilities diminishes. In 2004, the Centers for Disease Control and Prevention (CDC) reported that the number of emergency facilities decreased approximately 15% between 1992 and 2002. This is exacerbated by a recent report by the ACGME predicting that there would be a shortage of approximately 85,000 physicians by 2020. The end result, in trauma centers, is that trauma surgeons provide the overwhelming majority of day-to-day care for injured patients regardless of the fact that many of these patients have single system injuries that are within the scope of practice of a surgical specialist.

We have found that the best incentive to motivate orthopaedic and neurosurgical participation for patient care is to maintain the care of their patients under the trauma service. A strong case can be made that furnishing specialty care to an emergency patient leads to deferral or cancellation of elective surgery and office patients, which results in lost income. It is fitting that, in recognition of this lost revenue, a financial stipend for ER coverage is used as an effective means of increasing participation in the ER call schedule and responsiveness to trauma consultations. Instituting contractual agreements between the hospital and designated specialty groups is another alternative avenue that allows responsive care and, because the specialists practice together in focused groups, continuity of care is maintained. The complexity of ER coverage is such that on June 14, 2006, the Institute of Medicine (IOM) released three reports in Washington, D.C. where they addressed the future of emergency care in the United States Health System. The core of this study by the IOM addressed three key areas: 1) prehospital, 2) hospital based, and 3) adult and pediatric emergency and trauma care. They also provided an overview of the emergency care system in the United States.

THE MULTIDISCIPLINARY MANAGEMENT OF TRAUMA

Trauma patients present unique needs aside from the usual clinical care. These patients may require additional assistance due to social, financial, medical, and psychological needs. A multidisciplinary approach is fundamental to expedite acute clinical care, transfer to rehabilitation facilities, and to coordinate eventual discharge. Because an increased number of trauma patients carry inadequate or no insurance coverage, proper care beyond the acute care setting can be extremely challenging and compromised.[11] We will describe some of the alternatives currently used in different trauma centers to optimize acute clinical care and expedite patient disposition.

Members of the Team and Team Philosophy

Although multiple specialists are usually required to care for complex trauma patients, the basic principle of a "captain of the ship" remains as true now as when it was initially coined in the late 1970s. This term implies the clear need of a general surgeon with a strong trauma background as the responsible person to lead the team.

Since the early 1990s, trauma has been recognized as a discipline. Most new trauma surgeons complete formal preparation in an approved training center with the ultimate goal of obtaining a certification in Surgical Critical Care by the American Board of Surgery (ABS). Under a newly conceived early specialization program of the ABS, core training in general surgery may be reduced to 4 years. Specialization will consist of 2 additional years to achieve certification in both general surgery and surgical critical care. This concept is envisioned to further expand a potential concept for an "emergency care surgeon" that would incorporate trauma, surgical critical care, and emergency general surgery.[2,12] This work is in progress, with major changes anticipated in the way that trauma surgeons are trained and the boundaries of their specialty.

With the amended working hours and the use of physician extenders to provide first-line care for trauma patients, the concept of a team approach is better illustrated now than ever before. The need for continuous communication and well-organized "checkout" rounds between coming and going members of the team is crucial to avoid potential complications, missed injuries, and eventually missed patients altogether.

It has become evident in the last decade that with the multiple options available to care for some specific injuries (minimally invasive surgery, observation, selective angiography, and embolization, etc), it is paramount to have a strong leadership in trauma services at this point in time. It is apparent that with the accepted philosophic approach for nonoperative management, and the desire to "push the envelope" potentially exposing patients to unnecessary risks, a dedicated leadership by an experienced trauma surgeon is important.

Organizing the Initial Care of Trauma Patients

The initial care of trauma patients remains very straightforward in most trauma centers. The principles put forth by the Committee on Trauma of the American College of Surgeons on the Advanced Trauma Life Support (ATLS) protocols is what most trauma centers follow for initial resuscitation and management. The concept of hemorrhage control associated with an efficient and expeditious initial survey and resuscitation cannot be overemphasized.

As the quality and speed of the imaging technology has improved, most patients can be thoroughly evaluated in the first 15 minutes after arrival, as part of the initial "golden hour." Evolving concepts on evaluation and "clearing the spine"[13] also have expedited the initial evaluation of trauma patients. During bedside daily rounds in the intensive care unit (ICU), we routinely use a computer on wheels (COW) to review stored radiologic digital images, and to review our electronic database. While at the bedside, we check over our health informatics system for electronic results and clinical documentation. This avenue not only negates the need for a viewfinder but also provides real-time access to radiology images and information systems, expediting the patient's disposition.

In our unit, it is routine that a trauma attending completes a tertiary survey for those patients admitted longer than 24 hours. The survey is designed to perform a detailed physical examination of the trauma patient including review of all imaging studies to detect unrecognized injuries and expedite consultations if needed.

Role of Physician Extenders

Physician extenders do many of the same tasks as regular doctors, such as examining patients, taking medical histories, making diagnoses, and prescribing medications. They work in all areas of medicine. The scope of the physician extender's practice depends on state law, training and experience, and level of medical supervision (see Table 2). The need and importance of physician extenders has become more relevant since the new regulations for working hours for residents went into effect in 2003.

The presence of physician extenders in our unit has specifically provided us with the ability to provide continuity of care, and assists to expedite disposition of patients. Acting as a liaison between the trauma service, consultants, residents, and nursing staff, they ensure the necessary communication between these groups and the implementation of coordinated patient care. It is the attending trauma surgeon's responsibility to convey the continuity of care to families; however, physician extenders are in an excellent position to offer frequent bedside information and updates to families regarding their relative's condition.[14]

TABLE 2

PHYSICIAN EXTENDERS' SUPERVISED SKILLS IN A TRAUMA UNIT

1. Participation in morning and afternoon multidisciplinary rounds
2. Orientation of surgical residents and medical students to explain routines and protocols of the service
3. Assistance with resuscitation/evaluation of trauma alerts
4. Initiate airway control during emergencies
5. Placement of indwelling lines (arterial, venous, and pulmonary catheters)
6. Fluoroscopic transpyloric feeding tube placement
7. Assist with performance of bedside vena cava filters, and endoscopic placement of tracheostomies and gastrostomies
8. Guide pharmacologic management
   (a) Inotropes and vasodilators
   (b) Sedatives
   (c) Antibiotics
9. Weaning of patients from ventilators as per protocol
10. Initiate nutritional support
11. Thoracentesis and chest tube placement

Impact of Multidisciplinary Rounds

The increasing specialties, the lack of patient's resources, and the heavy workload of the different providers frequently compromise proper disposition of trauma patients. In a recent publication by the R. Adams Cowley Shock Trauma Center in Baltimore, Dutton et al. postulated that daily multidisciplinary rounds improve patient flow and increase readiness. Although there was no significant difference in mortality, potentially preventable deaths, and unexpected returns to the ICU, the authors were able to demonstrate that 1-hour multidisciplinary rounds daily resulted in a progressive decrease in the length of hospital stay by almost 2 days.[15]

The concept of multidisciplinary rounds is not new. Its relevance has been identified repeatedly due to the increasing multispecialty care of trauma patients. To maximize the benefit, experienced trauma surgeons must lead those rounds, since they have the expertise and knowledge of how to navigate the intricacies of trauma and coordinate multiple specialties.

In our unit, we conduct biweekly multidisciplinary rounds as well as daily checkout rounds as our standard of practice. This ability to concentrate multiple specialties clearly impacts our ability to formulate timely decisions and patient disposition (see Table 3). The most senior attending present leads these rounds, they are limited to 1 hour or less, and give the opportunity to participate to all those who attend. The goal of these rounds is early discharge planning, coordination of clinical care with other areas of expertise, and emphasis on patient prognosis.

TABLE 3
MEMBERS OF MULTIDISCIPLINARY ROUNDS

1. Trauma services
   (a) Senior trauma attending
   (b) Trauma attending
   (c) Trauma fellows
   (d) Residents
   (e) Physician assistants
   (f) Trauma program manager
   (g) Performance improvement nurse
   (h) Trauma research coordinator
   (i) Medical, physician assistant students
2. Rehabilitation
   (a) Physiatrist
   (b) Physical therapists
3. Nursing staff
   (a) ICU
   (b) Medical/surgical units
4. Pharmacists
5. Registered dietitian
6. Infection control nurse
7. Social and case worker(s)
8. Neuropsychologist/addiction specialist
9. Representative from hospital administration

ICU, intensive care unit.

TRAUMA AS A NONOPERATIVE SPECIALTY

A common reason given by surgical residents for not developing a life-term interest in trauma is because of the perception that trauma is a nonoperative specialty. According to Dr. C. William Schwab et al. from the University of Pennsylvania, dwindling surgical opportunities in trauma care have had a detrimental impact on career satisfaction among trauma surgeons and on career attractiveness to surgical trainees.[16] The significant decrease in the surgical management of injured patients is associated with considerable survival and organ preservation, as reflected by recently published data.[17] The nonoperative management of trauma patients with solid organ injuries, such as the liver and spleen and to some extent the pancreas, has changed dramatically in the last 2 decades because of our ability to image trauma patients in an efficient and expeditious manner. A better understanding of the role of ultrasonography and computed tomography scans in the initial evaluation of trauma patients has also been clarified. The use of handheld ultrasonographic devices that offer as good quality as conventional ultrasound devices has been demonstrated.[18] Also, in selected circumstances, there have been reports of conservative management of peripheral vascular injuries in patients without distal perfusion deficits.[19] This concept has also expanded to patients with blunt thoracic aortic injuries.[20]

Selective angiography and transcatheter embolization (SATE) has also become part of the armamentarium of trauma surgeons to expand the concept of nonoperative management of solid organ injuries.[21] Although its indications and limitations are still the subject of debate, there is no question that in selected patients (liver injuries, pelvic fractures, and to some extent splenic injuries) SATE is a well-accepted and effective alternative for hemorrhage control.

The impact of trauma as a nonoperative specialty is also reflected by the lack of experience in new graduates from general surgery programs. During the 1987 presidential address before the American Association for the Surgery of Trauma, Dr. Donald Trunkey commented on this issue. He reported that in a review of the 1980 surgical residents' applications to the ABS to take the qualifying examination, 18% had performed fewer than 10 surgeries for trauma and that 47% had performed fewer than 20. He further indicated that 75% of the provincial chairpersons of the Committee on Trauma of the American College of Surgeons believed that new surgeons were inadequately trained in trauma care.[22]

SPECIAL CONSIDERATIONS

Nutritional Support

Currently, the nutritional support of trauma patients should not be a subject of any controversy. It is well known and accepted that nutrition is part of the ongoing resuscitation process in trauma. The only discussion is whether to begin nutrition immediately after surgery, what is the best nutrient for a particular patient, and finally, what is the best test to determine the nutritional status of a patient. Clearly, these topics generate strong arguments from proponents of each theory and a definitive answer is beyond the objectives of this chapter. However, it is important to emphasize that the goal of nutritional support in patients sustaining severe trauma is to prevent malnutrition and its potential side effects such as sepsis, nonhealing wounds, multiple system organ dysfunction, and potentially death. Participation by a registered dietician with expertise in trauma is fundamental in the team approach of these patients. Immune-enhancing diets and hormone therapy remain highly debated nutritional topics at this point in time as well.

Substance Abuse and Chemical Dependence

The extent of substance abuse and chemical dependence impact in trauma patients cannot be overemphasized. Two reports from the Harborview Medical Center in Seattle, Washington, indicated that among 2,237 trauma patients, 47% tested positive for alcohol (mean level, 184 mg per dL). The highest alcohol level was documented among stab wound victims (mean level, 213 mg per dL). Furthermore, they identified that 45% of patients with positive alcohol tests were also positive for associated use of cocaine and marijuana.[23,24] Although there is no specific data across the country regarding the association of drugs, alcohol, and trauma, the Committee on Trauma of the American College of Surgeons suggests "as essential" routine alcohol and drug testing in Level I, II, and III trauma centers.

States such as Florida are preparing guidelines for the accreditation process of trauma centers, where an organized detection and treatment program needs to be in place to better screen and treat patients affected by alcohol and drugs. Besides the well-known complications of chronic alcohol abuse (pancreatitis, cirrhosis, malnutrition, etc.), there are recognized complications in trauma patients. The most common are associated with the actual critical care, relations to anesthesia and analgesia, withdrawal, and cardiovascular effects.

In critical care, it has been documented that alcohol modulates negatively the adrenergic response to blood loss and a shocklike presentation, even with minor injuries. Aside from the usual physiologic parameters in patients with acute alcoholic intoxication, measurement of serum lactate, arterial pH, and occasionally pulmonary artery pressures may be useful to properly resuscitate these patients. The clinician must be aware of other potential complications such as aspiration, baseline hypoxia, coagulopathies, hypothermia, abnormal drug metabolism, and immunosuppressive complications. Alcohol induces the inhibition of antidiuretic hormone (ADH); therefore, urinary output may not truly reflect normal perfusion or intravascular volume. Proper monitoring of serum electrolytes is crucial for an adequate resuscitation and also to minimize or prevent withdrawal syndromes.[25]

It is known that alcohol-intoxicated trauma patients require more anesthetic agents. Airway control can be a challenge, as well as proper sedation and analgesia in the postoperative period. There is no data to document the best manner to approach these patients; however, it is common practice to obtain early airway control in their care and continue its maintenance in the immediate postoperative period of patients undergoing emergency surgery.

Acute alcohol withdrawal significantly affects patient care. The clinical course varies from mild agitation, sleep deprivation, and irritability, to the full-blown syndrome of acute alcohol withdrawal *delirium tremens* (DTs). This is characterized by *delirium*, hallucinations, diaphoresis, and acute hyperdynamia. Seizure threshold decreases significantly and electrolyte abnormalities (specifically hypomagnesemia and hypocalcemia) are not uncommon.

Proper prophylaxis of alcohol withdrawal is controversial and deliberated among clinicians. What we know is that aggressive preventive measures are the most accepted course. The use of alcohol replacement (intravenously or orally) is strongly discouraged, although it is still common practice by many to provide alcohol replacement as a preventive and occasionally as a therapeutic measure.

Two other entities have also recently been recognized in patients testing positive for cocaine—malignant cardiac arrhythmias and the lethal effects of Taser guns. Within the last decade, there is an expressed concern that certain medical conditions, including drug use and heart disease, may increase the risk that Taser deployment may be lethal. It is felt that a device capable of depolarizing skeletal muscle could also depolarize heart muscle and cause fibrillation under certain circumstances. The use of Tasers may be generally safe in healthy adults; however, preexisting heart disease, psychosis, and the use of drugs including cocaine, phencyclidine (PCP), amphetamines, and alcohol may substantially increase the risk of fatality.[26]

Neuropsychological Support

The psychological impact of trauma is a phenomenon described mostly in military experiences. Trauma and the extent of its associated psychological side effects vary from individual to individual. In addition, a traumatic event can have immediate, short- and long-term consequences. It is not uncommon that patients subjected to severe trauma will not be able to express feelings and emotions being experienced.[27] This has been better documented in patients undergoing critical care with airway control and ventilatory support (see Table 4).

The psychological impact of trauma can also affect others close to the patient. These so-called secondary victims can also develop significant psychological needs as much as the victim. It is not unusual that a significant number of them will require some type of psychological support. In our unit, we have developed a support group for family members of critically ill trauma patients. Trauma can precipitate a crisis that upsets the equilibrium of the family system and immobilizes it. The event can cause a multitude of stressors

TABLE 4
CATEGORIES OF PSYCHOLOGICAL STRESS AFTER TRAUMA

1. Fear of strangers
2. Separation anxiety
3. Fear of rejection
4. Fear of control of basic functions (bladder, bowels, and privacy)
5. Fear and anger of loss of body parts
6. Reactivations of feelings of guilt and shame
7. Financial- and work-related concerns
8. Fear of disfigurement
9. Fear of findings by family and/or coworkers

Modified from Blumenfield M, Malt UF. Psychological issues. In: *The textbook of penetrating trauma.* Ivatury RR, Cayten CG, eds. Media: Williams & Wilkins; 1996:1113–1120.

such as separation, unfamiliar surroundings, and concern over progress and recovery. Our group participation offers the important support for information and relief of anxiety.

Interestingly, severe psychological disorders are rare in trauma care. However, evidence points to those patients who develop heightened psychological issues after traumatic injuries, maybe due to preexisting psychopathology. It is important to emphasize that in all cases of disruptive behavior, the key to a successful outcome is to continually orient the patients undergoing acute medical care.[27] The participation of a psychologist as part of the trauma team is crucial in expediting diagnosis and treatment of acute postinjury psychological reactions. In our biweekly multidisciplinary rounds, these specialists have become instrumental in optimizing the overall care of our patients.

Rehabilitation

The economic impact of carrying a trauma patient from injury to recovery is substantial. One third of the cost is spent toward the acute care hospitalization and the remaining two thirds toward the loss of wages and productivity of the disabled.[28] Rehabilitation of the trauma patient is significant. Additionally, it is an integral requirement to maintain Level I trauma center status. The institution must commit to prehospital and in-house care, as well as maximal recovery of the patients who survive. Spinal cord injury and traumatic brain injury result in the highest patient cost due to the extenuating long-term deficits.

The fundamentals of all rehabilitation units are guided by two standards of care. The first is to minimize complications in order to limit permanent damage. The second is to restore the remaining function to its full capacity. The object is not only to recapture physical mobility but also to embrace the patient in entirety. Restoration to personal autonomy encompasses not only the physical aspects of the injury but also the mental and social well-being of the individual. Unfortunately, because of rising costs of acute care and increasing involvement by third-party payers in the decision making to certify the need for specialized care, rehabilitation continues to be the forgotten offspring of the trauma system.

We focus on survival. However, we also need to place effort into achieving optimal functional outcomes and quality of life. Premorbid conditions, living environment, social issues, vocation, and previous substance abuse must be addressed; if not, the recovery will be compromised and less than ideal. Periodic progress assessment is usually necessary over a period of a year in order to shape an individualized approach for each patient. The need for financial and social support is common among these individuals and many require assistance to return to the workforce. The physician's role should be as the manager of the overall recovery plan. Once again, a team-oriented approach will bring the patient to his or her fullest potential.

FUTURE CHALLENGES OF TRAUMA CARE

There is no question that organizing trauma care has become a complicated and challenging part of the actual clinical care. Recent natural and man-induced disasters have not only exposed the strengths but also the significant weaknesses of our acute medical response in times of major emergencies. Trauma surgeons must redefine their overall role in patient care and resolve the paradigm of changes currently experienced by those practicing trauma. We have highlighted a new philosophy encompassing a constellation of issues confronting the trauma surgeon currently. Our colleagues ponder exactly what they are, as well as what they have become.

For those trying to gain or maintain trauma accreditation, it is strongly advised to reference the *Resources for Optimal Care of the Injured Patient* publication developed by the American College of Surgeons Committee on Trauma (ACS COT).[29] These guidelines are widely used to create optimal care for the trauma patient throughout the United States.

Level I trauma designation is granted by local and state government following a rigorous verification review. This evaluation involves the capabilities of the surrounding community and performance of the institution. Maintenance of trauma accreditation requires continued vigilance in trauma program performance, clinical qualifications, facility resources, performance improvement, rehabilitation services, and availability of specialists, research, community prevention, and outreach.

Current efforts by the Federal Trauma System's Development Act in conjunction with several other organizations including the American College of Surgeons, the Coalition for Trauma Care, and the American Trauma Society, and the Health Resources Service Administration (HRSA) will help better understand the needs and readiness of the different trauma systems across the United States.

It is clear that the organization of multispecialty management of trauma has become a complex and challenging endeavor. In depth, knowledge of finances, administration, and clinical care are paramount for a successful trauma program in the current health care environment.

ACKNOWLEDGMENT

The authors will like to thank Sally Bragg, RN, MSN, Trauma Research Nurse at Memorial Regional Hospital for her contributions and editorial assistance.

REFERENCES

1. Richardson JD, Miller FB. Will future surgeons be interested in trauma care? Results of a resident survey. *J Trauma.* 1992;32:229–235.

2. Shackford SR. The future of trauma surgery. A perspective. *J Trauma*. 2005;58:663–667.

3. Rodriguez A, Maull KI, Feliciano DV. Trauma care in the new millennium. *Surg Clin North Am*. 1999;79:1–16.

4. Nathens AB, Jurkovich GJ, Maier RV, et al. Relationship between trauma center volume and outcomes. *JAMA*. 2001;285:1164–1171.

5. Hoyt DB. What's new in general surgery: Trauma and critical care. *J Am Coll Surg*. 2002;194:335–351.

6. Franklin GA, Boaz PW, Spain DA, et al. Prehospital hypotension as a valid indicator of **trauma** team activation. *J Trauma*. 2000;48:1034–1039.

7. Tinkoff GH, O'Connor RE. Validation of new trauma triage rules for trauma attending response to the emergency department. *J Trauma*. 2001;49:1171–1175.

8. Durham R, Shapiro D, Flint L. In-house trauma attendings: Is there a difference? *Am J Surg*. 2005;190:960–966.

9. Glabman M. Specialist shortage shakes ERs; more hospitals forced to pay for specialist care. *Physician Exec*. 2005;31:6–11.

10. Silverman J. EMTALA panel ponders problems with on-call care. *Surg News*. 2005;1:1–3.

11. Selzer D, Gomez G, Jacobson L, et al. Public hospital-based Level I trauma centers: Financial survival in the new millennium. *J Trauma*. 2001;51:301–307.

12. Maier RV. Trauma: The paradigm for medical care in the 21st century. *J Trauma*. 2003;54:803–813.

13. Hauser CJ, Visvikis G, Hinrichs C, et al. Prospective validation of computed tomographic screening of the thoracolumbar spine in trauma. *J Trauma*. 2003;55:228–235.

14. Grabenkort WR. The use of physician assistants in the cardiothoracic intensive care unit. *Crit Connect*. 2007;4(1):7.

15. Dutton RP, Cooper C, Jones A, et al. Daily multidisciplinary rounds shorten length of stay for trauma patients. *J Trauma*. 2003;55:913–919.

16. Kimm PP, Dabrowski GP, Reilly PM, et al. Redefining the future of trauma surgery as a comprehensive trauma and general surgery service. *J Am Coll Surg*. 2004;199:96–101.

17. Richardson JD, Franklin GA, Lukan JK, et al. Evolution in the management of hepatic trauma: A 25-year perspective. *Ann Surg*. 2000;232:324–330.

18. Dumire RD, Doriac WC, Roth BJ, et al. Comparison of a hand portable ultrasound instrument to standard ultrasound for emergency department FAST exam. *J Trauma*. 2000;49:1174–1179.

19. Carrillo EH, Spain DA, Miller FB, et al. Femoral vessel injuries. *Surg Clin North Am*. 2002;82:49–65.

20. Kepros J, Angood P, Rabinovici R. Minor traumatic intimal flaps of the aorta: Natural history and nonoperative management. *J Trauma*. 2001;50:179–183.

21. Carrillo EH, Heniford BT, Senler SO, et al. Embolization therapy as an alternative to thoracotomy in vascular injuries of the chest wall. *Am Surg*. 1998;64:1142–1148.

22. Trunkey DD. Trauma care at mid-passage: A personal viewpoint. *J Trauma*. 1988;28:889–893.

23. Jurkovich GJ, Rivara FP, Gurney JG, et al. Effects of alcohol intoxication on the initial assessment of trauma patients. *Ann Emerg Med*. 1992;21:704–708.

24. Rivara FP, Mueller BA, Fligner CL, et al. Drug use in trauma victims. *J Trauma*. 1989;29:462–470.

25. Soderstrom CA, Smith TR. Alcohol. In: Ivatury RR, Cayten CG, eds. *The textbook of penetrating trauma*. Media: Williams & Wilkins; 1996:1033–1045.

26. Allen TB. Discussion of effects of the Taser in fatalities involving police confrontation. *J Forensic Sci*. 1992;37:956–958.

27. Blumenfield M, Malt UF. Psychological issues. In: Ivatury RR, Cayten CG, eds. *The textbook of penetrating trauma*. Media:Williams & Wilkins; 1996:1113–1120.

28. Morris, JA Jr, Limbird TJ, MacKenzie E. Rehabilitation of the trauma patient. In: Feliciano DV, Moore EE, Mattox KL, eds. *Trauma*, 3rd ed. Stamford: Appleton & Lange; 1996:1013–1022.

29. Committee on Trauma American College of Surgeons. *Resources for optimal care of the injured patient*. 1999. copyright 1998.

The Trauma Patient

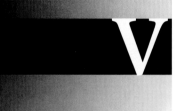

Prehospital Care

23

Alasdair K.T. Conn   Paul D. Biddinger

Since the publication of the landmark report titled, *Accidental Death and Disability: The Neglected Disease of Modern Society*—a report which detailed serious deficiencies in prehospital care—the prehospital management and development of established trauma systems have evolved to be recognized as one of the key links in the survival of the severely traumatized patient. This chapter will outline the levels of prehospital care and the capabilities of the prehospital provider to initiate care of the severely traumatized patient. All participants within an established trauma system should have knowledge of the capabilities and limitations of prehospital providers, so that recommendations for system change and individual quality improvement efforts can be appropriately targeted and monitored.

PREHOSPITAL PROVIDER LEVELS

Prehospital providers at all levels are certified or licensed at the individual state level. Although many states differ in exact requirements, most states have adopted the recommendations from the federal Department of Transportation (DOT) and specifically, the curricula developed by the National Highway Traffic Safety Administration (NHTSA). This federal agency, together with the Health Resources and Services Administration (HRSA), are the two agencies involved in monitoring and developing emergency medical service (EMS) systems. Prehospital providers may be classified as first responders, Emergency Medical Technician-Basic (EMT-B), Emergency Medical Technician-Intermediate (EMT-I), and Emergency Medical Technician-Paramedic (EMT-P). See Table 1 for a list of their capabilities. The exact capabilities may differ slightly from state to state, particularly at the paramedic level in terms of the medications that they are allowed to administer; some states may require that certain medications be given and procedures be performed on standing protocol and others may demand that paramedics speak with

a physician by radio (online medical direction) before they institute a specific therapy on a particular patient. The development of the standardized protocols and procedures is defined as *offline medical direction* and trauma surgeons should have input to the protocols for the trauma patient. Many states have adopted statewide trauma treatment and trauma protocols; these can often be upgraded at the regional or local level, but only with the appropriate state oversight and local quality assurance monitoring. In most states, emergency medical technicians (EMTs) and paramedics are required to obtain a certain number of continuing education credits and often to recertify by a practical and a written examination in order to maintain their certification.

The different levels of prehospital providers may be municipal employees, employees of an ambulance service providing EMS services to a local jurisdiction under contract, or volunteers or paid personnel from a local fire company or fire service jurisdiction. In all states, paramedics are required to have a medical director who is the physician legally responsible for the paramedics' practice. Complaints or concerns regarding an individual paramedic's performance should initially be directed to both the individual and the medical director level. All states will have a formal mechanism for investigating inappropriate and unprofessional conduct of prehospital providers at all levels.

ALTERNATIVE PREHOSPITAL CONFIGURATIONS

In many states, helicopter transport is available; some states have adopted licensing procedures to recognize the capability of providers, which are often above the EMT-paramedic level. Some programs fly with physicians and are, therefore, subject to the appropriate state licensing board—these physicians being capable of independent

TABLE 1
PREHOSPITAL RESPONDERS

Level of Provider	Skills	Comments
First responder	Bandaging, splinting, CPR, hemorrhage control. Approximately 40 hr of training	Examples: firefighters and police; they do not transport patients
Emergency Medical Technician-Basic (EMT-B)	Assess signs and symptoms; can give oxygen, immobilization skills, and triage; can often use automatic defibrillators (AEDs). Approximately 120–160 hr of training	Usually certified on a state level; in many states it is the minimal requirement to staff an ambulance; ambulances staffed by EMT-Bs are "BLS"
Emergency Medical Technician-Intermediate (EMT-I)	Trained in IV access, often in LMAs and other airway devices	Certified by state; do not usually give medications
Emergency Medical Technician-Paramedic (EMT-Paramedic)	Advanced airway management, endotracheal intubation, and ACLS protocols; can give medications; approximately. 500–2,000 hr of training	Certified by state; must have responsible medical director (MD); ambulances staffed by EMT-Ps are "ALS"
Flight nurse; flight paramedic, critical care transport nurse; critical care transport medic	Above paramedic; variable training/certification and skills	Highest level of nonMD found in prehospital phase; several states moving to Commission on Accreditation of Medical Transport Systems (CAMTS) as a state requirement

CPR, cardiopulmonary resuscitation; BLS, basic life support; LMA, laryngeal mask airway; ACLS, advanced cardiac life support.

practice. More than 90% of the US flight programs have flight nurses in their configuration; and these may operate using state-mandated protocols or protocols developed by the individual hospital or trauma center that is providing the helicopter service. Although certain components of the basic EMT, EMT-I, and paramedic course are specifically directed toward the initial care of the trauma patient, additional resources such as the Prehospital Trauma Life Support (PHTLS) course developed by the American College of Surgeons (ACS) are available in all states and provide additional information and training regarding the management of the trauma patient.

PREHOSPITAL CARE

Triage

Of all of the prehospital decisions and interventions that are to be provided to the multiply injured patient by the EMS provider, the most critical and most under-recognized is the initial recognition and triage of the trauma patient. States that have trauma systems have developed a specific definition of "the trauma patient" and direct the particular facility that such a trauma patient should be transferred. Transfer may be direct (by bypassing local facilities or using a helicopter to transfer directly from the scene) or by secondary triage—transferring patients to a local facility for initial resuscitation with subsequent transfer to the trauma center for definitive management and critical care. There are trauma triage guidelines that have been developed by the ACS, the American College of Emergency Physicians (ACEP),

and the National Association of Emergency Medical Service Physicians (NAEMSP); and most states have adopted these criteria (or a minor modification thereof) in developing their statewide trauma triage protocols. Such protocols usually involve physiologic criteria (hypotension, respiratory distress); anatomic criteria (amputations); mechanism of injury criteria (roll over, ejection from vehicle); as well as separate pediatric trauma triage criteria. These have recently been updated based upon a meeting sponsored by the CDC in 2005. Guidelines for helicopter activation to the scene have also been developed by the NAEMSP and are often adopted at the state, regional, or local level.

As standards are developed for the appropriate identification and prehospital management of the trauma patient within a developed trauma system, the prehospital provider is under an obligation to triage and treat these patients according to these standards. Prehospital providers and their respective agencies have been found liable for failure to identify a prehospital patient as a severe trauma patient, and if that patient is then transferred to a local jurisdiction and subsequently has an adverse outcome, the prehospital providers can be sued for failing to provide the standard of care.

Airway Management

An essential component of trauma prehospital management is the establishment of an appropriate airway and the administration of oxygen. First responders are trained to perform a jaw thrust and chin lift; in most states, oxygen can be administered at the first responder level. At the basic

EMT level, they are taught to use the nasopharyngeal airway (NPA) and the oral-pharyngeal airway (OPA), which are minimally invasive devices designed to keep the tongue off the base of the pharynx and maintain a patent airway. Semialert patients with an intact gag reflex can usually tolerate the NPA; most patients with an intact gag reflex will not tolerate an OPA. All patients who are apneic or hypoventilating should have respirations assisted with a bag-valve-mask (BVM) device until a more definitive airway can be obtained. BVM-assisted ventilation carries a risk of gastric insufflation with subsequent vomiting and aspiration. Overzealous hyperventilation may also produce prehospital hypocapnia.

Other Airway Adjuncts

Multiple adjunct devices to assist with airway management are available and can be used at either the basic, intermediate, or advanced level, depending on local protocols. These include the esophageal obturator airway (EOA); the pharyngeotracheal lumen airway (PTLA); the Combitube, and the laryngeal mask airway (LMA). The EOA has now fallen into disfavor because of the numerous reports of inadvertent esophageal intubation with esophageal rupture. The PTLA and Combitube are devices that are designed for blind insertion. The operator is expected to correctly identify which of the blindly inserted tubes is in the esophagus and which can be used to ventilate the trachea. The LMA can be blindly placed into the larynx and is relatively easy to use. It does have a decreased risk of gastric insufflation but does not protect the trachea from aspiration of blood or vomitus.

Endotracheal Intubation

Endotracheal intubation remains the gold standard of airway management and may or may not require the use of prehospital paralytic agents. Wherever it is practiced, prehospital endotracheal intubation must be performed under tight medical control; this is highlighted by the recent study from San Diego showing that prehospital endotracheal intubation performed by paramedics, as compared with BVM management of the prehospital airway, resulted in a higher mortality for seemingly matched prehospital trauma populations. A similar study in a pediatric population has again shown that endotracheal intubation of pediatric patients is associated with a higher mortality. Both these studies have served as a wake-up call to tighter medical control and oversight of these advanced airway techniques. Several studies have shown prehospital intubation rates of 96% to 98% success, compatible with in-hospital figures.

Nasotracheal intubation may be attempted for some patients who have spontaneous respiratory effort but still need definitive airway control. Success ranges from 48% to 84% in the prehospital setting. Confirmation of correct endotracheal tube (ETT) placement is mandatory, although the most specific method of confirming correct tube placement is documentation of exhaled CO_2. Other signs such as clinically symmetrical breath sounds, condensation within the ETT, or online measurement with a capnometer can be employed.

Advanced Rescue Airway Techniques

Cricothyrotomy is a mandated skill in the national paramedic curriculum; at this time, approximately 70% of the US ground paramedics and all aeromedical paramedics are allowed to perform this type of emergency surgical airway. The incidence for field cricothyrotomy is extremely low, although reported success rates in the field are from 82% to 100%. Additional airway procedures such as bougie-assisted or retrograde emergency tracheal intubation or the use of the lightwand are restricted to only a small number of prehospital services. Following establishment of the airway many programs rely on a manual oxygenation, although many helicopter units and an increasing number of ground advanced life support (ALS) units now carry mechanical ventilators.

Other Medical Field Care

Needle decompression of the chest for relief of a tension or a pneumothorax is a component of a national paramedic curriculum and is permitted in many states. In a typical protocol, a rescuer places a 14- or 16-gauge needle just above the second rib in the midclavicular line on the suspected side. As always, there should be radio communication to the receiving facility following needle decompression.

Prehospital Fluids

Intravenous (IV) access is performed at the paramedic and EMT-Intermediate level and a typical protocol would require the establishment of two large bore IVs in the severely traumatized patient and involve the administration of saline or Ringers lactate wide open if the blood pressure is below 90 systolic. The establishment of these IVs, often under less than ideal circumstances, can take 8 to 12 minutes and prehospital providers should weigh the delay in establishing these IVs with the potential benefit from the treatment of hypotension. The fluid volume is a matter of controversy following a publication in the *New England Journal of Medicine* from a Houston group demonstrating that aggressive prehospital fluid administration of hypotensive victims of penetrating trauma did not improve survival and increased blood loss when compared with delayed resuscitation when the patient arrived at the trauma center. The results of their study and its applicability to other settings are still vigorously debated.

Type of Fluid

In the United States, Ringers lactate and isotonic saline are the fluids of choice; a multicenter trial using prehospital administration of a blood substitute is under way. Hypertonic saline has been used in the prehospital arena in Europe for many years and has been advocated for more widespread use in the United States in the prehospital setting, particularly in patients with severe head injuries. Most EMS systems, however, have not adopted routine use of prehospital hypertonic saline at the time of writing.

Immobilization

All trauma patients should be appropriately immobilized in the prehospital environment. All patients with blunt injury should be brought in with a cervical collar and on a long backboard. For the best spinal immobilization, it has been shown that a well-trained EMT, a backboard, and cervical collar provide the most rigid immobilization of the injured spine. The scoop stretcher has been shown to be the most effective way of transferring the patient with a spinal injury, thereby minimizing spinal movement. Surgeons should be aware of an additional device called the Kendrick extrication device (KED), which is a vest-like device made up of a series of parallel splints longitudinally bound together, mostly seen on trauma patients. This device does not provide full spinal immobilization but is often used in pediatric patients who cannot or will not lie still on a stand-up backboard. The pneumatic antishock garment (PASG), formerly known as the military antishock trousers (MAST), was included in the mandatory equipment for ambulances until two outcome studies of the 1990s called its use into question. Many states have removed this from the mandatory requirements for essential ambulance equipment; the benefits to patient outcome are marginal, at best, not well-documented in clinical trials; and are probably only restricted to the benefits of splinting of a lower extremity fracture and possibly stabilization of an unstable pelvic fracture.

Splints

Various types of traction splints are utilized by the prehospital providers; by protocol, usually EMTs and above can straighten out a fractured limb but not a dislocated joint. If they do perform this realignment, documentation of distal, vascular, and neurologic function must be obtained before and after intervention and documented on the ambulance run report.

Wound Care

Prehospital providers are trained to provide hemorrhage control by direct pressure on the wound. Penetrating objects such as knives are often, by protocol, bandaged in place and should not be removed by prehospital providers.

Special Considerations

Separate triage criteria have been developed for pediatric trauma and for major burn injuries. Some states have developed destination protocols for spinal cord injury with paralysis and penetrating eye injuries to designated centers. Hand injuries with amputations are also triaged in several states to designated facilities; management of the finger of the digits or limbs are as per the ACS Committee on Trauma guidelines, which are adopted by many states. Surgeons should work with emergency medicine colleagues, prehospital medical directors, and outside agencies to optimize the prehospital care of the trauma patient. Protocols may also be developed for the very severely injured to bypass the emergency department and go "directly to the operating room (OR)." This is possible only in established, mature trauma systems; however, where it has been adopted, it is often associated with individual dramatic successes. Trauma surgeons should be reminded to be active participants in the clinical research, education, protocol development, and quality assurance of EMS providers at all levels; this is an essential component of trauma care for the severely injured patient.

SUGGESTED READINGS

EMS Systems

Ali J, Adam RU, Gana TJ, et al. Effect of the prehospital trauma life support program (PHTLS) on prehospital trauma care. *J Trauma.* 1997;42:786–790.

Eckstein M, Chan L, Schneir A, et al. Effect of prehospital advanced life support on outcomes of major trauma patients. *J Trauma.* 2000;48(4):643–648.

Liberman M, Mulder D, Sampalis J. Advanced or basic life support for trauma: Meta—analysis and critical review of the literature. *J Trauma.* 2000;49:584–599.

Marson AC, Thomson JC. The influence of prehospital trauma care on motor vehicle crash mortality. *J Trauma.* 2001;50:917–920, discussion 920–921.

Airway Management

Gerich TG, Schmidt U, Hubrich V, et al. Prehospital airway management in the acutely injured patient: The role of surgical cricothyrotomy revisited. *J Trauma.* 1998;45:312–314.

Orf J, Thomas SH, Ahmed W, et al. Appropriateness of endotracheal tube size and insertion depth in children undergoing air medical transport. *Pediatr Emerg Care.* 2000;16:321–327.

Thomas SH, Harrison T, Wedel SK. Flight crew airway management in four settings: A six-year review. *Prehosp Emerg Care.* 1999;3:310–315.

Wayne MA, Friedland E. Prehospital Use of Succinylcholine—a 20-year review. *Prehosp Emerg Care.* 1999;3(2):107–109.

Fluid Resuscitation

Novak L, Shackford SR, Bourguignon P. Comparison of standard and alternative prehospital resuscitation in uncontrolled hemorrhagic shock and head injury. *J Trauma.* 1999;47:834–844.

Spinal Immobilization

Cone DC, Wydro GC, Mininger CM. Current practice in clinical cervical spinal clearance: Implication for EMS. *Prehosp Emerg Care.* 1999;3:42–46.

Domeier RM. Indications for prehospital spinal immobilization. National Association of EMS Physicians Standards and Clinical Practice Committee. *Prehosp Emerg Care.* 1999;3:251–253.

Analgesia

DeVellis P, Thomas SH, Wedel SK. Prehospital fentanyl analgesia in air-transported pediatric trauma patients. *Pediatr Emerg Care.* 1998;14:321–323.

DeVellis P, Thomas SH, Wedel SK. Prehospital and E.D. analgesia for air-transported patients with fractures. *Prehosp Emerg Care.* 1998;2:293–296.

Air Transport

Thomas SH, Cheema F, Wedel SK et al. Trauma helicopter emergency medical services transport: annotated review of selected outcomes-related literature. *Prehosp Emerg Care* 2002;6(3):359–371.

Thomas SH. Helicopter EMS transport outcomes literature: annotated review of articles published 2004–06. *Prehosp Emerg Care* 2007; 11(4):477–488.

Thomas SH, Harrison TH, Buras WR, et al. Helicopter transport and blunt trauma outcome. *J Trauma.* 2002;52:136–145.

Thomas SH, Harrison T, Wedel SK, et al. Helicopter EMS roles in disaster operations. *Prehosp Emerg Care.* 2000;4:338–344.

Pediatric Care

Dieckmann RA, Athey J, Bailey B. A pediatric survey for the National Highway Traffic Safety Administration: Emergency medical services system re-assessments. *Prehosp Emerg Care.* 2001;5: 231–236.

Engum SA, Mitchell MK, Scherer LR. Prehospital triage in the injured pediatric patient. *J Pediatr Surg.* 2000;35:82–87.

Paul TR, Marias M, Pons PT, et al. Adult versus pediatric prehospital trauma care: Is there a difference? *J Trauma.* 1999;47: 455.

Triage

Bond RJ, Kortbeek JB, Preshaw RM. Field trauma triage: Combining mechanism of injury with the prehospital index for an improved trauma triage tool. *J Trauma.* 1997;43:283–287.

Field triage 2005: a meeting of experts. *Prehosp Emerg Care* 2006;10(3): 281–355.

Initial Resuscitation and Diagnosis

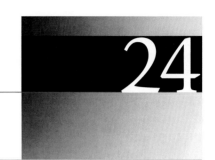

Andrew Rosenthal   *Grace S. Rozycki*

During the initial hospital phase, the injured patient is rapidly assessed and the treatments are prioritized based on the mechanism of injury and the patient's vital signs. The goal of the resuscitation is to improve organ and tissue perfusion by rapidly identifying and simultaneously treating life-threatening conditions. In most cases, the initial resuscitation of the patient is conducted in the trauma resuscitation area (the design of which is covered in Chapter 12 of this book), but there are select patients who should bypass the trauma resuscitation area and be taken directly to the operating room for lifesaving interventions (see Table 1). In either case, advance planning is needed so that all of the essential equipment and materials are immediately available to execute the American College of Surgeons' Advanced Trauma Life Support (ATLS) primary and secondary surveys.[1] Standard universal precautions (e.g., face mask, eye protection, water-impervious gown, leggings, and gloves) should be used even when evaluating patients who have seemingly minor injuries.[1] Additionally, because life-threatening procedures may need to be performed during the initial resuscitation, prepackaged trays with sterile contents such as airway, tube thoracostomy, open chest, and minor and major suture trays should be well stocked and immediately available. The trays should be easily accessible, consistently in the same place, and color-coded so that they can be identified and accessed instantly.

Medications frequently used in the trauma resuscitation area are listed in Table 2. Although the principles of resuscitation are based on the primary and secondary surveys, the resuscitating physician should keep in mind that treatment priorities are established on the basis of the patient's mechanism of injury, obvious injuries (on presentation or diagnosis soon thereafter), clinical examination, and vital signs. Furthermore, the resuscitating physician and trauma team members identify and treat life-threatening conditions simultaneously, but continually assess and reassess the patient's status.

PRIMARY SURVEY

A rapid assessment following the *A B C D Es* of trauma care provides a systematic method for simultaneously identifying and treating life-threatening conditions.

Airway (with cervical spine immobilization and protection)

Ensuring adequate oxygenation, ventilation, and protection from aspiration are the cornerstones of airway management and the first priority when treating trauma patients. All patients should receive supplemental oxygen by a secured

TABLE 1
INDICATIONS FOR DIRECT TRANSPORT TO THE OPERATING ROOM

- Systolic blood pressure ≤80 mm Hg
- Penetrating torso trauma
- Major limb amputation or mangled extremity
- Extensive soft tissue wounds
- Severe maxillofacial injury

Rhodes M, Brader A, Lucke J, et al. Direct transport to the operating room for resuscitation of trauma patients. *J Trauma*. 1989;29:907–915.[2]

TABLE 2

MEDICATIONS FOR THE TRAUMA RESUSCITATION AREA

Antitetanus

Tetanus may occur after minor wounds[a]

- 0.5 mL intramuscular tetanus toxoid vaccine for those immunized >10 years ago
- 250 U intramuscular tetanus immunoglobulin for the never-immunized and for grossly dirty wounds

Antibiotics

Generally a first-generation cephalosporin (e.g., 1 g cefazolin) intravenously, or clindamycin 600–900 mg IV for penicillin-allergic patients, for the following:

- Open fractures and joints
- Grossly contaminated wounds, major soft tissue injury
- Immunocompromised patients
- Patients with prosthetic cardiac valves

Analgesics (dose and frequency vary depending on patient status)

- Morphine 0.1 mg/kg intravenously
- Fentanyl 1 μg/kg intravenously
- Demerol 0.25–0.50 mg/kg intravenously

Anxiolytics (dose and frequency vary with patient status)

- Midazolam 2–4 mg intravenously
- Haloperidol 5–20 mg intravenously

---

[a]American College of Surgeons Committee on Trauma. *Advanced trauma life support program for doctors*, 7th ed. Chicago: American College of Surgeons Committee on Trauma; 2004; Rhee P, Nunley MK, Demetriades D, et al. Tetanus and trauma: A review and recommendations. *J Trauma.* 2005;58:1082–1088.[3,4]

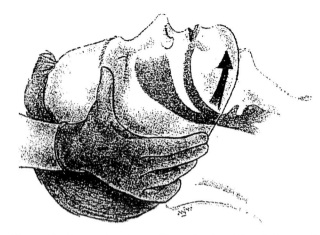

Figure 1 Trauma jaw thrust. (From Sanders MJ, ed. *Paramedic textbook*, 2nd ed, chapter 11, figure 1, St. Louis: Mosby; 2000: 397.)[5]

The absolute indications for immediate emergency intubation are the following:

1. Airway obstruction unrelieved with basic interventions (e.g., chin-lift and jaw-thrust maneuvers)
2. Apnea or near apnea
3. Respiratory distress
4. Severe neurologic deficits, such as a Glasgow Coma Score <9, or high (C1,C2) spinal cord injury

Urgent indications for intubation are the following:

1. Penetrating neck injury
2. Persistent or refractory hypotension
3. Chest wall injury or major pulmonary dysfunction such as flail chest with pulmonary contusion

oxygen reservoir face mask with a high flow rate. A pulse oximeter is applied to the patient's digit or ear lobe as a noninvasive method to measure oxygen saturation. If the patient is able to speak easily, then the airway is patent. A patient with facial fractures or tracheal/laryngeal injuries may have a patent airway but may have difficulty with secretions and therefore, may require a definitive airway in the form of a cuffed orotracheal or nasotracheal tube or by way of a surgical airway. In the unconscious patient, the tongue may fall backwards and obstruct the airway. While maintaining cervical spine immobilization, the chin-lift and jaw-thrust maneuvers (see Figs. 1 and 2) may be employed to relieve this obstruction. When performing the chin-lift maneuver in a trauma patient, the head is not tilted and the cervical spine is maintained in a neutral position. If the patient is not responsive, an oropharyngeal airway should be inserted to assist in bag-valve mask ventilation. The nasopharyngeal airway is reserved for the more awake patient with an intact gag reflex, but is not used as a definitive airway. Although other devices, such as the multilumen esophageal airway device or the laryngeal mask airway (LMA), may be used for temporary ventilation and oxygenation, they are not considered definitive airways because they do not provide secure long-term airway stabilization.

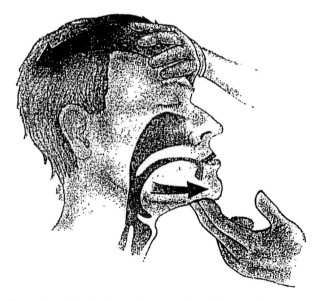

Figure 2 Chin lift. (From Sanders MJ, ed. *Paramedic textbook*, 2nd ed, chapter 11, figure 2, St. Louis: Mosby; 2000:397.)[6]

TABLE 3
DIFFICULT AIRWAY CART

Suction catheter
Endotracheal introducer and tube changer
Pediatric and adult laryngeal mask airway (sizes 1, 1.5, 2.0, 2.5, 3, 4, and 5)
Lighted laryngoscopes (Miller sizes 0, 1, 2, 3, and 4 and MacIntosh sizes 1, 2, 3, and 4)
Pediatric and adult endotracheal tubes (sizes 4.0 mm, 5.0 mm, 6.0 mm, 6.5 mm, 7.0 mm, 7.5 mm, and 8.0 mm)
Assorted Shiley tracheostomy tubes (sizes no. 4 and no. 6)
Oral airway
Nasopharyngeal airway
McGill forceps
14-gauge angiocatheter
10-mL syringe for cuff inflation
End-tidal CO_2 detector
Surgical airway tray (Table 5)

American College of Surgeons Committee on Trauma. *Advanced trauma life support program for doctors*, 7th ed, chapter 2, Airway and ventilatory management. Chicago: American College of Surgeons Committee on Trauma; 2004:53–68.[7]

4. Impending upper airway obstruction such as severe oral maxillofacial injury or laryngeal edema

In addition to standard intubation equipment, each trauma resuscitation area should have additional instruments that are used for "the difficult airway." The contents of a "difficult airway cart" are listed in Table 3. Rapid-sequence intubation is the accepted standard process for endotracheal intubation in a multitrauma patient who is assumed to have head injury, cervical spine injury, and a full stomach. The guidelines for rapid-sequence intubation are listed in Table 4. A surgical airway, that is, a cricothyroidotomy, is performed when there is an edematous glottis, severe oropharyngeal hemorrhage, or simply an inability to obtain an orotracheal airway expeditiously. A cricothyroidotomy is performed by making a small transverse incision through the cricothyroid membrane. Either the handle of the scalpel or a hemostat may be used to dilate the opening so that a small tracheostomy or endotracheal tube can be inserted (see Fig. 3). After the performance of a definitive airway, a CO_2 detector is used to ensure that the airway tube is within the tracheal lumen. Bilateral chest rise and breath sounds should be present. Additionally, the position of the tube is confirmed by a chest x-ray. Table 5 lists the equipment helpful in obtaining a surgical airway.

> **KEY POINTS**
> Although there are multiple guidelines for the indications of a definitive airway in the injured patient, the physician's clinical judgment remains the most important.

TABLE 4
RAPID SEQUENCE INTUBATION PROCEDURE

Preoxygenation with 100% oxygen
Cricoid cartilage pressure (Sellick maneuver) to compress the esophagus
Sedation (midazolam 3–5 mg or etomidate 0.3 mg/kg intravenously)
Succinylcholine (1–2 mg/kg, usually 100 mg dose intravenously)
Orotracheal intubation with inline stabilization of the cervical spine
Cuff inflation
Tube placement confirmation (ausculate, visualize chest rise, and confirm CO_2 return from exhaled air)
Release cricoid pressure
Ventilate and oxygenate the patient

American College of Surgeons Committee on Trauma. *Advanced trauma life support program for doctors*, 7th ed, chapter 2, Airway and ventilatory management. Chicago: American College of Surgeons Committee on Trauma; 2004:47–50.[8]

Breathing

Following the confirmation of a patent and functioning airway, adequate gas exchange involves oxygenation and ventilation. The lungs, chest wall, and diaphragm must be assessed as any respiratory organ injury limits gas exchange and overall tissue perfusion. Specifically, tension pneumothorax, open pneumothorax, flail chest with pulmonary contusion, and massive hemothorax should be identified and treated so that normal breathing can occur and gas exchange can be effective.

1. A *tension pneumothorax* is a clinical diagnosis. It develops when a one-way valve parenchymal air leak occurs, forcing air into the pleural space and completely collapsing the lung. Consequently, this increased intrathoracic pressure causes a decrease in venous return, marked hypotension, and cardiovascular collapse. The

TABLE 5
SURGICAL AIRWAY TRAY

Scalpels (no. 11 blade)
Hemostats
Tracheostomy hook
Respiratory suction catheter
Tracheostomy tube (Shiley no. 4 or no. 6)
Endotracheal tube 6.0 mm
Suture (Nylon 2-0)
Needle driver
Scissors
Tracheostomy-ventilator adaptor
10-mL syringe for cuff inflation
End-tidal CO_2 detector

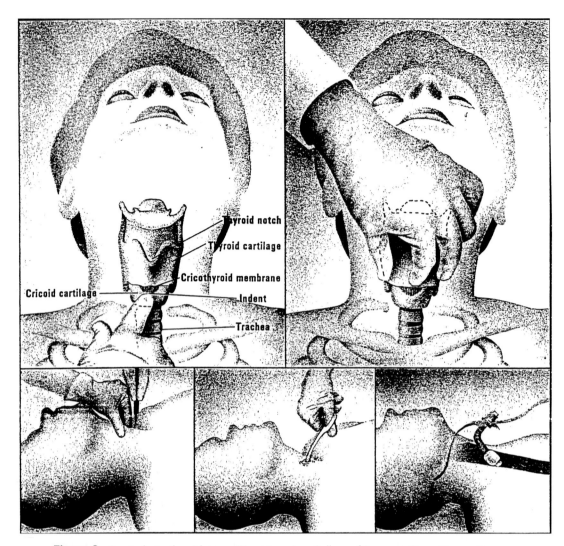

Figure 3 Surgical cricothyroidotomy. (From American College of Surgeons Committee on Trauma. *Advanced trauma life support program for doctors*, 7th ed, chapter 2, Chicago: American College of Surgeons Committee on Trauma; 2004:67.)[9]

signs and symptoms of a tension pneumothorax include severe "air hunger" (in the alert patient), respiratory distress, tachycardia, hypotension, tracheal deviation to the contralateral side, unilateral absence of breath sounds, percussion hyperresonance of the affected side, and neck vein distension. The treatment is immediate decompression with a large bore (14, 16, or 18 gauge) needle into the ipsilateral second intercostal space at the midclavicular line. This is followed by the insertion of a chest tube.

> **KEY POINTS**
> A simple pneumothorax may be converted to a tension pneumothorax if the patient is receiving positive pressure ventilation. Hence, *Airway* and *Breathing* should be assessed and reassessed during the initial resuscitation even if the patient is hemodynamically normal.

2. An *open pneumothorax* or "sucking chest wound" is the result of a large defect in the chest wall. Intrathoracic pressure and atmospheric pressure equilibrate. If the chest wall defect is approximately two thirds the diameter of the trachea, air will pass through the defect directly into the pleural space with inspiration (following the path of least resistance), limiting lung expansion and resulting in impaired ventilation and hypoxemia. A sterile occlusive dressing (e.g., petrolatum gauze) with one side open/untaped is placed over the defect and a chest tube is placed at a different site in the ipsilateral hemithorax. Surgical debridement and closure of the chest wall defect are commonly necessary.

TABLE 6
RESPONSE TO INITIAL FLUID RESUSCITATION

	Rapid Response	Transient Response	No Response
Vital signs	Return to normal	Transient improvement, recurrence of ↓ BP and ↑ HR	Remain abnormal
Estimated blood loss	Minimal (10%–20%)	Moderate and ongoing (20%–40%)	Severe (>40%)
Need for more crystalloid	Low	High	High
Need for blood	Low	Moderate to high	Immediate

BP, blood pressure; HR, heart rate.
American College of Surgeons Committee on Trauma. *Advanced trauma life support program for doctors*, 7th ed, chapter 3, Shock. Chicago: American College of Surgeons Committee on Trauma; 2004:79.[10]

3. A *flail chest* consists of two or more fractured ribs in two or more sites. The flail segment does not have bony continuity with the thoracic wall, and therefore, paradoxical chest wall movement occurs during respiration. The underlying segment of lung is invariably contused, thereby affecting both oxygenation and ventilation. Multiple signs and symptoms lead to the diagnosis including clinical examination, presence of paradoxical breathing, chest x-ray findings of multiple contiguous rib fractures in two places, and hypoxemia and hypercapnea on blood gas analysis. Treatment consists of supportive measures, that is, ensuring adequate oxygenation and ventilation accompanied by judicious fluid resuscitation. A tube thoracostomy may also be indicated if a pneumothorax or large hemothorax is found on imaging examinations.

4. A *massive hemothorax* results from the rapid accumulation of approximately one third of the patient's blood volume (∼1,500 mL) in the hemithorax. The patient is usually hypotensive and has diminished or absent breath sounds on the affected hemithorax. The treatment is decompression and drainage (by insertion of a 36 or 40 French chest tube) of the hemothorax with simultaneous restoration of the patient's blood volume. Both transfusion of autologous blood and autotransfusion of the patient's collected blood are indicated. If the patient's initial blood loss is 1,500 mL of blood, a thoracotomy is indicated, but 1.5 L is by no means an absolute rule. The indication for a thoracotomy is based on the clinician's judgment. Other strong indicators for a thoracotomy are continued blood loss of 200 mL per hour for 2 to 4 hours, persistent hypotension, massive air leak, or severe refractory acidosis despite ongoing resuscitation.

Circulation

"Stop the bleeding!" is the most essential part of assessing circulation, followed by the restoration of blood volume and the prevention or reversal of shock. The goal is to restore oxygen-carrying capacity to ensure end-organ perfusion. A rapid thready pulse, decreased level of consciousness, and cool pale skin may be observed when there is inadequate organ perfusion. Vital signs may be telling, and should be monitored with attention to their response to the initial fluid administration (see Table 6). Urine output, the most reliable marker of perfusion, is easily measured and underlies the need for early placement of an indwelling urinary catheter to monitor urine production when adequate circulation is suspect. Patients should have vascular access with several large bore (14 to 16 gauge) intravenous peripheral catheters and initiation of isotonic crystalloids. Although crystalloid is the fluid given initially, only approximately one third of the crystalloid fluid administered stays in the intravascular space. Depending on the patient's vital signs and overall status, blood may be indicated. Again, ATLS provides a standard classification for estimating blood loss and hypovolemia based on analysis of vital signs and this classification for shock is easily used in any environment (see Table 7).

The major sources of severe blood loss include external sources such as a major scalp laceration, a massive hemothorax, intra-abdominal hemorrhage (especially from a liver, spleen, or major mesenteric injury), and pelvic and long bone fractures. External bleeding should be controlled by direct manual pressure on the wound. Tourniquets should not be used generally because they crush tissue and cause distal ischemia.

1. Cardiac tamponade in trauma is secondary to the accumulation of blood in the pericardial sac leading to mechanical cardiac compression with limitation of ventricular filling and ejection, leading to hypotension and global hypoperfusion. The diagnosis is usually made by ultrasonographic evaluation of the pericardium through subxiphoid longitudinal view. The diagnosis is confirmed and temporized by decompression of the pericardial sac by either pericardiocentesis or

TABLE 7

ESTIMATED VOLUME AND BLOOD LOSS BASED ON PATIENT'S INITIAL PRESENTATION

	Class I	Class II	Class III	Class IV
Blood loss (mL)	Up to 750	750–1,500	1,500–2,000	>2,000
Blood loss (% blood volume)	Up to 15%	15%–30%	30%–40%	>40%
Pulse rate	<100	>100	>120	>140
Blood pressure	Normal	Normal	Decreased	Decreased
Pulse pressure (mm Hg)	Normal or increased	Decreased	Decreased	Decreased
Respiratory rate	14–20	20–30	30–40	>35
CNS/mental status	Slightly anxious	Mildly anxious	Anxious, confused	Confused, lethargic
Fluid replacement (3:1 rule)	Crystalloid	Crystalloid	Crystalloid and blood	Crystalloid and blood

CNS, central nervous system.
American College of Surgeons Committee on Trauma. *Advanced trauma life support program for doctors,* 7th ed, chapter 3, Shock. Chicago: American College of Surgeons Committee on Trauma; 2004:74.[11]

through subxiphoid pericardial window. Sternotomy or thoracotomy with cardiac repair is usually required.

2. The best candidates for a resuscitative thoracotomy are those who sustain penetrating thoracic trauma and arrive in the trauma resuscitation area pulseless, but have myocardial electrical activity. The procedure accomplishes the following:
   (a) Evacuation of the pericardial sac
   (b) Direct control of exsanguinating hemorrhage
   (c) Open cardiac massage
   (d) Cross-clamping of the descending thoracic aorta

Resuscitative thoracotomy in the trauma resuscitation area is reserved for patients who have arrested within 15 minutes of arrival in penetrating trauma or those who arrested within 5 minutes of arrival in blunt trauma. The best results have been reported with cardiac stab wounds, where thoracotomy allowed for relief and repair of cardiac tamponade.[12]

Disability (Neurologic Evaluation)

At the end of the primary survey, the physician performs a focused neurologic evaluation to establish the patient's level of consciousness. The Glasgow Coma Scale (GCS), pupillary size and reaction, motor and sensory examinations, and the presence of spinal cord injury are recorded. The GCS provides a quantitative and objective method for assessing and following the patient's mental status (see Table 8). All patients are presumed to have spinal cord instability until it is excluded and that is usually by physical examination and/or x-rays (or computed tomography [CT] scan). One cannot rely on radiography alone to rule out spine injury, and clinical examination is the most important

factor. If neurologic deficit secondary to spine injury is present, the level of spinal cord injury is carefully documented by the distribution of motor and sensory deficits. Spinal shock should be considered in the patient who is hypotensive but not tachycardic and who has warm skin and good perfusion. Other etiologies for hypotension, particularly hypovolemia, should be excluded first before spinal shock or neurologic shock is considered as the etiology.

Exposure/Environmental Control

The patient's clothes should be removed so that a thorough examination can be conducted. The patient's clothes should

TABLE 8

GLASGOW COMA SCALE (GCS)

Motor	Follows commands	6
	Localizes pain	5
	Withdrawal, normal flexion	4
	Decorticate, abnormal flexion	3
	Decerebrate, extension	2
	No movement, flaccid	1
Verbal	Oriented	5
	Confused conversation	4
	Inappropriate words	3
	Incomprehensible sounds	2
	No speech	1
Eye opening	Spontaneous	4
	To speech	3
	To pain	2
	None	1

GCS = Motor score + Verbal score + Eye-opening score.

not be discarded. External warming devices, such as warming blankets, should be applied to the patient as soon as possible. Furthermore, the thermostat in the trauma resuscitation area should be disengaged so that the room temperature is always 85°F. Hypothermia is much easier to prevent than to treat.

INTERVENTION AND ADJUNCTS

Monitoring

All patients should have electrocardiographic monitoring so that tachycardia and dysrhythmia can be readily detected. For example, pulseless electrical activity may be a sign of developing cardiac tamponade or tension pneumothorax. Bradycardia or premature ventricular beats may indicate hypoxia, global hypoperfusion, or a worsening traumatic brain injury.

Pulse oximetry should be used to measure the patient's oxygen saturation, but does not replace the arterial blood gas, as it neither measures the partial pressure of oxygen nor the partial pressure of carbon dioxide. The device depends on adequate blood flow to the region where it is placed, so no waveform or reading will be obtained if the extremity is ischemic or a tourniquet is used.

Catheters

The insertion of a urinary catheter should be considered in those patients whose volume status and overall perfusion is in question. If urethral injury is suspected, a retrograde urethrogram is performed before the insertion of the catheter. Insertion of a nasogastric or orogastric catheter is prudent to prevent gastric distention and to decrease the risk of aspiration. If the cribriform plate is fractured, the gastric tube should be inserted orally to prevent intracranial passage.

Diagnostic Studies

Because Chapter 25 of this book addresses diagnostic tests, only a brief discussion will be made here about the tests that may be useful during the initial resuscitation. It is crucial to remember that no imaging test replaces sound clinical examination and judgment.[13,14]

1. **Plain X-rays**
   (a) Cervical Spine
   If it shows a fracture (and other causes of shock are excluded), it may alert the clinician to spinal or neurogenic shock, especially in the multisystem injured patient)
   (b) Chest
   Detects pneumothorax, massive hemothorax, pulmonary contusion and assesses endotracheal, chest, and nasogastric tube placement

   (c) Pelvis
   Detects pelvic fracture which, if severe, may be a significant source of blood loss
2. **Ultrasonography**
   When used as an extension of the physical examination, this rapid, noninvasive test detects:
   (a) Hemopericardium
   (b) Pneumothorax
   (c) Hemoperitoneum
   (d) Sternal fracture
   The use of ultrasonography in the trauma setting is most accurate for the detection of hemopericardium and for its presence or absence in the hypotensive patient.[15–17]
3. **Diagnostic Peritoneal Lavage** (DPL)
   DPL is a rapid and sensitive diagnostic test for the detection of intra-abdominal hemorrhage. There is some surgical skill involved in performing a DPL, and meticulous hemostasis is important to minimize a false positive result. A positive DPL is indicated by the following:
   (a) A >10 mL of gross blood on the tap
   (b) Or if a diagnostic lavage (instilling 1 L of Ringer lactate into the peritoneal cavity) is performed:
       (i) More than 100,000 red blood cells per mm^3 (for blunt trauma)
       (ii) More than 10,000 red blood cells per mm^3 (for penetrating trauma)
       (iii) More than 500 white blood cells per mm^3
       (iv) Bacteria on Gram stain
       (v) Food fibers[18]

SECONDARY SURVEY

After the primary survey is completed and the patient is hemodynamically normal, the secondary survey is begun. This consists of a head to toe examination of the patient, further history taking, and a reassessment of the vital signs. During this time, a complete neurologic examination is performed and the GCS score is recorded. After the patient has been resuscitated, it is not unusual for the GCS to improve as the patient's overall perfusion (including cerebral perfusion) now improves. Indicated diagnostic studies and laboratory tests are now ordered. A condensed history (Allergies, Medication, Past illness/Pregnancy, Last meal and menstruation, Events/Environment related to the injury) is obtained.

Physical Examination

The survey of the head includes the scalp, eyes (including foreign bodies, lacerations, and testing of visual acuity), ears, mouth, and face with attention paid to fracture detection. Usually, the treatment of facial fractures is delayed until the more life-threatening or potentially life-threatening injuries are treated. If the patient is unable to maintain a secure airway, a cricothyroidotomy or tracheostomy may need to be performed depending on urgency and the patient's status. To fully assess the extent of facial fractures, a CT scan and/or panorex view of the mandible may be needed. Patients with maxillofacial or head injury are presumed to have unstable cervical spine injury. If the cervical collar is removed temporarily to examine the neck, another person should immobilize the neck until the collar is replaced.

Examination of the neck should include an evaluation for cervical spine tenderness, subcutaneous emphysema, tracheal deviation, and laryngeal trauma. The carotid arteries should be palpated and auscultated for bruits that, if detected, are a strong indicator for carotid occlusion or dissection. "Hard signs" mandating neck exploration include an expanding hematoma, airway compromise, bruits or thrills, or active arterial bleeding.

A complete evaluation of the chest requires inspection, auscultation, and palpation. Obvious injuries, such as an open pneumothorax, should have been treated during the primary survey. A small pneumothorax can rapidly develop into a tension pneumothorax if the patient is receiving positive pressure ventilation. Such changes underscore the importance of continually reassessing the patient and reevaluating the ABCs. A rapid bedside ultrasonographic examination can detect hemothorax, pneumothorax, and sternal fracture, but does not replace the chest x-ray that helps to detect rib fractures (especially flail segments), pulmonary contusions, widened mediastinum, and diaphragmatic rupture.

The following are the important principles regarding the evaluation of the abdomen. (i) In general, physical examination alone is insensitive for the detection of intra-abdominal injury, especially in patients who have an altered sensorium. Despite this fact, however, if peritonitis is present, an exploratory laparotomy is indicated and no other diagnostic tests for abdominal evaluation are needed. (ii) No diagnostic modality other than celiotomy consistently has a 100% sensitivity and specificity. (iii) Factors that influence the choice of diagnostic modality (CT scan, ultrasonography, and DPL) include the patient's age, hemodynamic stability, mechanism of injury, type of injuries, and select aspects of the history and physical examinations such as pregnancy status, current medications, and previous surgeries. (iv) Regardless of which diagnostic modality is used, the most important issue is to determine if the patient needs exploration, not the identification of a specific injury.

Included in an evaluation of the abdomen is an assessment of the perineum, rectum, and vagina. Especially in the presence of a pelvic fracture, detailed attention to these areas is critical as the detection of injury changes the management and increases the patient's morbidity. For example, vaginal laceration may connect with the pelvic fracture, making it an open pelvic fracture.

Some pelvic fractures can often be palpated by applying downward pressure to both anterior superior iliac spines,

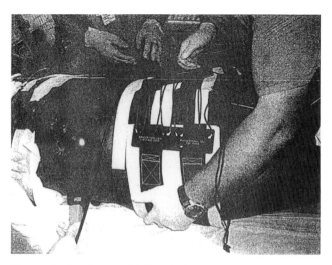

Figure 4 Application of Pelvic Binder.

and to the pubis. A careful genital and rectal examination should be performed to determine sphincter tone as well as the presence of blood, a high-riding or floating prostate, perineal or scrotal hematomas, and urethral injuries. Male patients with significant anterior pelvic fractures and pubic diastasis or straddle injuries are at risk for injury to the urethra and should have a retrograde urethrogram before the insertion of a urinary catheter. A cystogram is performed after the urethrogram (if normal) in order to evaluate bladder integrity. In the hypotensive patient, it may be useful to reduce pelvic volume by applying a pelvic stabilizing device, or even by just tightly wrapping a sheet around the patient's pelvis, to limit blood loss (usually venous in origin). This provides temporary immobilization for the fracture. A pelvic stabilizing device (see Fig. 4) is best applied in the hypotensive patient with an open-book fracture or vertical shear-type fracture, and should be avoided for those patients with lateral compression fractures.

The extremities are examined for contusions, lacerations, and hematomas. Palpation of the shafts of long bones will detect tenderness, crepitus, and abnormal motion. Simultaneously, the major peripheral pulses are also assessed. Open wounds and fractures are covered with sterile dressings, and bleeding wounds are controlled with sterile dressings and direct pressure. Multiple bilateral lower extremity fractures can be splinted and then reexamined later after the resuscitation is complete. Tight extremity compartments should alert the physician to the possibility of compartment syndrome and should prompt decompression or, at a minimum, compartment pressure measurement.

REEVALUATION

At the completion of the secondary survey, the patient is reevaluated beginning with the ABCs, progressing rapidly through the entire physical examination. Any problems that have been identified are reevaluated to rule out progression. Repeat ultrasonographic examinations of the pericardial area, the abdomen, and the sternum are performed and it is not uncommon to identify accumulated fluid at repeat ultrasound examination. Constant monitoring of the severely injured patient is required and may necessitate rapid transfer to the surgical intensive care unit or to the operating room.

SUMMARY

Resuscitation of the trauma patient is an intense, dynamic process in which the injured patient is assessed and re-assessed and where diagnoses evolve as the resuscitation progresses. A well-rehearsed protocol must meet impro-visation and a tailored approach is necessary for each individual. Suboptimal outcomes are usually the result of a failure to apply a systematic approach to diagnosing and treating life-threatening injuries, and are not secondary to a lack of advanced technology. Sound clinical judgment and experience in combination with an organized team approach and careful attention to detail will consistently provide for optimal patient outcomes.

REFERENCES

1. American College of Surgeons Committee on Trauma. *Advanced trauma life support program for doctors*, 7th ed. Chicago: American College of Surgeons Committee on Trauma; 2004.
2. Rhodes M, Brader A, Lucke J, et al. Direct transport to the operating room for resuscitation of trauma patients. *J Trauma.* 1989;29:907–915.
3. Rhee P, Nunley MK, Demetriades D, et al. Tetanus and trauma: A review and recommendations. *J Trauma.* 2005;58:1082–1088.
4. Moore EE, Feliciano DV, Mattox KL, eds. *Trauma*, 5th ed, chapter 47, New York: McGraw-Hill; 2004:1067–1068.
5. Sanders MJ, ed. *Paramedic textbook*, 2nd ed, chapter 11, figure 1, St. Louis: Mosby; 2000:397.
6. Sanders MJ, ed. *Paramedic textbook*, 2nd ed, chapter 11, figure 2, St. Louis: Mosby; 2000:397.
7. American College of Surgeons Committee on Trauma. *Advanced trauma life support program for doctors*, 7th ed, chapter 2, Airway and ventilatory management. Chicago: American College of Surgeons Committee on Trauma; 2004:53–68.
8. American College of Surgeons Committee on Trauma. *Advanced trauma life support program for doctors*, 7th ed, chapter 2, Airway and ventilatory management. Chicago: American College of Surgeons Committee on Trauma; 2004:47–50.
9. American College of Surgeons Committee on Trauma. *Advanced trauma life support program for doctors*, 7th ed, chapter 2, Chicago: American College of Surgeons Committee on Trauma; 2004:67.
10. American College of Surgeons Committee on Trauma. *Advanced trauma life support program for doctors*, 7th ed, chapter 3, Shock, Chicago: American College of Surgeons Committee on Trauma; 2004:79.
11. American College of Surgeons Committee on Trauma. *Advanced trauma life support program for doctors*, 7th ed, chapter 3, Shock, Chicago: American College of Surgeons Committee on Trauma; 2004:74.
12. Powell DW, Moore EE, Cothren CC, et al. Is emergency department resuscitative thoracotomy futile care for the critically injured patient requiring prehospital cardiopulmonary resuscitation? *J Am Coll Surg.* 2004;199:211–215.
13. Bokhari F, Brakenridge S, Nagy K, et al. Prospective evaluation of the sensitivity of physical examination in chest trauma. *J Trauma.* 2002;53:1135–1138.
14. Guillamondegui OD, Pryor JP, Gracias VH, et al. Pelvic radiogra-phy in blunt trauma resuscitation: A diminishing role. *J Trauma.* 2002;53:1043–1047.
15. Rozycki GS, Feliciano DV, Ochsner MG, et al. The role of ultrasound in patients with possible penetrating cardiac wounds: A prospective multicenter study. *J Trauma.* 1999;46:543–552.
16. Wherrett LJ, Boulanger BR, McLellan BA, et al. Hypotension after blunt trauma: The role of emergent abdominal sonography in surgical triage. *J Trauma.* 1996;41:815–820.
17. Dulchavsky SA, Schwarz KL, Kirkpatrick AW, et al. Prospective evaluation of thoracic ultrasound in the detection of pneumoth-orax. *J Trauma.* 2001;50:201–205.
18. Root HD, Hauser CW, McKinley CR, et al. Diagnostic peritoneal lavage. *Surgery.* 1965;57:633–637.

Diagnostic Imaging

William C. Chiu   *Thomas M. Scalea*

Continued advances in imaging technology and the application of existing techniques are at the forefront of the initial evaluation of the trauma patient, particularly in patients who are critically injured. Radiographic diagnostics must be rapid and accurate. The initial radiographic evaluation screens for immediate life-threatening conditions. More sophisticated diagnostics then identify organ-specific injury and characterize its severity.

There are a number of diagnostic and imaging techniques available; each has its advantages and disadvantages. No one technique will suffice in every patient. Imaging technology can be relatively expensive. While we once questioned how to obtain more information on patients, the current questions regard how much information we should obtain that are both clinically useful and will impact on patient care.

The utility of various diagnostic modalities depends on institutional resources, including physician, nursing, and technical support. In general, more advanced imaging modalities may require travel and extended time off-site, which may not be safe in unstable patients. Perhaps more importantly, someone at each institution must be able to rapidly and accurately interpret these images for them to be useful. All issues must be considered in order to choose a rational institutional algorithm.

DIAGNOSTIC SCREENING

Plain Radiography

The traditional teaching of radiologic screening in the multiply injured blunt trauma patient by the Advanced Trauma Life Support (ATLS) course has been to obtain initial radiographs of the lateral cervical spine, anteroposterior (AP) chest, and AP pelvis.[1] For the most part, this adage remains useful, as these initial films will identify the injuries that may require the most immediate attention following the primary survey. Following the secondary survey, thoracolumbar (T-L) spine radiographs and films of any extremities should then be obtained if there is any suspicion of injury to these areas.

The crosstable lateral cervical spine radiograph must include visualization of the base of the skull, all seven cervical vertebrae without overlying foreign bodies, and the top of the first thoracic vertebra. The initial lateral view should rapidly identify an unstable cervical fracture. Early knowledge of cervical spine injury may be especially important if respiratory insufficiency is present and intubation is needed. AP and open-mouth odontoid views or computed tomography (CT) scan can be obtained to supplement this view after the secondary survey.

The supine AP chest radiograph rapidly identifies potentially life-threatening injuries such as pneumothorax and hemothorax. The early detection of rib fractures, pulmonary contusion, or diaphragm rupture may also be made. The initial chest x-ray may explain asymmetric lung sounds, dyspnea, or hypoxia on initial presentation. It is often necessary to use an upright chest x-ray or CT to definitively exclude mediastinal hemorrhage from aortic injury.

The supine AP pelvic radiograph is used to identify obvious pelvic fractures or ring disruption from ligamentous injury. Abnormalities on this film may help explain any hemodynamic instability from potential pelvic hemorrhage. If any fracture is identified, a subsequent CT scan should be obtained. The initial trio of x-rays are most essential in patients in which hemodynamics or pulmonary function is unstable and the early diagnosis of life-threatening injuries is critical.

Statscan Radiography

The Statscan machine is a low-dose digital radiographic unit that can scan the entire body in <13 seconds. The device was developed in South Africa by LODOX Ltd.

(Johannesburg) and has since been used in a few centers in the United States. The physical unit appears somewhat similar to a CT scan device, but is somewhat smaller. The patient to be studied is transferred onto the Statscan table and scanning can be performed in the AP, lateral, or any oblique angle. The product of the scan is a full-body radiographic image of the patient projected electronically onto a local monitor or transmitted through an imaging network.

The utility of the Statscan in the initial evaluation for trauma is currently under investigation, but early results are promising for the technology. The most obvious benefit appears to be to expedite rapid radiographic evaluation, triage, and emergent management decisions in multiply injured trauma patients. In a prospective evaluation of the LODOX device, overall patient time required was only 5 to 6 minutes for LODOX compared to 8 to 48 minutes for conventional x-rays.[2]

The workflow advantage to an early full-body radiograph has considerable promise in the initial evaluation of trauma. Several patient situations would be most amenable to Statscan radiographic survey. The blunt multiply injured patient with altered sensorium, comatose, or intubated and sedated will have an unreliable history and physical examination. The blunt trauma patient who says "it hurts everywhere!" would otherwise require an extraordinary number of radiographic views. The patient with multiple gunshot or shotgun wounds in which the trajectory or number of remaining missiles must be assessed would otherwise have a risk of a missed injury with just a few conventional films.

Ultrasonography

The use of ultrasonography (US) by trauma surgeons and emergency physicians has clearly established a rapid noninvasive technique to make the diagnosis of hemoperitoneum and hemopericardium. US is portable, rapid, and can be interpreted in real time. The ability to repeat ultrasound, if indeterminate, is also quite attractive. US, however, must be carefully mastered before it is useful. Casual use of ultrasound imaging can produce disastrous results if false-negative studies are obtained. Practitioners should be adequately educated and obtain sufficient experience under supervision before utilizing ultrasound independently.

Computed Tomography

We have witnessed rapid improvements in CT technology. We have incorporated its diagnostic superiority to a vast array of disease processes, some of which we would never have traditionally evaluated by CT imaging (see Table 1). CT is able to identify organ-specific injury in virtually every body cavity. The ability to alter image windows allows vascular, bony, and soft tissue structures to be evaluated. Although the acquisition of the images may be rapid,

---

TABLE 1

ADVANCES AND IMPROVEMENTS IN COMPUTED TOMOGRAPHY (CT) TECHNOLOGY

- Helical/spiral continuous scanning data acquisition
- Thin-section multidetector row technology
- Focused timing power injection of contrast for CT angiography
- Digital reconstruction for up to 1 mm sections
- Two-dimensional digital reformation for sagittal and coronal planes
- Three-dimensional digital reformation for complex anatomic regions
- More rapid generation of images for viewing and analysis
- Ability to manipulate digital images for focused enhancement at workstation

---

complicated reconstruction does take some time. Transport to and from the scanner also requires time and the use of nursing resources. In most cases, torso CT scanning requires both oral and intravenous contrast with a small risk of aspiration and/or contrast allergic reaction.

The sensitivity of CT has improved and screening with CT has become increasingly popular. CT is no longer considered only an imaging modality for directed diagnosis. The multidetector format has made it more practical to perform scanning of larger body sections in relatively short periods of time, rather than scanning several focused and limited segments. The advantages of CT scanning are increasingly outweighing the disadvantages. In blunt, multiply injured patients, it is now common to obtain CT scans of the head, facial bones, cervical spine, chest, abdomen, and pelvis in a single setting for a relatively complete full-body survey.

CT angiography is also replacing conventional angiography as the initial method to evaluate the possibility of vascular injury in various sites in the body. It is less invasive than conventional angiography and many centers are gaining much more experience utilizing these studies. Conventional angiography is now used for therapeutic hemostasis, where we have expanded methods of embolization and angioplasty. Angiographic stenting for vascular injuries has increasing applicability, especially in high-risk surgical patients.

Magnetic Resonance Imaging

Magnetic resonance imaging (MRI) has a limited use for evaluation of the trauma patient. MRI may still be considered the definitive modality in the detection of acute spinal cord injury and the imaging test of choice for nonskeletal spinal support injuries. Magnetic resonance angiography still has a limited role in the vascular evaluation of trauma patients.

SPECIFIC REGIONS

Head

The radiologic assessment for traumatic brain injury is almost exclusively done with CT scan. The indications for obtaining a head CT should be relatively liberal, including any patient with a loss of consciousness, a significant external injury to the head, whether by blunt force or penetrating mechanism, or any patient with an altered sensorium. The noncontrast CT scan of the brain is ideal for detecting parenchymal lesions, extra-axial collections of blood, hematomas with mass effect, and skull fractures. Plain radiographic skull films are now obsolete.

MRI becomes relevant only when investigating for a predisposing lesion or infarct that may have contributed to the traumatic event. It is most useful in investigation of patients in which the clinical findings do not correlate with CT findings. CT is superior to MRI in the detection of acute trauma such as early extra-axial hematoma, skull fractures, and pneumocephalus, but MRI may better evaluate injuries to the brainstem and the multiple shearing injuries seen in the diffuse axonal injury syndrome. A specialized CT-perfusion study of the brain may also be performed as an adjunct.

The detection of skull base fractures is especially difficult on traditional CT scan of the head because the entire skull base may not be adequately imaged and the sections are not sufficiently narrow. The temporal bone CT scan provides more narrow sections at a section angle more suitable to detect skull base fractures.

Facial Bones

Any suspicion for facial trauma is an indication for CT scanning of the facial bones. The CT of facial bones should include the facial sinuses, orbital structures, and mandible. The superior sensitivity of CT with multiplanar reconstruction obviates any need for plain film radiography of the face to evaluate for trauma. CT provides all the detailed information important about fracture patterns, displacement, comminution, and associated soft tissue injury.

In the blunt multiply injured patient, facial fractures are at increased risk of being missed, especially in those patients with associated brain injury or altered sensorium. In a 5-year review of almost 5,000 patients undergoing head CT for trauma, 12% were found to have associated facial fracture.[3] This study advocated more liberal use of facial CT when performing head CT for blunt trauma.

Cervical Spine

Patients who are awake, alert, reliable, and lack any neck pain or tenderness may have the cervical spine cleared without any radiographic evaluation. Clearance of the cervical spine is one of the most controversial areas involving imaging in trauma. The inadequacy of the plain radiographic techniques and the need for clinical correlation has made this evaluation especially difficult. Still existing published protocols recommend that the initial studies performed should be plain radiographs. Various algorithms have been proposed to clear the cervical spine in trauma patients, with most requiring a minimum of three views.[4]

An adequate lateral view must portray the C7-T1 junction. It is typically necessary for someone to pull down on the patient's arms to clear the shoulders from obstructing the radiographic view. Even with the additional pulling, this image is frequently unable to project the cervicothoracic junction. The swimmer's view is a potential adjunctive view, but is also often limited in quality.

The open-mouth odontoid view is frequently a technical challenge to obtain an adequate view. Many trauma patients are simply not able to open their mouth for this view. Existing algorithms recommend supplementing the radiographic imaging with CT scanning directed at areas without adequate visualization. With multidetector CT technology, it is now common practice to scan the entire cervical spine.

MRI is reserved for those patients presenting with acute neurologic deficit that may be a result of a cervical spine injury. If the CT scan reveals the pathology, additional imaging may not be necessary before the initiation of treatment. MRI may still provide the additional information regarding the status of the spinal cord and vertebral ligaments. In those patients without overt spinal cord neurologic deficit, MRI scanning may still be important to definitively exclude ligamentous injury before removal of the hard cervical collar.[5]

For those who rely on MRI to definitively clear the cervical spine of ligamentous injury, the unreliable trauma patients present a significant challenge. It remains unclear at what time the MRI should be obtained to have the greatest sensitivity for ligamentous injury. Furthermore, trauma patients are a difficult group to obtain an adequate history to exclude the presence of metallic foreign bodies. Critically ill and hemodynamically unstable patients on moderate ventilator support may not be good candidates to go for MRI. Therefore, it may appear more practical to simply leave the cervical collar in place in these patients.

Previous studies performed have revealed that the incidence of isolated ligamentous cervical spine injury without fracture is low. In a study of 366 obtunded blunt trauma patients with normal cervical CT, MRI was negative for acute injury in 97%.[6] In this study, the negative predictive value for CT approached 99% for ligamentous injury.

Neck

Older algorithms to evaluate patients with penetrating neck injury stratify the approach based on the zone of injury. There has been a trend toward initial imaging to evaluate all patients without hard signs of vascular injury suggesting need for surgical exploration. The former standard diagnostic study to evaluate for cervical vascular injury was the conventional angiogram. The contrast esophagram remains the standard study to evaluate for esophageal injury, with or without esophagoscopy. In blunt trauma mechanisms, only patients with a very high index of suspicion for cervical vascular injury, such as those with neurologic deficit or those with direct evidence of neck trauma, should be subjected to diagnostic angiography.

The utility of CT angiography for the neck is still undergoing evolution but early studies have been favorable. CT angiography will almost certainly become the preferred initial study for penetrating neck trauma, with conventional angiography reserved for indeterminate cases. The trajectory of the injury occasionally allows confirmation that the esophagus is far remote from injury without further need for contrast esophagram.

With the increased application of CT angiography of the neck, a coincident increase in the incidence of carotid artery injuries are being diagnosed in blunt trauma patients. Grading systems for the severity of carotid injury exist and now the difficult task is to determine which lesions are clinically significant and what are the best ways to manage these lesions. The practical difficulty with this test is that it requires a separate power injection of contrast during scanning of the neck to obtain optimal imaging. CT imaging of the neck with contrast time for the chest may decrease the sensitivity for carotid artery lesions.

Chest

During the initial evaluation in trauma, and especially for those patients with penetrating injury, the Focused Assessment with Sonography for Trauma (FAST) examination should be performed to evaluate for pericardial tamponade. In patients with cardiac injury, hemopericardium should be detectable on this study and may warrant immediate surgical decompression. If no one capable of performing this procedure is immediately available, a temporizing pericardiocentesis may be helpful. The pericardial evaluation is somewhat problematic in the blunt trauma patient population. The incidence of sonographically detectable physiologic pericardial effusion may be greater than the incidence of clinically significant blunt traumatic hemopericardium.

The initial AP chest radiograph is recommended for most trauma patients. This study allows the clinician to rapidly exclude the presence of significant pneumothorax or hemothorax, check for major rib fractures, and make an assessment on the mediastinum. In any patient with a significant blunt trauma mechanism in which there is risk for thoracic aortic injury, the mediastinum must be cleared. In the initial evaluation for trauma, there are technical difficulties in obtaining optimal images of the mediastinum. These patients are admitted in the supine position and an erect posteroanterior view is not practical in most of these patients. It is now clear that the contrast-enhanced CT scan is the best way to evaluate the mediastinum for aortic injury.

Currently, the former standard of conventional aortography to evaluate the wide mediastinum on plain radiograph has been replaced by CT in many institutions. Sensitivity and negative predictive value for detecting aortic injury have been reported to be up to 100% and the convenience of using CT relative to angiography has led to increased acceptance and utility. In a prospective comparison between CT and aortography in 142 patients with potential aortic injury, it was found that the total cost of helical CT was approximately half that of performing aortography.[7] Another study showed that in 28 patients undergoing surgery after CT scan alone, there were no unexpected findings.[8] More importantly, the key finding in this study showed that the mean time from admission to definitive diagnosis was 5.7 hours for the angiography group, whereas the time was only 1.7 hours for the CT group.

There is controversy regarding the utility of routine thoracic CT in the evaluation of blunt trauma. CT has clearly been shown to be more sensitive than physical examination and plain radiography in detecting injuries. It may be thought that most occult injuries found on CT do not require treatment. In a prospective study of 375 patients with chest trauma, it was found that CT induced therapy change in 30% of patients.[9] This study demonstrated that CT was better than chest x-ray (CXR) in detecting pulmonary contusion, hemothorax, pneumothorax, and vertebral fractures.

Diaphragm

Diaphragmatic injury may still be an area in which CT scan has not clearly become the superior diagnostic study. Most blunt diaphragm ruptures are still diagnosed with plain radiography, in which the classic findings include the appearance of herniation of the stomach and other abdominal viscera into the chest, with the diagnosis often associated with findings of a gastric tube in the left chest and evidence for left hemopneumothorax. This lesion may be mistaken for elevated left hemidiaphragm or acute gastric dilatation.

Because the diaphragm is a thin structure, the axial sections of CT have difficulty in clearly depicting the location of the diaphragm relative to adjacent viscera. With increasing availability of digital reconstruction of images, the sagittal and coronal reconstructive images become crucial in evaluating for potential diaphragm injury. To facilitate the evaluation of the diaphragm, a special protocol would be necessary to include 5-mm thin sections from the lower chest to upper abdomen and patients should be encouraged to hold their breath for the critical portion of scanning to minimize the movement of the diaphragm.

Although CT is probably the more versatile study for the diaphragm, there may still be some utility in using MRI as an adjunctive test.[10]

Abdomen

In conjunction with the initial assessment for hemopericardium, the FAST examination should be performed initially to evaluate for potential intra-abdominal hemorrhage. The greatest utility for the FAST examination lies in those patients presenting with hypotension where the rapid identification of the source for hemorrhage is urgent. FAST has essentially replaced diagnostic peritoneal lavage (DPL) as the initial diagnostic study for the detection of hemoperitoneum. DPL is only indicated in those situations in which FAST is not available, FAST results are indeterminate, or when FAST appears negative, but the patient's unstable clinical condition warrants additional urgent diagnostic evaluation of the abdomen.

There remains debate on the utility of serial FAST in the observation of stable blunt trauma patients. When FAST is initially negative, clinical criteria may still warrant obtaining a CT scan. In a prospective study of 772 blunt trauma patients undergoing both FAST and CT, 29% of patients with abdominal injury had no initial free fluid on either study.[11] Furthermore, there is no consensus on when to perform the repeat FAST, or whether to even repeat the study at all in patients without clinical change that would indicate a need for a repeat study.

Although FAST has replaced DPL, FAST has not been able to decrease the use of CT in abdominal trauma. The reason for this appears to be that CT sensitivity has become so remarkable for detecting pathology and CT will be able to specify which organs are injured and to what extent (see Table 2). Therefore the mainstay for abdominal trauma imaging is the CT scan, especially adjunctive to any plans for nonoperative management of abdominal injury. The early concerns regarding the ability of CT to detect injuries of the diaphragm, bowel, and pancreas are beginning to abate as the evidence is now showing that new CT technology is very good at detecting all abdominal injuries. Following adequate FAST or DPL, CT scanning may still be beneficial to provide information regarding the retroperitoneum.

There remains some controversy regarding the utility or necessity for oral contrast administration for the trauma abdominal CT. If abdominal CT is only being used to evaluate the liver and spleen, then oral contrast administration has limited benefit. In the evaluation for abdominal trauma, oral contrast administration, even if only the stomach and duodenum are enhanced, provides substantial information. The critical peripancreatic, periportal, periduodenal, and central mesenteric regions are much easier to evaluate with oral contrast. The trauma protocol for oral contrast administration should provide that CT scanning must not be delayed to wait for contrast transit time. Once it is decided that an abdominal CT scan will be ordered, oral contrast should be provided to the patient or administered through an existing orogastric or nasogastric tube. Additional contrast administration may be given upon entry into the CT scan suite.

The sensitivity of CT in detecting bowel injury after blunt trauma has long been a concern. With the advent of helical technology, the role of CT for bowel and mesenteric injury has become more established. In a

---

TABLE 2

COMPARISON OF DIAGNOSTIC PERITONEAL LAVAGE (DPL), ULTRASONOGRAPHY (US), AND COMPUTED TOMOGRAPHY (CT) FOR THE EVALUATION OF ABDOMINAL TRAUMA

Factors for Comparison	DPL	US	CT
Transport	No	No	Yes
Invasive	Yes	No	No
Time	<1 hr	Fast	<1 hr
Repeatability	No	Yes	Possible
Contraindications	Previous surgery	None	Unstable, uncooperative
Sensitivity for fluid	Excellent	Excellent	Excellent
Sensitivity for injury	Excellent	Good	Excellent
Specificity for injury	No	No	Yes
Pneumoperitoneum	No	No	Yes
Retroperitoneum	No	No	Yes
Ongoing bleeding	No	No	Yes
Other regions	No	Yes	Yes
Complications	Visceral perforation	None	Contrast allergy, nephropathy

study of 150 blunt abdominal trauma patients, CT had 94% sensitivity for bowel injury and 96% for mesenteric injury.[12] This study showed the ability of CT to predict the need for surgery in bowel injury, but not so much for mesenteric injury.

With the improved sensitivity of CT scanning, it has become even more important to use intravenous contrast for abdominal CT in trauma. Arterial extravasation has previously been correlated with failure of nonoperative management in splenic injury. With the advent of angiography and embolization, these patients are increasingly successfully managed without splenectomy. In a multicenter study of 565 patients with abdominal visceral injury, arterial extravasation was noted in 18% of patients.[13] Almost 78% of patients with extravasation required surgery or embolization.

In penetrating trauma, there is evidence that the triple contrast-enhanced abdominal CT scan is an excellent way to evaluate patients who may not have significant intraperitoneal injury. Triple contrast adds rectal contrast administration to the intravenous and oral double contrast for standard abdominal CT scans, and facilitates the evaluation for colonic injury. While the triple-contrast CT scan has the greatest utility in patients with penetrating injury to the back and flanks, cautious application to those patients with potential superficial or tangential anterior abdominal wounds has been reported to be accurate.

Triple-contrast CT can accurately exclude peritoneal violation and predict need for laparotomy. In a prospective series of 75 patients with penetrating torso trauma evaluated with triple contrast-enhanced abdominopelvic CT, 96% of patients with negative findings had successful nonoperative management.[14] This study showed that CT was effective regardless of whether the mechanism was stab or gunshot wound and whether the injury site was toward the back or front.

Pelvis

There has also been debate regarding the utility of the initial AP pelvic radiograph that has traditionally been recommended by the ATLS course. Because of the increasing use of abdominopelvic CT scanning, the diagnosis of even the most subtle of pelvic fractures may be made by CT scan and an assessment on extent of pelvic hematoma, evidence for contrast blush, and associated visceral injury may be detected by CT. In a review of 311 pelvic fracture patients undergoing both pelvic radiography and CT, 55% had either additional fractures detected or an increase in the grade of fractures based on CT scan.[15] Despite the improved sensitivity of CT, some orthopaedic surgeons may still wish to have plain film radiography to evaluate the pelvis. They may still use the AP view in conjunction with Judet, inlet, and outlet projections to facilitate their decision-making on pelvic fracture management.

All patients found to have pelvic fracture on plain radiography should also have early CT scan performed. Ongoing hemorrhage in pelvic fracture is a significant cause of morbidity and mortality with hemodynamic alterations and need for blood transfusion. In a 5-year review of patients with pelvic fracture, 4.5% of pelvic CT scans identified contrast extravasation in which 69% were from hemodynamically unstable patients undergoing subsequent angiographic embolization.[16]

Thoracolumbar Spine

The diagnostic imaging evaluation for the T-L spine includes AP and lateral views of the thoracic and lumbar spine. Patients having a higher index of suspicion for fracture are those with pain or tenderness referable to the T-L spine. Those patients should undergo dedicated CT scanning of the entire thoracic or lumbar spine. Patients already having CT scanning of the chest or abdomen may have reformatted images of the thoracic and lumbar spine developed without additional patient scanning.

As with the evaluation of the cervical spine, those patients with focal neurologic deficit that may have resulted from spinal injury may benefit from directed MRI scanning to evaluate for spinal cord, ligamentous, or disc injury. Information from the MRI scan may help guide the management plan on whether operative or nonoperative therapy should be undertaken.

Pregnancy

Medically necessary diagnostic imaging should not be withheld from pregnant mothers because of concerns for the fetus. However, the selection of imaging studies should undergo more careful scrutiny in pregnant patients. Tests should be ordered judiciously, and mandatory shielding of the fetus for all except pelvic and lumbar spine radiographs should be performed. Redundancy and repeated examinations should be avoided.

The American College of Obstetricians and Gynecologists has set forth recommendations for diagnostic imaging during pregnancy. It states that there is no increased risk of fetal loss or birth defects with up to 5 rad fetal exposure, estimating fetal dose without shielding to be 30% that of the mother's dose (see Table 3). Furthermore, no study has shown any increase in teratogenicity at fetal exposures below 10 rad. The greatest fetal risk from ionizing radiation appears to be to the central nervous system from 8 to 15 weeks, and would require at least 20 to 40 rad.

Studies have suggested that there is a 6% to 8% increased risk for childhood cancer per 100 rad of fetal exposure. The Eastern Association for the Surgery of Trauma Practice Management Guidelines Committee has evaluated the body of evidence regarding the diagnosis of injury in the pregnant patient, and recommendations are currently published on their Web site (www.east.org).

TABLE 3

ESTIMATED FETAL EXPOSURE FOR VARIOUS RADIOGRAPHIC STUDIES

Examination Type	Estimated Fetal Dose Per Examination (Gy)
Plain films	
Cervical spine	0.00002
Chest (two views)	0.0000007
Pelvis	0.0004
Thoracic spine	0.00009
Lumbosacral spine	0.00359
CT scans (10 mm sections)	
Head	<0.0005
Chest	<0.001
Abdomen	0.026

CT, computed tomography.

Contemporary Algorithm

The current climate of the health care community increasingly demands nothing less than perfection from physicians and their medical management, regardless of cost. Although it remains a top priority to deal with the most urgent matters and decisions first, an important objective would be to subsequently identify all of a patient's injuries, using the combination of a thorough physical and imaging diagnostic strategy to limit the risk of having any missed injuries, however minor they may at first appear to you. A contemporary diagnostic imaging evaluation would include a full-body radiograph and a near full-body CT scan for this comprehensive examination in the multiply injured trauma patient (see Fig. 1). This is the style of practice that we have evolved into at the R Adams Cowley Shock Trauma Center in Maryland.

Future in Initial Diagnostic Imaging

It is likely that CT technology will continue to advance so that it may not only become the definitive diagnostic imaging study for the detection of injury but also become the best initial imaging study as well. Many factors have affected the increased utility of CT scanning. Helical technology and multidetector row scanning and routine two-dimensional sagittal and coronal reconstruction are now commonplace. The increased use of three-dimensional reconstruction may provide incremental sensitivity for injuries in certain difficult regions for diagnosis. This concept may prove to be advantageous for diagnosis and therapeutic planning for specific maxillofacial, orthopaedic, and spine fractures. The increased reliance on angiographic CT to improve the detection of vascular injuries or to detect areas of flow abnormality in the brain, neck, torso, and even extremities have seen increased usage.

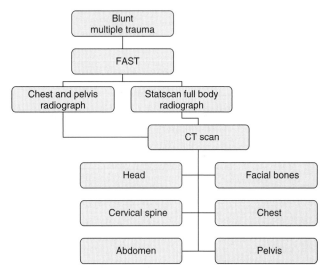

Figure 1 A contemporary algorithm for the radiologic evaluation of the blunt multiply injured trauma patient. Focused assessment with sonography for trauma (FAST) is typically performed with the secondary survey, but may be done in conjunction with initial resuscitation in unstable patients. Initial plain film radiography may consist of chest and pelvis x-ray or a Statscan radiograph. Liberal use of computed tomography (CT) enhances your ability to detect all traumatic injuries.

A study utilizing the portable CT scanner in an intensive care unit (ICU) setting showed that most portable scans performed were for head CT scans in unstable critically ill trauma patients, although chest, abdomen, and pelvis scans were also ordered portable.[17] This technology could potentially be a very useful device in institutions in which the fixed CT scanner was far remote from the emergency department. Because CT scanning has rapidly become the standard for the diagnosis of injury throughout the body, the portable CT scanner would most likely decrease the diagnostic time and would increase the CT utility in unstable patients.

There is increasing sentiment for performing urgent diagnostic CT scans in unstable patients. One example is the hypotensive blunt multiple trauma patient with lateralizing neurologic signs. It remains a judgment decision on whether this patient is too unstable to proceed to CT for an emergent diagnosis that may indicate life-saving craniotomy. There has even been discussion regarding early CT, in conjunction with initial resuscitation, rather than plain radiography for the initial imaging evaluation of the blunt trauma patient. The time advantage may be life saving in select situations.

REFERENCES

1. Alexander RH, Proctor HJ, eds. *Advanced trauma life support® course for physicians*, 5th ed. Chicago: American College of Surgeons; 1993.
2. Beningfield S, Potgieter H, Nicol A, et al. Report on a new type of trauma full-body digital X-ray machine. *Emerg Radiol.* 2003;10:23–29.

3. Holmgren EP, Dierks EJ, Homer LD, et al. Facial computed tomography use in trauma patients who require a head computed tomogram. *J Oral Maxillofac Surg.* 2004;62:913–918.

4. Chiu WC, Haan JM, Cushing BM, et al. Ligamentous injuries of the cervical spine in unreliable blunt trauma patients: Incidence, evaluation, and outcome. *J Trauma.* 2001;50:457–464.

5. Sliker CW, Mirvis SE, Shanmuganathan K. Assessing cervical spine stability in obtunded blunt trauma patients: Review of the medical literature. *Radiology.* 2005;234:733–739.

6. Hogan GJ, Mirvis SE, Shanmuganathan K, et al. Exclusion of unstable cervical spine injury in obtunded patients with blunt trauma: Is MR imaging needed when multi-detector row CT findings are normal? *Radiology.* 2005;237:106–113.

7. Parker MS, Matheson TL, Rao AV, et al. Making the transition: The role of helical CT in the evaluation of potentially acute thoracic aortic injuries. *Am J Roentgenol.* 2001;176:1267–1272.

8. Downing SW, Sperling JS, Mirvis SE, et al. Experience with spiral computed tomography as the sole diagnostic method for traumatic aortic rupture. *Ann Thorac Surg.* 2001;72:495–502.

9. Guerrero-Lopez F, Vazquez-Mata G, Alcazar-Romero PP, et al. Evaluation of the utility of computed tomography in the initial assessment of the critical care patient with chest trauma. *Crit Care Med.* 2000;28:1370–1375.

10. Shanmuganathan K, Mirvis SE, White CS, et al. MR imaging evaluation of hemidiaphragms in acute blunt trauma; ex-perience with 16 patients. *Am J Roentgenol.* 1996;167:397–402.

11. Chiu WC, Cushing BM, Rodriguez A, et al. Abdominal in-juries without hemoperitoneum: A potential limitation of fo-cused abdominal sonography for trauma (FAST). *J Trauma.* 1997;42:617–625.

12. Killeen KL, Shanmuganathan K, Poletti PA, et al. Helical computed tomography of bowel and mesenteric injuries. *J Trauma.* 2001;51:26–36.

13. Yao DC, Jeffrey RB, Mirvis SE, et al. *Using contrast-enhanced helical CT to visualize arterial extravasation after blunt abdominal trauma: Incidence and organ distribution.* AJR. 2002; 178: 17–20.

14. Chiu WC, Shanmuganathan K, Mirvis SE, et al. Determining the need for laparotomy in penetrating torso trauma: A prospective study using triple-contrast enhanced abdominopelvic computed tomography. *J Trauma.* 2001;51:860–869.

15. Guillamondegui OD, Pryor JP, Gracias VH, et al. Pelvic radiogra-phy in blunt trauma resuscitation: A diminishing role. *J Trauma.* 2002;1043–1047.

16. Pereira SJ, O'Brien DP, Luchette FA, et al. Dynamic helical computed tomography scan accurately detects hemorrhage in patients with pelvic fracture. *Surgery.* 2000;128:678–685.

17. McCunn M, Mirvis SE, Reynolds N, et al. Physician utilization of a portable computed tomography scanner in the intensive care unit. *Crit Care Med.* 2000;28:3808–3813.

Injury to the Brain

26

Jose L. Pascual *Vicente H. Gracias*
Peter D. LeRoux

Central nervous system (CNS) trauma is the most common cause of death from injury and accounts for a third of all trauma deaths.[1] Recent data show that in the United States, approximately 2% of the population (5.3 million citizens) lives with disability as a result of traumatic brain injury (TBI).[2] Approximately 50,000 deaths[1] and 1 million hospital visits each year are associated with head injury in North America.[3] Most patients are victims of a motor vehicle collision (MVC) and are aged between the ages of 16 and 30 years.[4] Gunshot wounds to the head also remain a common cause of brain injury.[5] During the last decade, greater awareness of the epidemiology of head injury and better understanding of its pathophysiology has led to the development of management guidelines. Implementation of these guidelines in patient care protocols appears to have improved outcomes.

ANATOMY

The brain is surrounded by several distinct layers (see Fig. 1). The bony skull is covered with muscle, subcutaneous fat, and skin. Beneath the skull are the leptomeninges including the outer dura mater (a fibrous membrane that adheres to the internal surface of the skull), the arachnoid, and the inner pia mater (which is intimately attached to the outer surface of the brain). Cerebrospinal fluid (CSF) circulates between the arachnoid membrane and pia mater in the subarachnoid space.

The cranial vault is divided into three regions: the anterior region covered by the frontal bone, the middle section or parietal region covered by the parietal and temporal bones and separated from the frontal bone by the coronal suture, and the posterior or occipital region covered by the occipital bone that contains the occipital lobe and in the suboccipital region, the cerebellum and lower brainstem. The bone is particularly thin in the temporal region and thick in the occiput.

The brain is formed by the cerebrum, which is divided into two hemispheres each with four lobes (frontal, parietal, temporal, and occipital), the cerebellum, and the brainstem. The brainstem is further divided into the midbrain, the pons, and the medulla. The reticular activating system (responsible for state of alertness) is within the midbrain and upper pons. The cardiorespiratory center resides in the medulla. Small lesions in the brainstem can cause profound neurologic deficit.

PHYSIOLOGY

To understand TBI management, two essential aspects of brain physiology must be understood—the Monro-Kellie Doctrine[6,7] and cerebral autoregulation. The Monro-Kellie Doctrine states that the total volume of intracranial contents is constant in an intact rigid cranial vault. Consequently, when there is an expanding mass lesion such as an ongoing hemorrhage, or edema, intracranial pressure (ICP) will only remain normal if there are concurrent reductions in the volume of other contents of the cranial vault, mainly CSF and blood.

When there is brain injury, cerebral edema usually ensues. This adds further to intracranial volume. This volume shift will continue until a reduction in blood/CSF volume can no longer occur, at which point ICP will begin to rise sharply. As ICP increases (>20 mm Hg), brain tissue begins to herniate from areas of high pressure to areas of low pressure.

ICP is sensitive to cardiac and respiratory functions that help to define its waveform when measured. Two other concepts are allied to ICP—elastance and its inverse, compliance. These concepts, in particular compliance, describe

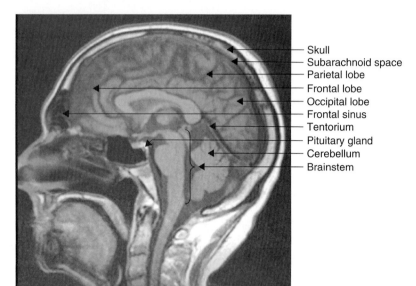

- Skull
- Subarachnoid space
- Parietal lobe
- Frontal lobe
- Occipital lobe
- Frontal sinus
- Tentorium
- Pituitary gland
- Cerebellum
- Brainstem

Figure 1 Sagittal magnetic resonance image (T1) of the skull and brain.

how the intracranial contents are able to compensate for changes in volume. When compliance is reduced, small changes in volume lead to large changes in ICP. It is important to understand this rightward shift of the pressure-volume index (PVI), (see Fig. 2) because even when ICP is normal, very small changes in volume can have disastrous effects by causing herniation through a rapid increase in ICP.

The concept of cerebral autoregulation refers to the ability of the brain to maintain a constant cerebral blood flow (CBF) despite changes in cerebral perfusion pressure (CPP) (see Fig. 3). CPP is defined as mean arterial pressure (MAP) minus intracranial pressure ($CPP = MAP - ICP$) and

normal CBF is approximately 50 mL/100 g brain/minute. CBF <20 mL/100 g brain/minute can lead to cerebral ischemia and CBF <5 mL/100 g brain/minute will result in cell death. There are both metabolic and pressure autoregulation. Metabolic autoregulation is influenced by cellular requirements. Pressure autoregulation refers to changes in vasomotor tone, which keep CBF constant over a range of mean arterial blood pressure. As CPP decreases or increases in the normal individual, vasoconstriction or dilation of the cerebral vasculature help maintain CBF constant across a broad range of perfusion pressures, which are believed to be between 50 and 150 mm Hg. Beyond these "breaking points," changes in CBF parallel changes in CPP and can result in inadequate or excessive (luxuriant) tissue oxygen and glucose delivery. Autoregulation is frequently impaired during the first 2 to 3 days following TBI. This can have deleterious effects on CBF but also allows certain therapies to be effective. When ICP equals CPP, CBF can no longer be maintained and vascular autoparalysis occurs.

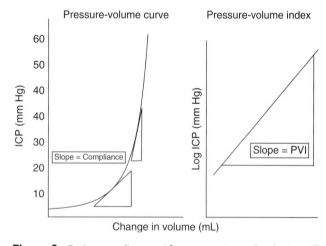

Figure 2 Brain compliance. After any injury, the brain will compensate for increases in pressure through elastance and compliance. As compliance is lost, small changes in volume can lead to large changes in pressure. In a patient who is on the right side of the curve, even with normal intracranial pressure (ICP), small changes in volume can precipitate large rises in pressure.

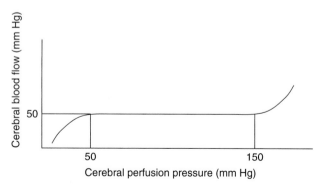

Figure 3 Cerebral autoregulation.

PATHOLOGY OF HEAD INJURY

Head injury can be classified as focal or diffuse. Focal injuries are typically associated with direct blows to the head and may cause fractures, hematomas, or contusions. The morbidity of focal injuries depends on their location as well as the magnitude of the applied force. Diffuse injury to the brain, often called *diffuse axonal injury* (DAI), is caused by inertial forces imparting acceleration/deceleration shearing within the brain tissue. Head injury can also be classified as open or closed. This depends on whether there is a fracture of the skull or sinuses that communicates with the external environment. A critical determinant of outcome and management of an open injury is whether the dura is intact or not.

Head injury can lead to brain injury through primary or secondary mechanisms. Primary brain injury results from the direct mechanical damage that occurs at the time of trauma. However, brain injury does not cease with the initial trauma but progresses over the subsequent hours, days, and even months. This continuing cerebral damage, known as *secondary brain injury*, is important and its identification and management are the basis of much of critical care for TBI. Several substances can contribute to secondary brain injury including excitatory amino acids, cytokines, and oxygen free radicals released during systemic inflammation.[8,9] In addition, systemic derangements can contribute to and aggravate secondary brain injury. In particular, hypotension and hypoxemia increase the risk of poor outcome following TBI.[10,11] A single hypotensive episode (systolic blood pressure [SBP] <90 mm Hg) results in a fourfold increase in the mortality risk of patients with TBI.[12] Other systemic abnormalities that contribute to secondary cerebral injury include hyperglycemia, hyperthermia, hypercapnea, and hypocapnea. In addition, seizures can contribute to secondary neuronal injury.

PATHOLOGIC SUBTYPES OF HEAD INJURY

Epidural Hematomas

Epidural (or extradural) hematomas (EDHs) are found in <1% of all patients with head injuries and 10% of those who are comatose.[13] On head computed tomography (CT) scan acute EDHs are typically hyperdense, lenticular, or biconvex in shape, and are formed by a pressure-driven separation of the dura mater from the overlying skull (see Fig. 4). The most common type of EDH occurs in the temporal region and is caused by a bleeding middle meningeal artery lacerated by a skull fracture. An EDH may present with a period of normal consciousness after an initial loss of consciousness. This can be followed by profound coma, that is, the "talk and die" phenomenon.

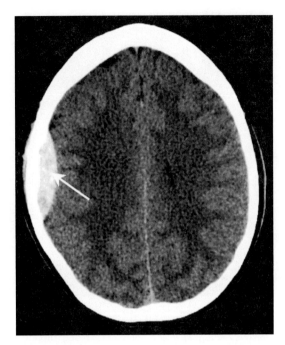

Figure 4   Right temporal epidural hematoma (*arrow*) on head computed tomography (CT). Note its smooth lentiform shape.

Subdural Hematomas

Acute subdural hematomas (SDHs) are the most common traumatic mass lesions and occur in 30% of patients with severe head injuries.[13] They usually result from a shearing disruption of the subdural bridging veins. Acute SDHs are most often crescent shaped, hyperdense on head CT, and are caused by passive filling of the subdural space with blood (see Fig. 5). In addition, SDHs are frequently associated with underlying brain injury (e.g., contusion, intracerebral hematomas [ICHs], or DAI) unlike EDH where there is generally no brain injury. It is the underlying brain injury that often determines the outcome of SDH and also helps explain why outcome is much worse after SDH than EDH. Chronic SDH may occur in individuals with brain atrophy (e.g., the elderly and alcoholics). Again, the subdural bridging veins are torn even after minor trauma. These bleeds can be subclinical initially but as the hematoma liquefies over the course of subsequent weeks, they can become symptomatic. These lesions are also crescenteric in shape but are usually iso- or hypodense on head CT scan. However, there can be mixed densities on head CT scan suggesting episodes of rebleeding within the same hematoma (i.e., acute or subacute on chronic SDH).

Intracerebral Hematomas and Contusions

ICHs and contusions are bleeding areas within the brain itself that appear as mass lesions. Brain tissue can be seen interspersed with hemorrhage on head CT scan (salt and pepper) in contusions. By contrast, the blood forms a

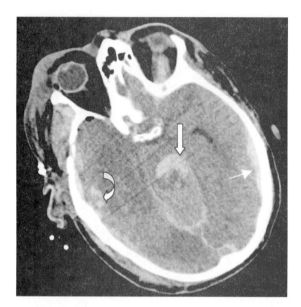

Figure 5   Subdural hematoma (SDH). Acute left temporal parietal subdural hematoma (*arrow*) and right temporal intraparenchymal contusion (*curved arrow*). In addition there is blood (subarachnoid) layering on the tentorium and involving the brainstem (*large arrow*).

coalesced mass in an ICH on CT scan. Contusions are often found in the frontal and temporal lobes because this tissue "glides" over the underlying rough bony surface of the skull base during impact and acceleration/deceleration of the head (see Fig. 6). The brain may also impact the inner table of the skull across from the area of impact, thereby causing

a contusion or hemorrhage. This is known as a *coup-contre-coup* lesion. ICH may also occur with penetrating injuries (e.g., stab wounds or gun shot wounds, see subsequent text). Finally, ICH may develop or progress ≥24 hours after injury (delayed traumatic ICH) and therefore, patients at risk require careful follow-up and repeat imaging.[14,15]

Traumatic Subarachnoid Hemorrhages/Intraventricular Hemorrhages

Subarachnoid hemorrhage (SAH) is often found following moderate or severe head injury. It is usually found in a diffuse pattern over the convexities and in the subarachnoid space. It is hyperdense on head CT scan (see Fig. 7), and is often associated with other intracranial pathology, in particular SDH or ICH. When SAH is found on imaging, it is important to determine whether it is traumatic or it arose from rupture of an aneurysm that then led to loss of consciousness, fall, and subsequent injury. This is important because SAH resulting from aneurysmal rupture may lead to vasospasm (delayed narrowing of cerebral vessels), which can cause delayed cerebral infarction and poor neurologic outcome.[16] For reasons that remain unknown vasospasm is not seen following traumatic SAH.

Intraventricular hemorrhage (IVH) is blood within the ventricles. This may occur with SAH, ICH, or SDH. Isolated IVH may also be seen in DAI. Patients with IVH are at increased risk for acute posttraumatic hydrocephalus[17] and more chronic hydrocephalus (i.e., enlargement of the ventricles).

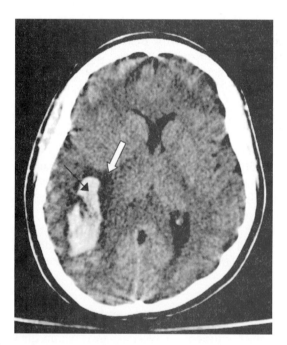

Figure 6   Intracerebral hemorrhage. Right temporal occipital lobe intracerebral hemorrhage (*arrow*) with associated vasogenic edema (*block arrow*). Note the compressed right occipital horn of the lateral ventricle.

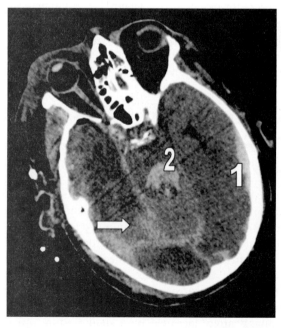

Figure 7   Subarachnoid hemorrhage (SAH). Different detail from the patient in Fig. 5 demonstrating extensive right posterior SAH (*arrow*). Note the accompanying left temporal subdural hematoma (*1*) and fourth ventricle blood (*2*).

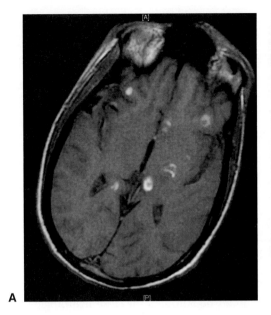
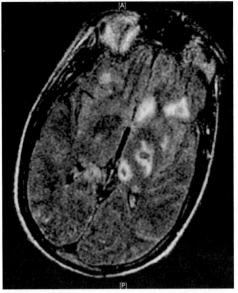

Figure 8 Diffuse axonal injury (DAI). **A:** T1 magnetic resonance imaging (MRI) demonstrating susceptibility artifact at the gray-white junction of the left thalamus, left internal capsule, right splenium, and corpus callosum. **B:** Equivalent image on flair MRI.

Diffuse Axonal Injury

DAI is considered the most common pathology in TBI. It is seen in mild, moderate, or severe TBI. It results from shearing forces that affect the axons.[18] These axons undergo sequential focal changes, which result in axonal cytoskeletal dysfunction followed by axonal swelling and disconnection in the hours that follow injury.[19] The corpus callosum, brainstem, white matter, and reticular activating system may be affected. The admission head CT scan may be normal but may also show small hemorrhages in the white matter, corpus callosum, deep basal ganglia, or brainstem. IVH may also occur. Acute SDHs are often associated with DAI. Depending on its severity, the prognosis of DAI can be poor and it is the leading cause of disability among TBI survivors. Brain magnetic resonance imaging (MRI) helps identify characteristics typical of the condition (see Fig. 8).

CLINICAL EVALUATION

Primary Survey

TBI requires prompt management but always after ensuring a secure airway with proper oxygenation and circulation (*Airway, Breathing, and Circulation* [ABCs]).[20] During the primary survey, one must determine whether all extremities are moving and if the pupils are equal and reactive. Pupils are an important element in the examination of patients with head injuries. A dilated pupil that does not react to light suggests ipsilateral uncal herniation and compression of the third cranial nerve.

The Glasgow Coma Scale (GCS)[21] is a standard score with excellent interobserver variability, which should be applied to all patients (see Table 1). The postresuscitation GCS is essential for subsequent management and prognostication and the *motor* score is the most predictive variable following TBI. When there is asymmetry in either eye opening or motor scores, the best score is used. The GCS should be obtained early in a patient's evaluation and preferably

TABLE 1
GLASGOW COMA SCALE

Signs	Score
Eye Opening	
Spontaneous	4
To verbal command	3
To pain	2
No response	1
Best motor response	
Obeys verbal commands	6
Localizes to pain	5
Withdraws to pain	4
Flexion response to pain	3
Extension response to pain	2
No response	1
Best verbal response	
Orientated	5
Confused	4
Inappropriate words	3
Nonspecific sounds	2
No response	1

TABLE 2

CLASSIFICATION OF TRAUMATIC BRAIN INJURY (TBI)

	Mild TBI	Moderate TBI	Severe TBI
GCS	13–15	9–12	≤8
Proportion of all TBI	80%	10%	10%
Sensorium	Transient confusion and retrograde amnesia, follows commands	Confused, can follow some commands	Unable to follow commands
Prognosis/mortality	Excellent/<1%	Good/<5%	Poor/30%–40%
Long-term recovery	Headaches, memory problems mostly in first month	Cognitive and behavioral deficits lasting months or permanently. Usually good recovery with treatment	Persistent coma, vegetative state; severe disability frequent

before administration of sedatives and/or paralytics. A GCS of ≤8 indicates coma and airway intubation, and ventilation should be considered early. If necessary, an emergency surgical airway (cricothyroidotomy, tracheostomy) may be required.

Secondary Survey

Once the primary survey is completed and immediate life-threatening conditions are managed or excluded, the secondary survey acts as a complete physical examination. A proper neurologic examination to evaluate motor and sensory deficits, reflexes, cranial nerves, and rectal tone should be included.

CLASSIFICATION OF TRAUMATIC BRAIN INJURY

TBI is categorized as mild, moderate, or severe according to the level of neurologic dysfunction at the time of initial evaluation (GCS 13 to 15; 9 to 12, and ≤8, respectively) (see Table 2). An advantage of using the GCS is that it can be repeated frequently to determine if there is any change in the patient's condition.

MILD AND MODERATE HEAD INJURY

The vast majority of head injuries are mild. Despite their names, both mild and moderate head injuries are not trivial conditions. The postconcussive symptoms following mild TBI are thought by some to be associated with shear stress at the gray-white cortical interface following sudden deceleration. The pathophysiologic correlation of these injuries may represent a part of the spectrum of DAI, and follow a similar mechanism of injury and pathology.

Which patients with mild or moderate TBI require hospital admission? Any patient with mild or moderate head injury and head CT abnormalities or a neurologic deficit should be admitted for close neurologic observation. An important question then is who needs a head CT scan? Some large emergency department (ED) studies suggest using certain guidelines to determine when to order a head CT in trauma patients with a GCS of 15. These guidelines, such as the Canadian Head CT Rules[22] and the New Orleans Criteria,[23] include criteria such as age older than 60 years, headache, vomiting, intoxication, retrograde amnesia, confusion, loss of consciousness, seizures, visible trauma above the clavicles, and mechanism of injury to indicate a need for a head CT scan in patients with mild TBI. A normal head CT scan, however, does not always exclude the need for neurosurgical consultation because 10% to 38% of mild TBI patients with normal initial head CT develop posttraumatic abnormalities on subsequent imaging, and 3% to 15% ultimately require a craniotomy for these lesions.[24] Most mild TBI patients with a *normal* head CT can be observed safely in the ED and subsequently discharged with a reliable adult.[24,25]

CONCUSSION

Mild TBI also includes concussion, which is defined as cerebral deficit (e.g., loss of consciousness, confusion, and amnesia) with a normal head CT scan. Concussion is often classified into three grades (see Table 3).[26-28] In large part, these classification systems are used to determine when athletes can return to sporting activities. This is important because repetitive minor head trauma is associated with long-term sequelae and may be an epigenetic marker for Alzheimer disease. Furthermore, mild TBI increases the risk of another such injury

Most "concussed" individuals recover completely but some may develop a postconcussive syndrome. Symptoms include vague cognitive impairment to persistent headaches, tinnitus, vertigo, gait unsteadiness, emotional lability, sleep disturbances, intermittent blurring of vision,

TABLE 3

SPORTS-RELATED HEAD INJURY GRADES AND RECOMMENDATIONS

Concussion	Grade I	Grade II	Grade III
	No LOC, PTA <1 hr Mild confusion	LOC <5 min, PTA or RA 1–24 hr Confusion	LOC >5 min, PTA >24 hr Obvious confusion
		Return to Sporting Activity	
Initial occurrence	1 wk after becoming asymptomatic	2 wks after becoming asymptomatic Must be asymptomatic for at least 1 wk	Must be asymptomatic for at least 2 wks and have normal head CT
First recurrence	2 wks after becoming asymptomatic Must be asymptomatic for at least 1 wk and have normal head CT	Must be asymptomatic for at least 1 month and have normal head CT	Terminate season
Second recurrence	Terminate season	Terminate season Indefinite end to contact sports	Terminate season Consider terminating career

LOC, loss of consciousness; PTA, posttraumatic amnesia; RA, retrograde amnesia. Adapted from Cushman JG, Agarwal N, Fabian TC, et al. *Practice management guidelines for the management of mild traumatic brain injury. The EAST Practice Management Guidelines Work Group.* Vol. available at http://www.east.org/tpg.asp. Eastern Association for the Surgery of Trauma. 2001[29]

and irritability. Symptoms may continue from weeks to years, but all tend to completely resolve. β-blocking agents, tricyclic antidepressants, nonsteroidal anti-inflammatory agents, psychotherapy, and physical therapy can be used to treat postconcussion syndrome.

IMAGING STUDIES

Skull X-rays

In the past, all patients with a suspected head injury underwent skull x-ray series (anterior-posterior [AP], Caldwell, Waters, and lateral). This practice is currently replaced by the use of CT scans. A skull series may, however, still be useful in skeletal surveys when child abuse is suspected, after some penetrating injuries, and to assess depressed skull fractures or craniofacial trauma.

Computed Tomography of the Head

Head CT scan is the emergency imaging technique of choice after head injury. This imaging study is done without contrast administration. Acute blood is visible as a hyperdensity. In some patients blood may be isodense or hypodense when imaging is hyperacute or if the patient is coagulopathic or anemic. Contusions can be hyperdense, hypodense, or may have a "salt and pepper" appearance, whereas air indicating an open skull fracture or craniofacial trauma is hypodense. It is important to determine whether the perimesencephalic cisterns are open, compromised, or closed and the degree of midline shift at the level of the

third ventricle. These factors are useful in surgical decision making or in estimating ICP. CT also allows the cranial vault and facial bones to be assessed for fractures, displacement of bone fragments, or penetrating objects.

Angiographic Studies

The cerebral vasculature can be evaluated using formal arteriography, CT angiography, or magnetic resonance (MR) angiography or venography. These studies may be useful when there is penetrating injury, a neurologic deficit that is not explained by head CT scan, fractures over the venous sinus, some neck injuries, or when a cause for the injury (e.g., aneurysm rupture) is suspected. Formal arteriography may also be therapeutic in allowing embolization of bleeding vessels or occlusion of carotid-cavernous fistulae.

Magnetic Resonance Imaging of the Head

MRI of the brain is rarely used acutely after head injury. It may be useful in the subacute or chronic phases after injury to look for suspected preexisting pathology, changes of DAI, or help explain failure to improve in the days after injury.

INITIAL MANAGEMENT OF PATIENTS WITH HEAD INJURIES

Patients with suspected head injury, particularly if confused or unresponsive, require emergency evaluation and treatment at a center with emergency neurosurgical capabilities. The goals of therapy are prompt diagnosis and appropriate evacuation of intracranial mass lesions with simultaneous management of extracranial injuries to avoid secondary brain injury from hypoxia and hypotension. In addition, other secondary insults such as hyperglycemia, hyperthermia, hypercapnea, and hypocapnea need to be prevented because all these may worsen outcome.

Trauma Bay Management of Head Injury

Like any other trauma patient, the first priority in brain-injured individuals is management of ABCs[20]—in large part to avoid secondary brain injury. Tracheal intubation or creation of a surgical airway should be established early in anyone with precarious breathing or with a depressed level of consciousness (GCS <8). It is preferable but not always possible to perform a focused neurologic examination, including assessment of the GCS, pupillary response, and extremity movement before pharmacologic sedation and/or paralysis for intubation. The cervical spine should be continuously protected by a rigid collar or manual in-line mobilization because cervical spine injuries occur in up to 10% of patients with head injuries.[30] Standard rapid sequence intubation (RSI) algorithms (e.g., etomidate/rocuronium) are preferable for intubation. Succinylcholine can be used although some studies suggest it increases ICP. Pretreatment with lidocaine may help reduce intracranial hypertension or prevent ICP spikes in some patients.[31] Once a secure airway has been obtained, 100% inspired oxygen should be administered until arrival to the intensive care unit (ICU). Routine hyperventilation to $Paco_2$ levels <35 mm Hg is not recommended because it may worsen cerebral ischemia through vasoconstriction.[32]

Large-bore venous access must be immediately obtained to help restore intravascular volume, blood pressure, and perfusion. Resuscitation is best performed with isotonic or hypertonic crystalloids because use of hypotonic dextrose-containing solutions can promote cerebral edema.[33] Until ICP (and therefore CPP) is measured, an initial MAP of ≥80 mm Hg is a reasonable goal although the optimal blood pressure levels for brain resuscitation remain in debate. However, higher target MAP may be associated with an increased risk of adult respiratory distress syndrome (ARDS).[34] Spinal cord injury should be suspected in those whose blood pressure does not respond to fluid resuscitation.

Pharmacologic sedation and paralysis are generally required following RSI, particularly when the patient is agitated or combative, or when elevated ICP is suspected. Short-acting agents (e.g., propofol, vecuronium bromide, and cisatracurium) are preferable to allow patient transport to and from the CT scanner. Pain may not be readily appreciable in a sedated/paralyzed patient but can be manifested by changes in blood pressure or pulse. Patients should receive opioid analgesia (fentanyl, morphine) as needed.

Blood pressure and blood oxymetry (Sao_2) should be monitored continuously because several substances (e.g., analgesics and sedatives) may decrease blood pressure in the setting of head injury. Blood should be obtained for electrolytes, renal function, complete blood count, osmolality, acoagulation profile, platelet count, and arterial blood gas. Correction of hypoxia and coagulation are necessary to prevent ongoing intracranial bleeding. A blood alcohol level can be useful in select patients. However, it should never be assumed that alcohol or other drugs are the cause for an altered neurologic state in head injury.

The next step is imaging. Chest and pelvic x-rays are usually obtained in the trauma bay during initial resuscitation. In some cases cervical spine x-rays are still obtained at the same setting, although most centers will defer to CT of the cervical spine when the head CT is performed. In the presence of suspected brain injury, management of other non–life-threatening injuries should be temporarily suspended to obtain an immediate head CT scan once the ABCs have been secured. The notable exception to this is the hypotensive hemorrhaging patient with signs of severe brain injury. In this instance, it may be reasonable to proceed directly to the operating room without a head CT and perform a laparotomy/thoracotomy with diagnostic burr holes and/or placement of an ICP monitor. A skull x-ray during resuscitation may be useful in these patients to decide where to place a burr hole. It should be placed ipsilateral to a fixed, dilated pupil. The diagnostic yield of burr holes and ultimate outcome in these patients is usually poor. If no CT capability exists in the facility, immediate referral to a neurosurgical center is preferable.

Mannitol (1 g/kg 20% solution) may be empirically administered to reduce ICP in patients with lateralizing motor signs or unequal pupillary dilation/nonreactivity. Otherwise mannitol should be given when there is >1 cm midline shift or significant sulci effacement on head CT.

The neurologic examination and GCS should be frequently repeated before, during, and after making management decisions and during resuscitation. When neurologic status deteriorates and in particular when there is clinical evidence of cerebral herniation, hyperventilation may be indicated for a short period of time. In addition, these patients should be checked for secondary cerebral insults and if necessary undergo additional imaging. Neurologic deterioration may occur because of seizures and therefore, anticonvulsants are also necessary in the first week following TBI.

INDICATIONS FOR INTRACRANIAL PRESSURE MONITORING

No randomized controlled study has ever demonstrated that use of an ICP monitor improves outcomes or survival of patients with head injuries. However, intensive neuromanagement protocols *including* ICP monitoring have been found to improve outcomes.[35] Furthermore, many clinical studies have demonstrated an inverse relation between outcome and time spent with ICP ≥20 mm Hg.[36] The Brain Trauma Foundation and American Association of Neurological Surgeons and Congress of Neurological Surgeons (AANS/CNS) Joint Section of Neurotrauma recommend that ICP monitors be inserted in all unexaminable patients with severe brain injury (GCS ≤8), particularly those with an abnormal head CT scan (hematoma, contusion, edema, and compressed basal cisterns). Severe TBI patients with a *normal* head CT should receive an ICP monitor if they fulfill two or more of the following criteria: age older than 40 years, unilateral or bilateral flexor or

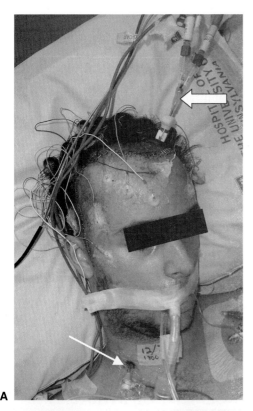

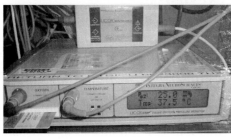

Figure 9 A: Patient with traumatic brain injury (TBI) with skull bolt (*block arrow*) with three intracerebral probes arising from it (intracranial pressure [ICP], temperature, and cerebral oxygenation). Note the right jugular venous bulb (*arrow*) and the multiple electroencephalography (EEG) leads for continuous cerebral activity measurement. **B:** Lycox unit attached to skull bolt displaying PbtO$_2$ and temperature.

extensor posturing, and SBP <90 mm Hg.[37] Patients with mild or moderate head injury may require an ICP monitor if they will be unexaminable for an extended period of time (e.g., general anesthesia for surgery and sedation for ventilatory care). Other monitors such as brain tissue oxygen monitoring, jugular bulb catheters, continuous electroencephalography (EEG), or assessment of CBF can be useful and supplement ICP monitors.[38-40] For example, the Licox system is a triple-lumen catheter that inserts through a skull bolt, and allows simultaneous placement of a fiber optic ICP, brain temperature, and brain oxygen tension (PbtO$_2$) probes (see Fig. 9). These probes should be inserted into normal appearing brain on CT to avoid placement within hematomas, contusions, or infarcted areas.[39]

SURGICAL MANAGEMENT

The decision to surgically evacuate an ICH depends on the patient's neurologic status and his/her CT scan findings. In general, all acute extra-axial hematomas ≥1cm, associated with ≥5 mm of midline shift should be evacuated regardless of the clinical condition.[13,41,42] ICH of >30 mL in volume or >3 cm in diameter, particularly with mass effect should also be evacuated. There are certain exceptions to this (e.g., advanced patient age, particularly when there are multiple premorbid or associated medical problems) that may be considered after neurosurgical consultation. In the posterior fossa, evacuation of smaller hematomas may be justified because even minimal expansion of a small lesion can cause sudden brainstem herniation and compression. Depressed skull fractures that are displaced greater than the thickness of the skull table and in particular, when open or compound generally require surgical repair.[13] An exception to this may be a depressed fracture immediately over a major venous sinus. Fractures of air sinuses, penetrating trauma, or craniofacial injuries all require specialized consideration. Decompressive craniectomy (DC), either a unilateral hemicraniectomy or bilateral frontal craniectomy, can be used to treat refractory, severe intracranial hypertension. Its use remains controversial and there are ongoing clinical trials to evaluate the role for DC in selected patients when maximal medical management has failed to control ICP. Surgical decision making and techniques are beyond the scope of this book but are reviewed elsewhere.[43]

INTENSIVE CARE MANAGEMENT OF BRAIN INJURY

Patients with severe brain injury (GCS ≤8) who do not require surgical intervention should be transferred immediately to an intensive care setting. Neuromonitoring (e.g., ICP and other modalities such as brain oxygen and continuous EEG) and neuro-observation are foundations of care and have two primary goals: (i) to rapidly identify neurologic deterioration and (ii) to avoid secondary brain injury (e.g., hypoxia, hypotension, hyperthermia, hypercapnea, hypocapnea, and hyperglycemia).

Optimal ICU management of the brain-injured patient involves the continuous monitoring of several extracranial physiologic parameters such as heart rate, electrocardiography (ECG), blood pressure, temperature, volume status, and pulse oximetry. End-tidal CO_2 can be monitored in ventilated patients. Ventilation should be titrated to a minimum Pco_2 of 35 mm Hg and to maintain an arterial saturation of 93% or greater. To help avoid cerebral hypoxia, arterial blood gases should be monitored frequently until a steady state is reached. Prophylactic hyperventilation (partial pressure of CO_2 ($Paco_2$) <35 mm Hg) may increase the risk of cerebral hypoxia through vasoconstriction and therefore it is not recommended.[32] Instead, hyperventilation (optimized hyperventilation) can be used when ICP is elevated immediately following TBI, provided no deleterious effect is observed on other monitoring (e.g., EEG and CBF suggestive of ischemia). The effect of hyperventilation on CBF and ICP is lost 2 to 3 days following TBI as autoregulation of blood flow is restored. Arterial blood pressure monitoring should be continuous, preferably through an arterial catheter. Mean arterial blood pressure should be maintained >80 mm Hg or to maintain CPP and $PbtO_2$ tailored to the patient's needs. The optimal CPP level remains debated and may be patient or pathology specific. Current guidelines suggest a CPP >60 mm Hg is adequate. Excess use of pressors or fluids to increase CPP can adversely affect lung function,[34,44] and so caution is necessary. An ICP <20 mm Hg and $PbtO_2$ >20 mm Hg are other treatment goals for most patients.[39,40] Patients should be kept euvolemic to avoid hypotension. Isotonic fluids are preferable because dextrose-containing hypotonic solutions may aggravate brain edema. Hypotonic fluids may be used to treat nephrogenic diabetes insipidus. When there is any question on the patient's fluid status, a pulmonary artery or central venous catheter can be inserted.

Blood should be sampled frequently for hemoglobin, platelet count, prothrombin time (PT), and partial thromboplastin time (PTT) to reduce the risk of further bleeding. Serum electrolytes (Na^+) and osmolality should be sampled every 6 hours if hyperosmolar therapy (mannitol and hypertonic saline [HTS]) is used. Desmopressin (DDAVP) may be needed to treat hypernatremia resulting from central diabetes insipidus. Hypomagnesemia may lower the seizure threshold and so calcium, phosphate, and magnesium levels should be monitored.[45]

Hyperthermia, either primary or secondary, can increase the cerebral metabolic rate and aggravate outcome. Shivering and profound hypothermia can aggravate ICP and so temperature control is important. The role for moderate hypothermia (33°C) in severe brain injury remains unclear.[46]

Patients with severe head injury are at increased risk for gastrointestinal (GI) ulceration,[47] deep vein thrombosis (DVT), and seizures. Patients therefore need GI ulcer prophylaxis (sucralfate or acid reducing therapy [H_2 blockade or proton pump inhibitors] and DVT prophylaxis (sequential compression devices). The timing for administration of pharmacologic agents (e.g., unfractionated or low molecular weight heparin) as phrophylaxis against DVT remains unclear. The role of prophylactic inferior vena cava (IVC) filters also remains unclear following TBI. Patients at risk for seizures (cortical contusions, extra-axial hematomas, penetrating head wounds, depressed skull fractures, and seizures within 24 hours of injury) should receive seizure prophylaxis (e.g., phenytoin) for 7 days following injury.[48,49] A repeat head CT scan is recommended within 24 hours of the initial scan to detect delayed posttraumatic abnormalities.

TBI is a catabolic state and increases caloric requirements by 25%. Nutritional supplementation should be initiated within 48 hours of injury with 25 to 30 kcal/kg/day through either enteral (preferred) or parenteral routes. Most patients will tolerate gastric or postpyloric feeding. This can benefit immunocompetence, and attenuate the stress response that leads to GI ulcers. Early enteral feeding in severely ill patients can help reduce infectious complications.[50]

Patients with TBI often have pulmonary injuries, other pathologies that limit lung function, or develop pulmonary problems (e.g., ventilator-associated pneumonia). Pulmonary care is therefore important. The role of early tracheostomy remains debated but tracheostomy and feeding access (e.g., gastrostomy or jejunostomy) should be considered when prolonged intubation and ventilation are expected.

Finally, the establishment and availability of dedicated head injury rehabilitation facilities can help improve long-term outcome for patients with severe head injury. Patients should be transferred to a rehabilitation facility for aggressive inpatient therapy once they are medically and neurologically stable.

MANAGEMENT OF INTRACRANIAL HYPERTENSION

Intracranial hypertension >20 mm Hg is associated with worse outcomes. ICP should therefore be monitored (see discussion on indications) and treated when elevated. Treatment of ICP can also be guided using other monitors (e.g., brain oxygen, jugular bulb, and transcranial Doppler) because every ICP treatment has potential deleterious effects. ICP can be measured using intraparenchymal or intraventricular (ventriculostomy) catheters. Fiberoptic parenchymal catheters are inserted through a skull bolt and, although more costly than ventriculostomies, are more accurate and can incorporate concurrent direct brain oxygen tension monitoring. It is easier to insert parenchymal probes than ventricular catheters. Parenchymal probes have a lower complication rate (1%) than ventriculostomies (5% to 10%). However, ventriculostomies can be used for CSF drainage, a useful, yet temporary treatment for intracranial hypertension. They are also particularly useful in hydrocephalus.

Jugular venous O_2 (Jvo_2) saturation or O_2 content may be monitored in cases of intractable ICP elevation, aiming for Jvo_2 >50% or O_2 content of 4 to 6 vol%. Brain O_2 extraction can also be calculated by substacting jugular O_2 content from the arterial O_2 content, normal O_2 extraction is 5 vol%. In one study, Jvo_2 <50% has been associated with a poor neurologic outcome after TBI.[51] The ultimate role or benefit of Jvo_2 monitoring remains unclear.[52] Adequate analgesia, sedation, correction of hyperthermia, and other physiologic derangements and mild head elevation (15 to 30 degrees) are the initial treatments for intracranial hypertension. Paralytics can be used to manage ICP; however, their routine use is associated with an increased risk of pneumonia and neuromuscular complications.[53,54]

Hyperosmolar therapy (mannitol and more recently HTS) is important in the management of intracranial hypertension. Bolus mannitol therapy (0.5 to 1.0 g per kg) should have an effect within 20 to 60 minutes of administration. The dose may be repeated if no effect occurs during that time. Most physicians will not administer mannitol if osmolality exceeds 310 to 320 mOsm. HTS solutions (HTS: 7.5%, 3%, 5%, 23.4% NaCl) have benefits resembling those of mannitol,[55–57] but are not associated with the diuresis, or in some patients the reverse osmotic shift that can increase ICP,[58] which follows mannitol administration. Recent reports suggest HTS administration can elevate $PbtO_2$ following severe head injury.[59] HTS may therefore be used to treat high ICP, particularly when there is hypotension.

In traditional ICP care, if head position, sedation, hyperosmolar therapy, or CSF drainage do not control ICP, secondary measures such as barbiturates, optimized hyperventilation, or DC are indicated. In several centers today, this traditional chair-step approach is not always followed. Instead targeted therapy is used on the basis of information from multimodality monitoring. High-dose barbiturate therapy can control elevated ICP.[60] Although ICP is controlled, the effect on outcome is less certain. When using barbiturates, patients should be monitored using a pulmonary artery catheter and EEG monitoring to reduce barbiturate-induced myocardial depression and confirm burst suppression. Optimized hyperventilation may be used *transiently* to treat some patients with high ICP, particularly those with hyperemia (elevated brain oxygen and decreased brain O_2 extraction). Use of hyperventilation requires that a monitor (e.g., brain oxygen or CBF) be in place to detect any potential adverse effects caused by vasoconstriction.

Decompressive hemicraniectomy is effective for ICP elevations. The precise use and timing of this procedure is debated. Many surgeons use decompressive hemicraniectomy when elevated ICP is unresponsive to maximal medical management.

PENETRATING BRAIN INJURIES

Penetrating cerebral injuries include high-velocity (gunshot wounds) and low-velocity (stab wounds) injuries. In a gunshot wound, the bullet causes a cylinder of tissue cavitation with a radius measuring up to ten times the diameter of the bullet as it traverses the brain.[61] Consequently intracranial hypertension is common. Patient prognosis depends on the cranial trajectory of the bullet and its velocity. If it traverses deep brain structures (basal ganglia, brainstem), the posterior fossa, or has a bihemispheric, multilobar or ventricular trajectory mortality is high[62] (see Fig. 10). Patients with a low (3 to 5) initial GCS score tend to have a high mortality (>80%), whereas 80% of patients who are awake and responsive on admission have mild or no disability at long-term follow-up. Prognosis may be difficult to estimate in young patients who are shot accidentally, particularly when there is no associated hypotension, respiratory distress, or coagulopathy and who have mid-range GCS with reactive pupils and normal ICP.[62] In those patients with a survivable injury (e.g., lobar injury and GCS ≥8), superficial debridement of the entrance and exit wounds is recommended.[61] Deep-seated bullet and bone fragments do not always have to be recovered

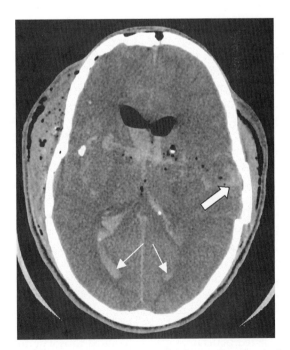

Figure 10 Penetrating injury to the brain. Transhemispheric gunshot wound from left to right with a trajectory of blood, gas, and missile fragments. Note blood in both lateral ventricles (*arrows*) as well as in the subarachnoid space (*block arrow*).

because the risk of neurologic damage from extensive brain exploration to remove all fragments usually exceeds the risk of abscess formation.[63] It is important, however, to achieve dural closure. Perioperative intravenous antibiotics and 7-day prophylactic anticonvulsant therapy are recommended.

The outcome after low-velocity missile wounds including stab wounds depends on the injury location in the brain. The missile should be removed under controlled conditions in the operating room because its removal may precipitate significant bleeding. In some stab wounds, the blade may break off in the skull and so this should be considered in all penetrating wounds. The broken blade will be identified on imaging including a skull x-ray. Broad-spectrum antibiotics and a tetanus booster should be given. Prophylactic anticonvulsants are also indicated for 7 days. A cerebral angiographic study should be considered following all penetrating head injuries to exclude a traumatic aneurysm. These lesions can often form within 7 days.

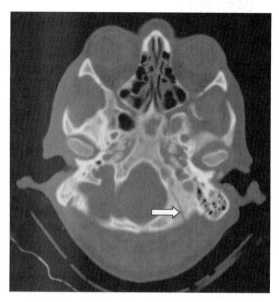

Figure 11 Basal skull fracture involving the left occipital bone (*arrow*).

SKULL FRACTURES

Linear skull fractures are common after head injury and occur most typically over the lateral convexities of the skull. This often involves the thin squamous portion of the temporal bone, which is closely associated with the middle meningeal artery. Fractures in this area can tear the artery and cause an EDH. The presence of skull fractures increases the likelihood of intracranial pathology 400-fold.[64] A linear skull fracture by itself rarely requires treatment. A nondepressed skull fracture rarely affects prognosis but the underlying brain injury may be severe and therefore it is important that all patients with suspected skull fractures undergo a head CT scan. Skull x-rays are rarely used now but can be useful to evaluate patients with some fractures (e.g., slot fractures after stab wound).

Skull fractures can be further classified as open (associated with an overlying scalp laceration) or closed, depressed or nondepressed, comminuted or not, or involving the skull base, air sinuses, or venous sinuses. Fractures that are depressed beyond the thickness of the inner cranial table often have an associated dural tear and should be elevated surgically. Other indications for operative management of skull fractures include evidence of CSF leak, cosmetic deformity, or contaminated bone or scalp fragments pushed into brain tissue. Fractures that involve air sinuses require special consideration. In particular, repair of the frontal bone should be considered if the posterior wall of the frontal sinus is fractured and there is associated pneumocephalus. This may also involve repair of craniofacial fractures. A vascularized pericranial graft is required to isolate the sinus from the dura. Fractures that involve a venous sinus need special caution because massive bleeding can occur at surgery. Consequently, not every fracture over a venous

sinus requires repair. Broad-spectrum antibiotics for 7 days are recommended for fractures that are open or involve air sinuses. Prophylactic anticonvulsant therapy should be continued for 7 days.

Basal Skull Fractures

Basal Skull Fractures (BSF) can involve the floor of the anterior cranial fossa and can therefore disrupt the orbital, sphenoid, occipital, and petrous temporal bones (see Fig. 11). CSF rhinorrhea can occur particularly when an anterior cranial fossa fracture involves the frontal sinus or ethmoid bones. In addition, BSF that involve the petrous bones can cause ipsilateral CSF otorrhea or rhinnorrhea (through the eustachian tube). Other clinical findings of BSF include Battle sign (subcutaneous hematoma overlying the mastoid bone), raccoon eyes (bilateral periorbital hematomas), and hemotympanum (blood in the middle ear). Injury to cranial nerves is common, particularly with petrous temporal fractures (e.g., facial palsy, numbness, or hearing loss). A careful examination of the cranial nerves is necessary with suspected BSF. Meningitis associated with a CSF leak is the major risk of BSF. Despite this risk, prophylactic antibiotic treatment is not recommended.[65] The leak can often be stopped by head elevation and bed rest. A lumbar CSF drainage catheter can be placed if the leak persists. If this fails to stop the leak within 72 hours, the patient should undergo surgical repair of the dural laceration.

REFERENCES

1. Sosin DM, Sniezek JE, Waxweiler RJ. Trends in death associated with traumatic brain injury, 1979 through 1992. Success and failure. *JAMA.* 1995;273(22):1778–1780.

2. Thurman DJ, Alverson C, Dunn KA, et al. Traumatic brain injury in the United States: A public health perspective. *J Head Trauma Rehabil.* 1999;14(6):602–615.

3. Guerrero JL, Thurman DJ, Sniezek JE. Emergency department visits associated with traumatic brain injury: United States, 1995–1996. *Brain Inj.* 2000;14(2):181–186.

4. Foulkes MA, Eisenberg HM, Jane JA, et al. The traumatic coma data bank: Design, methods, and baseline characteristics. *J Neurosurg.* 1991;75(5S):S8–S13.

5. Center for Disease Control. Surveillance data on traumatic brain injury. *MMWR Morb Mortal Wkly Rep.* 1997;46:8–11.

6. Monro A. *Observations on the structure and function of the nervous system.* Edinburg: Creech & Johnson; 1823.

7. Kellie G. An account of the appearances observed in the dissection of two of the three individuals presumed to have perished in the storm of the 3rd, and whose bodie were discovered in the vicinity of Leith on the morning of the 4th November 1821 with some reflections on the pathology of the brain. *Trans Med Chir Sci.* 1824;1:84–169.

8. Gourin CG, Shackford SR. Production of tumor necrosis factor-alpha and interleukin-1beta by human cerebral microvascular endothelium after percussive trauma. *J Trauma.* 1997;42(6):1101–1107.

9. Shohami E, Gallily R, Mechoulam R, et al. Cytokine production in the brain following closed head injury: Dexanabinol (HU-211) is a novel TNF-alpha inhibitor and an effective neuroprotectant. *J Neuroimmunol.* 1997;72(2):169–177.

10. Miller JD, Becker DP. Secondary insults to the injured brain. *J R Coll Surg Edinb.* 1982;27(5):292–298.

11. Chesnut RM, Marshall LF, Klauber MR, et al. The role of secondary brain injury in determining outcome from severe head injury. *J Trauma.* 1993;34(2):216–222.

12. Manley G, Knudson MM, Morabito D, et al. Hypotension, hypoxia, and head injury: Frequency, duration, and consequences. *Arch Surg.* 2001;136(10):1118–1123.

13. Marik PE, Varon J, Trask T. Management of head trauma. *Chest.* 2002;122(2):699–711.

14. Soloniuk D, Pitts LH, Lovely M, et al. Traumatic intracerebral hematomas: Timing of appearance and indications for operative removal. *J Trauma.* 1986;26(9):787–794.

15. Tabori U, Kornecki A, Sofer S, et al. Repeat computed tomographic scan within 24–48 hours of admission in children with moderate and severe head trauma. *Crit Care Med.* 2000;28(3):840–844.

16. Harders A, Kakarieka A, Braakman R. Traumatic subarachnoid hemorrhage and its treatment with nimodipine. German tSAH Study Group. *J Neurosurg.* 1996;85(1):82–89.

17. Matsushita H, Takahashi K, Maeda Y, et al. A clinical study of posttraumatic hydrocephalus. *No Shinkei Geka.* 2000;28(9):773–779.

18. Smith DH, Nonaka M, Miller R, et al. Immediate coma following inertial brain injury dependent on axonal damage in the brainstem. *J Neurosurg.* 2000;93(2):315–322.

19. Pettus EH, Christman CW, Giebel ML, et al. Traumatically induced altered membrane permeability: Its relationship to traumatically induced reactive axonal change. *J Neurotrauma.* 1994;11(5):507–522.

20. American College of Surgeons. *Advanced trauma life support faculty manual.* Chicago: American College of Surgeons; 2004.

21. Teasdale G, Jennett B. Assessment of coma and impaired consciousness. A practical scale. *Lancet.* 1974;2(7872):81–84.

22. Stiell IG, Wells GA, Vandemheen K, et al. The Canadian CT Head Rule for patients with minor head injury. *Lancet.* 2001;357(9266):1391–1396.

23. Haydel MJ, Preston CA, Mills TJ, et al. Indications for computed tomography in patients with minor head injury. *N Engl J Med.* 2000;343(2):100–105.

24. Stein SC, Ross SE. The value of computed tomographic scans in patients with low-risk head injuries. *Neurosurgery.* 1990;26(4):638–640.

25. Shackford SR, Wald SL, Ross SE, et al. The clinical utility of computed tomographic scanning and neurologic examination in the management of patients with minor head injuries. *J Trauma.* 1992;33(3):385–394.

26. Cantu RC. Return to play guidelines after a head injury. *Clin Sports Med.* 1998;17(1):45–60.

27. Quality Standards Subcommittee. Practice parameter: The management of concussion in sports (summary statement). Report of the Quality Standards Subcommittee. *Neurology.* 1997;48(3):581–585.

28. Colrado Medical Society Sports Medicine Committee. *Guidelines for the management of concussion in sports.* Denver, Colorado: Colrado Medical Society;1991.

29. Cushman JG, Agarwal N, Fabian TC, et al. *Practice management guidelines for the management of mild traumatic brain injury. The EAST Practice Management Guidelines Work Group.* Vol. available at http://www.east.org/tpg.asp. Eastern Association for the Surgery of Trauma. 2001.

30. Hills MW, Deane SA. Head injury and facial injury: Is there an increased risk of cervical spine injury? *J Trauma.* 1993;34(4):549–553; discussion 553–4.

31. Robinson N, Clancy M. In patients with head injury undergoing rapid sequence intubation, does pretreatment with intravenous lignocaine/lidocaine lead to an improved neurological outcome? A review of the literature 10.1136/emj.18.6.453. *Emerg Med J.* 2001;18(6):453–457.

32. The Brain Trauma Foundation, The American Association of Neurological Surgeons. The Joint Section on Neurotrauma and Critical Care. Hyperventilation. *J Neurotrauma.* 2000;17(6–7):513–520.

33. van den Brink WA, Santos BO, Marmarou A, et al. Quantitative analysis of blood-brain barrier damage in two models of experimental head injury in the rat. *Acta Neurochir Suppl (Wien).* 1994;60:456–458.

34. The Brain Trauma Foundation, The American Association of Neurological Surgeons. *The Joint Section on Neurotrauma and Critical Care. Guidelines for the management of severe traumatic brain injury: Cerebral perfusion pressure an update.* Available at: http://www2.braintrauma.org/guidelines/, 2003.

35. Colohan AR, Alves WM, Gross CR, et al. Head injury mortality in two centers with different emergency medical services and intensive care. *J Neurosurg.* 1989;71(2):202–207.

36. Marmarou A, Anderson RL, Ward JD, et al. Impact of ICP instability and hypotension on outcome in patients with severe head trauma. *J Neurosurg.* 1991;75(5S):S59–S66.

37. The Brain Trauma Foundation, The American Association of Neurological Surgeons. *The Joint Section on Neurotrauma and Critical Care. Management and Prognosis of Severe Traumatic Brain Injury.* 2000.

38. Stiefel MF, Spiotta A, Gracias VH, et al. Reduced mortality rate in patients with severe traumatic brain injury treated with brain tissue oxygen monitoring. *J Neurosurg.* 2005;103(5):805–811.

39. Gracias VH, Guillamondegui OD, Stiefel MF, et al. Cerebral cortical oxygenation: A pilot study. *J Trauma.* 2004;56(3):469–472; discussion 472–4.

40. van Santbrink H, Maas AI, Avezaat CJ. Continuous monitoring of partial pressure of brain tissue oxygen in patients with severe head injury. *Neurosurgery.* 1996;38(1):21–31.

41. Bullock MR, Chesnut R, Ghajar J, et al. Surgical management of acute subdural hematomas. *Neurosurgery.* 2006;58(Suppl 3):S16–S24; discussion Si-iv.

42. Bullock MR, Chesnut R, Ghajar J, et al. Surgical management of acute epidural hematomas. *Neurosurgery.* 2006;58(Suppl 3):S7–15; discussion Si-iv.

43. Winn H. *Richard youmans neurological surgery*, 5th ed. New York: Elsevier Science;2004.

44. Contant CF, Valadka AB, Gopinath SP, et al. Adult respiratory distress syndrome: A complication of induced hypertension after severe head injury. *J Neurosurg.* 2001;95(4):560–568.

45. Heath DL, Vink R. Neuroprotective effects of MgSO4 and MgCl2 in closed head injury: A comparative phosphorus NMR study. *J Neurotrauma.* 1998;15(3):183–189.

46. Clifton GL, Miller ER, Choi SC, et al. Lack of effect of induction of hypothermia after acute brain injury. *N Engl J Med.* 2001;344(8):556–563.

47. Cushing H. Peptic ulcer and the interbrain. *Surg Obst.* 1932;55:1–34.

48. Temkin NR, Dikmen SS, Wilensky AJ, et al. A randomized, double-blind study of phenytoin for the prevention of post-traumatic seizures. *N Engl J Med.* 1990;323(8):497–502.

49. Salazar AM, Aarabi B, Levi L, et al. Antiseizure prophylaxis for penetrating brain injury. *J Trauma.* 2001;51(Suppl 2):S41–S43.

50. Marik PE, Zaloga GP. Early enteral nutrition in acutely ill patients: A systematic review. *Crit Care Med.* 2001;29(12):2264–2270.

51. Sheinberg M, Kanter MJ, Robertson CS, et al. Continuous monitoring of jugular venous oxygen saturation in head-injured patients. *J Neurosurg.* 1992;76(2):212–217.

52. Cruz J. Relationship between early patterns of cerebral extraction of oxygen and outcome from severe acute traumatic brain swelling: Cerebral ischemia or cerebral viability? *Crit Care Med.* 1996; 24(6):953–956.

53. Hsiang JK, Chesnut RM, Crisp CB, et al. Early, routine paralysis for intracranial pressure control in severe head injury: Is it necessary? *Crit Care Med.* 1994;22(9):1471–1476.

54. Prough DS, Joshi S. Does early neuromuscular blockade contribute to adverse outcome after acute head injury? *Crit Care Med.* 1994; 22(9):1349–1350.

55. Ware ML, Nemani VM, Meeker M, et al. Effects of 23.4% sodium chloride solution in reducing intracranial pressure in patients with traumatic brain injury: A preliminary study. *Neurosurgery.* 2005;57(4):727–736; discussion 727–36.

56. Qureshi AI, Suarez JI, Bhardwaj A, et al. Use of hypertonic (3%) saline/acetate infusion in the treatment of cerebral edema: Effect on intracranial pressure and lateral displacement of the brain. *Crit Care Med.* 1998;26(3):440–446.

57. Suarez JI, Qureshi AI, Bhardwaj A, et al. Treatment of refractory intracranial hypertension with 23.4% saline. *Crit Care Med.* 1998;26(6):1118–1122.

58. Favre JB, Ravussin P, Chiolero R, et al. Hypertonic solutions and intracranial pressure. *Schweiz Med Wochenschr.* 1996; 126(39):1635–1643.

59. Pascual JL, Maloney-Wilensky E, Reilly PM, et al. The effect of an institutional pathway on TBI resuscitation with 7.5% hypertonic saline. *American Surgeon.* 2007. (in press).

60. Shapiro HM, Wyte SR, Loeser J. Barbiturate-augmented hypothermia for reduction of persistent intracranial hypertension. *J Neurosurg.* 1974;40(1):90–100.

61. Surgical management of penetrating brain injury. Part 1 *J Trauma.* 2001;51(Suppl 2):S16–S25.

62. Part 2: Prognosis in penetrating brain injury. *J Trauma.* 2001; 51(Suppl 2):S44–S86.

63. Brandvold B, Levi L, Feinsod M, et al. Penetrating craniocerebral injuries in the Israeli involvement in the Lebanese conflict, 1982–1985. Analysis of a less aggressive surgical approach. *J Neurosurg.* 1990;72(1):15–21.

64. Teasdale GM, Murray G, Anderson E, et al. Risks of acute traumatic intracranial haematoma in children and adults: Implications for managing head injuries. *Br Med J.* 1990;300(6721):363–367.

65. Management of cerebrospinal fluid leaks. Part 1 *J Trauma.* 2001;51(Suppl 2):S29–S33.

Injury to the Spinal Cord

27

Peter G. Thomas   *Neil R. Malhotra*   *M. Sean Grady*

Spinal cord injury (SCI) remains one of the most costly aspects of trauma currently, not just in terms of the financial burden but more importantly, in terms of the physical and emotional burden of the patient. Approximately 40 new cases of SCI are reported per million people each year. This equates to 11,000 cases per year and does not include those who died from their injuries at the scene.[1,2] These numbers represent data collected in the 1970s. No new nationwide incidence study has been conducted since then and as such, it is unknown if the incidence of SCI has changed. Significant improvement has however, been made in the survival rate of these patients. In 1970, 38% of patients with SCI died before hospital arrival.[3] This rate decreased to 15.8% between 1997 and 2000.[4] This reduction in injury has been attributed to increased seat belt and helmet use, improved auto design, improved swimming pool design, and improvements in the training of the prehospital personnel.[2,5,6] Advanced Trauma Life Support (ATLS) mandates that trauma patients be presumed to have a SCI until proved otherwise. Early and safe control of the airway, while protecting from further movement of a SCI, has been a major advance in the last 30 years along with complete spinal immobilization with rigid cervical collars and securing the patient to a full-length backboard.[7]

The age of the patient with SCI has risen over the last 3 decades. In the early 1970s, the average age of injury was approximately 29 years. Currently, the average age of injury is 38 years. In addition, the percentage of people older than 60 years of age with SCI has increased. Before 1980, 4.7% of the patients with SCI were older than 60 years of age but since 2000, this has increased to 11.5%.[1,2] Males comprise approximately 80% of SCI.[1] In 2000, motor vehicle crashes were responsible for 47% of the SCI followed by falls (21%), acts of violence (11%), and recreational sports (10%).[1,8,9] This order has been consistent throughout the last 30 years with the exception of the mid-1990s when gun violence caused more SCI than falls.[10]

ANATOMY

The spinal cord starts at the level of the distal brainstem and continues to the cauda equina, which usually terminates at L1-L2. It is divided into three regions: cervical, thoracic, and lumbosacral. The nerve roots from the cervical cord have a different function in the neck and arms at each level. The thoracic spinal cord supplies the nerve roots for the muscles of the chest and abdominal wall. The lumbosacral spinal cord and nerve roots are responsible for the functions of the pelvis, legs, bowel, bladder, and sexual function (see Fig. 1).

There are several different types of nerves within the spinal cord and each has a different function and hence a different injury pattern and treatment plan. The spinal cord contains both upper motor neurons (UMNs) and lower motor neurons (LMNs). UMN lesions (SCI) are located above the anterior horn cells and result in a spastic type of paralysis. LMN lesions (peripheral nerve injury) occur at or below the level of the anterior horn cells and these lesions tend to cause flaccid paralysis. UMN lesions carry a worse prognosis. There are also sensory nerves that are carried in the cord. These relay pain, temperature, vibration, and proprioception from the skin to the brain. For the purposes of this book, there are two main columns that relay this information. The spinothalamic column relays pain and temperature and it is located in the middle of the spinal

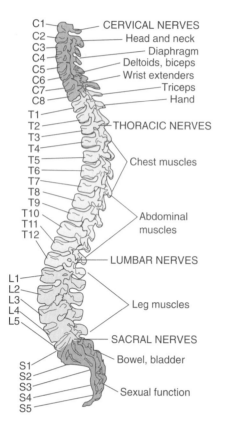

Figure 1   Structures affected by spinal nerves (From Timby B, Smith N. Instructor's resource CD-ROM to accompany essentials of nursing: care of adults and children. Philadelphia: Lippincott Williams & Wilkins, 2005.)

cord. The dorsal columns relay position and sensation or light touch and are located in the posterior portion of the cord (see Fig. 2).

The spinal cord also contains the autonomic nervous system (ANS). The ANS comprises the sympathetic and parasympathetic nervous systems. The sympathetic nerve fibers are located from the first thoracic nerve root to the third or fourth lumbar root. Two of the main functions of the sympathetic nervous system are to cause vasoconstriction of blood vessels and increase heart rate. The parasympathetic nerves are located in the cranial outflow tract and the sacral nerve roots. The cranial outflow tract includes the oculomotor, facial, glossopharyngeal, and vagus nerves. The parasympathetic system is responsible for vasodilating blood vessels and slowing the heart rate. Both systems help control the respiratory, digestive, and cardiovascular systems.[1,11,12] The anatomy of the spine will be discussed in Chapter 28.

EVALUATION/DIAGNOSIS OF INJURY

Physical examination is crucial to correctly determine the level of SCI. Whereas bony vertebral column injury is diagnosed with radiographs (see Chapter 28), SCI is diagnosed

with physical examination and supplemented with magnetic resonance imaging. As stated in the preceding text, all patients with a suspected SCI should be immobilized with a rigid cervical collar and spinal backboard. Rigid long boards should be removed as soon as possible and hard surfaces should be padded during resuscitation and in the operating room. Keep in mind that although a patient may have ambulated at the scene of the accident, it does not mean that serious cord or potential cord injury is not present. Patients may have either a spinal column injury or an SCI and each is neither inclusive nor exclusive of the other.

As with all trauma patients, ATLS protocol should be followed. The patient's airway must be secured, breathing must be adequate, and circulation intact. Full spinal immobilization is continued to prevent any further injury to the cord. Next, a thorough neurologic evaluation should be done. This evaluation should include a sensory and motor examination, a mental status examination, a reflex examination, and cranial nerve testing. The *mental status* can quickly and efficiently be evaluated with the Glasgow Coma Scale (GCS). The motor score is the patient's best movement of the upper extremity. If the patient is unable to move any extremity, but is following a command such as "stick out your tongue," the GCS would be incomplete or guarded with further more exact description of the deficit needed. The vertebral column is palpated feeling for deformities and step-offs. If the patient is alert, tenderness at a particular segment can be indicative of injury. Each extremity should be evaluated individually and each neurologic level assessed. The motor strength should be recorded according to the American Spinal Injury Association/International Medical Society of Paraplegia (ASIA/IMSOP) scoring system. The scale is from 0 to 5. Normal strength is given 5 points whereas some movement against resistance is given 4. Only within the 4 level of strength should a + or − be used to indicate near-normal strength or only slightly more resistance than gravity, respectively. Movement against gravity but not resistance receives 3 points and movement with gravity being eliminated is given 2. Finally, being able to feel muscle twitching is given 1 point and no movement is given 0 points.[13] Some key muscle groups can be quickly tested to determine the level of injury; C5 elbow flexors, C6 wrist extensors, C7 elbow extensors, C8 finger extensors, T1 small finger abductors, L2 hip flexors, L3 knee extensors, L4 ankle dorsiflexion, L5 long toe extensors, and S1 ankle plantar flexors (see Table 1).[14] Sensory testing is somewhat subjective. The scale is 0 to 2 with intact sensation being 2, decreased or hyperesthetic being 1 and no sensation being 0. The location of the dermatomes is shown in Fig. 3. A rectal examination is also a crucial part in evaluating the integrity of the spinal cord. The examination is done for two reasons. The first is to determine motor function of the sphincter muscle. The second is to determine perianal sensation. Presence of either of these demonstrates that there is sacral sparing, which indicates

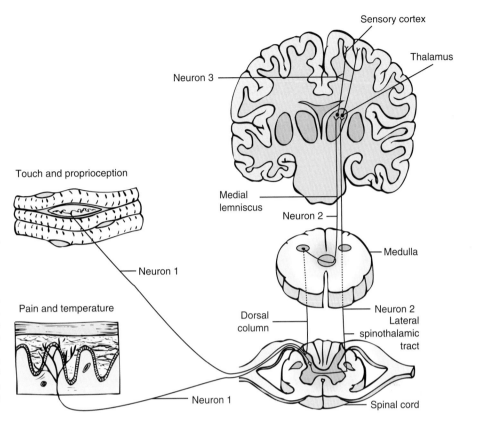

Figure 2 Pathways of ascending tracts. Sensory neurons enter the cord at the dorsal horn. Axons of sensory neurons for touch and proprioception ascend in the dorsal columns to the medulla, where they synapse with second-order projection neurons that cross (decussate) to the opposite side before ascending to the thalamus in the tract called the *medial lemniscus.* First-order neurons for pain and temperature enter the dorsal gray matter of the cord, where they synapse with second-order projection neurons that cross to the opposite side and ascend in the lateral spinothalamic tract to the thalamus. Third-order neurons connect both pathways from thalamus to the sensory cortex. (From Morton PG, Fontaine D, Hudak CM, et al. Instructor's resource CD-ROM to accompany critical care nursing: a holistic approach, 8e. Philadelphia: Lippincott Williams & Wilkins, 2005.)

TABLE 1
CHART OF MUSCLE GROUPS AND NERVE AND NERVE ROOT SUPPLY

Muscle	Nerve Root	Nerve
Cervical flexors	C1-C4	—
Cervical extensors	C1-C4	—
Trapezius	—	Cranial nerve XI
Sternocleidomastoid	—	Cranial nerve XI
Arm abduction		
0 to 15 degrees, supraspinatus	C4-C6	Suprascapular
15 to 90 degrees, deltoid	C5-C6	Axillary
>90 degrees, trapezius and serratus anterior	C5-C7	Long thoracic
Biceps	C5-C6	Musculocutaneous
Forearm supination	C5-C6	Musculocutaneous
Forearm pronation	C6-C7	Median
Wrist flexors	C7-C8, T1	Median
Wrist extensors	C6-C8	Radial
Hand intrinsics	C7-T1	Median and ulnar
Hip flexion	L1-L3	Femoral
Hip extension	L4-S1	Sciatic
Thigh abduction	L4-S2	Superior gluteal
Thigh adduction	L2-L4	Obturator
Leg flexion	L4-S2	Sciatic
Leg extension	L2-L4	Femoral
Foot plantar flexion	L5-S1	Superficial peroneal and tibial
Foot dorsiflexion	L4-L5	Deep peroneal
Great toe extension	L4-L5, S1	Deep peroneal
Foot inversion	L4-L5	Deep peroneal
Foot eversion	L5-L5	Superficial peroneal
Rectal sphincters	S2-S4	Pudendal

(From Welch WC, Donaldson WF, Marion DW. Injuries to the spinal cord and spinal column. *The trauma manual 2e.* Philadelphia: Lippincott Williams & Wilkins; 2002.)

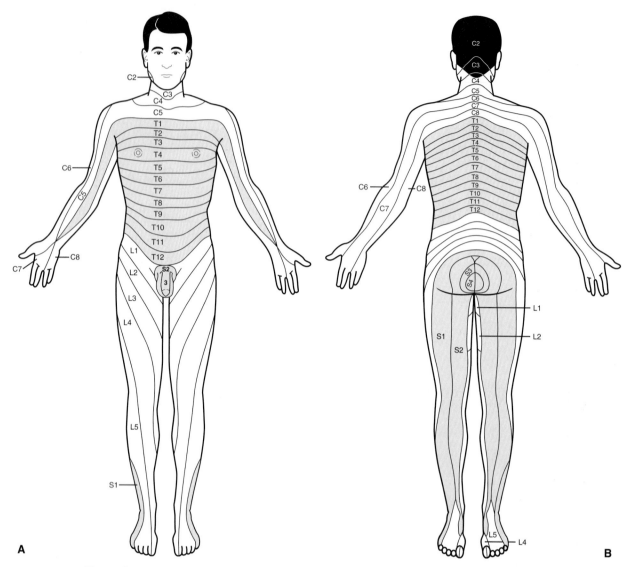

Figure 3   Anterior (A) and posterior (B) cervical, thoracic, lumbar, and sacral dermatomes. (From McDonald JV, Welch WC. Patient history and neurologic examination. In: Welch WC, Jacobs GB, Jackson RP, eds. *Operative spinal surgery*. Stamford: Appleton & Lange; 1999;3:15.)

that there is at least some integrity of the spinal cord because the sacral fibers travel along the periphery of the cord.

The patient can now be classified with the ASIA Impairment Scale; (A) through (E). Complete injury (A) indicates that the patient has no motor or sensory function preserved in the S4-S5 sacral segments. Incomplete injury (B) indicates that sensation is preserved below the neurologic level but motor function is not and this includes the S4-S5 segments. Incomplete injury (C) indicates that motor function is preserved below the injury but more than half of the key muscle groups have a muscle grade of <3. Incomplete injury (D) is the same as (C) but the muscle groups have a grade of ≥3. Classification (E) indicates a normal examination.[15]

Several clinical syndromes also play important roles when describing spinal cord injuries. These spinal cord syndromes are based on which columns of the spinal cord are affected. Central cord syndrome (CCS) primarily results secondary to cervical hyperextension. The classical finding is upper extremity weakness greater than lower extremity weakness. Decreased sensation is variable below the injury site. Patients may also experience bowel and bladder dysfunction. It tends to occur more frequently in the elderly population with cervical spondylosis but all age-groups are at risk. The pathophysiology is believed to be caused by either posterior compression of the cord by the ligamentum flavum or anterior compression from osteophytes. Central cord necrosis may also occur and this has a worse outcome.[16] Despite patients having significant motor and bladder dysfunction at the time of injury, independent ambulation was recovered in 86% of the patients whereas 81% recovered normal bladder and bowel continence.[17]

Anterior cord syndrome is caused by compression or disruption of the anterior spinal artery. The compression is usually caused by a bone fragment or disk in the canal. Clinically, the patient has complete paralysis and loss of pain and temperature but may retain position sense because of the sparing of the posterior spinal cord columns. It also tends to be due to significant hyperflexion of the spinal column. Recovery is generally poor.

Brown-Sequard syndrome occurs with the hemisection of the spinal cord. The patient has ipsilateral motor paralysis and loss of proprioception and contralateral loss of pain and temperature. The loss of pain and temperature is usually two to three segments below the injury whereas the loss of motor function is at the level of injury. The cause of the injury is usually from penetrating trauma or from a hyperflexion injury. Recovery is generally better than CCS and anterior cord syndrome.[18]

Conus medullaris syndrome and cauda equina syndrome occur when there is an injury from T12 to L2. Injury may be caused by either blunt or penetrating trauma. Symptoms encompass a large spectrum from complete paralysis, to perineal or saddle anesthesia to bladder and bowel incontinence. UMN injuries generally have a poorer prognosis.[19] In addition to the syndromes mentioned here, it is quite possible to have an injury pattern that has components of several different syndromes.

Patients may also have either spinal shock or neurogenic shock secondary to the SCI itself. Spinal shock is due to the loss of spinal reflex activity and sympathetic tone below the level of the injury. The patient may have a profound motor and sensory deficit below the area of injury. Initial hypertension may be followed by hypotension. Bladder and bowel function may also be lost and priapism may occur. The symptoms are usually transient and last hours to days. They resolve when the reflex arcs below the area of injury resume function.

Neurogenic shock presents with hypotension, bradycardia, and hypothermia. It generally occurs when the injury is above the level of T6. It occurs from disruption of the sympathetic system and the patient has unopposed vagal tone which reduces vascular resistance. Fluid resuscitation should be started immediately to restore intravascular volume. If hypotension persists, phenylephrine or dopamine may be required. The patient should have continuous venous and arterial monitoring. Consideration should also be given to a pulmonary artery catheter based on the patient's hemodynamics and comorbid conditions. The hypotension is usually self-limited and resolves within 24 to 72 hours.

MANAGEMENT

SCI management is determined upon the appropriate diagnosis. Each injury should be classified as either penetrating or blunt injury and either stable or unstable.

In general, unstable injuries relate to the vertebral column itself. These injuries will be discussed in Chapter 28. A key portion of SCI management is to prevent secondary injury to the spinal cord itself. Ascension of just a single level of SCI can have devastating consequences for the patient; for example, ventilator dependence versus unassisted ventilation or ambulation versus wheelchair dependence.

Spinal immobilization is the first step in SCI management in both penetrating and blunt trauma. This begins at the time of injury and continues until definitive spine stabilization is achieved. Definitive spinal stabilization is determined by the exact injury; however, there are essentially three different modalities: prolonged use of rigid cervical or thoracic/lumbar braces, application of a halo, or spinal surgery.[20] If the lesion is ascending based on physical examination, the patient may benefit from emergent surgical decompression of the cord to prevent further injury and loss of function. An emergent neurosurgical consult must be obtained for further evaluation.

High-dose steroids continue to be a controversial component of SCI management. The most recent recommendations are from the results of the National Acute Spinal Cord Injury Studies (NASCIS 2 and 3).[21,22] In the NASCIS 3, methylprednisolone was given as a bolus of 30 mg/kg body weight followed by 5.4 mg/kg body weight/hour for 23 hours if given within 3 hours of injury. This was extended to 48 hours if the bolus was initiated between 3 and 8 hours from the time of injury. These recommendations are Level II recommendations based on Class II data. The improvement of neurologic function after giving the corticosteroids is based on the theory that the steroids suppress the progressive tissue damage in the spinal cord over the next 1 to 2 days. In particular, the steroids suppress lipid peroxidation and hydrolysis at the injury site, enhance blood flow to the white matter of the spinal cord, and reduce vasoactive by-products from arachidonic acid.[23,24] Although attempts to reproduce these trials have been difficult and the design of the NASCIS studies have been challenged,[25–27] most trauma surgeons and emergency physicians, when surveyed, still consider high-dose steroids for blunt SCI as the standard of care even if they do not truly believe in its efficacy.[23,28] The primary reason cited for steroid use was medicolegal. This was, in part, caused by the release of the NASCIS 2 in 1990 to the media before a scientific review. The study was broadcast on national television and printed in a *New York Times* article that proclaimed the success of the trial and improvement of the patient's disability.[29] This essentially caused methylprednisolone to become the standard of care for SCI overnight.

Penetrating trauma to the spinal cord causes injury by two pathways. The first is by the direct pathway of the bullet and the second is caused by the concussive effects of the bullet.[10] The concussive effects of the bullet may cause injury in two ways; cord injury from the energy distribution of the bullet or vascular compromise of the spinal cord.[30]

LIFE EXPECTANCY FOR PERSONS WHO SURVIVE THE FIRST 24 HOURS

Age at Injury (yr)	No SCI	Motor Functional at any Level	Para	Low Tetra (C5-C8)	High Tetra (C1-C4)	Ventilator Dependent at any Level
20	58.4	52.8	45.6	40.6	36.1	16.6
40	39.5	34.3	28.0	23.5	23.8	20.2
60	22.2	17.9	13.1	10.2	7.9	1.4

SCI, spinal cord injury.
(From the National Spinal Cord Injury Statistical Center (NSCISC), www.spinalcord.uab.edu)

In general, penetrating wounds to the spinal cord are stable injuries and do not need surgical intervention.[31] There has also been no proven benefit of steroids for penetrating injury of the spinal cord.[32]

COMPLICATIONS

The complications of SCI can be many times more morbid than the injury itself. If a patient survives the initial insult, he will potentially have a life of complication after complication. Early recognition and management of these complications greatly improve the patient's quality of life and reduce the overall cost of the injury both to the patient and to society as a whole.

Respiratory complications are frequent in the patient with SCI; the higher the level the more likely it will be severe and require ventilator support. Patients are at greater risk of respiratory failure with some requiring intubation while others are at risk for pneumonia and atelectasis. Patients with combined head injuries have an increased risk of these complications.[33] Although many of the respiratory complications occur with cervical injuries, up to 51% of patients with T1 to T6 SCI and 34.5% with T7 to T12 SCI have respiratory complications.[34] Aggressive pulmonary support, with rotation must be considered immediately in the patient's care, and tracheostomy if ventilatory weaning is unsuccessful should be an early part of critical care management.

Skin breakdown is another significant cause of morbidity, both in the short term and the long term. In addition to the obvious discomfort, difficult dressing changes, and increased nursing care, decubitus ulcers can lead to potential limb loss, sepsis, and death. A single decubitus ulcer may add as much as $70,000 to a hospital bill and 4 to 7 days to the hospital stay.[35] Care involves turning the patient every 2 hours, pressure reducing surfaces, adequate nutrition, and preventing dry skin.

Bladder and bowel dysfunction are also frequent. Patients should be placed on bowel regimens and may need intermittent bladder catheterizations. Long-term catheters should be avoided secondary to the increased risk of urinary tract infections. Patients with SCI may have esophageal and swallowing dysfunction, increasing the risk of aspiration.[36] Aspiration precautions should be followed and a swallowing study should be obtained.

There is a high prevalence of deep venous thrombosis (DVT) and pulmonary embolism (PE) in SCI patients with 60% to 100% of patients developing DVTs and up to 10% developing PEs in patients without prophylaxis. Patients should be started on thromboprophylaxis as soon as possible. The American College of Chest Physician 2004 guidelines classify patients with SCI in the highest risk stratification. The recommended prophylaxis is low molecular weight heparin (LMWH), oral vitamin K antagonist or sequential compression devices (SCDs) in combination with low-dose unfractionated heparin (LDUH) or LMWH. LDUH or SCDs used alone have not been shown to be

LIFE EXPECTANCY FOR PERSONS WHO SURVIVE AT LEAST 1 YEAR POSTINJURY

Age at Injury (yr)	No SCI	Motor Functional at any Level	Para	Low Tetra (C5-C8)	High Tetra (C1-C4)	Ventilator Dependent at any Level
20	58.4	53.3	46.3	41.7	37.9	23.3
40	39.5	34.8	28.6	24.7	21.6	11.1
60	22.2	18.3	13.5	10.8	8.8	3.1

(From the National Spinal Cord Injury Statistical Center (NSCISC), www.spinalcord.uab.edu)

TABLE 4

AVERAGE YEARLY EXPENSES IN MAY 2006 (IN $)

Severity of Injury	First Year	Each Subsequent Year
High tetraplegia (C1-C4)	$ 741,425	$ 132,807
Low tetraplegia (C5-C8)	$ 478,782	$ 54,400
Paraplegia	$ 270,913	$ 27,568
Incomplete motor functional at any level	$ 218,504	$ 15,313

(From the National Spinal Cord Injury Statistical Center (NSCISC), www.spinalcord.uab.edu)

efficacious. Inferior vena cava (IVC) filters are not currently recommended as the primary prophylaxis against PEs.[37] Although there is no concrete evidence supporting IVC filters, most trauma centers are placing them in combination with SCDs to lower the potential risk of fatal PEs.

Spasticity is another painful complication of SCI. It is an exaggeration of the normal reflexes of the body and occurs below the level of the injury. It usually occurs in response to irritation or stretching of the muscles below the injury. Bladder infections, skin breakdown, and immobility can cause these spasms. Prevention starts with physical therapy and proper skin care. Muscle relaxants such as baclofen, dantrolene, and diazepam have been shown to give some relief.

Patients develop significant musculoskeletal problems as well. Osteoporosis and fractures are common from disuse. When bones no longer have to bear weight, they lose calcium and phosphorus and subsequently become brittle and break. Heterotopic ossifications (HO) are the abnormal deposition of bone in joints causing stiffness and ultimately fusion of the joint. The main therapy for prevention and treatment of both these conditions is aggressive physical therapy to prevent muscle and bone atrophy.

Autonomic dysfunction (AD) occurs in patients with injuries above T6. The patient has an unopposed sympathetic outflow with stimulation below the level of injury. Patients have severe hypertension due to the vasoconstriction of vessels. Below the level of injury, the skin is cool and clammy. The patient's brain tries to lower the blood pressure by increasing parasympathetic output above the injury. This causes bradycardia, flushing, and a crushing headache. The morbidity of AD includes all of the diseases associated with severe hypertension; stroke, myocardial infarction, seizures, renal failure, and death. The list of precipitating factors that cause AD is extensive. Bladder distension, fecal impaction, gallstones, gastritis, decubitus ulcers, menstruation, DVTs, PEs, HO, and pain have all been implicated. The main treatment of AD is prevention of the causative factors with aggressive physical, occupational, and respiratory therapy. If AD does develop, it is a medical emergency. The patient should be placed in the sitting position to help pool blood in the lower extremities and decrease blood pressure. Any restrictive clothing should be removed. A Foley catheter should be placed because bladder distension is the most common cause of AD. Fecal impaction is the second most common cause and as such, disimpaction may be necessary. If the patient remains hypertensive, a short-acting antihypertensive agent such as immediate release nifedipine should be given through the "bite and swallow" method. Other possible agents include hydralazine, nitroglycerin, nitropaste, and sodium nitroprusside. The patient should be monitored at least 2 hours after the hypertension resolves because if the precipitating event has not been treated, the hypertension may recur.[38]

CONCLUSION

SCI continues to be a significant cause of morbidity and mortality. In addition to the enormous physical costs, there is a tremendous financial cost. Tables 2 and 3 show the significant decrease in life expectancy. Tables 4 and 5 show the financial costs of SCI.

Clearly, prevention of the initial injury will have the greatest impact on overall survival and quality of life.

TABLE 5

ESTIMATED LIFETIME COSTS BY AGE AT INJURY (DISCOUNTED AT 2%)

Severity of Injury	25 years old	50 years old
High tetraplegia (C1-C4)	$ 2,924,513	$ 1,721,677
Low tetraplegia (C5-C8)	$ 1,653,607	$ 1,047,189
Paraplegia	$ 977,142	$ 666,473
Incomplete motor functional at any level	$ 651,827	$ 472,392

(From the National Spinal Cord Injury Statistical Center (NSCISC), www.spinalcord.uab.edu)

Once injury has occurred, the main goal is to stabilize the patient and prevent secondary injury of the spinal cord. Aggressive and early rehabilitation must be achieved to prevent the many complications of this devastating injury. To obtain these goals, care of the patient with SCI has to be a group effort by physicians, surgeons, nurses, physical and occupational therapists, rehabilitation therapists, and family members.

REFERENCES

1. National Spinal Cord Injury Statistical Center (NSCISC). *Facts and Figures at a Glance*, June 2006. The National SCI Statistical Center, University of Alabama; www.NSCISC@uab.edu, 2006.
2. Fisher CG, Noonan VK, Dvorak MF. Changing face of spine trauma care in North America. *Spine*. 2006;31:S2–S8.
3. Kraus JF, Franti CE, Riggins RS, et al. Incidence of traumatic spinal cord lesions. *J Chronic Dis*. 1975;28:471–492.
4. Dryden DM, Saunders LD, Rowe BH, et al. The epidemiology of traumatic cord injury in Alberta, Canada. *Can J Neurol Sci*. 2003; 30:113–121.
5. Tyrocj AH, Davis JW, Kaups KL, et al. Spinal cord injury: A preventable public burden. *Arch Surg*. 1997;132:778–781.
6. Kelly DF, Becker DP. Advances in neurosurgical trauma: USA and Canada. *World J Surg*. 2001;25:1179–1185.
7. Advanced trauma life support for Doctors, *Student Course Manual*, 7th ed, American College of Surgeons, 2004.
8. Fries JM. Critical rehabilitation of the patient with spinal cord injury. *Crit Care Nurs Q*. 2005;2:179–187.
9. Jackson AB, Dijkers M, Devivo MJ, et al. A demographic profile of new traumatic spinal cord injuries: Change and stability over 30 years. *Arch Phys Med Rehabil*. 2004;85:1740–1748.
10. Kitchel SH. Current treatment of gunshot wounds to the spine. *Clin Orthop Related Res*. 2003;408:115–119.
11. Ganong WF. *Review of medical physiology*. Norwalk: Appleton & Lange; 1993.
12. Peitzman AB, Rhodes M, Schwab CW, et al. eds. *The trauma manual*, 2nd ed. Philadelphia: Lippincott Williams & Wilkins; 2002.
13. Ditunno JF, Young W, Donovan WH, et al. The international standards booklet for neurological and functional classification of spinal cord injury. American Spinal Injury Association. *Paraplegia*. 1994;32:70–80.
14. Dawodu ST. Spinal cord injury: Definition, epidemiology, pathophysiology. *Emedicine*. 2005.
15. ASIA Impairment Scale, American Spinal Injury Association (ASIA). www.ASIA-spinalinjury.org, 2006.
16. Song J, Mizuno J, Nakagawa H. Clinical evaluation of traumatic central cord syndrome: Emphasis on clinical significance of prevertebral hyperintensity, cord compression, and intramedullary high-signal intensity on magnetic resonance imaging. *Surg Neurol*. 2006; 65:117–123.
17. Dvorak MF, Fisher CG, Hoekema J, et al. Factors predicting motor recovery and functional outcome after traumatic central cord syndrome. *Spine*. 2005;30:2303–2311.
18. Staffer ES. Neurologic recovery following injuries to the cervical spinal cord and nerve roots. *Spine*. 1984;9:532–534.
19. Harrop JS, Hunt GE, Vaccaro AR. Conus medullaris and cauda equina syndrome as a result of traumatic injuries: management principles. *Neurosurg Focus*. 2004;16:19–23.
20. Rechtine GR. Nonoperative management and treatment of spinal injuries. *Spine*. 2006;31:S22–S27.
21. Bracken MB, Shepard MJ, Collins WF, et al. A randomized controlled trial of methylprednisolone or naloxone in the treatment of acute spinal cord injury: Results of the second national acute spinal cord injury study. *N Engl J Med*. 1990;322:1405–1411.
22. Bracken MB, Shepard MJ, Holford TR, et al. Administration of methylprednisolone for 24 or 48 hours or tirilazad mesylate for 48 hours in the treatment of acute spinal cord injury. Results of the third National Acute Spinal Cord injury randomized controlled trial. *JAMA*. 1997;277:1597–1604.
23. Vellman WP, Hawkes AP, Lammertse DP. Administration of corticosteroids for acute spinal cord injury. *Spine*. 2003;28:941–947.
24. Amar AP, Levy ML. Pathogenesis and pharmacological strategies for mitigating secondary damage in acute spinal cord injury. *Neurosurgery*. 1999;44:1027–1039.
25. Trivedi JM. Spinal trauma: Therapy – options and outcomes. *Eur J Surg*. 2002;42:127–134.
26. Short DJ, El Masry WS, Jones PW. High dose methylprednisolone in the management of acute spinal cord injury. *J Spinal Disord*. 2000;38:273–286.
27. Coleman WP, Benzel D, Cahill DW, et al. A critical appraisal of the reporting of the National Acute Spinal Cord Injury Studies (II and III) of methylprednisolone in acute spinal cord injury. *J Spinal Disord*. 2000;13:185–199.
28. Eck JC, Nachitigall D, Hodges SD. Questionnaire survey of spine surgeons on the use of methylprednisolone for acute spinal cord injury. *Spine*. 2006;31:E250–E253.
29. Leary W. Treatment is said to reduce disability from spinal injury. *NY Times (Print)*. 1990;48:191.
30. Mirovsky Y, Shalmon E, Halperin N. Complete paraplegia following gunshot injury without direct trauma to the cord. *Spine*. 2005; 30:2436–2438.
31. Aryan HE, Amar AP, Ozgur BM, et al. Gunshot wounds to the spine in adolescents. *Neurosurgery*. 2005;57:748–752.
32. Heary RF, Vaccaro AR, Mesa JJ, et al. Steroids and gunshot wounds to the spine. *Neurosurgery*. 1997;41:576–584.
33. Como JJ, Sutton ER, McCunn M, et al. Characterizing the need for mechanical ventilation following cervical spinal cord injury with neurologic deficit. *J Trauma*. 2005;59:912–916.
34. Cotton BA, Pryor JP, Chinwalla I, et al. Respiratory complications and mortality risk associated with thoracic spine injury. *J Trauma*. 2005;59:1400–1409.
35. Reddy M, Sundeep SG, Rochon PA. Preventing pressure ulcers: A systematic review. *JAMA*. 2006;296:974–984.
36. Neville AL, Crookes P, Velmahos GC, et al. Esophageal dysfunction in cervical spinal cord injury: A potentially important mechanism of aspiration. *J Trauma*. 2005;59:905–911.
37. Geertz WH, Pineo GF, Heit JA, et al. Prevention of venous thromboembolism: The seventh ACCP conference on antithrombotic and thrombolytic therapy. *Chest*. 2004;126:338–400.
38. Karlsson AK. Autonomic dysfunction in spinal cord injury: Clinical presentation of symptoms and signs. *Prog Brain Res*. 2006; 152:1–8.

Injury to the Spine

28

Neil R. Malhotra　　*P. Thomas*　　*M.S. Grady*

EPIDEMIOLOGY

Significant advancements have been made at every level of care for the spine injured patient, from transport methodology to improved imaging modalities to diagnose injury to less invasive, more precise operative interventions. Despite remarkable progress in the care of the spine trauma patient, these injuries, especially when associated with neurovascular injury, remain a debilitating source of burden for the patient, the health care system, and the economy.

Spine and associated spinal cord injuries assail 180,000 to 230,000 males while in the prime of their lives.[1] The spine injury patient is most often male (81% male preponderance) and half of the time is between 16 and 30 years of age.[2] The spine injury is most often incurred in motor vehicle crash (43%), followed by violence (18.9%), falls (18.8%), and sport injury (11.1%).[2]

Safety advancements in car manufacturing can be attributed for a plateau in motor vehicle–related injuries although violence-related injury has expanded at an alarming rate.[3] Penetrating wounds, related to gunshot injury, are a common source of combined bone and cord injury. Substance abuse appears to have intimate connections to these violent, gun-induced, injuries.[4]

While ground was being lost to gun violence–related penetrating wounds during the 1990s, significant media attention was devoted to sports-related injury.[5,6] It is unclear if media attention reduced injury rates. Even if injury rates where reduced, it was likely a fleeting moment in the history of sporting as newly invented sports become progressively faster, less regulated, and more "extreme."

Ultimate solutions to the spine injury problem will not be found in our trauma bays but rather in political arenas where intervention can be directed at a point in the time line before the injury ever occurs. As patient care providers try to determine their role in the political process focused on improved safety for all, they must never lose sight of their role in the care of these patients late in the time line

when rigorous attention to detail can reduce morbidity and mortality. Understanding spine anatomy is the first step toward understanding spine injury and improving care of the spine injured patient.

SPINE ANATOMY

The human spine is composed of 31 segments including 8 cervical, 12 thoracic, 5 lumbar, and 6 sacrococcygeal segments (see Table 1). The adult spinal cord ends posterior to the L1-2 vertebral body. Neurologic examination should provide objective information related to lowest level of normal function and hence suggest anatomic site of injury.

TABLE 1

KEY SEGMENTAL SPINAL CORD LEVEL AND FUNCTION. LOCALIZATION OF INJURY BASED ON PHYSICAL EXAMINATION BEGINS WITH AN UNDERSTANDING OF NEUROLOGICALLY NORMAL FUNCTION ASSOCIATED WITH EACH SPINE LEVEL

Level	Function
C3, C4, C5	Supply to diaphragm
C5, C6	Shoulder movement, raise arm (deltoid), flexion of elbow (biceps)
C6	External arm rotation (supination)
C6, C7, C8	Extend elbow and wrist, (wrist pronation)
C7, C8, T1	Wrist flexion
C8, T1	Small musculature of hand
T1-T6	Intercostals and trunk above waist
T7-L1	Abdominal muscles
L1, L2, L3, L4	Thigh flexion
L4, L5, S1	Foot dorsiflexion
L5, S1, S2	Foot plantarflexion

Rapid, accurate neurologic assessment allows localization of possible fracture sites before any imaging. Spinal cord injury is often associated with head injury, which can complicate assessment and result in diminished reliance on physical examination with concomitant increase in reliance on imaging. Complete injury is often very clear and outcomes are well documented while incomplete injury results in a more complicated examination and a wider variety of outcomes. Effective care implemented at the first patient interface can significantly improve outcome in the incomplete injury.

In the cervical spine a few key findings allow localization and it is here that that one level of returned function from rapid effective care is most significant to outcome. Injuries to the level of C3 can often be clinically silent although cord injury here can result in diaphragm paralysis and ventilator dependence. With cord injury at the C4-5 level one may maintain some shoulder capability but wrist and hand function are eliminated. A functioning C6 level allows wrist function but no hand function. C7 permits arm straightening and hand use and is often regarded as the level that permits functional independence.

Thoracic fractures are rarely recognized before imaging. Cord injuries between T1 and T8 lead to lack of control of abdominal muscles making trunk control difficult whereas injury below T8 permits good sitting balance. Lumbar fractures are frequent but resultant neurologic injury is more difficult to predict than rostral levels given because nerve roots float freely and one may be injured while another escapes compression. Injury to lumbar nerve roots can lead to diminished control of the legs, hips, and anus. Neurologic examination and spine injury assessment should be assessed at each level of care, starting at the point of the patient's injury and retrieval.

PATIENT RETRIEVAL

Patient evaluation and spine protection begins at the site of patient retrieval. Increased awareness of potential spine injury, and proper immobilization, can prevent unnecessary cord damage and can significantly reduce further functional decline.[7] Unfortunately, all too often the Good Samaritan, unaware of spine injury, can make matters much worse before the arrival of emergency medical technicians (EMT).[8,9] *Airway, Breathing, and Circulation,* as with all trauma evaluations, start the course of treatment. Full spine immobilization should be implemented immediately. All accident victims must be assumed to have an unstable spine. History and physical examination are good and, if present, pain along the spine is indicative of a spinal column injury.

Head to toe secondary survey permits isolation of motor and sensory deficits that can provide clues to level of injury. Scalp lacerations, cervical spine tenderness, and obvious deformity suggest presence of cervical fracture. Cervical collar should not be considered to be complete immobilization as it permits significant translation especially in the high cervical spine where failed immobilization is most fatal.[10,11] The cervical soft collar, which permits neck movement in all directions, should never be considered for use in the trauma setting.[12] Securing the neck with parallel bilateral sand bags and silk tape is accepted as the most effective method of immobilization without airway obstruction and the addition of rigid collar eliminates the potential for hyperextension.[13] When turning is necessary, as in the case of emesis, the patient should be log rolled by three members of the team with the neck held in neutral position. Flat firm backboard is the standard of care for most patients but is not always ideal. Young children whose heads are proportionately larger than their body should be placed on back board with a hole for the head as boards without this feature result in an unacceptable amount of cervical flexion.[14] Rarely one is presented with an ankylosing spondilitis patient, who must be transported in the most comfortable position rather than risk inducing new fractures by forcing an abnormally fused spine into a "normal" position.[15] Once secured, the spine injury patient is brought to the closest trauma facility for further care.

TRAUMA/HOSPITAL EVALUATION

On arrival at the trauma center, the spine injury patient must be evaluated in the same detailed algorithm employed for all trauma patients. Evaluation must be repeated at multiple time points to catch progressive or ascending decline in neurologic function. All organ systems must be optimized to prevent secondary injury such as increase in spinal cord stroke from relative hypoxia. Subsequent to primary trauma survey, neurologic examination and external assessment for spinal deformity (e.g., spinous process step-off) radiologic evaluation should be initiated.

Physical examination in the trauma bay is critical to prioritization of care. Neurologic examination should include evaluation of lowest level of normal sensory and motor function. Neurologic motor examination is graded 1 to 5 in each major muscle group:

5—overcomes full resistance
4 (4+, 4, 4−)—overcomes some resistance
3—overcomes gravity but no resistance
2—does not overcome gravity but moves in the plain of gravity or
1—muscle twitch can be felt

The examiner should evaluate the patient for obvious deformity of the spinous processes. Neurologic examination and deformity assessment will guide selection of imaging studies. Physical examination is the guide that will direct selection of imaging studies and is most crucial when time, due to hemodynamic instability, or lack of facilities, necessitates limited imaging evaluation. As examination and evaluation progresses a member of the team should speak with emergency transport personal to determine the best examination in the field. A clear decline in neurologic function alters the course of further care and time line for interventions. In the stable patient, imaging studies immediately follow primary and secondary evaluation.

RADIOLOGY

Radiologic evaluation should be determined based on capabilities of the facility at hand to optimize amount of data gained in minimal time. Set algorithms designed by a multidisciplinary team within each center based on accepted guidelines is a most effective standard of practice[16-19] Trauma patients should undergo radiologic evaluation while still immobilized. Standard imaging modalities include computed tomography (CT), plain radiography, fluoroscopy, magnetic resonance imaging (MRI), and angiography. While CT has surpassed use of plain films in the evaluation of cervical spine injuries in many centers, plain films continue to serve as an excellent adjunct in the evaluation of this patient population, especially if CT is not immediately available.

The cervical spine series should include four views (i.e., lateral, open-mouth odontoid, anteroposterior, and oblique views).[20,21] Anterior, posterior, and lateral thoracic and lumbar films should also be attained. The plain films should be initially viewed for adequacy before evaluation for injury. If a patient is critically unstable, and time exists for only one film, one should acquire a lateral cervical spine film, which has a sensitivity of 70% to 80%.[21-25] Patient hemodynamic stability permitting, addition of open mouth and anteroposterior views will significantly improve sensitivity to cervical injury.[22,23,26,27] Insofar as the thoracic and lumbar spine is concerned, there are few clinically relevant fractures missed when standard trauma radiography protocols are followed.[28] CT has significantly enhanced the evaluation of spine injury in recent years.

When examination is limited by intubation and sedation or concomitant head injury, one must rely on available imaging and examination techniques until such time that a reasonable examination can be completed. The physical examination should include palpation of all spinous processes for clear step-off or fracture. Imaging studies that have shown promise for evaluation include helical CT. Helical CT offers nearly twice the sensitivity of plain films and rarely misses unstable fractures as opposed to plain radiography.[29] In situations where a patient is hemodynamically stable but without adequate neurologic examination, a combination of studies are commonly performed.

In situations in which only one modality of imaging will be permitted (e.g., multiple severe injuries, need for immediate surgery, etc.) CT has become the modality of choice for assessment of acute spinal trauma.[30] CT is appealing for its quick and effective assessment of bony abnormalities of the spine while securing crucial information about other organ systems in the multisystem trauma patient. When serving as a follow-up to plain radiography, thin slice CT can help clarify degree of abnormality.[8,30-32] In situations in which additional studies such as dynamic study (e.g., flexion extension) or angiographic study, in the setting of penetrating trauma, will be needed, CT should always precede such studies. When one is considering angiography for carotid or ventrical artery injury, one should consider CT angiography as it can provide information about possible vascular injury as well as bony abnormality in one study. CT angiography is particularly useful in assessment of penetrating injury.

Multiple modalities of imaging exist but everything beyond plain films and CT is to be considered secondary measures used for the evaluation of selected patients. MRI is especially valuable in assessing ligamentous injury, soft tissue pathology, and cord compression,[33-36] but its use is limited by inability to effectively assess bone pathology, and to provide adequate images in acutely injured, restless, unstable patients. Other imaging modalities, infrequently requested by the spine surgeon, include myelography and angiography. From a perspective of spine care, a rare exception of direct procession to CT is the patient with clear fracture/dislocation on plain films with progressing neurologic deficit. Rarely a patient will require implementation of closed reduction through traction before performance and evaluation of imaging studies beyond plain films.

CERVICAL TRACTION

Traction is applied in a variety of settings but early placement is most important with clear abnormality on plain films associated with concomitant acutely declining neurologic examination. Traction can play a major role in correction of cervical spine abnormalities but is ineffective in lower spine regions. The goal of early intervention is to reduce misalignment, resulting in decompression of neural elements, before the onset of irreversible deficit.[37,38] It has been argued that early reduction of compressive injury may confer recovery benefit.[39-41] It has been advocated that reduction not be delayed by waiting for MRI and further that this is a safe practice.[42] Early intervention consists of either surgical intervention or closed reduction by way of traction, at the discretion of the surgeon.

Accepted indications for cervical traction include facet joint subluxation (e.g., unilateral perched, or bilateral jumped facet), as well as burst type fractures.[43] Contraindications to cervical traction include certain skull fractures and distractive type of injuries,[44,45] as well as certain types of scalp injuries.[43]

Cervical traction is commonly achieved through Gardner-Wells tongs. One must always consider whether a halo would be more suitable for a given injury or patient. Halo traction seems most beneficial as a final treatment, when surgery will not be indicated, in the setting of pediatric spine trauma,[46] where more pins will lead to a lower skull fracture risk, and in cases of atlanto-occipital dislocation, to prevent distraction and high fatality risk. When weight-based traction is to be applied, the Gardner-Wells tongs are an excellent option for their ease of use, low cost, and reusability.

The Gardner-Wells tongs can be applied at the bedside with only local anesthetic and permit serial addition of weights to manifest reduction. The tongs are a semicircular rigid device that follows the contour of the calvarium. A torque-sensitive pin (one side) allows determination of degree of pressure displaced to the skull at insertion site, which is generally 2 cm above the pinna of the ear. Thirty lb of compressive force is applied to the skull at maximal setting and is confirmed again at 24 hours to ensure this is unchanged; thereafter no pressure adjustments are performed. Although anterior or posterior pin placement, to coincide with mechanism of injury, can be performed, we do not advocate this approach given the risk of miscalculation. Once securely in place, the tongs can be effectively employed for cervical reduction.

Slow, judicious, addition of weight is the most effective and safe approach to external reduction. Before weight addition, one must assure oneself that the mechanism of injury is not distractive with associated ligamentous injury. Failure to recognize occipitocervical dislocation, for example, would result in rapid patient demise on application of weight. Typically, traction would not be used in occipital-C1 dislocation cases. When mechanism of injury is clear, and traction indicated, it is always prudent to begin with a small amount of weight (e.g., 10 lb). Escalation of weight should be limited to 5 Lb increments and in general should not a exceed a total combined 5 Lbs per level (e.g. 25 Lbs max at C5). Muscle relaxants can be very affective in preventing failure of reduction due to muscle tension. Lateral radiograph should be completed for each incremental addition of weight to demonstrate correction or over distraction. Extensive distraction is a contraindication to further addition of weight, especially at sites away from the goal distraction site, and suggests that open correction of deformity will be required. Progression of neurologic deficit is a clear contraindication to continuance of cervical traction. Evaluation of imaging permits the surgeon to determine type of fracture or dislocation and thereby select appropriate surgical intervention.

COMMON ANATOMY INJURY/MECHANISM/EVALUATIONS OF IMAGING STUDIES

Working knowledge of spine anatomy, common types of injury, and associated mechanisms permits thorough trauma bay evaluation and guides further workup and treatment. Evaluation of imaging serves as a further guide to degree of instability and need for intervention, surgical or otherwise.

In the cervical spine, there is no one universally accepted fracture classification scheme. When evaluating imaging, one must divide the spine into regions for thorough evaluation. One must assess the craniocervical junction, the atlantoaxial junction, the subaxial cervical spine and the cervicothoracic junction. Denis three-column model of spine biomechanics offers definition of instability after injury.[47] While Denis' model was designed for the thoracolumbar spine, it is an effective adjunct in evaluation of cervical spine injuries as well. The posterior column consists of what Holdsworth described as the posterior ligamentous complex. The middle column includes the posterior longitudinal ligament, posterior annulus fibrosis, and posterior wall of the vertebral body.[48] The anterior column consists of the anterior vertebral body, anterior annulus fibrosis, and anterior longitudinal ligament.[48] A three-column analysis of the imaging findings serves as an initial assessment for stability.

Spine stability assessment by algorithm, in theory, is very specific; however, in application it can only really serve as a guide. Clinically cervical spine stability implies (a) there will not be excessive displacement or deformity under physiologic loading, (b) that deformity and abnormal displacement will not develop during the healing process, and (c) neural element compression does not exist and will not develop under normal physiologic loading.[15] Determination of stability begins with understanding of common fracture types.

FRACTURE TYPES

Each segment of the spine has a proclivity for certain types of fracture given the design and the most common mechanisms of injury. The spectrum of the most common injuries in the cervical and thoracolumbar spine include pathology that require morbid and extensive surgeries for injuries that require only immobilization in the cervical hard collar or thoracolumbar sacral orthosis (TLSO) brace. In a chapter of this nature, only the truly most common fractures can be covered briefly.

At the top of the cervical spine rests the atlas, providing articulation between the spine and occiput at the occipital condyle. Condylar fractures are commonly a result of axial load and are frequently missed on cervical radiograph.[49] Patients are usually neurologically intact, require CT scan for proper evaluation and rarely require anything more than cervical orthosis, except in the setting of avulsion of the alar ligament where halo vest or surgery may be indicated.[50,51] Atlanto-occipital (A-O) dislocation is probably a distraction type injury that can be fatal if unrecognized and is usually first documented as a large gap between the atlas and the occiput on lateral radiograph (see Fig. 1). A-O dislocation

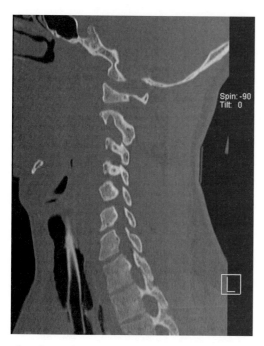

Spin: -90
Tilt: 0

L

Figure 1 Sagittal reconstruction of cervical spine computed tomography (CT) scan demonstrating increased gap between C1 and the occipital condyle, suggestive of atlanto-occipital dislocation. Additional imaging demonstrated increasing distance between basion and tip of dens.

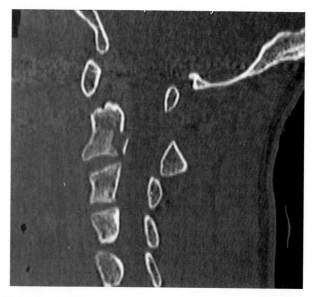

Figure 2 Sagittal reconstruction of cervical spine computed tomography (CT) scan demonstrating comminuted fracture of C2 consistent with Hangman type fracture.

is frequently associated with significant neurologic deficit, as opposed to atlas fractures, and requires fusion and halo vest placement.

Atlas fractures account for 10% of cervical spine fractures, are only rarely associated with neurologic deficit, and in 50% of cases are associated with other cervical spine fractures.[15,50] Injury to the transverse ligament, suggested by increasing atlanto-dens interval, imply instability and can lead to need for surgical stabilization. Below the atlas lies the axis, a site of many types of fractures.

Odontoid fractures make up 5% to 15% of cervical spine fractures and are associated with neurologic deficit in 25% of cases and mortality in 5% to 10% of cases.[50] The Anderson and D'Alonzo classification is a widely accepted assessment of odontoid fractures.[52] Type I fractures require orthosis if stable, type II fractures require halo vest stabilization or surgery, and type III fractures are treated with halo. These types of fractures have a high risk of nonunion especially type II fractures in patients older than 50 years and in cases of >5 mm of displacement. Other portions of the axis are also at risk of fracture in spine trauma.

Axis lateral mass fractures and traumatic spondylolisthesis fractures, commonly referred to as *Hangman*, are other types of common fractures seen in C2. Lateral mass fractures are commonly attributed to axial loading and frequently require no more than cervical orthosis. Hangman fractures involve bilateral pars interarticularis, are believed to result from hyperextension, and are rarely associated

with neurologic deficit (see Fig. 2). Traumatic spondylolisthesis is commonly treated with cervical orthosis.[15] The cervical spine below the axis is commonly evaluated together, rather than by vertebral level, because of similar anatomy and fracture types.

Allen et al., in 1982, developed a classification system for the subaxial cervical spine that is consistently applied now.[53] Compression fractures are usually associated with osteoporosis and are treated with immobilization in cervical collar. Cervical burst fractures involving all three columns are treated surgically if the patient is neurologically incomplete and on occasion with halo vest immobilization if complete (see Fig. 3). Teardrop fractures resulting from hyperflexion are commonly associated with neurologic deficit and require stabilization. Facet dislocation, while not a fracture, requires open or closed reduction; surgical fusion is highly advocated (see Fig. 4). C7 spinous process fractures are frequently referred to as *Clay Shoveler fracture* and thought to be stable although frequently painful. The Clay Shoveler fracture, like all spine fractures, suggests a severe mechanism and indicates need for aggressive search for other spine fractures and ligamentous injuries.

Thoracic and lumbar fractures are similar to the cervical subaxial spine in many ways. The multisystem trauma patient with head injury and extremity fracture will frequently have associated vertebral fracture[54] and will often complain of back pain. Wedge compression fractures are the most common major fracture seen in this region of the spine. Usually considered stable, a wedge fracture involves the anterior column alone most frequently. Posterior column involvement in wedge fractures through distraction can result in instability. Thoracolumbar burst fractures are similar to wedge fractures

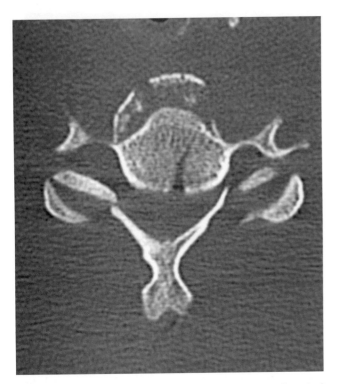

Figure 3   Axial computed tomographic (CT) image of cervical spine (C6) demonstrating burst fracture. Note bilateral laminar fractures that indicate fracture of all three columns.

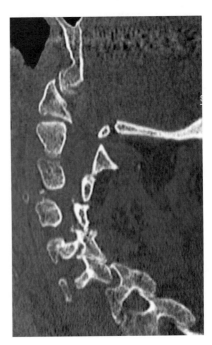

Figure 4   Sagittal reconstruction of cervical spine computed tomography (CT) scan demonstrating facet dislocation of C6 on C7. Note normal facet alignment at joint above and below the C6 on C7 "jumped" facet.

but result from both anterior and middle column failure from the addition of axial compression to the flexion of the wedge fracture. Although the Denis classification would rule the burst fracture, a two-column injury, unstable, these can commonly be braced without progressive deformity. In cases where posterior column fractures coexist, the burst fracture tends to reach criteria for instability and requires fusion. Another common fracture observed is the so-called seatbelt or Chance fracture, named respectively for the common mechanism and first to describe it. In the Chance fracture, the anterior column is preserved and serves as a sort of hinge whereas the posterior two have failed. Patients with these fractures are commonly neurologically intact; however, the spine is unstable and requires fusion. Fracture dislocation injuries account for approximately 20% of thoracolumbar injuries and must be addressed based on specifics of the injury.[47] Penetrating injuries can be considered to be in a separate category of fractures.

Penetrating injury, related to gunshot wound, and its role in spine injury is significant. Most civilian gunshot wounds are lower velocity and result in stable thoracolumbar spine fractures. Most of the time bullet fragments need not be removed. One must always assess wounds for cerebrospinal fluid drainage. Most authors have recommended surgical intervention only for stabilization.[55] Laminectomy for these wounds results in increased cerebrospinal fluid

leak, infection, and instability when compared to nonoperative management.[56] Penetrating, high-velocity gunshot, and shotgun injuries commonly require significant debridement and can bring about instability.[57] Clinical judgment in association with assessment of the spine with regard to accepted biomechanical models aid in determination of stability in this setting.

SURGICAL INTERVENTION

Surgical goals in all spine fracture include maximizing neurologic function while providing stability to the unstable spine. Stated simply, the goals of spine trauma surgery are to decompress neural elements and induce fusion. If decompression is not necessary, for example, stable neurologic condition, and the spine does not require man-made construct for support, arthrodesis is all that is needed. In the setting where requirements for surgery are met, careful evaluation of mechanistic details of injury, physical examination, appropriate imaging, and anatomy will guide the ideal operative intervention.

Starting at the time of extrication from the accident scene, the health care community can and must optimize care of the spine. A focus on spine care by multidisciplinary teams can significantly reduce the secondary injuries and thereby mitigate the potentially debilitating strain on society, our health care system, and lastly the suffering patient that results from spine and spinal cord injuries.

REFERENCES

1. Go BK, Richards JS. The epidemiology of spinal cord injury. *Spinal Cord Inj.* 1995;170–184.
2. Nepomuceno C, Fine PR, Richards JS, et al. Pain in patients with spinal cord injury. *Arch Phys Med Rehabil.* 1979;60(12):605–609.
3. Farmer JC, Vaccaro AR, Baldeston RA, et al. The changing nature of admissions to a spinal cord injury center: Violence on the rise. *J Spinal Disord.* 1998;11(5):400–403.
4. McKinley WO, Kolakowsky SA, Kreutzer JS. Substance abuse, violence, and outcome after traumatic spinal cord injury. *Am J Phys Med Rehabil.* 1999;78(4):306–312.
5. Torg JS, Naranja RJ Jr, Palov H, et al. The relationship of developmental narrowing of the cervical spinal canal to reversible and irreversible injury of the cervical spinal cord in football players. *J Bone Joint Surg Am.* 1996;78(9):1308–1314.
6. Tator CH, Carson JD, Edmonds VE. Spinal injuries in ice hockey. *Clin Sports Med.* 1998;17(1):183–194.
7. Gunby I. New focus on spinal cord injury. *JAMA.* 1981;245(12):1201–1206.
8. Gillingham J. The problem of head and spinal injuries: Prevention of the second accident. *Med Sci Law.* 1970;10(2):104–109.
9. Geisler WO, Wynne-Jones M, Jousse AT. Early management of the patient with trauma to the spinal cord. *Med Serv J Can.* 1966;22(7):512–523.
10. Johnson RM, Hart DL, Owen JR, et al. The Yale cervical orthosis: An evaluation of its effectiveness in restricting cervical motion in normal subjects and a comparison with other cervical orthoses. *Phys Ther.* 1978;58(7):865–871.
11. Johnson RM, Owen JR, Hart DL, et al. Cervical orthoses: A guide to their selection and use. *Clin Orthop Relat Res.* 1981;154:34–45.
12. Johnson RM, Hart DL, Simmons EF. Cervical orthoses. A study comparing their effectiveness in restricting cervical motion in normal subjects. *J Bone Joint Surg Am.* 1977;59(3):332–339.
13. Podolsky S, Baraff LJ, Simon RR, et al. Efficacy of cervical spine immobilization methods. *J Trauma.* 1983;23(6):461–465.
14. Boswell HB, Dietrich A, Shiels WE, et al. Accuracy of visual determination of neutral position of the immobilized pediatric cervical spine. *Pediatr Emerg Care.* 2001;17(1):10–14.
15. Jenkin AL, Eichler ME. Cervical spine trauma: Youmans neurological surgery. 2004;4:4885–4913.
16. Blackmore CC. Evidence-based imaging evaluation of the cervical spine in trauma. *Neuroimaging Clin N Am.* 2003;13(2):283–291.
17. Blackmore CC, Emerson SS, Mann FA, et al. Cervical spine imaging in patients with trauma: Determination of fracture risk to optimize use. *Radiology.* 1999;211(3):759–765.
18. Blackmore CC, Ramsey SD, Mann FA, et al. Cervical spine screening with CT in trauma patients: A cost-effectiveness analysis. *Radiology.* 1999;212(1):117–125.
19. Hanson JA, Blackmore CC, Mann FA, et al. Cervical spine injury: A clinical decision rule to identify high-risk patients for helical CT screening. *AJR Am J Roentgenol.* 2000;174(3):713–717.
20. Montgomery JL, Montgomery ML. Radiographic evaluation of cervical spine trauma. Procedures to avoid catastrophe. *Postgrad Med.* 1994;95(4):173–174, 177–179; passim.
21. Harris JH, Edeiken-Monroe B, Kopaniky DR Jr. A practical classification of acute cervical spine injuries. *Orthop Clin North Am.* 1986;17(1):15–30.
22. Blahd WH, Iserson KV, Bjelland JC Jr. Efficacy of the posttraumatic cross table lateral view of the cervical spine. *J Emerg Med.* 1985;2(4):243–249.
23. Gerrelts BD, Petersen EU, Mabry J, et al. Delayed diagnosis of cervical spine injuries. *J Trauma.* 1991;31(12):1622–1626.
24. Mace SE. Emergency evaluation of cervical spine injuries: CT versus plain radiographs. *Ann Emerg Med.* 1985;14(10):973–975.
25. Streitwieser DR, Knopp R, Wales LR, et al. Accuracy of standard radiographic views in detecting cervical spine fractures. *Ann Emerg Med.* 1983;12(9):538–542.
26. Doris PE, Wilson RA. The next logical step in the emergency radiographic evaluation of cervical spine trauma: The five-view trauma series. *J Emerg Med.* 1985;3(5):371–385.
27. Ross SE, Schwab CW, David ET, et al. Clearing the cervical spine: Initial radiologic evaluation. *J Trauma.* 1987;27(9):1055–1060.
28. Meldon SW, Moettus LN. Thoracolumbar spine fractures: Clinical presentation and the effect of altered sensorium and major injury. *J Trauma.* 1995;39(6):1110–1114.
29. Brohi K, Healy M, Fotheringham T, et al. Helical computed tomographic scanning for the evaluation of the cervical spine in the unconscious, intubated trauma patient. *J Trauma.* 2005;58(5):897–901.
30. Keene JS, Goletz TH, Lilleas F, et al. Diagnosis of vertebral fractures. A comparison of conventional radiography, conventional tomography, and computed axial tomography. *J Bone Joint Surg Am.* 1982;64(4):586–594.
31. Cacayorin ED, Kieffer SA. Applications and limitations of computed tomography of the spine. *Radiol Clin North Am.* 1982;20(1):185–206.
32. Ghoshhajra K, Rao KC. CT in spinal trauma. *J Comput Tomogr.* 1980;4(4):309–318.
33. Chakeres DW, Flickinger F, Bresnahan JC, et al. MR imaging of acute spinal cord trauma. *AJNR Am J Neuroradiol.* 1987;8(1):5–10.
34. Betz RR, Gelman AJ, DeFilipp GJ, et al. Magnetic resonance imaging (MRI) in the evaluation of spinal cord injured children and adolescents. *Paraplegia.* 1987;25(2):92–99.
35. Goldberg AL, Rothfus WE, Deeb ZL, et al. The impact of magnetic resonance on the diagnostic evaluation of acute cervicothoracic spinal trauma. *Skeletal Radiol.* 1988;17(2):89–95.
36. Kalfas I, Wilberger J, Goldberg A, et al. Magnetic resonance imaging in acute spinal cord trauma. *Neurosurgery.* 1988;23(3):295–299.
37. Bohlman HH. Acute fractures and dislocations of the cervical spine. An analysis of three hundred hospitalized patients and review of the literature. *J Bone Joint Surg Am.* 1979;61(8):1119–1142.
38. Sonntag VK, Hadley MN. Nonoperative management of cervical spine injuries. *Clin Neurosurg.* 1988;34:630–649.
39. Breig A, el-Nadi AF. Biomechanics of the cervical spinal cord. Relief of contact pressure on and overstretching of the spinal cord. *Acta Radiol Diagn (Stockh).* 1966;4(6):602–624.
40. Tarlov IM, Klinger H. Spinal cord compression studies. II. Time limits for recovery after acute compression in dogs. *AMA Arch Neurol Psychiatry.* 1954;71(3):271–290.
41. Tarlov IM, Klinger H, Vitale S. Spinal cord compression studies. I. Experimental techniques to produce acute and gradual compression. *AMA Arch Neurol Psychiatry.* 1953;70(6):813–819.
42. Vaccaro AR, Falatyn SP, Flanders AE, et al. Magnetic resonance evaluation of the intervertebral disc, spinal ligaments, and spinal cord before and after closed traction reduction of cervical spine dislocations. *Spine.* 1999;24(12):1210–1217.
43. Cree A, Bellabarba CJ, Mirza SK. Closed treatment of cevical spine injury. *Princ Pract Spine Surg.* 2003:415–439.
44. Gruenberg MF, Rechtine R, Chrin AM, et al. Overdistraction of cervical spine injuries with the use of skull traction: A report of two cases. *J Trauma.* 1997;42(6):1152–1156.
45. Jeanneret B, Magerl F, Ward JC. Overdistraction: A hazard of skull traction in the management of acute injuries of the cervical spine. *Arch Orthop Trauma Surg.* 1991;110(5):242–245.
46. Letts M, Girouard L, Yeadon A. Mechanical evaluation of four-versus eight-pin halo fixation. *J Pediatr Orthop.* 1997;17(1):121–124.
47. Denis F. The three column spine and its significance in the classification of acute thoracolumbar spinal injuries. *Spine.* 1983;8(8):817–831.
48. Denis F. Spinal instability as defined by the three-column spine concept in acute spinal trauma. *Clin Orthop Relat Res.* 1984;189:65–76.
49. Kelly A, Parrish R. Fracture of the occipital condyle: The forgotten part of the neck. *J Accid Emerg Med.* 2000;17(3):220–221.
50. Klein GR. Cervical spine trauma: Upper and lower. *Princ Pract Spine Surg.* 2003:441–461.
51. Anderson PA, Montesano PX. Morphology and treatment of occipital condyle fractures. *Spine.* 1988;13(7):731–736.

52. Anderson LD, D'Alonzo RT. Fractures of the odontoid process of the axis. 1974. *J Bone Joint Surg Am*. 2004;86-A(9):2081.

53. Allen BL Jr, Ferguson RL, Lehmann R, et al. A mechanistic classification of closed, indirect fractures and dislocations of the lower cervical spine. *Spine*. 1982;7(1):1–27.

54. Smith GR, Northrop CH, Loop JW. Jumpers' fractures: Patterns of thoracolumbar spine injuries associated with vertical plunges. *Radiology*. 1977;122(3):657–663.

55. Waters RL, Adkins RH. The effects of removal of bullet fragments retained in the spinal canal. A collaborative study by the National Spinal Cord Injury Model Systems. *Spine*. 1991;16(8):934–939.

56. Stauffer ES, Wood RW, Kelly EG. Gunshot wounds of the spine: The effects of laminectomy. *J Bone Joint Surg Am*. 1979;61(3):389–392.

57. Rechtine GRB, Vaccaro MJ. Fractures and dislocations of the thoracolumbar spine. *Princ Pract Spine Surg*. 2003;469–478.

SUGGESTED READING

Fox CJ, Gillespie DL, Weber MA, et al. Delayed evaluation of combat-related penetrating neck trauma. *J Vasc Surg*. 2006;44(1):86–93.

Comprehensive Management of Maxillofacial Injuries

Moises Salama   *Richard D. Klein*   *Brian M. Derby*

The treatment of facial trauma can be quite challenging. The goals of treatment are threefold. First, the establishment of the preinjury appearance or aesthetics is of paramount importance. Second, the function of the facial skeleton and soft tissues must be restored. The final goal is minimization of the disability period. The philosophy of treatment has shifted from that of the 1970s, where broad exposure and fixation of all buttresses were practiced to the current practice of minimizing approaches and potentially morbid exposures. Additionally, the advent of microvascular tissue transfer has made treatment of previously untreatable injuries possible. Further, the use of plate and screw rigid fixation has supplanted the use of cumbersome external fixation devices and the instability of interfragment wire fixation.[1]

GENERAL CONSIDERATIONS

Mechanisms of Injury

The most common cause of facial injuries is motor vehicle crashes. Other causes include fights, motorcycle and bicycle crashes, industrial mishaps, and athletic injuries. The use of seat belts and air bags has reduced the incidence of facial fractures associated with motor vehicle crashes. In a comprehensive review of 73,000 patients from 1983 to 1994, Lee et al. in 2000 published that the male to female ratio is 2:1, average age is 33, and the overall mortality is 5.9%. This mortality increases to 17% with a concomitant brain injury. The pattern of soft tissue injury was usually T-shaped involving the forehead, periorbital region, nose, lips, and chin. Lim et al. looked at concomitant injuries with facial fractures. He observed that in motor vehicle accidents, more than 50% of victims sustained injuries to the head, face, and cervical spine. Contributing factors included the use of alcohol and drugs and emotional problems. Eleven percent of patients had injuries other than the facial skeleton, 8% had injured extremities, 4% had ocular injuries, and 1% had spinal cord injuries.[1]

Associated Injuries

As with all trauma patients, victims of facial injuries need to be ruled out for concomitant injuries. A thorough physical examination and diagnostic workup is essential. This includes examining the airway, looking for significant blood loss, and diagnosing a brain or spinal cord injury.

The Airway

With extensive trauma to the mandible or midface asphyxia is a potential problem. The mouth and nasal passage should be cleared of foreign bodies, broken teeth or dentures, or blood clots, which may cause obstruction. Unstable mandibular fractures have the potential to push the tongue posteriorly and obstruct the airway. These patients may insist on sitting up and this is feasible if other injuries will not be exacerbated. Anterior traction on the jaw and tongue and placement of an oropharyngeal airway is an alternative if the patient cannot sit up or be placed prone. Patients with massive hemorrhage or fractures of the nose, maxilla, and mandible with resultant soft tissue edema are especially at risk. Endotracheal intubation or an emergency airway such as a cricothyroidotomy may be indicated, especially in patients with a head injury and blunted reflexes.

For surgical fixation of maxillary or mandible fractures, nasotracheal intubation is frequently used. However, orotracheal intubation can be used even in cases where maxillomandibular fixation (MMF) is necessary if the tube can be placed through a gap in the teeth or behind the last molar. Another technique used by some is to pass the tube through the floor of the mouth with an incision in the submental area. In patients with panfacial fractures where an endotracheal tube would interfere with the repair or those with head or chest injuries who cannot protect their airway, a tracheostomy is indicated. This also applies to patients with significant airway swelling who may or may not need intermaxillary fixation.

Hemorrhage

Displaced fractures and lacerations of the face can result in significant blood loss. Life-threatening hemorrhage can be seen in up to 5% of Le Fort type maxillary fractures. Seventy percent of these bleeds are from the internal maxillary artery and its branches. When the source is superficial, local pressure, packing, or ligation can be used for control. Temporary reduction of fractures can slow bleeding from fracture lines. For anterior nasal bleeds, nasal packing may be temporizing. If bleeding stops, nasal packing can be removed within 2 to 3 days. Deeper bleeding usually comes from the internal maxillary artery. This area can be difficult to access and control. The placement of Foley catheters, one in each nostril, with 30 to 50 mL balloons can temporize the bleeding along with nasal packing anterior to the balloons. The balloons are pulled snug against the posterior nasopharynx for maximal effect. This maneuver done for several hours with intermittently releasing the pressure usually stops the hemorrhage. Reported complications of this intervention include necrosis of the palate or columella (if the Foleys are secured against the columella).

Another method previously used to control bleeding is the use of external compression dressings or Barton bandages which encircle the head. These are rarely used now. For patients who continue to bleed despite more conservative measures, radiographic embolization is the next step. Complications from this procedure include facial nerve palsy, tongue necrosis, and stroke. Internal maxillary artery bleeds can be readily embolized with this technique. Bleeding that may not be embolized can be due to fractures in the anterior cranial fossa with transection through the carotid artery or veins such as the dural venous sinuses. These injuries can be defined by angiography and palliated with bilateral ligation of the external carotid arteries and superficial temporal arteries. Blood flow to the midportion of the face is diminished with this maneuver.

Brain Injury

When patients with facial fractures have concomitant head injuries, the focus of treatment should be to minimize secondary ischemia from brain edema, mass lesions, and hypothermia. Patients with head injury are stratified based on the Glasgow Coma Scale (GCS). This grading system has prognostic significance and patients with a GCS score of 3 have a very limited chance of survival. Prognosis also worsens with increasing age, decreasing mean arterial pressure, intracranial hypertension, and abnormal posturing. It should be noted though that even in patients in a coma, surgical treatment of facial injuries is not contraindicated. Patients can be monitored intraoperatively with intracranial pressure monitoring.

Cervical Spine Injury

Patients with multiple trauma, especially those with head and facial injuries, should be considered to have a spinal cord injury until proved otherwise. It is thought that approximately 10% of victims with facial injury have a concomitant cervical injury. The converse figure is 18%. Mandible fractures specifically are associated with upper cervical spine injuries. Studies indicate that these upper level injuries (C1-2) as well as lower C-spine injuries (C6-7) are the most commonly overlooked. This has been reported to occur in as many as 10% of cases. Therefore, it is imperative that these multitrauma patients be approached with a high level of suspicion.

Timing of Surgical Interventions

In the management of a multitrauma patient, the life-threatening injuries are treated first to optimize survival. Once these injuries are stabilized and the patient can tolerate surgical intervention, facial injuries and fractures should be treated as soon as possible. This optimizes aesthetic outcome, function, and makes fracture fixation easier. Other patients may not be able to tolerate surgery or may need definitive treatment for a graver injury. These patients should have their facial lacerations closed, their fractures grossly reduced, and may even be placed in temporary MMF. Many surgeons will subsequently wait until the edema subsides before attempting to operate on the facial skeleton. In any case, we do not recommend waiting any longer than 2 weeks postinjury before skeletal fixation to avoid having to deal with malunions, soft tissue contraction, and scar tissue.

Diagnostic Evaluation of the Facial Trauma Patient

The diagnosis of facial injuries relies on a thorough physical examination and a supplemental radiologic assessment. Although many radiologic views of the face and head have been described, all of the information needed can be obtained from a dedicated craniomaxillofacial computed

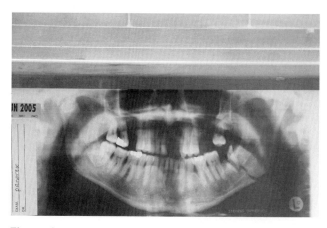

Figure 1 Mandibular panorex.

tomography (CT) scan with coronal, axial, and sagittal views. The only conventional radiographs which are still justifiable are the panorex mandible radiograph (see Fig. 1) and dental views.

The diagnosis of facial injuries is more difficult in children and the elderly.[1] Even with apparently minor external injuries such as abrasions or contusions, significant fractures may be present. This is why a good history and physical examination is of paramount importance. Treatment of facial lacerations should not be deferred and may even be done in the emergency department. Lacerations and wounds should be copiously irrigated, debrided, and closed with a layered closure to optimize aesthetic result.

Signs and symptoms of facial injuries include pain, tenderness, crepitus, paralysis of a specific motor nerve, hypo- or hyperesthesia, altered visual acuity, diplopia, dental malocclusion, facial deformity or asymmetry, lacerations, contusions, bleeding, edema, echymosis, and difficulty breathing. The examination should begin with inspection for facial asymmetry and deformity. Palpation should follow in a specific order. The bony prominences that should be palpated include the frontal bone, superior, lateral inferior and medial orbital rims, nose, zygomatic arches, malar eminence, maxilla, borders of the mandible, and alveolar ridges both maxillary and mandible (tooth-bearing segments).

Examination and palpation of the *periorbital region* should be carried out to check for tenderness, contour defects, and crepitus. One may find dystopia of the globes (unequal level), enophthalmos, proptosis, or diplopia, which may all indicate orbital, zygomatic, or maxillary fractures. Consultation with an ophthalmologist is indicated with injuries in this region to rule out globe injuries such as ruptures or retinal detachment. The eye examination should include visual acuity, extraocular movements, pupillary function, fundoscopic examination, and measurement of intraocular pressure. Extraocular movements may be assessed in the unconscious or sedated patient with

a forced duction test. This involves grasping the conjunctiva of the globe with fine-toothed Adson forceps rocking the globe up and down as well as side to side to rule out muscle entrapment from an orbital fracture. Other signs that should be assessed include eyelid excursion, double vision, enophthalmos, hyphema, and corneal abrasions. Enophthalmos can be assessed by asking the patient to tilt his/her head back and comparing the corneal planes by looking in a cephalad direction. Any loss of vision or acuity should be documented preoperatively. Pupillary reactivity is also important to assess and is thought to be the most reliable sign of optic nerve injury.

The nasal examination should include an intranasal examination to look for soft tissue lacerations or septal hematomas. Externally, nasal trauma documentation should include the presence of nasal dorsum deformity and/or tip deviation, nasal bone collapse or instability, and presence of any lacerations.

In the awake patient, the muscles of facial expression (cranial nerve [CN] VII) and tongue function (CN XII) can be easily assessed. In the unconscious patient, initial CN motor function evaluation is not possible. Therefore, serial physical examination over a period of days is required to document CN function once the patient has become awake and cooperative.

In the examination of *masticatory function*, the maxillary and mandibular dental arches are inspected and palpated to look for irregularities of bone, lacerations, loose teeth, hematomas, swelling, crepitus, or tenderness. Dental occlusion and the intercuspal relationship of the teeth are checked and may be the only evidence of a fracture. Trismus may also be seen with zygomatic, maxillary, or mandibular fractures. A careful dental examination is performed to document the condition and quality of the patient's dentition including the presence of decayed, fractured, or avulsed teeth. In condylar or subcondylar fractures, placing one finger in the ear canal and another over the condylar head may allow one to feel condylar movement or crepitus with jaw motion. In addition, one may see blood or fluid draining from the ear canal, which may indicate a laceration, a middle cranial fossa fracture with resultant cerebrospinal fluid (CSF) leak, or a condylar dislocation. Bleeding from the nasal passages may indicate nasal injuries, Le Fort fractures, orbital or nasoethmoid fractures, or anterior cranial fossa fractures. The mobility of the maxillary jaw should also be checked, for this also implies a Le Fort fracture. Finally, CSF rhinorrhea may be seen in anterior and middle basilar skull fractures, or cribriform plate fractures.

On *neurosensory* examination, one may find hypoesthesia or anesthesia in the distribution of one of the branches of the trigeminal nerve (CN V). This may indicate a fracture somewhere in the bony path of the nerve or injury from a soft tissue laceration. These nerves may be lacerated or just contused, implying neuropraxia. Neuropraxic nerves generally recover. These nerve branches travel through

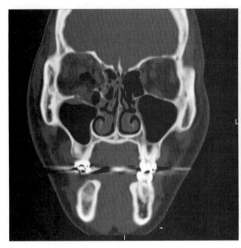
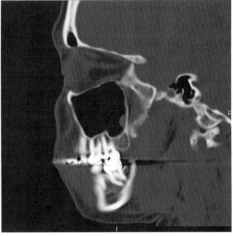

Figure 2 Computed tomography (CT) of the facial skeleton.

foramina, which are weak parts of the bone and can fracture thereby crushing the nerve. Cutaneous branches are small and generally do not warrant repair. Larger branches such as the supraorbital, infraorbital, inferior alveolar, or mental nerves can be primarily repaired.

Imaging

With the image resolution and quality available currently, the CT scan has supplanted plain radiographs in the diagnosis of maxillofacial trauma. The craniofacial CT must include axial, coronal, and sagittal sections with bone and soft tissue windows. This examination must be undertaken before any surgical intervention is commenced. Bone windows allow accurate visualization of fractures (see Fig. 2). Three-dimensional reconstructions can also be obtained to compare volume and symmetry between the two sides of the face. Further, special views such as the orbital apex view allow magnification into this area.

FACIAL SOFT TISSUE INJURIES

Etiopathogenesis

As previously mentioned, motor vehicle accidents are the most common source of facial soft tissue injury, with sports-related injuries, falls, altercations, and industrial accidents also contributing as common causes. These injuries include lacerations, abrasions, contusions, and avulsions. Treatment approach and potential complications are often dictated by type of injury encountered; therefore, accurate description of injury is imperative. Associated complications are also important to consider. Roughly 25% of facial lacerations resulting from motor vehicle accidents are accompanied by underlying facial bone fractures.[2] A sound knowledge of facial anatomy will assist in evaluation of soft tissue injuries potentially involving salivary ducts, CN V and VII, facial mimetic muscles, and significant vessels.

Anatomy

The management of facial soft tissue injuries requires a thorough knowledge of facial anatomy. From superficial to deep, facial layers include skin, subcutaneous tissue, superficial musculoaponeurotic system (SMAS), fine areolar tissue, and mucosa. Understanding this blueprint assists in identifying structures involved in injury, and ensures that wounds are closed properly. Layered closure is important for attainment of the ultimate treatment objective, functional and cosmetic restoration.

The facial nerve exits the skull at the stylomastoid foramen, enters the parotid gland, travels in the lateral aspect of the face deep to the facial mimetic muscles, and innervates them on the deep surface. Exceptions to this deep innervation include the buccinator, levator labii superioris, orbicularis oris, and the depressor angularis oris (see Fig. 3).

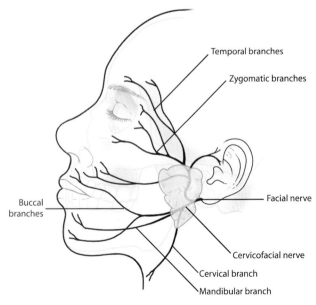

Figure 3 Facial nerves.

The parotid gland is located in the soft tissue of the lateral aspect of the face from the zygomatic arch superiorly to the mandibular angle inferiorly, and from the ear posteriorly to the midportion of the cheek anteriorly. The parotid duct travels along a transverse line from the tragus to the midportion of the upper lip and empties into the oral cavity, through the Stensen duct, opposite the second maxillary molar. The duct is often accompanied by the buccal branch of the facial nerve. Not uncommonly, both structures are simultaneously injured with lacerations to the lateral aspect of the face.

Blood supply is derived from branches of the external carotid artery—facial, internal maxillary, and superficial temporal (see Fig. 4). In the basilar skull region, tributaries of the internal jugular vein and intracranial circulation have valveless communication.

Lymphatics drain posteriorly and laterally. Avulsed tissue may have obstructed lymphatic drainage, frequently resulting in lymphedema. Trapdoor deformities, which are bulging soft tissue deformities that disrupt natural facial contours can result.

Diagnosis

Before the assessment of facial injury, the initial treatment of facial trauma patients focuses on management of life-threatening conditions. Following this initial evaluation, assessment of facial soft tissue injury can occur. A full facial examination is performed as previously described. This inspection should be performed in a systematic manner to avoid missing injuries. One can begin from the vertex of the head and proceed caudally from the top of scalp to the bottom of the neck.

The purpose of soft tissue wound inspection is to identify underlying damage and the presence of foreign material. The ends of transected structures, when isolated, can be made available for future repair. Foreign material serves to reduce the bacterial inoculum necessary to cause infection from 10^5 bacteria per gram of tissue to 10^2 per gram of tissue.

Bleeding, although initially best controlled with compression, is ultimately controlled with careful ligation. Recommendations for hemostasis caution against the use of cautery secondary to risk of damage to surrounding nerves, fat, and muscle. In the event that bleeding is slow to resolve, further investigation with arteriography may be required.

Insufficient hemostasis may result in hematoma. Like that found in any other region of the body, facial hematoma represents a nonvascularized region, inaccessible to antibiotics and white blood cells. Typically hematomas will resolve over time. The process may be expedited with application of warm, moist heat starting on day 3 after injury. Occasionally, a facial hematoma may be localized and considered fit for evacuation. This process is pursued under general anesthesia, with a suction tip advanced into the area of hematoma through a camouflaged incision. Patients must be warned of the risks of hyperpigmentation when hematomas are exposed to the sun.

General or local anesthesia is typically required during the inspection process, especially with pediatric patients.

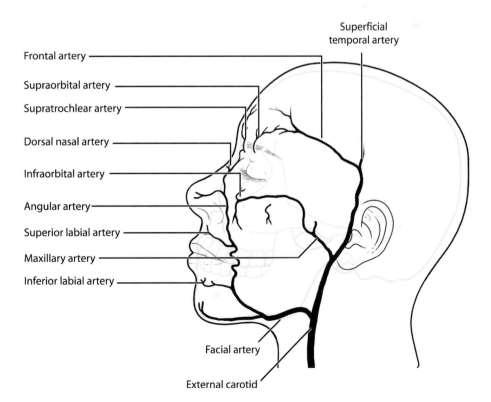

Frontal artery
Supraorbital artery
Supratrochlear artery
Dorsal nasal artery
Infraorbital artery
Angular artery
Superior labial artery
Maxillary artery
Inferior labial artery
Superficial temporal artery
Facial artery
External carotid

Figure 4   Facial blood supply.

One should also be sure to incorporate the use of extensive and accurate photographic documentation in their review. Photographs not only supplement and enhance medical documentation, but also enable the patient to appreciate the extent of injury and effectiveness of treatment.[2]

Contamination is dependent on time elapsed since injury. A direct relationship exists between the time elapsed from injury to cleansing and the risk of contamination.[2] Within the first few hours, inoculated organisms become encased in a protein-fibrin substrate that ultimately serves as a shield against antibiotics and dislodgment by normal irrigation fluids. More aggressive cleansing will require the use of surgical debridement, high-pressure irrigation, and scrubbing.

The surface of the skin, if contaminated by "traumatic tattoos," should be freed of all foreign particles. Primary surface dermabrasion may risk extension of the depth of cutaneous injury and result in more prominent, hypertrophic scarring.[2] Wound edges that are jagged and devitalized should be sharply excised. Typically, 1 to 2 mm of skin edge excision is all that is required to turn a traumatic wound into a surgically excised wound with improved cosmetic result upon closure. Very conservative excision is recommended in critical areas such as the eyelids, eyebrows, nostril rim, and the vermillion border, especially near the Cupid bow.[2]

Consideration of tetanus immunization status is also necessary, as all facial wounds are potentially contaminated. With obvious contamination, and no prior history of immunization, simultaneous injection of 250 IU of tetanus immune globulin and 0.5 mL of tetanus vaccine is recommended. The immunization is completed with two additional boosters at monthly intervals.

SPECIFIC FACIAL SOFT TISSUE INJURIES AND THEIR TREATMENT

Laceration Injury

Pertinent points to remember in repair of lacerated facial wounds are marginal edge excision and layered closure. Conversion of a crushed, devitalized, irregularly torn surface to a straight surgical incision enhances cosmesis upon closure while also reducing risk of infection. The basic sequence of facial closure entails repair of deeper structures—bone, glands, ducts, nerves—followed by approximation of muscle, fat, dermis, and epidermis. Fine grade absorbable sutures are used and should be strong enough to maintain dermal alignment after the skin sutures are removed on day 3 to 5. Early suture removal (within 5 to 7 postoperative days) prevents suture marks and further scarring. The physician should routinely inform a patient and his/her family about the possible need for future revision and/or reconstruction.

Bite Injury

Animal and human bites are not uncommon injuries. Significant points to remember with this injury are (a) the high likelihood of wound contamination secondary to extensive oral flora, and (b) the use of systemic antibiotic therapy is standard. Copious irrigation and sharp excision of contaminated wound edges is followed by prophylactic penicillin for potential *Pasteurella multocida* infection from cat bites, and broad-spectrum antibiotics for human bites (gram-positive, gram-negative, aerobic/anaerobic bacteria). The face is the only area where primary closure of bite wounds is considered, but debridement and irrigation must be thorough.

Facial Nerve Injury and Facial Muscle Injury

Wound inspection, combined with physical examination, may demonstrate laceration of the facial nerve. The extensive arborization and communication of the terminal branches of the facial nerve distal to a line drawn vertically from the lateral canthus may result in reduced functional deficit with injury to this region. Regardless, when able to be identified, transected nerve ends should be isolated and approximated with microsurgical techniques within 72 hours of injury.

Muscle realignment and approximation allows for some degree of nerve regeneration by neurotization of the muscle.[2] Additionally, balance and activity of facial movement is better restored when muscle edges are approximated.

Trigeminal Nerve Injury

Sensory nerves of the face arborize extensively, calling the practicality of repair into question. Exceptions are made when nerve laceration occurs in close proximity to skull foramina (supraorbital, infraorbital, mental). Most commonly, one undertakes sensory nerve repair to prevent the development of painful neuromas.[2]

Parotid Gland Injury

Evidence of parotid duct injury can be confirmed by retrograde irrigation of the Stensen duct while looking for extravasation of fluid into the wound. Should a bony fracture be a component of the injury, duct repair should follow bony repair. The parotid duct falls along the middle third of a line drawn from the tragus to the midpoint of the upper lip. The buccal branch of the facial nerve is in close proximity to the parotid duct in this region.

The sequence of parotid duct repair includes dilation of the intraoral orifice with a lacrimal dilator, insertion of small silicone tubing into the duct ends as a stent, and suturing of duct ends over the silicone tubing with fine 8.0 nonabsorbable suture.[3] Microsurgical technique should be used. Parotid duct ligation is not recommended for two reasons. First, considerable gland swelling with secondary atrophy can occur and second, chronic infection requiring parotidectomy may develop.[2] In contrast, damage to the submandibular gland or duct can be treated by duct ligation. Gland excision is another option for submandibular gland injury.

Eyelid Injury

Before eyelid repair, the importance of globe inspection and examination is paramount. This takes precedence over soft tissue restoration. Once assured, one proceeds with sequential conjunctival, tarsal, septal, levator, and orbicularis oculi repair with fine absorbable suture internally. Levator disruption may result in ptosis if not repaired. In closing external layers, sutures should be tied away from the globe to avoid corneal or conjunctival surface irritation.

Lid defects can be closed with lid mobilization and lateral canthotomy. This release allows for medial mobilization of the remaining lower lid.[2] Skin closure is performed with fine sutures. Proper alignment of the gray line, internal lid margin, and cilia is crucial to an esthetic and functional repair. In closing eyelid defects, one must be aware of the potential for development of ectropion. This occurs when the lid contracts from scarring and there is resultant scleral show. Techniques to prevent this complication include careful and meticulous closure of all anatomic layers after inferior orbital rim exposure as well as the application of Frost suture at the eyelid margin for 24 to 48 hours following the surgical intervention to maintain proper lid length (see Fig. 5). Participation in the care of these patients by plastic surgeon will help in obtaining optimal outcomes.

Lacrimal System Injury

Injury to the region of the medial canthus may result in damage to the lacrimal canaliculi or sac. This is assessed by cannulation of the puncta with a lacrimal probe. A laceration is proved by visualizing the probe in the wound. If an injury is present, the puncta are cannulated with Crawford tubes that are passed into the nose and are left in place for 4 weeks. If cannulation is not possible, lacerations are repaired and the patient may require a dacryocystorhinostomy if epiphora becomes problematic.[4]

Nasal Lacerations

Given its prominence, the nose is commonly involved with other soft tissue injuries of the face. Skin, cartilage, and mucous membrane defects must be managed separately in attempt to maintain nasal contour. In keeping with the concept of contour preservation, debridement should be kept to a minimum. Full-thickness lacerations are best repaired from the inside out. The nasal mucosa should be repaired with chromic sutures. The cartilage should be repaired with monofilament sutures. Lastly, the skin should also be repaired with monofilament sutures with good eversion of the skin edges.[4] Significant soft tissue avulsion can be reconstructed with local or regional flaps to restore the mucosa, framework, and external skin. The use of cartilage grafts is often necessary. Any septal hematoma should be evacuated to prevent potential septal perforation.

Lip Lacerations

The facial soft tissue repairs discussed to this point have highlighted a consistent theme of attention to layered closure and proper edge alignment. Perhaps nowhere on the face is attention to this detail more important than the vermilion border of the lip. Skin, orbicularis oris, and mucosa must be precisely aligned and repaired, especially the pars orbicularis (thick band of orbicularis muscle) underneath the vermilion of the lip. The vermilion should be marked with methylene blue before the administration of local anesthesia, which can distort the landmarks. Although proper vermilion positioning is essential, one should keep in mind that approximation of the orbicularis muscle sets up alignment of the vermilion. As stated previously, debridement in this region should be minimized, especially in the area of the Cupid bow. Uncorrectable deformity can result.

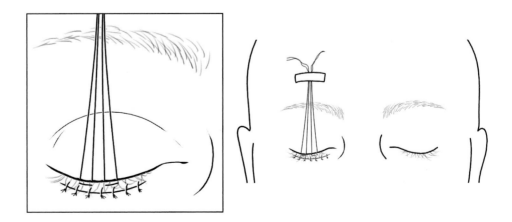

Figure 5 Frost sutures.

Eyebrow Injury

Similar to lip lacerations, eyebrow injuries should be treated with minimal debridement. The eyebrow varies in thickness along its length. Resection almost assures a step-off deformity. Such deformities are only reparable by hair unit transplantation. Anatomic proximity should trigger inspection for supraorbital nerve injury and repair when feasible.

Auricle Injury

Like the nose, auricular protrusion leads to its frequent involvement in trauma. Further, the injured auricle is prone to hematoma formation. Hematomas must be evacuated and bolsters applied to prevent them. Drains can also be placed for 24 hours to reduce hematoma formation. Undrained hematomas can result in fibrosis and a "cauliflower ear" deformity. Avulsed tissue should be wrapped in sterile saline-soaked gauze, and placed in a plastic bag in a container on ice. Before replantation, wound edges are debrided as is cartilage stripped of perichondrium. After replantation of avulsed tissue, leech therapy should be initiated for 3 to 5 days until venous connections begin to develop. This will aid with necrosis from venous congestion. If the ear canal is involved, lacerations are repaired and the canal is stented to prevent stenosis.[4] Secondary reconstruction may be necessary.

Significant Soft Tissue Defects

The scenario of avulsion injury or tissue loss that prevents primary closure may occur. These large wounds can be repaired with local undermining, local flaps, or skin grafting. Areas that may have compromised vascularity may be closed by delayed primary closure. This allows the wound to demarcate before definitive closure.

INJURIES TO THE FACIAL SKELETON

Frontal Sinus Fractures

Epidemiology

Frontal sinus fractures are relatively infrequent sequelae of facial trauma, occurring in approximately 5% to 15% of facial fractures.[5] Typically, 60% of frontal sinus injuries involve both anterior and posterior table injury. Anterior table fractures occur alone in 33% of cases, with the remaining frontal sinus fractures involving the posterior table alone.[1] Given the proximity of the posterior table to intracranial structures of the anterior cranial fossa, intracranial injury occurs in 33% to 70% of patients.[6]

Anatomy

The independently developing paired frontal sinuses are typically not pneumatized until the age of 2 years. Each approximates the size of a pea around the age of 4 years, and at about the age of 8 years become radiographically identifiable. Significant pneumatization does not occur until the age of 15 years, with maximal expansion not achieved until the age of 19. The paired structures are bound anteriorly by the anterior table, posteriorly by a posterior table, superiorly by the floor of the anterior cranial fossa, inferiorly by the orbital roof, and medially by the intersinus septum.

Identification of the involvement of the frontonasal duct (FND) in injury is essential. This structure is the most anterior and superior portion of the anterior ethmoidal complex. Its chief role is drainage of the frontal sinus into the middle meatus. Borders include the uncinate process anteriorly, the anterior ethmoidal air cells posteriorly, the medial portion of the middle turbinate medially, and the lamina papyracea or suprainfundibular plate laterally.

Arterial supply to the sinus involves contributions from the supraorbital, supratrochlear, and anterior ethmoidal arteries. Venous drainage can be divided into superficial and deep systems. Superficial drainage follows the angular vein, with deep drainage to the subdural venous system through foramina of Breschet. Lymphatic drainage follows meningeal and nasal cavity lymphatics. The complexity of the drainage system points to the risk of meningitis or brain abscess after a frontal sinus fracture, even in the absence of a posterior wall fracture

Diagnosis

Any laceration, hematoma, or ecchymoses of the forehead and glabellar region should heighten suspicion of an associated fracture. Subconjunctival ecchymosis and CSF rhinorrhea may also be present. If CSF leak is suspected, a halo test or laboratory analysis of fluid sampled from the nose for β-2 transferrin can be used to identify CSF. Additionally, the entire region should be palpated for bony irregularities (i.e., depressions, "step-offs," crepitus), with specific attention given to the superior orbital rims. Anesthesia in the distribution of the supraorbital nerve may be present. Associated swelling may obscure depression in the first few days after injury. Although good clinical examination skills can assist in the diagnosis, physical examination is not enough in determining the extent of injury to the frontal sinus and supplementation of the examination with imaging studies is essential.

Radiographic Analysis

Thin-section axial and coronal CT scans are the main imaging studies used for frontal sinus trauma assessment.[5] Complete evaluation involves determination of posterior and anterior wall involvement, fracture displacement, and associated intracranial or FND injury (see Fig. 6). The presence of air–fluid levels in the frontal sinus may imply absence of duct function.[1] Pathognomonic CT findings for FND involvement include associated fracture of the anterior ethmoid complex and a fracture of the floor of the frontal

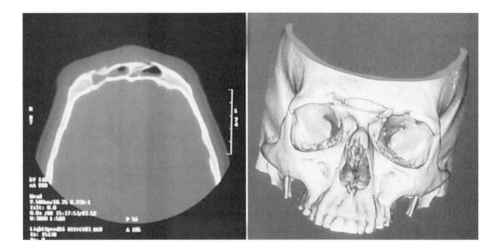

Figure 6 Frontal sinus fracture.

sinus.[6] Small fractures are not always readily identifiable radiographically, especially when nondisplaced.

Treatment

Surgical and nonsurgical management options exist. Independent assessment of the anterior and posterior tables and the FND will dictate the need for surgical intervention. Surgical intervention should take place within the first week if possible. Early treatment reduces incidence of long-term complications.[5]

Indications for surgical intervention include the following: depression of the anterior table, FND involvement on radiographic examination, FND obstruction identified by persistent air–fluid level or mucocele formation, displaced fractures of the posterior table that have presumably lacerated the dura, and CSF leak without resolution after 4 to 7 days. Nondisplaced, simple linear fractures are often managed nonoperatively.

Anterior Wall Fracture

Surgical intervention for anterior wall fracture is determined by the degree of bony displacement and comminution as well as the location of the fracture (e.g., fractures of the supraorbital rim). Nondisplaced anterior wall fractures are managed conservatively, with antibiotics administered for 7 days and follow-up CT scanning over a period of 12 months. Concern for late infection and formation of mucoceles dictates the need for long-term follow-up.

Typically, disruption of aesthetics, secondary to anterior table depression, necessitates surgical repair to restore forehead contour. Adequate exposure of the surgical field is essential for ensuring appropriate bony contouring. A coronal incision will allow for ample exposure down to the nasoglabellar region anteriorly and frontozygomatic junctions laterally.[5] Intraoperatively the fractured fragments of the anterior wall are removed, and the sinus cavity is explored for additional damage. In the absence of additional damage (i.e., FND), the bony fragments are carefully reassembled, replaced, and held in place with either titanium

screws and plates or resorbable screws and plates. The goal is to restore a proper aesthetic contour of the frontal bone and fronto-orbital bar. Split cranial bone graft may be necessary to restore the anterior wall if there is significant comminution and contamination of the fractured bone.

Posterior Wall Fracture

Isolated posterior wall fractures rarely occur. They are typically accompanied by anterior wall fractures. Should fracture of the posterior wall be nondisplaced, presence of FND damage and/or CSF leakage dictate the need for surgical intervention. Nondisplaced fractures without CSF leak are treated nonoperatively with close observation only. CSF rhinorrhea, if present, can be initially treated expectantly with elevation of the head of the bed to 30 degrees and the patient placed on mandated bed rest. For cases of leakage that extend beyond 4 days, spinal drainage may be considered to expedite resolution.

Significantly displaced posterior wall fractures, comminuted fractures, or nondisplaced fractures associated with persistent CSF rhinorrhea require a surgery. Treatment consists of cranializing the frontal sinus. The procedure involves removal of the entire posterior wall of the frontal sinus followed by repair of dural tears by a neurosurgeon.[5] The entire sinus mucosa is stripped and removed by mechanical abrasion using a fine bur. Subsequently, a galeal frontalis flap is placed to separate the intracranial cavity from the FNDs. The anterior table is then repaired and replaced and the frontal lobe expands and fills any remaining dead space.

Frontonasal Duct Fracture

The importance of identifying FND fracture in frontal sinus injury cannot be overemphasized as it is an absolute indication for surgical treatment. Further, because some extent of FND injury accompanies approximately 55% of all frontal sinus fractures, one must be cognizant of both radiographic and intraoperative tactics for FND injury identification. Radiographic findings were discussed previously. If the fractured segments are not easily observed intraoperatively, methylene blue or fluorescein dyes can be used to assess the drainage of the sinus through the duct into the nasal cavity. Significant FND injury, either isolated or in combination with anterior and/or posterior wall fracture, can be addressed in a variety of ways. A few authors recommend repairing the FND directly followed by stenting the duct open. Stenosis of the duct with potential mucocele formation is a possible long-term risk of this strategy. We recommend obliterating the frontal sinus. Obliteration involves exposing and opening the entire frontal sinus through a coronal approach. This is followed by complete removal of the entire sinus mucosa, closure of the FND with a galeal flap, and bone graft. The remaining dead space in the sinus can then be filled with either bone, fat, muscle, or some advocate leaving air in the sinus. Alloplastic material is not recommended as the rate of infection is significantly increased. If the posterior wall is significantly disrupted then cranialization is favored over obliteration. Long-term follow-up with serial CT scans is essential to rule out mucocele formation.

Complications

Complications of frontal sinus injury repair may include unaesthetic contour deformity, infection, mucocele formation, intracranial injury, CSF leak, and ophthalmic injuries.

Orbital Fractures

Anatomy

The orbit is made up of the maxilla, zygoma, ethmoid, frontal bone, lacrimal bone, greater and lesser wings of the sphenoid, and palatine bone. The orbital cavity resembles a cone but is thought of as having medial, lateral, superior, and inferior walls for ease of description (see Fig. 7). The superior wall is quite thin but isolated fractures in this area are rare due to the protection from the frontal bone and sinus, and thick supraorbital rim. Children are more predisposed to roof fracture because their cranium is proportionally bigger and the frontal sinus is not pneumatized. The frontal, zygomatic, and greater wing of the sphenoid bones make up the lateral wall. Its strength makes isolated fractures in this wall rare. It is commonly involved in zygomatic fractures. Here the zygoma articulates with the greater wing of the sphenoid.

The inferior wall is relatively weak and susceptible to fracture. Contributing to its weakness is the infraorbital canal, the thin maxillary roof, and the curvature of the floor. The anterior floor is concave and especially weak.

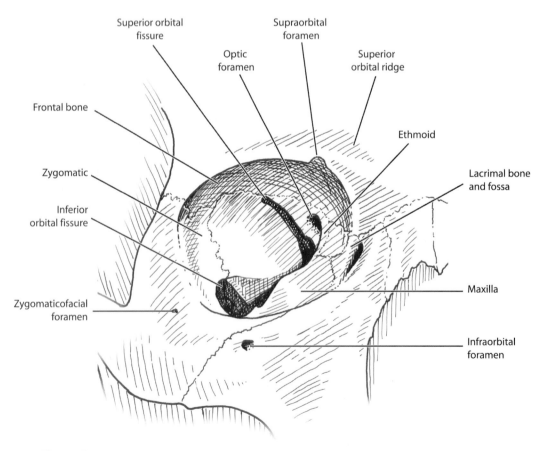

Figure 7 Bony orbit.

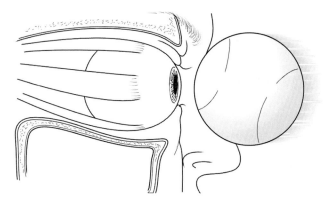

Figure 8 Orbital blowout.

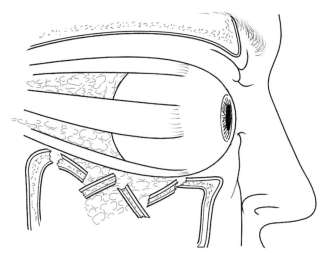

Figure 9 Increased orbital volume.

Similarly, the thin lacrimal bone and lamina papyracea of the ethmoid, which make up the medial wall, render it weak. In this area, the lacrimal sac, which is protected anteriorly by the frontal process of the maxilla, can be injured. The medial canthal tendon can also be avulsed or disrupted.

Biomechanics of Injury

Fractures of the floor and medial wall result from one of two mechanisms. One is the direct transmission of force to the orbital rim and the other is through transmission of force from the globe and other orbital contents. There has been much controversy as to which mechanism explains orbital blowout fractures but both likely play a role (see Fig. 8).

Clinical Evaluation

The most common clinical symptoms of blowout fractures are diplopia and enophthalmos. Diplopia is caused by restricted ocular motion. This is most common on upward gaze in blowout fractures. It can manifest on central vision, which is most problematic, or on peripheral gaze. Mechanical causes of diplopia include motion restriction due to entrapment of the intraorbital contents by the fracture, or from changes in the mechanical advantage of the inferior rectus muscle if the vector of pull or excursion changes. Entrapment of the orbital contents such as the inferior oblique or rectus muscles, Lockwood ligament, periorbital fat, or the Tenon capsule can be tested intraoperatively with the forced duction test. This test is performed by gently grasping the sclera with two Adson forceps and rocking the globe from side to side and up and down, being careful not to injure the cornea. Any entrapment becomes evident when the globe fails to move in any one direction. The medial rectus can become contused but rarely incarcerates. Nonmechanical causes of diplopia include extraocular muscle injury, nerve injury to these muscles, edema, or hematomas. The forced duction test is not always accurate in the acute setting, according to Hollier and Thornton.[7] Emery et al. observed that in blowout fractures diplopia resolved within 15 days in 55% of patients and persisted in 27%.[8]

Enophthalmos is gauged by the difference between the corneal surface and the lateral orbital rim. On examination, pseudoptosis and an exaggerated superior sulcus above the upper lid is seen. With pseudoptosis, the relationship of the upper lid and upper limbus is normal but the upper lid is more visible due to posterior positioning of the globe. Enophthalmos can be objectively measured using a Herthel exophthalmometer. A difference of 3 mm between eyes is considered significant. Posttraumatic enophthalmos is a consequence of inferior and posterior displacement of the globe. This can only occur if there is an increase in orbital volume. This change in volume must be posterior to the vertical axis of the globe to cause posterior displacement as concluded in Pearl's study (see Fig. 9).[9]

Other signs and symptoms that patients may have are epistaxis, orbital emphysema which can cause retinal artery occlusion, traumatic optic neuropathy, retrobulbar blindness, or hypo- or anesthesia in the infraorbital nerve distribution. Blood can accumulate in the maxillary sinus and lead to epistaxis. All these patients should receive a thorough ophthalmologic examination including visual acuity, pupil reactivity, eye motion, visual fields, intraocular pressure, and fundoscopic examination. A forced duction test with topical anesthesia should also be performed as previously mentioned if there is any evidence of abnormal eye movement so as to rule entrapment versus ocular muscle injury or CNs 3, 4, or 6 injuries.

On radiographic evaluation, a CT with axial and coronal cuts is imperative. This examination is the gold standard and other radiographs are not necessary. CT scans allow characterization of the fractures and visualization of injuries to the soft tissues such as the extraocular muscles. The images can be reformatted to give saggital views. These cuts allow the surgeon to visualize the relationship of the fracture to the axis of the globe (see Fig. 10). In the case of a blowout fracture, this relationship will influence whether the patient is predisposed to enophthlamos. Orbital

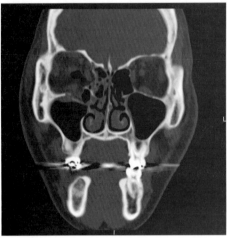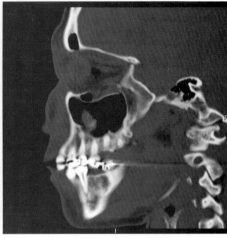

Figure 10 Orbital floor blowout.

volume has also been estimated with CT scans.[10] Surgical repair has been recommended for floor defects >1 cm^2.

Treatment

Indications for surgery in orbital fractures include enophthalmos >2 mm, persistent diplopia (>2 weeks), evidence of soft tissue entrapment by CT or forced duction test, a large orbital floor defect (>1 cm^2), and significant hypoglobus.

The common approaches used now are through the transconjunctival, subciliary, or subtarsal incisions. The orbital floor can also be reached through the Caldwell-Luc approach, which involves an upper gingivobuccal incision and accessing the floor through a maxillary antrotomy. This approach can be used in endoscopic repair of the orbital floor (see Fig. 11). The subtarsal incision involves making a skin incision in a natural crease of the lower lid, dissecting through the orbicularis oculi to the septum, and following the septum to the arcus marginalis, where the floor is entered. After a subciliary incision, the same plane of dissection can be used as in the subtarsal incision. This incision can be extended laterally, and the lateral canthus can be taken down to access the lateral orbital wall and zygomaticofrontal suture. A transconjunctival incision is made below the tarsus and carried through the lower lid

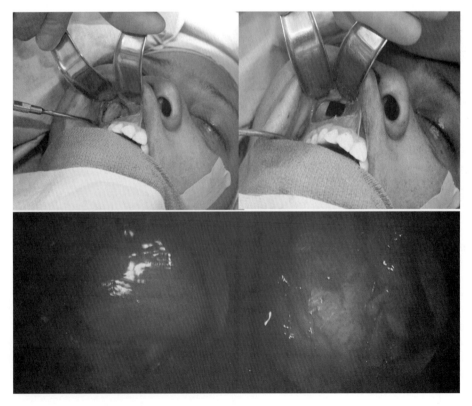

Figure 11 Endoscopic floor repair.

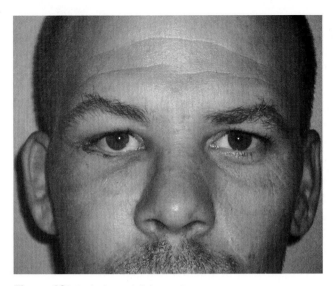

Figure 12 Right lower lid shortening.

retractors to the plane between the septum and orbicularis oculi. Dissection is then carried out in this plane to the orbital floor. This incision leaves no external scar but vertical shortening of the lower lid and entropion can occur (see Fig. 12).

The primary method to fix orbital floor fractures is to reconstruct the floor with bone or alloplastic materials. Autogenous graft materials include split cranium membranous bone, iliac bone, split rib, cartilage, and fascia lata.[11-19] These grafts have a lower infection rate but have donor site morbidity and can resorb. Alloplastic implants include titanium mesh, absorbable polymers, nonabsorbable polymers, Teflon, Supramyd, Silastic, Gelfilm, and others.[20-24] These grafts have no donor site morbidity.

Complications

Implants that have a pseudocapsule, which prevents vascular ingrowth, are at higher risk of becoming infected. These include silicone or Teflon implants. On the other hand, high-density porous polyethylene (MedPor[2]) and coralline hydroxyapatite allow for vascular ingrowth. Implants can also become extruded.

Diplopia can persist after surgical therapy from incomplete release of the entrapped soft tissues, re-entrapment, or from adhesions between the soft tissues and the reconstruction graft. This complication had an incidence of 37% at 6 months in one study.[25] A forced duction test should be performed at the end of surgery to rule out residual or new entrapment. If this has been done, postoperative diplopia is probably due to edema or neuropraxia and can be treated conservatively. Neuropraxia can take several months to resolve.

Orbital fractures can also result in enophthalmos that is persistent in the postoperative period. Contributing factors include scar contracture, loss of supporting ligaments, fat

atrophy, and timing of repair. Timing of repair appears to be important because late repairs may have more fibrosis of the extraocular muscles, which limits the ability to adjust the anteroposterior dimension of the eye.[26] Preoperatively placing traction on the medial and lateral bulbar conjunctiva may help predict this problem. Manson[27] advocates reconstruction of the missing volume with bone grafts.

With transcutaneous approaches to the orbital floor, the lower lid can become retracted due to scarring of the lid to the orbital rim. Frost sutures in the ciliary area of the lower lid taped to the forehead for 24 to 48 hours can help prevent this complication. Once the complication presents, aggressive lid massage can alleviate and even solve this problem. If the ectropion persists for 4 to 6 months, the scar can be released through various techniques. Earlier release is justified if corneal exposure is a problem.

Another well-known complication is the superior orbital fissure syndrome (SOFS). This results from extension of the fracture into the superior orbital fissure and injury to CNs III, IV, V1, and VI. Symptoms include ophthalmoplegia, proptosis, upper lid ptosis, decreased sensation in the V1 distribution, and a fixed and dilated pupil. The contralateral eye has a consensual response but the affected eye has no direct response to light. Conservative treatment is advocated. An orbital apex syndrome can also occur which is similar with the additional involvement of the optic nerve, producing blindness. This can be due to direct trauma or ischemic optic neuropathy from a retrobulbar hemorrhage.

Nasal Fractures

The structural components of the nose can be divided into upper, middle, and lower vaults. The upper vault is composed of the nasal bones, the upper edge of the septum, the ethmoid, and vomer. The middle vault is made up of the upper lateral cartilages, the septum, and the frontal processes of the maxilla. The lower vault is the lower border of the septum and the lower lateral cartilages. Stranc and Robertson classified nasal fractures as those resulting from frontal impact and those resulting from lateral impacts.[28] Frontal impact injuries are more likely to damage the septum which must be repaired and the nasoorbitoethmoid (NOE) complex may be involved. These are categorized by the anteroposterior plane of injury.

Nasal fractures are diagnosed through physical examination. X-rays are usually not necessary. If a CT is obtained to assess for other injuries, this study will complement the examination. An intranasal examination should be performed after vasoconstricting the mucosa with a topical agent. Septal hematoma should be promptly drained to prevent cartilage resorption and a saddle nose deformity.

Most surgeons will reduce nasal fractures in a closed manner, reserving open reduction for noses with extensive lacerations. Reduction should be performed in the first

2 hours before swelling has occurred or definitely within 2 weeks of the trauma after the edema has subsided. The reduction is performed with intravenous sedation and local anesthesia or with general anesthesia. Four percent cocaine pledgets can be used for the hemostatic and anesthetic effects. A blunt tip elevator or a scalpel handle is introduced and the depressed fragments are elevated and septum is repositioned.

If the fragments are unstable postreduction, the nose can be packed with antibiotic-impregnated packing for a few days. An external splint is placed for 1 week to protect the nose from further trauma. Intranasal splints may also be used if much manipulation was performed on the septum. These patients should be advised that they might need rhinoplasty surgery in the future. One study looked at 107 patients with closed nasal reductions. Seventy percent looked deviated and 50% had abnormal breathing.[29]

Nasoorbitoethmoid Fractures

Anatomy
The NOE complex has distinct anatomic borders. Anteriorly, it is defined by the nasal processes, the frontal process of the maxilla, and the frontal bone spine. Inferiorly, it is bordered by the lower border of the ethmoidal labyrinths and laterally by the lamina papyraceae and lacrimal fossa (see Fig. 13). The vessels commonly torn in NOE fractures exit the anterior and posterior ethmoidal foramina at the upper border of the lamina papyraceae. The lamina papyracea is a very thin bone that sits behind the lacrimal fossa. NOE fractures result from a blow to the upper bridge of the nose. Once the nasal bones are fractured in this area, the NOE complex also usually fractures.

Diagnosis
Patients usually present with a flattened upper nose and swelling in the medial canthal area. Telecanthus may be masked by significant swelling. Palpation of the upper nose may reveal crepitus and loss of support. Involvement of the medial canthal tendon should be ascertained and is examined by grasping the lower eyelid and gently tugging laterally. Disruption is suspected if the medial canthal tendon cannot be pulled taut. This can be confirmed intraoperatively by inserting a clamp intranasally and pushing out on the medial canthal region while palpating the area externally.

Classification
Three types of NOE fractures have been classified by Markowitz et al.[30] Type I fractures involve a single fractured segment. Type II fractures involve a comminuted central segment and in type III fractures, the medial canthal tendon is avulsed (see Fig. 14). This classification is helpful to the surgeon in stratifying treatment.

Treatment
Exposure of the NOE complex necessitates a coronal incision with scoring of the periosteum over the nasal radix to further release the soft tissues and improve visualization of the fracture fragments. The "open sky" approach or transverse incision across the root of the nose is no longer recommended.[7] Type I injuries necessitate stabilization of the bony segment to relocalize the medial canthal tendon. Type II and III injuries necessitate a transnasal canthopexy. During this procedure, the canthal tendon should be pulled to a point posterior to the apex of the lacrimal fossa. Fixation should be kept below the anterior and posterior ethmoidal vessels, along the frontoethmoidal suture, because they mark the inferior border of the cranial cavity. The posterior ethmoidal foramen is adjacent to the optic canal and care should be taken near this area. Type I injuries should be fixated with miniplate fixation. Type II injuries may require fixation with interfragment wiring or miniplates and then junctional plating to the frontal bone, infraorbital rim, and Le Fort I level of the maxilla. In

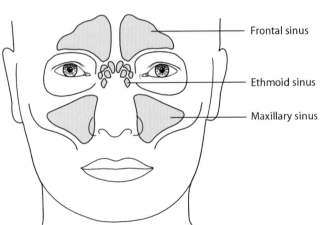
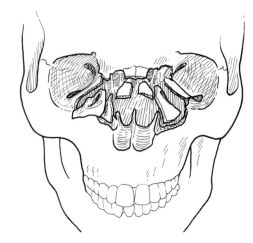

Frontal sinus

Ethmoid sinus

Maxillary sinus

Figure 13 Nasoorbitoethmoid (NOE) anatomy.

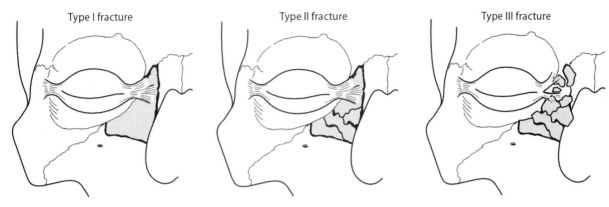

Type I fracture   Type II fracture   Type III fracture

Figure 14   Nasoorbitoethmoid (NOE) fractures.

type III injuries, the canthal tendon must be detached for reduction because the fracture fragments are small. The canthal tendon is reattached with a transnasal wire and bony reduction of the intercanthal distance should be 5 to 7 mm less than the soft tissue distance for each side.

The lacrimal system can be injured with these fractures. If it is lacerated, it should be repaired. The internal orbit should also be reconstructed by placing bone grafts behind the orbital rim. These grafts may be stacked against the displaced ethmoidal bones until the appropriate contour is achieved. Some authors advocate fixating the skin to the nasal bones after repair with bolsters transfixed by two transnasal wires.[2] Close observation should be exercised to prevent skin necrosis.

Complications

Posttraumatic telecanthus is seen with increased intercanthal distance, nasal root flattening, and lacrimal system dysfunction (see Fig. 15). Clinically, the palpebral openings are narrowed, the medial canthi are rounded, and epiphora is present.[7] Lateralization of the medial canthal tendon can be ascertained by comparing the injured to the uninjured side. Secondary correction shows poorer results than primary treatment.

NOE fractures can disrupt the lacrimal system by direct obstruction or by avulsion of the tendon–orbicularis

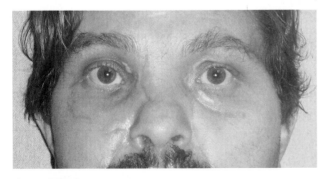

Figure 15   Telecanthus.

oculi muscle pump in 20% of patients. With persistent obstruction or dacryocystitis, a dacryocystorhinostomy or conjunctivodacryocystorhinostomy may be indicated.

Zygomatic Fractures

Anatomy

The zygomatic bone gives prominence to the cheek. It articulates with the maxilla, the greater wing of the sphenoid, and frontal and temporal bones (see Fig. 16). The bone has a lateral or malar surface and a medial orbital surface. The masseter, temporalis, zygomaticus, and zygomatic head of the quadratus labii superioris muscles attach at the zygomatic bone. The masseter attaches to the inferior border of the zygomatic arch and is the predominant deforming force in zygomatic fractures. The temporal fascia attaches to the superior border.

The term *tripod* is frequently used to refer to the zygoma and was coined by Ungley and Suggit in 1944. This is an incorrect description based on faulty knowledge of the true anatomy and should no longer be used to describe this type of fracture. The zygoma is more properly described as a pentapod for it has five main articulations (see Fig. 17). Further, in zygomatic fractures, it is usually not the zygomatic bone itself that is fractured; rather, it is separated from articulating bones at the suture lines or through fractures of the adjacent bones. As such, the zygoma has a profound effect on the position of the globe because it constitutes a large portion of the lateral wall and floor of the orbit. Even small displacement of the zygoma can result in enophthalmos.

Diagnosis

Patients with zygomaticomaxillary complex (ZMC) fractures frequently complain of numbness in the territory of the infraorbital nerve. They most commonly show periorbital edema. As the swelling subsides, step-offs can sometimes be palpated at the infraorbital rim or frontozygomatic suture. The malar area may also be depressed compared to the contralateral side. Trismus secondary to

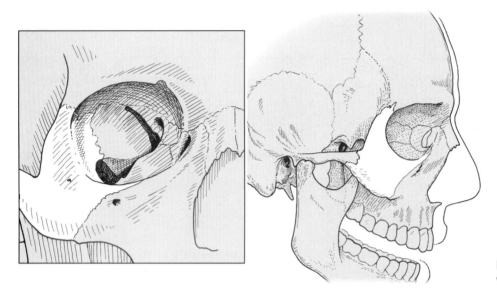

Figure 16 Zygomaticomaxillary complex (ZMC) anatomy.

the impingement of the zygoma on the coronoid process can also be seen.

A careful ocular examination is key in ZMC fractures. If the orbital volume is increased, enophthalmos will result. This is tested by comparing corneal planes on basal view. This may cause diplopia on examination. If the zygomatic contribution to the orbital floor is inferiorly displaced, hypoglobus or inferior globe displacement will result. The extraocular muscles or globe can also be injured.

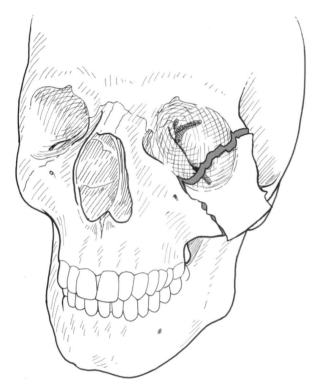

Figure 17 Zygomaticomaxillary complex (ZMC) fracture.

On radiographic examination, the role of plain x-rays is controversial. The Waters view, taken in 30-degree occipitomental projection, shows the zygomatic buttresses. With the advent of high-resolution CT, all patients with facial fractures should undergo a CT scan. Cuts measuring 1.5 mm should be used in axial and coronal views. Coronal views may need to be reconstructed from axial images, because these views require the head to be hyperextended. This is not always possible in trauma patients. In complex fractures, three-dimensional reconstructions may aid in the diagnosis and treatment plan.

Treatment

As with other fractures in the body, nondisplaced fractures are usually treated nonoperatively and displaced fractures are treated surgically. Comminution, another important factor, may require wider exposure or multiple approaches. Patients with nondisplaced fractures are observed closely, put on a soft diet, and instructed to protect the malar region for 6 weeks, especially during sleep. With isolated zygomatic arch fractures, indications for surgery include trismus and facial asymmetry with the contralateral side. The Gillies temporal approach can be used for isolated noncomminuted arch fractures.[31] This involves an incision through the temporoparietal and temporalis fascias behind the temporal hairline. An elevator is placed behind the temporalis fascia and depressed arch, and the arch is manually reduced with outward pressure. Alternatively, this can also be done through a gingivobuccal sulcus incision. The reduced fragments are maintained in position by tying a splint to the skin with sutures placed percutaneously deep to the arch on each side of the fracture and placement of a modified Glascok external ear dressing over the arch.

For displaced malar fractures, multiple approaches are often necessary.[7] The lower lid incision exposes the inferior orbital rim and floor. This incision can be transconjunctival, subciliary, or subtarsal and the decision on which to use depends on the surgeon's experience. The gingivobuccal incision exposes the zygomaticomaxillary suture and the anterior maxilla. The upper lid incision accesses the zygomaticofrontal suture as a lateral extension of the upper blepharoplasty incision. Comminuted arch fractures require a coronal approach for adequate exposure and repair. Additionally, coronal incisions may be indicated for high-impact injuries where comminution is present and wide exposure is necessary. In such cases, reduction of the arch first may provide a clue to the proper alignment of the zygoma. Approach to the arch can also be performed endoscopically.

Hollier and Thornton believe that the zygomaticofrontal region should be plated first with a 1.0-mm plate to establish the correct vertical position of the zygoma.[7] The infraorbital rim is then plated with a 1.0- or 1.5-mm plate. After this plate is placed, the position of the fracture fragments is secured so the alignment of the zygoticomaxillary buttress should be checked first. The zygomaticomaxillary buttress is plated with a 1.5- or 2.0-mm L plate. Most authors agree that at least two points of fixation are necessary to achieve stability, although three-point fixation is preferred.

After surgical fixation, the malar soft tissues are resuspended to the inferior orbital rim with suture. This allows repositioning of the soft tissues and avoids a postoperative flattened appearance to the cheek. This also supports the lower lid in the postoperative period to decrease the risk of lower lid retraction and ectropion.

Complications

On reviewing the literature on zygomatic fractures, Barclay concluded that approximately 10% of patients have diplopia initially and it persists in half of the patients (5%).[32,33] Permanent diplopia is usually experienced on upward gaze on either side. The most common cause is inferior rectus muscle entrapment when the orbital floor is involved. Other causes include injury to the extraocular muscles or the nerves or scarring of the muscles to the bony fragments. Patients with diplopia postoperatively should be followed closely as most will improve. If symptoms persist after 4 to 6 months, rebalancing of the extraocular muscles may be indicated.

The incidence of enophthalmos following zygomatic fractures is 3%.[34] Any increase in orbital volume from lateral rotation of the lateral wall will result in posterior displacement of the globe. To treat this problem, the fracture must be recreated with a saw and the zygoma must be moved superiorly, anteriorly, or medially.[35] Another approach is to just deal with the enophthalmos by augmenting the orbital floor. The periorbita are released to allow the globe to move anteriorly and graft is placed within the floor through a lower lid incision or an antral approach. The position of the globe should appear overcorrected and proptotic in the postoperative period. Once the edema

recedes, the globe will come to sit just posteriorly in a more natural position.

Fractures through the nerve foramen for the infraorbital nerve are common, for this area is weakened by the foramen. Patients complain of numbness in the cheek and upper lip. An incidence of 24% has been reported in the Zingg series.[36] This complication usually resolves as the nerve is rarely transected. Resolution may take several weeks.

Through the oculocardiac reflex, patients with zygomatic fractures can experience bradycardia, nausea, and syncope. This is mediated through the ophthalmic division of the trigeminal nerve, which passes through the reticular formation to the vagus nerve. Patients with intraoperative bradycardia should be suspected of having entrapment of the intraorbital fat or muscles in the orbital floor and prompt release is indicated. Without release, life-threatening arrhythmias can result.

MAXILLARY FRACTURES

Introduction

The maxilla has been termed the *central keystone of the face*,[37] as it connects the cranial base with the mandible inferiorly. The early methods of fixation included external fixation, internal wiring, and suspension techniques. In the 1970s, Ferraro and Berggren introduced rigid internal fixation with bone grafting for repair of complex facial fractures. This has become the standard of care. The principles of repair currently include[1] early single-stage repair,[2] accurate anatomic reduction,[3] rigid fixation,[4] wide exposure of fracture,[5] immediate autogenous bone grafting,[6] and definitive soft tissue repair. In their studies of midfacial skeletal anatomy, Manson, Hoopes, and Su identified three vertical pillars of the maxilla. These include the nasomaxillary, zygomaticomaxillary, and the pterygomaxillary buttresses (see Fig. 18). These buttresses resist vertical stresses during trauma. Perpendicular forces, though, produce "disjunctions of the maxilla."[38,39] Manson et al. described horizontal buttresses which include the frontal bar, infraorbital rims, zygomatic arches, and mandibular body.[39,40] Midfacial width and projection is determined by these horizontal pillars and the NOE complex, maxillary arch, and palate. The horizontal buttresses are coronal or sagittal but the midface lacks good sagittal buttresses except for the zygomatic arch. Unlike the mandible, the buttresses of the midface are relatively thin and fragile.

Epidemiology

Approximately 40% of facial fractures involve the midface.[38,41–47] This does not include nasal fractures which account for one third of cases. Large series of facial fractures show that Le Fort II fractures are more common than

Lateral

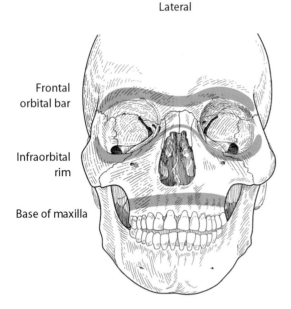

Frontal
orbital bar

Infraorbital
rim

Base of maxilla

Vertical

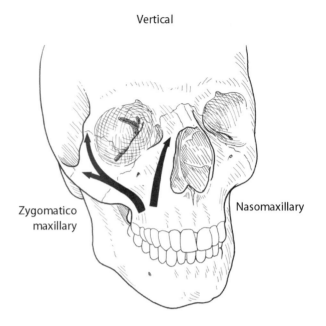

Zygomatico
maxillary

Nasomaxillary

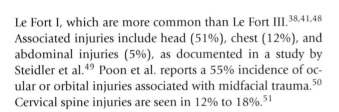

Figure 18   Maxillary buttresses.

Le Fort I, which are more common than Le Fort III.[38,41,48] Associated injuries include head (51%), chest (12%), and abdominal injuries (5%), as documented in a study by Steidler et al.[49] Poon et al. reports a 55% incidence of ocular or orbital injuries associated with midfacial trauma.[50] Cervical spine injuries are seen in 12% to 18%.[51]

Biomechanics

In a biomechanical study by Nahum, the following conclusions were reached regarding the vulnerability of facial bones to impact force:[1] women have a lower impact tolerance than men;[2] the soft tissue envelope helps to absorb some of the impact energy;[3] the nasal bones are the most fragile followed by the zygomatic arch;[4] the maxilla is sensitive to localized horizontal trauma;[5] the mandible is less resistant to lateral forces than to frontal ones. High-energy fractures are seen in the frontal bone, maxilla, and anterior mandible. Low-energy fractures are seen in the nasal bones, zygoma, frontal sinus, and nasoethmoid region. Still, it is interesting to note that a 30-mph crash will exceed the impact tolerance of most facial bones.[52]

Clinical Evaluation

In Le Fort I fractures, edema of the midface can be seen and the patient may complain of pain and tenderness in the area. This type of fracture is through the maxilla and results in a floating palate. Le Fort II fractures extend through the orbits and nasoethmoid region separating the midface. Le Fort III fractures separate the face from the cranium by also extending through the lateral orbital walls (see Fig. 19). Most complex midface fractures, though, do not fall into

one particular category but into a combination of more than one type. Le Fort II and III fractures show periorbital and subconjunctival echymosis, edema and lengthening of the face, and malocclusion. These findings constitute the "panda facies." Palpation of the maxilla should be carried out with one hand on the anterior maxilla and the other on the nasal root. In Le Fort I fractures, the lower maxilla and palate move but the nasal root does not. Le Fort II fractures have nasal root motion and a fracture can be felt at the infraorbital rim. Le Fort III fractures also have nasal root motion and movement of the lateral orbital rim.

Treatment

After the airway is secured and potentially life-threatening injuries are treated, the goal of treatment is to establish preinjury occlusion, mastication, facial height, facial width, and the ability to communicate. Access to the anterior buttresses and to the inferior orbital rim can be obtained through the upper gingivobuccal sulcus. The inferior orbital rims can also be reached through transconjunctival, subciliary, or subtarsal incisions. The choice of incision depends on surgeon preference and care should be taken not to injure the infraorbital nerve. Nasoethmoid fractures can be exposed through a coronal incision or through a traumatic skin laceration. A lateral canthotomy incision or a laterally extended upper blepharoplasty incision can be used to access fractures at the zygomaticofrontal suture line. This injury can also be reached through a coronal incision if it is being performed for another injury.

In the past, midfacial fracture treatment consisted of MMF and craniofacial suspension. Currently, the mainstay of treatment involves rigid fixation. Plate fixation

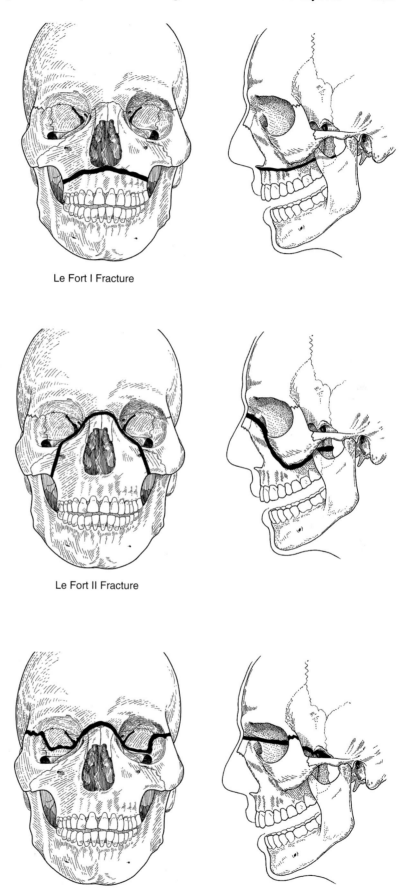

Le Fort I Fracture

Le Fort II Fracture

Le Fort III Fracture

Figure 19 Le Fort fractures.

must prevent six different motions. These include three translational and three rotational motions along the x, y, and z axes. To prevent rotation, plates must fixate fractures in three points that are not in the same line.[53] Bony compression is not necessary for healing and small bone gaps (<5 mm) are acceptable. At least two screws should be placed on either side of the fracture and the bone will heal with direct bony union. Comminuted buttress fracture should be bone grafted. Manson has written that the midface should be stabilized in MMF with the mandible before plate fixation of the midface. This will assure preinjury occlusion and avoid midfacial retrusion.

Hendrickson describes six types of *palatal fractures:*[54]

Type I, anterior and posterolateral alveolar; Type II, sagittal; Type III, parasagittal; Type IV, para alveolar; Type V, complex; Type VI, transverse. Thornton and Hollier feel that fractures with anterior–posterior orientation and with no comminution should be internally fixated.[37] Otherwise, comminuted or complex fractures should be managed with palatal splints. Care should be taken not to devascularize the buccal, gingival, or palatal mucosa during surgical access. Sometimes, the gingivobuccal incision must be oriented vertically in line with a traumatic laceration. In the palatal vault, incisions should be directed longitudinally and located centrally to avoid injuring the greater palatine artery, which runs anteroposteriorly above the palatal mucoperiosteum. For alveolar fractures, closed reduction and immobilization for 4 to 6 weeks is often adequate. Adequate reduction mandates that the dental arch, palatal vaults, and four anterior vertical buttresses be reduced and stabilized. Intraoral splints are also useful to supplement stabilization of the palate after reduction and fixation.

Complex midface fractures are usually caused by high-velocity mechanisms such as gunshot wounds or motor vehicle crashes. These fractures are usually comminuted and unstable. A low GCS is not a contraindication to surgical intervention unless the prognosis is very poor. The intracranial pressure, though, must be monitored and should be kept <25 mm Hg.

To adequately treat complex midfacial fractures, diagnostic imaging should be used to create a three-dimensional configuration of the fractures. Well-established treatment principles should be used as outlined by Marciani and Gonty.[55] These include[1] early definitive repair,[2] anatomic repair of NOE injuries,[3] wide exposure of the fracture,[4] and stable fixation in all planes. Pollock and Gruss recommend the following sequence for management of complex midfacial fractures.[56,1] The mandible is stabilized first and any fractures rigidly fixated.[2] The maxilla is placed in proper occlusion in relation to the mandible and stabilized with arch bars.[3] Zygomatic fractures and any fragments that may interfere with the reduction of maxillary fragments are reduced and plated.[4] The maxillary buttresses are reduced and rigidly fixated with miniplates.[5] Orbital fractures are reduced through an open approach.[6] The NOE complex

is reconstructed and the medial canthal tendon is reattached if indicated.[57] Nasal fractures are reduced and any nasofrontal separation is reduced.[58] Frontal bone and sinus fractures are treated.[7] Facial lacerations and soft tissue avulsions are repaired.

After surgical fixation, MMF is released unless bony stabilization is difficult to obtain because of comminution or a complex fracture. Releasing MMF simplifies airway management and may eliminate the need for tracheostomy.

Fractures in Children

In children younger than five years, facial fractures are relatively rare (<1% of facial trauma). As children enter school, this incidence increases steadily into young adulthood. There is a preponderance of these fractures in males compared to females. Parker and Lehman[59] have postulated reasons for the difference of anatomic distribution of facial fractures in children as compared to adults. Newborns have a much smaller bony volume of the face in relation to the cranium. The cranial sutures are not fused and the bone is pliable. The midface is foreshortened and the sinuses are small. Children between the ages of 6 and 12 years have mixed temporary and permanent dentition. Therefore, fractures of the midface are rare.

The assessment of midface fractures in children often requires sedation and sometimes, general anesthesia. Plain films are less useful than with adults and CT scans are usually necessary for evaluation. Children may be prone to vomiting and aspiration from gastric distension so the airway must be assessed and secured early. Fractures that are minimally displaced can be treated nonoperatively. Displaced or comminuted fractures should be treated expeditiously as children's bones heal faster than that of adults. MMF or fixation hardware should not be placed near tooth buds to avoid damage to the developing teeth. MMF can be accomplished with acrylic splints and piriform aperture or circummandibular wires. After plate and screw fixation, many authors recommend[60] the removal of hardware after the fracture has healed. Some clinicians prefer to use splints or nonrigid systems for fracture repair.

Complications

Patients with midface fractures often complain of numbness and paresthesias in the infraorbital nerve distribution. This is the most common nerve problem in facial trauma. This is especially true with zygomatic fractures. Ocular problems are also common from 17% to 55% of the time. These problems include diplopia, enophthalmos, blindness, blurred vision, telecanthus, and epiphora. The incidence of blindness in the literature is 1%.[43]

CSF rhinorrhea is also relatively common in severe facial fractures. In a study by Morgan the incidence was found to be 35%.[41] In his study, the rhinorrhea resolved in 66% of patients by the fifth day and persisted >10 days in

13%. Surgical repair of the dura is indicated when the drainage lasts >2 weeks, is significant, or persists even with placement of a lumbar drain.

Infections are relatively rare in facial fractures. Meningitis was seen in 1 in 240 patients in Steidler's study.[61] Sinusitis was seen in 1.7% of patients. With surgical fixation, fixation hardware can become infected, prominent, exposed, or migrate from its intended position. A large retrospective study of 1,112 fractures showed a 12% incidence of complications requiring hardware removal.[62] This can be decreased with perioperative antibiosis, adequate placement of hardware, and good soft tissue coverage. Other complications include malocclusion as in mandibular fractures. Careful attention to occlusal relationships before fixation can minimize this problem.

MANDIBULAR FRACTURES

Epidemiology

Mandibular fractures are common injuries due to the prominence of this bone and its susceptibility to external trauma. More than half of mandibular fractures are caused by assaults or altercations. Motor vehicle crashes also cause a significant number of these injuries. In decreasing order or incidence, fractures occur in the body, angle, condyle, ramus, symphysis, alveolar process, and coronoid process.

Anatomy

The mandible is a long U-shaped bone with tooth-bearing and non–tooth-bearing portions. The tooth-bearing portion has a thick and compact anterior border supporting the alveolar process. The mandible can be divided into the symphysis, body, angle, ascending ramus, coronoid process, and condylar process (see Fig. 20). The mandibular angle, ramus, coronoid process, and condyle are points of attachment for the muscles of mastication. The condyle

articulates with the cranium at the temporomandibular joint (TMJ). This joint is a compressed fibrous disc interposed between the condyle of the mandible and the temporal fossa.

The blood supply to the mandible arises from the inferior alveolar artery, which is a branch of the maxillary artery, and from the muscular attachments through perforating periosteal arterioles. The artery enters the mandibular foramen and exits the mental foramen as does the inferior alveolar nerve and mental nerve. The artery sends apical and periodontal branches within the mandibular canal. The inferior alveolar nerve innervates the mandible and mandibular teeth.

A key component of managing mandibular trauma is the maintenance of the occlusal relationships of the mandibular and maxillary teeth. The Angle classification stratifies the normal and abnormal relationships. This classification is based on the relationship of the mesial buccal cusp of the maxillary first molar to the mesial buccal groove of the mandibular first molar. Class I or normal occlusion is one where the mesial buccal cusp sits on the mesial buccal groove. In class II or distal occlusion, the mesial cusp sits anterior to the mesial buccal groove giving a retrusive or underdeveloped appearance to the mandible. Class III malocclusion gives a protruding appearance and the mesial buccal cusp sits posterior to the groove (see Fig. 21). In addition, abnormalities of occlusion in the lateral direction, which are termed *crossbite* or *laterognathism*, or an *absence to contact in any area*, should be noted. These relationships are very important to note both pre- and postoperatively so that previous dental occlusion can be established.

Biomechanics

For normal mandibular development, the bone must have an adequate soft tissue and muscular envelope and must undergo proper functional loading. If these are not present, deformation can occur. In general, tensile forces

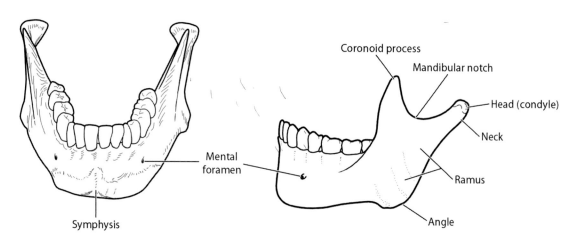

Figure 20 Mandible anatomy.

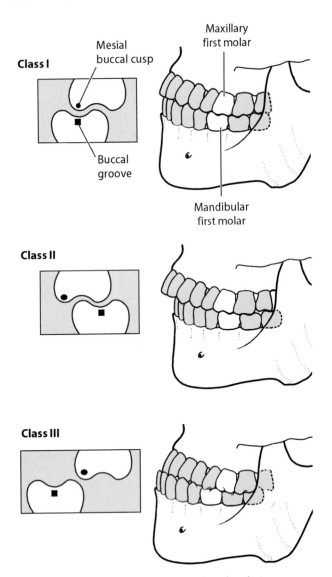

Class I

Mesial buccal cusp

Maxillary first molar

Buccal groove

Mandibular first molar

Class II

Class III

Figure 21 The Angle classification of dental occlusion.

the fracture ends. This type of healing only occurs with absolute stability of the fracture site as seen with rigid plate or screw fixation. Secondary healing occurs through stages, which include bone resorption, callus formation, and differentiation of osteogenic cells into osteoblasts and chondroblasts that form cartilage. This cartilage is ultimately replaced by bone. This type of bone healing is not slower and occurs when there is relative fracture instability such as in MMF or wire fixation.

Fracture Classification

Fractures of the mandible are classified as open or closed, displaced or nondisplaced, linear or comminuted, and complete or incomplete. Open fractures are those that communicate with the environment, although a tear in the mucosa or skin or if it communicates with a tooth socket clinically or radiographically. Fractures may be displaced or nondisplaced depending on the level of comminution and the orientation of the fracture with respect to the muscles of mastication. Muscle contraction or the nature of the trauma can be responsible for the displacement. For example, the lateral pterygoid muscle is responsible for displacing the superior component of a subcondylar fracture anteriorlly and medially.

Clinical Evaluation

The signs and symptoms of mandibular injuries include pain, tenderness, trismus, malocclusion, edema, paresthesia, anesthesia, echymosis, and hemorrhage. Function is assessed by looking at teeth opening and lateral excursion. On opening of the mouth, protrusion and deviation of the jaw indicates limited translation of the ipsilateral condyle, which may be due to a condylar fracture. The TMJ can be palpated in the preauricular area through the external auditory canal. In an intraoral examination, any fractured, avulsed, or loose teeth should be documented. Malocclusion should also be documented and compared to the preinjury occlusion. Malocclusion is not always the result of injury and is often present in the general population. Preinjury occlusion is estimated by matching the wear facets of the maxillary and mandibular teeth. Sometimes dental models are needed to determine the preinjury occlusion.

Treatment

The goals of treatment of mandibular fractures are[1] to achieve anatomic reduction and stabilization,[2] to establish preinjury occlusion,[3] to restore facial height and projection,[4] and to achieve a balanced facial contour and symmetry.[37] Nonoperative treatment is indicated when the fracture is non- or minimally displaced, when mandibular range of motion is normal, and when preinjury occlusion is maintained. This subset of patients should be followed

predominate along the alveolus and superior border, whereas compressive forces predominate on the inferior border. These forces affect the displacement and stability of different fracture patterns.

The TMJ functions both as a hinge but also translates. Early in mandibular opening, the condyle rotates like a hinge. With wider opening, the condyle moves anteriorly and inferiorly along the temporal fossa. Mandibular function and strength are also greatly affected by the presence or absence of teeth. Without teeth, the functional stimulus is absent and the alveolar bone will resorb. This will decrease the vertical dimension of the mandible and will weaken the involved portion.

After a mandibular fracture, the type of bony healing that occurs depends on both bone contact and degree of movement. Primary bone healing consists of direct bone formation without differentiation of connective tissue and cartilage. There is no callus formation or resorption of up closely and should be restricted to a liquid-only or soft diet for 30 days. Mouth opening should be restricted and good oral hygiene should be maintained.[63]

The goal of surgical intervention should be to establish preinjury occlusion. Closed reduction may be appropriate when the fracture is minimally displaced. These fractures may require MMF for 3 to 6 weeks. More displaced fractures require open reduction with internal fixation. Fractures should be reduced as soon as possible to prevent infection and minimize pain. If surgery must be delayed, then the fracture should be stabilized with MMF or bridle wires to the adjacent teeth. Open fractures should be treated within 72 hours. If this does not occur, some advocate placing the patient in MMF on intravenous antibiotics before definitive repair. Loose teeth or those that prevent reduction should be removed. Edentulous patients can be stabilized with a cervical collar or with external dressings such as a Barton bandage.

Fracture Reduction by Dental Fixation

Fractures of the mandible can alter the occlusal relationship of the maxillary and mandibular teeth. It is essential that the teeth be brought into the best occlusion possible to facilitate a good chewing surface and joint function after healing of the fracture. There are several methods to establish intermaxillary fixation. The most common is the arch bar method. The arch bar is fixed to the outer surface of the teeth by securing it with a 24- or 26-gauge steel wire to the necks of the teeth. All teeth are ligated but care should be used with the incisors, which can be extruded with aggressive tightening. Extrusion can particularly be a problem in children because their teeth are not as well grounded. Arch bars can also be secured to the facial skeleton if dentition is incomplete. They are usually applied at the beginning of fracture fixation to establish good occlusion and removed after rigid fixation. Arch bars can also be used exclusively to treat certain mandibular or maxillary fractures. Rubber orthodontic bands can be used following the removal of wires or instead of wires as they exert a constant traction and help maintain the teeth in proper occlusion during the healing process.

Intermaxillary fixation with screws provides a rapid technique for stabilization. This method should be used in patients with good dentition and uncomplicated fractures. Screws are positioned superior and inferior to the maxillary and mandibular tooth roots, respectively, to avoid injury. Mandibular screws are also placed lateral to the canines to avoid injury to the mental nerves. The number and location of screw placement depends on the fracture type, location, and surgeon preference. The focused points of force can be disadvantageous and can produce a posterior open bite.

Acrylic splints are also very useful and can be wired to the teeth or used as palatal or lingual splints to specific fractures. This technique requires detailed dental knowledge and the use of models for splint construction. They are particularly useful in complex fractures such as mandibular fractures with an alveolar component or in fractures with segments of missing teeth. Splints can be used at the beginning of rigid fixation or throughout the healing period. Other techniques that are used include the application of orthodontic bands, and the Gilmer and eyelet methods.

Mandibular body fractures can sometimes be treated closed if the fracture is reducible, isolated, and the associated teeth are intact. If there is significant displacement or comminution, open treatment is indicated. The approach is usually through an intraoral incision although an extraoral Risdon incision will also provide good access. A plate is applied to the inferior border of the mandible to avoid injury to the inferior alveolar nerve within the mandibular canal. A second monocortical plate or tension band is placed on the superior border to prevent distraction of the superior border. Arch bars can also be used as a tension band. In the past, severely comminuted fractures were treated closed to avoid devascularization with periosteal stripping. In a review by Smith and Johnson, ten comminuted fractures were treated with plate fixation and all went on to heal without bone grafting.[64] With adequate reduction and internal fixation postoperative MMF is not required.

Angle fractures are commonly associated with a fracture on the contralateral side. This area is susceptible to fracture because of the presence of third molars that weakens the area, thinner bone, and the lever function of the angle. These fractures are associated with the highest complication rates. They are best managed by open reduction internal fixation (ORIF) because the proximal segment tends to displace. The intraoral approach is again more common. An extraoral approach may be used but care must be taken not to injure the marginal mandibular nerve, a branch of the facial nerve. This incision is more advantageous for severely comminuted fractures where stabilization of the fragments may pose a problem. With the intraoral approach, a transcutaneous trocar may be necessary to place the screws. Ellis concluded in 1999 based on a 10-year study that the use of a single noncompression 2.0 miniplate placed intraorally had the lowest complication rate.[65] The use of lag screws has also been described but is more technically challenging.

In patients with normal occlusion, stable *symphyseal or parasymphysial* fractures can be treated closed. With unstable fractures or abnormal occlusion an intraoral incision is commonly used for symphyseal or parasymphyseal exposure and internal plate fixation. Care must be taken not to injure the mental nerves during dissection of the soft tissues from the mandible. After reducing the fragments with a reduction clamp and ensuring preinjury occlusion, the fracture is stabilized with plates or lag screws. The inferior plate is placed at the inferior border and a tension band is placed superiorly.

Fractures of the *coronoid process* or *ramus* are usually nondisplaced because they are splinted by the masseter, temporalis, and medial pterygoid muscles. These injuries are usually treated by closed reduction with MMF. Isolated coronoid fractures rarely require any treatment.

The mandibular *condyle* can be fractured at the head, neck, and subcondylar region. The condylar neck has a small diameter and is therefore vulnerable. Condylar head fractures are intracapsular and have a tendency to produce ankylosis. In the absence of malocclusion, the patient can be placed on a soft diet and watched closely. Malocclusion mandates that preinjury occlusion should be established and the patient be placed in MMF. It is essential that the patient undergo physiotherapy after fixation with stretching and lateral excursion exercises. ORIF of condylar fractures is more controversial. Joos and Kleinheinz have written that the absolute indication to nonoperative treatment include condylar neck fractures in children, high condylar neck fractures without dislocation, and intracapsular fractures.[66] On the other hand, Zide and Kent list absolute indications to ORIF which include inability to obtain preinjury occlusion with closed maneuvers, displacement of the condyle into the middle fossa, lateral extracapsular displacement of the condyle, and the presence of a foreign body, such as a bullet, in the condyle.[67] Endoscopic assisted fracture fixation has also been described for these injuries.[68–71]

Mandibular Fractures in Children

Mandibular fractures can account for as many as 50% of pediatric facial fractures. Most frequently, the cause is motor vehicle crashes. The pediatric mandible is relatively weak because it has less bone content as unerupted teeth are developing. However, the fractures tend to be incomplete and minimally displaced because the mandible has less cortical bone and is more elastic. In children younger than 10 years, condylar fractures constitute two thirds of mandibular fractures. Fracture treatment differs in children because of the presence of deciduous and unerupted teeth. Most fractures are treated with closed reduction also because children heal fast and there is a risk of interrupting mandibular growth with surgical intervention. Stabilization can be achieved with MMF or lingual splints. Care should be exercised in applying MMF wires in children because teeth can be extracted with tightening of the wires. Condylar and subcondylar fractures should especially be treated nonoperatively because of the risk of ankylosis and growth retardation. Conversely, comminuted or displaced fractures may require ORIF in the pediatric population.

The Edentulous Patient

Treating edentulous patients is challenging because[1] they lack teeth with which to support MMF;[2] the edentulous mandible is made primarily of cortical bone and has little potential for repair;[3] the alveolar ridge is atrophic and the fragments are easily displaced by pull from the musculature;[4] the edentulous patient is usually older and has other comorbidities. Fracture stabilization can be achieved by using the patient's dentures, Gunning splints, or external fixation such as the Morris appliance. Still, Thornton and Hollier advocate rigid fixation with plates and screws because it eliminates the need for splints, it has improved healing and shorter disability time, and is associated with better function.[37]

Postoperative Care and Complications

Patients with MMF should not be extubated until they are wide awake. Further, their stomachs should be aspirated before extubation to prevent aspiration. Presumptive antibiotics are recommended in patients with open facial wounds. MMF patients should be instructed to maintain good nutrition with a high-protein full liquid diet. This population can lose significant weight if nutrition is poor. MMF is maintained for a minimum of 3 weeks postoperatively.

The most common complications after mandibular fractures include malocclusion, infection, malunion, nonunion, nerve injury, and plate exposure. The incidence of nonunion is approximately 3.2% and it occurs most frequently in the mandibular body.[37] Causes include inadequate fracture alignment and stabilization, interposition of tissue, segmental bone loss, infection, and incorrect plate application. In addition, alcoholics and patients who abuse drugs are at higher risk. The treatment for nonunion is removal of infected teeth, fracture debridement, and rigid internal fixation with or without bone grafting.

Inferior alveolar nerve sensory deficits were documented in 56% of patients before surgery in one study by Marchena et al.[72] This deficit persisted in 19% of patients. Malocclusion is usually caused by poor placement of the fixation plate, which results in improper reduction of the bone and teeth movement. Once surgery is finished and MMF is released, if occlusion is off, the surgeon should remove the plate, reapply MMF, and reestablish plate fixation. Surgeons should not rely on MMF or elastics to correct this problem.

CONCLUSION

Indeed, the treatment of the patient with maxillofacial trauma not only requires the team approach, but it also requires a thorough understanding of the anatomy and mechanisms of injury involved. Primary attention should first be given to ruling out life-threatening injuries. Although, most maxillofacial injuries are not life threatening, they can cause significant disfigurement and loss of function. As such, treatment should be guided so that preinjury form and function is reestablished.

REFERENCES

1. Manson PN. Facial Fractures. *Plastic surgery.* 2006:77–381.
2. McCarthy JG, Galiano RD, Boutros SG. *Current therapy in plastic surgery.* WB Saunders; 2006:215–270.
3. Hochberg J, Ardenghy MA, Toledo S, et al. Soft tissue injuries to face and neck: Early assessment and repair. *World J Surg.* 2001;25:1613–1625.
4. Potter JK. Facial soft tissue trauma. *Essentials of plastic surgery: a UT southwestern medical center handbook.* Quality Medical Publishers; 2007:243–248.
5. Yavuzer R, Sari A, Kelly C, et al. Management of frontal sinus fractures. *Plast Reconstr Surg.* 2005;115:6.
6. Chen K, Chen C, Mardini S, et al. Frontal sinus fractures: A treatment algorithm and assessment of outcomes based on 78 clinical cases. *Plast Reconstr Surg.* 2006;118:2.
7. Hollier L, Thornton JF. Facial fractures I: Upper two thirds. *Selected Read Plast Surg.* 2002;9(26):1–34.
8. Emery JM, von Noorden GK, Schlernitzauer DA. Orbital floor fractures: Long-term follow-up of cases with and without surgical repair. *Trans Am Acad Ophthalmol Otolaryngol.* 1971;75:802.
9. Pearl RM. Surgical management of volumetric changes in the bony orbit. *Ann Plast Surg.* 1987;19:349.
10. Raskin EM, Millman AL, Lubkin V, et al. Pediction of late enophthalmos by volumetric analysis of orbital fractures. *Ophthalmic Plast Reconstr Surg.* 1998;14:19.
11. Zins JE, Whitaker LA. Membranous versus endochondral bone: Implications for craniofacial reconstruction. *Plast Reconstr Surg.* 1983;72:778.
12. Antonyshyn O, Gruss JS, Galbraith DJ, et al. Complex orbital fractures: A critical analysis of immediate bone graft reconstruction. *Ann Plast Surg.* 1989;22:220.
13. Spaeth EB. *The principles and practice of plastic surgery.* Philadelphia: Lea & Febiger; 1939.
14. Constantian MB. Use of auricular cartilage in orbital floor reconstruction. *Plast Reconstr Surg.* 1982;69:951.
15. Stark RB, Frileck SP. Conchal cartilage grafts in augmentation rhinoplasty and orbital floor fractures. *Plast Reconstr Surg.* 1969;43:591.
16. Bartkowski SB, Krzystkowa KM. Blow-out fracture of the orbit: Diagnostic and therapeutic considerations, and results in 90 patients treated. *J Maxillofac Surg.* 1982;10:155.
17. Converse JM, Smith B. Reconstruction of the floor of the orbit by bone grafts. *Arch Ophthalmol.* 1950;44:1.
18. Costa EA, Pitanguy I, Fontoura LFS. Reconstruction of the orbital floor with rib graft. *Rev Bras Cir.* 1977;67:55.
19. Wheeler JM. *Collected papers of John M. Wheeler on opthalmic subjects.* New York: Columbia University Press; 1939.
20. Freeman BS. The direct approach to acute fractures of the zygomatic-maxillary complex and immediate prosthetic replacement of the orbital floor. *Plast Reconstr Surg.* 1962;29:587.
21. Polley JW, Ringler SL. The use of Teflon in orbital floor reconstruction following blunt facial trauma: A 20-year experience. *Plast Reconstr Surg.* 1987;79:39.
22. Browning CW. Alloplast materials in orbital repair. *Am J Ophthalmol.* 1967;63:955.
23. Converse JM. *Kazanjian and converse's surgical treatment of facial injuries,* 3rd ed. Baltimore: Williams & Wilkins; 1974.
24. Burres SA, Cohn AM, Mathog RH. Repair of orbital blow-out fractures with marlex mesh and gelfilm. *Laryngoscope.* 1981;91:1881.
25. Biesman BS, Hornblass A, Lisman R, et al. Diplopia after surgical repair of orbital floor fractures. *Ophthalmic Plast Reconstr Surg.* 1996;12:9.
26. Dulley B, Fells P. Long-term follow-up of orbital blow-out fracture with and without surgery. *Mod Probl Ophthalmol.* 1975;14:467.
27. Manson PN, Ruas EJ, Iliff NT. Deep orbital reconstruction for correction of post-traumatic enophthalmos. *Clin Plast Surg.* 1987;14:113.
28. Stranc MF, Robertson GA. A classification of injuries of the nasal skeleton. *Ann Plast Surg.* 1979;2:468.
29. Mayell MJ. Nasal fractures, their occurrence, management, and some late results. *J R Coll Surg Edinb.* 1973;18:31.
30. Markowitz BL, Manson PN, Sargent L, et al. Management of the medial canthal tendon in nasoethmoid orbital fractures: The importance of the central fragment in classification and treatment. *Plast Reconstr Surg.* 1991;87:843.
31. Feinstein FR, Krizek TJ. Fractures of the zygoma and zygomatic arch. In: Fostor CA, Sherman JE, eds. *Surgery of facial bone fractures.* New York: Churchill Livingstone; 1987:136.
32. Barclay TL. Diplopia in association with fractures involving the zygomatic bone. *Br J Plast Surg.* 1958;11:147.
33. Barclay TL. Some aspects of the treatment of traumatic diplopia. *Br J Plast Surg.* 1963;16:214.
34. Crumley RL, Leibsohn J, Krause CJ, et al. Fractures of the orbital floor. *Laryngoscope.* 1977;87:934.
35. Longaker MT, Kawamoto HK. Enophthalmos revisited. *Clin Plast Surg.* 1997;24(3):531.
36. Zingg M, Laedrach K, Chen J, et al. Classification and treatment of zygomatic fractures: A review of 1,025 cases. *J Oral Maxillofac Surg.* 1992;50:778.
37. Thornton JF, Hollier L. Facial fractures II: Lower third. *Selected Read Plast Surg.* 2002;9:27.
38. Manson PN, Hoopes JE, Su CT. Structural pillars of the facial skeleton: An approach to the management of Le Fort fractures. *Plast Reconstr Surg.* 1980;66:54.
39. Markowitz BL, Manson PN. Panfacial fractures: Organization of treatment. *Clin Plast Surg.* 1989;16(1):105.
40. Manson PN, Clark N, Robertson B, et al. Subunit principles in midface fractures: The importance of sagittal buttresses, soft-tissue reductions, and sequencing treatment of segmental fractures. *Plast Reconstr Surg.* 1999;103:1287.
41. Morgan BDG, Madan DK, Bergerot JPC. Fractures of the middle third of the face – a review of 300 cases. *Br J Plast Surg.* 1972; 25:147.
42. Manson PN, Shack RB, Leonard LG, et al. Sagittal fractures of the maxilla and palate. *Plast Reconstr Surg.* 1983;72:484.
43. McCoy FJ, Chandler RA, Magnan CG, et al. An analysis of facial fractures and their complications. *Plast Reconstr Surg.* 1962; 29:381.
44. Kelly DE, Harrigan WF. A survey of facial fractures: Bellevue Hospital, 1948–1974. *J Oral Surg.* 1975;33:146.
45. Turvey TA. Midfacial fractures: A retrospective analysis of 593 cases. *J Oral Surg.* 1977;35:887.
46. Afzelius LE, Rosen C. Facial fractures: A review of 368 cases. *Int J Oral Surg.* 1980;9:25.
47. Schultz RC, Carbonell AM. Midfacial fractures from vehicular accidents. *Clin Plast Surg.* 1975;2:173.
48. Gwyn PP, Carraway JH, Horton CE, et al. Facial fractures – associated injuries and complications. *Plast Reconstr Surg.* 1971;47:225.
49. Steidler NE, Cook RM, Reade PC. Incidence and management of major middle third facial fractures at the Royal Melbourne Hospital: A retrospective study. *Int J Oral Surg.* 1980;9:92.
50. Poon A, McCluskey PJ, Hill DA. Eye injuries in patients with major trauma. *J Trauma.* 1999;46:494.
51. Manson P. Management of facial fractures. *Perspect Plast Surg.* 1988;2(2):1.
52. Huelke DF, Harger JH. Maxillofacial injuries: Their nature and mechanism of production. *J Oral Surg.* 1969;27:451.
53. Rudderman RH, Mullen RL. Biomechanics of the facial skeleton. *Clin Plast Surg.* 1992;19(1):11.
54. Hendrickson M, Clark N, Manson PN, et al. Palatal fractures: Classification, patterns, and treatment with rigid internal fixation. *Plast Reconstr Surg.* 1998;101:319.
55. Marciani RD, Gonty AA. Principles of management of complex craniofacial trauma. *J Oral Maxillofac Surg.* 1993;51:535.
56. Pollock RA, Gruss JS. Craniofacial and panfacial fractures. In: Foster CA, Sherman JE, eds. *Surgery of facial bone fractures.* New York: Churchill Livingstone; 1987: 235–253.
57. Kirk NJ, Wood RJ, Goldstein M. Skeletal identification using the frontal sinus region: A retrospective study of 39 cases. *J Forensic Sci.* 2002;47:2.
58. Lynham AJ, Hirst JP, Cosson JA, et al. Emergency department management of maxillofacial trauma. *Emerg Med Australas.* 2004;16.

59. Parker MG, Lehman JA. Management of facial fractures in children. *Perspect Plast Surg.* 1989;3:1.
60. Posnick JC, Wells M, Pron GE. Pediatric facial fractures: Evolving patterns of treatment. *J Oral Maxillofac Surg.* 1993;51:836.
61. Steidler NE, Cook RM, Reade PC. Residual complications in patients with major middle third facial fractures. *Int J Oral Surg.* 1980;9:259.
62. Francel TJ, Brent CB, Ringleman PR, et al. The fate of plates and screws after facial fracture reconstruction. *Plast Reconstr Surg.* 1992;90:586.
63. Guerrissi JO. Fractures of the mandible: Is spontaneous healing possible? Why? When? *J Craniofac Surg.* 2001;12(2):157.
64. Smith BR, Johnson JV. Rigid fixation of comminuted mandibular fractures. *J Oral Maxillofac Surg.* 1993;51:1320.
65. Ellis E III. Treatment methods for fractures of the mandibular angle. *Int J Oral Maxillofac Surg.* 1999;28:243.
66. Joos U, Kleinheinz J. Therapy of condylar neck fractures. *Int J Oral Maxillofac Surg.* 1998;27:247.
67. Zide MF, Kent JN. Indications of open reduction of mandibular condyle fractures. *J Oral Maxillofac Surg.* 1983;41:89.
68. Jacobovicz J, Lee C, Trabulsy PP. Endoscopic repair of mandibular subcondylar fractures. *Plast Reconstr Surg.* 1998;101:437.
69. Lauer G, Schmelzeisen R. Endoscope-assisted fixation of mandibular condylar process fractures. *J Oral Maxillofac Surg.* 1999;57:36.
70. Lee C, Mueller RV, Lee K, et al. Endoscopic subcondylar fracture repair: Functional, aesthetic, and radiographic outcomes. *Plast Reconstr Surg.* 1998;102:1434.
71. Troulis MJ, Kaban LB. Endoscopic approach to the ramus/condyle unit: Clinical applications. *J Oral Maxillofac Surg.* 2001;59:503.
72. Marchena JM, Padwa BL, Kaban LB. Sensory abnormalities associated with mandibular fractures: Incidence and natural history. *J Oral Maxillofac Surg.* 1998;56:822.

Ocular Injuries

30

Adrienne L. West   Erika M. Levin

Ocular trauma is one of the leading causes of visual impairment in the United States. It is frequently accompanied by other injuries; it is imperative to assess patients for periocular and retrobulbar trauma, intracranial injury, facial and skull fractures, and injuries to the rest of the body as pertains to the mechanism of the injury. While taking a history, specific visual symptoms such as diplopia, decreased vision, flashes of light, and floaters are helpful. Visual acuity should be measured with the patient's corrective eyewear in place, and measured one eye at a time. If unable to read the largest print on the chart, measure the ability to count fingers, perceive hand motion, or light. Horizontal and vertical motility should be assessed. Confrontation visual fields are tested monocularly. The pupils should be examined for shape as well as function. External and slit lamp examinations are helpful in diagnosing many injuries. Dilated fundus examination is typically performed by an ophthalmologist. One should not dilate an eye if a ruptured globe is suspected, and it may be contraindicated in some head injury patients. Additional studies may be beneficial in certain circumstances, including ocular ultrasonography, plain radiographs, computed tomography (CT) (with a maximum of 3-mm orbital cuts and dedicated axial and coronal images), and less often magnetic resonance imaging (MRI).

EYELID LACERATIONS

Lacerations to the eyelids may need specialized repair by an ophthalmologist. If not properly closed, wounds that involve the eyelid margin may result in a notched appearance. All patients with lid lacerations should be evaluated for injuries to the globe. When the medial one third of either eyelid is affected, the lacrimal drainage system may be damaged. Probing and irrigation through the punctum aid in the diagnosis of canalicular lacerations. These are repaired with placement of a silastic stent into

the nasolacrimal duct. Yellow fat visible in the wound signifies that the orbital septum has been violated, which may result in significant scarring and/or ptosis. In these cases, exploration and repair by an oculoplastic surgeon or an ophthalmologist with extensive knowledge of the orbit is recommended.

CHEMICAL INJURIES

Chemical injuries are ocular emergencies. In particular, alkali burns quickly penetrate the eye and can be devastating. Irrigate immediately with saline or water before obtaining a history or checking visual acuity. Topical anesthetic may be used before irrigation to facilitate patient cooperation. The patient should be placed in such a position that the irrigating solution will not drain into the unaffected eye. Irrigation should continue until the pH level reaches neutral. Sweep the fornices with a moistened cotton tip applicator to remove any precipitated chemicals. Mildly damaged eyes are typically red and irritated. More severe burns cause conjunctival ischemia, corneal opacification, and glaucoma. Whitening of the eye is an ominous predictor of long-term complications.

SUBCONJUNCTIVAL HEMORRHAGE

Subconjunctival hemorrhage is a collection of blood underneath the conjunctiva. No treatment is necessary other than to evaluate the integrity of the globe and to lubricate eye when the hemorrhage interferes with eyelid closure.

SUPERFICIAL FOREIGN BODIES

Foreign bodies of the cornea and conjunctiva cause a variety of symptoms such as pain, tearing, photophobia, and irritation. Corneal foreign bodies are diagnosed by direct examination with a slit lamp and subsequent fluorescein administration. Metallic foreign bodies frequently leave rust rings in the cornea, which rarely cause visual complaints. Palpebral conjunctival foreign bodies may cause vertical or oblique scratches on the cornea. Superficial foreign bodies can be removed with irrigation or rolling a moistened cotton-tipped applicator over the particle. Deep or embedded foreign bodies should be removed by an ophthalmologist with a needle or fine forceps. Topical antibiotics should be prescribed, and follow-up ophthalmic examination is recommended to ensure that the foreign body has been completely removed and no infection is present. Topical anesthetics should never be prescribed to patients as they are associated with an increased risk of corneal perforation and mask symptoms of infection.

CORNEAL ABRASIONS

Corneal abrasions present with symptoms similar to foreign bodies. Clear corneas that stain with fluorescein dye are diagnostic of abrasions. White spots or opacifications of the cornea that stain suggest ulcers or infections, which need urgent ophthalmic consultation. A simple abrasion should be treated with topical ophthalmic antibiotics. Large abrasions may be treated with a pressure patch for 24 hours. Children should not be patched because of the risk of amblyopia, nor should contact lens wearers due to the increased risk of infection. Patients should be seen by an eye care specialist the next day to assess healing and check for infection.

HYPHEMA

Blood present in the anterior chamber of the eye is referred to as a hyphema (see Fig. 1). A hyphema results from the tearing of blood vessels of the iris or the ciliary body. It may be seen at the slit lamp as red blood cells floating in the aqueous fluid, layered blood in front of the iris, or filling the entire anterior chamber. Blood cells can block the outflow of aqueous through the trabecular meshwork, resulting in elevation of intraocular pressure, that is, glaucoma. Patients with sickle cell disease or trait are especially at risk for glaucoma. Patients are kept at bedrest to minimize rebleeding, a shield is placed over the eye, and topical corticosteroid and dilating drops are given. Anticoagulants should be avoided when possible. Controversy exists whether to treat with systemic steroids or aminocaproic acid (Amicar) to prevent rebleeding.[1] Patients are followed up daily for 5 days with intraocular pressure checks, and then as needed. Patients should be reexamined a month after the injury to stratify the risk of future glaucoma development.

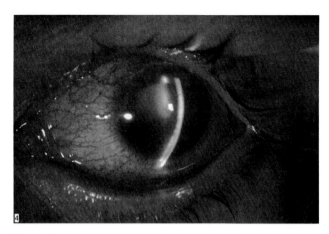

Figure 1 Anterior chamber hyphema. (Photo courtesy of WK Kellogg Eye Center.)

RUPTURED GLOBE

Physical signs of a ruptured or lacerated globe include a peaked or teardrop-shaped pupil, iris or brown uveal tissue protruding through the cornea or sclera, subconjunctival or intraocular hemorrhage, or a physically distorted eye. If a foreign body is present, it is better to leave the object in place to avoid further trauma to the eye. No pressure should be exerted onto the globe. Visual acuity, pupil response, and presence or absence of a red reflex should be measured as this may be helpful in counseling the patient on postoperative visual prognosis. Defer measurements of intraocular pressure and do not patch the eye. Instead, place a metal shield or plastic cup over the eye and orbit, securing it with tape at the brow and cheek. Ophthalmology consultation should occur in a timely manner. Tetanus booster and intravenous antibiotics should be administered in the emergency department. Surgical exploration and repair are recommended as soon as possible, hence standard preoperative orders should commence. These eyes are at high risk for infectious endophthalmitis (8%) and ultimate enucleation (11%).[2,3]

IRIS INJURIES

Trauma to the iris results in a peaked or irregular-shaped pupil, peripheral tears causing an additional red reflex (iridodialysis), or hyphema. Three potential problems exist for these patients: secondary glaucoma, glare, and diplopia. Secondary glaucoma occurs when the anterior chamber angle is sufficiently traumatized to interfere with outflow of aqueous through the trabecular meshwork, resulting in increased intraocular pressure and optic nerve damage. Medical or surgical management may be required to maintain adequately low intraocular pressure. Damage to the iris sphincter muscles can result in a large or irregularly-shaped pupil. Photosensitivity may be a problem for these patients. Peripheral tears cause the iris to dehisce from the sclera, creating another opening in the iris. These patients may also suffer extreme photosensitivity or diplopia as a result of having images pass through this second pupil. Both conditions may be managed with specialty colored contact lenses to mask the abnormality. Surgical correction may be warranted.

LENS INJURIES

Lens damage can be caused by blunt or penetrating trauma, chemicals, radiation, or electrical currents. A cataract is an opacification of some or all of the layers of the lens. Lens material may leak from the capsule, with resultant intraocular inflammation and glaucoma, requiring urgent cataract surgery. If the capsule remains intact, cataract extraction may not be necessary. Significant loss of zonular integrity can cause subluxation or even complete dislocation of the lens within the eye, causing decreased or fluctuating vision. Lenses dislocated into the anterior chamber frequently cause acute glaucoma, requiring urgent removal, whereas lenses in the posterior vitreous cavity will ultimately require lensectomy by vitreoretinal techniques.[4]

VITREORETINAL TRAUMA

Any tear to a blood vessel of the ciliary body or retina can cause a hemorrhage into the vitreous cavity and subsequently obscure vision. Small hemorrhages may resorb on their own, whereas large, persistent hemorrhages may require surgical evacuation.[5] The vitreous may also separate from the optic nerve, retina, and/or vitreous base. One needs to carefully examine patients with intraocular hemorrhage or complaints of flashes of light and/or floaters in the vision for retinal detachment. Simple retinal tears without an associated buildup of fluid under the retina can usually be repaired with laser retinopexy or cryotherapy to create scar tissue surrounding the tear. If the retina is detached, more complicated surgical interventions including scleral buckling or pars plana vitrectomy need to be performed to achieve anatomic reattachment with the hope of visual recovery. Intraocular foreign bodies may be present in the vitreous cavity and can be directly visualized or seen on imaging studies. Vitrectomy techniques using magnets or forceps are applied. Blunt impact to the eye may result in edema of the retina (commotio retinae), with possible decreased vision. Commotio frequently resolves with restoration of normal vision and appearance of the retina; however, some patients may have permanent visual loss.[5]

OPTIC NERVE INJURIES

Direct or indirect trauma to the optic nerve may result in an optic neuropathy with decreased visual acuity or complete loss of vision. An afferent pupillary defect is present on the affected side. Initial examination usually shows a normal optic nerve head, but edema and/or hemorrhages may be present. Optic disc pallor takes several weeks to develop. Visual recovery is highly variable. Management for traumatic optic neuropathy is controversial, varying from no treatment to high-dosage intravenous methylprednisolone.[6] Rapid deceleration forces can cause complete avulsion of the optic nerve. This is typically painful, and the patient has no light perception in the involved eye. The affected eye shows a fixed pupil while the uninvolved side dilates when the light is shone in the traumatized eye. Fundus examination reveals a hole where the optic nerve head used to be located, hemorrhage, and retinal pallor. These eyes are enucleated.

ORBITAL FRACTURES

Orbital fractures may result in enophthalmos or exophthalmos, double vision, and/or limited extraocular movement. The thin medial and inferior walls are most often affected. Clinical signs of an inferior rim fracture include hypesthesia of the cheek and upper teeth, crepitus of the lower eyelid, and a palpable step-off of the orbital rim. It is important to check pupil response to light and visual acuity to assess the possibility of optic nerve damage. Plain x-rays may show fluid in the maxillary sinus in orbital floor fractures, but CT is best at diagnosing bony and soft tissue abnormalities. If the superior wall is fractured, one should check for intracranial air. Orbital fractures are usually treated conservatively with oral antibiotics, cool compresses, decongestant nasal spray, and instructions for the patient to not blow his/her nose. If either a large fracture or diplopia with soft tissue prolapse/entrapment exists, surgical repair by an orbital specialist is performed within the first 2 weeks.[7]

RETROBULBAR HEMORRHAGE

Large hemorrhages within the orbit are dangerous. As there is no natural mechanism for decompression, a compartment syndrome may develop. The elevated pressure cuts off blood flow to the optic nerve, resulting in vision loss. Clinically, one should suspect retrobulbar hemorrhage in a patient complaining of eye pain and decreased vision with a large subconjunctival hemorrhage, afferent pupillary defect, or orbital fractures. Patients using anticoagulant medications are at very high risk for retrobulbar hemorrhage with regional trauma. If a retroorbital hemorrhage is noted on CT or MRI scans, immediate examination of the patient is required. Elevated ocular pressure with decreased vision requires a lateral canthotomy and cantholysis with a hemostat and scissors. A successful procedure is recognized by the sudden outflow of accumulated blood and a lowering of the intraocular pressure readings. If performed expediently, vision loss may be averted.

REFERENCES

1. Walton W, Von Hagen S, Grigorian R, et al. Management of traumatic hyphema. *Surv Ophthalmol.* 2002;47:297–334.
2. Lieb DF, Scott IU, Flynn HW Jr, et al. Open globe injuries with positive intraocular cultures: Factors influencing final visual acuity outcomes. *Ophthalmology.* 2003;110:1560–1566.
3. Dunn ES, Jaeger EA, Jeffers JB, et al. The epidemiology of ruptured globes. *Ann Ophthalmol.* 1992;24:405–410.
4. Mian SI, Azar DT, Colby K. Management of traumatic cataracts. *Int Ophthalmol Clin.* 2002;42:23–31.
5. Pieramici DJ. Vitreoretinal trauma. *Ophthalmol Clin North Am.* 2002;15:225–234.
6. Steinsapir KD. Traumatic optic neuropathy. *Curr Opin Ophthalmol.* 1999;10:340–342.
7. Chang EL, Bernardino CR. Update on orbital trauma. *Curr Opin Ophthalmol.* 2004;15:411–415.

Injuries to the Neck

31

Arvin Chun-Yin Gee   *Kelli D. Salter*
Donald B. McConnell   *Donald D. Trunkey*

The optimal management and care of both blunt and penetrating neck trauma has undergone significant evolution in the last few decades. However, optimal management of some injuries remains unclear and is the subject of active investigation. Many of the changes have been spurred by the development of new diagnostic and therapeutic technologies that have increased the safety and efficacy of nonsurgical management.

Historically the management of neck trauma has been influenced by military experience with high-energy missile and blast injuries. This generated protocols that mandated surgical neck exploration, which lowered the rate of missed injuries but increased the number of nontherapeutic surgeries. However, in this age of "cost-containment" and evidence-based medicine, the economic cost, resource utilization, and high morbidity of exploratory neck surgery has led to some authors and trauma centers questioning this management protocol in civilian practice.

As with all other anatomic locations, blunt and penetrating injuries often require different management approaches. Considering the plethora of vital structures that reside in this compact anatomic region, neck injuries can result in significant morbidity and mortality. Seemingly innocuous wounds may not manifest clear signs or symptoms, and potentially lethal injuries could be easily overlooked or discounted. Therefore the surgeon faced with initially managing a traumatically injured person must be cognizant of the currently recommended guidelines for the evaluation and the management of neck injuries.

In this overview, we review, in a systems fashion, the diagnosis and management of the various blunt and penetrating injuries encountered by the surgeons managing these patients. This chapter provides practical guidelines and algorithms for the safe evaluation and management of civilian patients, with soft tissue injuries of the neck.

Cervical spinal cord injuries and cervical spine fractures will not be addressed in this chapter.

EPIDEMIOLOGIC FEATURES

Most neck trauma is due to a penetrating mechanism. As shown in Fig. 1, most of the penetrating neck trauma in the United States occurs as a result of interpersonal violence with firearms being the most common weapon of choice. These injuries most often affect the vascular system or results in injury of the great vessels or lung apices (see Fig. 2). Blunt neck trauma stems from a variety of etiologies. Motor vehicle crashes, falls, hangings, and chiropractic neck manipulations have all been documented to lead to blunt injuries.

Penetrating neck trauma represents approximately 5% to 10% of all trauma cases that present to the emergency department. Approximately 30% of these cases are

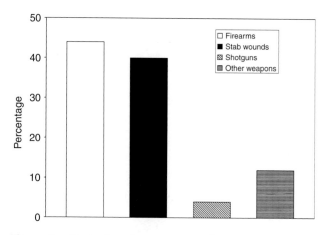

Figure 1   Mechanism of penetrating neck injuries in the United States.

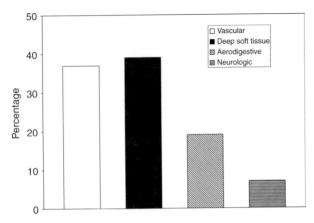

Figure 2   Distribution of systems injured by penetrating neck injury. (From Bell RB, Osborn T, Dierks EJ, et al. Management of penetrating neck injuries: A new paradigm for civilian trauma. *J Oral Maxillofac Surg.* 2007;65:691–705.)

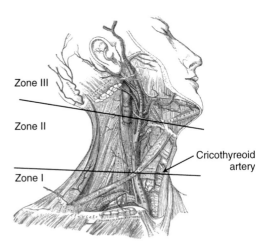

Figure 4   Zones of the neck. Zone I: thoracic inlet to the cricoid cartilage; zone II: cricoid cartilage (highlighted by the arrow) to the mandibular angle; zone III: mandibular angle to the skull base. (Adapted from Gray H. Anatomy of the human body, 20th ed. Philadelphia: Lea & Febiger; 1918. Bartleby.com, 2000. http://www.bartleby.com/br/107.html.)[3]

accompanied by injury outside of the neck zones as well. The current mortality rate in civilians with penetrating neck injuries ranges from 3% to 6%. Whereas blunt neck trauma is fairly common, actual soft tissue injuries from blunt trauma is relatively rare and has been estimated to be <1% of all neck injuries.[1] Despite its relative rarity, blunt laryngotracheal (LT) trauma carries a mortality rate that can be as high as 40%, whereas the mortality rate of penetrating LT injuries is approximately 20%.[2]

ANATOMIC FEATURES

Successful management of neck injuries depends on a clear understanding of the anatomy of the neck. The close

proximity of vital structures with the anterior third of the neck is clearly demonstrated in the cross-sectional view of the neck as shown in Fig. 3.

For the purposes aiding clinical decisions for diagnostic testing and management, surgeons have described the neck by dividing it into three anatomic zones in the caudal to cranial orientation as shown in Fig. 4. The six organ systems within these neck zones include vascular, respiratory, digestive, neurologic, endocrine, and skeletal. The vascular system includes the innominate, subclavian, axillary, carotid, jugular, and vertebral vessels. The respiratory system includes the larynx, trachea, and the lung. The

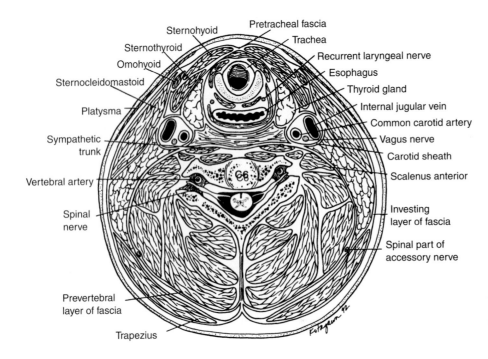

Figure 3   A cross-section drawing of the neck anatomy. (From McConnell DB, Trunkey DD. Management of penetrating trauma to the neck. *Adv Surg.* 1994;27:97–127.)

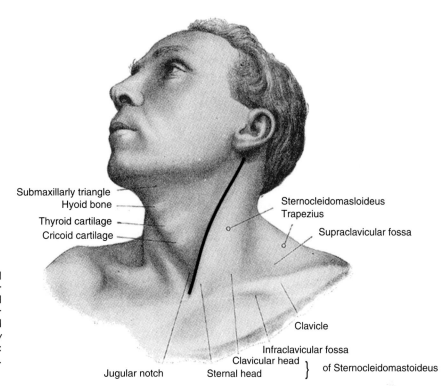

Figure 5   Surface anatomy of the head and neck with the incision for an anterior sternocleidomastoid approach. The solid black line indicates the anterior border of the patient's left sternocleidomastoid muscle. (Modified from Gray H. *Anatomy of the human body*, 20th ed. Philadelphia: Lea & Febiger; 1918. Bartleby.com, 2000. http://www.bartleby.com/br/107.html.)[3]

digestive system includes the pharynx and esophagus. The neurologic system includes the spinal cord, brachial plexus, cranial nerves, and the sympathetic chain. The endocrine system includes the thyroid and parathyroid. The skeletal system includes the cervical spine, clavicle, upper rib cage, and skull base.

Serving as the line of demarcation, the sternocleidomastoid muscle separates the neck into anterior and posterior triangles. Most of the important vascular and visceral organs lie within the anterior triangle bounded by the sternocleidomastoid posteriorly, the midline anteriorly, and the mandible superiorly. Except for individual nerves to specific muscles, few vital structures cross the posterior triangle, which is delineated by the sternocleidomastoid, the trapezius, and the clavicle (with the exception of the region just superior to the clavicle). The area of injury depends on the mechanism of injury. Overall, zone II is the most commonly injured area (see Fig. 5).[4]

Zone I, the base of the neck, is demarcated by the thoracic inlet inferiorly and the cricoid cartilage superiorly. Vascular structures at greatest risk in this zone include the innominate vessels, jugular veins, common carotid artery origin, subclavian vessels, and vertebral artery. Other important nonvascular structures located within this zone include the brachial plexus, trachea, esophagus, apices of the lungs, thoracic duct, cervical spine, and cervical nerve roots. Surgical exposure of these structures, particularly the vascular structures, is difficult because of the presence of the clavicle. Furthermore, signs of a significant injury in the zone I region may be hidden from inspection by residing within the chest or the mediastinum.

Zone II encompasses the midportion of the neck and is defined as the region between the cricoid cartilage and the angle of the mandible. Important structures in this region include the carotid and vertebral arteries, jugular veins, pharynx, larynx, trachea, esophagus, and cervical spine and spinal cord. Zone II, in comparison with zones I and III, is the most easily accessible region for clinical examination and surgical exploration. Therefore, zone II injuries are likely to be the most apparent on physical examination and are also the easiest to evaluate intraoperatively without the aid of preoperative diagnostic testing.

Zone III defines the superior aspect of the neck and is bounded by the angle of the mandible and the base of the skull. Diverse structures, such as the salivary and parotid glands, cervical spine, the distal extracranial carotid arteries, jugular veins, and major nerves (including cranial nerves IX-XII), traverse this zone. Zone III is not amendable to easy physical examination or surgical exploration; therefore, injuries in zone III can require special diagnostic studies to aid in management.

PREHOSPITAL MANAGEMENT

The evaluation of a patient with penetrating neck trauma should always begin with Advanced Trauma Life Support, a paradigm that starts with a directed primary survey emphasizing airway, breathing, and circulation. However, attempts to manage the airway and resuscitate the patient in the field are ill advised and potentially dangerous. Therefore, the scene time should be kept to a minimum, especially if there is a short transport time to the nearest designated trauma center.

Bleeding control can be achieved by direct pressure and the risk of an air embolism can be reduced by the placement of patient in the Trendelenburg position. Placement of intravenous (IV) lines can be attempted *en route* to the hospital. Oxygen can be administered by mask or nasal cannula. However, assisted ventilation with bag-valve-mask may be contraindicated because it may result in massive subcutaneous emphysema or air embolus in patients with an open LT injury. Furthermore, prehospital endotracheal intubation should be attempted only in patients in extremis, have a compromised airway, or have anticipated prolonged transport times. Most low-velocity gunshots and stab wounds do not result in airway compromise, but high-velocity gunshot and shotgun wounds and severe blunt trauma will often necessitate emergent airway management.

Traumatized airways are usually challenging to intubate because of the primary injury, blood, tissue, local edema, and debris. Blind intubation can result in the endotracheal tube creating a false passage or complete the transection of an injured trachea resulting in severe morbidity. Blind intubation should not be attempted because of its inherent low success rate and the high mortality of a failed blind intubation. It is important to remember that a surgical airway is sometimes needed and prehospital personnel must be prepared for this scenario before any attempts at endotracheal tube placement.

Cervical spine protection by means of a neck collar remains a common practice during the prehospital transportation. Given the high incidence of cervical spine fracture associated with high-energy penetrating neck injuries, cervical immobilization should be attempted when feasible.[5] However, it should be abandoned if it would cause an undue delay or hindrance to emergent management of the patient and may, in fact, be harmful in patients with an expanding hematoma that may cause respiratory obstruction.

Zone I injuries can have a concomitant pneumothorax, which can be simply treated during transport by placing a large-bore needle and IV catheter into the pleural space. Additionally, if a large venous injury is suspected, peripheral IV line placement should be on the contralateral side to the injury to minimize fluid extravasation and to maximize the ability to replete the patient's intravascular volume.

EMERGENCY DEPARTMENT/TRAUMA BAY MANAGEMENT

Airway Management

Upon arrival at the emergency department, the patient should be surveyed and treated for immediate life-threatening conditions as delineated in the Advanced

Trauma Life Support protocols.[6] Airway management is the first and most challenging priority in the management of severe penetrating neck injury. In a review by Vassiliu et al., 29% of patients with LT trauma and 41% of patients with pharyngoesophageal (PE) trauma required emergency intubation.[7]

Airway compromise may arise due to direct trauma or severe edema to the larynx or trachea or from external compression by a stable or expanding hematoma. Management of airway in patients with penetrating neck injury should be individualized according to the condition of the patient, the nature of the injury, and the experience of the trauma team.

Ideally, there is an experienced anesthesiologist on the trauma team to assist with advanced airway management. A surgeon should always be present in case an emergent surgical airway is warranted because up to one fourth of patients with aerodigestive tract trauma have failed rapid sequence induction intubation.[7] If a surgical airway is required and there is an obvious LT wound, the endotracheal tube can be carefully inserted under direct vision into the distal airway. Creation of surgical airway in these challenging conditions requires a closely coordinated team effort between the surgeons and the anesthesiologists.

In most emergent situations a cricothyrotomy is the surgical airway of choice rather than a tracheostomy. The more inferior placement of a tracheostomy has a lower rate of tracheal stenosis than with cricothyrotomies. However, the exposure required for a tracheostomy is often more technically challenging due to the location of the anterior jugular veins and the thyroid gland and its associated vasculature. A cricothyrotomy safely avoids the thyroid gland and most of the anterior vessels of the neck. The higher rate of late complications associated with cricothyrotomy can be avoided by electively converting it to a tracheostomy 1 to 2 days after the patient's condition allows for the procedure.

Circulation Management

As in the prehospital setting, the patient should be placed in the Trendelenburg position when there is active bleeding to reduce the risk of air embolism from venous injuries. Hemorrhage control can often be achieved simply by direct pressure in most patients. However, in the event that external pressure is not effective, as in the case of bleeding from the vertebral or subclavian vessels, digital compression with a gloved index finger inserted into the wound may be more effective in temporizing the bleeding *en route* to the operating room.

Regardless of the zonal location of injury, exsanguinating hemorrhage, expanding hematoma, refractory shock, airway compromise, and severe subcutaneous emphysema (see Table 1) are all indications for immediate surgical exploration and intervention.[8] Finally, for those patients in cardiac arrest or imminent cardiac arrest, an anterior

TABLE 1

INDICATIONS FOR EMERGENT NECK EXPLORATION

Indication for Emergent Exploration

Exsanguinating hemorrhage
Expanding hematoma
Shock refractory to resuscitation
Airway compromise
Severe subcutaneous emphysema

---

resuscitative thoracotomy may be indicated if an injury to zone I vasculature is suspected.[9] The thoracotomy exposure should allow for intrathoracic direct control of zone I vascular injuries. However, the survival rate following resuscitative thoracotomy for penetrating neck injury is very poor.

SECONDARY SURVEY

History and Physical Examination

Following airway management and circulation stabilization, the secondary survey should be conducted to evaluate for concomitant injuries. Especially in instances where a neck injury is present or suspected, a thorough head and neck examination is mandatory. Clinical examination has been shown to have good sensitivity for detecting clinically significant vascular injury in cases of zone II penetrating injuries.[10,11]

Particular attention should be given to the LT, vascular, and PE systems to evaluate for "hard" signs, which are pathognomonic of injury, and "soft" signs, which are suspicious but not diagnostic of significant injury (Table 1). These steps, together with the laboratory and diagnostic studies, are used to identify the likely injury complex and direct further treatment or diagnostic testing. In general, "hard" signs usually warrant a surgery without specific diagnostic studies, whereas "soft" signs require further diagnostic evaluation to identify those patients with significant injuries requiring surgical repair. The clinical examination should also include assessment of the nervous system through the use of the Glasgow Coma Scale, localizing signs, pupils, cranial nerves, spinal cord, brachial plexus, phrenic nerve, and the sympathetic chain.

Diagnostic Imaging

The mechanism of injury and clinical examination should determine the need and type of diagnostic imaging. As was stated earlier, patients with "hard" signs of major vascular or LT injuries, summarized in Table 2, need to undergo a surgery without delay for definitive investigations.

Chest Radiograph
A chest radiograph should be obtained in all trauma patients but is of particular importance in patients with penetrating injuries to zone I or those with any other wounds that may violate the chest cavity. Furthermore, chest and neck radiographs may be helpful in locating foreign bodies in other zones of the neck or parts of the chest cavity.

Angiography, Color Flow Doppler, and Helical Computed Tomography
Angiography has been advocated since the 1970s for the diagnosis of cervical vascular injury, particularly for injuries

TABLE 2

CLINICAL SIGNS OF NECK INJURIES

	Hard Signs	Soft Signs
Laryngotracheal	Respiratory distress	Subcutaneous emphysema
	Air bubbling	Hoarseness
	Major hemoptysis	Minor hemoptysis
Vascular	Severe hemorrhage	Stable small-moderate hematoma
	Large or expanding hematoma	Minor hemorrhage
	Absent/diminished peripheral pulses	Mild hypotension
	Bruits on auscultation	Proximity wound
	Unexplained hypotension	
Pharyngoesophageal		Painful swallowing
		Subcutaneous emphysema
		Hematemesis

(From Bell RB, Osborn T, Dierks EJ, et al. Management of penetrating neck injuries: A new paradigm for civilian trauma. *J Oral Maxillofac Surg.* 2007;65:691–705; Demetriades D, Salim A, Brown C, et al. Neck Injuries. *Curr Probl Surg.* 2007;44:13–85.)

in zones I and III. The gold standard has been catheter-based four-vessel digital subtraction angiography (DSA). DSA potentially allows for the immediate endovascular repair of an injury. However, angiography is often not readily available at most institutions during off-hours and it carries an estimated 2% risk of significant complications, including arterial dissection, thrombosis, embolism, and vasospasm.[12] Additionally, recent evidence suggest that routine angiography in asymptomatic patients with penetrating neck injuries is unnecessary, has a low yield, and does not offer any benefit over physical examination and other noninvasive investigations.[13,14]

Color flow Doppler (CFD) with a careful physical examination was then proposed as a safe, cost-effective, and reliable alternative to angiography. However, CFD has the disadvantage of being operator dependent and being technically difficult due to open wounds, pain, hematomas, and subcutaneous emphysema. CFDs are also limited in their ability to adequately visualize the proximal left subclavian artery, the internal carotid artery near the base of the skull, and the segments of the vertebral artery under the bony part of the vertebral canal.[4] As with catheter-based angiography, CFD studies are unavailable in many institutions at night and on weekends. Therefore, some surgeons continued to promote a policy of routine angiography for injuries in zones I and III, regardless of the clinical findings, as well as penetrating injuries with specific diagnosis or therapeutic indications.

More recently, helical computed tomographic angiography (CTA) has emerged as a fast, minimally invasive, and accurate alternative study to conventional angiography for the screening and evaluation of cervical vascular injury. Important advantages of CTA are that it is readily available at most trauma centers regardless of the time of day and that it provides evaluation of the soft tissues, skeletal structure, and vasculature structures in <5 minutes. Several authors have advocated the liberal use of CTA in the evaluation of blunt cervical trauma because it simultaneously evaluates the vasculature and skeletal structures of the neck.[15] It has been reported to have positive and negative predictive values as high as 100% and 93%, respectively, for blunt cervical vascular injury (BCVI).[13] Use of CTA in the evaluation of penetrating neck trauma can lead to a reduction in the rate of negative neck explorations.[14,16] A distinct disadvantage of CTA is that the quality of the study can be severely degraded by metallic debris that is embedded in the soft tissue following penetrating trauma, as is often seen after high-velocity missile injuries.[17,18]

Esophageal and Laryngotracheal Evaluation

Aerodigestive injuries are rare in blunt cervical trauma (~1% incidence) and slightly more common following penetrating neck injuries (~5% to 15% incidence).[2,7] Despite their relative rarity, missed injuries to the aerodigestive tract carry a high mortality rate.

Physical findings that are suspicious for aerodigestive tract injury include hemoptysis, hematemesis, malocclusion, hoarseness, subcutaneous emphysema, and evidence of a missile trajectory tract toward the larynx or trachea. Subcutaneous or mediastinal emphysema seen on radiographic studies are concerning for aerodigestive injuries. Distal tracheal injuries may in fact manifest as a pneumothorax.[2] Any of these described findings mandates further LT and PE evaluation.

LT evaluation through flexible fiberoptic endoscopy is indicated in all patients with suspected LT injuries. Injuries can be directly visualized or be heralded by bleeding, cord motion abnormality, or edema. It has been estimated that only approximately 20% of patients with endoscopic findings suggestive of LT injury required surgical intervention.[4]

Both contrast esophagography and esophagoscopy are recommended to evaluate for potential injury to the pharynx and cervical esophagus. It is believed that the combination of the two studies can overcome the limitations of the individual studies.[7] Esophagography has the benefit of allowing for the detection of small leaks that may not be visualized through endoscopy. Esophagoscopy has the advantage that it can be used in nearly all patients regardless of their level of consciousness and can also be performed intraoperatively.

PENETRATING NECK INJURIES

Little controversy exists concerning the management of hemodynamically unstable patients, or those who present with direct evidence of vascular or aerodigestive tract injury. In such cases, surgical exploration is warranted without debate. However, the management of patients with stable vital signs continues to be controversial. Routine neck exploration of all wounds penetrating the platysma muscle was traditionally performed. However, such practice is no longer recommended secondary to the high percentage of nontherapeutic explorations and the significant associated morbidity of the exploration. An exploration of a zone II injury may have minimal morbidity, but indiscriminate exploration of any neck zone is associated with a significant economic and personnel cost. Although it may be tempting, there is no indication for probing or locally exploring the neck outside of the operating room because this may dislodge a clot and initiate uncontrolled hemorrhage.[19]

The selection of patients for surgery or observation is based on clinical examination and interpretation of the appropriate investigations. However, the indication for and selection of the most appropriate investigation varies between centers and remains a controversial issue. Our algorithm for the selective management of penetrating neck injuries is summarized in Fig. 6.

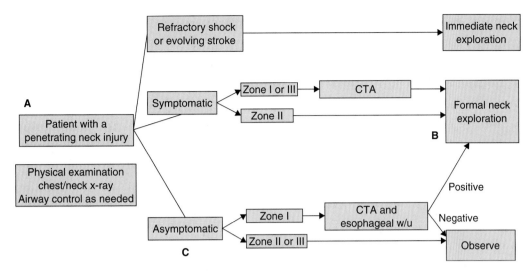

Figure 6 Algorithm for the selective management of penetrating neck trauma. **A:** Airway and circulatory management are the priority at this point in the algorithm. **B:** Intraoperative endoscopy can be used as an adjunct during the neck exploration to evaluate for laryngotracheal or pharyngoesophageal injuries. **C:** Endoscopy and/or contrast studies can be considered at this point to evaluate for occult laryngotracheal or pharyngoesophageal injuries, CTA, computed tomographic angiography; w/u, workup.

MANAGEMENT OF SPECIFIC PENETRATING INJURIES

Certain steps in the management of penetrating neck trauma have remained unchanged. These include cervical spine immobilization, establishment of a secure airway, and circulatory support with intravenous fluids, and/or direct pressure for hemorrhage control.[8,19,20] Although mandatory neck exploration was previously accepted for any neck wound penetrating the platysma, even in asymptomatic patients, this practice has recently been modified, especially in zone I and III injuries. A large number of studies since the 1970s have shown that selective versus mandatory surgical management of patients with certain penetrating neck wounds had similar or less mortality.[21–27] These findings revolutionized the management of penetrating neck injuries. Further changes in practice management has occurred secondary to the increased availability and high accuracy of diagnosis with both CTA and DSA. Currently, mandatory neck exploration is no longer recommended for civilian trauma, especially for injury in zones I and III.[8] A more aggressive surgical approach may be needed in the military combat setting where diagnostic equipment may not be immediately available. Preliminary data from the current conflicts in Iraq and Afghanistan have suggested that selective delayed evaluation of penetrating neck trauma *may* be safe in stable patients.[18]

The nature of penetrating neck trauma makes multiple simultaneous combinations of injuries more likely than isolated injuries. Surgical access to zones I and III can be difficult. Therefore, immediate control through angiography and embolization or balloon occlusion may be life saving. Mandatory laryngoscopy, bronchoscopy,

esophagoscopy, and/or a contrast study are warranted in these zones to evaluate for potentially devastating aerodigestive injuries. Endoscopy studies can be conducted intraoperatively. Patients with penetrating zone II injuries who are symptomatic should undergo neck exploration (see Fig. 7). Asymptomatic patients with penetrating zone II injuries may be treated with either neck exploration or directed evaluation and serial examinations. Whether one takes the selective or the mandatory approach to neck exploration for neck trauma, it is imperative that surgeons avoid missed injury and delay of needed treatment that inevitably leads to increased morbidity and mortality.

As previously discussed, any of the injuries or surgical manipulation of the traumatized area may create an emergency or an impending airway compromise. Therefore, the initial priority in any patient with penetrating neck injury should be to ensure a secure airway. In true emergencies, a cricothyrotomy should be done which can later be revised electively to a standard tracheostomy.[6] When the airway may be compromised but not emergent then a tracheostomy created. On rare occasions, injury to the distal, cervical, or proximal intrathoracic trachea may occur. In such circumstances, a median sternotomy for left-sided injuries or a right thoracotomy is necessary to provide access to the more distal intrathoracic trachea.

SURGICAL ACCESS (ZONE II AND III)

Nonvascular Injuries

Exposure to the larynx can best be achieved through a transverse collar incision, approximately 2 cm above

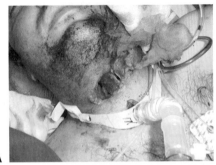
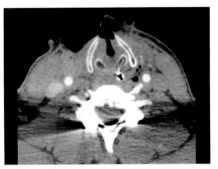
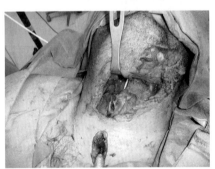

Figure 7   Case Study: A 28-year-old male patient sustained a zone II penetrating injury to the larynx, trachea, and pharynx and was transferred to Oregon Health and Science University Hospital after stabilization at a regional hospital in Oregon. The patient was using a concrete saw when it struck a rebar and kicked back into his neck resulting in a significant zone II injury. Before transport, a tracheostomy was created and the left external carotid artery was ligated. **A:** Clinical appearance of the patient's anterior neck on arrival at the intensive care unit. A complex fracture of the thyroid cartilage is clearly visible in the wound bed. **B:** Computed tomographic (CT) scan of the patient's neck at the level of the thyroid cartilage injury. **C:** An intraoperative view of the full-thickness pharyngeal injury. A Dobhoff feeding tube is visible within the pharynx.

the sternal notch. A midline thyrotomy may be required in patients with significant endolaryngeal injuries.[8,9,19] For proximal tracheal, pharyngeal, or cervical esophageal injuries, a transverse collar or anterior sternocleidomastoid incision (as described in the subsequent text) can be utilized. The omohyoid muscle located in the pretracheal fascia can be retracted or divided to improve exposure. While the inferior thyroid artery and middle thyroid vein can be divided, care should be taken to avoid injury to the recurrent laryngeal nerves located in the tracheoesophageal groove. Distal tracheal or esophageal injuries may require a median sternotomy for exposure.

Vascular Injuries—Penetrating

Most vascular injuries located in the anterior neck compartment can be accessed through an oblique incision along the anterior border of the sternocleidomastoid muscle from the angle of the mandible to the sternoclavicular joint (Fig. 5). Retraction of the sternocleidomastoid muscle laterally exposes the internal jugular vein and the carotid artery (lying medial and deep to the vein). When gaining surgical access, care should be taken not to injure the vagus nerve that is located posterior to the carotid sheath. Division of the facial vein will expose the carotid bifurcation and allow mobilization and control of the internal and external carotid arteries. The cervical incision can be extended superiorly into the posterior auricular area to improve access when injury occurs in zone III. To further improve exposure in this area, the digastric muscle can be divided but care should be taken to avoid injury to the hypoglossal, glossopharyngeal, and facial nerves. Neurosurgical or maxillofacial consultation may be required to assist with exposure of the internal

carotid at the skull base. Separate incisions should be made when bilateral neck exploration is warranted.

For vertebral artery injuries, initial exposure can be achieved through an anterior sternocleidomastoid incision as described in the preceding text. This approach will allow exposure of both the proximal and the distal vertebral artery. The vertebral arteries enter into their bony canal at C6 and control of the vessel can be gained proximal to this through a transverse supraclavicular incision on the ipsilateral side of the neck. Alternatively, a no. 3 Fogarty catheter can be advanced either proximally or distally to occlude the vertebral artery and facilitate repair of the vascular injury. The carotid sheath should be incised at the lateral margin of the internal jugular vein and the contents of the carotid sheath retracted medially to allow exposure to the plane just superficial to the prevertebral muscles. When possible, care should be taken to locate and protect the cervical sympathetic chain ganglia that are located between the carotid sheath and the prevertebral muscles. A longitudinal incision should be made in the anterior longitudinal ligament, located deep in the medial aspect of the wound. The ligament, the underlying periosteum, and the overlying longus colli and longissimus capitis are then mobilized anterolaterally with a periosteal elevator. The transverse process tips demarcate the posterolateral extent of the dissection. The elevation is carried laterally along the margin of the bodies and along the anterior aspect of the transverse processes of the cervical vertebrae.

A small rongeur can be used to remove the transverse processes of the cervical vertebrae located distal to the area of injury. Blind clamping or clipping should be avoided because the cervical roots are located behind the artery. Finally, access of the vertebral artery through the space between the transverse processes should be avoided to prevent injury to the venous plexuses that are intimately associated with the vertebral artery. If rapid control of the vertebral artery is required, an approach at the base of the neck at the vertebral artery origin at the subclavian artery can be performed. This access can be achieved through one of two ways. The anterior sternocleidomastoid incision can be extended toward the clavicle to allow transection of the muscle off the clavicle. The subclavian vein is retracted caudal and the anterior scalene retracted laterally to allow access to the first portion of the vertebral artery as it branches off the subclavian artery. Alternatively, a cut down directly on the clavicle can be performed to allow disarticulation of the bone at the sternoclavicular joint.

ISOLATED AERODIGESTIVE TRACT INJURIES—PENETRATING

Laryngotracheal—Penetrating

Injuries to the trachea or larynx from penetrating wounds can be subtle or obvious. Overt injuries require immediate surgical attention. Unlike blunt LT trauma, penetrating LT injury is more commonly associated with injury to adjacent organs. Therefore, preoperative or intraoperative laryngoscopy, bronchoscopy, and esophagoscopy are essential in evaluating patients with LT injuries.[2] Furthermore, injuries to the larynx that result in airway compromise require immediate creation of a surgical airway. Minimal debridement of laryngeal structures should be performed at the initial surgery. An otolaryngologist should be consulted to assist with definitive repair of all but small injuries without tissue loss or injury to the laryngeal skeleton.

Small injuries to the trachea can be repaired primarily by reapproximating the mucosa with a single layer absorbable monofilament suture. Again, tissue debridement should be minimized.[2] A protective tracheostomy is not warranted if the defect is small and repaired successfully. Similarly, lateral and posterior injuries can be repaired primarily but may require tracheostomy for protection. Large anterior defects, however, should not be repaired primarily and require immediate conversion to tracheostomy. LT injuries generally do not require routine drainage unless associated with injury to pharynx or esophagus. Patients with laryngeal injuries should be monitored carefully postoperatively for signs of mediastinitis, which may result from persistent airway leak or a missed LT injury.

Pharyngoesophageal—Penetrating

The need to identify patients with esophageal injury from penetrating neck trauma is critical because mortality significantly increases when the diagnosis is delayed.

When the site of perforation is difficult to localize, either air in the nasogastric tube or extravasation of barium or methylene blue can be utilized to assist in injury localization.

An attempt, independent of injury severity, should be made to repair nearly all injuries to the pharynx and the esophagus with either one or two layers using absorbable sutures and either open or closed drainage. In those patients with associated LT injuries, a vascularized local tissue flap should be interposed between the tracheal and esophageal injuries to help prevent tracheoesophageal fistula formation. In extreme cases of very large injuries or very delayed surgical intervention, wide drainage of the neck with conversion to a cervical esophagostomy may be necessary to ensure drainage. Injuries very low in the neck of in the thoracic esophagus may require esophageal diversion with distal esophageal ligation, leaving definitive repair for later. Patients with PE injuries should receive postoperative antibiotics appropriate for oral flora for several days. Before removal of the drains, a radiographic contrast study should be performed to evaluate for extravasation indicating an incompetent repair. Nutrition parenterally or through an enteral feeding tube is warranted until a contrast study demonstrates no leak, usually at a minimum of 5 to 7 days after the last repair. Missed or inadequate drained injuries may result in profound infection and a septic response. A high index of suspicion for mediastinitis should always be maintained during the immediate postoperative period.

VASCULAR INJURIES—PENETRATING

Internal Jugular Vein

Simple injuries to the internal jugular vein should be repaired. Large injuries, however, should be repaired only if the patient's general condition and associated injuries allow for the procedure; otherwise the veins should be ligated. In the rare instance that both internal jugular veins have been injured, an attempt should be made to repair at least one vessel. If such a case is not possible, bilateral internal jugular vein ligation may be necessary and is usually tolerated.

Carotid Artery

The objective of surgical care in patients with carotid artery injury is to arrest hemorrhage while maintaining flow to preserve neurologic function. Management of external carotid artery injuries, in general, is governed by the extent of injury to the artery, the associated other organ injuries, and the overall hemodynamic and neurologic status of the patient. Simple injuries to the external carotid artery likely can be repaired, whereas in the setting of complex injuries, hemodynamic instability or profound neurologic deficits, the artery should be ligated. In the setting of neurologic deficits, the decision to repair versus ligate is difficult. Earlier reports warned against revascularization in the presence of neurologic deficits secondary to conversion of an ischemic infarct to a hemorrhagic infarct.[19,28] Subsequent studies, however, have shown improvement with revascularization in preoperative weakness or paralysis without significant conversion of infarct type.[28–30] Revascularization did not improve but often exacerbated cerebral edema and intracranial hypertension in patients with prolonged (>4 hours) ischemia.

Whereas external carotid injuries may be ligated without significant consequence, injuries to the common carotid and internal carotid are more problematic and depend on the degree of injury, the amount of back bleeding, and the hemodynamic stability of the patient. Devastating neurologic sequelae can occur in the presence of inadequate collateral circulation. Carotid ligation should be reserved in patients with minimal back bleeding, injuries at the base of the skull or in patients with established ischemic infarction. A temporary intraluminal carotid shunt should be considered in patients who are hemodynamically unstable but may later benefit from delayed carotid artery reconstruction. The internal carotid artery should be repaired in the setting of a hemodynamically stable patient with minimal or moderate artery injury. As in elective vascular surgery, carotid artery injury with minimal vascular wall loss can be repaired primarily. A patch repair, either venous or synthetic, should be performed on arteries with injuries longer than 1 to 2 cm. Use of a shunt should be strongly considered when primary repair of the artery is performed. Completion angiography should be done after interposition graft placements and complex repairs of the common or internal carotid arteries.

It is useful to remember to prepare both lower extremities for possible saphenous vein harvest for use as a vein graft. This is important as nearly the entire extracranial internal carotid can be replaced by a saphenous vein graft.

Angiography with possible endovascular intervention is an alternative approach to hemodynamically stable patients with distal internal carotid artery injury, an arteriovenous or carotid-cavernous sinus fistula, ongoing facial or intraoral hemorrhage from external carotid branches, or small intimal defects or pseudoaneurysms in surgically inaccessible locations.

Vertebral Artery

In rare instances patients who present with a penetrating neck injury, especially in the posterior triangle of the neck, will have an injury to the vertebral artery. Most such injuries that occur in stable patients are asymptomatic and require no intervention. Most of the vertebral artery injuries are discovered on angiography. Such injuries can usually be managed with embolization. However, in urgent circumstances, an angiographic approach may not be practical thereby warranting a direct surgical approach. Surgical management can be very difficult. Following the dissection described earlier, the proximal and distal vertebral artery can be exposed through an anterior sternocleidomastoid incision. In contrast to injuries of the carotid arteries, in which either repair or ligation is an option, injuries to the vertebral arteries should always be treated with ligation.

BASE OF THE NECK INJURY (ZONE I)

Unlike penetrating injuries in zones II and III, penetrating injuries involving zone I of the neck are more likely to be lethal because of the potential for injury to the great vessels of the neck and mediastinum, as well as the cervical and thoracic esophagus. Hemodynamically unstable patients with injury to the base of the neck frequently require a median sternotomy for exposure of the most likely injured vessels, namely the innominate or right subclavian artery. Extension of the median sternotomy into the right neck may be necessary to obtain adequate distal control of the arteries. Injuries to the base of the left neck may require a left thoracotomy for adequate exposure of the left subclavian artery. Distal control of the vessel can be achieved through a left supraclavicular incision. Further exposure of the left subclavian artery can be achieved by resection of the medial one third to one half of the left clavicle. Primary repair of the subclavian artery should be attempted. However, branches of the artery should be divided and ligated as necessary to gain mobility and adequate exposure. Minimal injury to the innominate and subclavian veins can be repaired by lateral venorrhaphy. Complex injuries to either vein warrants suture ligation.[19]

Management of hemodynamically stable patients is variable. Approximately one third of patients with a clinically significant zone I injury may be asymptomatic at initial presentation. Therefore, most trauma centers advocate routine angiography of the aortic arch and great vessels, along with an esophageal evaluation.

BLUNT NECK INJURIES

Although the mechanisms of injury are vastly different between blunt and penetrating neck trauma, the initial management priorities are the same, as they are for all traumas. Our algorithm for the management of blunt neck trauma is summarized in Fig. 8.

MANAGEMENT OF SPECIFIC INJURIES

Blunt Aerodigestive Injuries

Blunt aerodigestive injuries compromise 1.2% of all blunt traumas and can be divided into two anatomic groups: LT

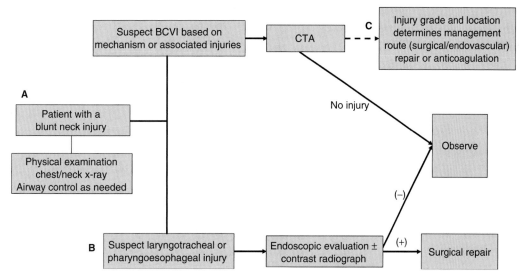

Figure 8   Algorithm for management of blunt neck trauma. **A:** Airway and circulatory management are the priority at this point in the algorithm. **B:** If there is obvious injury and/or airway compromise, then immediate exploration with intraoperative endoscopy may be warranted. **C:** As shown in Table 4, the management route of blunt cervical vascular injury (BCVI) is dependent on the grade and location of injury. Endovascular management may or may not be appropriate depending on the location and nature of the lesion, CTA, computed tomographic angiography.

and cervical PE.[1,7] Early in the clinical course, any significant trauma can lead to compromise of the airway, either by compressive hematomas or by direct occlusion or laceration from fractured tracheal cartilage. Late complications primarily manifest as cervical esophageal leaks.

Blunt Laryngotracheal Injuries

Blunt LT injury can be due to a direct blow, a sudden deceleration leading to shear injury at the cricoid or carina, or by compressive chest trauma in the presence of a close glottis resulting in the pressure-driven perforation of the posterior membranous trachea.[31] Several studies have demonstrated that patients with minimal blunt LT trauma can often be managed nonoperatively, although as many as 70% will need advanced airway management at the initial presentation.[31,32] These minimal injuries include nondisplaced fractures of the LT cartilage, minor trachea mucosa lacerations, or lacerations that are less than one third the circumference of the tracheal itself.[9] Patients must be closely observed initially in the intensive care unit to facilitate the emergent intubation or surgical airway creation. Demetriades et al. recommend that serial flexible endoscopy be incorporated as an integral part of this observation strategy.[2,31] There is no clear evidence supporting the use of corticosteroids to reduce airway swelling in the setting of blunt trauma.

If surgical intervention is required for the repair of blunt LT injury, consultation with a head and neck surgeon may be warranted, particularly if the injury is extensive or involves significant soft tissue loss. Simple repairs of the larynx can be performed through a transverse

"collar" incision made approximately 2 cm superior to the sternal notch. Proximal tracheal injuries can also be approached in this same manner or through an anterior sternocleidomastoid incision. More distal tracheal injuries require exposure through a median sternotomy or right posterolateral thoracotomy. Disruptions of the membranous trachea in the neck should be approached through an anterior tracheotomy. Care must be exercised to minimize injury to the recurrent laryngeal nerves.

Tracheal wounds can be reapproximated with interrupted 3-0 synthetic absorbable monofilament sutures. The cartilaginous tracheal rings may be reapproximated with perichondrial nonabsorbable suture. If possible, buttressing the repair with an adjacent strap muscle or other soft tissue flap is helpful in protecting the repair. Buttressing the repair is essential in the repair of the membranous trachea because the suture or wound can erode into the esophagus resulting in a tracheal-esophageal fistula.

Tracheostomy after simple repairs does not appear to improve outcomes, and may increase the infection rate. Conversely, tracheostomy is likely to be required after a more extensive injury. If one is deemed necessary, it should be placed at least two tracheal rings inferior to the repaired portion of the trachea.

Blunt Pharyngoesophageal Injuries

PE injury due to blunt trauma is exceedingly rare and was present in 0.08% of blunt trauma admissions at one institution.[7] Any significant leaks in the pharynx or cervical esophagus that are detected upon workup of the patient mandates surgical repair. If left alone, leaks in the region

TABLE 3

INJURIES THAT ARE SUSPICIOUS FOR CONCOMITANT BLUNT CERVICAL VASCULAR INJURY

Injury

Hyperextension, -flexion, -rotational injuries (especially if associated with severe Le Fort fractures, mandibular fractures or diffuse axonal injury)

Near-hangings

Shoulder-belt abrasions with neurologic symptoms or local swelling

Basilar skull fractures (especially if the carotid canal is involved)

Cervical spine fracture involving the transverse foramina

Any cervical spine distraction injury

(Adapted from Biffl WL, Moore EE, Offner PJ, et al. Optimizing screening for blunt cerebrovascular injuries. *Am J Surg.* 1999;178:517–522.)

will form neck abscesses or potentially drain into the mediastinum leading to mediastinitis. The surgical approach and repair for blunt injuries are identical to that described earlier for penetrating PE injuries. Similarly, any injury that is not amenable to immediate repair can be delayed by the creation of a diverting cervical esophagostomy.

Blunt Cervical Vascular Injuries

The diagnosis and management of cervical vascular injuries, both blunt and penetrating, have undergone significant changes over the last several years with the advent of CTA and endovascular therapies. Although controversial, it has been suggested that any patient with a suspected BCVI requires further diagnostic evaluation.[15] However, it must be noted that this approach is resource intensive. A recent review by Mayberry et al. has suggested that aggressive blunt carotid injury screening is not warranted because of both the rarity of the presence of an injury (0.16% incidence) and of the small percentage of those injuries in which intervention would lead to a change in outcome.[9,33]

In general, patients should be suspected of harboring a BCVI if they have any of the injuries listed in Table 3.[34,35] Any patient with neurologic deficits or otherwise is strongly suspected of having sustained a BCVI, should have further radiologic workup beginning with CTA to evaluate for the presence of vascular injury (see Fig. 9). Once an injury has been diagnosed, the best management strategy for BCVI remains controversial. The several strategies most often used are open surgical repair, observation, endovascular repair/embolization, or anticoagulation therapy. Biffl et al. have developed a grading scale for blunt carotid injuries to aid in the management decision-making process.[36] Although the scale was initially developed for the description of carotid injuries, its use has been extended, by many authors, to describe blunt vertebral artery injuries.

The scale has been used to formulate treatment recommendations for carotid injury (see Table 4).[35] Grade I injuries rarely worsened, but there is an estimated 3% stroke rate with this injury. Retrospective studies have suggested that there is no difference in outcome regardless of the type of anticoagulation (including antiplatelet therapy) used for treatment. Grade II injuries had high rate of progression onto pseudoaneurysm or occlusive thrombus formation. This propensity has lead Biffl et al. to recommend surgical repair or systemic anticoagulation to minimize the risk of further complications. Grade III injuries require surgical intervention as studies have suggested that anticoagulation may worsen the lesion.[37,38] Lesions that are not easily accessed surgically may be amenable to endovascular repair as will be discussed shortly. With the complete occlusion of lumen in a grade IV injury, anticoagulation is the recommended treatment. Revascularization has not been shown to lead to changes in outcome. Grade V injuries are potentially amenable only to surgical repair, but are most often associated with lethal outcomes.

Blunt vertebral artery injuries are slightly more common than blunt carotid injuries. They have been estimated to have an incidence of 0.2% to 0.71%.[39-41] In general, vertebral arteries are injured by high-energy trauma that generates significant rotational shear or cervical spine bony injury that secondarily injures the arteries.[35] Cothren et al. found that 70% of all blunt vertebral artery injuries were associated with a cervical spine fracture, and that more than 80% of these injuries had a fracture or subluxation that involved the transverse foramina.[39] It is because of these associated injuries that mortality rate in patients with a blunt vertebral artery injury is approximately 20%.[42]

Unlike blunt carotid injuries, there is somewhat less controversy on the management of blunt vertebral artery injuries. The primary indication for surgical intervention is life-threatening hemorrhage, again, due to the inherent morbidity of the exposure required to gain proximal and distal control and to repair the lesion itself. The recommendation for nontransecting injuries has been systemic anticoagulation to minimize the risk (or extent) of vertebrobasilar ischemia. A newer treatment approach to managing these injuries is endovascular embolization or stenting.

Despite the development of injury grading, the management of BCVI remains a clinical decision that needs to integrate the injury location and grade, neurologic symptoms, concomitant injuries, and the overall condition of the patient.

SURGICAL MANAGEMENT

Zone II injuries are amenable to exploration and direct management of carotid and jugular vessels. The surgical approach to the repair of zone II vascular injuries is the same as was described earlier in the management of penetrating injuries. However, most blunt carotid injuries involve the internal branch at or above the base of the

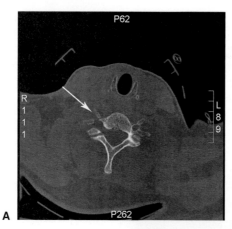

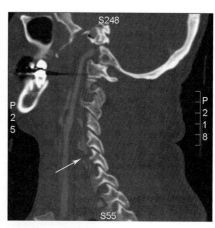

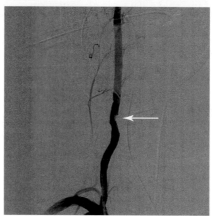

Figure 9 Case Study: A 58-year-old male bicyclist was struck by a motor vehicle. The patient sustained a fracture of the right C6 facet with extension into the right foramen transversarium. A right vertebral artery dissection was subsequently diagnosed by computed tomography (CT) angiography. The patient underwent conventional angiography in an attempt to retrieve a thrombus in the basilar artery. **A:** Axial CT image showing the facet fracture (*arrow*) that extends into the foramen transversarium. **B:** CT angiogram of the neck demonstrating an intraluminal defect in the right vertebral artery (*arrow*). **C:** Digital subtraction angiography of the right vertebral artery. The arrow highlights a contour irregularity suggestive of vessel injury.

skull.[35] This relatively inaccessible location often precludes direct surgical repair and therefore nonsurgical treatment is the preferred strategy.

ANTICOAGULATION

Several groups have advocated systemic intravenous anticoagulation as the mainstay for surgically inaccessible BCVI.[34,37] These groups have noted that there was significant improvement in neurologic symptoms in patients who received systemic therapy. The protocol used by Biffl et al. is to start the heparin infusion at 15 units/kg/hour without any initial bolus, then the partial thromboplastin time (PTT) is measured at 6-hour intervals and the heparin drip rate is titrated for a PTT of 40 to 50 seconds.[35] This protocol requires that there is no contraindication to

TABLE 4

BLUNT CAROTID ARTERY INJURY GRADING SCALE

Injury Grade	Description	Recommended Treatment
I	Irregular lumen or dissection with <25% narrowing	Observation ± minimal anticoagulation
II	Dissection or intramural hematoma with 25% narrowing, intraluminal thrombus, or raised intimal flap	Surgical repair OR anticoagulation
III	Pseudoaneurysm	Surgical repair
IV	Occlusion	Anticoagulation
V	Transection with free extravasation	Surgical repair OR balloon occlusion if the lesion is not accessible

(Adapted from Biffl WL, Moore EE, Offner PJ, et al. Blunt carotid arterial injuries: Implications of a new grading scale. *J Trauma.* 1999;47:845–853; Biffl WL, Moore EE, Offner PJ, et al. Blunt carotid and vertebral arterial injuries. *World J Surg.* 2001;25:1036–1043.)

TABLE 5

CONTRAINDICATIONS TO SYSTEMIC ANTICOAGULATION

Contraindication for Systemic Heparinization

Intolerance to heparin (e.g., history of heparin-induced thrombocytopenia)
Concurrent traumatic brain injury
Need for other surgeries
Ongoing hemorrhage

heparin therapy, as listed in Table 5. There is no consensus on the duration of anticoagulation.

Observation of blunt vertebral artery injuries alone is generally an unacceptable management strategy in patients with symptomatic injuries because of the known high rate of morbidity (53%) and mortality (28%) in BCVI.[35] Only if the artery is completely thrombosed at the time of evaluation can observation alone be considered, but there is anecdotal evidence that anticoagulation leads to an increased rate of recannulization. Anticoagulation and expectant management is appropriate in asymptomatic blunt vertebral artery injuries. Often these are found incidentally on radiographic evaluation for suspected cervical spine injury. Unfortunately, systemic anticoagulation may be problematic due to the multiple injuries that are often sustained by trauma patients.

ENDOVASCULAR REPAIR

Endovascular repair of the vascular injuries does not replace immediate open surgical management, but rather adds to the armamentarium available to the trauma surgeon in the management of these injuries. For example, zone I injuries with signs of acute hemorrhage or clinical instability will often involve major vascular injuries. These injuries would not be amenable to an endovascular approach and would in fact mandate an emergent anterior thoracotomy to gain both proximal and distal control. Similarly, zone III injuries with ongoing acute hemorrhage associated with clinical instability would mandate surgical intervention to repair the vascular injury or at a minimum temporizing the hemorrhage until definitive repair can be attempted. As with DSA, endovascular interventional teams may not be readily available at night or weekends because of individual institutional policies.

Endovascular repair of blunt cervical vascular injuries have been generally reserved for symptomatic patients with hemorrhage, pseudoaneurysm, or arteriovenous fistula, although their use has been slowly liberalizing. Injuries that are within 2 cm of the artery origin or within a short distance to the posterior inferior cerebellar artery are not

endovascular candidates.[44,45] There have been descriptions of successful stent deployment into the vertebral artery in the setting of trauma, but no long-term follow-up studies are currently available.[46] As with carotid artery injuries, coil embolization is rarely used, except in the setting of a grade V injury, because of fears of distal coil migration resulting in a stroke. Caution is still advised for carotid stent placement due to minimal long-term safety data and the observation of an increased stroke rate in patients undergoing carotid balloon and stent placement for atherosclerotic disease.

REFERENCES

1. Pierre EJ, McNeer RR, Shamir MY. Early management of the traumatized airway. *Anesthesiol Clin.* 2007;25:1–11.
2. Atkins BZ, Abbate S, Fisher SR, et al. Current management of laryngotracheal trauma: Case report and literature review. *J Trauma.* 2004;56:185–190.
3. Gray H. *Anatomy of the human body,* 20th ed. Philadelphia: Lea & Febiger; 1918. Bartleby.com, 2000. http://www.bartleby.com/br/107.html.
4. Demetriades D, Theodorou D, Cornwell E, et al. Evaluation of penetrating injuries of the neck: Prospective study of 223 patients. *World J Surg.* 1997;21:41–47; discussion 478.
5. Medzon R, Rothenhaus T, Bono CM, et al. Stability of cervical spine fractures after gunshot wounds to the head and neck. *Spine.* 2005;30:2274–2279.
6. Committee on Trauma, American College of Surgeons. *Advanced trauma life support instructors manual.* Chicago: American College of Surgeons; 2005.
7. Vassiliu P, Baker J, Henderson S, et al. Aerodigestive injuries of the neck. *Am Surg.* 2001;67:75–79.
8. Bell RB, Osborn T, Dierks EJ, et al. Management of penetrating neck injuries: A new paradigm for civilian trauma. *J Oral Maxillofac Surg.* 2007;65:691–705.
9. Demetriades D, Salim A, Brown C, et al. Neck Injuries. *Curr Probl Surg.* 2007;44:13–85.
10. Atteberry LR, Dennis JW, Menawat SS, et al. Physical examination alone is safe and accurate for evaluation of vascular injuries in penetrating zone II neck trauma. *J Am Coll Surg.* 1994;179:657–662.
11. Jarvik JG, Philips GR III, Schwab CW, et al. Penetrating neck trauma: Sensitivity of clinical examination and cost-effectiveness of angiography. *Am J Neuroradiol.* 1995;16:647–654.
12. Willinsky RA, Taylor SM, TerBrugge K, et al. Neurologic complications of cerebral angiography: Prospective analysis of 2,899 procedures and review of the literature. *Radiology.* 2003;227:522–528.
13. Eastman AL, Chason DP, Perez CL, et al. Computed tomographic angiography for the diagnosis of blunt cervical vascular injury: Is it ready for primetime? *J Trauma.* 2006;60:925–929; discussion 929.
14. Woo K, Magner DP, Wilson MT, et al. CT angiography in penetrating neck trauma reduces the need for operative neck exploration. *Am Surg.* 2005;71:754–758.
15. Biffl WL, Egglin T, Benedetto B, et al. Sixteen-slice computed tomographic angiography is a reliable noninvasive screening test for clinically significant blunt cerebrovascular injuries. *J Trauma.* 2006;60:745–751; discussion 751–2.
16. Ofer A, Nitecki SS, Braun J, et al. CT angiography of the carotid arteries in trauma to the neck. *Eur J Vasc Endovasc Surg.* 2001;21:401–407.
17. Fox CJ, Gillespie DL, O'Donnell SD, et al. Contemporary management of wartime vascular trauma. *J Vasc Surg.* 2005;41:638–644.
18. Fox CJ, Gillespie DL, Weber MA, et al. Delayed evaluation of combat-related penetrating neck trauma. *J Vasc Surg.* 2006;44:86–93.
19. McConnell DB, Trunkey DD. Management of penetrating trauma to the neck. *Adv Surg.* 1994;27:97–127.

20. Kendall JL, Anglin D, Demetriades D. Penetrating neck trauma. *Emerg Med Clin North Am.* 1998;16:85–105.

21. Biffl WL, Moore EE, Rehse DH, et al. Selective management of penetrating neck trauma based on cervical level of injury. *Am J Surg.* 1997;174:678–682.

22. Insull P, Adams D, Segar A, et al. Is exploration mandatory in penetrating zone II neck injuries. *ANZ J Surg.* 2007;77:261–264.

23. Klyachkin ML, Rohmiller M, Charash WE, et al. Penetrating injuries of the neck: Selective management evolving. *Am Surg.* 1997;63:189–194.

24. Narrod JA, Moore EE. Selective management of penetrating neck injuries. A prospective study. *Arch Surg.* 1984;119:574–578.

25. Narrod JA, Moore EE. Initial management of penetrating neck wounds – a selective approach. *J Emerg Med.* 1984;2:17–22.

26. Nason RW, Assuras GN, Gray PR, et al. Penetrating neck injuries: Analysis of experience from a Canadian trauma centre. *Can J Surg.* 2001;44:122–126.

27. Roden DM, Pomerantz RA. Penetrating injuries to the neck: A safe, selective approach to management. *Am Surg.* 1993;59:750–753.

28. Thal ER, Snyder WH III, Hays RJ, et al. Management of carotid artery injuries. *Surgery.* 1974;76:955–962.

29. Brown MF, Graham JM, Feliciano DV, et al. Carotid artery injuries. *Am J Surg.* 1982;144:748–753.

30. Liekweg WG Jr, Greenfield LJ. Management of penetrating carotid arterial injury. *Ann Surg.* 1978;188:587–592.

31. Demetriades D, Velmahos GG, Asensio JA. Cervical pharyngoesophageal and laryngotracheal injuries. *World J Surg.* 2001;25: 1044–1048.

32. Gold SM, Gerber ME, Shott SR, et al. Blunt laryngotracheal trauma in children. *Arch Otolaryngol Head Neck Surg.* 1997;123:83–87.

33. Mayberry JC, Brown CV, Mullins RJ, et al. Blunt carotid artery injury: The futility of aggressive screening and diagnosis. *Arch Surg.* 2004;139:609–612; Discussion 612–3.

34. Biffl WL, Moore EE, Offner PJ, et al. Optimizing screening for blunt cerebrovascular injuries. *Am J Surg.* 1999;178:517–522.

35. Biffl WL, Moore EE, Offner PJ, et al. Blunt carotid and vertebral arterial injuries. *World J Surg.* 2001;25:1036–1043.

36. Biffl WL, Moore EE, Offner PJ, et al. Blunt carotid arterial injuries: Implications of a new grading scale. *J Trauma.* 1999;47: 845–853.

37. Fabian TC, Patton JH Jr, Croce MA, et al. Blunt carotid injury. Importance of early diagnosis and anticoagulant therapy. *Ann Surg.* 1996;223:513–522; discussion 522–5.

38. Mokri B. Traumatic and spontaneous extracranial internal carotid artery dissections. *J Neurol.* 1990;237:356–361.

39. Cothren CC, Moore EE, Biffl WL, et al. Cervical spine fracture patterns predictive of blunt vertebral artery injury. *J Trauma.* 2003;55:811–813.

40. Inamasu J, Guiot BH. Vertebral artery injury after blunt cervical trauma: An update. *Surg Neurol.* 2006;65:238–245; discussion 245–6.

41. Miller PR, Fabian TC, Croce MA, et al. Prospective screening for blunt cerebrovascular injuries: Analysis of diagnostic modalities and outcomes. *Ann Surg.* 2002;236:386–393; discussion 393–5.

42. Peck MA, Rasmussen TE. Management of blunt peripheral arterial injury. *Perspect Vasc Surg Endovasc Ther.* 2006;18:159–173.

43. Cogbill TH, Moore EE, Meissner M, et al. The spectrum of blunt injury to the carotid artery: A multicenter perspective. *J Trauma.* 1994;37:473–479.

44. Mwipatayi BP, Jeffery P, Beningfield SJ, et al. Management of extra-cranial vertebral artery injuries. *Eur J Vasc Endovasc Surg.* 2004;27:157–162.

45. Starnes BW, Arthurs ZM. Endovascular management of vascular trauma. *Perspect Vasc Surg Endovasc Ther.* 2006;18:114–129.

46. Lee YJ, Ahn JY, Han IB, et al. Therapeutic endovascular treatments for traumatic vertebral artery injuries. *J Trauma.* 2007;62: 886–891.

Thoracic Injuries—Overview

32

Edward Hal Kincaid   *J. Wayne Meredith*

Because of the relative size of the thorax and convexity of the diaphragm, most victims of torso trauma will sustain some degree of associated injury to the chest. Thoracic injuries are therefore common in both blunt and penetrating trauma, and are a primary or contributing cause of death in approximately half of all cases.[1] Fortunately, many thoracic injuries can be treated effectively and often definitively by relatively simple maneuvers that can be learned and performed by most physicians involved in the early care of trauma patients. Approximately one in six patients, however, will require urgent operative repair of life-threatening injuries. These extremes in injury severity are relatively unique to the chest, and require a corresponding broad range of knowledge and skills that often must be applied rapidly.

INITIAL ASSESSMENT

Chest injuries often produce life-threatening derangements of ventilation or perfusion. An orderly, well-defined process for the initial evaluation and treatment of patients with thoracic injury is guided by the same principles and priorities as for patients with other injuries. The evaluation begins with an organized and rapid primary survey designed to recognize and treat immediately life-threatening problems. The first priority is to ensure an adequate airway. An airway can often be established by clearing any blood or debris from the oropharynx and pulling the mandible or tongue forward. Severely injured patients commonly require nasotracheal or orotracheal intubation. Cricothyroidotomy or tracheostomy is necessary occasionally, especially in patients with severe maxillofacial trauma. The second priority

is to ensure adequate ventilation. If the patient is not breathing, intubation must be performed promptly. If ventilation is inadequate because of open or tension pneumothorax, these problems should be addressed at this stage of care. The next consideration is control of external hemorrhage and restoration of circulation. External hemorrhage is controlled best by direct pressure. Inadequate perfusion generally results from either hypovolemia or pump (cardiac) problems. Operation is often required as part of the resuscitative effort to control hemorrhage that is producing hypovolemia. Pump problems can be recognized by distended neck veins and are caused by one of four conditions: (i) tension pneumothorax, (ii) pericardial tamponade, (iii) coronary air embolism, or (iv) cardiac contusion/myocardial infarction. These conditions should be addressed sufficiently to provide adequate perfusion early in the initial treatment of the injured patient. For most patients suffering blunt trauma, urgent treatment of thoracic injury is accomplished during the primary survey because the most common blunt chest injuries can be controlled by endotracheal intubation or tube thoracotomy. In this setting, thoracotomy is indicated for cardiac tamponade, a massive hemothorax, or uncontrolled massive air leaks. Neither pulmonary nor cardiac contusions mandate delay in the diagnosis or definitive treatment of extrathoracic injuries resulting from blunt trauma.

Focused assessment sonography for trauma (FAST) has become routine as part of the secondary survey at many institutions and may be a valuable tool to assess for thoracic injuries. For example, extended FAST diagnoses clinically occult pneumothoraces with greater efficacy than plain x-ray.[2] Additionally, the ability to evaluate for blood in the pericardial space is excellent with reported sensitivities of 96% to 100% and a specificity of 100%, or essentially equivalent to pericardial window.[3] Cardiac ultrasonography may also be used for evaluating the hemodynamic effects of a pericardial effusion and for diagnosing structural injuries to the heart. The complete echocardiographic examination, however, requires much more time and expertise and should therefore be relegated to appropriate personnel in the later stages of evaluation.

TUBE THORACOSTOMY: INDICATIONS AND TECHNIQUE

During the initial resuscitation, placement of chest tubes can serve as both therapeutic and diagnostic procedures. Although the two most common indications for chest tube placement in this setting are pneumothorax and hemothorax, signs and symptoms of these conditions may not be readily apparent. Additionally, in the patient in shock, inadequate breathing or circulation may preclude taking time to differentiate between various causative conditions. Because the procedure is quick, relatively safe, and simple, the liberal use of chest tubes for patients in extremis is encouraged. Tension pneumothorax, the most common and easily treated immediately life-threatening thoracic injury, may accompany blunt or penetrating trauma. It results from a disruption in the respiratory system that allows air to escape from the lung parenchyma or tracheobronchial tree into the pleural space, thereby increasing intrathoracic pressure. This increased pressure is transmitted to all the cardiac chambers and retards venous return to the heart, resulting in hypotension. The classic signs of tension pneumothorax, which include decreased breath sounds, percussion tympany on the ipsilateral side, tracheal shift, and distended neck veins, are commonly absent or manifested incompletely in a busy emergency department. The diagnosis is often suspected on the basis of presence of shock with evidence of adequate venous filling on physical examination and recognition of asymmetric motion of the two sides of the chest. Treatment of suspected tension pneumothorax should not be delayed in patients with hemodynamic compromise.

The technique for chest tube placement is straightforward in the trauma setting. The chest is prepared and draped in a sterile manner. A local anesthetic such as 1% lidocaine is not required in an unconscious patient, but should be used in an alert patient. The appropriate location is the midaxillary line in approximately the fifth interspace. A scalpel is used to make a 2- to 3-cm incision through all layers of the skin and subcutaneous tissue. The incision should be oriented in the direction of the interspace. A finger or blunt clamp is used to penetrate the intercostal muscles and parietal pleura. The wound should be explored with an index finger in adults or a fifth finger in children. This ensures that the pleural space has been entered and allows exploration of the chest cavity. In adults, a 36 French

chest tube should then be inserted and directed posteriorly and toward the apex. This tube position is best achieved by appropriate orientation of the skin incision relative to the entrance into the chest cavity. The straight line between these two points will define the direction of the tube once in the chest. A posterior, apically directed tube allows for effective drainage of air and blood, which commonly accompanies traumatic pneumothoraces. The tube should be attached to 20 cm of suction with a water seal and collection chamber. Visual inspection of air passing through the water seal gives some estimation of the magnitude of the air leak, an important factor in assessment of suspected airway injuries. Collection chambers for hemothoraces should be of the same design. Those associated with autotransfusion devices such as cell savers have immense theoretic potential for rapid retrieval and processing of shed blood. In actual practice, however, their use is limited. For example, in a small- to moderate-sized hemothorax (<1,000 mL), the red-cell yield of an autotransfusion device would be small and not worth the associated time and expense. In a large hemothorax, the most important goal of therapy is to control bleeding, and arranging for autotransfusion may delay and obscure this most important principle. Additionally, products of autotransfusion may contain harmful cytokines, damaged cells and debris, and lack platelets and other important proteins and coagulation factors. The use of prophylactic antibiotics after tube thoracostomy is controversial. However, most clinicians would recommend use of a first-generation cephalosporin for 24 hours, ideally started before the initial tube placement.

After the primary survey, less dramatic pneumothoraces may be diagnosed, along with hemothoraces, on various imaging studies. The treatment of the occult pneumothorax, that is those seen only on computed tomography (CT) scan, deserves special mention. Placement of a chest tube in this condition requires use of good clinical judgment. Patients requiring positive pressure ventilation, those with hypotension or respiratory distress of any etiology, and those with associated complex injuries or associated hemothorax should generally be treated with tube thoracostomy. Patients with occult pneumothoraces treated without tube thoracostomy should be observed for at least 24 hours, and have a repeat pulmonary artery (PA) and lateral chest radiograph obtained.

RETAINED HEMOTHORAX AND EMPYEMA

When treating a hemothorax with tube thoracostomy, the goal is complete removal of blood. Complications such as atelectasis and empyema after chest trauma are clearly related to residual blood, fluid, and air, as can occur secondary to inadequate positioning of the tube (i.e., within a fissure), obstruction of a tube, or blood clot or loculated fluid within the chest. A persistent or clotted hemothorax is suggested by the presence of a persistent opacification in the pleural space in a patient with a known previous hemothorax. This radiodensity can be confused with adjacent pulmonary contusion or atelectasis. Chest CT can be quite helpful in this situation. Because retained blood serves as a nidus for infection and empyema,[4] aggressive attempts at removal are justified. Occasionally, this can be accomplished with placement of more chest tubes, but often an operative approach is needed. Video-assisted thoracoscopic surgery (VATS) may be useful for small, clotted hemothoraces and free flowing blood in patients that can tolerate single-lung ventilation.[5] For most operators, VATS also limits ability to control bleeding and perform definitive repair of injuries. In patients with ongoing bleeding or with large, clotted hemothoraces, posterolateral thoracotomy or muscle-sparing lateral thoracotomy is generally required.

Empyema thoracis is a relatively common complication after chest trauma, occurring in 5% to 10% of patients.[6,7] Etiologies of posttraumatic empyema include retained hemothorax, parapneumonic, persistent foreign body, ruptured pulmonary abscess, bronchopleural fistula, esophageal leak, and tracking through the intact or injured diaphragm from an abdominal source. The diagnosis of empyema may be difficult, and one must differentiate from pleural thickening, pulmonary contusion, and an uninfected effusion. Chest CT with intravenous (IV) contrast will usually demonstrate a fluid collection with loculations or an enhancing rim. Such radiographic findings coupled with a clinical scenario of low-grade sepsis or failure to thrive is diagnostic. Analysis and culture of fluid obtained at thoracentesis or chest tube placement confirms the diagnosis, but the fluid may appear sterile if the patient is already on antibiotics. Culture-directed (usually gram-positive organisms) or broad-spectrum antibiotics are certainly an important component of therapy, but the primary goal is removal of the infection while the fluid is still thin. The benefits associated with this principle include performance of a simpler therapeutic procedure, less risk of developing a restrictive pulmonary peel, and faster overall recovery of the injured patient. In early stages, this procedure may simply be tube thoracostomy. However, if the infected pleural process cannot be completely evacuated by chest tubes because of thicker fluid, loculations, or pleural adhesions, a formal thoracotomy with decortication is generally required.

Decortication should not be undertaken in the face of severe sepsis. Instead, antibiotics and chest drainage with tube thoracostomy, CT directed catheters, or open rib-resection drainage should be employed until sepsis is controlled. For early empyema, VATS has been successfully used for lysis of adhesions and fluid removal.[8,9] Because of limited ability to perform pleurectomy with this procedure, VATS should not be used when thick peel or trapped lung is present. For adult patients with posttraumatic empyema, there is no proven role for intrapleural fibrinolytic therapy.

EMERGENCY DEPARTMENT THORACOTOMY

Emergency department thoracotomy is a drastic step in the treatment of an injured patient. If possible, the patient should be stabilized and transported to the operating room, where better facilities are available for definitive care. Patients who arrive at the emergency department and deteriorate rapidly and those who have undergone cardiac arrest just before arrival are candidates for emergency department thoracotomy. The results of this procedure are dismal in patients who have had cardiac arrest before arriving at the hospital and have required cardiopulmonary resuscitation for more than a few minutes. Victims of blunt trauma who have sustained cardiopulmonary arrest at the scene should not be subjected to thoracotomy either at the scene or in the emergency department.[10] Similarly, patients who are found at emergency thoracotomy to have no cardiac activity, and those who fail to respond with improvement of the systolic blood pressure after aortic occlusion have a dismal prognosis. In general, patients undergoing emergency department thoracotomy for blunt trauma have a survival rate of <10%. For penetrating trauma, the reported survival rate ranges from 16% to 57%, and that for cardiac wounds ranges from 57% to 72%. The technique of emergency department thoracotomy is straightforward. Preparatory solution may be splashed on the chest, but skin preparation is not required. An incision is made from the sternal border to the midaxillary line in the fourth intercostal space. A chest retractor is inserted and opened widely. The costochondral junctions of the fifth, fourth, and, sometimes, third ribs can be divided quickly with the scalpel to provide excellent exposure. Attention is directed first to the injury. If there is exsanguination from a great vessel, the hemorrhage is controlled using pressure. If air embolism is the cause of the arrest, the hilum of the lung is clamped and air is evacuated from the ascending aorta. Otherwise, the pericardium is opened anterior and parallel to the phrenic nerve. The hemopericardium is evacuated, the cardiac injury is controlled with digital pressure, and a temporary repair is performed. After the cause of the arrest has been addressed, the descending thoracic aorta can be occluded with a vascular clamp or digital pressure and intrathoracic cardiac compression can be initiated. The patient's intravascular volume is restored, electrolyte imbalances are corrected, and, if the patient can be saved, he or she is transported to the operating room for definitive repair and closure.

SECONDARY SURVEY AND DEFINITIVE DIAGNOSIS

The secondary survey with respect to the chest should focus on more subtle evidence of injury that may be detected on physical examination and chest x-ray. Simple rib fractures are clinically relevant when associated with pain and are better diagnosed by palpation than by most imaging studies. Pneumothorax and hemothorax often go undetected during the primary survey but are common findings later in the workup. Only rarely should these conditions be observed in the trauma setting. Echocardiography can be an important adjunct for wounds in proximity to the heart or for evaluation of a new murmur. Because of continuing improvements in CT scanning technology, this modality is being more often used in the evaluation of the widened mediastinum.[11] Indeed, definitive diagnosis of aortic injuries is now routine with the use of CT angiography, obviating the need for standard angiography in most cases.[12]

INDICATIONS FOR OPERATION AND CHOICE OF INCISION

Indications for surgery on thoracic injuries generally fall into several categories: (i) hemorrhage, (ii) major airway disruption, (iii) heart/vascular injuries, (iv) esophageal disruption, and (v) diaphragm disruption. For hemorrhage, bleeding amounts and location can be detected from open wounds but are more often determined after chest tube insertion. Upon insertion, initial amounts of blood of 1,500 mL or ongoing bleeding of 300 mL per hour for 3 hours are indications for thoracotomy.[13] Massive air leak and the presence of gastric or esophageal contents are also chest tube findings necessitating surgical intervention. The severity of air leak can be estimated by the amount of air traversing the water seal on a tube thoracostomy suction/collection chamber. An intermittent bubble is defined as small, whereas a continuous leak is defined as large. A continuous leak, coupled with an inability to completely expand the lung or with inadequate tidal volumes, is a massive air leak. In stable patients without evidence of bleeding, specific diagnostic measures may be performed to evaluate the thoracic viscera. The likelihood of associated intra-abdominal injuries must not be overlooked.

The choice of thoracic incision obviously depends on many factors including the indication, urgency, associated injuries, mechanism, and information from preoperative studies. For injuries that are suspected or diagnosed preoperatively, approaching the affected thoracic structure is relatively straightforward (see Table 1). For exploratory surgery, the choice of incision should depend on the mechanism, instrument, location, and symptoms. The appropriate approach depends on the location of the entire injury, not just the site of entry. Stab wounds generally have a lower potential for deep penetration than do missile injuries. One of the more versatile of thoracic incisions is the median sternotomy. Compared to a thoracotomy, this incision is quicker to open and close, is associated with less postoperative pain, and may be associated with less

TABLE 1

SURGICAL APPROACHES FOR TRAUMATIC INJURIES TO THORACIC VISCERA

Site	Sternotomy	Right Thoracotomy	Left Thoracotomy
R atrium	+++	++	0
R ventricle	+++	+	+
L atrium	+++	+	+
L ventricle	++	0	+++
SVC	+++	++	0
Azygos vein	++	+++	0
IVC	+++	++	0
Aortic root	+++	+	0
Aortic arch	+++	0	++
R subclavian	++	++	0
Proximal R carotid	+++	+	0
Innominate	+++	++	0
L subclavian	+	0	+++
Proximal L carotid	++	0	++
Descending aorta	0	+	+++
Main PA	+++	0	++
R PA	++	+++	0
L PA	++	0	+++
RUL	++	+++	0
RML	++	+++	0
RLL	+	+++	0
LUL	+	0	+++
LLL	0	0	+++
R hilum	++	+++	0
L hilum	++	0	+++
Pericardium	+++	++	++
R IMA	++	+++	0
L IMA	++	0	+++
Proximal esophagus	0	+++	0
Distal esophagus	0	++	+++
Proximal trachea	++	+	+
Carina	0	+++	+
R mainstem	0	+++	0
L mainstem	0	++	++
R hemidiaphragm	+	+++	0
L hemidiaphragm	+	0	+++
CPB	+++	++	++

+++, preferred; ++, acceptable; +, with difficulty; 0, not accessible; R, right; L, left; SVC, superior vena cava; IVC, inferior vena cavae; PA, pulmonary artery; RUL, right upper lobe; RML, right middle lobe; RLL, right lower lobe; LUL, left upper lobe; LLL, left lower lobe; IMA, internal mammary artery; CPB, cardiopulmonary bypass.

contamination of the dependent lung as can occur through the trachea during a thoracotomy with the patient in the lateral decubitus position.

In general, the median sternotomy provides the best exposure to right-sided cardiac chambers, ascending aorta, aortic arch, and arch vessels (excluding the left subclavian artery), along with adequate exposure to both lungs and hemidiaphragms. For exploratory surgery, the median sternotomy is the best incision for mantel stab wounds and some precordial gunshot wounds whose trajectory can be reliably determined. The main limitation of this incision is its lack of exposure to the posterior mediastinal structures and the left lobe of the lung.

The posterolateral thoracotomy on the side of the injury is the best choice of incision for exploration of lateral stab or gunshot wounds. This incision performed through the fifth interspace is most useful for exploration and is the most versatile choice of interspace overall. The exposure can be markedly enhanced through the removal of the fifth rib, as this provides an incision the length of the rib, as high as the fourth interspace, and as low as the fifth interspace. In general, it is usually unwise to perform an exploratory thoracotomy higher than the fourth interspace or lower than the sixth. The transverse anterior thoracotomy or "clamshell" incision is occasionally useful for undetermined or transmediastinal injuries in the urgent setting. In the nonurgent setting, staged bilateral posterolateral thoracotomies are preferred when both hemithoraces require operation because of much better exposure.

In the trauma setting, the role of VATS continues to be defined. VATS is useful in the acute setting for ruling out diaphragm injury and may be preferable to laparoscopy because of less risk of tension pneumothorax. VATS may also have a role in the management of persistent intercostal or internal mammary artery bleeding, but this application requires some degree of experience with thoracoscopic surgery. Later postinjury, VATS can be useful for evacuation of retained hemothorax and in the early stages of empyema.

DAMAGE CONTROL TACTICS

In contrast to patients with abdominal trauma, there are only limited applications to the concept of damage control in patients with thoracic injuries. Although serious bleeding from most thoracic structures is unlikely to be controlled with packing, occasionally severe coagulopathy will prevent definitive repair and necessitate abbreviation of surgery and temporary closure of the chest by suturing or stapling of the skin incision only.[14] The two most common locations of injury in this scenario are the lung and chest wall. Hemorrhage from lung lacerations in patients with metabolic exhaustion generally should not be treated with formal anatomic resections; stapled wedge resections, tractotomies, and simple suture repair are more appropriate. In patients with persistent chest wall bleeding not associated with a major vessel, usually lung reexpansion for local tamponade and correction of coagulopathy will suffice. In rare circumstances, complex esophageal injuries may be associated with extensive loss of tissue and will require rapid exclusion and proximal diversion. However, attempts at closure of the injury, buttressing the repair with autologous tissue, and wide drainage should be employed in most patients with any chance of survival because of the high rate of ultimate success with this technique and the high rate of late complications with exclusion and diversion.

ANESTHETIC CONSIDERATIONS

Airway management can be extremely complex in patients with thoracic injuries, especially when injury to the trachea or bronchi is present. When operative management is required for any patient with thoracic trauma, planning of the operation should include a discussion with the anesthesiology team about airway issues. Double-lumen and bronchial blocker endotracheal tubes, which allow for better exposure by partial or complete deflation of a selected lung, should be strongly considered for any thoracic operation. For any given patient, the advantages of better exposure possible with use of these tubes must be weighed against the disadvantages. These include the additional time needed for placement and the requirement that single-lung ventilation must be tolerable from a cardiopulmonary standpoint. Hemodynamic stability, therefore, is usually a prerequisiste for their use. The amount of advantage gained by lung isolation must also be considered. For example, surgery on the mediastinum or hilum is greatly facilitated by lung deflation, whereas surgery on the chest wall is not. When needed, these tubes can often be placed in the emergency department when a secure airway is required and a thoracotomy or thoracoscopy is expected.

For patients with an otherwise adequate airway upon presentation, signs of airway injury such as massive air leak, subcutaneous air, or hemoptysis should be further evaluated with bronchoscopy in the operating room. This examination should be performed before replacing an existing adequate airway. In the absence of a massive air leak, bronchial tear, or hemorrhage into one mainstem bronchus, a double-lumen tube should be placed into the left mainstem bronchus. Otherwise, the tube should be placed to protect the uninjured side.

Postoperatively, for patients requiring continued intubation, a double-lumen tube must generally be replaced with a standard endotracheal tube or tracheostomy because of the inability to perform adequate pulmonary toilet through a double-lumen tube. In contrast, a suction catheter will pass down a bronchial blocker tube, which may therefore be left in place after surgery. A disadvantage with the bronchial blocker tube, however, is that intraoperative lung isoloation may be less complete than that obtained with a double-lumen tube. For patients requiring a thoracic surgery who have an inadequate airway on presentation, specific airway management depends on the nature of the injuries. Most of these patients can be intubated in a standard manner. If this is unsuccessful, however, attempts at cricothyroidotomy should not be delayed. In cases of tracheal transection, the distal segment must be controlled quickly through a neck incision and selectively intubated through the wound. For patients with known or suspected thoracic airway injuries, an endotracheal tube should be inserted over a bronchoscope past the injury or into an uninjured mainstem bronchus.

The intraoperative management of the airway in patients with complex tracheobronchial injuries can be challenging and is discussed in detail later. Injuries to the thoracic trachea may require creative placement of temporary tubes within the operative field to provide ventilation. After repair of a tracheobronchial injury, extubation should be performed if at all possible to prevent stress on the repair.

Other anesthestic considerations include placement of arterial catheters. In general, radial arterial lines should be placed in the extremity opposite the side of intended thoracotomy and obviously not in vessels distal to anticipated cross clamps. Epidural catheters for postoperative pain management should also be considered in patients undergoing thoracotomy in the nonurgent setting.

Control of body temperature is an extremely important component of operative and nonoperative management of injuries. Most patients are hypothermic and require a warm operating room, warm IV fluids, and warming blankets. Occasionally, controlled hypothermia is a useful adjunct to procedures on the thoracic aorta when spinal cord injury and paraplegia are risks. For patients with severe coagulopathy and a core temperature <33.5°C, extracorporeal warming can be life saving. This procedure involves placement of a 21 French femoral venous cannula, a 17 French internal jugular cannula, and use of a centrifugal pump and heat exchanger. Heparin is not necessary because of the intrinsic coagulopathy already present.

REFERENCES

1. Kemmerer WT, Eckert WJ, Gathwright JB, et al. Patterns of thoracic injuries in fatal traffic accidents. *J Trauma*. 1961;1:595.

2. Kirkpatrick AW, Sirois M, Laupland KB, et al. Hand-held thoracic sonography for detecting post-traumatic pneumothoraces. The extended focused assessment with sonography for trauma (EFAST). *J Trauma*. 2004;57:288–295.

3. Rozycki GS, Feliciano DV, Ochsner MG, et al. The role of ultrasound in patients with possible penetrating cardiac wounds. A prospective multicenter study. *J Trauma*. 1999;46:543–552.

4. Aguilar MM, Battistella FD, Owings JT, et al. Posttraumatic empyema. Risk factor analysis. *Arch Surg*. 1997;132:647–651.

5. Meyer DM, Jessen ME, Wait MA, et al. Early evacuation of traumatic retained hemothoraces using thoracoscopy: A prospective, randomized trial. *Ann Thorac Surg*. 1997;64:1396–1401.

6. Wilson JM, Boren CH Jr, Peterson SR, et al. Traumatic hemothorax: Is decortication necessary? *J Thorac Cardiovasc Surg*. 1989;77:489–495.

7. Mandal AK, Thadepalli H, Mandal AK, et al. Posttraumatic empyema thoracis: A 24-year experience at a major trauma center. *J Trauma*. 1997;43:764–771.

8. O'Brien J, Cohen M, Solit R, et al. Thoracoscopic drainage and decortication as definitive treatment for empyema thoracis following penetrating chest injury. *J Trauma*. 1994;36:536–540.

9. Scherer LA, Battistella FD, Owings JT, et al. Video-assisted thoracic surgery in the treatment of posttraumatic empyema. *Arch Surg*. 1998;133:637–642.

10. Hopson LR, Hirsh E, Delgado J, et al. National Association of EMS Physicians; American College of Surgeons Committee on Trauma. Guidelines for withholding or termination of resuscitation in prehospital traumatic cardiopulmonary arrest: Joint position statement of the National Association of EMS Physicians and the American College of Surgeons Committee on Trauma. *J Am Coll Surg*. 2003;196:106–112.

11. Exadaktylos AK, Sclabas G, Schmid SW, et al. Do we really need routine computed tomographic scanning in the primary evaluation of blunt chest trauma in patients with "normal" chest radiograph? *J Trauma*. 2001;51:1173–1176.

12. Fabian TC, Davis KA, Gavant ML, et al. Prospective study of blunt aortic injury: Helical CT is diagnostic and antihypertensive therapy reduces rupture. *Ann Surg*. 1998;227:666–676.

13. Karmy-Jones R, Jurkovich GJ, Nathens AB, et al. Timing of urgent thoracotomy for hemorrhage after trauma. A multicenter study. *Arch Surg*. 2001;136:513–518.

14. Vargo DJ, Battistella FD. Abbreviated thoracotomy and temporary chest closure. An application of damage control after thoracic trauma. *Arch Surg*. 2001;136:21–24.

Chest Wall Injury

33

Jordan A. Weinberg   **Martin A. Croce**

Thoracic injuries occur commonly as a result of both blunt and penetrating trauma, and are implicated in 50% of all trauma deaths.[1] In general, thoracic injury must be identified and managed expediently because such injuries are often associated with early mortality. Injuries to the chest wall that may be immediately life threatening include open pneumothorax and flail chest. Other chest wall injuries, although not as obviously critical, can result in significant morbidity and mortality if not appreciated and managed appropriately. In this chapter, the management of common chest wall injuries will be presented, including rib fractures, sternal fractures, flail chest, open pneumothorax, and chest wall defects.

RIB FRACTURES

Rib fractures occur commonly as a result of blunt trauma, and have been documented in up to two thirds of thoracic injury cases.[2,3] In one center's experience, rib fractures were radiographically present in 10% of total trauma admissions.[4] Isolated or multiple rib fractures are among the most common injuries in the elderly, with an incidence of approximately 12%.[5] The true incidence of rib fractures, however, is likely underreported, given that up to 50% of rib fractures are not visualized on initial plain x-ray.[6]

Although rib fractures tend to be uncomplicated skeletal injuries requiring no specific orthopaedic treatment, they are associated with significant pulmonary morbidity. Rib fractures are a marker for serious injury, with an 84% to 94% incidence of associated injury including hemothorax, pneumothorax, and pulmonary contusion.[3,4] Fractures of the lower ribs are associated with abdominal injury, with lower right-sided fractures having a 19% to 56% risk of liver injury, and lower left-sided fractures having a 22% to 28% risk of spleen injury.[7,8] Although often disseminated, there is actually no demonstrated association between first and second rib fractures and blunt aortic injury.[7,9] Overall, rib

fractures portend a 12% mortality risk and 33% incidence of pulmonary complications.[4]

Advancing age has been considered to be a significant comorbidity in the setting of rib fractures. Bergeron et al., in a prospectively studied group of 405 patients with rib fractures, demonstrated a five times greater risk of mortality in patients older than 65 years.[10] Bulger et al. also demonstrated an increased mortality rate among patients older than 65 years (22% vs. 10%), as well as an associated increase in the incidence of pneumonia (31% vs. 17%).[11] Also, they demonstrated that mortality and pneumonia risk correlated with the number of rib fractures. Each additional fracture was associated with an approximately 20% increase in mortality and pneumonia.

Children, on the other hand, have a much lower incidence of rib fracture given the relative compliance of the pediatric skeleton. The presence of rib fracture suggests a high-energy mechanism. Rib fractures in an infant or toddler in the absence of such mechanism should warrant an investigation into abuse. In children younger than 3 years, rib fracture has been demonstrated to have a positive predictive value of 95% for determining nonaccidental trauma.[12]

Rib fracture generally results from compression on the thoracic cage. Fractures often occur at a 60 degree rotation from the sternum because this area is one of mechanical weakness relative to other locations.[13] Rib fractures are often segmental, with one break at 60 degrees and the other posterior.[14] A flail segment is created by the segmental fracture of two or more contiguous ribs. The phenomenon of flail chest is discussed in the subsequent text.

It is unusual for rib fractures to require treatment directed at the fractures themselves, such as operative stabilization. Rib fractures tend to heal with good result. Therapy is directed toward the prevention of respiratory embarrassment that may occur. Pulmonary morbidity may result from pain interfering with pulmonary toilet, underlying pulmonary injury such as contusion, or a combination of the two. Initial therapy consists of pain control, chest physiotherapy, and mobilization. Modalities for pain control include systemic therapies such as narcotics and nonsteroidal antiinflammatory drugs (NSAIDs), and regional therapies including local rib blocks, pleural infusion catheters, and epidural analgesia.

Intravenous narcotics have historically been the mainstay of pain therapy for chest wall trauma, and patient-controlled anesthesia (PCA) has emerged as the most efficacious method to deliver narcotics. The advantages of narcotic analgesia, including ease of administration and monitoring, are tempered by inconsistent efficacy and the tendency of narcotics to cause sedation, cough suppression, and respiratory depression, all detrimental to pulmonary toilet.

Epidural analgesia is the most common regional therapy used for chest wall pain management. Narcotics, anesthetics, or a combination of the two are introduced into the spinal epidural space through a catheter inserted at the thoracic or lumbar level. The main advantages of epidural analgesia are its superior efficacy and absence of side effects detrimental to pulmonary toilet. When compared to intravenous narcotic analgesia, epidural analgesia is associated with improved pain perception and improved performance of pulmonary function tests.[15,16] There is also evidence that the benefit of epidural analgesia

may translate into decreased ventilator days, pulmonary complications, and mortality.[17] The prime disadvantage of epidural analgesia is its relative invasiveness, subjecting the patient to the small but serious risks of epidural infection, epidural hematoma, and direct spinal cord trauma. The contraindications to epidural analgesia are numerous, including coagulopathy, infection, altered mental status, and spinal fracture, limiting its applicability in the multi-injured patient. In a recent study, 64% of patient candidates for epidural analgesia had contraindications to epidural placement as a result of associated injuries.[17]

Other regional modalities include intercostal nerve block, intrapleural analgesia, and thoracic paravertebral block (see Fig. 1). Intercostal nerve block involves injection of local anesthetic regionally in the intercostal spaces involving the rib fracture(s). Intrapleural analgesia involves the placement of local anesthetic into the pleural space through an indwelling catheter, producing analgesia by gravity-dependent retrograde diffusion of the anesthetic across the parietal pleura. Paravertebral block involves the injection of local anesthetic in close proximity to the thoracic vertebrae, resulting in a unilateral somatic and sympathetic block. Each of these modalities has their inherent advantages and disadvantages. Overall, there is a relative paucity of reported experience with these techniques in trauma patients, making it difficult to make strong conclusions regarding their relative efficacies.

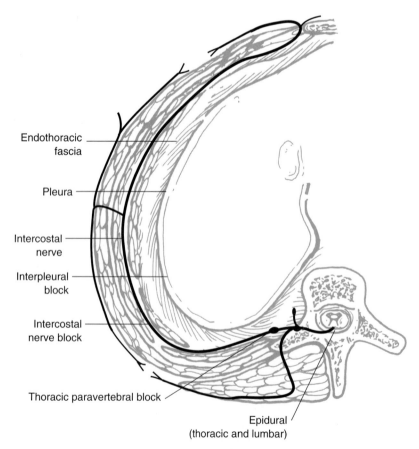

Endothoracic
fascia

Pleura

Intercostal
nerve

Interpleural
block

Intercostal
nerve block

Thoracic paravertebral block

Epidural
(thoracic and lumbar)

Figure 1   The anatomic location of delivery for the various modalities of regional thoracic analgesia. (Modified from Karmakar MJ, Anthony MH. Acute pain management of patients with multiple rib fractures. *J Trauma*. 2003:54:615–625.)

In 2003, the Eastern Association for the Surgery of Trauma reported practice guidelines on pain management in blunt thoracic trauma, attempting to identify both the optimal method of pain control in blunt chest trauma and the patient group particularly at risk for pulmonary morbidity.[18] Following a thorough evaluation of the existing literature, the authors concluded that epidural analgesia is the optimal modality of pain relief for blunt chest wall injury and is the preferred technique after severe blunt thoracic trauma. Patients with four or more rib fractures who are 65 years and older should be provided with epidural analgesia barring any contraindications. Younger patients with four or more rib fractures or patients 65 years and older should also be considered for epidural analgesia.

FLAIL CHEST

A flail segment results when two or more contiguous ribs are fractured segmentally (see Fig. 2). Although this may be evident radiographically, a true flail chest is a clinical diagnosis, where the flail segment moves paradoxically during spontaneous negative pressure ventilation. With spontaneous inspiration, the flail segment is pulled inward by negative intrathoracic pressure, while on expiration the segment protrudes outward as a result of positive intrathoracic pressure. This paradoxical movement may be masked, however, by positive pressure mechanical ventilation or muscle splinting.

Flail chest is an immediately life-threatening injury, associated with acute respiratory failure if not rapidly identified and treated. Mortality from isolated flail chest has

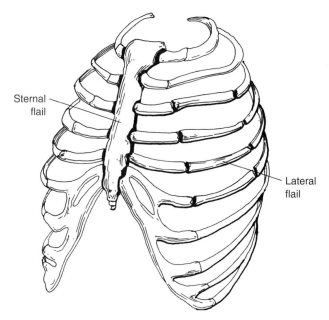

Figure 2 Two types of chest flail: sternal and lateral. (Modified from Mayberry JC, Trunkey DD. The fractured rib in chest wall trauma. *Chest Surg Clin N Am.* 1997;7:239–61.)

been reported to be as high as 16%.[8] The observed respiratory failure was initially attributed to the flail segment itself causing ineffective gas exchange, but it is now accepted that the pathophysiology of this injury is largely secondary to the associated pulmonary contusion. The age of the patient and the severity of associated injuries are strongly associated with outcome in flail chest. After age 55, the likelihood of death increases 132% for every decade increase in age and 30% for each unit increase in injury severity score.[19]

Management of flail chest is directed toward respiratory support with analgesia, pulmonary toilet, and positive pressure mechanical ventilation when warranted. The physician should have a low threshold for endotracheal intubation and mechanical ventilation in patients with flail chest, particularly for the multi-injured and the elderly. Early intubation in patients 30 years or older with moderate to severe injury resulted in 6% mortality, compared to 50% mortality associated with delayed intubation.[20]

Generally, no therapy such as chest wall stabilization need be directed at the flail segment; the fractures will heal without intervention, save for rare occasions. Many institutions, particularly in Europe, have documented their respective experiences with operative stabilization of flail chest.[21-23] Voggenreiter et al., in their review of 42 patients with flail chest, found that operative stabilization contributed to fewer ventilator days compared to no stabilization in the absence of radiographic pulmonary contusion (6.5 vs. 26.7 days). When pulmonary contusion, however, was present, no difference in ventilator days was observed. Most centers in North America favor supportive care over operative stabilization with the underlying philosophy that the lung injury, and not the flail segment, is responsible for the associated morbidity and mortality. Highly select patients, however, may benefit from internal fixation of the flail segment. Such patients would be those failing to wean from the ventilator clearly as a result of chest wall instability and not the underlying lung injury.

STERNAL FRACTURE

Fracture of the sternum generally occurs as a result of direct frontal impact. Sternal fracture following motor vehicle collision, usually as a result of sternal impact against the steering column, should be considered a marker for associated injuries. In a review of 60 patients with sternal fracture, associated injuries included rib fractures in 40%, long bone fractures in 25%, and head injuries in 18%.[24] Although blunt cardiac injury may occur concomitantly with sternal fracture, the presence of a sternal fracture does not predict the presence of blunt cardiac injury, and in and of itself, does not warrant monitoring for blunt cardiac injury.[25] In fact, patients with isolated sternal fracture and an otherwise unremarkable evaluation do not require hospital admission.[26,27] Management of the sternal fracture is symptomatic, but operative reduction and fixation are occasionally indicated for significantly displaced fractures.

OPEN PNEUMOTHORAX AND CHEST WALL DEFECTS

The open pneumothorax, or "sucking chest wound," is usually the result of a large destructive penetrating wound, resulting in equilibration of intrathoracic and atmospheric pressure through the chest wall defect. If the opening is more than two thirds the diameter of the trachea, then atmospheric air follows the path of least resistance (i.e., the chest wall defect) on inspiration, resulting in significant deficiency of alveolar ventilation. When such an injury is encountered in the prehospital setting, it may be treated with a dressing taped on three sides to achieve a valve mechanism whereby gas may exit the pleural space to prevent tension pneumothorax. Caution must be exercised to prohibit the inadvertent creation of an occlusive dressing (i.e., tight dressings and petrolatum gauze should be avoided). This type of management is only a bridge to definitive care. Once the patient arrives in the hospital setting, a chest tube should be immediately placed on the side of the wound, and the wound itself should be occluded completely. Often such patients, as a result of pulmonary embarrassment and associated injuries, will require endotracheal intubation in the emergency room. Once the airway is secured and positive pressure ventilation initiated, the pathophysiology of the open pneumothorax becomes inconsequent.

Large chest wall defects require immediate establishment of positive pressure ventilation to restore alveolar ventilation. Occlusive dressings and chest tubes have little immediate applicability in the presence of massive tissue loss. Initial operative management usually involves thoracotomy with the goal of achieving hemostasis. Some form of temporary closure of the wound is necessary, and we have found in recent experience that prosthetic polyglactin 910 mesh in combination with a negative pressure vacuum dressing achieves a durable temporary closure. Following hemostasis and debridement of devitalized skin and soft tissue, the mesh is secured to the chest wall with monofilament absorbable suture. The vacuum sponge dressing may then be applied over the mesh and connected to suction. Chest tubes are also placed at this time. Once the patient has stabilized and recovered sufficiently, definitive wound closure may be entertained. This may involve flap reconstruction requiring the participation of thoracic and/or reconstructive surgeons.

REFERENCES

1. LoCicero J, Mattox KL, III. Epidemiology of chest trauma. *Surg Clin North Am.* 1989;69:15–19.
2. Newman RJ, Jones IS. A prospective study of 413 consecutive car occupants with chest injuries. *J Trauma.* 1984;24:129–135.
3. Shorr RM, Crittenden M, Indeck M, et al. Blunt thoracic trauma. Analysis of 515 patients. *Ann Surg.* 1987;206:200–205.
4. Ziegler DW, Agarwal NN. The morbidity and mortality of rib fractures. *J Trauma.* 1994;37:975–979.
5. Palvanen M, Kannus P, Niemi S, et al. Epidemiology of minimal trauma rib fractures in the elderly. *Calcif Tissue Int.* 1998;62:274–277.
6. Trunkey DD. *Cervicothoracic Trauma.* New York: Thieme; 1986.
7. Shweiki E, Klena J, Wood GC, et al. Assessing the true risk of abdominal solid organ injury in hospitalized rib fracture patients. *J Trauma.* 2001;50:684–688.
8. Clark GC, Schecter WP, Trunkey DD. Variables affecting outcome in blunt chest trauma: Flail chest vs. pulmonary contusion. *J Trauma.* 1988;28:298–304.
9. Lee J, Harris JH Jr, Duke JH Jr, Williams JS. Noncorrelation between thoracic skeletal injuries and acute traumatic aortic tear. *J Trauma.* 1997;43:400–404.
10. Bergeron E, Lavoie A, Clas D, et al. Elderly trauma patients with rib fractures are at greater risk of death and pneumonia. *J Trauma.* 2003;54:478–485.
11. Bulger EM, Arneson MA, Mock CN, et al. Rib fractures in the elderly. *J Trauma.* 2000;48:1040–1046; Discussion 1046–7.
12. Ricci LR. Positive predictive value of rib fractures as an indicator of nonaccidental trauma in children. *J Trauma.* 2004;56:721; Author reply 721–2.
13. Viano DC, Lau IV, Asbury C, et al. Biomechanics of the human chest, abdomen, and pelvis in lateral impact. *Accid Anal Prev.* 1989;21:553–574.
14. Wanek S, Mayberry JC. Blunt thoracic trauma: Flail chest, pulmonary contusion, and blast injury. *Crit Care Clin.* 2004;20:71–81.
15. Mackersie RC, Karagianes TG, Hoyt DB, et al. Prospective evaluation of epidural and intravenous administration of fentanyl for pain control and restoration of ventilatory function following multiple rib fractures. *J Trauma.* 1991;31:443–449; Discussion 449–51.
16. Moon MR, Luchette FA, Gibson SW, et al. Prospective, randomized comparison of epidural versus parenteral opioid analgesia in thoracic trauma. *Ann Surg.* 1999;229:684–691; Discussion 691–2.
17. Bulger EM, Edwards T, Klotz P, et al. Epidural analgesia improves outcome after multiple rib fractures. *Surgery.* 2004;136:426–430.
18. Simon BJ, Cushman J, Barraco R, et al. Pain management guidelines for blunt thoracic trauma. *J Trauma.* 2005;59:1256–1267.
19. Albaugh G, Kann B, Puc MM, et al. Age-adjusted outcomes in traumatic flail chest injuries in the elderly. *Am Surg.* 2000;66:978–981.
20. Sankaran S, Wilson RF. Factors affecting prognosis in patients with flail chest. *J Thorac Cardiovasc Surg.* 1970;60:402–410.
21. Balci AE, Eren S, Cakir O, et al. Open fixation in flail chest: Review of 64 patients. *Asian Cardiovasc Thorac Ann.* 2004;12:11–15.
22. Voggenreiter G, Neudeck F, Aufmkolk M, et al. Operative chest wall stabilization in flail chest – outcomes of patients with or without pulmonary contusion. *J Am Coll Surg.* 1998;187:130–138.
23. Mouton W, Lardinois D, Furrer M, et al. Long-term follow-up of patients with operative stabilisation of a flail chest. *Thorac Cardiovasc Surg.* 1997;45:242–244.
24. Buckman R, Trooskin SZ, Flancbaum L, et al. The significance of stable patients with sternal fractures. *Surg Gynecol Obstet.* 1987;164:261–265.
25. Pasquale MD, Nagy K, Clarke J. Practice management guidelines for screening of blunt cardiac injury. In: Kurek S Jr, ed. *Trauma practice guidelines*: Eastern Association for the Surgery of Trauma; 1998.
26. Hills MW, Delprado AM, Deane SA. Sternal fractures: Associated injuries and management. *J Trauma.* 1993;35:55–60.
27. Jackson M, Walker WS. Isolated sternal fracture: A benign injury. *Injury.* 1992;23:535–536.

Penetrating Pulmonary Injuries

34

Juan A. Asensio   Luis M. García-Núñez   Patrizio Petrone

"War surgery has rendered surgery of the lung easy and without any particular danger. It is our earnest hope that the new field opened by the horrors of war may be utilized for the benefit of mankind."

–Pierre Duval, MD
France 1919

Thoracic trauma accounts for approximately 20% to 25% of all trauma deaths; however, most of the thoracic injuries can be managed nonoperatively with insertion of chest tubes. Approximately 10% to 15% will require operative intervention to control life-threatening hemorrhage. What is not known is the true incidence of pulmonary injuries requiring operative intervention. Most of the thoracic injuries requiring surgical intervention will be due to penetrating mechanisms of injury such as gunshot wounds (GSW), stabwounds (SW), and shotgun wounds (SGW). Much less common are blunt thoracic injuries requiring operative intervention. Similarly, a significant number of pulmonary injuries occur in association with injuries to thoracic vascular structures or the heart. Thoracoabdominal injuries represent a difficult dilemma for the trauma surgeon in deciding which cavity to access and when.

Factors associated with survival for penetrating pulmonary injuries requiring surgical intervention include the type of wounding agents, that is, GSW versus SW or SGW, prehospital transport time, presence of shock at the scene or upon arrival, loss of the airway, and number of associated injuries. Patients sustaining penetrating pulmonary injuries arriving in cardiopulmonary arrest at a trauma center which require emergency department thoracotomy (EDT) have an extremely poor prognosis.

CLINICAL DIAGNOSIS

The clinical presentation of patients sustaining penetrating pulmonary injuries ranges from hemodynamic stability to cardiopulmonary arrest. Patients with penetrating pulmonary injuries may present with symptoms and signs of pneumohemothorax or an open pneumothorax with a partial loss of the chest wall; or may also present with a tension pneumothorax or hemothorax.

Patients with penetrating pulmonary injuries may rarely present with a pneumomediastinum upon auscultation. The Hamman crunch—a systolic crunch may be detected upon auscultation in these patients. Similarly, they may also present with a pneumopericardium, detected by auscultating Brichiteau's windmill bruit (*bruit de moulin*). Patients with penetrating pulmonary injuries may rarely present with true hemoptysis; they may also present with symptoms and signs of associated cardiac injuries.

During the evaluation of these patients, the trauma surgeon must be cognizant that the thoracic cavity is composed of both a right and left hemithoracic cavity as well as an anterior, posterior, and superior mediastinum because missiles or other wounding agents may often traverse one or more of these cavities. Similarly, missile trajectories are often unpredictable and frequently create secondary missiles if they impact on hard bony structures such as the ribs, spine, and sternum thereby creating the potential for associated injuries and greater damage.

CLINICAL INVESTIGATIONS

Patients presenting with penetrating thoracic trauma may be studied by invasive and noninvasive means.

Noninvasive Techniques

Noninvasive techniques include:

- Trauma ultrasonography (focused assessment with sonography for trauma [FAST])—will reliably diagnose and exclude an associated cardiac injury and can also diagnose the presence of a hemothorax
- Chest x-ray—will provide an assessment of the following:
  - Both hemithoracic cavities
  - Mediastinum
  - Pericardium
  - Extra-anatomic air: peneumomediastinum, pneumopericardium, or subcutaneous air
- Electrocardiogram (ECG)

Invasive Techniques

Invasive techniques can be both diagnostic and therapeutic.

- Insertion of chest tubes in one or both hemithoracic cavities will serve to:
  - Evacuate air
  - Evacuate and quantify blood, evaluate whether it is arterial or venous
  - Detect massive air leaks
- Establish an indication for thoracotomy

SURGICAL DECISIONS IN THE EMERGENCY DEPARTMENT

For patients that present in cardiopulmonary arrest, it will be necessary to proceed to EDT. With the simultaneous insertion of a large-bore chest tube in the right hemithoracic cavity, the left anterolateral thoracotomy may be extended into bilateral anterolateral thoracotomies if required. For patients who present with systolic blood pressure (BP) ≤80 mm Hg, insert bilateral chest tubes and resuscitate per Advanced Trauma Life Support (ATLS) protocol. If patient remains unstable, transport immediately to the operating room (OR). If patient stabilizes, institute an investigative workup. For patients presenting with thoracoabdominal injury, insert chest tube or tubes. Transfer expediently to OR for abdominal exploration and reassess the need for thoracotomy.

OPERATIVE MANAGEMENT

Indications

Indications for thoracotomy in patients sustaining penetrating thoracic injuries include the following:

- Cardiopulmonary arrest
- Impending cardiopulmonary arrest upon arrival in the emergency department (ED)
- Evacuation of 1,000 to 1,500 mL of blood upon initial placement of chest tube
- Evacuation of ≥1,000 mL of blood upon placement of chest tube and ongoing blood loss
- Tension hemothorax
- Large retained hemothorax
- Massive air leak from chest tube

Settings

Thoracotomy may be performed in the ED or in the OR. For patients presenting with cardiopulmonary arrest proceed immediately to EDT. The objectives of EDT include the following:

- Resuscitation of agonal patients with penetrating cardiothoracic injuries
- Evacuation of pericardial tamponade if there is an associated cardiac injury
- Direct repair of cardiac injuries, if there is an associated cardiac injury
- Control of thoracic hemorrhage
- Prevention of air embolism
- Perform cardiopulmonary resuscitation, which may produce up to 60% of the normal ejection fraction (EF)
- Control pulmonary hemorrhage
- Crossclamp pulmonary hilum
- Crossclamp descending thoracic aorta

Adjunct Surgical Maneuvers

The trauma surgeon must be cognizant of the physiologic effects of some of the adjunct surgical techniques employed to deal with cardiopulmonary injuries. Each of these maneuvers may be instituted in the ED or in the OR. Each has both positive and negative effects.

Pulmonary Hilar Crossclamping

The positive effects of pulmonary hilar crossclamping include the following:

- Preservation and redistribution of remaining blood volume
- Improvement in perfusion to contralateral uninjured lung
- Control of hilar hemorrhage
- Prevention of air emboli

The negative effects of pulmonary hilar crossclamping include the following:

- Rendering crossclamped lung ischemic
- Imposing a great afterload onto the right ventricle (RV)
- Decreasing oxygenation and ventilation to crossclamped lung

The unknown effects of pulmonary hilar crossclamping include the following:

- Length of safe crossclamp time
- Incidence of pulmonary reperfusion injury to both the injured and uninjured lung

Thoracic Aortic Crossclamping

The positive effects of thoracic aortic crossclamping include the following:

- Preservation and redistribution of remaining blood volume
- Improvement of coronary/carotid arterial perfusion
- Reduction of subdiaphragmatic blood flow
- Increases in the left ventricular stroke work index (LVSWI)
- Increased myocardial contractility

The negative effects of thoracic aortic crossclamping include the following:

- Decreasing blood flow to the abdominal viscera to approximately 10%
- Decreasing renal blood flow to approximately 10%
- Decreasing blood flow to the spinal cord to approximately 10%
- Inducing anaerobic metabolism
- Inducing hypoxia/lactic acidosis
- Imposing a great afterload onto the left ventricle (LV)
- May rarely cause paraplegia

The unknown effects of thoracic aortic crossclamping include the following:

- Length of safe crossclamp time
- Incidence of reperfusion injury

Emergency Department Thoracotomy

The technique for EDT may be used for patients sustaining penetrating pulmonary injuries arriving in cardiopulmonary arrest. This technique is outside of the scope of this chapter and is described in another chapter in the textbook.

Operating Room

The trauma surgeon must be familiar with the use of these special instruments that are needed to access the thoracic cavity as well as to retract, manipulate, and surgically intervene in the thoracic structures and lung (see Fig. 1). These instruments include the following:

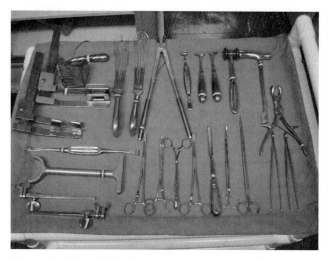

Figure 1   Thoracic instrument tray.

- Doyen costal elevators (right and left) (see Fig. 2)
- Alexander periostotome (see Fig. 2)
- Cameron-Haight periosteal elevator (see Fig. 2)
- Bethune rib shears (see Fig. 3)
- Stille-Horsley bone cutting rongeurs (see Fig. 3)
- Lebsche knife and mallet (see Fig. 3)
- Rib raspatory
- Finochietto retractor
- Davidson scapular retractor (see Fig. 4)
- Allison lung retractors (see Fig. 4)
- Semb lung retractors
- Nelson lung dissecting lobectomy scissors (see Fig. 5)
- Metzenbaum long dissecting scissors (see Fig. 5)
- Tuttle thoracic tissue forceps (see Fig. 5)
- Duval lung forceps (see Fig. 6)
- Davidson pulmonary vessel clamps

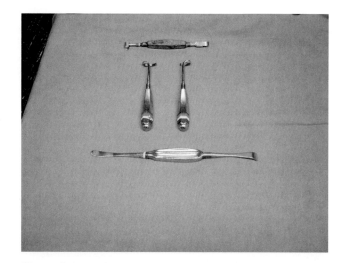

Figure 2   Alexander periostotome. Right and left Doyen costal elevators and Cameron-Haight periosteal elevator.

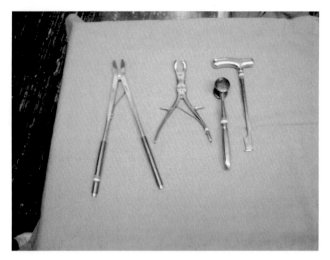

Figure 3   Bethune rib shears, Stille-Horsley bone cutting rongeurs, and Lebsche knife and mallet.

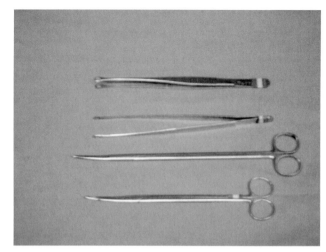

Figure 5   Tuttle thoracic tissue forceps. Nelson lung dissecting lobectomy scissors and Metzenbaum long dissecting scissors.

- Sarot bronchus clamps (right and left)
- Bailey rib approximator (see Fig. 7)
- Berry sternal needle holder
- Vascular clamps

Adjuncts

Double-Lumen Tubes

Double-lumen tubes are invaluable adjuncts in the management of penetrating pulmonary injuries. Although more difficult to insert by the anesthesiologists, double-lumen tubes are designed to ventilate either the right or left lung selectively. There are two types of double-lumen tubes, one designed for the left and one designed for the right mainstem bronchus (see Fig. 8). By inflating the balloon that occludes either the right or left mainstem bronchus, the lung can be collapsed, thereby allowing the trauma surgeon to operate on a collapsed and still lung.

Bronchoscopy

Bronchoscopy is also an invaluable adjunct when utilized intraoperatively. It can serve as a diagnostic tool by locating injured bronchi at the lobar and even segmental levels. It can also be therapeutic by removing blood within the tracheobronchial tree which tends to cause bronchospasm (see Fig. 9).

Ventilation

There are two types of ventilation that can be employed in the OR. The conventional method intermittently allows for a periodic inflation and deflation of the lung or high-frequency jet ventilation that allows the trauma surgeon to operate on a nonmoving still lung (see Fig. 10).

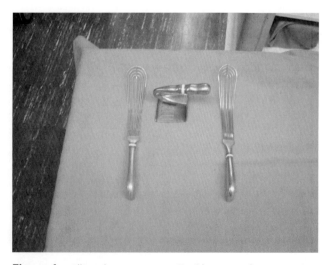

Figure 4   Allison lung retractors. Davidson scapular retractor.

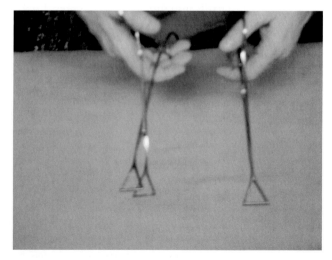

Figure 6   Duval lung forceps.

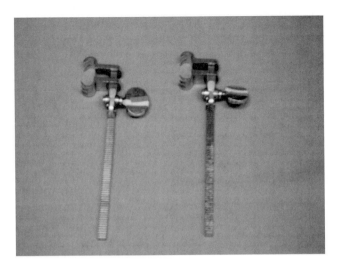

Figure 7 Bailey rib approximator.

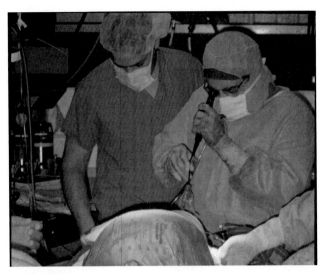

Figure 9 Bronchoscopy being performed before closure of left anterolateral thoracotomy and left lower lobectomy on patient that sustained multiple thoracoabdominal gunshot wounds. Notice prosthetic abdominal wall closure with IV bag after damage control laparotomy.

Surgical Incisions and Exposures

The thoracic cavity is composed of both the right and left hemithoracic cavity as well as an anterior, posterior, and superior mediastinum. Not one single incision will allow the surgeon to access all of them. The incisions used to access the thorax for the management of penetrating pulmonary injuries are mentioned in the subsequent text.

Anterolateral Thoracotomy (Spangaro Incision)

This is the most frequently used incision to access either the right or left hemithoracic cavity because most of these patients will be transported to the OR with some degree of hemodynamic instability. This incision will allow the trauma surgeon to operate on either the right or left lung although it provides for a much more limited operating field. It does not allow for access to the posterior structures of either the right or left hemithoracic cavity.

The left anterolateral thoracotomy will provide access to the heart and the descending thoracic aorta should crossclamping be necessary if the patient's hemodynamic instability and/or cardiopulmonary arrest demands it. It is also the incision of choice when the thoracic cavity needs

to be accessed in the presence of an associated abdominal injury because it can be extended into bilateral anterolateral thoracotomies if associated pathology is found in the contralateral hemithoracic cavity.

Posterolateral Thoracotomy

It provides for the very best exposure for the management of penetrating pulmonary injuries. The disadvantage of this incision is that it is time consuming as it requires a special positioning of the patient on the operating table. Most of these patients are usually transported to the OR with hemodynamic instability and cannot afford the luxury of being placed in this position. This incision provides suboptimal access for the management of associated cardiac injuries.

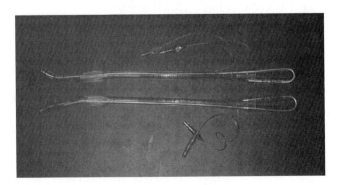

Figure 8 Double-lumen endotracheal tubes.

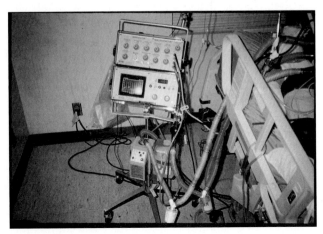

Figure 10 High-frequency jet ventilator (Percussonator).

A right posterolateral thoracotomy provides access to the right lung, the thoracic esophagus up to its most distal portion when it crosses anterior to the thoracic aorta into the left hemithoracic cavity, and is found superior to the descending thoracic aorta. It provides access to the azygos and hemiazygos veins and is the incision of choice for the management of most, if not all, tracheal injuries.

A left posterolateral thoracotomy will provide access to the left lung, descending thoracic aorta, and the distal-most portion of the esophagus as it crosses from the right into the left hemithoracic cavity and it is found superior to the descending thoracic aorta.

Median Sternotomy (Duval-Barasty Incision)

This is the incision of choice for the management of patients with associated cardiac injuries who arrive with vital signs in the OR. The right or left hemithoracic cavities can be accessed if the mediastinal pleura is sharply transected. This provides access to the anterior portions of either the right or left lung although exposure of the posterior aspects of the pulmonary lobes is suboptimal. Care must be exercised when a significant portion of the lung is mobilized medially into this incision because the pulmonary hilar vessels can be rotated at a 90-degree angle occluding both the inflow and outflow and causing significant hemodynamic compromise to the patient. Similarly, extreme caution must be exercised when mobilizing the inferior pulmonary ligaments because an inadvertent iatrogenic injury to the inferior pulmonary vein may ensue.

Adjunct Maneuvers—Technical Aspects

Important associated maneuvers utilized in the management of pulmonary injuries include the following:

Aortic Crossclamping

The aorta can be crossclamped only through a left anterolateral thoracotomy. This requires a meticulous combination of sharp and blunt dissection of this vessel before its entrance into the abdominal cavity through the aortic hiatus. The aorta should be digitally encircled; however, lateral digital dissection must be gentle and limited to prevent iatrogenic injuries to the intercostal arteries. The esophagus, which lies immediately superior to the anterior border of the aorta, must be separated before placement of a Crafoord-DeBakey aortic crossclamp. Esophageal identification is facilitated by the prior insertion of a nasogastric tube.

Pulmonary Hilar Crossclamping

This maneuver is utilized when there is a central hilar hematoma or active bleeding from the pulmonary hilum. The hilum of the lung can be isolated utilizing a meticulous combination of sharp and blunt dissection of the perihilar tissues to allow for the digital encirclement of all the structures. A Crafoord-DeBakey aortic crossclamp is then placed as close to the pericardium as possible.

Complete Inflow Occlusion

The Shumacker maneuver may occasionally be required if there is an associated cardiac injury either to the lateral-most aspects of the right atrium and/or atriocaval junction. This involves placement of Crafoord-DeBakey aortic crossclamps in the intrapericardial portions of the superior vena cava as well as the inferior vena cava at the space of Gibbons. This will allow for immediate emptying of the heart. Although it is estimated that the safe period for this maneuver ranges from 1 to 3 minutes, the actual safety period is unknown.

Pulmonary Hilar Vessel Control

This maneuver is necessary to control hemorrhage from either the pulmonary artery or vein. The dissection and ligation or stapling of pulmonary arteries and veins requires a different technique than for systemic vessels. The pulmonary vessels are thin walled and fragile. They tear easily and cannot be clamped with standard hemostats. The dissection must be gentle and meticulous. There is almost always a perivascular plane that permits rapid and safe dissection in a vascular area. This plane must be sought and identified. Before encirclement of either the pulmonary artery or vein, three sides of the vessels should be dissected completely before an attempt is made to pass a Mixter right angle forceps beneath the vessel. If this is not done, perforation is likely. Pulmonary vessels should not be held with vascular forceps because they may tear; only the adventitia should be grasped. Either of these vessels may be held or retracted with Cushing vein retractors or Kittner dissectors safely.

- Control of the main right or left pulmonary artery can be in an extrapleural location at the hilum or intrapericardial, which requires lateral cardiac displacement and occasionally transection of the pericardium.
- Pulmonary vein control can either be extrapleural at the hilum or intrapericardial although this maneuver is quite difficult.

UNIFORM APPROACH TO THE MANAGEMENT OF PULMONARY INJURIES

This includes the following steps:

- Evacuate blood and clots from the thoracic cavity
- Expose the injured lung
- Pack if necessary to allow for restoration of depleted intravascular blood volume
- Evaluate for evidence of a hilar and/or central hematoma or hemorrhage
- Decide whether pulmonary hilar crossclamping is necessary. If this is necessary, place a Crafoord-DeBakey aortic crossclamp across the pulmonary hilum

- Proceed to identify bleeding structures within the pulmonary parenchyma and control hemorrhage proceeding to sequential declamping of the pulmonary hilum
- If the pulmonary parenchymal hemorrhage is away from the hilum, clamp the pulmonary injury with Duval lung forceps
- Evaluate pericardium and mediastinum
- Proceed to repair

SURGICAL TECHNIQUES FOR THE MANAGEMENT OF PENETRATING PULMONARY INJURIES

The surgical armamentarium to manage penetrating pulmonary injuries can be divided into tissue sparing and resectional procedures.

Tissue Sparing Procedures

- Suture pneumonorrhaphy
- Stapled pulmonary tractotomy with selective vessel ligation
- Clamp pulmonary tractotomy with selective vessel ligation
- Nonanatomic resection

These procedures are indicated for the following:

- Control of hemorrhage
- Control of small air leaks
- Preservation of pulmonary tissue
- When the pulmonary injury is amenable to reconstruction

It is estimated that approximately 85% of all penetrating pulmonary injuries can be managed with these techniques.

Resectional Procedures

- Formal lobectomy
- Formal pneumonectomy

These procedures are indicated for the following:

- Control of hemorrhage
- Resection of devitalized or destroyed pulmonary tissue
- Control of major air leaks from lobar bronchi and/or mainstem bronchi not amenable to repair.
- Control of life-threatening hemorrhage

Useful Intraoperative Tools

- Argon beam coagulator
- Tissue sealants—Fibrin glue

Description of Surgical Techniques

Suture Pneumonorrhaphy

The lung is stabilized with Duval lung forceps. Stay sutures of 3-0 chromic or other absorbable sutures are placed in the superior and inferior aspect of the wound as well as in the lateral aspects. These stay sutures are used to gently retract the edges. Very fine malleable ribbon retractors are placed to separate the wound and to provide for visualization of the injured vessels, which are then selectively ligated with 3-0 chromic sutures or other similar size absorbable sutures. The same is done for small bronchi. The edges of the wound are then approximated with a running locked suture of 3-0 chromic.

Stapled Pulmonary Tractotomy

The lung is stabilized with Duval lung forceps. Orifices of entrance and exit are defined. If need be, the overlying visceral pleura is sharply incised with Nelson scissors. A GIA 55 or 75 stapler with 3.8 mm staples are placed through the orifices of entrance and exit and fired. This will open the tract traversed by the missile or other wounding agent effectively exposing the injured vessels and bronchi, which are then selectively ligated utilizing 3-0 chromic or the same size absorbable suture. The lung parenchyma can then be approximated with a single running locked suture of 3-0 chromic or the same size absorbable suture. The orifices of entry and exit are left open for the egress of air and/or blood. The integrity of the suture line is tested by having the anesthesiologist inflate the lung. Air leaks are then detected and repaired (see Figs. 11 to 13).

Clamp Pulmonary Tractotomy

The same technique as stapled pulmonary tractotomy is followed; however instead of a stapler, two Crafoord-DeBakey clamps are placed through the orifices of entrance and exit and the pulmonary tissue between the clamps is sharply transected with either Nelson or Metzenbaum scissors.

Nonanatomic Resection

This procedure is indicated when a very small and peripheral portion of a lobe or a segment is devitalized. The area of resection is stabilized between Duval lung forceps and a GIA 55 or 75 stapler with 3.8 mm staples is fired across, thereby resecting the injured portion of the lung. The staple line may be oversewn with a running locked suture of 3-0 chromic or the same size absorbable suture although this is not generally necessary. Nonanatomic resections can also be complex and require resections of major segments with complex reconstruction. This procedure will require meticulous attention in the reconstruction of an injured lobe.

Formal Lobectomy

This is indicated when there is total lobar tissue destruction, uncontrollable hemorrhage from the lobar vessels, or a

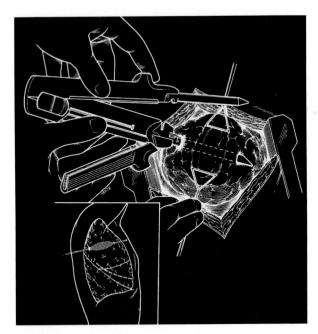

Figure 11 The cavitary effect created by a missile traversing the lung. The GIA-55 is then inserted through the orifices of entry and exit. (From Asensio JA, Demetriades D, Berne JD, et al. Stapled pulmonary tractotomy: A rapid way to control hemorrhage in penetrating pulmonary injuries. *J Am Coll Surg.* 1997;185(5):486–487.)

large lobar bronchial injury that is destructive and not amenable to repair.

To perform a lobectomy the fissures must be separated. In the case of the right lung, the oblique fissure separates the upper and middle lobe from the lower lobe whereas the horizontal fissure separates the upper lobe from the middle lobe. In the left lung, the oblique fissure divides the left upper from the left lower lobe. The lingula of the left upper lobe corresponds to the middle lobe on the right, but it is fused with the upper lobe in most instances.

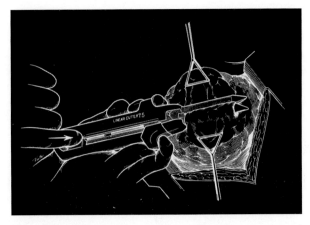

Figure 12 The GIA is closed and fired to open up the missile tract. (From Asensio JA, Demetriades D, Berne JD, et al. Stapled pulmonary tractotomy: A rapid way to control hemorrhage in penetrating pulmonary injuries. *J Am Coll Surg.* 1997;185(5):486–487.)

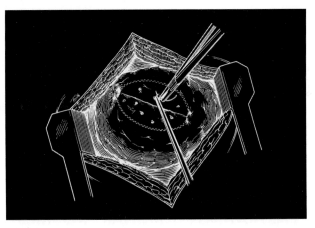

Figure 13 The tract is open and the deep bleeding vessels are ligated. (From Asensio JA, Demetriades D, Berne JD, et al. Stapled pulmonary tractotomy: A rapid way to control hemorrhage in penetrating pulmonary injuries. *J Am Coll Surg.* 1997;185(5):486–487.)

Vascular dissection should be initiated extrapleurally at the hilum through a perivascular plane to find the major pulmonary vessels. Vascular dissection in the fissures identifies the lobar vessels. Transection of the inferior pulmonary ligament distally will allow greater mobility of the lower lobes of both lungs. All pulmonary vessels whether they are the main lobar vessels or segmental vessels can be ligated in continuity and transfixed with nonabsorbable sutures. Alternatively they may be stapled with a TA-30, TA-45, or TA-90 with 3.5 mm staples or an endovascular stapler. All pulmonary vessels may also be oversewn with 4-0, 5-0, or 6-0 monofilament polypropylene sutures.

The bronchi, whether they are the main, lobar, or segmental bronchi should be stapled and transected with either a TA-30, TA-45, or TA-90 stapler with 4.8 mm staples. This is the preferred method for handling all bronchial structures. Bronchi may also be transected utilizing Sarot lung clamps and sutured with 4-0 Tev-Dek synthetic sutures. Should a suture technique be chosen, the trauma surgeon should avoid grasping the cut end of a bronchus with any instrument.

The suture technique involves clamping the bronchus distal to the intended point of transection. The bronchus is cut transversely for 4 to 5 mm, and the cut end is sutured with a 4-0 Tev-Dek. These sutures should be tied very carefully to avoid cutting or unnecessary devascularization. After placement of two sutures, the cut end is extended and additional sutures are placed. The sutures should be 2 to 3 mm apart. For a main bronchus, seldom are more than six sutures required. For a lobar bronchus three to four sutures are usually enough. Too many sutures devascularize the transected bronchus. After closure is complete, the suture line is immersed in saline and the lung is inflated by the anesthesiologist with up to 45 cm of inflation pressure. Additional sutures are placed if an air leak is detected. Tissue sealants may be utilized as an adjunct in the bronchial suture line.

After a lobectomy is performed, the remaining lobes are pexed to the thoracic wall with 2-0 chromic sutures to prevent lung torsion. This is very important. The bronchial stump may be covered with a pleural flap or pericardial fat-Brewer patch. These techniques are of unproven value. An intercostal pedicled muscle flap is probably superior but it is time consuming.

Right Upper Lobectomy

To perform a right upper lobectomy, both the pulmonary artery and the vein are dissected peripherally toward the right upper lobe to carefully delineate the individual blood supply of the lobe. First, the anterior and apicoposterior segmental branches of the main pulmonary artery to the upper lobe are ligated in continuity with 2-0 silk sutures, divided, and transfixed proximally with 3-0 silk suture ligatures. Within the major fissure, the posterior segmental branch of the upper lobe is identified, ligated, transfixed, and divided in a similar manner. Within the minor fissure that exists between the upper and middle lobes, the pulmonary venous drainage from the upper lobe is identified and carefully dissected. The vein is ligated in continuity with 0 silk sutures, transfixed with 2-0 silk sutures, and divided. At this point, the lung is retracted forward to gain access to the posteriorly placed bronchus. The right mainstem bronchus and the carina are identified. The upper lobe bronchus is identified and transected with a TA-30 or TA-45 stapler with 4.8 mm staples.

Right Middle Lobectomy

For a right middle lobectomy, the pulmonary artery branch to the middle lobe is identified, ligated with 0 silk sutures, transfixed with 2-0 silk sutures, and divided. The middle lobe division of the superior pulmonary vein is similarly ligated with 0 silk sutures, transfixed with 2-0 silk sutures, and divided. With these two vessels addressed, the trauma surgeon carefully isolates the middle lobe bronchus, which is then transected with a TA-30 or TA-45 stapler with 4.8 mm staples.

Right Lower Lobectomy

To perform a right lower lobectomy, the main pulmonary artery is followed in the major fissure, and the segmental branches to the lower lobe are identified. The superior and basal segmental branches to the lower lobe are carefully identified, ligated in continuity with 0 silk sutures, transfixed with 2-0 silk sutures, and divided. Particular care is taken to avoid injury to the middle lobe arteries. Next, attention is directed to the inferior pulmonary vein where, after the surgeon has ensured that any drainage from the middle lobe is protected, the inferior pulmonary vein is ligated in continuity with 0 silk sutures and transfixed with 2-0 silk sutures and transected. Again, within the same major fissure, the superior segmental and

the basal segmental bronchi are individually identified and transected with a TA-30 or TA-45 stapler with 4.8 mm staples.

Left Upper Lobectomy

To perform a left upper lobectomy, the interlobar fissure is separated by a meticulous combination of sharp and blunt dissection. If the interlobar fissure is not complete, it can be divided with a TA-30 or TA-45 with 3.8 mm staples. Arterial dissection is begun at the junction of the upper third with the middle third of the fissure. The artery is exposed. The perivascular plane is entered and the individual segmental branches to the upper lobe are identified, carefully dissected, ligated in continuity with 0 silk sutures and then transfixed with 2-0 silk sutures. Similarly the superior pulmonary vein and branches to the left upper lobe are identified, ligated in continuity with 0 silk sutures, and transfixed with 2-0 silk sutures. The left upper lobar bronchus is then identified and transected with a TA-45 with 4.8 mm staples.

Left Lower Lobectomy

To perform a left lower lobectomy, the same steps are taken as for a left upper lobectomy; however, the arterial and venous dissection are directed toward the appropriate left lower lobar vessels. The lingular artery or arteries, because there may be two, are identified, ligated in continuity with 0 silk sutures, and transfixed with 2-0 silk sutures. The left lower lobar bronchus is then identified and transected with a TA-30 or TA-45 with 4.8 mm staples.

Pneumonectomy

Right Pneumonectomy

A thorough exploration of the right hemithoracic cavity is carried out. The azygos vein is identified and the right pulmonary hilum located. Utilizing a meticulous combination of sharp and blunt dissection the right main pulmonary artery is identified and encircled with a vessel loop. Avoidance of undue traction is key. The right inferior pulmonary ligament is sharply transected. Both superior and inferior pulmonary veins are identified and encircled with vessel loops. All vessels may be either ligated in continuity or stapled individually utilizing a TA-30 or TA-45 stapler with 3.5 mm staples or an endovascular stapler. The right mainstem bronchus is then identified and encircled. The trauma surgeon must be careful not to apply undue traction to avoid tearing subcarinal structures. The bronchus is then transected with a TA-30 or TA-45 stapler with 4.8 mm staples.

Left Pneumonectomy

A thorough exploration of the left hemithoracic cavity is carried out. The phrenic, vagus, and left recurrent laryngeal nerves are identified and preserved. The left pulmonary hilum is located. Utilizing a meticulous combination of sharp and blunt dissection the left main pulmonary artery is identified and encircled with a vessel loop. Avoidance of undue traction is key. The left inferior pulmonary ligament is sharply transected. Both superior and inferior pulmonary veins are identified and encircled with vessel loops. All vessels may be either ligated in continuity or stapled utilizing a TA-30 or TA-45 stapler with 3.5 mm staples or an endovascular stapler. The left mainstem bronchus is then identified and encircled. The trauma surgeon must be careful not to apply undue traction to avoid tearing subcarinal structures. The bronchus is then transected with a TA-30 or TA-45 stapler with 4.8 mm staples.

Alternate Technique for Pneumonectomy (Either Right or Left)

If the patient is exsanguinating from a central hilar vascular injury the pulmonary hilum may be digitally encircled and compressed to allow the anesthesiologist to replace the lost intravascular volume. A Crafoord-DeBakey aortic crossclamp is then placed a few centimeters from the mediastinal pleura. If this maneuver controls the life-threatening hemorrhage, extrapleural dissection of hilar vessels may be carried out and individual vessels ligated. If this maneuver cannot be performed, if it does not contain the hemorrhage, or if the crossclamp is required in a very proximal location, the pericardium may have to be opened to control the pulmonary artery and the pulmonary veins. Intrapericardial control of the pulmonary veins is quite difficult and requires lateral displacement of the heart. This can be accomplished using a Satinsky clamp placed in the right auricle. It may even require total inflow occlusion with a Shumacker maneuver.

Alternatively a TA-90 stapler with 4.8 mm staples may be placed across the pulmonary hilum and fired transecting the pulmonary artery, pulmonary veins, and mainstem bronchus. In most cases, this controls the hemorrhage if the injuries to the pulmonary artery or veins are found in an extrapericardial location. If this does not control the bleeding then intrapericardial control of the pulmonary vessels will be needed.

POSTOPERATIVE MANAGEMENT

Virtually all of these patients require admission to a surgical intensive care unit because their postoperative management can be very complex. Patients will usually require conventional mechanical ventilation and occasionally high-frequency jet ventilation. Hemodynamic invasive monitoring with a Swan-Ganz catheter is usually recommended to guide fluid therapy because the injured lung is very sensitive to under- and overperfusion. At times, vasoactive agents may be infused into the pulmonary artery to control pulmonary hypertension, such as nitroglycerin, isoproterenol, and morphine sulfate as a drip.

MORBIDITY

- The key to prevent complications is to avoid extensive resections
- Be a pulmonary tissue sparer
- It is not what you resect, it is what you leave behind
- Intraoperative complications
  - Univentricular failure; usually right ventricular failure
  - Biventricular failure

Postoperative complications can be temporarily divided into short and long term. Immediate postoperative complications can be both technical and physiological.

POSTOPERATIVE COMPLICATIONS—SHORT TERM

- Technical
  - Lung hernia
  - Lung torsion
  - Bronchopleural fistulas
  - Arteriovenous fistulas
  - Bronchial stump leaks
  - Bronchial stump blow-outs
- Physiologic
  - Right ventricular failure
  - Pulmonary artery hypertension
  - "Runaway" pulmonary artery hypertension
  - Biventricular failure

POSTOPERATIVE COMPLICATIONS—LONG TERM

These complications can be quite devastating and will often require reintervention. Fortunately, they are infrequent.

- Persistent bronchopleural fistula
- Bronchial stenosis
- Empyema
- Lung abscess
- Bronchiectasis
- Arteriovenous fistula

MORTALITY

The estimated mortality for those procedures is listed here:

Procedure	Mortality (%)
Stapled procedures	10
Nonanatomic resections	20
Lobectomies	30–50
Pneumonectomies	50–100

CONCLUSIONS

Pulmonary injuries that require operative surgical intervention can be quite challenging; trauma surgeons must possess superb knowledge of thoracic anatomy as well as excellent technical skills. Fortunately, most of these injuries can be managed with pulmonary tissue sparing techniques such as stapled pulmonary tractotomy.

SUGGESTED READINGS

Asensio JA, Demetriades D, Berne JD, et al. Stapled pulmonary tractotomy: A rapid way to control hemorrhage in penetrating pulmonary injuries. *J Am Coll Surg.* 1997;185:486–487.

Asensio JA, McDuffie L, Petrone P, et al. Reliable variables in the exsanguinated patient which indicate damage control and predict outcome. *Am J Surg.* 2001;182(6):743–751.

Gasparri M, Karmy-Jones R, Kralovich KA, et al. Pulmonary tractotomy versus lung resection: Viable options in penetrating lung injury. *J Trauma.* 2001;51:1092–1097.

Karmy-Jones R, Jurkovich GJ, Shatz DV, et al. Management of traumatic lung injury: A western trauma association multicenter review. *J Trauma.* 2001;51:1049–1053.

Wall MJ Jr, Villavicencio RT, Miller CC III, et al. Pulmonary tractotomy as an abbreviated thoracotomy technique. *J Trauma.* 1998;45:1015–1023.

Thoracic Vascular Injury

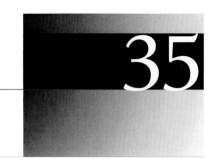

35

Matthew J. Wall, Jr.   *Tammy Zapalac*   *Bradford G. Scott*

PATHOPHYSIOLOGY

More than 90% of thoracic great-vessel injuries are caused by penetrating external or iatrogenic trauma.[1] Aortic injuries have caused or contributed to 15% of deaths following motor vehicle accidents (MVAs).[2–4] Blunt injuries to the innominate artery are actually aortic arch injuries. At the aortic plate, the innominate artery may be "pinched" between the sternum and the vertebral column during anterior sternal impact.

Owing to the high density of vascular structures in the upper midline mediastinum, a common presentation for brachiocephalic vessel injuries is either a stab wound or gunshot wound to the suprasternal notch traversing the upper mediastinum. As expected, stab wounds most commonly injure the ascending aorta, whereas gunshot wounds injure the descending thoracic aorta. Lacerations of the thoracic great vessels, including the arch of the aorta, are reported complications of percutaneous central venous catheter placement.[5,6]

INITIAL EVALUATION AND MANAGEMENT

The patient with penetrating thoracic vascular trauma is often hemodynamically unstable, with hemorrhage into either pleural cavities or the mediastinum. These patients are rapidly taken for an urgent thoracotomy and the diagnosis of a vascular injury is made intraoperatively. Fortunately, in many patients with either penetrating or blunt trauma, a contained hematoma of the mediastinum develops. This permits the evaluation and planning of the operative approach.

For patients with penetrating thoracic trauma, information regarding the length of the knife, the firearm type and number of rounds fired, the patient's distance from the firearm, and a history of previous gunshot wounds, although not always reliable, may be helpful if obtained from the patient or accompanying persons.

Historical information relating to potential blunt injury to the innominate artery/transverse arch include deceleration injury, fall from a significant height, the magnitude of energy transfer, vehicle crash dynamics, cockpit intrusion, and the amount of vehicle deformity. Emergency medical personnel can also provide medical information that is important in evaluating the potential for a thoracic great-vessel injury, such as the amount of hemorrhage at the scene, any history of neurologic deterioration following the accident, and hemodynamic instability during transport.

Physical Examination

The patient is evaluated using the standard Advanced Trauma Life Support approach. Specific findings such as hypotension; decreased, absent, or unequal peripheral pulses; unequal blood pressures in the extremities; expanding hematoma of the thoracic outlet or base of the neck; palpable fracture of the sternum; or proximity of missile or knife path to the brachiocephalic vessels. External signs of major chest trauma may increase suspicion for brachiocephalic vessel injury.

Chest Roentgenograms

In many cases of brachiocephalic injury, the radiologic findings on a supine film may be sufficient to warrant immediate arteriography. For penetrating injuries, it may be helpful to reconstruct trajectory by placing radiopaque markers to identify the entrance and exit sites. Radiographic findings that suggest penetrating thoracic great-vessel injury are noted in Table 1.

Fluid Resuscitation

The treatment of significant shock may include blood transfusion. However, rapid infusion of significant volumes of either blood or crystalloid before surgery may elevate the blood pressure. This may dislodge a protective clot and cause further exsanguination resulting in a cyclic hyper-resuscitation.[7] The principles of permitting moderate hypotension (systolic blood pressure of 70 to 90 mm Hg) and limiting fluid administration until operative control of bleeding are principles established for ruptured abdominal aortic aneurysms, which may equally apply to acute thoracic vascular injury because the pathophysiology is remarkably similar.[8,9] With both penetrating and blunt chest trauma, associated pulmonary contusion occur and provide additional rationale for limiting perioperative fluid administration.

Emergency Department Thoracotomy

Emergency department thoracotomy in patients presenting with signs of life and hemodynamic collapse may reveal injuries to major thoracic vessels. These injuries require rapid control of bleeding, allowing transfer to the operating room for definitive repair. For example, subclavian vessel injuries can be controlled by packing the apex of the chest or inserting a large balloon catheter. Major hemorrhage from the pulmonary hilum can be managed temporarily by clamping the entire hilum or twisting the lung 180 degrees after releasing the inferior pulmonary ligament.[10] Fortunately, the brachiocephalic vessels are relatively anterior and accessible by extending the left thoracotomy into a clamshell incision. The goal is rapid vascular control so the patient can be moved to the operating room. Emergency center thoracotomies for brachiocephalic vessel injures are daunting procedures with a high mortality.

ADVANCED DIAGNOSTIC STUDIES

Computed Tomography/Transesophageal Echocardiography/Magnetic Resonance Imaging

Conventional computed tomography (CT) may demonstrate hemomediastinum but has not demonstrated the diagnostic capability of aortography. Therefore, we have reserved CT for patients who have a "normal"-appearing mediastinum on chest x-ray, a suggestive mechanism, and require a CT for other reasons such as a concomitant head injury. If a mediastinal hematoma is visualized on CT, formal aortography is still obtained to determine the site(s) of injury and to identify any vascular anomalies that may require a different operative approach.

Helical CT angiography may provide images that may be as accurate as arteriograms.[11,12] Three-dimensional reconstruction of these images can produce representations of the vascular anatomy and pathology. This is being utilized by some to evaluate the aorta. Although compelling, technical limitations and artifacts occur often enough to currently limit its use for brachiocephalic vessels. Currently, its reliability is being evaluated.

Magnetic resonance angiography can generate similar images, but unfortunately its application in these potentially unstable trauma patients is not currently practical due to the difficulty in monitoring and managing the patient in the magnetic resonance imaging (MRI) coil. Transesophageal echocardiography has not been helpful in the management of brachiocephalic vessel injuries because it provides limited views of the aortic arch and brachiocephalic vessels.[13,14]

Arteriography

In penetrating thoracic trauma, if the patient is hemodynamically stable, arteriography is indicated for suspected innominate, carotid, or subclavian arterial injuries. Information gained from arteriography is important because different thoracic incisions are required for vascular control of each of these brachiocephalic vessels (see Fig. 1). The proximity of a missile trajectory to the brachiocephalic vessels, even without any physical findings of vascular injury, can be an indication for arteriography. Although arteriography of the aorta may be useful in hemodynamically stable patients with suspected penetrating aortic injuries, its limitations due to the large dye column obscuring small injuries in this setting must be recognized. Therefore, if performed, an effort must be made to

---

TABLE 1

X-RAY FINDINGS THAT SUGGEST PENETRATING BRACHIOCEPHALIC VESSEL INJURIES

Widened upper mediastinum
Large hemothorax
A trajectory with proximity to the thoracic outlet
Foreign bodies (bullets or shrapnel) in proximity to the great vessels
"Missing" missile in a patient with a gunshot wound to the chest, suggesting distal embolization

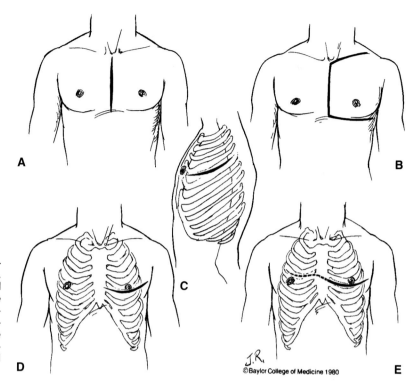

Figure 1 Multiple thoracic incisions may be employed to manage brachiocephalic vessel injuries. **A:** Median sternotomy. **B:** Combined anterolateral thoracotomy and supraclavicular incision (can be connected with sternotomy to form "book thoracotomy"). **C:** Posterolateral thoracotomy. **D:** Anterolateral thoracotomy—the utility incision for the patient in extremis. **E:** Extension of left anterolateral thoracotomy to the right to form "clamshell incision."

obtain views tangential to possible injuries for penetrating trauma.

Following blunt trauma, the need to proceed with arteriography can be determined on the basis of (i) the history/mechanism of injury, (ii) physical examination, and (iii) the chest radiograph. Because each of these is seldom absolute, all three must be considered in context. One half of patients with blunt thoracic vascular injuries present without any external signs of injury.[3] Seven percent of patients with blunt injury to the aorta and brachiocephalic arteries have a normal-appearing mediastinum on admission chest radiography.[15] Therefore, arteriography can be considered if either historical, physical, or radiographic findings are suggestive of a blunt vascular injury.

Arteriography remains the "gold standard" imaging study for evaluation of suspected blunt aortic and brachiocephalic vessel injuries. It allows precise localization of the injury and provides information regarding vascular anomalies and other factors that influence operative strategy. Other diagnostic techniques currently under investigation will have to match its accuracy and availability before replacing it as the imaging study of choice.

TREATMENT OPTIONS

Endovascular Stenting

Because many of these patients have concomitant injuries, a less invasive means of repairing major vascular injuries

would be attractive. Data regarding endovascular graft repairs in trauma patients are primarily anecdotal. A recent report by Patel of six patients with penetrating subclavian artery injuries describes early success in the application of endovascular stenting.[16]

Unfortunately, randomized trials are needed to further define the indications in the trauma population. Because many trauma patients are young, the long-term results of stenting have not been established. However, because the incisions to manage brachiocephalic vessel injuries can have their own morbidity, stenting potentially permits repair while avoiding these complications.

Surgical Repair

Indications for urgent transfer to the operating room for thoracotomy include hemodynamic instability, significant hemorrhage after tube thoracostomy, and radiographic evidence of a rapidly expanding mediastinal hematoma. Whenever possible, patients and particularly their families should be made aware of the potential for neurologic complications following surgical reconstruction of the thoracic great vessels. These include paraplegia, exacerbation of head injury, stroke, and brachial plexus injuries. If possible, careful documentation of preoperative neurologic defects should be obtained. During the induction of anesthesia, wide swings in blood pressure should be avoided. Although profound hypotension is clearly undesirable, hypertensive episodes can have equally significant adverse consequences.

Preparation/Patient Positioning

The initial steps of patient positioning and incision are important in surgery for great-vessel injuries, as adequate exposure is required for proximal and distal control. Prepping and draping of the patient should provide access from the chin to the knees to allow management of all contingencies. For the hypotensive, unstable patient with an undiagnosed injury, the empiric incision is the left anterolateral thoracotomy with extension into a clamshell incision with the patient in the supine position. In stable patients, preoperative arteriography may dictate an operative approach by another incision. For subclavian injuries, it can be helpful to prepare the arm first so it can be manipulated during the procedure.

Instrumentation

Thoracic vascular injuries occur at unplanned times, and the surgeon may not be working with the usual team. It is therefore extremely helpful to confer with the surgical technologists who will scrub the case regarding the possible procedures and needed instrumentation. The need for the sternal saw, specific retractors, and the surgeon's preferred vascular instrumentation can be discussed. Specifically, useful instruments to achieve vascular control include Craaford and DeBakey aortic clamps, various sizes of partial occluding clamps, and DeBakey peripheral vascular clamps, as well as moist umbilical tape and snare tourniquets. Experienced vascular surgeons try to keep this list as simple as possible when operating. It is often helpful for the surgeon to pick from the shelves a selection of possible vascular grafts that may be needed. Adjuncts such as shunts or balloon catheters can be procured. The surgeon should not allow an assistant to stand between the surgeon and the scrub technician, so the technician can follow the surgery and anticipate the next step. In the operating room, an autotransfusion device should be prepared and appropriate blood products made available.

Damage Control

Patients in critical condition may require a damage control approach. Damage control philosophies for thoracic injuries include (i) the definitive repair of injuries using simpler techniques during a single surgery, or (ii) an abbreviated thoracotomy approach that achieves a survivable physiology, which then requires a planned reoperation for definitive repairs.[10] Temporary vessel ligation or placement of intravascular shunts can control bleeding until subsequent correction of acidosis, hypothermia, and coagulopathy allow the patient to undergo definitive repair. Although towel clips can be used to rapidly close and terminate the surgery, *en masse* closure of the chest wall muscles is often more hemostatic. A "Bogota bag" or patch closure can be used as temporary closure of a thoracic incision in cases with associated cardiac dysfunction.

ARTERIAL INJURIES

Traverse Aortic Arch

For an injury to the transverse aortic arch, extension of the median sternotomy to the neck allows complete exposure of the arch and brachiocephalic branches. If necessary, exposure can be further enhanced by division of the innominate vein. Simple lacerations may be repaired by lateral aortorrhaphy. With difficult lesions, such as posterior lacerations or those with concomitant pulmonary artery injuries, cardiopulmonary bypass can be employed. Survival rates approach 50% for patients having stable vital signs on arrival at a trauma center.[3,17,18]

Innominate Artery/Left Intrathoracic Common Carotid Artery

Median sternotomy with right carotid extension is used to access innominate artery injuries. Exposure is enhanced by division of the innominate vein. Blunt injuries typically involve the proximal innominate artery/aortic arch and require obtaining proximal control at the transverse aortic arch. In contrast, penetrating injuries of the innominate artery may occur throughout its course.

In selected patients with limited penetrating injuries, a lateral arteriorrhaphy using a fine polypropylene suture is occasionally possible. More commonly, injuries to the innominate artery are managed using the bypass exclusion technique[3,19] (see Fig. 2). A graft is placed from the ascending aorta to the distal innominate artery (immediately proximal to the bifurcation of the subclavian and right carotid arteries) using a 10-mm Dacron tube graft. Proximal control is obtained with a large partial occluding clamp on the arch of the area of injury. The aortic defect is oversewn once the bypass is performed. Neither hypothermia, systemic anticoagulation, nor shunting is required. If concomitantly injured or previously divided, the innominate vein may be ligated or repaired. Injuries to the left common carotid artery are managed in a similar manner.

Subclavian Artery

A median sternotomy with a right supraclavicular extension is employed for exposure of right-sided subclavian injuries. For left subclavian artery injures, proximal control is obtained through a third intercostal space anterolateral thoracotomy, whereas a separate supraclavicular incision provides distal control. Although these incisions can be connected to create a formal "book" thoracotomy, this carries significant morbidity.[3,20] Intrathoracic proximal left subclavian artery injuries can be managed by a fourth left posterolateral thoracotomy.

In subclavian vascular trauma, a high associated rate of brachial plexus injury is seen; therefore, documentation of

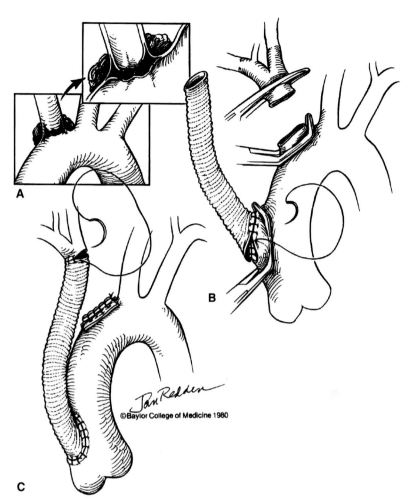

Figure 2   Bypass exclusion principle to address innominate artery injuries. The chest is opened by a median sternotomy. **A:** A 10-mm Dacron graft is sewn end-to-side to the aorta with a partial occluding clamp avoiding the hematoma. **B:** The aortic arch is controlled with a large partial occluding clamp. The distal innominate artery is isolated just proximal to its bifurcation. This is divided and sewn end-to-end to the graft without heparin, shunts, or cardiopulmonary bypass. **C:** After restoration of flow, the aortic arch sis oversewn.

©Baylor College of Medicine 1980

preoperative neurologic status is important. In obtaining exposure, it is important to avoid injuring the phrenic nerve that lies anterior to the scalenus anticus muscle.

Achieving proximal and distal control of a subclavian artery injury reduces bleeding from massive to just bothersome due to the large number of collaterals. After control, injuries at the thoracic outlet can be approached through the supraclavicular incision. If more distal, any difficulty in exposure can be managed with division or resection of the clavicle exposing the more distal subclavian.

Injuries distal to the clavicle can be managed with combined supraclavicular and infraclavicular incisions sparing the clavicle. Repair can usually be accomplished with either lateral arteriorrhaphy or graft interposition. It is unusual that an end-to-end anastomosis can be performed because of the difficulty in mobilizing the fragile artery. Reconstruction commonly requires the use of a graft with our preference, a knitted Dacron, although for the soft, small subclavian artery, a saphenous vein graft is often used. For the patient in extremis, flow can be reestablished with the use of a shunt or the artery can be ligated as a life saving measure. There is a frequent associated injury to the lung. These associated through-and-through lung injuries

can be managed with pulmonary tractotomy[21] (see Fig. 3). An overall mortality of 4.7% has been reported by Graham for patients with subclavian artery injuries.[20]

The operative exposure of the subclavian veins is similar to that described for subclavian artery injuries. Although isolated venous injuries occur, they are most often encountered during the management of arterial injuries. In most instances, repair can be accomplished with either lateral venorrhaphy or ligation.

POSTOPERATIVE MANAGEMENT

A significant portion of the in-hospital mortality associated with great-vessel injury is secondary to multiorgan failure. Careful hemodynamic monitoring, with avoidance of both hypertension and hypotension, is optimal. Although urinary output is generally a good indicator of cardiac function, for the patient with massive injuries Swan-Ganz catheter monitoring is often helpful.

Various pulmonary problems, including atelectasis, pneumonia, respiratory insufficiency, and adult respiratory distress syndrome (ARDS), represent the primary

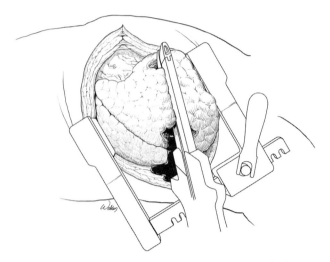

Figure 3   Pulmonary tractotomy with selective vascular ligation can be used to manage a concomitant lung injury. The tract is opened with the linear cutter stapler or between vascular clamps and bleeding/air leaks directly controlled with fine suture.

postoperative complications in this group of patients. The presence of pulmonary contusion and the possibility of ARDS suggest that fluid administration be carefully monitored. Coagulation abnormalities are corrected with administration of appropriate blood products. Blood draining through chest tubes can be collected and autotransfused. Prophylactic antibiotics are given for a short period of time postoperatively, particularly if a vascular graft is placed. Patients with recent vascular grafts are counseled regarding the necessity of antibiotic prophylaxis during invasive procedures, including dental manipulations.

For the management of pain related to a thoracotomy or multiple rib fractures, postoperative thoracic epidural anesthesia can be considered in appropriate patients; alternatively, intercostal nerve blocks can be performed intraoperatively and repeated in the intensive care unit.

CONCLUSION

Patients with brachiocephalic vascular injuries fall into two groups—those that are exanguinating and require an empiric surgery with a high mortality and those with contained injuries that permit preoperative evaluation. The unstable group requires an empiric position, exposure, and surgery. Multiple thoracic incisions are available to access and achieve vascular control of thoracic vascular injuries. Therefore, a stable patient may benefit from preoperative imaging, which can then suggest an optimal surgical approach.

Obtaining appropriate imaging studies, choosing an operative strategy to achieve proximal and distal control, careful operative technique of these soft vessels, and avoiding cyclic hyper-resuscitation can optimize the outcome of these challenging patients.

REFERENCES

1. Mattox KL, Feliciano DV, Burch JM, et al. Five thousand seven hundred sixty cardiovascular injuries in 4,459 patients epidemiologic evolution 1958–1987. *Ann Surg.* 1989;209(6):698–707.
2. Williams JS, Graff JA, Uku JM, et al. Aortic injury in vehicular trauma. *Ann Thorac Surg.* 1994;57:726–730.
3. Mattox KL. Approaches to trauma involving the major vessels of the thorax. *Surg Clin North Am.* 1989;69:77–91.
4. Feczko JD, Lynch L, Pless JE, et al. An autopsy case review of 142 nonpenetrating (blunt) injuries of the aorta. *J Trauma.* 1992;33:846–849.
5. Feliciano DV, Mattox KL, Graham JM, et al. Major complications of percutaneous subclavian catheters. *Am J Surg.* 1979;138:869–874.
6. Childs D, Wilkes RG. Puncture of the ascending aorta: A complication of subclavian venous cannulation. *Anesthesia.* 1986;41:331–332.
7. Bickell WH, Wall MJ Jr, Pepe PE, et al. Immediate versus delayed fluid resuscitation for hypotensive patients with penetrating torso injuries. *N Engl J Med.* 1994;331:1105–1109.
8. Crawford ES. Ruptured abdominal aortic aneurysm: An editorial. *J Vasc Surg.* 1991;13:348–350.
9. Aronstam EM, Gomez AC, O'Connell TJ Jr, et al. Recent surgical and pharmacologic experience with acute dissecting and traumatic aneurysms. *J Thorac Cardiovasc Surg.* 1970;59:231.
10. Wall MJ Jr, Soltero E. Damage control for thoracic injuries. *Surg Clin North Am.* 1997;77(4):863–878.
11. Gavant ML, Menke PG, Fabian T, et al. Blunt traumatic aortic rupture: Detection with helical CT of the chest. *Radiology.* 1995;197:125–133.
12. Trerotola SO. Can helical CT replace aortography in thoracic trauma? *Radiology.* 1995;197:13–15.
13. Ben-Menachem Y. Assessment of blunt aortic-brachiocephalic trauma: Should angiography be supplanted by transesophageal echocardiography? *J Trauma.* 1997;42:969–972.
14. Vignon P, Ostyn E, Francois B, et al. Limitations of transesophageal echocardiography for the diagnosis of traumatic injuries to aortic branches. *J Trauma.* 1997;42:960–963.
15. Woodring JH. The normal mediastinum in blunt traumatic rupture of the thoracic aorta and brachiocephalic arteries. *J Emerg Med.* 1990;8:467–476.
16. Patel AV, Marin ML, Veith FJ, et al. Endovascular graft repair of penetrating subclavian artery injuries. *J Endovasc Surg.* 1996;3:382–388.
17. Reyes LH, Rubio PA, Korampai FL, et al. Successful treatment of transection of aortic arch and innominate artery. *Ann Thorac Surg.* 1975;19:468–471.
18. Pate JW, Cole FH, Walker WA, et al. Penetrating injuries of the aortic arch and its branches. *Ann Thorac Surg.* 1993;55:586–592.
19. Johnston RH, Wall MJ Jr, Mattox KL. Innominate artery trauma: A 30-year experience. *J Vasc Surg.* 1993;17:134–139.
20. Graham JM, Feliciano DV, Mattox KL, et al. Management of subclavian vascular injuries. *J Trauma.* 1980;20:537–544.
21. Wall MJ, Hirshberg A, Mattox KL. Pulmonary tractotomy with selective vascular ligation for penetrating injuries to the lung. *Am J Surg.* 1994;168:665–669.

Cardiac Injuries

36

Edward H. Kincaid   *J. Wayne Meredith*

The incidence of traumatic injuries to the heart continues to rise with increases in urban violence and improved detection, and a larger percentage of patients with cardiac injuries are arriving at trauma centers alive. This improvement in prehospital transport, along with improvements in diagnostic, surgical, and anesthetic techniques has contributed to an increase in overall survival in patients with injuries to the heart. Although the overall mortality of these injuries remains high, survival rates of 50% to 95% are not uncommon in patients with cardiac injuries who arrive to the hospital with vital signs.[1-4]

PENETRATING CARDIAC TRAUMA

Stab and gunshot wounds frequently cause injury to the heart, with an incidence of 10% to 20% for proximity wounds. Patients with penetrating cardiac injuries generally present in one of three clinical patterns. In approximately 20% of patients, the injury will be clinically silent, at least initially, and is subsequently diagnosed at surgery or by an imaging study. Approximately 50% of patients will present with evidence of pericardial tamponade, including one or more signs in the Beck triad (hypotension, distended neck veins, and muffled heart sounds). In the remaining patients, the presentation is of hemorrhagic shock following free bleeding from an atrial or ventricular wound into one, or both, hemithoraces.

The diagnosis of penetrating injuries to the heart often requires a high index of suspicion. Location of entrance and exit wounds, trajectory path, and location of retained missiles on radiographs are helpful criteria in predicting heart injuries. Proximity wounds to the heart are defined as those which penetrate the chest wall in the area bounded superiorly by the clavicles, laterally by the midclavicular lines, and inferiorly by the costal margins. Any missile or instrument that traverses the anterior mediastinum is also considered a proximity wound. Because cardiac injuries are present

in 15% to 20% of patients who present with proximity wounds, cardiac injuries must be definitively excluded.

Physical examination is often unreliable for the detection of pericardial tamponade. The presence of all three signs in the Beck triad is rarely found, and, in fact, any two of the three signs are present in only about half the number of patients with tamponade. Additionally, detecting muffled heart sounds and distended neck veins amidst the commotion in the trauma bay, and in the often agitated or intoxicated patient, can be extremely difficult. Because of this, additional diagnostic modalities must be used whenever any suspicion exists. As more surgeons are becoming familiar with the use of ultrasonography in the trauma setting, two-dimensional surface echocardiography is an accepted technique for diagnosing cardiac injuries. When performed by appropriately trained surgeons, the test detects blood within the pericardial sac with a sensitivity of 96% to 100% and a specificity of 100%, or essentially equivalent to pericardial window.[5] When equipment is readily available, this noninvasive test can be performed in approximately 2 minutes. It is of vital importance that the trauma surgeon who is attending to the patient perform and interpret the examination. This allows for the quickest results, best clinical correlation, and most rapid use of the information in treatment decisions. The limitations of this test are the expense of the equipment and the specialized training required.

Although cardiac ultrasonography has many advantages, subxiphoid pericardial window remains the gold standard for exclusion of cardiac injury. In patients with equivocal ultrasonographic findings, or where ultrasound is unavailable, it should be considered in otherwise stable patients with proximity wounds and/or suggestive signs and symptoms. This procedure is usually performed in the operating room with general anesthesia, often in combination with abdominal exploration. A subxiphoid pericardial window is performed through a 10-cm vertical, midline incision over the xiphoid, slightly favoring the epigastrium. The xiphoid is grasped with a clamp, and, after dissecting the xiphoid free from the abdominal fascia and diaphragmatic fibers, the substernal plane is accessed. While elevating the inferior portion of the sternum, the prepericardial adipose tissue is dissected to gain exposure of the acute margin of the pericardium. The pericardium can then be retracted inferiorly into the wound and incised sharply. The presence of blood or clot within the pericardial sac indicates a positive result, necessitating immediate repair of the injury. Pericardial window can also be accomplished during thoracoscopy of the left hemithorax.

The use of pericardiocentesis is advocated by some for the detection of cardiac injuries, especially where rapid access to the operating room, trauma surgeons, and anesthesiologists is not available. Problems with pericardiocentesis include the high rate of false positives, false negatives, and potential for iatrogenic cardiac injuries. Furthermore, this technique has limited use in the treatment of tamponade because, often, blood within the pericardial sac is clotted and not amenable to removal through a needle.

The treatment of penetrating cardiac wounds depends on the urgency of the presentation. In patients in shock from suspected cardiac injuries, the distinction between the two most likely etiologies, pericardial tamponade or free hemorrhage, is important. Patients with distended neck veins and a distinctive plethoric, dusky facial expression should undergo immediate placement of bilateral chest tubes to relieve possible tension pneumothorax, which can clinically mimic cardiac tamponade. If this fails to resolve the shock, the diagnosis of tamponade should be presumed, and pericardial window performed, either in the emergency room with local or no anesthesia, or in the operating room as previously described. Patients with shock and suspected free hemorrhage into one or both hemithoraces, which can be usually detected by physical examination, chest radiograph, or chest tube output, should be transported to the operating room for definitive treatment. In patients in extremis from either condition, or who suffer cardiac arrest while in the emergency room, an emergency left anterior thoracotomy should be performed.

In planning the surgical approach for the repair of cardiac injuries, the location of the entrance and exit wounds, trajectory path, type of wound, associated signs and symptoms, and suspicion for other thoracic vascular or visceral injuries are important considerations. The median sternotomy is a logical extension of the subxiphoid pericardial window and provides access to all four chambers of the heart. This approach is appropriate for most precordial stab wounds and some low-caliber gun shot wounds. The main limitations of this incision are that it does not allow for repair or cross-clamping of the descending aorta, examination or repair of the esophagus and bronchi, and provides limited exposure to the lower lobes of the lungs and hemidiaphragms. In the setting of suspected penetrating injury to the heart, a left

thoracotomy should be performed in any patient who may require cross-clamping of the distal aorta, and in patients with suspected cardiac injuries along with other complex thoracic visceral injuries. Only occasionally is a right thoracotomy required in this setting because this approach generally does not provide adequate exposure of the heart. An anterior left thoracotomy may be extended across the sternum into a "clamshell" thoracotomy to provide excellent exposure of the heart and anterior mediastinum. The internal mammary arteries must be controlled and divided bilaterally to accomplish this exposure.

Atrial wounds lend themselves well to early control by finger pressure or by exclusion with a vascular clamp followed by simple oversewing. Right or left ventricular free wall injuries away from the coronary arteries may be treated with digital pressure over the entrance wound for hemostasis, and horizontal mattress sutures under the wound reinforced with epicardial running suture along the site of injury. All left ventricular wounds require pericardial-pledgetted reinforcement at the sutures. Many right ventricular stab wounds can be closed primarily without pledgets if the sutures are tied accurately. Injuries near coronary arteries must be closed without encompassing the coronary artery within the suture. This can be accomplished by placing horizontal mattress sutures lateral and deep to the coronary artery across the cardiac laceration. Tying these sutures with attention to the function of the myocardium distal to the injury and attention to the electrocardiogram (ECG) allows closure of the laceration without coronary artery occlusion and subsequent ischemia. An alternative method of temporary repair of cardiac lacerations uses a skin stapler, which is successful in controlling hemorrhage from stab injuries and low velocity gun shot wounds.[6] The stapler can be used on all chambers of the heart, and in some instances, may be quicker than suture repair.

With all penetrating cardiac wounds, it is important to recognize the possibility of associated intracardiac injuries. The surgeon should palpate the heart along the pulmonary outflow tract for a thrill that indicates a traumatic ventricular septal defect. This diagnosis can be confirmed by performing co-oximetry evaluation of blood aspirated from the pulmonary artery and right atrium, and demonstrating a step up. Digital palpation through atrial wounds should be used routinely to identify atrioventricular valvular insufficiency or, occasionally, an atrial septal defect. Intraoperative surface echocardiography and transesophageal echocardiography are also excellent at diagnosing intracardiac pathology but are not readily available in the urgent trauma setting.

Postoperatively, all patients with cardiac wounds should receive a thorough cardiovascular examination to assess for murmurs or evidence of cardiac failure, and undergo echocardiography if either is detected. Intracardiac lesions can usually await repair until the patient's condition is stable and a cardiac catheterization has been performed, although some patients have such profound heart failure that immediate surgical repair, using cardiopulmonary bypass, must be performed.

BLUNT CARDIAC TRAUMA

Blunt cardiac injuries range from disruption of the myocardium, septum, or valvular structures to cardiac contusion. Both cardiac disruption, also known as *cardiorrhexia*, and cardiac contusion are common. The former is seen most often in patients who die at the scene of injury and the latter in those who survive to reach the hospital. The pathophysiology of blunt cardiac injury consists of a direct blow to the chest, usually sustained in a motor vehicle collision or a fall. Cardiac injuries are generally associated with sternal or rib fractures, but may occur in the absence of any chest wall fracture. Conversely, a sternal fracture does not mandate the presence of blunt cardiac injury. The most common location of blunt cardiac injury is the anterior heart, which consists primarily of the right ventricle. A blow that causes the sternum to impact directly against the myocardium may result in direct injury to myocardial cells, sometimes leading to cell death, mechanical dysfunction, or arrhythmias. The diagnosis of myocardial contusion is elusive. Many tests have been proposed, but none has been proved definitive except direct visualization of the heart at surgery or autopsy.

In practical terms, myocardial arrhythmias and pump failure must be considered as the clinically significant sequelae of myocardial contusion, and both require treatment regardless of whether the diagnosis of blunt cardiac injury can be made. Nevertheless, guidelines have been proposed to assist with the workup of this condition.[7] As an initial test, a 12-lead ECG should be obtained on any patient in whom blunt cardiac injury is suspected. A patient who exhibits a normal ECG requires no further workup for cardiac contusion. Those who have some abnormality of the ECG that does not require treatment (e.g., nonspecific ST-T wave changes) should undergo monitored observation for 12 hours and be discharged if they exhibit no arrhythmias and have a normal ECG at that time. Patients with more serious ECG abnormalities, such as arrhythmias, ST elevation, or heart block, require observation for at least 24 to 48 hours and may require further testing and treatment depending on the sequelae of the electrical abnormality. In patients with hemodynamic instability and suspected blunt cardiac injury, echocardiography should promptly be performed. There is no role for the use of cardiac enzyme analysis including creatinine phosphokinase or cardiac troponins. Although the latter test may detect myocardial injury, this information is not complimentary to ECG and echocardiography, and has no clinical utility. Similarly, there is no role for nuclear medicine studies.

Pump failure associated with cardiac contusion usually results from right heart failure, because most hemodynamically significant cardiac contusions are caused by injury to the anterior right ventricular free wall. The treatment of right heart failure resulting from cardiac contusion consists of inotropic support and reduction of right ventricular afterload. The treatment of arrhythmias secondary to cardiac contusion is the same as that of arrhythmia with any other etiology.

The commonly repeated adage that cardiac contusion should be treated similar to myocardial infarction is misleading. Therapy for myocardial infarction is based on the premise that the patient is likely to have concomitant coronary artery disease and that increased myocardial oxygen demand may result in extension of the evolving infarct or the production of an additional infarction. Most young, injured patients have normal coronary arteries, and cardiac contusion is unlikely to be extended by increased myocardial oxygen demand unless an additional blow is administered to the heart. The goal in resuscitation of the injured patient generally is to increase systemic oxygen delivery, which may increase cardiac work. Additionally, in contrast to patients with myocardial infarction, patients with myocardial contusion appear to have no increased risk for cardiac complications with general anesthesia and surgery.

In the rare patient with cardiorrhexia who presents to the hospital with signs of life, the most common injury is right atrial perforation. Other lesions seen in patients who reach the hospital with vital signs, in order of decreasing incidence, are left atrial perforation, right ventricular perforation, atrial septal perforation, ventricular septal perforation, coronary artery thrombosis, and valvular insufficiency, most commonly of the tricuspid and mitral valves. Patients with cardiac rupture generally present with signs of pericardial tamponade requiring rapid decompression. Placement of an intra-aortic balloon pump is often an effective temporizing measure while preparing for definitive repair. Patients with blunt cardiac trauma who lose vital signs in the field or suffer prehospital cardiac arrest generally should not be subjected to emergency room thoracotomy because essentially none of these patients can be salvaged. The survival rate, however, for patients admitted with vital signs after suffering blunt cardiac rupture is approximately 50%, and much of the mortality in these patients is due to associated injuries.

REFERENCES

1. Lancey RA, Monahan TS. Correlation of clinical characteristics and outcomes with injury scoring in blunt cardiac trauma. *J Trauma.* 2003;54:509–515.
2. Henderson VJ, Smith RS, Fry WR, et al. Cardiac injuries: Analysis of an unselected series of 251 cases. *J Trauma.* 1994;36:341–348.
3. Henderson VJ, Smith RS, Fry WR, et al. Cardiac injuries: Analysis of an unselected series of 251 cases. *J Trauma.* 1994;36:341–348.
4. Fulda G, Brathwaite CE, Rodriquez A, et al. Blunt traumatic rupture of the heart and pericardium: A 10-year experience (1979-1989). *J Trauma.* 1991;31:167–172.
5. Rozycki GS, Feliciano DV, Ochsner MG, et al. The role of ultrasound in patients with possible penetrating cardiac

wounds. A prospective multicenter study. *J Trauma*. 1999;46: 543–552.

6. Macho JR, Markison RE, Schecter WP. Cardiac stapling in the management of penetrating injuries of the heart: Rapid control of hemorrhage and decreased risk of personal contamination. *J Trauma*. 1993;34:711–716.

7. Pasquale MD, Nagy K, Clarke J. *Practice management guidelines for screening of blunt cardiac injury. Eastern Association for the Surgery of Trauma Practice Parameter Workgroup for Screening of Blunt Cardiac Injury. 1998.* Available at http://www.east.org/tpg/chap2.pdf. Accessed Frebruary 19, 2004.

Injury to the Diaphragm

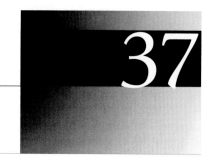

Thérèse M. Duane   **Rao R. Ivatury**   **Michel B. Aboutanos**
Ajai K. Malhotra

INTRODUCTION

Diaphragmatic injuries are often occult and easily over-looked in the acutely injured trauma patient. Both blunt as well as penetrating trauma can result in injury to the diaphragm with significant associated morbidity and mortality. Ideally, these injuries should be identified and repaired early to avoid immediate and delayed complications. Never is the trite concept of "high index of suspicion" more true than when dealing with these patients. This chapter will review the anatomic and physiologic considerations specific to the diaphragm and then provide an approach to the blunt and penetrating trauma patient.

Anatomic and Physiologic Considerations

The diaphragm is an extremely resilient dome-shaped muscle. The fibers of the diaphragm surround the central tendon, which is an aponeurotic sheath that separates the abdominal and thoracic cavities. Arching from the first through third lumbar vertebrae posteriorly, the diaphragm attaches to the ribs laterally and to the posterior aspect of the lower sternum. The crura of the diaphragm decussate to form the aortic and esophageal hiatus through which passes the aorta, thoracic duct, azygos vein, esophagus, and the vagi. The caval hiatus is located laterally to the right and transmits the inferior vena cava (IVC) at approximately the eighth thoracic vertebral level. The liver is adjacent to the undersurface of the diaphragm on the right along with the right kidney, whereas the spleen, stomach, and left kidney border the inferior aspect of the diaphragm on the left. Multiple branches from the aorta,

pericardiophrenic arteries, and the intercostals supply the diaphragm. The phrenic nerves innervate the diaphragm arising from the third through the fifth cervical roots and travel along the lateral aspect of the mediastinum on the right and the pericardium on the left.

There is significant variability in the location of the diaphragm during the respiratory cycle. It fluctuates between the fourth and eighth intercostal spaces during inspiration and expiration—a fact of vital importance in trauma. As the diaphragm moves so does the closely associated organs, putting them at risk with trauma to the lower chest. Because of this risk, the space from the costal margin up to thoracic spine 4 (T4) anteriorly, T6 laterally, and T8 posteriorly is considered the thoracoabdominal region. This region requires evaluation for both abdominal and thoracic injury as well as injury to the diaphragm.

Physiologically, the diaphragm is an integral part of the respiratory cycle. By its motion, the diaphragm creates a negative intrathoracic pressure that enhances the tidal volumes generated by the lung. In this function, the diaphragm has more contribution than the rib cage. The creation of negative intrathoracic pressure also allows the diaphragm to play a major role in the venous return to the right heart. The fall in pressure during inspiration decreases right atrial pressure, which enhances both superior vena cava (SVC) and IVC blood flow. Because of the ability of the abdominal venous compartment to be a capacitor when hypervolemic but collapsible when hypovolemic, inspiration does not always result in increased flow to the heart. Increases in abdominal pressures produced by active diaphragmatic descent can increase the total IVC venous return by enhancing the splanchnic IVC flow under relatively hypervolemic conditions, but decrease the total IVC venous return by impeding the nonsplanchnic IVC flow under hypovolemic conditions.

Injury to the diaphragm can therefore interfere with the normal physiology of this organ. Defects resulting from penetrating trauma may produce hemopneumothoraces, which impairs the ability of the diaphragm to appropriately contract and produce negative pressure. Herniation of abdominal contents into the thoracic cavity after rupture of the diaphragm can increase pressure on the IVC as it traverses the hiatus. Such pressure can lead to impaired venous return to the heart and cardiovascular collapse. Of interest is the observation that in a patient mechanically ventilated with positive pleural pressure, there is no pressure gradient so intra-thoracic migration may not occur and the diaphragmatic rupture may be missed. The remainder of the chapter focuses on the identification of such injuries after both blunt and penetrating trauma and the treatment options.

BLUNT DIAPHRAGM INJURIES

Incidence

Blunt trauma accounts for 10% to 30% of traumatic diaphragmatic ruptures in North American urban trauma centers.[1] Overall, its incidence is rather low and ranges substantially depending on the series. It has been reported as low as 0.8% to as high as 7%.[2,3] The left side is affected more often than the right side. The reasoning for this is not clear and it may be due to a combination of under diagnosis, underreporting, true congenital weakening, or effective and protective buffering by the liver. In a recent review of 65 patients with traumatic rupture of the diaphragm, Mihos et al. reported left-sided ruptures in 43 patients (66%) with 86% of the ruptures resulting from blunt trauma.[4] Similar results were seen by Shah et al. in a review of 980 patients, where left-sided rupture was reported in 68.5% of patients.[5]

Motor vehicle collisions and falls from heights are the most common cause of blunt diaphragmatic injuries (BDIs).[6,7] An acute increase in intra-abdominal pressure results in rupture of the diaphragm. Such forces are quite severe, which explains the significant association with other injuries. In a series of 52 patients with blunt diaphragmatic injury, blunt thoracic injuries (multiple rib fractures and pneumothoraces) accounted for the most frequent associated injuries (90%). Long bone fractures and closed head injuries were seen in 75% and 42% of the patients, respectively. Intra-abdominal injuries that were identified included splenic in 60% of patients, hepatic in 35% of patients, and to the kidney, pancreas, and small bowel in 10% to 12% of patients.[8] Moreover, right side diaphragm injuries were more commonly associated with other injuries compared to the left. In one series, there was

a 100% incidence on the right.[9] All these factors can assist in making the diagnosis of a BDI in these patients.

Diagnosis

The diagnosis of BDI is very difficult even with the highest index of suspicion. Previously, these injuries were diagnosed intraoperatively or at postmortem. Up to two thirds of conservatively managed patients had a missed diaphragm injury. In the largest reported series (160 patients) of blunt diaphragmatic ruptures from six university centers in Canada, the rupture was diagnosed preoperatively in only 37.1% of patients operated for other indications.[6] The goal of early diagnosis is to avoid the significant morbidity and mortality from visceral herniation and strangulation.

When possible, a thorough history and physical examination can assist with this challenging diagnosis. It is useful to recall that most ruptures are associated with crush, falls, and particularly side impact motor vehicle collisions. This history of the trauma along with patient complaints of upper abdominal pain and possibly shortness of breath should stimulate one to consider the diagnosis of BDI. It is also important to remember that these patients may have no complaints at all or may be in shock. Physical findings of decreased breath sounds or decreased chest expansion or the detection of bowel sounds in the chest should heighten one's concern. Once the diagnosis is entertained, then further radiographic studies and interventions can assist to confirm the diagnosis.

Currently, there is no ideal radiologic tool for the diagnosis of the occult diaphragmatic insult. The diagnosis relies on the demonstration of visceral herniation rather than the actual visualization of the diaphragmatic tear. Options that are currently available to evaluate for diaphragm injuries include chest x-rays, upper and lower gastrointestinal contrast studies, thoracoabdominal computed tomography (CT), sonography, diagnostic peritoneal lavage, liver scintigraphy, contrast or air peritoneography, and magnetic resonance imaging (MRI). Other than the first three modalities, there is little evidence to support the use of any of the latter interventions. Sonography is operator dependent and therefore, unreliable, and MRI tends to be impractical in the acute trauma setting. The focus of this chapter is on the plain film, contrast studies, and CTs.

The radiographic workup for a blunt diaphragm injury should always begin with a plain chest x-ray because this is quick and easily obtained in the trauma bay. The initial chest x-ray may show visceral herniation, elevation of the diaphragm, loss of the diaphragmatic shadow, irregularity of the apparent contour of the diaphragm, or a pleural effusion. A nasogastric tube should be placed because its presence in the left chest cavity is pathognomonic for left diaphragmatic rupture and gastric eventration into the left thorax. Unfortunately, up to half the number of the patients with this injury will have a normal chest x-ray. Those patients with abnormal chest radiographs may have other chest pathology such as pulmonary contusions and hemothoraces that can mimic a diaphragm injury. Therefore, if there continues to be suspicion for a BDI then further evaluation should be pursued.

Contrast studies may be helpful in both the acute and chronic situations. Both the upper gastrointestinal series and barium enema can identify visceral herniation through a diaphragm injury. Unfortunately, injuries may be missed if the bowel contents remain intraperitoneal. Consequently, CT has found a role in the diagnosis, given its overall increased sensitivity after blunt trauma.

CT scan is currently the diagnostic modality of choice in stable patients with blunt thoracoabdominal injuries. It has the benefit of evaluating for other chest or abdominal pathology that may require surgical intervention. Its specific accuracy in identifying BDI, however, is variable and often disappointing especially when typical chest x-ray findings are absent.[10,11] The sensitivity suffers on the right side because the liver obscures the view and often precludes visceral herniation. It remains to be seen whether the advent of helical (spiral) CT with three-dimensional reconstruction can enhance its diagnostic utility for blunt diaphragmatic injury. Until studies are performed to determine the reliability of the helical CT, further interventions must be pursued if the diagnosis of diaphragm injury is still being entertained.

Currently, either thoracoscopy or laparoscopy remains the diagnostic tool of choice for diaphragmatic injuries, both being much more reliable than nonoperative modalities.[4,12] Thorocoscopy is mainly helpful in the chronic situation or when abdominal injuries have been ruled out. If any question remains about intra-abdominal pathology, then laparoscopy is more appropriate. Tension pneumothorax remains the main potential complication in the use of laparoscopy in patients with diaphragmatic injuries. Fundamentally, the comfort level of the surgeon should dictate which approach is taken.

Treatment

Prompt repair is indicated for BDI to avoid the morbidity and potential mortality from visceral herniation, strangulation, and cardiorespiratory compromise. Acute BDI is generally repaired using an abdominal approach, with abdominal exploration and repair of any associated visceral injuries. Delayed repair may be better pursued through a thoracic approach where retracted tissues and adhesions are easier to handle. Ultimately, the personnel preference of the surgeon should dictate the approach with a combined approach occasionally being necessary in the face of extensive adhesions and chronic visceral eventration.

There are a number of ways to repair the diaphragmatic defect. Because of its dome shape, there is often a fair amount of redundant tissue that easily allows for primary repair. Primary repair is usually carried out in one or two layers depending on the size and integrity of the tissue. A nonabsorbable monofilament suture such as zero polypropylene works well in an interrupted figure-of-eight pattern. The suture line can also be done in a running manner. In the face of significant tissue loss, the diaphragm can be reconstructed with the use of a prosthetic nonabsorbable material such as Marlex mesh. Given the risk of infection with this type of mesh, it is best avoided if there is concomitant gastrointestinal injury. In this scenario, the use of autologous tissue such as omentum, tensor fascia lata, or a latissimus dorsi flap may be preferable. Another option that is under investigation is the use of a biological tissue grafting material such as AlloDerm (human acellular tissue matrix; Life Cell Corp.). This material is purportedly resistant to infection and can be utilized if autologous tissue is not available.[13]

Laparoscopic or thoracoscopic repair is another option but is dependent on surgical expertise in minimally invasive surgery. Such an approach has no role in the acutely injured unstable trauma patient. Regardless of the surgical skill, it is too time consuming to deal with all of the potentially life-threatening injuries in that setting. It should be reserved for the technically proficient surgeon in minimally invasive surgery on a stable trauma patient, ideally for the chronic diaphragmatic hernia. Careful selection of the patients is vital.

PENETRATING INJURIES TO THE DIAPHRAGM

Incidence

Penetrating injury to the thoracoabdominal region is more likely to result in a diaphragm injury than blunt trauma. Such injuries are more common after gunshot wounds (GSWs) than stabs and more common on the left than the right side. Similar to patients with blunt trauma, those with penetrating injuries are frequently asymptomatic. The group from University of California, Los Angeles (UCLA) found that 26% of their patients had an occult diaphragm injury.[14] Because of the frequency and the insidiousness of its presentation, emphasis must be placed on appropriate and timely diagnosis.

Diagnosis

It is incumbent on the trauma surgeon to rule out a diaphragm injury when treating a patient with a thoracoabdominal wound. Diagnostic tools are similar to those of blunt trauma although there tends to be less of a role for simple observation. Other diagnostic options include radiography, surgical exploration either through the chest or abdomen, or a minimally invasive approach.

A plain chest x-ray is part of the standard evaluation for a stable trauma patient with this type of injury. These films identify the presence of a hemo- or pneumothorax secondary to penetration of the pleural space. Neither a normal nor an abnormal chest x-ray accurately assists in the diagnosis of a penetrating injury to the diaphragm, yet plain radiographs have been used over the years to evaluate patients for diaphragmatic injury. In 1988, Demetriades et al.[15] looked at 163 patients with penetrating trauma to the diaphragm and found the chest x-ray to be diagnostic in only 13% of patients, abnormal but not diagnostic in 76% of patients, and completely normal in 11% of patients. The earlier the diagnosis, the better the outcome with a 3.2% mortality rate for patients diagnosed early versus 30% mortality for those diagnosed late. Given the need to promptly identify these injuries, plain radiographs are inadequate to provide conclusive evidence of a diaphragmatic injury after penetrating trauma. Most of these patients have ambiguous findings[15,16] and interventions such as positive pressure ventilation interfere further with the ability to diagnose this problem.

Other nonsurgical options for evaluation include sonography, CT, and MRI. Like blunt trauma, these modalities are quite disappointing in their ability to diagnose this problem. Udobi et al.[17] prospectively evaluated the focused assessment with sonography for trauma (FAST) after penetrating abdominal trauma and had 13 false-negative studies out of 75 patients. Three of these 13 patients had diaphragm injuries missed. CT and MRI did not fare any better in their current state of the art.

Although there is no good radiographic means of diagnosing a penetrating diaphragm injury, there should be a healthy reluctance to force a negative laparotomy in an otherwise stable patient without any other indication for exploration. Ivatury et al.[18] reviewed 657 laparotomies for penetrating trauma and found 78 of these were nontherapeutic. Almost half of these were from thoracoabdominal wounds and three fourths of these were stab wounds. These patients could have benefited from a minimally invasive approach to the diagnosis.

Thoracoscopy has been studied since the early 1990s and has consistently been found to be both accurate and safe. Freeman et al.[19] published the largest series to date with the use of video-assisted thoracoscopic surgery (VATS) after penetrating chest trauma. Out of 171 patients who underwent a VATS, 60 had a diaphragm injury. Not only were they able to accurately diagnose these injuries, but they also did so with few complications. On the basis of their study, they identified five independent risk factors for diaphragm injuries including abnormal chest x-ray, right-sided entrance wound, entrance inferior to the nipple line, velocity mechanism of injury, and associated intra-abdominal injuries. The main shortfall of thoracoscopy is its inability to evaluate the abdominal cavity for pathology.

Laparoscopy provides another minimally invasive alternative to thoracoscopy for the evaluation of the diaphragm. It has the added benefit over thoracoscopy to evaluate the intra-abdominal cavity for associated injuries. Therefore, it should be the minimally invasive approach of choice when intra-abdominal pathology is a possibility. Ivatury et al.[19] helped define its role in the evaluation of diaphragm injuries when they evaluated 100 hemodynamically stable patients by laparoscopy. A total of 43 patients had no peritoneal penetration, which was evenly divided between stabs and GSWs. Most (75%) of these patients had thoracoabdominal or epigastric injuries. All 17 patients with diaphragm lacerations were accurately identified at the time of laparoscopy. Those patients who were able to avoid a laparotomy had a significantly lower hospital stay than those who underwent exploratory laparotomy for nonpenetrating GSW, and there were no laparoscopy-related complications in this series. A number of other trials have replicated sensitivities of more than 80% and usually closer to 100% for thoracoabdominal penetrating trauma. They have also had very few complications. Consequently, laparoscopy is the evaluation modality of choice for penetrating thoracoabdominal trauma in patients without an immediate indication for exploration.

Treatment

Treatment should focus on early identification and repair of the diaphragm. Some animal studies suggest that after low-velocity injury to the muscular portion of the diaphragm, it heals spontaneously. Such findings have not been replicated in humans and are not the safe approach to a trauma patient with a thoracoabdominal wound. Therefore, there is no role for mere observation of this patient population.

With the increased use of the laparoscope and thoracoscope in the diagnosis of diaphragm injuries, it stands to follow that more attempts would be made to repair these injuries with the less invasive approach when other indications for open exploration are not present. Again, animal studies have found the repair to be as sturdy as with an open approach. The obvious benefit would be less postoperative complications and shorter lengths of stay in the hospital.

Matthews et al.[20] had a series of 17 patients of whom 8 had penetrating trauma. Only 13 were repaired through the laparoscope and 4 were converted to open. The four patients requiring open technique all suffered from a blunt trauma. Their eight penetrating trauma victims were successfully repaired with the laparoscope with no documented recurrence at a mean follow-up of 7 to 9 months.

Thoracoscopy has also been successful in select patients. Martinez et al.[21] looked at patients with penetrating trauma, of whom 80% were stab victims. They identified 35 with diaphragm injuries. All of these patients were successfully repaired thoracoscopically without complications.

Of all the treatment options, the gold standard still remains an open repair. As surgeons become more proficient with minimally invasive surgery, open repair may be replaced by these newer techniques. However, just as with the blunt trauma victim, there is no role for a minimally invasive approach in the unstable trauma patient.

These injuries may be approached either through the thorax or the abdomen. The decision on which approach to take is similar to that as in blunt trauma patients. For patients who have an acute injury, the most reasonable option is an abdominal exploration to allow for evaluation of the intra-abdominal structures. For those patients who have a chronic injury the technique is based on personal preference, most surgeons favoring laparotomy.

The major difference in the actual repair after penetrating trauma versus blunt trauma is the size of the injury. Blunt trauma more commonly results in larger defects. Often

there is a small hole in the diaphragm after a stab or even a low-velocity GSW. Consequently, primary repair is easily performed. Acute injuries to the diaphragm may be fixed using interrupted figure-of-eight or horizontal mattress suture with a zero nonabsorbable suture. A two-layer closure is an option for defects longer than 2 cm. The inner layer is an interlocking horizontal mattress reinforced by a running zero nonabsorbable suture. For chronic injuries, care must be taken to reduce the hernia and perform adhesiolysis. Larger defects that cannot be repaired primarily can be patched with a mesh with the same caveats as in blunt injury. Contamination cannot be present if a prosthetic is used. In this situation, autologous tissue as described in the blunt injury section may be used.

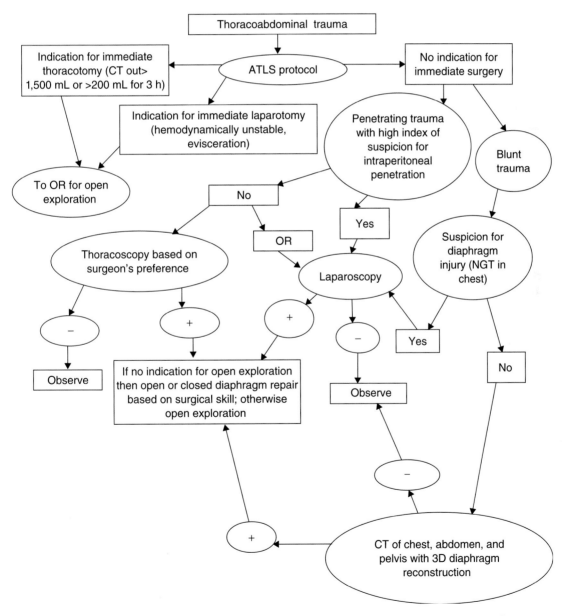

Figure 1   Management algorithm for thoracoabdominal trauma. CT, computed tomography; ATLS, Advanced Trauma Life Support; OR, operating room; NGT, nasogastric tube.

OUTCOMES

Morbidity

Morbidity from diaphragm injuries can be divided into complications of the acute phase or consequences of the chronic phase. Initially these patients are predisposed to the usual postoperative complications such as infections and postoperative ileus. Respiratory compromise may result from poor function or delayed function of the repaired diaphragm. Aggressive pulmonary toilet is vital especially if a thoracic approach has been used. They are also at risk for complications from their other injuries. Associated injuries may range from a small pneumothorax with little associated morbidity to an organ injury with some morbidity to a major vessel injury with significant morbidity. It is often difficult to attribute perioperative problems directly to the diaphragm itself. In a series that evaluated only penetrating trauma, complications seen in up to half of the patients included wound infections, subdiaphragmatic abscess, respiratory insufficiency, hypotension, small bowel obstruction, and bronchopleural fistula.[22]

Chronic phase morbidity results from unrecognized injury to the diaphragm. This problem tends to be higher in the blunt trauma victims who have a greater likelihood of being observed than penetrating trauma patients who are more likely to be explored. However, if an injury is missed, the complications are the same regardless of whether the patient suffered blunt or penetrating trauma. Herniation is the main complication that can occur within days or up to years of injury. Herniation can cause pulmonary compromise and intermittent obstruction. The most feared sequela is incarceration with strangulation of the contents. When this occurs, the patient is at significant risk of death.

Mortality

Death can result from the initial trauma or from long-term complications from missed injury. Mortality ranges from 0% to 42%. In both blunt and penetrating trauma, the high initial morbidity and mortality is from associated injuries. Williams et al.[23] reviewed 731 patients with blunt and penetrating trauma to the diaphragm. Gunshot wounds had the highest mortality at 42%. Blood transfusions of >10 units, revised trauma score, and need for thoracotomy predicted mortality. Therefore, they emphasized early identification of associated injuries and control of bleeding to improve survival.

It is more difficult to discern the mortality associated with chronic disruption of the diaphragm. First of all, most of the missed injuries are secondary to a blunt cause and secondly, they may not be identified as directly resulting in death. There are few series available that evaluate this question, but the ones that do show a mortality anywhere from 2% to 10%. The usual cause of death in these circumstances is from perforation of the viscus and

subsequent infection. Clearly, it is beneficial to identify these injuries at the time of the trauma to prevent such complications.

CONCLUSIONS

History and physical examination alone are inadequate to make the diagnosis of diaphragm injury but can provide clues to its presence depending on the type of blunt trauma or the location of a penetrating injury. Current radiographic techniques are too inaccurate to be relied on safely to exclude this diagnosis. For the unstable trauma patient with a clear indication for exploration, the diaphragm should be thoroughly explored and no injuries missed. For patients without another indication for exploration, thoracoscopy is a reasonable option when the injury is higher in the chest and from a low-velocity mechanism or when intra-abdominal injuries are thought unlikely. Laparoscopy is a better choice when one has a high index of suspicion for an intraperitoneal injury and can be done safely with the elimination of a large number of laparotomies.

If a surgeon has the capabilities and resources, then a closed repair is appropriate. If any question exists regarding one's ability to repair the injury or there is concern for other injuries, then an open exploration is mandatory.

Fundamentally, these patients should be managed using standard trauma protocols to ensure that all injuries are identified. Morbidity and mortality are closely related to these associated injuries, so they should be considered when management decisions are made. Early,

TABLE 1

BLUNT TRAUMA RECOMMENDATIONS

	Class Data	Recommendations
Computed tomography	III	Level III
Thoracoscopy	III/Expert opinion	Level II
Laparoscopy	III/Expert opinion	Level II

TABLE 2

PENETRATING TRAUMA RECOMMENDATIONS

	Class Data	Recommendations
Computed tomography	III	Not recommended
Thoracoscopy	III/Expert opinion	Level II
Laparoscopy	II/III/Expert opinion	Level II

aggressive treatment of diaphragm injuries results in minimal complications and good long-term outcomes and should be the goal when caring for this patient population. Figure 1 provides an algorithm for the approach to these patients. Tables 1 and 2 provide a description of the evidence available for our recommendations.

REFERENCES

1. Johnson CD. Blunt injuries of the diaphragm. *Br J Surg.* 1988; 75:226–230.
2. Rodriguez-Morales G, Rodriguez A, Shatney CH. Acute rupture of the diaphragm in blunt trauma: Analysis of 60 patients. *J Trauma.* 1986;26:438–444.
3. Rosati C. Acute traumatic injury of the diaphragm. *Chest Surg Clin N Am.* 1998;8:371–379.
4. Mihos P, Potaris K, Gakidis J, et al. Traumatic rupture of the diaphragm: Experience with 65 patients. *Injuiry Int J Care Injured.* 2003;34:169–172.
5. Shah R, Sabanathan S, Mearns AJ, et al. Traumatic rupture of diaphragm. *Ann Thorac Surg.* 1995;60:1444–1449.
6. Bergeron E, Clas D, Ratte S, et al. Impact of deferred treatment of blunt diaphragmatic rupture: A 15-year experience in six trauma centers in Quebec. *J Trauma.* 2002;52:633–640.
7. Reiff D, McGwin G, Metzger J, et al. Identifying injuries and motor vehicle collision characteristics that together are suggestive of diaphragmatic rupture. *J Trauma.* 2002;53:1139–1145.
8. Ilgenfritz FM, Stewrat DE. Blunt trauma of the diaphragm: A 15 county private hospital experience. *Am Surg.* 1992;58:334–338.
9. Boulanger BR, Milzman DP, Rosati C, et al. A comparison of right and left blunt traumatic diaphragmatic rupture. *J trauma.* 1993;35:255–260.
10. Beal SL, Mckennan M. Blunt diaphragmatic rupture: A morbid injury. *Arch Surg.* 1988;123:828–832.
11. Jones TK, Walsh JW, Maull KI. Diagnostic injury in Blunt trauma of the abdomen. *Surg Gynecol Obstet.* 1983;157:389.
12. Patselas T, Gallagher E. The diagnostic dilemma of diaphragm injuries. *Am Surg.* 2002;68:633–639.
13. Hirsch EF. Repair of an abdominal wall defect after a salvage laparotomy for sepsis. *J Am Coll Surg.* 2004;198:324–328.
14. Murray JA, Demetriades D, Cornwell EE III, et al. Penetrating left thoracoabdominal trauma: the incidence and clinical presentation of diaphragm injuries. *J Trauma.* 1997;43:624–626.
15. Demetriades D, Kakoyiannis S, Parekh D, et al. Penetrating injuries of the diaphragm. *Br J Surg.* 1988;75:824–826.
16. Wiencek RG Jr, Wilson RF, Steiger Z. Acute injuries of the diaphragm. An analysis of 165 cases. *J Thorac Cardiovasc Surg.* 1986;92(6):989–993.
17. Udobi KF, Rodriguez A, Chiu WC, et al. Role of ultrasonography in penetrating abdominal trauma: A prospective clinical study. *J Trauma.* 2001;50:475–479.
18. Ivatury RR, Simon RJ, Weksler B, et al. Laparoscopy in the evaluation of the intrathoracic abdomen after penetrating injury. *J trauma.* 1992;33:101–109.
19. Ivatury RR, Simon RJ, Stahl WM. A critical evaluation of laparoscopy in penetrating abdominal trauma. *J Trauma.* 1993;34:822–827.
20. Matthews BD, Bui H, Harold KL, et al. Laparoscopic repair of traumatic diaphragmatic injuries. *Surg Endosc.* 2003;17: 254–258.
21. Martinez M, Briz JE, Carillo EH. Video thoracoscopy expedites the diagnosis and treatment of penetrating diaphragmatic injuries. *Surg Endosc.* 2001;15:28–33.
22. Freeman RK, Al-Dossari G, Hutcheson KA, et al. Indications for using video-assisted thoracoscopic surgery to diagnose diaphragmatic injuries after penetrating chest trauma. *Ann Thorac Surg.* 2001;72:342–347.
23. Williams M, Carlin AM, Tyburski JG, et al. Predictors of mortality in patients with traumatic diaphragmatic rupture and associated thoracic and/or abdominal injuries. *Am Surg.* 2004;70:157–163.

Selective Nonoperative Management of Abdominal Injury

38

S. Peter Stawicki   **John P. Pryor**

Over the last two decades, one of the most important developments in the care of the trauma patient has been the use of selective nonoperative management (SNOM) of significant injuries. Pediatric surgeons were the first to pioneer nonoperative care for splenic and hepatic injuries in children. The success in children prompted the adaptation of selective management in adult patients. Subsequent experience and research has demonstrated that nonoperative techniques are applicable to most types of blunt injuries, and a small proportion of penetrating type injuries. Although many agree that the techniques have greatly reduced morbidity from unnecessary surgeries, new complications and management challenges have arisen that must be understood if these techniques are to be applied correctly.[1]

Often nonoperative is equated with "conservative" management. However, the reality is that nonoperative management is often more resource demanding, with more complex decision making, than performing a surgery. The nonoperative approach relies heavily on the availability of trauma-trained surgeons, modern radiographic imaging such as computed tomography (CT), accurate interpretation of such high-quality radiographic images, as well as the presence of appropriate supporting infrastructure and ancillary services such as intensive care units and interventional radiology.[1]

Although initially met with some resistance, SNOM of penetrating injury is being practiced in a very limited way in some experienced centers.[2,3] Although clearly applicable in stab wound injury, the role of SNOM in gunshot wounding is still controversial and must be applied with the utmost care by experienced surgeons.

HISTORICAL BACKGROUND

Nonoperative management of penetrating abdominal trauma remained the standard of care throughout most of the 19th century due to the lack of anesthesia, antibiotics, and therefore poor outcomes after attempted surgical procedures. This paradigm began to change after 1887, when the American Surgical Association recommended exploration of civilian penetrating abdominal wounds.[2] Owing to high mortality associated with nonoperative management of penetrating abdominal injuries, a policy of routine surgical exploration evolved during World War I, and became policy during World War II.[2] Mandatory exploration became surgical dictum when surgeons coming back from World War II advocated mandatory surgical exploration for all gunshot wounds in the civilian setting.[3] This approach appeared to be associated with significant reductions in mortality and remained the standard of care until the 1960s and 1970s when a trend toward SNOM of stab wounds to the abdomen began to emerge.[2] Mandatory exploration of all gunshot wounds to the abdomen remained the standard practice until the 1990s, when trauma centers in the United States and South Africa published their experiences on SNOM of those injuries.[2]

The concept of nonoperative management of blunt abdominal injuries has been evolving slowly throughout this century. However, SNOM did not become popularized until the 1970s, when better imaging techniques, improvement in nonoperative interventional techniques, refinement of intensive care of the critically ill, and increasing number of clinical studies that proved this approach is safe and effective.[4,5] During the 1980s and 1990s, the nonoperative management of blunt abdominal trauma (BAT) underwent a maturation process through multiple clinical investigations, trial and error, and detailed scrutiny. As a result, the modern application of SNOM is based largely on the evidence-based approach, with known benefits, risks, indications, and contraindications (see Table 1).[4]

TABLE 1

SUCCESS OF NONOPERATIVE MANAGEMENT STRATEGY FOR DIFFERENT ORGAN/ANATOMIC LOCATION INJURIES (IN ALPHABETICAL ORDER) AND MECHANISM OF INJURY (BLUNT VS. PENETRATING)

Blunt[a]	
Adrenal	80% [b]
Aortic (selective initial medical management)	>80%
Bowel (hematoma)	10%–15%
Duodenum (hematoma)	50%–60%
Esophagus	Rarely
Kidney	85%[c]
Liver	80%
Pancreas	Low-grade injuries only
Spleen	80%–90%
Urinary bladder (extraperitoneal)	>75%
Penetrating[d]	
Overall	20%
Back and flank	60%
Extremity	Variable, case by case
Kidney	15%
Liver	20%–30%
Neck (selective nonoperative management)	Variable, case by case
Pelvic/gluteal area	65%–70%
Spleen	<5%

[a]Schwab CW. Selection of nonoperative management candidates. *World J Surg.* 2001;25:1389–1392.
[b]Stawicki SP, Hoey BA, Grossman MD, et al. Adrenal gland trauma is associated with high injury severity and mortality. *Curr Surg.* 2003;60:431–436.
[c]Hagiwara A, Sakaki S, Goto H, et al. The role of interventional radiology in the management of blunt renal injury: A practical protocol. *J Trauma.* 2001;51:526–531.
[d]Pryor JP, Reilly PM, Dabrowski GP, et al. Nonoperative management of abdominal gunshot wounds. *Ann Emerg Med.* 2004;43:344–353.

TABLE 2

UNNECESSARY LAPAROTOMY—STATISTICS

Percentage of unnecessary laparotomies	1.7%–38% (average 20%)
Associated early complications	8.6%–25.6%
Associated late complications	2.4%–5%
Hospital cost difference	$10,000 more for operative management

---

THE BENEFIT OF SELECTIVE NONOPERATIVE MANAGEMENT—PREVENTING UNNECESSARY SURGERY

One clear benefit to SNOM is avoiding an unnecessary surgery. A laparotomy is classified as unnecessary, if the exploration reveals either no pathology (negative) or a minor injury that requires no surgical treatment (nontherapeutic).[2] The reported incidence of unnecessary laparotomies for trauma varies from 1.7% to 38%, and depends on the experience and practice patterns of the individual trauma center.[2] The rates were highest during the era of mandatory exploration for penetrating injuries, as well as solid organ injuries found on CT scan.[6–13] In contrast, centers that practiced a policy of SNOM demonstrated a significantly lower rate of unnecessary laparotomies (3.2% to 10%).[14–19]

Exploratory laparotomy is associated with significant morbidity and costs (see Table 2). The reported incidence of laparotomy or anesthesia-related early complications varies between 8.6% and 25.6%.[12,20] For late complications, such as bowel obstruction or incisional hernia, the reported overall incidence is between 2.4% and 5%.[13,21] In addition, the cost and hospital stay for patients undergoing laparotomy are significantly higher than for patients successfully managed nonoperatively.[15,17] In one study, the mean hospital charges for patients with abdominal gunshot wounds successfully managed nonoperatively were nearly $10,000 less than those for patients who underwent unnecessary surgeries.[15] In fact, a policy of SNOM for abdominal gunshot wounds has been shown to save both significant amount of hospital days and hospital-related charges.[17]

THE RISKS OF SELECTIVE NONOPERATIVE MANAGEMENT—DELAYS, MISSED INJURY, AND COMPLICATIONS

The benefits of SNOM should be weighed against the consequences of missed injuries and delayed diagnosis. Several reports have shown that when SNOM schemes are used by experienced practitioners, the risks of delay in diagnosis are minimal.[2,22] The delay beyond which the

TABLE 3

TYPES OF MINIMALLY INVASIVE PROCEDURAL INTERVENTIONS IN TRAUMA PATIENT MANAGEMENT

- Arteriographic interventions, including embolization, stenting, and diagnostic applications.
- Percutaneous drainage of bile collections, urinomas, abscesses, and hematomas.
- Endoscopic stenting of bile duct injuries and selected urinary tract injuries.
- Minimally-invasive endoscopic-guided placement of various adjunctive devices, including percutaneous gastrostomy (PEG) or percutaneous jejunostomy (PEJ) enteric access tubes, and percutaneous endoscopically-guided tracheostomy placement.

morbidity increases is not precisely known, but some have suggested a time frame of 6 to 12 hours.[2] The injured organ, the length of delay, and the degree of peritoneal contamination are all likely to play a role in the incidence and severity of complications related to delay in diagnosis and/or treatment.

Missed injury is a significant risk when undertaking SNOM. Approximately 5% of patients with BAT managed in a nonoperative manner will have a delay in diagnosis or a missed injury.[23] Although the resultant mortality is very low, a variety of complications (abscesses, pseudocysts, bile collections, etc) necessitate a careful follow-up that extends beyond the initial postinjury period.[23]

In many ways, the use of SNOM has traded one set of potential morbidities for another. For example, nonoperative management of liver injuries has clearly shown to decrease overall blood loss and transfusion requirements.[24] However, a number of significant injuries will develop bile leaks from the fractured surface of

the organ. Therefore, the decreased blood loss and complications of the laparotomy are exchanged for the risk of undrained biloma. Fortunately, as with this example, many of the complications of SNOM are amendable to minimally invasive techniques such as percutaneous drainage and ductal decompression with endoscopic retrograde cholangiopancreatography (ERCP) (see Table 3). Surgeons who endeavor to practice SNOM must be aware of, and ready to handle these specific types of complications (see Table 4).

PRINCIPLES OF SELECTIVE NONOPERATIVE MANAGEMENT

Nonoperative management of various injuries has certain unifying principles that must be followed for clinical success (see Table 5). The first tenet is that there must be hemodynamic stability to pursue SNOM. Unstable patients are assumed to have ongoing bleeding and need surgical control of the hemorrhage. Potential exceptions to this are those with lesions not amenable to surgery such as pelvic fractures; however, the number of patients like this is small compared to the many that have unyielding hemorrhage. A corollary to the first rule is that generalized peritonitis denotes the possibility of bowel perforation, and remains an indication for surgical exploration.

The next step is to define and characterize the injury that will be treated nonoperatively. This was a challenge years ago where nonspecific tests for injury such as diagnostic peritoneal lavage (DPL) were utilized. However, with excellent cross-sectional imaging capabilities, injuries can be anatomically identified and graded. The success of SNOM for many organs is directly related to the grade of injury. In addition, imaging is used to look for variants that are associated with SNOM failure and make an educated

TABLE 4

SYNOPSIS OF COMPLICATIONS ASSOCIATED WITH NONOPERATIVE MANAGEMENT OF INJURIES

- Missed injuries
- Delay in diagnosis
- Delay in treatment
- Inadequate/delayed resuscitation
- Retained hematomas (at risk for infection/abscess)
- Iatrogenic injuries secondary to minimally invasive treatment
- Abdominal sepsis and/or abscess
- Biliary/pancreatic leaks secondary to biliary/pancreatic injury
- Urinary collection secondary to renal/ureteral/bladder injury
- Delayed rupture of pseudoaneurysms
- Delayed aortic rupture
- Complications of delayed treatment of vascular injury (thrombosis, compartment syndrome, potential limb loss)

TABLE 5

SYNOPSIS OF GENERAL PRINCIPLES OF NONOPERATIVE MANAGEMENT

- Clearly define the injury
- Assure the patient is examinable, with clear mental status
- Assure patient is hemodynamically stable, with no obvious surgical indications
- Use caution when committing to nonoperative management in multiply injured patients
- Insist that adequate health care team resources are available to perform frequent physical examinations and re-imaging as needed
- Provide an appropriate setting for nonoperative observation such as observation ward, intensive care unit, or monitored emergency department bed
- Be prepared to provide surgical management promptly if indicated by a change in the signs or symptoms

decision about whether or not a particular patient will be successfully managed. Such a situation exists with the finding of a "blush" on CT scan indicating active extravasation, and the need for hemorrhage control.[25]

The third tenet is to make a decision about nonoperative management in the context of the whole patient, taking into account all of the injuries, not each one in isolation. This is particularly important in multiply injured patient where there are competing priorities. For example, an otherwise nonoperative grade III spleen injury may be treated differently if there is an associated severe pelvic fracture. In this case, it may be difficult to determine if a subsequent drop in hemoglobin is due to ongoing pelvic bleeding or hemorrhage from the spleen. Alternatively, a lower grade spleen injury may need removal if there is a concomitant severe head injury where hypotension would lead to undue neurologic morbidity. Many such conflicts can occur from the permutations of multiple injuries in different organ systems.

The keystone of SNOM is the obligation of the surgical team to admit the patient into a highly monitored setting where continuous reassessment of the clinical situation is assured. This not only requires a monitored bed but also trained nursing staff who understand the signs and symptoms of failing SNOM, and the availability of surgeons to reexamine the patient on a regular basis. It is easy to see how resources to meet these requirements can quickly disappear in a busy trauma unit where residents and surgeons are caring for multiple patients, or in smaller hospitals where physicians may not be available in-house at night. SNOM is a safe technique only if clinical deterioration is noted promptly and laparotomy is immediately available if needed.

Lastly, factors beyond the host and the injury need to be considered. It may not be plausible to treat a homeless patient with a known substance addiction with SNOM, knowing that after a few days in the hospital he/she would be released into an environment with a high risk of reinjury. Therefore, in addition to the whole patient, the entire social situation must be considered in the decisions for SNOM.

THE DECISION TO PURSUE SELECTIVE NONOPERATIVE MANAGEMENT

Hemodynamics

As stated previously, the first requirement of attempting SNOM is hemodynamic stability. Although there is some debate about what the optimal blood pressure is for a patient with acute injury, most believe that a systolic blood pressure below 90 mm Hg is concerning. The constellation of hypotension, tachycardia, and systemic signs such as pallor, diaphoresis, and mental status changes are late indications that the patient is in shock. These patients are characterized as hemodynamically unstable. It is clear from clinical experience and a vast body of literature that patients who are hemodynamically unstable have ongoing bleeding that needs control and are not candidates for nonoperative management.

There is a subset of patients who may present as initially hemodynamically unstable but rapidly improve with minimal resuscitation to a *metastable* state. Patients who are metastable have likely lost a volume of blood, but have perhaps stopped actively bleeding. Using nonoperative techniques in *metastable* patients is done with great caution, and with the understanding that if there is renewed bleeding, chances are that the patient will become unstable again.

During the course of nonoperative management, vital signs are recorded frequently. An increased temperature or respiratory rate can indicate a hollow visceral perforation or early abscess formation. Pulse and blood pressure can also change with sepsis or intra-abdominal bleeding. Adjunctive laboratory testing, such as serial determination of white blood cell count, hemoglobin and hematocrit levels, and serum lactic acid level and base deficit can also help to determine whether failure of nonoperative management is occurring.

Physical Examination

Physical examination remains the cornerstone of the triage of traumatic injuries. Peritonitis or hemodynamic instability with other signs of abdominal injury constitutes a strong indication for emergency laparotomy. Unfortunately, the physical findings of significant abdominal injury can be subtle and the diagnosis of intra-abdominal injury uncertain. Moreover, between 20% and 40% of patients with significant hemoperitoneum have a benign abdominal examination upon initial assessment.[9]

The physical examination can have significant limitations in certain situations, including the older trauma patient population, where the effect of medications such as β-blockers may effectively mask manifestations of shock.[2] Similarly, young patients, especially with short prehospital transport times, may not exhibit signs or symptoms of shock despite the presence of significant internal bleeding.[2] Patients with associated severe head or spinal injury may not have reliable examinations. Clouded sensorium due to alcohol or other substance use may further confound the accuracy of clinical assessment. Combative and intoxicated patients pose further diagnostic dilemma, not only due to the lack or reliable physical examination findings but also due to the potential danger to the health care personnel and inability to cooperate during imaging studies, which require the patient to remain still.

Especially challenging is the evaluation of a hemodynamically unstable patient with multiple injuries and competing priorities, such as a concurrent head injury, aortic injury, pelvic fractures, or extremity trauma. In patients for whom clinical examination is not reliable, special investigations can be crucial in early and accurate triage. Lack of reliable physical examination may constitute a relative contraindication to nonoperative management of traumatic injuries in patients who fall into this "gray" zone.

Imaging

The condition of the patient and the specific pattern of injury that is suspected will determine the imaging modality most appropriate in the given traumatic injury. An armamentarium of radiographic studies exists including plain radiograms, CT, magnetic resonance imaging, as well as a wide spectrum of ultrasonographic techniques. Imaging has become the integral part of the early decision-making process as to whether to proceed to the operating theater, interventional radiology suite, the trauma-surgical floor or the intensive care unit (see Table 6).

The location of the imaging equipment and the clinical capabilities of the supporting health care team staff and facilities should always be considered. Regardless of the type of radiographic investigation, the trauma patient who is undergoing the study should always be monitored appropriately. In addition, the trauma team should carefully plan the sequence of the resuscitation in order to minimize the loss of time and avoid radiographs that are technically impaired or have low diagnostic yield.

Plain Radiography

The overall value of plain films in the evaluation of patients with BAT is limited. The chest roentgenogram is paramount in diagnosing pneumothorax, hemothorax, and widened mediastinum in the trauma bay. Rarely, the chest radiograph may also aid in the diagnosis of abdominal injuries such as ruptured hemidiaphragm or pneumoperitoneum.

TABLE 6

IMPACT OF RADIOGRAPHIC IMAGING ON NONOPERATIVE TRAUMA MANAGEMENT

- Plain films remain valuable in chest, pelvic, and penetrating injury
- High-resolution computed tomography allows accurate organ injury assessment
- Ultrasonography is a fast and reliable adjunct in determining intra-abdominal hemorrhage
- Every trauma practitioner should be intimately familiar with FAST ultrasonography
- Interventional radiology techniques are used to treat acute hemorrhage as well as late complications of solid organ injury
- Advanced image reconstructions may be helpful when dealing with suspected aortic, spinal, and diaphragmatic injuries

FAST, focused assessment with sonography for trauma.

The pelvic or chest radiograph can demonstrate fractures of the thoracolumbar spine. The presence of transverse fractures of the vertebral bodies (i.e., Chance fractures) suggests a higher likelihood of blunt injuries to the bowel. In addition, free intraperitoneal air, or trapped retroperitoneal air from duodenal or colonic injury, may be seen. Penetrating wounds should have a radiopaque marker placed over each penetration site and radiographs obtained to determine trajectory and retained bullets or fragments.

Ultrasonography

The American College of Surgeons included the use of ultrasonography in the Advanced Trauma Life Support secondary survey since 1999. The focused assessment with sonography in trauma (FAST) examination can be repeated as many times as needed, providing an excellent adjunct to serial physical examinations in the nonoperative management of traumatic injury.[26] In many centers, the FAST examination has virtually replaced DPL as the procedure of choice in the evaluation of hemodynamically unstable trauma patients.

The FAST examination is based on the assumption that all immediately life-threatening abdominal injuries are associated with hemoperitoneum or pericardial tamponade. The current examination protocol consists of the pericardial, perihepatic, perisplenic, and pelvic acoustic windows performed with the patient supine. The detection of free intraperitoneal fluid is based on factors such as the body habitus, injury location, presence of clotted blood, position of the patient, and amount of free fluid present. The FAST examination is interpreted as positive if fluid is found in any of the four acoustic windows and is interpreted as negative if no fluid is seen. An examination is deemed indeterminate if any of the windows cannot be adequately assessed. Studies show that as little as 30 to 70 mL of blood can be detected with ultrasonography, with a small anechoic stripe in the perihepatic space representing approximately 250 mL of fluid, and 0.5- to 1-cm stripes represent approximately 500 mL to 1 L of free fluid, respectively.[27,28]

Reported sensitivities and negative predictive values for ultrasonography in the detection of hemoperitoneum are 78% to 99% and 93% to 99%, respectively. Ultrasonographic examination relies on hemoperitoneum to identify patients with injury. However, the reliance on hemoperitoneum as the sole indicator of abdominal visceral injury limits the utility of FAST as a diagnostic screening tool in hemodynamically stable patients with BAT, and CT scanning may be necessary to further delineate the nature and severity of injuries and reduce an otherwise unacceptably high laparotomy rate.[29,30]

Computed Tomography

CT in trauma has evolved to the point of nearly becoming a universal part of the initial trauma patient evaluation, and is arguably the most valuable and most widely used tool in the initial evaluation of the hemodynamically stable patient with BAT. Modern helical CT technology has improved the speed and accuracy of the image acquisition process, which can now be performed in potentially unstable, or metastable patients who might not have been able to tolerate the long scanning times of the older imaging machines. The presence of the CT scanner in the emergency department, within seconds of the trauma bay, may enable the speedy evaluation of critically injured patients.

CT can provide highly reliable information about the presence and size of hemoperitoneum, the extent or grade of solid-organ injuries, and retroperitoneal injuries. The evolution of high-quality, multidetector, CT scanners allow accurate assessment of ongoing bleeding by showing a "blush" which represents active extravasation of blood from a vessel. CT scan is much less sensitive in many cases of hollow visceral perforation and in the diagnosis of diaphragm injury. In addition, the CT will characterize associated fractures, especially vertebral and pelvic fractures, as well as injuries within the thoracic cavity. CT scans, unlike DPL or FAST examinations, have the capability to define the specific source of hemorrhage. In addition, many retroperitoneal injuries that are missed on DPL and FAST examinations, are easily detected on CT scans.[31,32]

Spleen

Splenic injury is common, and it is still the most common indication for laparotomy following BAT. However, the vast majority of spleen injuries in children and adults are now managed nonoperatively.[1] Currently there is controversy as to whether age older than 55 years and preexisting splenic disease truly entail increased risk of failure of nonoperative management.[25] The success of SNOM is related to grade, with approximately 95% success in grades I and II. Grade III splenic injuries can be treated nonoperatively, based on patient stability and reliability of the physical examination. The presence of significant hemoperitoneum is not a contraindication *per se*, although the failure rate in this group is as high as 20%.[33] In addition, there is emerging evidence that patients who are metastable, who rapidly stabilize with fluid or blood replacement, have SNOM success rates as high as 80% to 90%.[33,34]

Failure of SNOM of splenic injury is also related to presence of a contrast "blush" on CT scan.[25] A radiographic "blush" represents a focal area where extravasation of radiodense contrast material has occurred and is a sign of ongoing bleeding. Currently there are two options for splenic injuries with active extravasation: splenectomy or selective angioembolization. The decision to attempt embolization is complex and relies on an experienced surgeon weighing the hemodynamic stability, associated injuries, availability of interventional resources, and other logistic factors that are specific for each patient.

A formal protocol incorporating splenic angioembolization for severe splenic injuries has been shown to be successful in splenic salvage in more than 90% of grade III to V injuries.[35] There is a risk of rebleeding, subsequent psuedoaneurysm formation, and splenic infarction with angioembolization. It is unclear how many patients after splenic embolization experience complete splenic infarction and are rendered asplenic, making prophylactic vaccination necessary.

Overall approximately 10% to 20% of adult patients will fail SNOM of splenic injuries. Therefore, patients with significant splenic injuries treated nonoperatively should be observed in the intensive care unit and have immediate access to CT imaging, surgical staff, and an operating suite. Institutional protocols allowing for orderly and systematic treatment of splenic injuries may allow more consistent and evidence-based approach to these injuries and consequently higher success rates of SNOM.

Liver

Although hepatic and splenic injuries still represent the most common injuries in BAT, the liberal use of advanced high-resolution imaging techniques such as CT scanning has revealed that the liver and not the spleen is the most common solid organ injured in BAT (see Fig. 1).[8,34] The frequency of blunt hepatic and splenic injuries appears to be fairly constant, while the percentage of patients managed nonoperatively has increased dramatically since the 1990s.[1]

The vast majority of hemodynamically stable patients with low-grade hepatic injuries can be treated nonoperatively, provided that no other injuries that require laparotomy are present.[33] Grade IV or V hepatic injuries, with associated large-volume hemoperitoneum or some degree of transfusion requirement, can be managed nonoperatively with consideration of hepatic angiography with possible embolization.[33,36] In addition, there is emerging evidence that nonoperative management of hepatic injury that rapidly stabilizes with little fluid or blood replacement is successful in more than 80% of cases.[33,34,37] Moreover, it seems that neither advanced patient age nor higher grade of injury appears to correlate with the incidence of failure of nonoperative therapy.[1] Predictors of decreased success of nonoperative management include large hemoperitoneum, arterial blush, or pooling of contrast, as well as high-grade (IV and V) injuries.

The criteria for nonoperative treatment of blunt hepatic trauma include hemodynamic stability, absence of peritonitis, reliable examination in a neurologically intact patient, delineation of the injury by CT, and radiographic absence of other surgical injuries, <2 units of packed red blood cells transfused for the injury, as well as CT documentation of resolution of the injury. In addition, posterior right hepatic lobe and "split liver" injuries (where seemingly extensive injury occurs along a relatively avascular plane) can usually be managed nonoperatively.

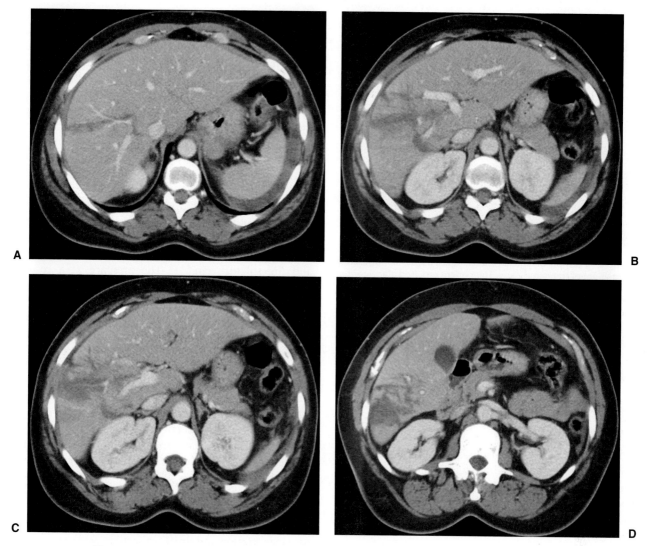

Figure 1 Example of high-grade hepatic injury managed nonoperatively. In the absence of other surgical indications, such injuries can routinely be managed without surgery, with or without interventional radiologic techniques.

Observation of patients with blunt hepatic injury depends mainly on injury grade. Grade I and II injuries can generally be observed on the ward. Injuries of grade III and above should be observed in the intensive care unit for the first 24 to 48 hours. Observation includes serial abdominal examinations and hematocrit determinations over a 3- to 5-day period of bed rest. Obtaining a follow-up CT scan at approximately 48 hours postinjury for injuries of grade III or higher is advocated by some groups, although it is not considered mandatory. Most liver injuries treated nonoperatively usually heal by 8 to 12 weeks.

Complications of nonoperative management of liver injuries include intrahepatic vascular fistulae (hemobilia) in up to 3%; delayed hemorrhage in <3%; liver abscess and perihepatic sepsis in up to 20%; hyperpyrexia, biliary fistulae, and extrahepatic ductal disruption; bile collection; and posttraumatic liver cysts

(see Fig. 2).[4] Many of these complications are amenable to percutaneous or endoscopic interventions and do not require formal surgical exploration. For example, biliary leaks and bile collections can be successfully managed by combining ERCP with sphincterotomy and stenting to decrease bile duct pressure, with percutaneous drainage of bile collections.[38]

Although many perihepatic hematomas resolve spontaneously, percutaneous techniques may be of therapeutic and diagnostic value, and may obviate surgical intervention if successful. The benefits of percutaneous drainage of hematomas (ability to obtain fluid Gram stain and cultures, relief of compressive symptoms, potential cure) must be weighed in the context of associated risks (more bleeding, introducing infection, damage to surrounding structures). Infections prevail as one of the most common causes of morbidity in patients with liver injuries treated

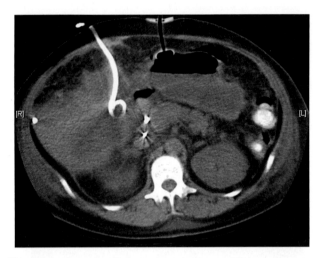

Figure 2 Example of adjunctive techniques used in nonoperative management of traumatic injury. This patient required placement of a percutaneous drain to evacuate posttraumatic biliary collection. In addition, a percutaneous endoscopic gastrostomy tube was placed to facilitate administration of enteral nutrition.

with SNOM. Suspicion of perihepatic or hepatic abscess should be treated aggressively with percutaneous drainage and antibiotic therapy guided by cultures.

Duodenum and Bowel

Nonoperative management of duodenal injuries is largely limited to isolated contusions due to blunt trauma. Although more common in children, isolated intramural duodenal hematomas are amenable to nonoperative management in most cases.[39] In these patients, a follow-up upper gastrointestinal series with gastrograffin should be performed every 7 days if the obstruction persists clinically. Other components of therapy in these nonoperatively treated duodenal injuries include nasogastric suction and intravenous alimentation. However, the usually accepted time limit to nonoperative management is a 2- to 3-week time frame.

Small or large bowel injury that appears to be limited to a bowel wall hematoma on advanced imaging studies can potentially be observed. Frequent clinical reexaminations should be performed, up to and including repeating the CT scan. Mesenteric hematomas, in the asymptomatic patient, can be observed. If the hematomas are large, or involve main visceral vessels, progressive ischemia of the adjacent bowel wall may occur. This may manifest as delayed onset of abdominal pain and peritoneal signs. Therefore if any evidence of clinical worsening or peritonitis develops during the observation period, the patient should undergo prompt laparotomy.

Pancreas

Isolated pancreatic injuries resulting from nonpenetrating trauma are rare. Less than 10% of all major trauma events include injury of the pancreas, and most of them are associated with other solid organ injuries. Several series report a range of 1.6 to 4.5 associated injuries per patient, including associated injuries to the numerous adjacent vascular structures. Rarely, the pancreas is the sole organ injured.[40–42]

If the patient is stable enough to undergo imaging, the initial test of choice is a CT scan, performed with intravenous contrast. The findings on CT which may indicate pancreatic injury include (a) peripancreatic fluid in the lesser sac; (b) pancreatic hematoma or laceration; (c) diffuse gland enlargement with pancreatitis or focal edema at the site of injury; and (d) thickening of the left anterior renal fascia. These findings are unusual and often subtle. An additional finding which is easy to recognize is the presence of fluid interdigitating between the pancreas and the splenic vein.[43,44] The presence of a complete pancreatic fracture is usually, but not always, associated with a concomitant main duct transection.[45–47]

One CT grading scheme, which has recently been suggested, parallels the surgical classification of Moore, without including direct evaluation of pancreatic duct integrity:[47] grade A, pancreatitis or superficial laceration (<50% pancreatic thickness); grade B1, deep laceration (>50% pancreatic thickness) of the pancreatic tail; grade B2, transection (entire thickness) of the pancreatic tail; grade C1, deep laceration of the pancreatic head; and grade C2, transection of the pancreatic head. The difficulties involved in initial CT scan grading of pancreatic injury highlight the need to proceed with great caution if the nonoperative path is taken. False-negative results or underestimation of initial CT scan grading may be associated with unopacified bowel loops adjacent to the pancreas, motion and streak artifacts, as well as suboptimal bolus enhancement. In grade B or C injuries, the pancreatic fracture line is not easily detected when the separation of the fractured pancreatic fragments is minimal or nonexistent.[46] Furthermore, overestimation on CT could occur in grade C injuries because deep lacerations through the proximal pancreas are sometimes not associated with disruption of the proximal main duct, and transections through the proximal pancreas may merely disrupt the minor duct.[47] CT scans can also be useful in demonstrating complications such as abscesses, fistulae, pancreatitis, and pseudocysts.

There seems to be a strong trend in the frequency of pancreatic-specific complications in patients requiring delayed surgical intervention versus continued observation.[48] The reasons for the delay in diagnosis and treatment of isolated pancreatic trauma include the fact that pancreatic injury can be asymptomatic in up to 20% of patients, laboratory findings are often nonspecific (in particular, initial serum amylase levels may be normal in approximately 25% of patients), and underestimation of the severity of pancreatic injury on the initial computed tomogram is possible.[48,49] Lastly, it is possible for low severity BAT to be associated with isolated pancreatic injury.

Initially, it is important to separate the patients into two groups: those who need immediate surgery and those who qualify for nonoperative observation. Although nonoperative management of other solid organs (spleen, liver) is an accepted practice, nonoperative management of pancreatic injuries is more controversial. The integrity or disruption of the pancreatic duct is the principal determinant in the management of pancreatic injuries. Because prompt surgical intervention is usually undertaken in patients with penetrating injuries or multiple organ involvement, delay in the diagnosis of a pancreatic duct injury most commonly occurs in patients with BAT isolated to the pancreas. Some authors claim that CT grading of the degree of severity of blunt pancreatic trauma can be useful in predicting ductal integrity or disruption, although this is not universal.[45,48,50]

In the case of an isolated pancreatic injury, serial physical examinations and repeated CT scans may be a determinant in the diagnosis and grading of pancreatic injury if nonoperative management is to be undertaken.[50] One has always to keep in mind that the initial CT scan will sometimes miss or underestimate pancreatic injuries that ultimately require surgical treatment and may cause a false sense of security and delay of surgery.

Certain complications of nonoperative management of pancreatic injuries may also require further invasive treatment. These include pancreatic fistulae, pancreatic ascites, and posttraumatic pancreatitis with potential for pseudocyst formation. Although many of these injuries can be treated with a combination of ERCP and percutaneous techniques, some may require surgical intervention.

Kidney

Approximately 80% of renal injuries in the United States are due to blunt mechanism, and are associated with a loss of the kidney in 5% of cases. Blunt renal injury is suggested by the mechanism of injury, the presence of hematuria, as well as physical findings and radiography. CT of renal injuries has evolved to a point where renal injury staging can be done almost exclusively by CT criteria.

In the setting of blunt renal trauma and selected instances of penetrating renal trauma, a nonoperative approach may be chosen, beginning with careful patient selection as the preliminary step. One series, with predominantly blunt mechanisms of injury, documented that 85% of patients were treated successfully without surgery. Ultimately, the exclusion of concurrent injury may be the key in treating patients nonoperatively.

The anatomic structure of the kidney lends itself well to nonoperative management in the setting of blunt trauma. The kidney has an end artery blood supply with a segmental pattern of division that supplies the renal parenchyma. When subjected to blunt force, renal lacerations tend to occur through the parenchyma. The resulting hematoma may displace renal tissue, but the segmental vessels themselves are often not lacerated. The closed retroperitoneal space around the kidney also promotes tamponade of bleeding renal injuries. Finally, the kidney is rich in tissue factor, further promoting hemostasis after injury through activation of the extrinsic coagulation pathway.

Nonoperative treatment of renal trauma (grades I to III) has become standard. If the injury is properly staged, nonoperative management is successful for contusions, contained lacerations, and even lesions with moderate amount of extravasation of urine or blood in the hemodynamically stable patient.

Traumatic renal arterial thrombosis usually results in renal loss. Renal salvage is unusual if the warm ischemia time exceeds 30 minutes. Nonoperative management is usually recommended in stable patients, with the understanding that late nephrectomy may be required for control of hypertension or sequelae of renal infarction.

Interventional radiology has extended the applicability of the nonoperative approach. Percutaneous drainage of perinephric fluid collections or urinomas has been used to address one clinical complication of nonoperative management. In addition, angiography with selective embolization has been used in the setting of isolated renal trauma. Another method to enhance nonoperative approach includes endourologic stenting. With these strategies, successful nonoperative management of renal lacerations may be achieved in a greater number of patients.

Bladder

Bladder injuries following blunt trauma are rare, constituting <2% of abdominal injuries requiring surgery. The relative rarity of these injuries has been attributed to the protected position of the bladder deep in the bony pelvis. This, in part, makes bladder injury a marker for other severe injuries with significant associated mortality.[51] Bladder injuries following blunt trauma are significantly associated with pelvic fractures, with more than 80% of patients with bladder injuries having a pelvic fracture, and approximately 10% of patients with pelvic fractures having a bladder injury.[52,53]

Most patients with bladder injury will present with gross hematuria, although a small minority will only have microscopic hematuria.[51,52] Gross hematuria is felt to be associated with more significant injury (i.e., bladder rupture) whereas microscopic hematuria is seen more commonly with bladder contusions.[52]

Evaluation of suspected bladder injury starts with a proper history and physical examination. Lower abdominal pain, tenderness, and bruising over the lower abdominal and perineal area may be present. However, these signs and symptoms may be difficult to discern from the findings associated with pelvic fractures. Some intraperitoneal bladder injuries are discovered when a urethral catheter fails to return urine. In patients with a delayed diagnosis of bladder injury, fever, absence of voiding, peritoneal irritation, and elevated blood urea nitrogen may be observed. Any patient with these signs and symptoms should have formal cystography to rule out bladder injury.

Inspection for blood at the urethral meatus should be performed during routine trauma evaluation. This sign is present in approximately half of significant urethral injuries.[54] Passage of a urinary catheter should not be attempted in these patients, but rather an immediate retrograde urethrogram should be obtained to rule out urethral injury. Between 10% and 17% of patients with bladder injuries will have associated urethral injury.[52,54] If findings on urethrography are normal, a urinary catheter can be placed. However, if these findings are abnormal, suprapubic urinary catheter, bladder exploration, and repair should be considered.

If no urethral injury is present, retrograde cystography with plain abdominal roentgenographic imaging has been shown to be very accurate in determining whether there is an intraperitoneal or extraperitoneal bladder rupture.[51] The technique has two important technical considerations. First, the bladder needs to be filled completely. Second, a postdrainage film is essential. Approximately 300 mL of diluted contrast medium is infused into the bladder by gravity.

Given the widespread utilization of CT in modern trauma practice, CT cystography has gained popularity as a study of choice for evaluation of potential bladder trauma. Diluted contrast medium is infused into the bladder, and pelvic tomography is subsequently performed.

The management of intraperitoneal bladder ruptures is surgical, and will be described in detail in the chapter on urologic injuries. Extraperitoneal ruptures, which are found alone in approximately two thirds of cases, may be amenable to nonoperative management.[51] They can most commonly be managed with urinary catheter drainage alone, although some argue that a bone fragment projecting into the rupture (a rare occurrence), open pelvic fracture, and rectal perforation may constitute a contraindication to nonoperative management.[55] Open pelvic fracture and rectal perforation are associated with high risk of serious infection if managed conservatively.[56] Others suggest that if clots obstruct the urinary catheter within 48 hours of injury, then open repair should be undertaken and a suprapubic tube placed.[57] A relative indication for surgical repair of extraperitoneal ruptures is found in patients undergoing exploratory laparotomy for other reasons.[57]

In extraperitoneal bladder ruptures, antimicrobial agents are instituted on the day of injury and continued until 3 days after the urinary catheter is removed.[57] Follow-up cystography should be performed in cases of extraperitoneal bladder rupture at 10 to 14 days postinjury.[58] Most ruptures will heal by 10 days, and nearly all heal by 3 weeks.[57,58] If the cystogram shows no extravasation, the catheter can be removed. Otherwise, cystography is repeated at 21 days.[58] Most authors report few complications with nonoperative management of extraperitoneal bladder rupture.

PRINCIPLES OF SELECTIVE NONOPERATIVE MANAGEMENT IN PENETRATING INJURY

Unlike blunt injury, the vast majority of penetrating injuries will require surgical management. Therefore, application of SNOM in the setting of penetrating injury requires significant experience with this kind of management and is best done at high volume penetrating trauma centers (see Table 7). The factor most strongly linked to the appropriate application of SNOM in the setting of penetrating injury at high volume centers is the adequacy of resources available to emergently "convert" SNOM to surgical management if the nonoperative approach fails.

Selective management of penetrating abdominal wounds involves several important principles. First, adequate resources have to be present in order to provide continued and timely monitoring of injured patients, providing immediate feedback when failure of nonoperative therapy is suspected. Second, adequate high-quality imaging modalities have to be readily available for the purpose of initial definition of the path of the projectile as well as for the reimaging (if appropriate) when failure of nonoperative management is suspected. Third, adequate resources (operating surgeon, operative suite, nursing staff, and house staff) need to be in place in order to expeditiously institute operative therapy if needed.

When a patient is being evaluated for possible nonoperative management of penetrating torso injury, two questions must be asked by the treating physician. First, did the projectile enter the thoracic, peritoneal, retroperitoneal, or pelvic cavity? And second, if it did, is there an injury that will require a surgery? Accurate determination of the projectile trajectory can help answer both of these

---

TABLE 7

IMPORTANT CONSIDERATIONS WHEN TREATING PENETRATING TRAUMA NONOPERATIVELY

- Nonoperative approach is employed *selectively* in the setting of penetrating traumatic injury
- Patients who sustained penetrating trauma and are being treated nonoperatively must be hemodynamically stable, and must be able to give reliable serial physical examinations
- Establish accurate trajectory of the penetrating injury
- Use computed tomography to determine accurate missile trajectory and facilitate nonoperative management
- Adequate resources have to be present in order to provide continued and timely monitoring of injured patients, providing immediate feedback when failure of nonoperative therapy is suspected
- Adequate resources (operating surgeon, operative suite, nursing staff, and house staff) need to be in place in order to expeditiously institute operative therapy, if needed

questions. Therefore, the decision about whether a patient can undergo nonoperative management depends on the clinical evaluation and determination of trajectory, and trajectory determination equates with injury identification (Fig. 3).[3] To simplify the decision-making process, hemodynamically unstable patients with penetrating injury are not candidates for SNOM.

In a hemodynamically stable patient, trajectory of the projectile that has been documented to be clearly extraperitoneal should result in clinical observation and/or hospital discharge. The choice of whether to observe the patient should be based on the proximity of the bullet tract to other organs (i.e., possibility of "proximity" injury to vessels, bowel, bladder, etc.) and on whether there are other factors that could result in need for delayed treatment (i.e., presence of hematoma or radiographic "blush" in the bullet tract). If the trajectory appears to be intraperitoneal, the default pathway should be to perform an exploratory laparotomy. Rarely, nonoperative management of isolated hepatic injuries has been undertaken following penetrating trauma, keeping in mind that potential exists for both delay in treatment (if another injury is missed) or for complications of nonoperative management (bile collection, bile duct injury, hemobilia, etc.). Similar principles can be applied to isolated renal injuries from penetrating wounds. Again, one must be cognizant of possibility of missed injury and complications of SNOM (urine collection, ongoing or delayed bleeding, etc.).

Penetrating Injuries: Mechanism-Based Considerations

There are several factors that differentiate penetrating military and civilian wounds. Civilian injuries tend to be caused by handguns with low-caliber missiles and with muzzle velocities between 800 and 1,400 ft per second.[59]

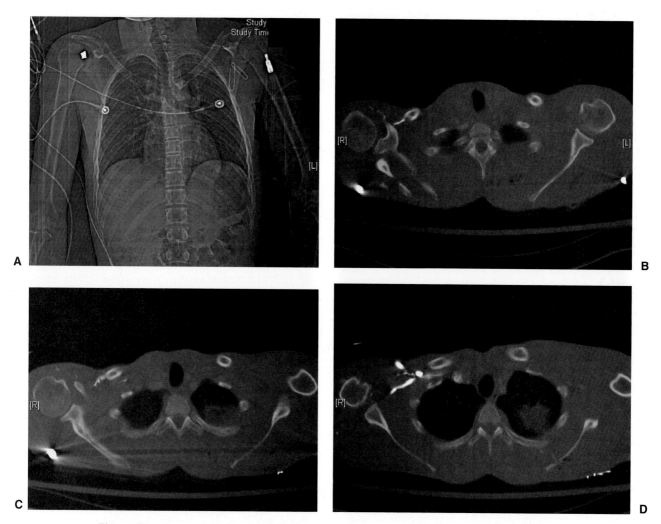

Figure 3 Utilization of computed tomography to determine penetrating injury trajectory following a gunshot wound to left posterior shoulder area. **A:** The paperclip seen on the left indicates the entrance wound, with the bullet seen in the right shoulder area. **B–D:** The bullet trajectory is seen posteriorly, with an area of left pulmonary contusion and left scapular fracture. The patient did not require any surgical interventions.

Typically, these weapons cause a relatively small wound associated with minimal damage caused by blast or cavitation effect. Tissue damage is limited to a small area around the missile path, and usually only organs directly in the path of the projectile will be injured.[59] In contrast, blast injury and cavitation are more significant with high-velocity missiles, such as those originating from rifles and military weapons, or in shotgun wounds.[60] These projectiles cause much more widespread tissue destruction along a missile path significantly wider than the actual projectile. The tissue destruction often involves large areas of necrosis, and most surgical interventions for these wounds involve exploration and debridement, even without signs of peritonitis or evidence of peritoneal penetration.

Stab wounds can be broadly divided into those with wider blades (knives, bayonets, etc.), and those with long punctate objects (ice picks, screwdrivers, etc.). Stab wounds tend to cause direct damage around the wound, with less damage to surrounding tissues. Special attention should be paid to the exact mechanism of stabbing, the suspected path, and depth of the stabbing blade, as imaging techniques will not be as useful as they are in injuries caused by bullets.

SELECTIVE NONOPERATIVE MANAGEMENT IN PENETRATING INJURY: REGIONAL APPROACH

The evolution of the nonoperative approach to penetrating traumatic injury can be divided into regional and anatomic considerations of the injury mechanism as well as the patient's clinical stability. The following section will focus on regional anatomy in relation to injury in an attempt to simplify the overall approach to the penetrating trauma patient.

Abdomen

Evidence dating back to the 1990s supports that selected patients with abdominal gunshot wounds can be successfully treated utilizing the nonoperative approach. In one study, approximately 80% of patients exhibited peritonitis and were taken directly to the operating room, while 20% of patients were treated nonoperatively and did not require a laparotomy.[61] In that study, among the patients who were observed, eight were believed to have negative physical examination results, even with indirect evidence of peritoneal penetration (i.e., by estimation of trajectory by surface wounds). The negative and nontherapeutic laparotomy rates were 5% and 1%, respectively. Selection was based entirely on physical examination and plain radiographs. Advanced imaging technology, such as CT scan, was not utilized.

Demetriades et al. confirmed the utility of physical examination in evaluation of intra-abdominal injury in a prospective evaluation of 146 patients with abdominal gunshot wounds.[62] Similar to prior studies, most patients (72%) had a positive clinical examination on admission, prompting an immediate laparotomy. Of the 41 (28%) patients who were observed, 7 eventually underwent delayed laparotomy, with no apparent added morbidity or mortality.

In the largest series of nonoperative management of abdominal gunshot wounds, 1,856 patients from the Los Angeles/University of Southern California medical center were evaluated.[17] A total of 792 (42%) patients were initially triaged to nonoperative observation, of whom 712 were eventually discharged without a surgery. Of the 80 patients who failed nonoperative management and underwent a delayed laparotomy, 57 had injuries requiring surgical repair. Although the primary tool of triage determination was the physical examination, most patients chosen for nonoperative management also underwent a CT scan. The combined negative and nontherapeutic laparotomy rate was 13% in patients undergoing immediate exploration and 29% in those receiving a delayed surgery. There were five complications, including three intra-abdominal abscesses, one ileus, and one acute respiratory distress syndrome, that were attributed to a delay in treatment among the 80 patients who underwent delayed exploration, but no deaths. Combined, this and the other studies support the physical examination as a sensitive indicator of intra-abdominal injury after penetrating trauma.

In stab wounds, trajectory determination by imaging techniques is more difficult, and adjunctive techniques such as local wound exploration and diagnostic laparoscopy may be of benefit when determining the applicability of SNOM. Penetration of the anterior abdominal fascia constitutes the traditional indication for abdominal exploration, but this has been questioned by numerous studies due to high percentage of nontherapeutic laparotomies associated with stab wounds. Again, repeated physical examinations and high index of clinical suspicion are important in determining the failure of SNOM, and nonoperative management of stab wounds is best performed at high volume penetrating trauma centers where significant experience and adequate clinical resources are available to approach these types of injuries.

Thoracoabdominal Area

The thoracoabdominal area extends from the nipple line to the costal margins bilaterally. This region represents a space that can be filled by thoracic and abdominal contents. The difficulty in determining trajectory in this region is partly caused by the diaphragmatic mobility and the changing relationship of the internal structures to surface landmarks. The right side of this region is mostly occupied by the liver, whereas the left side contains the spleen, stomach, colon, and small bowel. Because of these anatomic relationships, injuries to this region are treated differently, depending on which side the injury is found.[3]

Isolated penetrating injuries to the right thoracoabdomen will generally involve the liver and diaphragm. Although it has been postulated that diaphragm injuries to the right side are less severe because the liver acts to obturate the defect and prevent herniation of bowel contents, this theory may not be true.[63] Overall, right thoracoabdominal gunshot injuries account for <7% of all abdominal gunshot wounds.[64] A nonoperative approach to this specific injury has evolved from the high incidence of unnecessary laparotomies where the only findings have been nonbleeding injuries confined to the liver. In one series of right thoracoabdominal gunshot injuries, most patients had both a chest injury (hemothorax, pulmonary contusion) and a solid organ injury (liver, kidney). The chest injuries were treated with tube thoracostomy only, and the solid organ injuries were observed without the need for intervention.[64] In another series of 33 patients with right thoracoabdominal gunshot wounds treated nonoperatively, only 1 underwent a laparotomy for worsening clinical symptoms, which proved to be nontherapeutic.[65] Another study of 16 hemodynamically stable patients with a right thoracoabdominal gunshot injury were treated nonoperatively after evaluation with abdominal CT.[66] In this group of patients, five underwent a delayed laparotomy for developing peritonitis or abdominal compartment syndrome. In the remaining 11 patients treated nonoperatively, 1 patient developed a biloma that was treated with percutaneous drainage.

In contrast to the right side, injury to the left thoracoabdomen has a higher chance of diaphragmatic and hollow visceral penetration. Because abdominal CT is not sensitive or specific for determining diaphragmatic injury, other methods must be utilized.[67] Murray et al. reported the incidence of diaphragmatic injury with left thoracoabdominal gunshot wounds at 42%.[68] In that study, all patients underwent diagnostic laparoscopy to rule out diaphragmatic injury. In patients who were determined to have a diaphragmatic defect, 31% had no signs of peritonitis and 40% had a normal chest radiograph. Because of these findings, the authors recommend diagnostic laparoscopy for all patients with left thoracoabdominal gunshot injuries.

Back and Flank

The surface landmarks for the flank region include the tips of the scapulae superiorly, the iliac crests inferiorly, the anterior axillary lines, and the posterior axillary lines. The back region is bounded by the posterior axillary line bilaterally, the scapular tip superiorly, and the iliac crest inferiorly. Evaluating patients with penetrating injuries to these areas is especially difficult. First, there is paucity of literature supporting nonoperative management in this anatomic area, and studies that do exist have small numbers of patients. Also, there is the clinical challenge of penetrating injuries involving only the retroperitoneum, which can cause the classic signs of peritoneal irritation to be delayed or missing altogether. Finally, some adjuncts, such as laparoscopy, FAST ultrasonography, and DPL, are of limited value in evaluating the retroperitoneum.

Abdominal CT has been shown to be sensitive and specific for diagnosing injuries in this area and is considered the test of choice for wounds thought to be limited to the retroperitoneum. A variation of the standard CT scan is performed with "triple contrast." In addition to the standard oral and intravenous contrast, soluble contrast is placed into the colon by the way of an enema. Proponents of this type of preparation believe that it can help identify subtle injuries to the retroperitoneal colon. The disadvantages are the inconvenience, delay that the preparation necessitates, and added cost. Injuries to the colon by posterior wounds are rare, comprising only 1% of patients at risk for such injury.[69] After studying 145 patients with posterior stab wounds, one study failed to find a single patient in whom colonic contrast helped to identify an injury.[70]

Velmahos et al. reviewed an extensive clinical experience with back and flank gunshot wounds.[16] According to clinical examination alone, without utilizing abdominal CT or DPL, patients were selected for nonoperative treatment. Overall, 130 (69%) of 206 patients studied were treated by observation. There were 4 (3%) delayed laparotomies, all of which were nontherapeutic. The authors concluded that SNOM of back and flank gunshot wounds is appropriate and safe. Ginzburg et al. used abdominal CT to characterize 45 gunshot injuries to the flank.[71] Of these, 40 patients had negative abdominal CT results, were observed for 24 hours, and had no delayed laparotomies or complications.

Pelvis

The pelvis is an anatomically restricted space with densely crowded internal structures. A study from the University of Pennsylvania demonstrated that transpelvic penetrating injuries have an 85% chance of causing an internal organ injury.[72] However, this group was able to use a selective nonoperative approach similar to the one used in abdominal and back wounds (Fig. 4). Unique adjuncts in pelvic injury included urinalysis to diagnose injury to the urethra and bladder and rigid proctoscopy to identify rectal injury. Gross hematuria or hematochezia are both clinical findings that have a high predictive value of pelvic organ injury.[73]

Velmahos et al. applied a selective surgical approach to evaluate 59 patients with pelvic or gluteal gunshot wounds.[73,74] According to physical examination, adjunct examinations, and in some cases CT scan, 40 (67.8%) patients underwent nonoperative management. There were no delayed explorations in this group of patients, and the authors concluded that the clinical examination alone was 100% sensitive and 95.3% specific for identifying internal organ injuries after pelvic gunshot wounds.

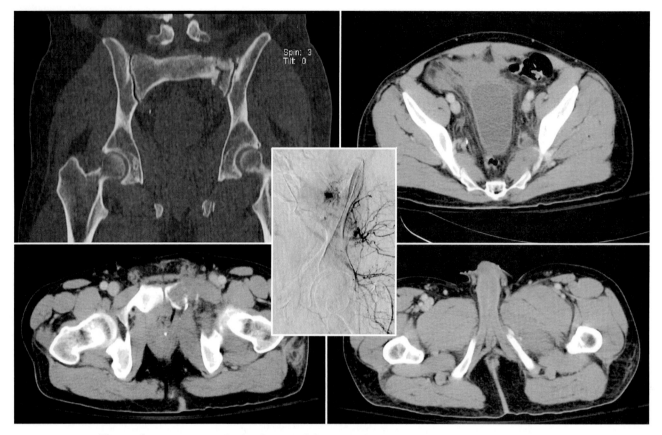

Figure 4   Management of pelvic fractures following high-speed motor vehicular crash. The patient was taken to interventional radiology and underwent embolization of branches of the left internal iliac artery. No surgical intervention was required.

CONCLUSIONS

The application of SNOM to all types of blunt and penetrating injury has become a large part of the modern care of the trauma patient. By avoiding unnecessary surgeries, the short-term morbidity is decreased. In some cases, late complications are directly related to the nonoperative management early on in the hospital course, but most are amendable to treatment with minimally invasive techniques and minor surgery. The role and execution of SNOM for penetrating injuries is less accepted and more difficult to perform. Unlike patients with blunt injuries, most patients with stab and gunshot wounding will require surgery to control hemorrhage and contain contamination. The use of SNOM will continue to evolve as new noninvasive diagnostic and therapeutic modalities become available.

REFERENCES

1. Schwab CW. Selection of non-operative management candidates. *World J Surg.* 2001;25:1389–1392.
2. Demetriades D, Velmahos G. Technology-driven triage of abdominal trauma: The emerging era of non-operative management. *Annu Rev Med.* 2003;54:1–15.
3. Pryor JP, Reilly PM, Dabrowski GP, et al. Non-operative management of abdominal gunshot wounds. *Ann Emerg Med.* 2004;43:344–353.
4. Carrillo EH, Wohltmann C, Richardson JD, et al. Evolution in the treatment of complex blunt liver injuries. *Curr Probl Surg.* 2001;38:9–60.
5. Rance CH, Singh SJ, Kimble R. Blunt abdominal trauma in children. *J Paediatr Child Health.* 2000;36:2–6.
6. McAnena OJ, Moore EE, Marx JA. Initial evaluation of the patient with blunt abdominal trauma. *Surg Clin North Am.* 1990;70:495–515.
7. Davis JJ, Cohn I, Nance FC Jr. Diagnosis and management of blunt abdominal trauma. *Ann Surg.* 1976;183:672–678.
8. Knudson MM, Maull KI. Non-operative management of solid organ injuries-past, present and future. *Surg Clin North Am.* 1999;79:1357–1371.
9. McConnell DB, Trunkey DD. Non-operative management of abdominal trauma. *Surg Clin North Am.* 1990;70:677–688.
10. Christmas AB, Wilson AK, Manning B, et al. Selective management of blunt hepatic injuries including non-operative management is a safe and effective strategy. *Surgery.* 2005;138:606–610.
11. Rutldege R, Hunt JP, Lentz CW, et al. A statewide, population based time-series analysis of the increasing frequency of non-operative management of abdominal solid organ injury. *Ann Surg.* 1995;222:311–326.
12. Renz BM, Feliciano DV. Unnecessary laparotomies for trauma: A prospective study of morbidity. *J Trauma.* 1995;38:350–356.
13. Leppaniemi A, Salo J, Haaipainen R. Complications of negative laparotomy for truncal stab wounds. *J Trauma.* 1995;38: 54–58.
14. Demetriades D, Rabinovitz B. Indications for operations in abdominal stab wounds. *Ann Surg.* 1987;205:129–132.

15. Demetriades D, Velmahos GC, Cornwell EE, et al. Selective non-operative management of gunshot wounds of the anterior abdomen. *Arch Surg.* 1997;132:178–183.
16. Velmahos GC, Demetriades D, Foianini E, et al. A selective approach to the management of gunshot wounds of the back. *Am J Surg.* 1997;174:342–346.
17. Velmahos GC, Demetriades D, Toutouzas KG, et al. Selective non-operative management in 1856 patients with abdominal gunshot wounds: Should laparotomy still be the standard of care? *Ann Surg.* 2001;234:395–403.
18. Henderson VJ, Organ CH, Smith RS. Negative trauma celiotomy. *Am Surg.* 1993;59:365–370.
19. Miller FB, Cryer HM, Chilikuri S, et al. Negative findings on laparotomy for trauma. *South Med J.* 1989;82:1231–1234.
20. Hasaniya N, Demetriades D, Stephen A, et al. Early morbidity and mortality of nontherapeutic operations for penetrating trauma. *Am Surg.* 1994;60:1–4.
21. Weigelt JA, Kingman RG. Complications of negative laparotomy for trauma. *Am J Surg.* 1998;156:544–548.
22. Bensard DP, Beaver BL, Berner GE, et al. Small bowel injury in children after blunt abdominal trauma: Is diagnostic delay important? *J Trauma.* 1996;41:476–483.
23. Yoo SY, Lim KS, Kang SJ, et al. Pitfalls of non-operative management of blunt abdominal trauma in children in Korea. *J Pediatr Surg.* 1996;31:263–266.
24. Pryor JP, Stafford PW, Nance ML. Severe blunt hepatic trauma in children. *J Pediatr Sur.* 2001;36:974–979.
25. Ochsner MG. Factors of failure for non-operative management of blunt liver and splenic injuries. *World J Surg.* 2001;25:1393–1396.
26. Scalea TM, Rodriguez A, Chiu WC, et al. Focused Assessment with Sonography for Trauma (FAST): Results from an international consensus conference. *J Trauma.* 1999;46:466–472.
27. Kawaguchi S, Toyonaga J, Ikeda K. Five point method: An ultrasonographic quantification formula of intra-abdominal fluid collection. *Jpn J Acute Med.* 1987;7:993–997.
28. Tiling T, Boulion B, Schmid A, et al. Ultrasound in blunt abdominothoracic trauma. In: Border JR, ed. *Blunt multiple trauma: comprehensive pathophysiology and care.* New York: Marcel Dekker Inc; 1990:415–433.
29. Chiu WC, Cushing BM, Rodriguez A, et al. Abdominal injuries without hemoperitoneum: A potential limitation of Focused Abdominal Sonography for Trauma (FAST). *J Trauma.* 1997;42:617–623.
30. Rozycki GS, Ballard RB, Feliciano D, et al. Surgeon-performed ultrasound for the assessment of truncal injuries: Lessons from 1540 patients. *Ann Surg.* 1998;228:557–567.
31. Demetriades D, Gomez H, Velmahos G, et al. Routine helical computed tomographic evaluation of the mediastinum in high-risk blunt trauma patients. *Arch Surg.* 1998;133:1084–1088.
32. Velmahos G, Demetriades D, Chan L, et al. Predicting the need for thoracoscopic evacuation of residual traumatic hemothorax: Chest radiograph is insufficient. *J Trauma.* 1999;46:65–70.
33. Goan Y, Huang M, Lin M. Non-operative management for extensive hepatic and splenic injuries with significant hemoperitoneum in adults. *J Trauma.* 1998;45:360.
34. Meredith JW, Young JS, Bowling J, et al. Non-operative management of blunt hepatic trauma: The exception or the rule. *J Trauma.* 1994;36:529–535.
35. Gaarder C, Dormagen JB, Eken T, et al. Non-operative management of splenic injuries: Improved results with angioembolization. *J Trauma.* 2006;61:192–198.
36. Daphne AL. American Association for the Surgery of Trauma. AAST injury scaling and scoring system; 1998, http://www.aast.org/injury/injury.html. Last accessed February 25, 2007.
37. Croce MA, Fabian TC, Menke PG, et al. Non-operative management of blunt hepatic trauma is the treatment of choice for hemodynamically stable patients: Results of a prospective trial. *Ann Surg.* 1995;221:744.
38. Jaik NP, Hoey BA, Stawicki SP. Evolving role of endoscopic retrograde cholangiopancreatography in management of extrahepatic hepatic ductal injuries due to blunt trauma: diagnostic and treatment algorithms. *HPB Surgery.* 2008; in press.
39. Huerta S, Bui T, Porral D, et al. Predictors of morbidity and mortality in patients with traumatic duodenal injuries. *Am Surg.* 2005;71:763–767.
40. Akhrass R, Yaffe MB, Brandt CP, et al. Pancreatic trauma: A ten-year multi-institutional experience. *Am Surg.* 1997;63:598–604.
41. Glancy KE. Review of pancreatic trauma. *West J Med.* 1989;151:45–51.
42. Ivatury RR, Nallathambi M, Rao P, et al. Penetrating pancreatic trauma: Analysis of 103 consecutive cases. *Am Surg.* 1990;56:90–95.
43. Gay SB, Sistrom CL. Computed tomography evaluation of blunt abdominal trauma. *Radiol Clin North Am.* 1992;30:367–388.
44. Lane MJ, Mindelzun RE, Sandhu JS, et al. CT diagnosis of blunt pancreatic trauma: Importance of detecting fluid between the pancreas and the splenic vein. *Am J Roentgenol.* 1994;163:833–835.
45. Gupta A, Stuhlfaut JW, Fleming KW, et al. Blunt trauma of the pancreas and biliary tract: A multimodality imaging approach to diagnosis. *Radiographics.* 2004;24:1381–1395.
46. Soto JA, Alvarez O, Munera F, et al. Traumatic disruption of the pancreatic duct: Diagnosis with MR pancreatography. *Am J Roentgenol.* 2001;176:175–178.
47. Wong YC, Wang LJ, Lin BC, et al. CT grading of blunt pancreatic injuries: Prediction of ductal disruption and surgical correlation. *J Comput Assist Tomogr.* 1997;21:246–250.
48. Bradley EL IIIrd, Young PR Jr, Chang MC, et al. Diagnosis and initial management of blunt pancreatic trauma: Guidelines from a multiinstitutional review. *Ann Surg* 1998;227:861–869.
49. Leppaniemi AK, Haapiainen RK. Risk factors of delayed diagnosis of pancreatic trauma. *Eur J Surg.* 1999;165:1134–1137.
50. Akhrass R, Kim K, Brandt C, et al. Computed tomography: An unreliable indicator of pancreatic trauma. *Am Surg.* 1996;62:647–651.
51. Carroll PR, McAninch JW. Major bladder trauma: Mechanisms of injury and a unified method of diagnosis and repair. *J Urol.* 1984;132:254–257.
52. Cass AS. The multiply injured patient with bladder trauma. *J Trauma.* 1984;24:731–734.
53. Hochberg E, Stone NN. Bladder rupture associated with pelvic fracture due to blunt trauma. *Urology.* 1993;41:531–533.
54. Cass AS, Gleich P, Smith C. Simultaneous bladder and prostatomembranous urethral rupture from external trauma. *J Urol.* 1984;132:907–908.
55. Corriere JN, Sandler CM Jr. Mechanisms of injury, patterns of extravasation and management of extraperitoneal bladder rupture due to blunt trauma. *J Urol.* 1988;139:43–44.
56. Cass AS, Luxenberg M. Management of extraperitoneal ruptures of bladder caused by external trauma. *Urology.* 1989;33:179–183.
57. Kotkin L, Koch MO. Morbidity associated with non-operative management of extraperitoneal bladder injuries. *J Trauma.* 1995;38:895–898.
58. Corriere JN, Sandler CM Jr. Management of extraperitoneal bladder rupture. *Urol Clin North Am.* 1989;16:275–277.
59. Bellamy RF, Zajtchuk R, eds. *Conventional warfare: ballistic, blast and burn injuries.* Washington, DC: Office of the Surgeon General, Department of the Army; 1990.
60. Swan KG, Swan RC. Principles of ballistics applicable to the treatment of gunshot wounds. *Surg Clin North Am.* 1991;71:221–239.
61. Muckart DJ, Abdoul-Carrin ATO, King B. Selective conservative management of abdominal gunshot wounds: A prospective study. *Br J Surg.* 1990;77:652–655.
62. Demetriades D, Charalambides D, Lakhoo M, et al. Gunshot wounds of the abdomen: Role of selective conservative management. *Br J Surg.* 1991;78:220–222.
63. Zierold D, Perlstein J, Weidman ER, et al. Penetrating trauma to the diaphragm: Natural history and ultrasonographic characteristics of untreated injury in the pig model. *Arch Surg.* 2001;136:32–37.
64. Renz BM, Feliciano DV. The length of hospital stay after an unnecessary laparotomy for trauma: A prospective study. *J Trauma.* 1996;40:187–190.

65. Chmielewski GW, Nicholas JM, Dulchawsky SA, et al. Non-operative management of gunshot wounds of the abdomen. *Am Surg.* 1995;61:665–668.

66. Demetriades D, Gomez H, Chahwan S, et al. Gunshot wounds to the liver: The role of selective non-operative management. *J Am Coll Surg.* 1999;188:343–348.

67. Guth AA, Patcher HL, Kim U. Pitfalls in the diagnosis of diaphragmatic injury. *Am J Surg.* 1995;170:5–9.

68. Murray JA, Demetriades D, Cornwell EE, et al. Penetrating left thoracoabdominal trauma: The incidence and clinical presentation of diaphragm injuries. *J Trauma.* 1997;43:624–626.

69. Phillips T, Scalafani SJA, Goldstein A, et al. Use of contrast enhanced CT enema in the management of penetrating trauma to the flank and back. *J Trauma.* 1986;26:593–596.

70. Kirton OC, Wint D, Thrasher B, et al. Stab wounds to the back and flank in the hemodynamically stable patient: A decision algorithm based on contrast-enhanced computed tomography with colonic opacification. *Am J Surg.* 1997;173:189–193.

71. Ginzburg E, Carillo EH, Kopelman T, et al. The role of computed tomography in selective management of gunshot wounds to the abdomen and flank. *J Trauma.* 1998;45:1005–1009.

72. DiGiacomo JC, Schwab CW, Rotondo MF, et al. Gluteal gunshot wounds: Who warrants exploration? *J Trauma.* 1994;37:622–628.

73. Velmahos GC, Demetriades D, Cornwell EE, et al. Gunshot wounds to the buttocks: Predicting the need for operation. *Dis Col Rectum.* 1997;40:307–311.

74. Velmahos GC, Demetriades D, Cornwell EE. Transpelvic gunshot wounds: Routine laparotomy or selective management? *World J Surg.* 1998;22:1034–1038.

SUGGESTED READINGS

Bowlanger BR, Kearney PA, Tsuei B, et al. The routine use of sonography in penetrating torso injury is beneficial. *J Trauma.* 2001;51:320–325.

Coley BD, Mutabagani KH, Martin LC, et al. Focused Abdominal Sonography for Trauma (FAST) in children with blunt abdominal trauma. *J Trauma.* 2000;48:902–906.

Thurani VH, Pettitt BJ, Schmidt JA, et al. Validation of surgeon-performed emergency abdominal ultrasound in pediatric trauma patients. *J Pediatr Surg.* 1998;33:322–328.

Udobi KF, Rodriguez A, Chin WC, et al. Role of ultrasonography in penetrating abdominal trauma: A prospective clinical study. *J Trauma.* 2001;50:475–479.

Injuries to the Esophagus and Stomach

39

Niels D. Martin   *Babak Sarani*

ESOPHAGEAL TRAUMA

Introduction

Injury to the esophagus is very rare, with the overwhelming majority of trauma being caused by penetrating injury. Iatrogenic injuries from foreign bodies or forceful vomiting are far more common but will not be discussed in this chapter. Although infrequent, a complete understanding of the diagnosis and management of esophageal trauma is essential to minimize the morbidity and mortality associated with esophageal injuries. Time from injury to definitive management and the degree of soilage to surrounding tissues are the most important factors for morbidity. The most important difference between traumatic injury and other forms of esophageal perforation is the high incidence of concomitant injury. Often, the underlying cause of morbidity or mortality in trauma patients is not the esophageal injury itself, but rather the constellation of other injuries sustained. For these reasons, the trauma surgeon must be aware of how esophageal injuries can present and expedite their evaluation.[1]

Anatomy and Mechanism of Injury

The esophagus can be divided into three anatomic regions: cervical, thoracic, and abdominal. These regions differ in the associated injury pattern and also in the approach to the diagnosis and management of the esophageal injury itself. The cervical esophagus borders the trachea anteriorly, the spine posteriorly, and the carotid sheaths laterally. Cervical esophageal injuries are the most common overall and are the least lethal. Thoracic esophageal injuries are the second most common and carry the highest morbidity and mortality due to their proximity to other vital structures and the risk of severe mediastinal sepsis. The abdominal esophagus is the least commonly injured. The Organ Injury Scaling Committee of the American Association for the Surgery of Trauma has created a standardized grading system for esophageal injuries based on the degree of injury ranging from contusion to laceration to segmental loss (see Table 1).[2]

Injury patterns in esophageal trauma vary based on mechanism. As already noted, most esophageal injuries involve penetrating trauma, but the specific cause of penetrating esophageal injury (gunshot vs. stab wound) may differ based on the common type of weapons used in a particular area. For example, gunshot wounds are more common in the United States whereas stab wounds are more prevalent in other areas of the world. Penetrating cervical esophageal injury is present in <1% of all penetrating trauma, but is found in 5% to 12% of all penetrating trauma to the neck.[3–5] Conversely, penetrating thoracic esophageal trauma has a reported incidence of <1% of all penetrating wounds to the chest.[6]

Depending on muzzle velocity, bullet characteristics, and the attitude of the projectile, gunshot wounds can cause significant shearing, stretch, and blast injury to surrounding tissues. Therefore, ischemia and full-thickness

TABLE 1

THE ORGAN INJURY SCALING COMMITTEE OF THE AMERICAN ASSOCIATION FOR THE SURGERY OF TRAUMA GRADING SCALE OF ESOPHAGEAL INJURY

Grade	Description
I	Contusion/hematoma
II	Laceration <50%
III	Laceration >50%
IV	<2 cm disruption of tissue or vasculature
V	>2 cm disruption of tissue or vasculature

Moore EE, Jurkovich GJ, Knudson MM, et al. Organ injury scaling. VI: Extrahepatic biliary, esophagus, stomach, vulva, vagina, uterus (nonpregnant), uterus (pregnant), fallopian tube, and ovary. *J Trauma-Injury Infect Crit Care*. 1995;39(16):1069–1070.

TABLE 2

INCIDENCE OF CONCOMITANT INJURIES IN PATIENTS WITH ESOPHAGEAL INJURY

Injury	Incidence (%)
Vascular	5–40
Lung	5–35
Trachea	15–64
Spinal cord	8–16
Diaphragm	10–20
All injuries	88

Asensio JA, Chahwan S, Forno W, et al. Penetrating esophageal injuries: Multicenter study of the American Association for the Surgery of Trauma. *J Trauma-Injury Infect Crit Care*. 2001;50(2):289–296; Glatterer MS Jr, Toon RS, Ellestad C, et al. Management of blunt and penetrating external esophageal trauma. *J Trauma-Injury Infect Crit Care*. 1985;25(8):784–792; Armstrong WB, Detar TR, Stanley RB. Diagnosis and management of external penetrating cervical esophageal injuries. *Ann Otol Rhinol Laryngol*. 1994;103(11):863–871; Attar S, Hankins JR, Suter CM, et al. Esophageal perforation: A therapeutic challenge. *Ann Thorac Surg*. 1990;50(1):45–51; Ngakane H, Muckart DJ, Luvuno FM. Penetrating visceral injuries of the neck: Results of a conservative management policy. *Br J Neurosurg*. 1990;77(8):908–910; Richardson JD, Tobin GR. Closure of esophageal defects with muscle flaps. *Arch Surg*. 1994;129(5):541–548; Winter RP, Weigelt JA. Cervical esophageal trauma. Incidence and cause of esophageal fistulas. *Arch Surg*. 1990;125(7):849–852.

necrosis may evolve with time resulting in a delay in presentation of significant injury. Stab wounds, on the other hand, generally cause minimal injury to surrounding tissues. As will be discussed further, using advanced imaging for trajectory determination, especially for the path of a bullet, is a key aid to help determine esophageal injury.[7] However, it should be remembered that using imaging for this process is less reliable following stab injury because surrounding tissues are less disturbed or disrupted.

Blunt esophageal injury most commonly affects the abdominal esophagus. Such injury results from the sudden application of a blunt force to the abdomen, usually with a full stomach. This causes the gastroesophageal (GE) junction to stretch against the hiatal crura, which in turn act as a guillotine.[8] The lack of a serosal layer on the esophagus makes an injury more likely to result in perforation. Motor vehicle collisions are the most common cause.[9]

Esophageal injury can also result from trauma to other structures. For example, vertebral column injuries associated with bony fragmentation can injure the esophagus—especially where the esophagus lies in very close proximity to the spine at C5 and T3-T4.[10] Mediastinal hematomas have also been described to cause external compression on the esophagus and become clinically symptomatic from compression.[11]

It is crucial to understand that most traumatic esophageal injuries are not isolated injuries; therefore once noted, investigation of adjacent and associated structures should be undertaken to rule out concomitant injuries. In the largest study to date, Asensio et al. performed a multicenter retrospective review and reported 88% of patients with esophageal trauma had associated injuries. In this review, Asensio et al. found significant associations with tracheal, vascular, pulmonary, diaphragmatic, and spinal cord injuries.[12] In a similar study, Glatterer et al. reported on 26 patients with esophageal trauma, noting 24 had associated injuries, 14 of which involved the trachea.[13] Table 2 summarizes the incidence of concomitant injuries in patients with esophageal injury.

Presentation and Diagnosis

A high index of suspicion coupled with accurate, timely, and high-resolution imaging is necessary because injury to the esophagus commonly presents with nonspecific signs and symptoms or can be totally asymptomatic. Notably, Smakman et al. found that <10% of patients presented with bloody nasogastric aspirate, hematemesis, or pneumomediastinum.[14] Clinical examination was negative in 80% of all esophageal injuries.[5] Signs and symptoms that are associated with esophageal injury can include pain, fever, dysphagia, odynophagia, hematemesis, hoarse voice, subcutaneous emphysema/crepitus, mediastinal crunch (Hamman sign), oropharyngeal blood, hemoptysis, and dyspnea (see Table 3).[15-18] Most series of esophageal perforation have reported the most common symptoms to be chest pain (71% to 85%), followed by fever (51% to 90%) and dyspnea (24% to 40%).[19,20] However, these data generally include all esophageal injury modalities of which only 20% to 25% of the cohort is traumatically injured.

Various modalities, including chest x-ray (CXR), esophagography, esophagoscopy, and computed tomography (CT) scan can be used to image the esophagus. Chest x-ray and lateral C-spine films are usually the first images obtained in a trauma patient but are also the least specific. Air in the soft tissues of the neck or mediastinum mandates

TABLE 3

COMMON SIGNS AND SYMPTOMS OF ESOPHAGEAL PERFORATION (%)

Sign/Symptom	Smakman et al.	Goudy et al.
Prevertebral air	48	—
Fever	—	—
Pain/odynophagia	21	—
Blood in NG tube	10	—
Hoarseness	10	—
Hematemesis	6	—
Hemoptysis	6	—
Mediastinal air	—	—
Dysphagia	29	63
Hemothorax	33	—
Widened mediastinum	10	—
Crepitus/subcutaneous emphysema	46	21
Dyspnea	—	—

NG, nasogastric.
Smakman N, Nicol AJ, Walther G, et al. Factors affecting outcome in penetrating oesophageal trauma. *Br J Neurosurg.* 2004;91(11): 1513–1519; Goudy SL, Miller FB, Bumpous JM. Neck crepitance: Evaluation and management of suspected upper aerodigestive tract injury. *Laryngoscope.* 2002;112(5):791–795.

further evaluation of the aerodigestive system, especially in the absence of pneumothorax.

CT is much more sensitive than plain films in noting air and fluid collections around the esophagus. Although pneumomediastinum and/or pleural effusions are associated with esophageal injury, the lack of these findings does not adequately exclude injury and their presence does not definitively diagnose injury. CT is also helpful for determining bullet trajectory but less so for tracts created by stab wounds. Further invasive studies can often be eliminated from the diagnostic workup if CT scan demonstrates trajectories remote from the esophagus.[21] Trajectory determination on CT is much more difficult for stab wounds because of the minimal blast effect, hemorrhage, and deposition of air along the wound tract.[22,23] In conjunction with clinical examination, CT can help determine whether further directed workup is necessary. As stated previously, even small amounts of air within the mediastinum or neck, especially in the absence of pneumothorax, mandate full evaluation of the aerodigestive system.

Formal evaluation of the esophagus is reserved for patients who are suspected of having an esophageal injury. This entails laryngoscopy for proximal injuries and esophagoscopy with or without esophagography for the remainder of the esophagus. The decision as to whether to use rigid or flexible endoscopy for trauma patient evaluation is controversial, although most centers now rely mainly on flexible endoscopy due to its ease of use at the bedside, lack of need for general anesthesia, and safety in patients who remain in cervical spine precautions.[17,24]

Endoscopy is usually the first tool used after radiographic imaging. It is available, simple, and in trained hands, technically easy. However, flexible endoscopy alone must be used with caution. Flexible esophagoscopy has been shown to have a 40% to 100% sensitivity and 66% to 100% specificity with a positive predictive value of 33% and negative predictive value of 100%.[5,20,24,25] Flexible esophagoscopy has a lower sensitivity in the cervical esophagus as compared to the thoracic esophagus, and rigid esophagoscopy remains the preferred endoscopic modality for diagnosis of proximal esophageal injury.

Esophagography, utilizing water-soluble followed by barium contrast, was historically the gold standard in evaluating esophageal injury. Unfortunately, the patient's clinical status may not allow for contrast imaging; for example, a patient with a decreased mental status at risk of aspiration or an intubated patient who cannot actively swallow contrast. Esophagography may be more sensitive than flexible endoscopy in evaluating the cervical esophagus, but the two modalities are equivalent in evaluating the thoracic esophagus.[20]

The most recent literature suggests that the new gold standard is the combination of both flexible esophagoscopy and esophagography.[5,26,27] Combining both modalities results in almost 100% sensitivity and specificity in detecting all esophageal injuries, although many trauma surgeons suggest this is needed only in cases where either study alone is technically limited.

Management Options

The management of esophageal injuries depends on location, time of diagnosis, associated injuries, and general medical condition. In general, the earlier esophageal injuries are addressed, the better. This is especially true in thoracic esophageal injuries where continued soilage of the mediastinum can cause severe sepsis and impede healing of a future repair. It should be remembered that the lack of a serosal layer makes esophageal repair far more tenuous than that of other parts of the gastrointestinal (GI) tract. Although attention to more life-threatening injuries or other pressing medical conditions may take precedence, the potential morbidity of waiting to repair an esophageal injury is significant. Definitive closure and drainage are best carried out as soon as possible.

Nonoperative Management

Nonoperative management is possible in patients who have contained leaks and few signs/symptoms or those who are moribund and unable to survive surgery. These patients generally have had a significant delay in diagnosis and have a high mortality rate. A contained leak is best described as extravasation of contrast on esophagography, but the contrast "goes-out and back-in" the esophagus.[28]

This is usually a small area not associated with a standing fluid collection, mediastinal inflammation, or pleural effusion. If any of these criteria are violated, serious consideration should be given to invasive treatment.[28] Esophagography can be repeated in several days to document resolution before starting a soft diet. Patients not fit for operative intervention because of severe sepsis or pulmonary compromise should undergo wide chest drainage at the bedside using more than one large chest tube.

Operative Management

Although there are no prospective studies defining a safe period during which preoperative testing can be completed before operative intervention, there is general agreement that esophageal injury is a surgical emergency and preoperative testing must be expedited to facilitate a timely repair. Frequently, the severity of concomitant injuries necessitates delay of esophageal repair. Recently, it has been shown that morbidity is more accurately predicted by the degree of soilage. There is a preponderance of recent literature that states the degree of inflammation in surrounding tissues, and not time since injury *per se*, should dictate whether primary repair or simply drainage should be performed.[8,13,14,29,30] Repairs can be accomplished, even at delayed time periods, in select patients with minimal soilage at time of surgery. It should be noted, however, that morbidity and mortality is mainly related to anastomotic failure, and breakdown of the esophageal repair is associated with at least 50% mortality.[1]

Location of the injury is another factor that dictates the surgical approach and repair options (see Table 4). Cervical injuries are best approached from the left neck where the recurrent nerve can be more easily identified and preserved. The incision should be placed at the anterior border of the sternocleidomastoid muscle and carried down through the soft tissues between the trachea and the carotid sheath. The esophagus can be mobilized bluntly with a finger circumferentially with careful attention not to injure either recurrent nerve or the membranous portion of the trachea. Thoracic esophageal injuries are best approached from a right posterolateral thoracotomy. Appropriate positioning is imperative to optimize visualization, and therefore fashion a better technical repair. The intercostal muscle bundle should receive careful attention and be preserved when entering the chest, as it is a potential repair-buttressing flap. The distal third of the thoracic esophagus actually lies more to the left and can be accessible either from a left posterolateral thoracostomy or from the abdomen after appropriate mobilization. Lastly, the intra-abdominal esophagus is best accessed by an upper midline laparotomy. This should be carried up to the xiphoid process and down to at least just below the umbilicus.

TABLE 4

SURGICAL REPAIR OPTIONS FOR ESOPHAGEAL INJURY

Surgery	Comments
Primary repair	Preferred approach in 70%–80% of patients, two-layer repair, buttress with intercostal flap or stomach
Diversion/ exclusion	Can result in bacterial overgrowth and sepsis, makes subsequent reconstruction difficult
T-tube	Used mostly in distal esophageal injury in the area of the GE junction; can be a good temporizing measure for a difficult area to expose and repair
Esophagectomy	Poorly tolerated during initial surgery, but removes source of ongoing mediastinal sepsis

GE, gastroesophageal.

Primary Repair

Primary repair of an esophageal injury requires attention to several important tenets. First, the tissues must be fully debrided to healthy tissue. Use of necrotic or devascularized tissue will result in failure of the repair. Second, esophageal injuries are largest at the mucosa. Therefore, simply identifying and repairing the muscular portion of the injury will inevitably result in nonclosure of the mucosal defect. The muscular defect should be enlarged until the ends of the mucosal injury are identified. Next, the repair must be tensionfree, mobilization of the esophagus should be minimized because its blood supply is segmental and overmobilization can make the anastomosis ischemic and result in a postoperative leak. Finally, the esophagus should be repaired in a two-layer manner utilizing an inner, running, absorbable suture and an outer interrupted nonabsorbable suture.

Repairs should be buttressed with local tissue and muscle flaps, especially if repair is delayed (longer than 8 to 12 hours since injury) or if there is a concomitant injury with an adjacent suture line.[14] For example, injury to both the esophagus and trachea with parallel suture lines should be separated by a tissue flap to help prevent fistula formation. These muscle flaps can potentially improve the vascular supply in contaminated fields, and thereby expedite healing and lower bacterial counts.[31] The choice of tissue flap is dictated by location and the flap's inherent vascular supply. Commonly used flaps include latissimus dorsi, serratus anterior, or intercostal muscles. Pericardium or pleura may be too weak and avascular to serve as an adequate tissue flap, although this may change in late repairs when these tissues are inflamed and have increased blood flow.

In the neck, the sternocleidomastoid muscle can be placed between adjacently injured structures or to reinforce a tenuous repair. Owing to its abundant blood supply and location, the sternocleidomastoid is a reliable and convenient flap.[31] Wrapping the esophagus with a platysma flap has also been described.[32] In the chest, the intercostal muscle flap is the simplest and most reliable tissue flap. Careful attention to preserving this flap must be maintained when entering the chest. Other options in the chest include the latissimus dorsi, the rhomboid, and the diaphragm. In the abdomen, a Thal patch (gastric fundus) or various types of fundoplications can be performed.

Appropriate drainage should accompany all repairs so that in the event of an anastomotic breakdown, the leak can be potentially noted earlier and hopefully contained. This is especially important in the chest as an undrained mediastinal collection can lead to severe sepsis and carries a significant mortality rate. Utilized appropriately and performed in a timely manner, primary repair of the esophagus has the lowest morbidity and mortality of any treatment modality for esophageal injury.

Wide Chest Drainage

Wide chest drainage alone can be utilized as a "damage control" option in patients who are not candidates for primary repair or diversion. This may be due to other more pressing injuries, preterminal comorbid conditions, or in cases of heavily inflamed and soiled tissues where the esophagus cannot be manipulated. This type of damage control drainage can be performed in the intensive care unit (ICU) in patients who are too unstable to withstand formal operative drainage; however, operative placement of drains is much more effective. Beyond initial management, if wide chest drainage is to become primary management, it is usually combined with esophageal diversion and/or exclusion as described in the subsequent text. Generally, wide chest drainage alone is utilized in moribund patients and therefore portends an exceedingly high mortality.

Diversion and Exclusion

Esophageal diversion and exclusion allow for decreased flow of oral secretions and reflux of gastric contents across an injury. A diverting cervical esophagostomy should be performed in all patients where reliable primary repair is not feasible and wide drainage is the definitive treatment. Esophageal exclusion (diversion plus closure of the gastroesophageal junction) is performed for extensive esophageal injuries or those diagnosed late with significant tissue contamination and swelling. These injuries are usually in the mid to distal esophagus.

Patients with a delayed diagnosis of esophageal injury can present with marked inflammation of the upper mediastinum that can preclude mobilization and thereby creation of a proximal loop esophagostomy. In such cases an end cervical esophagostomy can be formed, but if combined with a distal exclusion a blind loop of esophagus is created. This is an acceptable treatment strategy for 2 to 7 days while the mediastinal sepsis resolves. Careful attention must be given for the development of blind loop

syndrome once the esophageal injury seals. Bacterial stasis and overgrowth within the excluded esophagus can result in sepsis. CT imaging will usually display a grossly dilated and enhancing esophagus. Drainage of the loop is adequate temporizing therapy until the inflammation resolves to a point where resection and reconstruction are possible.

T-tube diversion of the esophagus can be used for smaller distal injuries in patients who are not candidates for primary repair, and where formal diversion and exclusion may not be needed.[33] The T-tube is placed directly through the injury into the esophagus and kept on constant suction to create a controlled fistula. The tube is kept in place for several weeks to allow a tract to form. This approach may be especially useful for small injuries near the GE junction. Placement of large-bore mediastinal and pleural tubes should accompany the T-tube. Once resuscitated, the patient will need a decompressing gastrostomy tube and feeding jejunostomy tube.

In patients with significant comorbid conditions, intra-luminal stenting has been described as a means to prevent swallowed material from contacting the esophageal wall as it heals.[32] This technology is still in its infancy, but may play more of a role in the future.

Esophagectomy

Esophagectomy is rarely required as therapy for esophageal injuries but is occasionally required if primary repair fails or after damage control using diversion/exclusion. Esophagectomy in these circumstances should always be performed using the Ivor-Lewis technique because the mediastinum will be too inflamed to allow a transhiatal approach. Because of the difficult technical nature of the surgery, it should be carried out in conjunction with experienced thoracic or esophageal surgeons.

Reconstruction after esophagectomy can be performed using a colonic interposition (usually transverse colon), a Roux-en-Y jejunal limb or a gastric pull-up. Often, the decision as to which conduit to use depends on the concomitant injuries sustained and subsequent availability of noninjured, well-perfused organs. By far, the simplest technical repair, resulting in only one anastomosis, is the gastric pull-up.[34] Because the stomach is usually the conduit of choice, gastrostomy tubes should not be placed in patients with esophageal injuries. Feeding access should always be through a jejunostomy tube.

Postoperative Care

Postoperative care involves appropriate monitoring in an ICU setting. Early recognition and treatment of sepsis is paramount. Early nutrition also plays an important role in recovery. Total parenteral nutrition or jejunostomy feeding should be started as soon as possible—jejunal feeds may be superior to parenteral feeds. Contrast swallow evaluations should take place 5 to 7 days postprimary repair if no clinical signs of a leak are present. All drains should be maintained until contrast radiography documents healing.

Complications

Anastomotic breakdown is unfortunately not a rare occurrence after repair of an esophageal injury. Depending on location, these leaks can subsequently cause wound infection, mediastinitis, abscess, empyema, pneumonia, and sepsis. Of all these complications, sepsis carries the highest mortality. The goal of therapy should be prevention of sepsis by maintenance or establishment of wide drainage.[17]

Fistula formation between the repaired esophagus and adjacent structures can present in the postoperative period or in a delayed manner. Their incidence increases when an adjacent structure also requires surgical repair. Cutaneous and vascular fistulas have been described, but the most common fistula is a tracheal-esophageal fistula. These fistulae usually form at or just above the carina, and present with pneumonia or cough after swallowing.[18]

Longer-term complications include stricture formation at the anastomotic sites. These strictures can usually be treated with endoscopic dilations, although some may require esophagectomy. Diverticulum formation has also been noted after repair; treatment of which depends on size, location, and clinical circumstance.

Summary

Esophageal injuries can result from both penetrating and blunt trauma. The need to screen for injury is based on a high degree of suspicion. Many patients may be asymptomatic initially. Imaging using CT scan is helpful to determine the potential for injury, especially in penetrating injury. Further workup should be timely, as an early diagnosis can help prevent further soilage and subsequent morbidity and mortality. Flexible endoscopy and contrast esophagography are complementary and together give the highest diagnostic yield. Primary repair with suture line reinforcement using muscle flaps and wide drainage affords the patient the best outcome. Early enteral nutrition through jejunostomy is preferred to parenteral nutrition. Overall, the morbidity and mortality of esophageal trauma are high and a high index of suspicion and aggressive treatment plan is required to optimize outcome.

GASTRIC TRAUMA

Introduction

Surgical repair of penetrating injuries to the abdominal cavity were first reported by the ancient Greek civilization. Nollenson was the first to successfully surgically repair a gastric wound in 1765, and Theodore Kocher reported the first successful repair of a gunshot wound to the stomach in the late 19th century. The mortality of gastric injury decreased in the 20th century from 29% during World War I to <5% after World War II.[35] Such a dramatic decrease is most likely due to improvements in surgical technique, perioperative care, and expediency in transport of the injured patient to a surgical facility.

The stomach is unique in that it has three layers of muscle. As such, blunt perforation of the stomach requires a large transfer of energy. Therefore, isolated gastric injuries resulting from blunt trauma are exceedingly rare and much of the associated morbidity and mortality are due to other concomitant injuries.[36] Similarly, because the stomach is located in the center of the epigastric region, isolated gastric injuries are also rare. However, its ability to distend markedly renders it susceptible to injury from various trajectories resulting from penetrating trauma.

The stomach is anchored superiorly by the GE junction and the gastrohepatic and gastrophrenic ligaments, laterally at the greater curve by the short gastric arteries which attach it to the spleen, medially by the pylorus/duodenum, and inferiorly by the greater omentum and transverse colon. Of note, posteriorly the stomach abuts the pancreas, left kidney, and left adrenal gland. Anteriorly, the left lobe of the liver covers the proximal stomach. Variable portions of the stomach can move into an intrathoracic position above the left hemidiaphragm, as with various types of hiatal herniae, thereby rendering the stomach potentially susceptible to injury from thoracic trauma. As discussed in subsequent text, high-energy blunt trauma can result in rupture of the left hemidiaphragm and herniation of the stomach and the viscera to which it is attached to the left hemithorax.

The stomach has a rich arterial supply: the right and left gastroepiploic, right and left gastric, and short gastric arteries. Therefore, the stomach can heal most suture lines but can also be the site for life-threatening hemorrhage if hemostasis is not complete. The stomach needs only one of its four main arteries to remain viable and tolerate surgical repair, resection, and reconstruction.[37]

Incidence and Mechanism of Injury

Gastric trauma can manifest as contusion, intramural hematoma, penetration, or perforation. Table 5 depicts the Organ Injury Scale (OIS) grading system of the stomach and surgical repair options. This chapter will only address traumatic injury to the stomach and will not discuss iatrogenic injuries or perforation due to other causes.

Perforation of the stomach due to blunt injury is extremely rare, with an incidence of 0.02% to 1.7%.[36,38] The incidence of gastric contusion or hematoma is not known as these injuries are not easily detectable radiographically and are most often diagnosed incidentally during laparotomy. As such, the true incidence of all gastric injury, including contusion and hematoma, is most likely underreported in the literature. However, the total incidence of injury may

TABLE 5

GRADE OF GASTRIC INJURY

Grade	Extent of Injury	Surgical Repair
I	Intramural hematoma OR superficial laceration	Observe or drain with Lembert, imbricated repair
II	<2 cm laceration of pylorus or GE junction OR	Primary repair
	<5 cm laceration of proximal one third of stomach OR	—
	<10 cm laceration of distal two thirds of stomach	—
III	>2 cm laceration of pylorus or GE junction OR	Primary repair
	≥5 cm laceration of proximal one third of stomach OR	Close pylorus as pyloroplasty
	≥10 cm laceration of distal two thirds of stomach	Consider total gastrectomy for GE[a] junction injury
IV	Perforation or devascularization of less than two thirds of stomach	Subtotal/total gastrectomy with either Roux-en-Y or Billroth II reconstruction
V	Perforation or devascularization of more than two thirds of stomach	Gastrectomy with Roux-en-Y reconstruction

[a]GE, gastroesophageal.

not be clinically relevant in the absence of perforation or other concomitant injuries because most gastric contusions and hematoma will be asymptomatic and resolve over time. As previously noted, the thick muscular wall of the stomach and its ability to distend prevents most OIS grade I injuries from resulting in either obstruction or perforation—the possible exception being large hematoma of the distal stomach which may cause luminal narrowing.

Although the exact mechanism for gastric rupture from blunt trauma has not been elucidated, gastric distension is known to increase the risk of perforation.[38–40] The site of perforation is most commonly the anterior wall of the stomach, and Table 6 lists the areas prone to rupture with their reported incidence.[41] The law of LaPlace states that tension across the wall of a hollow viscus is greatest in areas with the largest radius. This may explain the reason for such an injury pattern, especially if the force is transmitted at a time when the pylorus and lower esophageal sphincters are both closed. Another proposed mechanism involves crushing of the distended stomach against the spine.

Blunt gastric perforation is most often due to sudden deceleration, although other mechanisms whereby significant kinetic energy is transmitted to the abdomen can also tear the stomach. Most commonly, this involves high energy transfer, such as a pedestrian struck by a motor vehicle or a motor vehicle collision, either with ejection of the occupant or an improperly worn lap belt. Alvarez and Bruscagin found in independent, retrospective studies that 75% to 85% of gastric perforations from blunt trauma were due to one or another of these mechanisms.[38,41] Much less commonly, direct blows to the abdomen, such as a kick by a horse or handle bar injury, can also result in gastric injury.

As stated in preceding text, blunt injury to the stomach requires great force, and has a high association with other concomitant injuries. Bruscagin found a mean injury severity score of 17 (range 4 to 50) when blunt trauma resulted in gastric perforation.[41] He also found that 95% of patients had at least one other major injury. The most common concomitant injuries involved the spleen (27% to 43%) and the left chest (18% to 29%), followed by the liver (18%) and small bowel (18%).[38,41]

Penetrating injury to the stomach is more common and must be evaluated if the site of skin penetration is inferior to the nipples (or fourth intercostal space) anteriorly or the tips of the scapulae posteriorly. As

TABLE 6

THE REPORTED INCIDENCE OF GASTRIC RUPTURE/PERFORATION BY LOCATION

Location	Incidence (%)
Anterior wall	40
Greater curve	23
Lesser curve	15
Posterior wall	15

Bruscagin V, Coimbra R, Rasslan S, et al. Blunt gastric injury. A multicentre experience. *Injury.* 2001;32(10):761–764; Yajko RD, Seydel F, Trimble C. Rupture of the stomach from blunt abdominal trauma. *J Trauma.* 1975;15(3):177–183.

discussed elsewhere, gunshot trajectory can be determined by radiographic imaging to determine the possibility of gastric (or other abdominal) injury. In all patients, skin markers and plain film x-ray are helpful and in stable patients contrast-enhanced CT scan, if necessary, is more precise.[42] Furthermore, in addition to assessing the other organs in the abdomen, injury to the left hemidiaphragm and pancreas must specifically be evaluated when assessing for possible penetrating trauma to the stomach. Gunshot wounds to the stomach usually cause two perforations, and the entire stomach including the posterior wall and the GE junction must be thoroughly visualized to prevent missed injuries.

Diagnosis

Penetrating injury to the stomach may be asymptomatic initially, especially if the time from injury to presentation to the hospital is short and other organs have not been injured. However, gastric perforation from blunt trauma is rarely asymptomatic because of the large energy transfer required to cause such injury. The extent of the perforation or rupture is usually large with excessive spillage of acid and food contents and resultant chemical peritonitis. Table 7 depicts the reported symptom(s) patients may have on arrival at the emergency department. Caution must be used in evaluating patients with traumatic brain injury, distracting injury, or patients who have ingested illicit substances or excessive amounts of alcohol as the clinical diagnosis of hollow viscus injury may be falsely negative in 50% of these patients.[43,44]

Multiple tests are available to assess for possible gastric or other hollow viscus injury. Although the presence of

TABLE 7

SYMPTOMS OF GASTRIC RUPTURE/PERFORATION ON ARRIVAL TO THE EMERGENCY DEPARTMENT

Sign	Incidence (%)
Abdominal pain	45–90
Hematemesis or bloody nasogastric tube aspirate	29
Peritonitis	33
Shock	25–43

Brunsting LA, Morton JH. Gastric rupture from blunt abdominal trauma. *J Trauma.* 1987;27(8):887–891; Bruscagin V, Coimbra R, Rasslan S, et al. Blunt gastric injury. A multicentre experience. *Injury.* 2001;32(10):761–764; Bergqvist D, Hedelin H, Karlsson G, et al. Abdominal trauma during thirty years: Analysis of a large cases series. *Injury.* 1981:13(2):93–99; Hockerstedt K, Airo I, Karaharju E, et al. Abdominal trauma and laparotomy in 158 patients. A comparitive study of penetrating and blunt injury. *Acta Chir Scand.* 1982;148(1):9–14; Knottenbelt JD, Van AS S, Volschenk S. Gastric rupture from blunt trauma: Two unusual presentations. *Injury.* 1993;24(1):65–66.

subdiaphragmatic free air on CXR has a high positive predictive value for perforated hollow viscus, its absence does not rule out such injury. Frequently, the time from injury to evaluation in the trauma center is not sufficient to allow for accumulation of intraperitoneal air, and the initial CXR is most often a supine view where air may not be evident in the upper abdomen. Focused assessment by sonography for trauma (FAST) is used to assess for the presence of free fluid in the abdominal cavity. Although there are no controlled, prospective studies assessing its role in detecting gastric perforation, its sensitivity and specificity for small bowel injury after blunt trauma is 84% and 100%, respectively, although this technique is highly operator dependent.[45] In a retrospective study over 14 years, Bruscagin reported a sensitivity of 60% using FAST to diagnose gastric perforation in a retrospective study involving 33 patients with gastric perforation after blunt trauma, although only 5 out of 33 underwent testing with ultrasonography.[41] There was no protocol to guide which patients were evaluated with FAST as opposed to other modalities, and the authors do not state what factor(s) led the use of ultrasonography in evaluating these five patients. Because of this, FAST alone cannot be used to determine if the gastric injury exists and other modalities are needed for definitive diagnosis.

Diagnostic peritoneal lavage (DPL) is no longer commonly used but remains very useful in determining hollow viscus injury. Most often, either bloody turbid fluid or particulate matter is noted after lavage. Biochemically, alkaline phosphatase level >10 IU per L, amylase >20 IU per L, and white blood cell count >500 cells per mL have been shown to result in a sensitivity of 95% to 100%.[36,41,46] However, DPL is invasive and may require 1 to 2 hours to complete laboratory analysis of the effluent.

Although CT scan of the abdomen has become an indispensable tool in the evaluation of the stable trauma patient, there are no studies evaluating its ability to detect traumatic gastric perforation or rupture. However, findings of free intraperitoneal fluid without solid organ injury or stranding in the epigastric or peripancreatic region should raise strong concern for gastric or bowel injury. Administration of oral contrast may assist in diagnosing gastric perforation, although it also increases the risk of vomiting and aspiration.[47] To date, there are no studies defining the sensitivity and specificity of CT scan for detecting gastric perforation after blunt abdominal trauma.

Diagnostic laparoscopy can be used to determine the nature of free fluid noted on CT scan or to further evaluate for injury in easily visualized organs. To date, studies have not supported laparoscopic evaluation of the small bowel itself or laparoscopic repair of noted injuries.[48,49] Until studies validate its safety, laparoscopic evaluation of the posterior wall of the stomach or retroperitoneal structures and repair of injuries is not recommended. Patients with actual or suspected injury to these regions should undergo prompt conversion to open surgery and complete exploration for associated injuries. Complete gastric inspection requires mobilization of many structures and entrance into the lesser sac. Both the anterior and posterior walls of the stomach must be inspected up to the esophageal hiatus. This is best done using laparotomy, which remains the gold standard method to evaluate for and repair gastric injuries. In cases where a hole is found in the stomach, it is important to search rigorously for another perforation on the posterior wall, both curvatures, duodenum, and distal esophagus.

Surgical Repair

In general, an isolated gastric contusion is diagnosed as an incidental finding intraoperatively and can be managed expectantly. Intramural hematomas can be diagnosed by CT scan or during laparotomy. Although most hematomas can be observed, large intramural hematomas at the distal stomach can cause obstruction. Therefore, many trauma surgeons recommend drainage and imbrication of the wall of the stomach if laparotomy is required for other reasons.

As with other gastric surgeries, a nasogastric tube should be placed preoperatively to decompress the stomach. Occasionally, a larger than standard nasogastric tube is needed with repeated lavage to clear solid food material. The left lobe of the liver must be mobilized to allow for exposure of the proximal stomach. The short gastric arteries may have to be ligated to allow exposure of the greater curve of the proximal stomach, especially the posterior aspects of the fundus and cardia. Iatrogenic injury to the spleen during this maneuver is common and can be avoided by stretching the stomach medially and then individually ligating the short gastric vessels or cauterizing the vessels using an ultrasonic shear or vessel sealing system. The lesser sac and posterior wall of the stomach are most easily visualized by incising the avascular plane in the greater omentum (gastrocolic ligament). Care must be taken during this maneuver to prevent opening of the transverse mesocolon and ligation of the middle colic artery. Reverse Trendelenburg positioning is helpful.

Although most gastric injuries can be repaired primarily, some may require more sophisticated intervention. In general, the vast majority of gastric injuries can be repaired primarily; resection and complex reconstruction is seldom needed. Table 5 lists the most commonly used procedures by grade of injury. Grade I injuries can be either observed or reenforced with Lembert sutures. Grade II injuries can be repaired in one or two layers, although the authors prefer a two-layer technique consisting of an inner running, absorbable suture, and an outer, interrupted permanent suture. Grade III injury near the pylorus may require converting the injury into a pyloroplasty by extending it longitudinally and closing the pylorus transversely. Grade III injury near the GE junction can usually be

closed primarily and buttressed with a fundoplication. Very rarely, either total gastrectomy with Roux-en-Y esophagojejunostomy or proximal hemigastrectomy with esophagogastrostomy may be needed if the injured area is large or extensive devascularization is found. Although there is no outcome data in the trauma population, the latter option may result in significant postoperative reflux, and most authors recommend total gastrectomy for patients who have proximal gastric lesions (such as tumors). Regardless, wide drainage near the repair and GE junction with multiple suction drains is mandatory. The decision to reconstruct a grade IV injury with Billroth II or Roux-en-Y gastro-jejunostomy depends on whether there is concomitant duodenal injury. Although this specific intervention has not been studied, a Roux-en-Y repair is the treatment of choice to minimize retrograde flow of gastric juice into the duodenum if it has also been injured. Finally, a grade V repair will mandate a total gastrectomy and Roux-en-Y reconstruction. Such patients will usually be unstable, and the surgeries may require staging, following the principles of damage control laparotomy that are discussed elsewhere.

A unique but not uncommon set of injuries are rupture of the left hemidiaphragm and stomach with contamination in the left hemithorax and pleural space. Although this can occur with penetrating injury, larger diaphragmatic rupture and massive contamination are seen more frequently with high-energy blunt trauma. They are associated with concomitant and significant thoracic and intra-abdominal injury. After controlling leak from the GI tract, the left chest should be copiously irrigated and chest tubes placed. Even with such lavage, some patients will retain food materials within the pleural space and develop an empyema requiring subsequent thoracotomy. At times, left anterolateral thoracotomy for direct inspection and lavage is indicated to minimize the possibility of empyema.

As noted previously, patients with gastric injury almost always have other associated injuries. The principles of "damage control" must be remembered when treating the multiply injured patient, and it is prudent to perform a temporizing procedure to control bleeding and contamination and defer reconstruction in patients who are cold, coagulopathic, and acidemic. Such patients have improved outcome if the surgery is staged such that definitive reconstruction is performed after the patient has been resuscitated and homeostasis restored.

Postoperative Complications

The mortality and morbidity rates of gastric injury after blunt abdominal trauma are ill defined due to the rarity of the disorder. Many series have reported mortality rates of 0% to 65%, with a significant decrease noted most recently.[36,38,39,41] Mortality is due to concomitant injury(ies) and most commonly occurs in the perioperative period. Morbidities can be grouped into abdominal sepsis/inflammation, fistula formation, and GI hemorrhage. As noted in the preceding text, there is also the risk of empyema with left chest gastric contamination.

Postoperative morbidity is mainly related to chemical peritonitis and/or infectious complications. The degree of peritonitis is related to the severity of injury, timing of last meal (and therefore degree of contamination), and time to definitive control of the injury in the operating room.[36,50] It has been shown that abscess formation is much more likely in multisystem injury, especially if the colon has also been injured.[51,52] Recently, blood transfusion has also been shown to be an independent risk factor for morbidity, especially infectious complications, in traumatized patients.[53-57]

Fistula formation from a gastric wound is rare because of the stomach's rich blood supply and ability to heal. Because the fistula will often seal with nonoperative management, the treatment principles are essentially the same as with other fistulae: expectant management with fluid, electrolyte, and nutritional support. Skin care and control of effluent are keys to successful nonoperative management. If surgery is needed, resection of the involved portion of the stomach (if possible) and wide drainage are imperative.

Postoperative bleeding can be due to bleeding from the short gastric vessels after gastrectomy, or from anastomotic or repair suture lines. Bleeding from a short gastric artery is usually a technical problem and requires reoperation and surgical control. Bleeding from a gastroenteral or gastrorrhaphy suture line is often self-limited and can be addressed endoscopically as needed. There are no studies on when it is safe to perform an upper endoscopy after gastric surgery, and the decision to proceed with this modality in a patient with postoperative GI hemorrhage must be weighed against the possibility of disrupting the surgical repair.

REFERENCES

1. Andrade-Alegre R. Surgical treatment of traumatic esophageal perforations: Analysis of 10 cases. *Clinics.* 2005;60(5):375–380.
2. Moore EE, Jurkovich GJ, Knudson MM, et al. Organ injury scaling. VI: Extrahepatic biliary, esophagus, stomach, vulva, vagina, uterus (nonpregnant), uterus (pregnant), fallopian tube, and ovary. *J Trauma-Injury Infect Crit Care.* 1995;39(6):1069–1070.
3. Bladergroen MR, Lowe JE, Postlethwait RW. Diagnosis and recommended management of esophageal perforation and rupture. *Ann Thorac Surg.* 1986;42(3):235–239.
4. Meyer JP, Barrett JA, Schuler JJ, et al. Mandatory vs. selective exploration for penetrating neck trauma. A prospective assessment. *Arch Surg.* 1987;122(5):592–597.
5. Weigelt JA, Thal ER, Snyder WH III, et al. Diagnosis of penetrating cervical esophageal injuries. *Am J Surg.* 1987;154(6):619–622.
6. Cornwell EE III, Kennedy F, Ayad IA, et al. Transmediastinal gunshot wounds. A reconsideration of the role of aortography. *Arch Surg.* 1996;131(9):949–953.
7. Grossman MD, May AK, Schwab CW, et al. Determining anatomic injury with computed tomography in selected torso gunshot wounds. *J Trauma-Injury Infect Crit Care.* 1998;45(3):446–456.
8. Fernandez-Llamazares J, Moreno P, Garcia F, et al. Total rupture of the gastro-oesophageal junction after blunt trauma. *Eur J Surg.* 1999;165(1):73–74.
9. Beal SL, Pottmeyer EW, Spisso JM. Esophageal perforation following external blunt trauma. *J Trauma-Injury Infect Crit Care.* 1988;28(10):1425–1432.
10. Nakai S, Yoshizawa H, Kobayashi S, et al. Esophageal injury secondary to thoracic spinal trauma: The need for early diagnosis and aggressive surgical treatment. *J Trauma-Injury Infect Crit Care.* 1998;44(6):1086–1089.
11. Park NH, Kim JH, Choi DY, et al. Ischemic esophageal necrosis secondary to traumatic aortic transection. *Ann Thorac Surg.* 2004;78(6):2175–2178.
12. Asensio JA, Chahwan S, Forno W, et al. Penetrating esophageal injuries: Multicenter study of the American Association for the Surgery of Trauma. *J Trauma-Injury Infect Crit Care.* 2001;50(2):289–296.
13. Glatterer MS Jr, Toon RS, Ellestad C, et al. Management of blunt and penetrating external esophageal trauma. *J Trauma-Injury Infect Crit Care.* 1985;25(8):784–792.
14. Smakman N, Nicol AJ, Walther G, et al. Factors affecting outcome in penetrating oesophageal trauma. *Br J Neurosurg.* 2004;91(11):1513–1519.
15. Goudy SL, Miller FB, Bumpous JM. Neck crepitance: Evaluation and management of suspected upper aerodigestive tract injury. *Laryngoscope.* 2002;112(5):791–795.
16. Campisi P, Stewart C, Forte V. Penetrating esophageal injury by ingestion of a wire bristle. *J Pediatr Surg.* 2005;40(10):e15–e16.
17. Thompson EC, Porter JM, Fernandez LG. Penetrating neck trauma: An overview of management. *J Oral Maxillofac Surg.* 2002;60(8):918–923.
18. Euathrongchit J, Thoongsuwan N, Stern EJ. Nonvascular mediastinal trauma. *Radiol Clin North Am.* 2006;44(2):251–258.
19. Nesbitt JC, Sawyers JL. Surgical management of esophageal perforation. *Am Surg.* 1987;53(4):183–191.
20. White RK, Morris DM. Diagnosis and management of esophageal perforations. *Am Surg.* 1992;58(2):112–119.
21. Gracias VH, Reilly PM, Philpott J, et al. Computed tomography in the evaluation of penetrating neck trauma: A preliminary study. *Arch Surg.* 2001;136(11):1231–1235.
22. Shanmuganathan K, Matsumoto J. Imaging of penetrating chest trauma. *Radiol Clin North Am.* 2006;44(2):225–238.
23. Gonzalez RP, Falimirski M, Holevar MR, et al. Penetrating zone II neck injury: Does dynamic computed tomographic scan contribute to the diagnostic sensitivity of physical examination for surgically significant injury? A prospective blinded study [see comment]. *J Trauma-Injury Infect Crit Care.* 2003;54(1):61–64; discussion 4–5.
24. Flowers JL, Graham SM, Ugarte MA, et al. Flexible endoscopy for the diagnosis of esophageal trauma. *J Trauma-Injury Infect Crit Care.* 1996;40(2):261–265; discussion 5–6.
25. Srinivasan R, Haywood T, Horwitz B, et al. Role of flexible endoscopy in the evaluation of possible esophageal trauma after penetrating injuries. *Am J Gastroenterol.* 2000;95(7):1725–1729.
26. Cordero JA, Kuehler DH, Fortune JB. Distal esophageal rupture after external blunt trauma: Report of two cases. *J Trauma-Injury Infect Crit Care.* 1997;42(2):321–322.
27. Nagy KK, Roberts RR, Smith RF, et al. Trans-mediastinal gunshot wounds: Are stable patients really stable? *World J Surg.* 2002;26(10):1247–1250.
28. Cameron JL, Kieffer RF, Hendrix TR, et al. Selective nonoperative management of contained intrathoracic esophageal disruptions. *Ann Thorac Surg.* 1979;27(5):404–408.
29. Armstrong WB, Detar TR, Stanley RB. Diagnosis and management of external penetrating cervical esophageal injuries. *Ann Otol Rhinol Laryngol.* 1994;103(11):863–871.
30. Port JL, Kent MS, Korst RJ, et al. Thoracic esophageal perforations: A decade of experience. [see comment]. *Ann Thorac Surg.* 2003;75(4):1071–1074.
31. Losken A, Rozycki GS, Feliciano DV. The use of the sternocleidomastoid muscle flap in combined injuries to the esophagus and carotid artery or trachea. *J Trauma-Injury Infect Crit Care.* 2000;49(5):815–817.
32. Zhou JH, Jiang YG, Wang RW, et al. Management of corrosive esophageal burns in 149 cases. *J Thorac Cardiov Sur.* 2005;130(2):449–455.

33. Andrade-Alegre R. T-tube intubation in the management of late traumatic esophageal perforations: Case report. *J Trauma-Injury Infect Crit Care.* 1994;37(1):131–132.
34. Victorino GP, Porter JM, Henderson VJ. Use of a gastric pull-up for delayed esophageal reconstruction in a patient with combined traumatic injuries of the trachea and esophagus. *J Trauma-Injury Infect Crit Care.* 2000;49(3):563–564.
35. Ferrada R, Garcia A. Stomach and small bowel. In: Ivatury R, Cayten C, eds. *Textbook of penetrating trauma.* Philadelphia: Williams & Wilkins; 1996:598–607.
36. Brunsting LA, Morton JH. Gastric rupture from blunt abdominal trauma. *J Trauma.* 1987;27(8):887–891.
37. Barlow T, Bentley F, Walder D. Arteries, veins, and arteriovenous anastomoses in the human stomach. *Surg Gynecol Obstet.* 1951;130:608.
38. Tejerina Alvarez EE, Holanda MS, Lopez-Espadas F, et al. Gastric rupture from blunt abdominal trauma. *Injury.* 2004;35(3):228–231.
39. Siemens RA, Fulton RL. Gastric rupture as a result of blunt trauma. *Am Surg.* 1977;43(4):229–233.
40. Talton DS, Craig MH, Hauser CJ, et al. Major gastroenteric injuries from blunt trauma. *Am Surg.* 1995;61(1):69–73.
41. Bruscagin V, Coimbra R, Rasslan S, et al. Blunt gastric injury. A multicentre experience. *Injury.* 2001;32(10):761–764.
42. Grossman MD, May AK, Schwab CW, et al. Determining anatomic injury with computed tomography in selected torso gunshot wounds. *J Trauma.* 1998;45(3):446–456.
43. Kemmeter PR, Senagore AJ, Smith D, et al. Dilemmas in the diagnosis of blunt enteric trauma. *Am Surg.* 1998;64(8):750–754.
44. Pikoulis E, Delis S, Psalidas N, et al. Presentation of blunt small intestinal and mesenteric injuries. *Ann R Coll Surg Engl.* 2000;82(2):103–106.
45. Rozycki GS, Ballard RB, Feliciano DV, et al. Surgeon-performed ultrasound for the assessment of truncal injuries: Lessons learned from 1540 patients. *Ann Surg.* 1998;228(4):557–567.
46. Fakhry SM, Watts DD, Luchette FA. Current diagnostic approaches lack sensitivity in the diagnosis of perforated blunt small bowel injury: Analysis from 275,557 trauma admissions from the EAST multi-institutional HVI trial. *J Trauma.* 2003;54(2):295–306.
47. Tsang BD, Panacek EA, Brant WE, et al. Effect of oral contrast administration for abdominal computed tomography in the evaluation of acute blunt trauma. *Ann Emerg Med.* 1997;30(1):7–13.
48. Elliott DC, Rodriguez A, Moncure M, et al. The accuracy of diagnostic laparoscopy in trauma patients: A prospective, controlled study. *Int Surg.* 1998;83(4):294–298.
49. Guth AA, Pachter HL. Laparoscopy for penetrating thoracoabdominal trauma: Pitfalls and promises. *JSLS.* 1998;2(2):123–127.
50. Leddy JE, Frew EM. Complete transection of the body of the stomach resulting from blunt trauma. *Can J Surg.* 1977;20(3):264–266.
51. Croce MA, Fabian TC, Patton JH Jr, et al. Impact of stomach and colon injuries on intra-abdominal abscess and the synergistic effect of hemorrhage and associated injury. *J Trauma.* 1998;45(4):649–655.
52. O'Neill PA, Kirton OC, Dresner LS, et al. Analysis of 162 colon injuries in patients with penetrating abdominal trauma: Concomitant stomach injury results in a higher rate of infection. *J Trauma.* 2004;56(2):304–312; discussion 12–3.
53. Agarwal N, Murphy JG, Cayten CG, et al. Blood transfusion increases the risk of infection after trauma. *Arch Surg.* 1993;128(2):171–176; discussion 6–7.
54. Croce MA, Tolley EA, Claridge JA, et al. Transfusions result in pulmonary morbidity and death after a moderate degree of injury. *J Trauma.* 2005;59(1):19–23; discussion -4.
55. Dunne JR, Riddle MS, Danko J, et al. Blood transfusion is associated with infection and increased resource utilization in combat casualties. *Am Surg.* 2006;72(7):619–625; discussion 25–6.
56. Edna TH, Bjerkeset T. Association between blood transfusion and infection in injured patients. *J Trauma.* 1992;33(5):659–661.
57. Malone DL, Dunne J, Tracy JK, et al. Blood transfusion, independent of shock severity, is associated with worse outcome in trauma. *J Trauma.* 2003;54(5):898–905; discussion -7.
58. Attar S, Hankins JR, Suter CM, et al. Esophageal perforation: A therapeutic challenge. *Ann Thorac Surg.* 1990;50(1):45–51.
59. Ngakane H, Muckart DJ, Luvuno FM. Penetrating visceral injuries of the neck: Results of a conservative management policy. *Br J Neurosurg.* 1990;77(8):908–910.
60. Richardson JD, Tobin GR. Closure of esophageal defects with muscle flaps. *Arch Surg.* 1994;129(5):541–548.
61. Winter RP, Weigelt JA. Cervical esophageal trauma. Incidence and cause of esophageal fistulas. *Arch Surg.* 1990;125(7):849–852.
62. Yajko RD, Seydel F, Trimble C. Rupture of the stomach from blunt abdominal trauma. *J Trauma.* 1975;15(3):177–183.
63. Bergqvist D, Hedelin H, Karlsson G, et al. Abdominal trauma during thirty years: Analysis of a large case series. *Injury.* 1981;13(2):93–99.
64. Hockerstedt K, Airo I, Karaharju E, et al. Abdominal trauma and laparotomy in 158 patients. A comparative study of penetrating and blunt injury. *Acta Chir Scand.* 1982;148(1):9–14.
65. Knottenbelt JD, Van As S, Volschenk S. Gastric rupture from blunt trauma: Two unusual presentations. *Injury.* 1993;24(1):65–66.
66. Theunis P, Coenen L, Brouwers J. Gastric rupture from blunt abdominal trauma. *Acta Chir Belg.* 1988;88(5):309–311.

Injuries to the Duodenum and Pancreas

40

Benjamin Braslow   *George Joseph Koenig, Jr.*

PANCREATIC INJURIES

In comparison to injury to other visceral organs from both blunt and penetrating trauma, injury to the pancreas is far less common probably secondary to its retroperitoneal location. Likewise, isolated pancreatic injury with major duct disruption is exceptionally rare and is associated with injury to other organs, most commonly liver, stomach, spleen, or colon, in up to 98% of cases.[1] Pancreatic injury has been reported to occur in only 3% to 12% of patients presenting with abdominal injuries.[1,2] Two thirds of these injuries are penetrating in nature with gunshot wounds being most common followed by stabbings.[3] In fact, pancreatic injury has been reported to occur in 1.1% of all patients presenting with penetrating torso traumas, as opposed to 0.2% of all blunt trauma patients.[4] Regarding blunt pancreatic injury, motor vehicle accidents are by far the most common causative mechanism, being reported in approximately 65% of such patients. Most pancreatic traumas are observed in unrestrained drivers secondary to direct abdominal impact with the steering wheel or by the handle bars during a motorbike crash.[4] Although proved to save lives by preventing ejection from the vehicle, seat belts are also often implicated in abdominal visceral trauma during a crash. The so-called seat belt syndrome is characterized by the presence of abdominal wall contusions or abrasions associated with lumbar spine compression fracture (most commonly at L1 or L2 secondary to hyperflexion) and visceral injury.

Here the organ is compressed against the vertebral body by the force of the belt against the abdominal wall.[5] Airbag deployment during a crash does not entirely rule out the possibility of such injury.[6]

Despite the infrequent nature of pancreatic injuries, when present, the associated morbidity is exceptionally high often because identification is a diagnostic challenge and delays in diagnosis are common.

Pancreatic Anatomy and Physiology

The pancreas lies transversely across the retroperitoneum at the level of the pylorus and crosses the anterior body of the first and second lumbar vertebrae. It measures roughly 15 to 20 cm in length, 3 cm in width, and up to 1.5 cm in thickness and weighs an average of 90 g.[7] The head of the pancreas is nestled within the concavity of the second and third portion of the duodenum with which it shares its blood supply through the pancreaticoduodenal arcades. The body crosses the spine obliquely headed in a superior direction toward the left shoulder. The tail ends in close proximity to the splenic hilum. The splenic artery arises from the celiac plexus and takes a tortuous course along the upper border of the pancreas whereas the splenic vein courses medially behind the pancreas just above its inferior edge. Both vessels give off multiple branches into the body and tail of the pancreas that must be ligated in spleen-sparing procedures. The superior mesenteric vein and artery lie just behind the neck of the pancreas and are partially enclosed posteriorly by an extension of the pancreatic head known as the *uncinate process*.

The main pancreatic duct of Wirsung usually traverses the entire length of the pancreas just above the midline of the gland and opens into the posterior medial wall of the second portion of the duodenum, at the ampulla of Vater along with the common bile duct. The accessory duct of Santorini usually arises from the main pancreatic duct in the neck of the pancreas and empties into the duodenum proximal to the ampulla of Vater. Pancreatic ductal anatomy is highly variable and intraoperative pancreatography is often necessary to determine the status of the pancreatic duct following injury.

At the microscopic level, the pancreas is organized into exocrine and endocrine units called *acini* and *islets of Langerhans*, respectively. The acini and related ductal system produce up to 2 L per day of pancreatic juice, which is not only rich in digestive enzymes necessary for the breakdown of proteins (i.e., trypsinogen, chymotrypsinogen, and procarboxypolypeptidase), carbohydrates (amylase), and fats (lipase) but also contains large quantities of bicarbonate necessary to neutralize the acid chyme emptied from the stomach into the duodenum. The islets of Langerhans are distributed throughout the pancreas but seem to be most concentrated in the pancreatic tail area. These islets are composed primarily of α, β, δ, and F or pancreatic polypeptide (PP) cells which produce glucagon, insulin, somatostatin and PP, respectively with β cells being the most prevalent (60%) cell type. It has been shown that excision of >90% of the pancreas substance is required to produce a state of endocrine deficiency, if the pancreas is otherwise normal. This is likely a result of islet hypertrophy and increased activity following partial resection. Remarkably, even after removal of 90% to 95% of the pancreas following trauma, digestion and absorption of food may be unimpaired.

Diagnosis

Outcome following pancreatic injury is directly linked to the accurate and timely diagnosis of major pancreatic duct injury.[8,9] Patients with isolated pancreatic injuries often present with vague or totally absent abdominal complaints and frequently lack any physical signs.[2,10] The retroperitoneal position of the pancreas accounts for most of the delay in symptoms. Also, most of the caustic pancreatic enzymes released at the site of injury are in their inactivated form and surrounding tissue destruction is limited. Usually when a patient does have symptoms, they may be related to coexisting visceral or boney injuries. A high index of suspicion is reasonable in any patient who has sustained a direct high-energy blow to the epigastrium. For adults, this is most often a result of chest wall impact with the steering wheel of a car during a crash, whereas children often suffer a spearing type insult from the handlebars of a bicycle. For patients with blunt trauma, the presence of soft tissue contusion or abrasion in the upper abdomen or epigastric pain out of proportion to the abdominal examination should prompt suspicion of retroperitoneal injury. If the patient has a clear indication for laparotomy, and the suspicion of pancreatic injury is present, preoperative evaluation directed at identifying a possible pancreatic injury is usually not indicated and would lead to unwarranted delays in definitive patient care. Here, the diagnosis of pancreatic injury should be made intraoperatively after hemorrhage control and control of abdominal contamination has been achieved. Without a clear indication for exploratory laparotomy, the physician has several diagnostic modalities available to help in identifying injury to the pancreas.

Despite the fact that the highest concentration of amylase in the human body is in the pancreas, hyperamylasemia is not a reliable indicator of pancreatic trauma but its presence should raise the index of suspicion for pancreatic injury and warrant further evaluation.[11,12] Other sources of hyperamylasemia following trauma include salivary gland injury, bowel injury, and even brain injury although the etiology for this is not clear.[13] The spectrum of the sensitivity and specificity of the serum amylase assay in multiple studies has been quite varied; however, the accuracy of the assay seems to be time dependant. Takishima et al. found that when the blood specimen was drawn later than 3 hours after injury, the accuracy of the test was significantly increased.[14] On a more useful note, after blunt trauma the negative predictive value of a normal serum amylase level has been shown to be approximately 95%.

Diagnostic peritoneal lavage (DPL), although useful in the abdominal investigation of the unexaminable, unstable blunt trauma patient, has not been proved to be useful in diagnosing significant injury to the pancreas. The retroperitoneal location of the pancreas renders DPL inaccurate in the prediction of isolated pancreatic injury. Also the estimation of amylase levels in the DPL fluid, even if >20 IU/L, is unreliable leading to both false-positive and false-negative results.[15]

The central retroperitoneal position of the pancreas also renders ultrasonographic evaluation of the gland following injury very difficult and inaccurate. The large amount of air-containing bowel overlying the pancreas interferes with the transmission of ultrasonographic waves and obscures the view generated by this modality.

To date, contrast-enhanced computed tomography (CT) is generally accepted as the imaging modality of choice for evaluating the retroperitoneum in a hemodynamically stable patient following trauma. Sensitivities and specificities between 70% and 80% have been reported with factors including the experience of the interpreter, the quality of the scanner, and the time elapsed since injury all playing an important role.[16] Characteristic CT findings associated with pancreatic injury include (a) fracture of the pancreas with or without separation of the fractured fragments, (b) enlargement of the pancreas or presence of hematoma in or around the gland, (c) fluid separating the splenic vein and pancreas, (d) increased attenuation of the peripancreatic fatty tissue, (e) thickening of the anterior renal fascia, (f) fluid accumulation in the lesser sac, and (g) retroperitoneal fluid or hematoma. Often these findings are subtle and rarely are they all present at a single scan. The sensitivity of CT increases with time as the injury evolves.[17] This accounts for the false-negative CT scans reported in as many as 30% of patients with significant pancreatic injuries and indicates the utility of repeat scans if symptoms persist.[17] Bradley et al. found CT to be sensitive in approximately 72% of cases of pancreatic trauma but noted that CT did not accurately estimate the grade of injury and showed only a 43% sensitivity for the prediction of ductal injury.[18]

Endoscopic retrograde cholangiopancreatography (ERCP) is a very accurate method of defining pancreatic duct anatomy and integrity, especially in patients with blunt abdominal trauma, but has no role in the acute evaluation of hemodynamically unstable patients.[19] This modality offers both the ability to diagnose and occasionally treat pancreatic duct disruption by stent placement either across the zone of injury or at the ampulla to decrease the pressure within the ducts and allow for healing of ductal lesions.[20-22] ERCP can preclude laparotomy in stable patients with suspected pancreatic injury by demonstrating an intact pancreatic duct or a stentable lesion in the absence of peritonitis. It is an invasive procedure associated with limited but real morbidity including pancreatitis, hemorrhage, and gastrointestinal (GI) perforation in up to 5% of patients. Although limited, there is occasionally a role for intraoperative ERCP to evaluate the pancreatic duct when injury determination is equivocal. This is only an option in a hemodynamically stable patient with limited other injuries. Often coordinating an ERCP during an emergency surgery is difficult and limited by the timely availability of the appropriate personnel and equipment.[23] Intraoperative ERCP can eliminate morbidity associated with duodenotomy or distal pancreatectomy in order to gain access to the pancreatic duct for pancreatography.[24]

Magnetic resonance imaging, more specifically, magnetic resonance cholangiopancreatography (MRCP), is emerging as a valuable modality for the evaluation of the pancreatic duct following suspected injury. Several recent studies have touted its accuracy and low morbidity profile.[25-27] Unlike CT technology, MRCP depicts the pancreatic duct and biliary tract as high signal intensity or bright structures without the use of contrast material. It has been shown to be diagnostic in 95% to 99% of cases.[28] In addition to delineating the pancreatic duct, MRCP detects pancreas-specific complications such as pseudocysts that may not opacify at ERCP. Because MRCP is performed without instrumentation, it avoids the above-mentioned risks of ERCP but does not offer the possibility of being a therapeutic modality.

Intraoperative Evaluation

The presence of an upper abdominal central retroperitoneal hematoma, edema around the pancreatic gland and the lesser sac, and retroperitoneal bile staining and/or the presence of saponification of the retroperitoneal fat mandate thorough pancreatic inspection. More simply stated, if there are any of the "3 Bs" (bile, blood, and bubbles) present around the peripancreatic area, the local structures should be meticulously explored.[29] Inspection of the pancreas requires complete exposure of the gland. Entering the lesser sac through an opening in the gastrocolic omentum allows visualization of the anterior surface of the body and tail of the pancreas to be explored. The stomach is retracted upward while the transverse colon is retracted in a caudal direction. Frequently, there are some adhesions between the posterior wall of the stomach and the anterior surface of the pancreas that must be lysed. Next, a generous Kocher maneuver is performed including mobilization of the hepatic flexure of the colon. This provides adequate visualization of the pancreatic head and the uncinate process both anteriorly and posteriorly and allows for bimanual examination of the head and neck of the gland. Injury to the tail requires mobilization of the spleen and left colon to allow medial reflection of the pancreas by creating a plane between the kidney and the pancreas with blunt finger dissection. Division of the ligament of Treitz and reflection of the fourth portion of the duodenum can enhance exposure of the inferior aspect of the pancreas.

Most pancreatic duct injuries, regardless of mechanism, can be diagnosed through careful inspection of the injury tract following adequate exposure. With most penetrating wounds to the periphery of the gland, the pancreas can be inspected directly and the likelihood of duct disruption ruled out. With penetrating wounds to the head, neck, or central portion of the pancreas, however, further evaluation is often required. Occasionally, intravenous (IV) injection of 1 to 2 μg of cholecystokinin pancreozymin (CCK-PZ) may stimulate pancreatic secretions enough to allow for visualization of pancreatic duct leakage from an otherwise occult ductal injury. Several options exist for intraoperative imaging of the pancreatic duct. These include intraoperative ERCP, direct open ampullary cannulation through lateral duodenostomy, needle cholangiopancreatography, or antegrade pancreatography through transaction of the tail of the pancreas and distal ductal cannulation. Remember that in unstable (hypotensive, cold, coagulopathic, and acidotic) patients for whom damage control principles are indicated, prolonged techniques of evaluating the pancreatic duct integrity at the initial surgery are not appropriate. Here the peripancreatic region is packed and widely drained. Postoperative duct interrogation is performed following physiologic resuscitation. For stable patients, as stated in the preceding text, intraoperative ERCP is often logistically too difficult to organize during an emergency surgery especially at night in most hospitals. Much has been written about duodenotomy and direct ampullary cannulation or transaction of the tail of the pancreas and distal duct cannulation in the past. These techniques are very invasive, requiring iatrogenic injury to an otherwise uninjured section of the bowel or pancreas and have largely been abandoned by most surgeons as a consequence of advances in less invasive perioperative imaging techniques such as ERCP and MRCP. Needle cholecystocholangiopancreatography remains a useful intraoperative adjunct in the evaluation of the injured pancreatic duct. This technique involves cannulating the gallbladder with an 18-gauge angiocatheter and injecting 30 to 75 mL of water-soluble contrast material under fluoroscopic guidance. In a recent study, this technique visualized the pancreatic duct in 64% of patients.[30] The administration of IV morphine, which promotes contracture of the sphincter of Oddi, may enhance the likelihood of pancreatic duct visualization. If the gallbladder is surgically absent then the common bile duct can be directly cannulated using a short "butterfly" needle for injection. Some operative dissection of the hepatoduodenal ligament is usually required here to expose the duct and a smaller caliber needle is necessary to minimize ductal trauma and limit leakage once the needle is removed. This can limit contrast flow and decrease the accuracy of the study.

Classification of Pancreatic Injuries

Classification of pancreatic injuries is based on the status of the pancreatic duct and the site of the injury relative to the neck of the pancreas or the superior mesenteric vein. Currently, the system devised by the American Association for the Surgery of Trauma (AAST) (see Table 1) is most widely used.[31] Management strategies for pancreatic trauma vary greatly and are guided by the grade of pancreatic injury and the presence of associated injuries.

Operative Management

Grades I and II Pancreatic Injuries
Contusions and lacerations without duct injury are treated with hemostasis and adequate external drainage.[32–34] Approximately 75% of all pancreatic injuries fall into these two categories. Closing the pancreatic capsule is ill advised as this might lead to pseudocyst formation whereas a controlled pancreatic fistula is usually self-limiting. Soft closed suction drains (i.e., 10 F Jackson-Pratt) are preferred over Penrose drains or sump drains (Davol) because they provide more complete removal of secretions, offering decreased intra-abdominal abscess formation, fewer infectious complications, and less skin excoriation at the drain exit site.[35] Duration of drainage remains a matter of controversy. Most authors recommend drainage until the patient is tolerating an oral diet or gastric feeds and the concentration of amylase in the effluent is equal to or less than that of serum. Others advocate earlier drain removal if output is minimal or ceases outright before a feeding challenge.[36]

Grade III Pancreatic Injuries
Distal transection or distal parenchymal injury with duct disruption are best treated by distal pancreatectomy and drainage.[10,35,37–40] Following mobilization of the distal pancreas, a large (4.8 mm) TA-55 stapler can be used to divide the gland or some surgeons prefer to ligate the duct individually and place full thickness nonabsorbable mattress sutures through the cut parenchyma (anterior capsule to posterior capsule) to minimize leakage. A small omental patch may be used to buttress the cut surface of

---

TABLE 1

AMERICAN ASSOCIATION FOR THE SURGERY OF TRAUMA (AAST) GRADING OF PANCREAS INJURY

Pancreas Injury Scale

Grade[a]	Type of Injury	Description of Injury	AIS-90 Score
I	Hematoma	Minor contusion without duct injury	2
	Laceration	Superficial injury without duct injury	2
II	Hematoma	Major contusion without duct injury or tissue loss	2
	Laceration	Major laceration without duct injury or tissue loss	3
III	Laceration	Distal transection or parenchymal injury with duct injury	3
IV	Laceration	Proximal transection or parenchymal injury with probable duct injury (not involving ampulla)[b]	4
V	Laceration	Massive disruption of pancreatic head	5

[a]Advance one grade for multiple injuries up to grade III.
[b]Proximal pancreas is to the patient's right of the superior mesenteric vein.
AIS, Abbreviated Injury Scale.

the pancreas and a closed suction drain placed nearby. Placement of fibrin sealant over the cut surface of the gland might add some additional leak protection,[41] but not much has been written in the trauma literature to confirm its efficacy. If there is any question regarding the integrity of the more proximal duct, intraoperative pancreatography can be performed through the open lumen of the proximal duct. However, locating the aperture is not always an easy task especially if a stapling device is used to transect the gland.

Concerns for the development of overwhelming post-splenectomy infection (OPSI) and the potential for left subphrenic abscess have prompted several authors to recommend splenic preservation during distal pancreatectomy.[39,42–46] This is only considered an option in the traumatized patient provided the spleen is not severely injured and the patient's condition is stable. This procedure requires complete mobilization of the distal pancreas and spleen. There are on average 22 tributaries of the splenic vein and 7 branches of the splenic artery that must be ligated to separate the structures.[47] This maneuver has been shown to increase operative times by approximately 1 hour (37 to 80 minutes).[45] Meticulous technique is mandated to prevent injury to the splenic hilum and thrombosis of the splenic vein.

Procedures associated with resection of >80% of the pancreatic tissue can be associated with a risk of endocrine or exocrine pancreatic insufficiency.[48] Even resection of all pancreatic tissue left of the superior mesenteric vein, or roughly left of the spine, leaves roughly 45% to 50% of the gland *in situ*,[49] and safely avoids pancreatic insufficiency.[50]

Grade IV Pancreatic Injuries

Proximal transection or parenchymal injury to the pancreatic head with probable duct disruption can be the most difficult pancreatic injuries to manage. More often then not, injuries to this portion of the pancreas are associated with injuries to adjacent structures such as the duodenum and great vessels and are therefore associated with very high morbidity and mortality rates.[10] Once bleeding and local contamination are controlled, defining the anatomy of the pancreatic duct becomes paramount. If the patient is unstable, damage control principles should prevail. The pancreatic bed is packed and drained widely and ductal interrogation is delayed. For the stable patient, local exploration is initially performed to evaluate the integrity of the duct. If after careful inspection of the gland there is still a question of ductal injury, more extensive intraoperative diagnostic procedures can be attempted (see preceding section on interoperative assessment). Generally there is a trend toward a more conservative approach with proximal pancreatic injuries, including wide external drainage and limited use of pancreaticoenteric anastomosis even in the presence of injury to the main pancreatic duct. The morbidity associated with proximal pancreatic resection is high. Some authors have concluded that the morbidity

associated with a moderately high rate of fistula formation is more easily managed than the potential early and late complications of major proximal pancreatic resection.[40] Nevertheless, in the presence of proximal pancreatic ductal disruption without injury to the ampulla or duodenum (an albeit rare scenario) two operative options exist. The first option is extended distal pancreatectomy, resulting in subtotal gland removal. Here, the proximal residual gland drains into the duodenum in a normal manner. If, however, by this approach a >90% distal pancreatectomy ensues, endocrine and exocrine pancreatic insufficiency is bound to develop. Alternatively, preservation of the distal pancreas with a Roux-en-Y jejunal anastamosis to the distal pancreatic stump has been proposed.[51,52] This technique involves division of the pancreas at the site of injury, debridement of injured retained parenchyma, closure of the proximal duct and cut edge of proximal parenchyma, and anastamosis of the open end of the distal pancreas to the Roux jejunal limb. The benefits of this technique are, however, debatable as it has been demonstrated that obstructive fibrotic lesions often develop in the preserved distal pancreatic segment, which results in gradual loss of its endocrine and exocrine function.[53]

Historically, in cases of incomplete pancreatic parenchymal transection, surgeons have tried end-to-side jejunopancreatic anastamosis. This technique is no longer recommended as anastomotic failure rates were extremely high as were mortality rates.[54] Often the extent of parenchymal injury is not fully appreciated at the initial inspection and debridement and progressive destruction compromises the suture line of the anastamosis.[55]

Grade V Pancreatic Injuries

Massive disruption of pancreatic head or combined pancreatic-duodenal injuries are discussed in the latter portion of this chapter.

Morbidity Associated with Pancreatic Injury

Morbidity after pancreatic trauma is high, ranging between 20% and 65% in several published series.[38,56–58] It is mainly influenced by the grade on the AAST scale of the injury and the presence and number of associated intra-abdominal injuries.[36] The most common of these complications are pancreatic fistula, pancreatic pseudocysts, pancreatitis, hemorrhage, intra-abdominal abscesses, wound complications, and pancreatic exocrine and endocrine insufficiency.[3,4,10,18] Fistula and pseudocysts formation are dependent on the presence of pancreatic duct injury while septic complications seem related to the presence of concomitant hollow viscus injuries, particularly colonic injuries.[2,18] Although almost all pancreas-related posttraumatic complications are treatable or self-limiting, very often they could have been completely avoided by a more accurate and timely assessment of whether the pancreatic duct was damaged.[9,58–60]

Pancreatic Fistula

In general, any measurable amylase-rich abdominal drainage persisting for longer than 7 to 10 days should be considered a fistula and thoroughly investigated. It is the most common complication after pancreatic duct injury, occurring in 7% to 20% of patients (26% to 35% of patients with combined pancreatic-duodenal injury).[30,39,40,61] Most pancreatic fistulas develop within the first 3 weeks of injury, are considered minor (drain output <200 mL per day) and spontaneously resolve within 2 weeks of injury, provided they are adequately drained externally. However, high-output fistulas (>700 mL per day) may require operative intervention for closure or prolonged drainage. Here, ERCP is indicated if technically possible to help elucidate the cause of the persistent fistula and guide further intervention. The type of surgery depends on the anatomy. Fistulas arising from the body or tail of the pancreas are best managed by distal pancreatectomy, provided that the remaining portion of the gland is not severely injured. Fistulas arising from the proximal pancreas are best treated by internal drainage procedures, utilizing a Roux limb of jejunum.

Nutritional support must be provided during this period. For this reason, it is often encouraged to place a feeding jejunostomy tube at the time of the initial celiotomy if possible or during a subsequent take-back procedure. Post ligament of Treitz elemental or short-chained polypeptide formula feedings provide the most physiologic and economical nutritional support in this instance. These types of feedings cause less pancreatic stimulation than standard enteral formulas delivered through the gastric route. Overall, enteral nutrition not only prevents intestinal nutritional atrophy but helps to restore immune competence and is therefore the preferred form of nutritional support over total parenteral nutrition (TPN) when possible.[62]

Somatostatin and its synthetic analog, octreotide, have been shown to inhibit pancreatic exocrine secretion by inhibition of certain GI hormones (i.e., cholecystokinin, secretin, and neurotensin).[63] After pancreatic surgery, somatostatin can reduce the output from a pancreatic fistula, but whether it hastens fistula closure is still not determined.[64,65] Despite some reports that somatostatin does prevent some postoperative complications in elective pancreatic surgery, several nonrandomized studies of its efficacy in pancreatic trauma have yielded conflicting results.[66–68] Therefore, further investigation is necessary to define the role of somatostatin and its analogs in pancreatic trauma.

Pancreatic Pseudocysts

Assuming accurate diagnosis and appropriate operative intervention, the postoperative rate of pseudocyst formation following pancreatic trauma should be quite low (2% to 3%).[2] Psuedocysts most commonly occur in cases of blunt pancreatic trauma managed nonoperatively.[69] Unresolved pseudocysts should be treated to avoid hemorrhage, perforation, infection, gastric outlet obstruction, or bile duct obstruction.[70] The status of the duct determines the best treatment plan. If the pancreatic duct is intact, percutaneous drainage of the pseudocysts is often successful and definitive. If the pseudocyst connects to a major duct disruption, however, percutaneous drainage will not be curative and merely converts the pseudocyst into a chronic fistula. ERCP should therefore precede any attempt at percutaneous drainage. If pancreatic duct stenosis or injury is found during ERCP, current options for treatment include cystgastrostomy (open or endoscopic), internal jejunal Roux-en-Y pseudocyst drainage, endoscopic transpapillary stenting of the duct,[70,71] or resection distal to the zone of injury including the pseudocyst.

Pancreatitis

Posttraumatic pancreatitis has been defined as persistent serum amylase elevation persisting for more than 3 days.[38] This may be anticipated in 8% to 18% of post operative patients and carries a high mortality rate.[3,9,72] Treatment is conservative consisting of nasogastric tube decompression and IV hydration. Bowel rest and TPN used to be an integral part of this schema, but much has been written recently to combat this approach. Patients with severe acute pancreatitis are frequently hypercatabolic and nutritional support must be started early to avoid a malnourished state. Accumulating evidence strongly supports enteral feeding over the parenteral route (TPN). It is now recommended that enteral nutrition be initiated after initial resuscitation through the nasojejunal route, if possible, but nasogastric is also acceptable. Parenteral nutrition should be implemented when attempts at enteral nutrition have failed after a 5- to 7-day trial secondary to proximal obstruction or ileus. Regardless of the route of nutritional support, supplemental glutamine and tight glycemic control have also been associated with decreased complication rates. Clinical trials of agents that inhibit activated pancreatic enzymes (gabexate mesilate, aprotinin), inhibit pancreatic secretions (somatostatin, octreotide), or blunt inflammation (lexipafant, anti-tumor necrosis factor α [TNF-α]) have failed to demonstrate improved outcomes in patients with acute pancreatitis.[73,74] A more common but far more deadly complication is hemorrhagic pancreatitis whereby the inflammatory process may erode into an adjacent vessel and result in severe bleeding, often heralded by an acute change in pancreatic drain effluent from serous to sanguinis. Generally this requires emergent operative repair but immediate angiography and embolization is sometimes a viable option if the patient is at least quasi stable.

Intra-abdominal Abscess

The incidence of abscess formation after pancreatic injury ranges from 10% to 34%.[2,9,58,61] Most abscesses are peripancreatic and usually develop as a result of contamination from adjacent hollow viscus injuries, especially the colon, and are often associated with gram-negative enteric organisms.[40] Infrequently, they may develop as a result of drain tract contamination with skin flora. CT or ultrasonographic-guided drainage is frequently effective in evacuating these abscesses. A true pancreatic abscess is rare and usually results from inadequate debridement of necrotic tissue or inadequate initial drainage.[10,38,61] Often true pancreatic abscesses are not amenable to percutaneous drainage secondary to the bulky material contained within and must be treated with operative debridement and drainage. Mortality rates from posttraumatic pancreatic abscess may be as high as 20% because of the high association with multisystem organ failure.[75]

Exocrine and Endocrine Insufficiency

Exocrine or endocrine insufficiencies are quite rare after pancreatic injury. As long as 10% to 20% of the pancreas is left *in situ* following pancreatic resection, normal pancreatic function is expected. Any resection left of the superior mesenteric vessels is therefore safe. Patients who have procedures that leave less functioning tissue will require exogenous endocrine and exocrine enzyme replacement.[38,76]

DUODENAL INJURIES

Duodenal injuries are relatively uncommon. The incidence of duodenal trauma is estimated to occur between 3% and 5%.[77] Owing to the infrequent nature of this injury and the anatomic location of the duodenum, it remains a challenge to the surgeon to diagnose and treat. The diagnosis relies heavily on an understanding of the mechanism of injury in the case of blunt trauma or on the proper identification of the trajectory in penetrating trauma. Penetrating injuries are generally caused by stab and gunshot wounds that traverse the peritoneal cavity. Blunt injuries result from motor vehicle collisions, falls, or assaults.

The mechanism of blunt injury is related to a direct force causing compression of the duodenum against the adjacent vertebral body. Typically, blunt duodenal injury is a result of the crushing of the duodenum between a steering wheel or the handlebar of a bicycle and the L1 vertebral body. Injuries sustained from physical assault usually spare the duodenum due to its anatomic location in the retroperitoneum. However, the retroperitoneal location can mask injury because of the delayed onset of physical signs or symptoms.

The leading cause of duodenal injury seen in urban trauma centers is penetrating trauma. The incidence of blunt versus penetrating mechanisms is directly related to the geographic location of the receiving hospital (i.e., rural vs. urban). One review from an urban center reported the incidence of duodenal injury resulting from penetrating injury as high as 77% versus 23% from a blunt mechanism.[78]

The morbidity of these injuries is reported at 48% with a mortality of 19%.[79] The time from injury to surgery impacts outcome. Lucas and Ledgerwood reported a mortality of 11% for patients who were operated on within 24 hours of injury versus a mortality of 40% when operated on after 24 hours.[80] Delay in the identification and control of the leakage of activated enzymes and bowel contents into the retroperitoneal and peritoneal space results in a greater likelihood of anastomotic dehiscence and infectious complications. The failure of the repair is the primary determinant of outcome related to the injury.[81]

Anatomy and Physiology

The duodenum is the first portion of the small intestine. It is mostly a retroperitoneal organ except for the anterior half of its most proximal segment. It extends from the pylorus to the ligament of Treitz and curves around the head of the pancreas. For descriptive purposes, it can be divided into four portions—superior, descending, transverse, and ascending—and spans approximately 25 cm in length.

The first portion starts at the pyloric ring, which can be identified by the pyloric vein of Mayo. It passes laterally (right), superiorly and posteriorly, before making a sharp curve inferiorly into the superior duodenal flexure. It ends at the common bile duct superiorly and the gastroduodenal artery inferiorly. The second portion forms an angle and descends into the retroperitoneum. It passes inferiorly to the lower border of vertebral body L3, before making a sharp turn medially into the inferior duodenal flexure. The entry of the common bile duct and pancreatic duct marks the end of the second portion of the duodenum. The third portion passes transversely to the left crossing the inferior vena cava, aorta, and the vertebral column. It continues to the mesenteric vessels, which cross anteriorly over the junction of the third and fourth portion. The fourth portion extends from these vessels to where the duodenum emerges from the retroperitoneum marked by the ligament of Treitz to connect to the jejunum.

The duodenum and head of the pancreas share a common blood supply. The gastroduodenal artery, which arises from the common hepatic artery, gives off the superior anterior and posterior pancreaticoduodenal arteries. These arteries anastomose with the inferior anterior and posterior pancreaticoduodenal arteries which branch from the superior mesenteric artery. The right gastric artery and the gastroepiploic artery also supply the duodenum.

The duodenum is the site where partially digested chyle and proteolytic/lipolytic enzymes are combined. More than 6 L of fluid pass through the duodenum per day. This fluid contains active digestive enzymes, including lipase, trypsin, amylase, elastase, peptidases, and bile. A breach in the wall would cause large amounts of these enzymes to be liberated into the retroperitoneal and peritoneal space. The resulting inflammatory response and destructive effects of the enzymes would cause severe illness and significant morbidity.[82]

Diagnosis

Isolated injury to the duodenum is rare due to its retroperitoneal location and its proximity to vascular and visceral structures.[83] Diagnosis is generally made in the operating room during abdominal exploration. The evidence of bile, blood, or air bubbles around the pancreas, duodenum, or base of the ligament of Treitz warrants thorough investigation of the retroperitoneum. Evaluation of the duodenum requires mobilization of the entire duodenum (i.e., Kocharization), because subtle injuries may be easily missed especially posteriorly and laterally.

Blunt injury poses more of a diagnostic dilemma. The retroperitoneal location often masks symptoms of perforation or injury and can lead to a delay in diagnosis. Although physical examination is the first step in evaluating any injury, in the case of evaluating blunt trauma it can be misleading.[84] It is often confounded by other factors such as the presence of alcohol, illicit drugs, or a decreased level of consciousness. Common physical findings include tachycardia, right upper quadrant tenderness, vomiting, and a progressive rise in temperature and heart rate. However, these signs are subtle, nonspecific, and may present with a multitude of other injuries. They are frequently overlooked and the injury is not recognized until peritonitis develops several hours later secondary to delayed extravasation of the duodenal contents.[85]

In theory, when a full thickness injury to the duodenum occurs, serum amylase levels should increase as amylase and other digestive enzymes extravasate and get absorbed systemically. Several retrospective studies have correlated an increase in serum amylase to duodenal injury.[86,87] However, serum amylase has not proved helpful in diagnosing duodenal injuries because the test lacks sensitivity.[11] Serial determinations of serum amylase are more sensitive, but serial determinations delay diagnosis and treatment. In addition, normal amylase levels do not exclude significant duodenal injury.

DPL is also not reliable in detecting duodenal injury or any retroperitoneal injury for that matter. Although DPL has been shown to be positive in 35% of patients with duodenal injury, the result is usually related to other associated injuries.[88] Likewise, a negative DPL does not exclude duodenal injury.

In hemodynamically stable patients, a suspicion of duodenal injury can usually be excluded or confirmed by abdominal CT scan. It is recommended that both IV and oral contrast be given. However, in high volume centers with radiologists experienced in interpreting trauma abdominal CT scans without oral contrast, the results of identifying GI injuries without oral contrast are comparable.[89] The subtle findings of small amounts of retroperitoneal air, blood, duodenal wall thickening, or hematoma should raise suspicion for duodenal injury.[90] Even with careful evaluation of CT findings, false-negative results occur.[91]

Injury Classification

Physical examination findings, laboratory data, or diagnostic data that suggest a duodenal injury warrant operative evaluation. Diagnostic laparoscopy is not recommended at the present time. The anatomic location of the duodenum does not lend itself to easy visualization by laparoscopy and diagnostic laparoscopy does not confer any improvement over traditional methods.[92]

Abdominal injuries should be explored through a generous midline incision. As for all trauma laparotomies, hemorrhage control takes immediate priority, followed by control of contamination. Even when duodenal injury is suspected, a thorough sequential abdominal and retroperitoneal exploration is performed before more formal duodenal mobilization and exploration. Suspicious findings of duodenal injury include a right-sided retroperitoneal hematoma or perinephric hematoma, bile staining, air bubbles, or crepitus.

The duodenum should be fully mobilized to allow full visualization of its four anatomic zones.[93] A Kocher maneuver involves the dissection of the lateral peritoneal attachments of the duodenum displacing the duodenum medially. This maneuver should expose the first and second portion of the duodenum. The third portion can be visualized by mobilizing the hepatic flexure medially using the Cattell-Braasch maneuver. The fourth portion can be inspected by transecting the ligament of Treitz.

Several classifications systems exist for categorizing duodenal injury. Snyder et al. identified several important factors that allowed the classification of the severity of injury.[87] This classification provided guidance in determining whether a duodenal wound should be primarily repaired. Injuries were classified by the agent of entry, the size and site of injury, the injury to repair interval, and associated injury to the common bile duct. Injuries were classified as mild on the basis of the following: (a) agent of entry consisted of a stab wound, (b) the size of injury encompassed <75% of the duodenal wall, (c) the site of injury was located in the third or fourth portion of the duodenum, (d) the interval of time of injury to repair was <24 hours, and (e) there was no adjacent common bile duct injury. Severe injuries were classified on the basis of the following: (a) the agent of entry was blunt trauma or a missile, (b) the size encompassed more than 75% of the duodenal wall, (c) the site of injury was located in the first or second portion of the duodenum, (d) the interval of time of injury to repair was >24 hours, and (e) there was adjacent common bile duct injury.

In their review of 247 patients treated for duodenal trauma, they demonstrated that patients presenting with a "mild" duodenal injury had 0% mortality and 2% duodenal fistula rate. In comparison, those presenting with a "severe" injury had 6% mortality and 10% fistula rate. They concluded that patients with "mild" injury and no pancreatic injury could be primarily repaired. Patients with more severe duodenal injury may require more complex operative management.

The AAST proposed a classification system grading injury from I to V increasing in order of severity (see Table 2). One multicenter trial graded 164 duodenal injuries. In this study, the mortality rates for classes I, II, III, IV, and V were 8, 19, 21, 75, and 25%, respectively. The mortality did not correlate with severity and the authors concluded that the anatomic features of injury were only a part of the overall morbidity and mortality.[94] Nevertheless, the classification system allows for comparison between different types of injuries to the duodenum and operative interventions.

Operative Management

There are several key considerations when determining the operative course for duodenal injury. These factors are the severity or extent of the injury, the involved circumference of the duodenum, and the involvement of vascular, pancreatic, or common bile duct injury.[95] In addition, the condition of the patient at the time of surgery must be taken into account. Complex reconstructive procedures may not be optimal with other associated abdominal injuries and signs of shock. In this case, a staged procedure should be considered.

Intramural Hematoma

An intramural hematoma is a rare injury of the duodenum. It is most common in children and caused by blunt trauma to the upper abdomen. Fifty percent of these cases have been attributed to child abuse.[96] This condition can also occur in adults. The hematoma develops in the submucosal or subserosal layers of the duodenum. Typically, it presents with symptoms of gastric outlet obstruction occurring approximately 48 hours after injury. The diagnosis can be made with either a contrast-enhanced CT or an upper GI contrast study. Particular attention should be directed toward excluding pancreatic injuries. Pancreatic injuries have been identified in approximately 20% of patients with a duodenal hematoma.[97]

The management is usually nonoperative and responds to conservative therapy. Continuous nasogastric suction and administration of total parental nutrition should be initiated. If signs of obstruction do not resolve, the patient should be reevaluated with imaging studies at 5- to 7-day intervals. If the obstruction has not resolved after 2 weeks, the hematoma should be surgically evacuated and the area should be explored for pancreatic injury, duodenal perforation, or strictures.[98] There have been several case reports of percutaneous drainage but the accepted standard is operative.[99]

Duodenal Perforation

Most duodenal perforations can be closed primarily with a simple operative technique. Several studies have shown that primary repair can manage 60% to 85% of duodenal injuries.[94,100,101] Primary repair should be performed on duodenal perforations that are <50% of the circumference injured, short interval between injury and surgeries, and no associated pancreatic or biliary injuries.[102] The repair should be performed in a transverse manner using single- or

---

TABLE 2

AMERICAN ASSOCIATION FOR THE SURGERY OF TRAUMA (AAST) GRADING OF DUODENAL INJURY

Duodenum Injury Scale

Grade[a]	Type of Injury	Description of Injury	AIS-90 Score
I	Hematoma	Involving single portion of duodenum	2
	Laceration	Partial thickness, no perforation	3
II	Hematoma	Involving more than one portion	2
	Laceration	Disruption <50% of circumference	4
III	Laceration	Disruption 50%–75% of circumference of D2	4
		Disruption 50%–100% of circumference of D1, D3, and D4	4
IV	Laceration	Disruption >75% of circumference of D2	5
		Involving ampulla or distal common bile duct	5
V	Laceration	Massive disruption of duodenopancreatic complex	5
	Vascular	Devascularization of duodenum	5

AIS, Abbreviated Injury Scale; D1, first position of duodenum; D2, second portion of duodenum; D3, third portion of duodenum; D4, fourth portion of duodenum.
[a]Advance one grade for multiple injuries up to grade III.

double-layer suture technique. This provides a tension-free repair and prevents vascular compromise and luminal narrowing.

A Roux-en-Y jejunal limb technique has been used to repair perforation of 50% to 75% of the circumference of the duodenum. The limb of the jejunum is sutured directly to the site of the perforation in an end-to-side manner. This technique has been utilized with large defects in the second portion of the duodenum in close proximity to the ampulla. In the case of complete transection, it is preferred to primarily anastomose the two ends after debridement and mobilization.[103]

Primary repair should be considered in cases with complete transection of the duodenum as long as the injury does not involve the region of the ampulla. In cases where it is not possible to mobilize the two ends of the duodenum or when the injury is near the ampulla and mobilization could cause common bile duct injury, a Roux-en-Y jejunal limb anastomosis to the proximal duodenal site of injury should be completed and the distal end is oversewn.

Other methods have been described to repair larger defects such as a mucosal or serosal patch or pedicled grafts. However, the experience with these methods has been limited and neither has proved to be efficacious. Pancreatoduodenectomy is rarely required for duodenal injuries unless there is massive duodenal disruption, uncontrollable pancreatic hemorrhage, or combined duodenal and distal common bile duct or pancreatic duct trauma.

Various methods have been suggested to safeguard the duodenal closure. Simple techniques include buttressing the repair with a tongue of omentum or a serosal patch from a loop of jejunum.[104] Other procedures for duodenal decompression such as tube duodenostomy or pyloric exclusion have also been described. Controversies surround the use of these additional techniques to safeguard the closure.

Several different techniques for tube duodenostomy have been detailed in the literature to protect a tenuous closure. In primary duodenostomy, the tube is placed through a separate incision in an uninjured portion of duodenum.[105] The goal is to decompress the duodenum and protect the suture line. This technique does not totally divert gastric contents. Other techniques such as antegrade and retrograde tube duodenostomy have been proposed to further decrease the flow of gastric contents. In antegrade tube duodenostomy, a nasogastric tube is passed through the pylorus beyond the point of injury.[106] In retrograde tube duodenostomy, a proximal tube is threaded retrograde past the duodenal repair and a distal tube is placed for use as a feeding jejunostomy. Some advocate adding a gastric tube to accomplish further decompression.

Stone and Fabian reported in their experience of 237 patients treated with retrograde duodenostomy tubes that <0.5% had fistula formation in contrast to a 19.3% incidence of duodenal complications when not utilized.[107] Their observations were also supported by Hasson et al. in their review of penetrating trauma

and tube duodenostomy.[108] They reported an overall mortality of 19.4% and a fistula rate of 11.8% without decompression, compared to 9% mortality and 2.3% fistula rate with decompression. However, other clinical reviews disagree and suggest that decompression does not decrease complications and may increase them.[94,109] To date, there has not been a prospective, randomized analysis of the efficacy of tube duodenostomy.

Diversion of gastric contents is another option to protect the duodenal repair. Originally, this was accomplished by complete duodenal diverticulization. In the early 1900s, Summers described this technique to divert the gastric and billiary flow by antrectomy, vagotomy, end-to-side gastrojejunostomy, T-tube common bile duct drainage, and lateral tube duodenostomy. In the 1960s, Berne and Donovan advocated using it for duodenal and pancreatic injury.[110,111]

The most common technique currently used is the pyloric exclusion technique originally described by Vaughan and later advocated by others.[112-115] Pyloric exclusion can be accomplished through a gastrotomy. The pylorus is grasped with a Babcock clamp and sutured closed using slow absorbable suture. Then, a loop gastrojejunostomy is constructed to divert the flow of gastric contents. Several weeks later the pylorus opens and the gastrojejunostomy functionally closes. Another option is to fire a thoracoabdominal stapling device across the stomach just proximal to the pylorus. In time, this staple line will open spontaneously secondary to the muscular contractions of the gastric wall. Although no prospective, randomized trails have been performed, several reports support the use of pyloric exclusion with severe duodenal injuries or in the case of delayed diagnosis.[116-118]

Marginal ulceration at the site of the gastrojejunostomy has been reported between 5% and 10%.[112,116] However, one study suggested that the incidence of a marginal ulcer to be as high as 33%.[113] This finding prompted some to recommend the addition of truncal vagotomy to the procedure. Currently, most surgeons do not include a truncal vagotomy with pyloric exclusion because most of the pyloric closures open within a few weeks and the ulcers can be medically managed until that time.

Mortality directly related to duodenal injury has been reported between 2% and 5% of patients.[82,86,87,94,109,119] The cause of mortality in these reports was due to duodenal dehiscence which led to sepsis and subsequent multiple system organ failure. The knowledge that mortality is directly linked to dehiscence fuels the debate of pyloric exclusion, buttressing, or duodenostomy to repair grade III or IV duodenal injuries. In the case of combined duodenal and pancreatic injury, most will add pyloric exclusion to the procedure. In a case study of 40 patients with penetrating duodenal injuries, there were 14 patients with combined pancreatic and duodenal injuries.[120] Five patients had primary repair of the duodenum, and two incurred leaks. Three patients had pyloric exclusion, and none had duodenal leaks.

COMBINED PANCREATIC-DUODENAL INJURIES

Combined pancreatic and duodenal injuries have been associated with high morbidity and mortality rates, ranging from 20% up to 100% depending on the extent of injury and operative intervention.[121,122] Controversy exists as to the optimal management of combined pancreatic and duodenal injuries. Clinical experience is limited due to the low incidence of combined injury and the lack of consistency in the repair modality chosen amongst surgeons and centers.[115,123,124] Recent studies have supported a trend toward the simplification of treatment.[40]

In a review of eight studies with 1,407 patients, operative intervention was related to mortality.[125] The overall mortality rate was 16.8%. Total pancreatectomy resulted in mortality rates of 100%. Patients who were not operated on and had pancreatic injury detected at autopsy or during a later procedure had a mortality rate of 89.7%. Patients undergoing pancreatoduodenectomy with a Roux-en-Y anastomosis to the distal pancreas had a mortality rate of 38.2%. Intermediate mortality rates were seen for suture and drainage of the pancreas (19.3% mortality), Roux-en-Y anastomoses with either a single loop to the left end of the pancreas or a double loop interposed between transected segments of the pancreas (16.7% mortality), distal pancreatectomy (14.3% mortality), and duodenal exclusion (12.5% mortality). Most of the patients (60.8%) only had a drainage procedure. The mortality in this group was the lowest at 10.9%.

Owing to the large variation of injuries to the pancreas and duodenum, it is not possible to determine one specific therapy appropriate for all situations. The determination of the best treatment option should be based on the condition of the patient and the integrity of the distal common bile duct and ampulla. An intraoperative cholangiogram, pancreatogram, and visualization of the ampulla can assist in determination of injury. If there is unobstructed flow into the duodenum, it can be assumed that the common bile duct and ampulla are intact.

In this case, the duodenal injury can be primarily closed and the pancreatic injury can be treated conservatively. If it is not possible to determine the status of the pancreatic duct intraoperatively, it is recommended to perform wide external drainage of the pancreatic head and leave closed suction drains. A resulting fistula due to an unrecognized duct injury can be managed at a later surgery.[126] The development of a postoperative enterocutaneous fistula, a pancreatic fistula, or an intra-abdominal abscess suggests a major pancreatic duct leak requiring a pancreatoduodenectomy.[127]

With severe duodenal and pancreatic head injury, it may be warranted to divert gastric contents from the duodenal repair. This can be accomplished as previously discussed by tube duodenostomy or pyloric exclusion. These techniques have proved useful in combined pancreatic and duodenal injuries not requiring a pancreatoduodenectomy. However, with massive injuries to the head of the pancreas, ampulla, proximal pancreatic duct, or distal common bile duct it may not be possible to complete a primary reconstruction. This is further complicated by the head of the pancreas and duodenum sharing a common blood supply. In these cases, a pancreatoduodenectomy is required. In the extremely unstable patient, the completion of a pancreatojejunostomy or pancreatogastrotomy may not be possible. Gentilello et al. suggest the ligation of the distal pancreatic duct as an option. Their experience, based on a small case study of 13 pancreatic duct ligations, indicate that ligation is a viable option.[128] They reported a 54% mortality rate, 50% fistula rate, 10% pancreatitis rate, and a 7.7% pancreatic remnant–related mortality.

Mortality ranges from 31% to 36% in patients undergoing pancreatoduodenectomy for trauma.[129] Between 1961 and 1994, 184 pancreatoduodenectomy performed for traumatic injuries have been reported in the literature. There were 26 operative deaths (14%) and 39 delayed deaths, for an overall survival rate of 64%. However, some investigators suggest that with appropriate selection criteria similar morbidity and mortality, as described in resections for cancer, can be achieved.[128,130–132]

Associated injuries continue to influence morbidity and mortality in patients with combined pancreas and duodenal injuries. The most common cause of early mortality is due to major vascular injury in the vicinity of the head of the pancreas. One study reviewed 33 patients, between 1997 and 2001, that had combined pancreatoduodenal injuries.[133] In this series, 9 (27%) of the patients had a portal vein injury, 8 (24%) had an injury to the superior mesenteric artery, and 7 (21%) sustained an injury to their inferior vena cava. If immediate control of hemorrhage and resuscitation can be achieved, pancreatoduodenectomy remains the procedure of choice in those patients with unreconstructable injury to the ampulla or proximal pancreatic duct, or severe injury to the duodenum and pancreatic head. Lengthy procedures should be avoided in patients with hemodynamic instability and developing acidosis, hypothermia, and coagulopathy. These patients should be treated with a staged "damage control" procedure.[126] Arrest of active hemorrhage should be the primary goal at the initial surgery with subsequent control of GI contamination. Following resuscitation and physiologic capture in the intensive care unit, these patients should be brought back to the operating room for definitive repairs.

REFERENCES

1. Jurkovich GJ, Carrico CJ. Pancreatic trauma. *Surg Clin North Am.* 1990;70:575–593.
2. Wilson RH, Morehead RJ. Current management of trauma to the pancreas. *Br J Surg.* 1991;78:1196–1202.
3. Akhrass R, Yaffe MB, Brandt CP, et al. Pancreatic trauma: A ten-year multi-institutional experience. *Am Surg.* 1997;63: 598–604.

4. Timberlake GA. Blunt pancreatic trauma: Experience at a rural referral center. *Am Surg.* 1997;63:282–286.
5. Cushing BM, Clark DE, Cobean R, et al. Blunt and penetrating trauma - has anything changed? *Surg Clin North Am.* 1997;77:1321–1332.
6. Augenstein JS, digges KH, Lombardo LV, et al. Occult abdominal injuries to airbag-protected-crash victims: A challenge to trauma systems. *J Trauma.* 1995;38:502–508.
7. Innes J, Carey L. Normal pancreatic dimensions in the adult human. *Am J Surg.* 1994;167:261–264.
8. Heitsch RC, Knutson CO, Fulton RL, et al. Delineation of critical factors in the treatment of pancreatic trauma. *Surgery.* 1976;80:523.
9. Smego DR, Richardson JD, Flint LM. Determinents of outcome in pancreatic trauma. *J Trauma.* 1985;25:771.
10. Patton JH, Fabian TC. Complex pancreatic injuries. *Surg Clin North Am.* 1996;76:783–795.
11. Olsen W. The serum amylase in blunt abdominal trauma. *J Trauma.* 1973;13:200.
12. Moretz JA, Campbell DP, Parker DE, et al. Significance of serum amylase level in evaluating pancreatic trauma. *Am J Surg.* 1975;150:698.
13. Liu KJ, Atten MJ, Lichtor T, et al. Serum amylase and lipase elevation is associated with intracranial events. *Am Surg.* 2000;67:215.
14. Takishima T, Hirata M, Kataoka Y, et al. Pancreatographic classification of pancreatic ductal injuries caused by blunt injury to the pancreas. *J Trauma.* 2000;48:745.
15. Wisner DH, Wold RL, Frey CF. Diagnosis and treatment of pancreatic injuries: An analysis of management principals. *Arch Surg.* 1990;125:1109–1113.
16. Ilahi O, Bochicchio GV, Scalea TM. Efficacy of computed tomography in the diagnosis of pancreatic injury in adult blunt trauma patients: A single-institutional study. *Am Surg.* 2002;68:704.
17. Akhrass R, Kim K, Brandt C. Computed tomography: An unreliableindicator of pancreatic trauma. *Am Surg.* 1996;62:647–651.
18. Bradley EL, Young PR, Chang MC, et al. Diagnosis and initial management of blunt pancreatic trauma: Guidelines from a multiinstitutional review. *Ann Surg.* 1998;227:861–869.
19. Harrell DJ, Vitale GC, Larson GM. Selective role for endoscopic retrograde cholangiopancreatography in abdominal trauma. *Surg Endosc.* 1998;12:400–404.
20. Wolf A, Bernhardt J, Patrzyk M, et al. The value of endoscopic diagnosis and treatment of pancreas injuries following blunt abdominal trauma. *Surg Endosc.* 2005;19:665–669.
21. Lin BC, Liu NJ, Fang JF, et al. Long term results of endoscopic stent in the management of blunt major pancreatic duct injury. *Surg Endosc.* 2006;20:1551–1555.
22. Huckfeldt R, Agee C, Nichols WK, et al. Nonoperative treatment of traumatic pancreatic duct disruption using endoscopically placed stent. *J Trauma.* 1996;41:143.
23. Laraja RD, Lobbato VJ, Cassaro S, et al. Intraoperative endoscopic retrograde cholangiopancreatography (ERCP) in penetrating trauma of the pancreas. *J Trauma.* 1986;26:1146.
24. Blind PJ, Mellbring G, Hjertkvist M, et al. Diagnosis of traumatic pancreatic duct rupture by on-table endoscopic retrograde pancreatography. *Pancreas.* 1994;9:387–389.
25. Soto JA, Alvarez, O, Munera, F, et al. Traumatic disruption of the pancreatic duct: Diagnosis with MR pancreatography. *AJR Am J Roentgenol.* 2001;176:175–178.
26. Ragozzino A, Manfredi R, Scaglione M, et al. The use of MRCP in the detection of pancreatic injuries after blunt trauma. *Emerg Radiol.* 2003;10(1):14–18.
27. Fulcher AS, Turner MA, Yelon JA, et al. Magnetic resonance cholangiopancreatography (MRCP) in the assessment of pancreatic duct trauma and its sequelae: Preliminary findings. *J Trauma.* 2000;48(6):1001–1007.
28. Fulcher AS, Turner MA, Capps GW, et al. RARE MR cholangiopancreatography in 300 subjects. *Radiology.* 1998;207:21–32.
29. Carrillo EH, Richardson JD, Miller FB. Evolution in the management of duodenal injuries. *J Trauma.* 1996;40:1037–1045.
30. Kao LS, Bulger EM, Parks DL, et al. Predictors of morbidity after traumatic pancreatic injury. *J Trauma.* 2003;55:426.
31. Moore EE, Cogbill TH, Malangoni MA, et al. Organ injury scaling II: Pancreas, duodenum, small bowel, colon, and rectum. *J Trauma.* 1990;30:1427.
32. Madiba TE, Mokoena TR. Favourable prognosis after surgical drainage of gunshot, stab or blunt trauma of the pancreas. *Br J Surg.* 1995;82:1236–1239.
33. Nowak M, Baringer D, Ponsky J. Pancreatic injuries: Effectiveness of debridement and drainage for nontransecting injuries. *Am Surg.* 1986;52:599.
34. Jurkovich GJ, Carrico CJ. Pancreatic trauma. *Surg Clin North Am.* 1994;70:575–593.
35. Fabian TC, Kudsk KA, Croce MA, et al. Superiority of closed suction drainage for pancreatic trauma: A randomized, prospective study. *Ann Surg.* 1990;211:724–730.
36. Vasquez JC, Coimbra R, Hoyt DB, et al. Management of penetrating pancreatic trauma: An 11-year experience of a level-1 trauma center. *Injury, Int J Care Injured.* 2001;32:753–759.
37. Buccimazza I, Thomson SR, Anderson F, et al. Isolated pancreatic duct injuries spectrum and management. *Am J Surg.* 2006;191:448–452.
38. Cogbill TH, Moore EE, Morris JA, et al. Distal pancreatectomy for trauma: A multicenter experience. *J Trauma.* 1991;31:1600–1606.
39. Farrell RJ, Krige JEJ, Bornman PC, et al. Operative strategies in pancreatic trauma. *Br J Surg.* 1996;83:934–937.
40. Patton JH, Lyden SP, Croce MA, et al. Pancreatic trauma: A simplified management guideline. *J Trauma.* 1997;43(2):234–241.
41. Marczell AP, Stierer M. Partial pancreaticoduodenectomy (Whipple procedure) for pancreatic malignancy: Occlusion of a non-anastomosed pancreatic stump with fibrin sealant. *HPB Surg.* 1992;5:251–259.
42. Robey E, Mullen JT, Schwab CW. Blunt transection of the pancreas treated by distal pancreatectomy, splenic salvage and hyperalimentation: Four cases and review of the literature. *Ann Surg.* 1982;196:695–699.
43. Aldridge MC, Williamson RCN. Distal pancreatectomy with and without splenectomy. *Br J Surg.* 1991;78:976–979.
44. Warshaw AL. Conservation of the spleen with distal pancreatectomy. *Arch Surg.* 1988;123:550–553.
45. DeGiannis E, Levy RD, Potokar T, et al. Distal pancreatectomy for gunshot injuries of the distal pancreas. *Br J Surg.* 1995;82:1240–1242.
46. Pachter HL, Hofstetter SR, Liang HG, et al. Traumatic injuries to the pancreas: The role of distal pancreatectomy with splenic preservation. *J Trauma.* 1989;29:1352–1355.
47. Dawson D, Scott-Conner C. Distal pancreatectomy with splenic preservation: The anatomic basis for a meticulous operation. *J Trauma.* 1986;26:1142.
48. Kendall DM, Sutherland DE, Najarian JS, et al. Effects of hemipancreatectomy on insulin secretion and glucose tolerance in healthy humans. *N Engl J Med.* 1990;322:898–903.
49. Innes J, Carey L. Normal pancreatic dimensions in the adult human. *Am J Surg.* 1994;167:261.
50. Hutchins RR, Hart RS, Pacifico M, et al. Long-term results of distal pancreatectomy for chronic pancreatitis in 90 patients. *Ann Surg.* 2002;236:612.
51. Warshaw AL, Rattner DW, Fernandez-del Castillo C, et al. Middle segment pancreatectomy: A novel technique for conserving pancreatic tissue. *Arch Surg.* 1998;133:327–331.
52. Thanh LN, Duchmann JC, Latrive JP, et al. Conservation of the left pancreas in rupture of the pancreatic isthmus. Apropos of 3 cases. *Chirurgie.* 1999;124:165–170.
53. Wind P, Tiret E, Cunningham C, et al. Contribution of endoscopic retrograde pancreatography in management of complications following distal pancreatic trauma. *Am Surg.* 1999;65:777–783.
54. Stone HH, Fabian TC, Satiani B, et al. Experiences in the management of pancreatic trauma. *J Trauma.* 1981;21:257.
55. Jurkovich GJ. Injuries to the duodenum and pancreas.In: Souba WW, Fink MP, Jurkovich GJ, et al. eds. *ACS surgery: principals and practice 2005.* New York: WebMD; Nov 2005.

56. Leppaniemi A, Haapiainen R, Kiviluoto T, et al. Pancreatic trauma: Acute and late manifestations. *Br J Surg.* 1988;75: 165–167.

57. Lin BC, Chen RJ, Fang JF, et al. Management of blunt major pancreatic injury. *J Trauma.* 2004;56:774–778.

58. Young PR, Meredith JW, Baker CC, et al. Pancreatic injuries resulting from penetrating trauma: A multi-institution review. *Am Surg.* 1998;64:838–844.

59. Lane MJ, Mindelzun RE, Jeffrey RB. Diagnosis of pancreatic injury after blunt abdominal trauma. *Semin Ultrasound CT MR.* 1996; 17:177–182.

60. Craig MH, Talton DS, Hauser CJ, et al. Pancreatic injuries from blunt trauma. *Am Surg.* 1995;61:125–128.

61. Jones R. Management of pancreatic trauma. *Am J Surg.* 1985; 150:698.

62. Kudsk KA, Croce MA, Fabian TC, et al. Enteral versus parenteral feeding. Effects on the septic morbidity after blunt and penetrating abdominal trauma. *Ann Surg.* 1992;215:503–513.

63. Williams ST, Woltering EA, O'Dorisio TM, et al. Effect of octreotide acetate on pancreatic exocrine function. *Am J Surg.* 1989; 157:459–462.

64. Barnes SM, Kontny BG, Prinz RA. Somatrostatin analogue treatment of pancreatic fistulas. *Int J Pancreatol.* 1993;14: 181–188.

65. Martineau P, Shwed JA, Denis R. Is octreotide a new hope for enterocutaneous and external pancreatic fistulas closure? *Am J Surg.* 1996;172:386.

66. Berberat PO, Friess H, Uhl W, et al. The role of octreotide in the prevention of complications following pancreatic resection. *Digestion.* 1999;60:15.

67. Nwariaku FE, Terracina A, Mileski WJ, et al. Is octreotide beneficial following pancreatic injury? *Am J Surg.* 1995;170:582.

68. Amirata E, Livingston DH, Elcavage J. Octreotide acetate decreases pancreatic complications after pancreatic trauma. *Am J Surg.* 1994;168:345–347.

69. Kudsk KA, Temizer D, Ellison EC, et al. Post-traumatic pancreatic sequestrum: Recognition and treatment. *J Trauma.* 1986; 26:320.

70. Lin BC, Fang JF, Wong YC, et al. Blunt pancreatic trauma and pseudocyst: Management of major pancreatic duct injury, *Injury.* 2007;38(5):588–593.

71. Kozarek RA, Ball TJ, Patterson DJ, et al. Endoscopic transpapillary therapy for disrupted pancreatic duct and peripancreatic fluid collections. *Gastroenterology.* 1991;100:1362.

72. Moore JB, Moore EE. Changing trends in the management of combined pancreatoduodenal injuries. *World J Surg.* 1984; 8:791–797.

73. Heinrich S, Schafer M, Rousson V, et al. Evidence-based treatment of acute pancreatitis. A look at established paradigms. *Ann Surg.* 2006;243:154–168.

74. Nathens AB, Curtis JR, Beale RJ, et al. Management of the critically ill patient with severe acute pancreatitis. *Crit Care Med.* 2004;32:2524–2536.

75. Wynn M, Hill DM, Miller DR, et al. Management of pancreatic and duodenal trauma. *Am J Surg.* 1985;150:327–332.

76. Balasegaram M. Surgical management of pancreatic trauma. *Curr Probl Surg.* 1979;16:1.

77. Carrillo EH, Richardson JD, Miller FB. Evolution in the management of duodenal injuries. *J Trauma.* 1996;40(6):1037–1046.

78. Asensio JA, Feliciano DV, Britt LD, et al. Management of duodenal injuries. *Curr Probl Surg.* 1993;11:1026–1092.

79. Huerta S, Bui T, Porral D, et al. Predictors of morbidity and mortality in patients with traumatic duodenal injuries. *Am Surg.* 2005;71(9):763–767.

80. Lucas C, Ledgerwood A. Factors influencing outcome after blunt duodenal injury. *J Trauma* 1975; 15:839–846.

81. Weigelt JA. Duodenal injuries. *Surg Clin North Am.* 1990;70(3): 529–539.

82. Flint LM, McCoy M, Richardson JD, et al. Duodenal injury: Analysis of common misconceptions in diagnosis and treatment. *Ann Surg.* 1980;191(6):697–701.

83. Degiannis E, Boffard K. Duodenal injuries. *Br J Surg.* 2000;87: 1473–1479.

84. Schurink GW, Bode PJ, vanLuijt PA, et al. The value of physical examination in the diagnosis of patients with blunt abdominal trauma: A retrospective study. *Injury.* 1997;28(4):261–265.

85. Aherne NJ, Kavanagh EG, Condon ET, et al. Duodenal perforation after a blunt abdominal sporting injury: The importance of early diagnosis. *J Trauma.* 2003;54:791–794.

86. Levison MA, Peterson SR, Sheldon GF, et al. Duodenal trauma: Experience of a trauma center. *J Trauma.* 1984;24:475–480.

87. Snyder WH, Weigelt JA, Watkins WL, et al. The surgical management of duodenal trauma: Precepts based on a review of 247 cases. *Arch Surg.* 1980;115:422–429.

88. Lucas CE, Dulchavsky SA, Ledgerwood AM. Pancreaticoduodenal injury. In: Hurst JM, ed. *Common problems in trauma.* Chicago: Year Book Medical Publishers; 1987:204–212.

89. Holmes JF, Offerman SR, Chang CH, et al. Performance of helical computed tomography without oral contrast for the detection of gastrointestinal injuries. *Ann Emerg Med.* 2004; 43(1):120–128.

90. Kunin JR, Korobkin M, Ellis JH, et al. Duodenal injuries caused by blunt abdominal trauma: Value of CT in differentiating perforation from hematoma. *AJR Am J Roentgenol.* 1993;163: 1221–1223.

91. Sherck J, Oakes D. Intestinal injuries missed by computed tomography. *J Trauma.* 1990;30(1):1–7.

92. Brooks AJ, Boffard KD. Current technology: Laproscopic surgery in trauma. *Trauma.* 1999;1:53–60.

93. Cattell RB, Braasch JW. A technique for exposure of the duodenum. *Surg Gynecol Obstet.* 1954;98:376–377.

94. Cogbill TH, More EE, Feliciano DV. Conservative management of duodenal trauma: A multicenter prespective. *J Trauma.* 1990; 30:1469–1475.

95. Blocksom JM, Tyburski JG, Sohn RL, et al. Prognostic determinants in duodenal injuries. *Am Surg.* 2004;70(3):248–255.

96. Wooley M, Mahour G, Sloan T. Duodenal hematoma in infancy and childhood. *Am J Surg.* 1978;136(8):1978.

97. Jewett TC, Caldarola V, Karp MP. Intramural hematoma of the duodenum. *Arch Surg.* 1988;123(1):54–58.

98. Touloukian R. Protocol for the nonoperative treatment of obstructing intramural duodenal hematoma. *Am J Surg.* 1983;145: 330–334.

99. Gullotto C, Paulson EK. CT-guided percutaneous drainage of a duodenal hematoma. *AJR Am J Roentgenol.* 2005;184: 231–233.

100. Ivatury RR, Gaudino J, Ascer E. Treatment of penetrating duodenal injuries. *J Trauma.* 1985;25:337–341.

101. Seamon MJ, Pieri PG, Fisher CA, et al. A ten-year retrospective review: Does pyloric exclusion improve clinical outcome after penetrating duodenal and combined pancreaticoduodenal injuries? *J Trauma.* 2007;62(4):829–833.

102. Kraus M, Condon RE. Alternative techniques of duodenotomy. *Surg Gynecol Obstet.* 1974;139:417–419.

103. Ivatury RR, Nassoura ZE, Simon R, et al. Complex duodenal injuries. *Surg Clin North Am.* 1996;76:797–812.

104. McInnis WD, Aust JB, Cruz AB. Traumatic injuries of the duodenum: A comparison of primary clousre and the jejunal patch. *J Trauma.* 1975;15:847–853.

105. Welsh CE. Treatment of acute, massive gastroduodenal hemorrhage. *JAMA.* 1949;141:1113–1123.

106. Smith AD, Woolverton WC, Weichert RF. Operative management of pancreatic and duodenal injuries. *J Trauma.* 1971;14: 570–579.

107. Stone H, Fabian T. Management of duodenal wounds. *J Trauma.* 1979;19(5):334–339.

108. Hasson J, Stern D, Moss G. Penetrating duodenal trauma. *J Trauma.* 1984;24(6):471–474.

109. Ivatury R. Penetrating duodenal injuries: An analysis of 100 consecutive cases. *Ann Surg.* 1985;202(2):154–158.

110. Berne C. Duodenal "diverticulization" for duodenal and pancreatic injury. *Am J Surg.* 1974;127:503–505.

111. Donovan A, Hagen W, Berne D. Traumatic perforations of the duodenum. *Am J Surg.* 1966;111:341–350.

112. Vaughan G. The use of pyloric exclusion in the management of severe duodenal injuries. *Am J Surg.* 1977;134:785–790.

113. Buck JR. Severe pancreatico-duodenal injuries: The effectiveness of pyloric exclusion with vagotomy. *Am Surg.* 1992;58(9):557–560.

114. Cogbill T, Moore E, Kashuk J. Changing trends in the management of pancreatic trauma. *Arch Surg.* 1982;117:722–728.

115. Feliciano DV. Management of combined pancreatoduodenal injuries. *Ann Surg.* 1987;205(6):673–679.

116. Martin T. Severe duodenal injuries: Treatment with pyloric exclusion and gastrojejunostomy. *Arch Surg.* 1983;118:631–635.

117. Kashuk J, Moore E, Cogbill T. Management of the intermediate severity duodenal injury. *Surgery.* 1982;92:758–764.

118. Cone JB, Eidt JF. Delayed diagnosis of duodenal rupture. *Am J Surg.* 1994;168(6):676–678.

119. Shorr R, Greaney G, Donovan A. Injuries of the duodenum. *AJR Am J Roentgenol.* 1987;154(7):93–98.

120. McKenny MG. Evaluation of minor penetrating duodenal injuries. *Am Surg.* 1996;62(11):952–955.

121. Flynn WJ. Reappraisal of pancreatic and duodenal injuries management based on injury severity. *Arch Surg.* 1990;125:1539–1541.

122. Kerry RL, Glas WW. Traumatic injuries of the pancreas and duodenum. *Arch Surg.* 1962;85:813–816.

123. Mansour MA. Conservative management of combined pancreatoduodenal injuries. *AJR Am J Roentgenol.* 1989;158:531–535.

124. Burrus GR, Howell JF, Jordan GL. Traumatic duodenal injuries: An analysis of 86 cases. *J Trauma.* 1961;1:96–104.

125. Glancy KE. Review of pancreatic trauma. *West J Med.* 1989;151(1):45–51.

126. Rickard M, Brohi K, Bautz PC. Pancreatic and duodenal injuries: Keep it simple. *ANZ J Surg.* 2005;75:581–586.

127. Heimansohn DA. The role of pancreaticoduodenectomy in the management of traumatic injuries to the pancreas and duodenum. *Am Surg.* 1990;56(8):511–514.

128. Gentilello LM, Cortes V, Buechter KJ, et al. Whipple procedure for trauma: Is duct ligation a safe alternative to pancreaticojejunostomy? *J Trauma.* 1991;31(5):661–668.

129. Asensio JA, Demetriades D, Hanpeter DE. Management of pancreatic injuries. *Curr Probl Surg.* 1999;36:325–420.

130. Oreskovich M, Carrico C. Pancreaticoduodenectomy for trauma: A viable option? *AJR Am J Roentgenol.* 1984;147(5):618–623.

131. Delcore R. The role of pancreatogastrostomy following pancreatoduoenectomy for trauma. *J Trauma.* 1994;37(3):395–400.

132. McKone T, Bursch L, Scholten D. Pancreaticoduodenectomy for trauma: A life saving procedure. *Am Surg.* 1988;54(6):361–364.

133. Lopez PP, Benjamin R, Cockburn M, et al. Recent trends in the management of combined pancreatoduodenal injuries. *Am Surg.* 2005;71(10):847–852.

Injuries to the Liver and Spleen

41

William J. Mileski

INTRODUCTION AND HISTORICAL PERSPECTIVE

The liver and spleen are the most commonly injured abdominal organs.[1,2] Few areas of trauma care have evolved so dramatically over the last 4 decades as has the management approaches to hepatic and splenic injuries. The change from early surgery and emphasis on resectional and devascularization techniques to nonoperative approaches has been driven by the understanding that spontaneous hemostasis occurs in at least 50% of patients with injury to the liver or spleen. For example, Walt[3] reviewed approximately 1,500 patients with liver injuries from a single trauma center and found that spontaneous hemostasis occurred in more than 50% of the patients. The converse of this concept is that injured patients who are going to bleed sufficiently from the injured liver or spleen to require surgery will manifest their bleeding clinically; the overwhelming majority of the patients requiring surgery will present to the trauma resuscitation area with signs of major blood loss and clinical evidence that the blood loss is intraperitoneal in location. For those patients who are initially stable, the success of nonoperative therapy depends on the knowledge that dangerous bleeding will be detectable in time to perform the necessary surgery before blood loss becomes life threatening.

For patients with liver injury, the conditions for consistently successful nonoperative management have been documented. The main historical reasons for early surgery, control of bleeding, debridement of devitalized liver tissue, and drainage have included fear of infection, bile leak, hemobilia, and late bleeding from hepatic venous injury. Some of these complications do occur but not often

enough to threaten the patient's life while nonoperative therapy is undertaken. Richardson[4] described changes in management of liver injury over a 25-year time interval and noted that the use of nonoperative management was associated with improved outcomes in terms of mortality; declines in the rates of septic complications, particularly associated with the cessation of the practice of placing drains; and a reduced frequency of exsanguination from hepatic venous injuries. Walt[3] also noted that hepatic venous and retrohepatic vena cava injuries were associated with spontaneous hemostasis. Although management of liver and spleen injuries is predominantly nonoperative, it is critical to remember that the liver and the spleen are both highly vascular, and can be the sources of major abdominal hemorrhage following either blunt or penetrating injuries and may require rapid operative intervention.

Close observation of hemodynamically stable patients with liver injury is now widely practiced and the success of this approach has been documented.[5-7] Technologic advances have occurred as clinical experience has increased. Computed tomographic (CT) scans permit visualization of the injury (see Fig. 1) and assist in clinical decision making.[8] Although the use of sequential CT scans to document liver healing is intellectually appealing, the utility of this approach has been controversial.[9,10] Selective angiographic embolization has become the main means of controlling liver bleeding that occurs during nonoperative management in initially stable patients.[11]

Success of nonoperative management of liver injury also depends on the recognition that failures of this approach occur.[12,13] Successful management of treatment failures depends heavily on recognition of high-risk comorbidities such as liver cirrhosis and severe associated injuries as

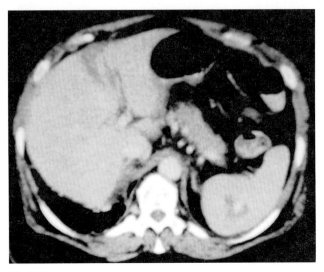

Figure 1   Liver injury visualized by computed tomographic (CT) imaging.

well as readily available methods of rapid detection of the need for surgery and the necessary institutional infrastructure such as available surgeons, operating rooms and equipment, radiology services, critical care units, and a responsive blood bank.[14,15]

The change to mainly nonoperative management of spleen injuries also occurred because surgeons recognized the capacity for spontaneous hemostasis, especially in children.[16] Another important influence was the description of serious, sometimes fatal infections in asplenic children.[17–20] Fear of infection stimulated the expansion of nonoperative management to adults.[21,22] Inconsistency of patient compliance with vaccination and postsplenectomy antibiotic prophylaxis has provided further impetus to efforts to conserve the injured spleen prompting the development of methods of splenic repair or embolization for preservation of splenic mass.[23,24] The actual risk of life-threatening postsplenectomy infection in adults undergoing splenectomy for injury has been difficult to document.[25,26] Similarly, the risk of life threatening delayed bleeding has been a controversial topic with some authors concerned that delayed bleeding is underreported.[26] Nonetheless, nonoperative therapy for spleen injury in stable children and adults is the most often practiced approach.

MECHANISMS OF INJURY

Blunt trauma due to motor vehicle crashes, auto-pedestrian collisions, falls, and sports injuries is the most common cause of both liver injury and spleen injury and as already noted both types of injury are most frequently managed nonoperatively in *hemodynamically normal/stable patients.* Penetrating injuries of both the liver and spleen

are generally treated surgically to ensure rapid control of bleeding as well as the identification and repair of any associated abdominal injuries.

ANATOMIC CONSIDERATIONS

The potential for exsanguination and death in patients who sustain liver and spleen injuries requires an understanding of anatomy and the emergent maneuvers to allow rapid control of severe hemorrhage.

Liver

The liver is tethered superiorly by attachments to the diaphragm and the anterior parietal peritoneum through the coronary ligaments, triangular ligaments, and the falciform ligament. Inferiorly the liver is connected to the porta hepatis, including the portal vein, hepatic artery, and common bile duct, and to the lesser curve of the stomach, by the lesser omentum. Posteriorly the liver is connected to the inferior vena cava by numerous very short direct venous branches arising primarily from the caudate lobe. The hepatic veins—superior, middle, and inferior—are located in the central aspect of the coronary ligaments. They are short broad structures that empty directly into the vena cava and require careful attention when mobilizing the coronary ligament. Up to a dozen small venous channels empty into the inferior vena cava from the caudate lobe of the liver. The concept of segmental anatomy of the liver based on the locations of the portal vein branches and the hepatic veins has been eloquently reviewed by Bismuth.[27,28] Figure 2 is an illustration of the segmental liver anatomy described in Bismuth's articles. Liver injury results from compression of the hepatic parenchyma by blunt forces and penetration/cavitation of the parenchyma when penetrating mechanisms occur. Disruption of the liver occurs across segmental boundaries and, when bleeding occurs, multiple arterial and venous branches are involved. Anatomic liver resection is not often feasible for the bleeding patient with liver injury. Nonetheless, knowledge of the locations of inflow and outflow vessels facilitates management.

An important maneuver to achieve immediate control of hepatic hemorrhage is manual compression followed by perihepatic packing. Patients who undergo exploratory laparotomy for liver bleeding have the liver laceration compressed manually as quickly as possible. Then, the spaces above and below the liver are packed with gauze pads. Packing allows for freeing of the surgeon's hands for additional exploration and hemorrhage control from other injuries. Packing may serve as the definitive means for controlling hemorrhage. Packing and temporary abdominal closure provide time for resuscitation and measures for prevention of coagulopathy and maintenance of body temperature (see the following text).

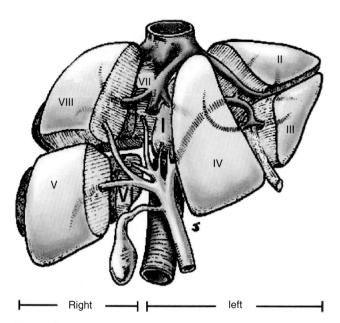

Right ———— left ————

Figure 2   Hepatic segmental anatomy.

Another useful maneuver for temporary control of major hemorrhage associated with hepatic injures is occlusion of the hepatic artery and portal vein in the porta hepatis (Pringle Maneuver). This can be initially accomplished manually by placement of the index finger of the left hand in the epiploic foramen of Winslow followed by compression of the entire porta between the index finger and thumb. Manual control can be replaced with either a vascular clamp or Rommel tourniquet. Total vascular isolation of the liver is obtained by isolating the infrahepatic inferior vena cava superior to the renal and adrenal veins and inferior to the diaphragm using Rommel tourniquets. Extension of the midline abdominal incision to a median sternotomy may be necessary to gain exposure. On occasion, exposure of the intrapericardial inferior vena cava is the most expeditious method for encircling the vena cava above the liver.

Spleen

The vascular supply of the spleen is composed primarily of the splenic artery and vein and the short gastric vessels. Primary anatomic considerations in treating spleen injuries are related to immediate packing of the left upper quadrant to control ongoing bleeding followed by early control of the short gastric arteries and mobilization of the retroperitoneal attachments of the spleen, the splenocolic, splenorenal, and splenophrenic ligaments. These lateral, posterior, and superior retroperitoneal attachments can be sharply divided with scissors and rapidly released so that a retropancreatic/prenephric plane of dissection can be entered allowing the spleen to be retracted caudally and medially into the midline incision. Caution is required because of the ease of entering the plane between the

splenic capsule and the parenchyma of the spleen. Active bleeding can be easily controlled with manual compression of the splenic hilum, or application of vascular clamps to the hilum. If clamps are used it is important to exercise care to avoid injury to the tail of the pancreas, which is always in close proximity to the splenic hilum. Several laparotomy pads can be packed behind the spleen to tamponade bleeding and support the spleen while the lesser sac is opened on the proximal aspect of the greater curve of the stomach and the short gastric vessels ligated. At this point, the spleen can be freely mobilized along with the tail of the pancreas to the midline. Splenic arterial branches and venous branches are individually isolated and controlled with suture ligatures followed by free ligatures.

INITIAL ASSESSMENT

The initial management of all injured patients should follow the principles outlined in the Advanced Trauma Life Support course sponsored by the American College of Surgeons. In patients who are *hemodynamically unstable,* early identification of intra-abdominal hemorrhage may be obvious based on physical examination but most often is identified by focused abdominal sonogram for trauma (FAST) supplemented, in selected patients, with diagnostic peritoneal lavage (DPL). Under such circumstances the specific identification and management of hepatic and/or splenic injury will occur at the subsequent exploratory laparotomy.

DIAGNOSIS AND SEVERITY GRADING

CT scanning is an increasingly integral part of the assessment of trauma patients and is highly sensitive and specific in the assessment of injuries to the liver and spleen in hemodynamically stable patients. The American Association for the Surgery of Trauma has developed organ injury severity scaling systems, based on CT scan imaging, as well as intraoperative observations that are helpful in making decisions regarding operative management of injuries of the liver and spleen.[29,30] Table 1 represents the 1994 revision of the liver injury scale whereas Table 2 is the 1994 revision of the spleen injury scale.

PATIENT SELECTION AND CONDUCT OF NONOPERATIVE MANAGEMENT

The last 20 years of experience with increased use of nonoperative management of liver and spleen injuries has established the safety and efficacy of this approach in most cases. Patients with isolated liver injuries encompassing all injury grades that are hemodynamically stable and who

TABLE 1

LIVER INJURY GRADING SCALE (AMERICAN ASSOCIATION FOR THE SURGERY OF TRAUMA, 1994 REVISION)

Grade	Injury Type	Description	ICD-9 Code	AIS Score
I	Hematoma	Subcapsular, <10% surface area	864.01	2
	Laceration	Capsular tear, <1 cm parenchymal depth	864.11	2
II	Hematoma	Subcapsular, 10%–50% surface area intraparenchymal <10 cm in diameter	864.02	2
	Laceration	Capsular tear 1–3 cm parenchymal depth, <10 cm in length	864.12	2
III	Hematoma	Subcapsular, >50% surface area of ruptured subcapsular or parenchymal hematoma; intraparenchymal hematoma >10 cm or expanding	864.03	3
	Laceration	>3 cm parenchymal depth	864.13	3
IV	Laceration	Parenchymal disruption involving 25%–75% hepatic lobe or 1–3 Couinaud segments	864.04 864.14	4
V	Laceration	Parenchymal disruption involving >75% of hepatic lobe or >3 Couinaud segments within a single lobe	864.04	4
	Vascular	Juxtahepatic venous injuries; i.e., retrohepatic vena cava/central major hepatic veins	864.14	5
VI	Vascular	Liver avulsion		6

ICD, International Classification of Diseases; AIS, Abbreviated Injury Scale.

have no history of underlying cirrhosis or portal hypertension may be safely managed nonoperatively in an intensive care unit (ICU) using hemodynamic monitoring, abdominal physical examinations at two-hourly intervals for the first 24 hours and twice daily subsequently and twice-daily assessments of hemoglobin level to assess for development of peritonitis or progressive blood loss. When signs of bleeding emerge, angioembolization may also be used to control hemorrhage. Liver injuries that are grade 4 and grade 5, those with contrast extravasation consistent with arterial bleeding, those with significant free fluid in the abdomen as evidenced by large amounts of fluid in the pelvis and surrounding small bowel loops, equivalent to approximately 1000 mL, are more likely to fail attempts at nonoperative management and require angiography with embolization or operative intervention. Traditionally, blunt liver injuries have been treated nonoperatively whereas penetrating injuries due to stab wounds have been treated selectively and abdominal or thoracoabdominal gunshot wounds have been treated with mandatory laparotomy. The frequent finding of a nonbleeding liver injury needing no repair when right-sided abdominal and thoracoabdominal gunshot wounds are explored led to several reports documenting the safety of nonoperative

TABLE 2

SPLEEN INJURY SCALE (AMERICAN ASSOCIATION FOR THE SURGERY OF TRAUMA, 1994 REVISION)

Injury Grade	Injury Type	Description of Injury	ICD-9	AIS-90
I	Hematoma	Subcapsular, <10% surface area	865.01	2
	Laceration	Capsular tear <1 cm parenchymal depth	865.11	2
II	Hematoma	Subcapsular, 10%–50% of surface area	865.01	2
	Laceration	Intraparenchymal, <5 cm in diameter	865.11	2
III	Hematoma	Capsular tear 1–3 cm parenchymal depth not involving a trabecular vessel; subcapsular >50% of surface area or expanding; ruptured subcapsular or parenchymal hematoma; intraparenchymal hematoma ≥5 cm or expanding	865.02 865.12	2
	Laceration	>3 cm parenchymal depth or involving trabecular vessels	865.03	3
IV	Laceration	Laceration involving segmental or hilar vessels producing major devascularization (>25% of spleen)	865.13	4
V	Laceration	Completely shattered spleen	865.04	5
	Vascular	Hilar vascular injury which devascularizes spleen	865.14	5

therapy for gunshot wounds of the liver and this practice is becoming commonplace. No increase in mortality or morbidity have been observed but decreased hospital length of stay has been reported.[31,32] Nonoperative management of penetrating injuries to the spleen which have been documented by CT scan has been reported in a small number of patients.[33,34] This approach cannot be recommended at this time outside of a prospective study protocol. Necessary resources for successful practice of this approach include ready availability of surgeons, operating rooms, anesthesia support, blood bank support, interventional radiology capability, and critical care.

When isolated spleen injuries are assessed, decisions to intervene operatively are also based principally on the patient's hemodynamic status and assessment of ongoing hemorrhage and transfusion requirements, even in the face of grade 4 and 5 injuries. Age older than 55 years, severe comorbid conditions, multiple injuries, and the presence of a large hemoperitoneum are findings associated with failure of nonoperative management of spleen injuries and early surgery is indicated where these signs are present. Figure 3 is the CT scan of a 58-year-old patient with spleen injury and large hemoperitoneum. The patient had a history of coronary artery disease. Splenectomy was chosen over nonoperative therapy for this patient.

Angiographic embolization is a valuable adjunct to nonoperative management protocols. When this intervention is chosen, careful monitoring and support of the patient while in the angiography suite is critical. The level of support is chosen on the basis of an assessment of the patient's hemodynamic status and risk of a sudden increase in the rate of bleeding. For critically ill patients, the same level of anesthesia and critical care support provided for the patient in the operating room is necessary for safe angioembolization.

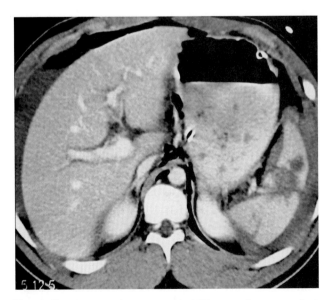

Figure 3   Computed tomographic (CT) scan of severe splenic injury with large hemoperitoneum.

Anesthesiologists should be physically present along with equipment for monitoring, infusion of warm blood, and fluids. Success of angiographic control of bleeding has been documented in a wide variety of hepatic injuries.[35,36] Although our preference for splenic preservation is splenic repair, angioembolization has proved successful for the management of selected patients with spleen injuries where preservation of splenic mass is important. The findings of angiography may also disclose high-risk vascular injuries within the spleen that will respond to embolization.[37]

OPERATIVE MANAGEMENT

Because the patients operated on with liver and spleen injuries are those that present as hemodynamically unstable with severe hemorrhage or have failed attempts at nonoperative management, the approach to surgery is generally of an emergent nature and requires direct and rapid control of hemorrhage. The torso should be widely prepped and draped, and a generous midline incision carried from the xiphisternum to just above the pubis. The patient should be prepared so that the abdominal incision can be extended as a median sternotomy. The use of table-mounted self-retaining retractors aids in retraction of the costal margins and lateral abdominal walls resulting in improved exposure.

In some patients, opening of the peritoneum may result in decompression of tamponade and result in severe hypotension; in these instances, temporary compression of the aorta at the diaphragmatic hiatus either manually, with an aortic compression device, or the end of a small Richardson retractor can provide for improved cardiac function and partial distal hemostasis while the anesthesia personnel restore intravascular volume. Ledgerwood and Lucas[38] described preabdominal exploration left thoracotomy with control of the distal thoracic aorta to achieve hemodynamic improvement and partial distal hemostasis. Upon evacuation of the hemoperitoneum, the right upper and left upper quadrants of the abdomen can be initially packed with laparotomy pads and the source of hemorrhage determined.

Liver

When the source of hemorrhage is identified as primarily from the liver it is important to determine whether the injury is amenable to repair or if a damage control approach that involves packing of the hepatic injury should be pursued.[39] This determination requires consideration of the patient's hemodynamic status, the degree of shock, acidosis, coagulopathy, hypothermia, associated injuries, and the severity of the liver injury itself.

If bleeding is not controlled by compression of the porta hepatis (Pringle maneuver), the suspicion of a retrohepatic venous injury should be high and damage control and packing of the liver performed rapidly. Similarly, in patients with grade 4 or 5 injuries associated with massive hemoperitoneum, profound shock, coagulopathy, or severe acidosis (pH, 7.0), a damage control approach with early control of bleeding from the liver by hepatic packing should be considered. Prevention of trauma and shock-related coagulopathy by the use of early packing and damage control is crucial to patient survival. Garrison has recently reported the clinical findings that suggest that damage control approaches should be used.[40]

Several (three to six) laparotomy pads should be placed superior and posterior to the right lobe of the liver and several more placed inferior to the right lobe. This should be followed with two to three laparotomy pads being placed superior to the left lobe and inferior to the left lobe. This can be furthered by manual compression to control hemorrhage.

Following packing of the liver and control/repair of other life-threatening injuries, the abdomen can be closed in a temporary manner, using any number of widely described techniques that employ a temporary prosthetic barrier to limit contamination of the peritoneal contents as well as to collect peritoneal fluid losses which may, on occasion, be massive. The patient is transported to the critical care unit for correction of coagulopathy, hypothermia, and hypoperfusion. Replacement of coagulation proteins using fresh frozen plasma (1 unit for every unit of packed red blood cells transfused) is aggressively pursued as described by Lucas et al.[41] Exogenous platelets are administered if the platelet count is <100,000 per mm.[3] Cryoprecipitate may be needed if the fibrinogen level is depressed. Activated factor VII may also be used in selected patients.[42,43] Typically the damage control resuscitation period requires 24 to 48 hours. During this interval, adjunctive therapies including angioembolization may be considered to aid in control of hemorrhage. When the patient has been resuscitated and acidosis and coagulopathy reversed, reexploration will most often involve removal of the perihepatic packing. Although management of liver and spleen injuries is predominantly nonoperative, it is critical to remember that the liver and the spleen are both highly vascular, and can be the sources of major abdominal hemorrhage following either blunt or penetrating injuries and may require rapid operative intervention.

Repacking, simple ligation or clamp control of persistently bleeding vessels, and filling of the injury cavity with vascularized omentum are potentially valuable maneuvers.[44,45]

In cases where the patient rapidly responds to resuscitative measures and the liver injury appears amenable to repair, several techniques can be employed to establish hemostasis.

It is essential to have good exposure and mobilization of the injured area of the liver; in the case of the most frequently injured right lobe, this is accomplished by mobilization of the falciform and triangular ligaments

allowing medial rotation of the right lobe of the liver. From this point, combinations of direct suture ligation, electrocautery, argon beam coagulation and packing with topical hemostatic agents are employed. Topical cellulose fabric, spray thrombin, and tissue glues have been employed alone and in various combinations with success. Rarely, extension of a hepatic laceration or missile injury with a finger fracture technique may be required for exposure and control of active hemorrhage. Upon control of hepatic bleeding, the omentum can be used as an additional packing and closed suction drains placed in the suprahepatic and infrahepatic areas in the event of bile leak.

Retrohepatic Venous Injuries

When hepatic venous injuries and retrohepatic injuries are encountered, the patients are most often in profound shock and the damage control approach is used at first surgery. The definitive approach to these injuries can then be made at a second or third surgery.

Preparation for entry into the chest and abdomen should be made and the availability of rapid infusion devices and cell saver machines ensured. Assistance from an experienced liver surgeon or liver transplant surgeon may be valuable. The approach to these injuries requires vascular isolation of the liver, which consists of controlling the suprahepatic or intrapericardial inferior vena through median sternotomy, the suprarenal inferior vena cava, and the porta hepatis. The use of Rommel tourniquets for these maneuvers is most helpful. This produces near-complete hepatic vascular isolation and ischemia and every effort should be made to limit its duration (<60 minutes is generally recommended). The venous injuries can than be exposed, usually within the liver substance and repaired by primary lateral venorrhaphy or, if necessary, the hepatic vein involved ligated. Formerly, the placement of intracaval plastic shunts was recommended for these injuries.[46] Contemporary management with nonoperative means and damage control interventions has reduced the need for these devices. Most of these injuries can be managed with compression and/or suture without shunting.[47] These injuries are still associated with mortality rates that exceed 30%.

Spleen

Following release of the retroperitoneal attachments, the splenocolic, splenorenal, and splenophrenic ligaments, and mobilization of the spleen to the midline it can be rapidly determined if the injury has active hemorrhage that will require splenectomy or a more modest injury amenable to splenorrhaphy.[23,48] If the patient is hypotensive, coagulopathic, acidotic, hypothermic, or has multiple other injuries that contribute to or are worsened by ongoing hemorrhage (closed head injury) the decision to control hemorrhage by splenectomy is straightforward and should be made rapidly.

In patients who respond to control of the bleeding and resuscitation, splenorrhaphy remains an option. This can be accomplished with topical hemostatic agents, suture ligature with or without pledgets, and in some cases wrapping of the spleen in absorbable mesh.

NONOPERATIVE MANAGEMENT

Nonoperative management of liver and spleen injuries is applicable to most of the patients who present in *hemodynamically stable* condition, and the diagnosis of injury is most often made as a result of CT scanning. Under these conditions the success rates for nonoperative therapy is very high >80% in most modern series. Patients should be placed at bed rest in the ICU, serial hemoglobin levels are assessed, and serial abdominal examinations performed in an ICU for 24 to 48 hours. Hemodynamic deterioration or the development of peritonitis is typically considered an indication to switch to an operative treatment mode. Some centers have reported success in controlling hemorrhage from both liver and spleen injuries with angioembolization, but this requires prompt availability of the interventional radiologists which may not be applicable in many situations. There is no clear definition of what transfusion requirement merits abandonment of nonoperative treatment, or how far to allow the hemoglobin to fall in these cases before transfusion and/or operative intervention. In most instances, however, persistent hemorrhage is manifest in the first 24 hours with progressive reduction in hemoglobin levels at 6, 12, and 18 hours post injury or episodes of hypotension. The development of peritonitis is another clear indication for operative intervention.

One controversial area of the management of patients with spleen and liver injuries is the duration of the period of limited activity following successful nonoperative therapy. Our practice has been to urge young patients who play competitive sports to forego competition for 3 months following a liver injury and for 6 months following spleen injury. Patients who are not athletes and who are not employed in jobs with fall or contact hazards may return to work 1 month following injury.

There are caveats associated with nonoperative management of liver and spleen injuries:

1. It cannot be overemphasized that nonoperative treatment is only applicable when the patient is hemodynamically stable.
2. Patients who have evidence of significant hemoperitoneum including significant free fluid surrounding loops of small intestine, those with contrast blush on the CT scan, those on anticoagulants (warfarin, clopidogrel), those with portal hypertension, with multiple injuries that may increase the risk from hemorrhage or intracranial injury, and the elderly are at increased risk of ongoing hemorrhage and failure of nonoperative treatment.
3. Careful attention to serial abdominal examination and early identification of peritonitis, should it develop, are essential.
4. Deep venous thrombosis (DVT) prophylaxis should be restricted to sequential compression devices for 48 to 72 hours, after heparin prophylaxis using a standard protocol is added.

COMPLICATIONS

Hemorrhage is a worrisome complication of nonoperative management; however, when proper patient selection is performed at the outset and only hemodynamically stable patients are treated nonoperatively the risk of uncontrolled bleeding is <20% and generally occurs in the first 48 to 72 hours of injury. There are numerous reports of delayed "splenic rupture" even beyond 2 and 3 weeks; a large subcapsular hematoma is a specific risk factor for delayed bleeding.

Delayed diagnosis of a hollow viscous injury remains a prominent concern when the decision is to follow a nonoperative course of management for liver and spleen injuries, particularly when there is free intraperitoneal fluid on the CT scan. Despite appropriate initial reservations when nonoperative management was in its early evolution, it is now clear from large prospective reports that the risk of a delayed recognition of a hollow viscus injury is <1%. It remains essential to ensure careful serial examinations, however, to identify evolving peritonitis as early as possible.

Bile leaks are a frequent complication in the nonoperative management of liver injuries occurring in upward of 20% of cases, and these can generally be managed with CT or ultrasound-guided percutaneous drainage. Rarely, a large or persistent bile leak may require endoscopic retrograde cholangiopancreaticography (ERCP) and stenting to facilitate closure.

Abscesses are much less common as a complication of nonoperative management of both liver and spleen injuries than once thought, and can also be managed successfully with guided percutaneous drainage in most instances.

Pancreatic fistula may occur following splenectomy as a result of pancreatic trauma or iatrogenic injury. Careful inspection of the tail of the pancreas and care to avoid pancreatic injury while ligating the vasculature of the spleen are the best preventative measures. If there is concern that the tail of the pancreas might be damaged at the time of surgery, a closed suction drain should be left and effluent assayed for amylase and lipase levels before the drain is removed.

Gastric fistula following splenectomy is a recognized complication that can be avoided by careful ligation of the short gastric vessels without including any of the gastric serosa, or, if necessary, imbricating the short gastric ligatures.

Overwhelming Postsplenectomy Sepsis

The spleen contributes to immune competence in a variety of ways including opsonization and phagocytosis. Asplenic patients are at increased risk of overwhelming postsplenectomy infection from encapsulated bacteria such as *Streptococcus pneumoniae*, *Neisseria meningitidis* and *Haemophilus influenzae*.[49] Following splenectomy, patients should be counseled regarding the increased susceptibility to infections and vaccinated against these potential infections before discharge from the hospital. The effectiveness of vaccination alone in very young patients is not completely documented and additional prophylaxis with amoxicillin may be helpful.[50-52]

REFERENCES

1. Velmahos GC, Toutouzas KG, Radin R, et al. Nonoperative treatment of blunt injury to solid abdominal organs: A prospective study. *Arch Surg.* 2003;138(8):844–851.
2. Knudson MM, Maull KI. Nonoperative management of solid organ injuries. Past, present, and future. *Surg Clin North Am.* 1999;79(6):1357–1371.
3. Walt AJ. Founder's lecture: The mythology of hepatic trauma-or Babel revisited. *Am J Surg.* 1978;135(1):12–18.
4. David Richardson J, Franklin GA, Lukan JK, et al. Evolution in the management of hepatic trauma: A 25-year perspective. *Ann Surg.* 2000;232(3):324–330.
5. Duane TM, Como JJ, Bochicchio GV, et al. Reevaluating the management and outcomes of severe blunt liver injury. *J Trauma.* 2004;57(3):494–500.
6. Pachter HL, Spencer FC, Hofstetter SR, et al. Significant trends in the treatment of hepatic trauma. Experience with 411 injuries. *Ann Surg.* 1992;215(5):492–500; discussion 500–492.
7. Velmahos GC, Toutouzas K, Radin R, et al. High success with nonoperative management of blunt hepatic trauma: The liver is a sturdy organ. *Arch Surg.* 2003;138(5):475–480; discussion 480–471.
8. Meyer AA, Crass RA, Lim RC Jr, et al. Selective nonoperative management of blunt liver injury using computed tomography. *Arch Surg.* 1985;120(5):550–554.
9. Cuff RF, Cogbill TH, Lambert PJ. Nonoperative management of blunt liver trauma: The value of follow-up abdominal computed tomography scans. *Am Surg.* 2000;66(4):332–336.
10. Cox JC, Fabian TC, Maish GO III, et al. Routine follow-up imaging is unnecessary in the management of blunt hepatic injury. *J Trauma.* 2005;59(5):1175–1178; discussion 1178–1180.
11. Mohr AM, Lavery RF, Barone A, et al. Angiographic embolization for liver injuries: Low mortality, high morbidity. *J Trauma.* 2003;55(6):1077–1081; discussion 1081–1072.
12. Moulton SL, Lynch FP, Hoyt DB, et al. Operative intervention for pediatric liver injuries: Avoiding delay in treatment. *J Pediatr Surg.* 1992;27(8):958–962; discussion 963.
13. Shilyansky J, Navarro O, Superina RA, et al. Delayed hemorrhage after nonoperative management of blunt hepatic trauma in children: A rare but significant event. *J Pediatr Surg.* 1999;34(1):60–64.
14. Fang JF, Chen RJ, Lin BC, et al. Liver cirrhosis: An unfavorable factor for nonoperative management of blunt splenic injury. *J Trauma.* 2003;54(6):1131–1136; discussion 1136.
15. Coughlin PA, Stringer MD, Lodge JP, et al. Management of blunt liver trauma in a tertiary referral centre. *Br J Surg.* 2004;91(3):317–321.
16. Ein SH, Shandling B, Simpson JS, et al. Nonoperative management of traumatized spleen in children: How and why. *J Pediatr Surg.* 1978;13(2):117–119.
17. King H, Shumacker HB Jr. Splenic studies. I. Susceptibility to infection after splenectomy performed in infancy. *Ann Surg.* 1952;136(2):239–242.
18. Linet MS, Nyren O, Gridley G, et al. Causes of death among patients surviving at least one year following splenectomy. *Am J Surg.* 1996;172(4):320–323.
19. Eraklis AJ, Filler RM. Splenectomy in childhood: A review of 1413 cases. *J Pediatr Surg.* 1972;7(4):382–388.
20. Eraklis AJ, Kevy SV, Diamond LK, et al. Hazard of overwhelming infection after splenectomy in childhood. *N Engl J Med.* 1967;276(22):1225–1229.
21. O'Neal BJ, McDonald JC. The risk of sepsis in the asplenic adult. *Ann Surg.* 1981;194(6):775–778.
22. Malangoni MA, Dillon LD, Klamer TW, et al. Factors influencing the risk of early and late serious infection in adults after splenectomy for trauma. *Surgery.* 1984;96(4):775–783.
23. Burrington JD. Surgical repair of a ruptured spleen in children: Report of eight cases. *Arch Surg.* 1977;112(4):417–419.
24. Haan JM, Biffl W, Knudson MM, et al. Splenic embolization revisited: A multicenter review. *J Trauma.* 2004;56(3):542–547.
25. Luna GK, Dellinger EP. Nonoperative observation therapy for splenic injuries: A safe therapeutic option. *Am J Surg.* 1987;153(5):462–468.
26. Richardson JD. Changes in the management of injuries to the liver and spleen. *J Am Coll Surg.* 2005;200(5):648–669.
27. Bismuth H. Surgical anatomy and anatomical surgery of the liver. *World J Surg.* 1982;6(1):3–9.
28. Bismuth H, Houssin D, Castaing D. Major and minor segmentectomies "reglees" in liver surgery. *World J Surg.* 1982;6(1):10–24.
29. Moore EE, Cogbill TH, Jurkovich GJ, et al. Organ injury scaling: Spleen and liver (1994 revision). *J Trauma.* 1995;38(3):323–324.
30. Moore EE, Shackford SR, Pachter HL, et al. Organ injury scaling: Spleen, liver, and kidney. *J Trauma.* 1989;29(12):1664–1666.
31. Demetriades D, Gomez H, Chahwan S, et al. Gunshot injuries to the liver: The role of selective nonoperative management. *J Am Coll Surg.* 1999;188(4):343–348.
32. Renz BM, Feliciano DV. Gunshot wounds to the right thoracoabdomen: A prospective study of nonoperative management. *J Trauma.* 1994;37(5):737–744.
33. Velmahos GC, Demetriades D, Toutouzas KG, et al. Selective nonoperative management in 1,856 patients with abdominal gunshot wounds: Should routine laparotomy still be the standard of care? *Ann Surg.* 2001;234(3):395–402; discussion 402–393.
34. Demetriades D, Hadjizacharia P, Constantinou C, et al. Selective nonoperative management of penetrating abdominal solid organ injuries. *Ann Surg.* 2006;244(4):620–628.
35. Denton JR, Moore EE, Coldwell DM. Multimodality treatment for grade V hepatic injuries: Perihepatic packing, arterial embolization, and venous stenting. *J Trauma.* 1997;42(5):964–967; discussion 967–968.
36. Croce MA, Fabian TC, Menke PG, et al. Nonoperative management of blunt hepatic trauma is the treatment of choice for hemodynamically stable patients. Results of a prospective trial. *Ann Surg.* 1995;221(6):744–753; discussion 753–745.
37. Davis KA, Fabian TC, Croce MA, et al. Improved success in nonoperative management of blunt splenic injuries: Embolization of splenic artery pseudoaneurysms. *J Trauma.* 1998;44(6):1008–1013; discussion 1013–1015.
38. Ledgerwood AM, Kazmers M, Lucas CE. The role of thoracic aortic occlusion for massive hemoperitoneum. *J Trauma.* 1976;16(08):610–615.
39. Shapiro MB, Jenkins DH, Schwab CW, et al. Damage control: Collective review. *J Trauma.* 2000;49(5):969–978.
40. Garrison JR, Richardson JD, Hilakos AS, et al. Predicting the need to pack early for severe intra-abdominal hemorrhage. *J Trauma.* 1996;40(6):923–927; discussion 927–929.
41. Harrigan C, Lucas CE, Ledgerwood AM. The effect of hemorrhagic shock on the clotting cascade in injured patients. *J Trauma.* 1989;29(10):1416–1421; discussion 1421–1412.
42. Boffard KD, Riou B, Warren B, et al. Recombinant factor VIIa as adjunctive therapy for bleeding control in severely injured trauma patients: Two parallel randomized, placebo-controlled, double-blind clinical trials. *J Trauma.* 2005;59(1):8–15; discussion 15–18.
43. Rizoli SB, Boffard KD, Riou B, et al. Recombinant activated factor VII as an adjunctive therapy for bleeding control in severe

trauma patients with coagulopathy: Subgroup analysis from two randomized trials. *Crit Care.* 2006;10(6):R178.

44. Stone HH, Lamb JM. Use of pedicled omentum as an autogenous pack for control of hemorrhage in major injuries of the liver. *Surg Gynecol Obstet.* 1975;141(1):92–94.

45. Carrillo EH, Spain DA, Miller FB, et al. Intrahepatic vascular clamping in complex hepatic vein injuries. *J Trauma.* 1997;43(1):131–133.

46. Schrock T, Blaisdell FW, Mathewson C Jr. Management of blunt trauma to the liver and hepatic veins. *Arch Surg.* 1968;96(5):698–704.

47. Bethea MC. A simplified approach to hepatic vein injuries. *Surg Gynecol Obstet.* 1977;145(1):78–80.

48. Beal SL, Spisso JM. The risk of splenorrhaphy. *Arch Surg.* 1988;123(9):1158–1163.

49. Hansen K, Singer DB. Asplenic-hyposplenic overwhelming sepsis: Postsplenectomy sepsis revisited. *Pediatr Dev Pathol.* 2001;4(2):105–121.

50. Cullingford GL, Watkins DN, Watts AD, et al. Severe late postsplenectomy infection. *Br J Surg.* 1991;78(6):716–721.

51. Green JB, Shackford SR, Sise MJ, et al. Late septic complications in adults following splenectomy for trauma: A prospective analysis in 144 patients. *J Trauma.* 1986;26(11):999–1004.

52. Waghorn DJ. Overwhelming infection in asplenic patients: Current best practice preventive measures are not being followed. *J Clin Pathol.* 2001;54(3):214–218.

Evaluation and Management of Small Bowel, Colon, and Rectal Injuries

42

Glenda G. Quan   **Melanie S. Morris**   **Donald D. Trunkey**

PENETRATING ABDOMINAL TRAUMA

The most commonly injured intra-abdominal organs in penetrating trauma are the small bowel and the colon. One prospective study of 309 gunshot wounds to the anterior abdomen demonstrated that the small bowel was injured in 37.7% of patients and the colon in 27.3%, followed in frequency by the liver (27.2%), the kidney (15.7%), the diaphragm (15.2%), the abdominal vasculature (14.3%), the stomach (12.4%), the spleen (6.9%), and the bladder (6.5%).[1]

The goal of the evaluation of penetrating abdominal trauma is to reliably detect intra-abdominal organ injury requiring operative management while avoiding unnecessary celiotomy. The obvious benefits of early detection must be balanced against the morbidity associated with unnecessary operative intervention.

Before the 1960s, celiotomy was the gold standard for the evaluation of all cases of penetrating injuries to the abdomen. However, negative explorations are associated with significant morbidity. In one prospective study of 938 trauma patients undergoing celiotomy, unnecessary surgery was performed in 254 patients for an overall unnecessary celiotomy rate of 27%.[2] This rate was similar between patients with stab wounds and gunshot wounds. Forty-one percent of these patients developed a complication attributed to the negative celiotomy. The complications included atelectasis (15.3%), postoperative hypertension requiring medical management (11.0%), pleural effusion (9.8%), pneumothorax (5.1%), prolonged ileus (4.3%), pneumonia (3.9%), surgical wound infection (3.2%), small bowel obstruction (2.4%), and urinary tract infection (1.9%).

Approximately 20% of patients who did not have an associated injury and underwent completely negative celiotomy experienced a perioperative complication.[2] Subanalysis of this data revealed that the mean length of stay was 8.2 and 5.5 days, respectively, for patients with gunshot wounds and stab wounds after negative celiotomies. The overall mean length of stay for patients who had no associated injuries and on whom completely negative celiotomies were performed was 4.7 days. Postoperative complications increased this mean length of stay to 9 days.[3] This increased length of stay was associated with significantly higher hospital costs compared to those patients with similar wounds that were managed nonoperatively.

Patients who are hemodynamically unstable or who have diffuse abdominal tenderness after penetrating abdominal trauma should undergo emergent operative exploration. A patient with an unreliable clinical examination due to severe head injury, spinal cord injury, severe intoxication, or the need for sedation or intubation should have operative exploration or undergo further diagnostic evaluation for the presence of an intraperitoneal injury.[4]

EVALUATION OF STAB WOUNDS TO THE ABDOMEN

Stab wounds to the abdomen are associated with a lower incidence of intra-abdominal injury than gunshot wounds. On the basis of this observation, there has been a shift toward selective nonoperative management of anterior abdominal stab wounds since the 1960s, and cautious conservatism is now the standard of care. Evidence suggests that selective operative management of stab wounds based on physical examination, local wound exploration, laparoscopy, computed tomography (CT), or some combination of these diagnostic modalities is safe and effective. Because no single technique has been proved to be adequate for all patients with anterior abdominal stab wounds, no standard of care regarding the most appropriate management exists.

There are some patients with abdominal stab injuries who may qualify for initial nonoperative management based on benign abdominal examination findings. These patients should be closely observed and serial examinations should be performed. In those patients who are selected for initial observation, exploratory celiotomy should be performed if peritonitis develops or an unexplained drop in blood pressure or hematocrit occurs.

Demetriades et al. performed a prospective study of 651 patients with anterior abdominal stab wounds. Patients were selected for operative or nonoperative management based on physical findings alone. Those who presented with peritoneal signs (tenderness, guarding, rebound tenderness, and absent bowel sounds) underwent immediate celiotomy; all other patients were selected for observation with serial physical examinations. These authors found that of the 306 patients who were initially managed nonoperatively only 11 (3.6%) required subsequent operative exploration. Of those who underwent delayed operative management, two patients had negative celiotomies. In total, 27.5% of patients with abdominal stab wounds were successfully managed nonoperatively without any deaths or major complications. The sensitivity of the initial physical examination to detect the need for operative management was 97.1%.[5] Another group reported similar results in a study of 330 patients with anterior abdominal stab wounds. On the basis of physical examination, they were able to select 176 patients for nonoperative management with three (1.7%) missed injuries.[6] Physical examination of the patient's abdomen is highly sensitive and specific for intra-abdominal injury and is extremely cost effective.

Some centers use the presence of peritoneal penetration as an indication for operative management of hemodynamically stable patients with abdominal stab wounds. In cases of obvious peritoneal penetration, such as omental or bowel evisceration, celiotomy is used to completely evaluate the peritoneum for intra-abdominal injury. According to several series, evisceration of any organ is associated with a 75% to 100% incidence of intra-abdominal injury requiring operative management.[7] In addition, evisceration indicates the presence of a fascial defect large enough to allow bowel herniation and requires repair. Most would agree that omental or hollow viscus evisceration mandates operative evaluation.

For stable patients in whom peritoneal penetration is in question, local wound exploration may be employed to evaluate for penetration of the anterior abdominal fascia. This may be performed in the emergency department using local anesthetic and sterile technique. The wound should be surgically extended to facilitate visualization of the anterior fascia. If fascial penetration is confirmed, celiotomy is performed. Some centers advocate the additional step of laparoscopy to confirm peritoneal penetration before celiotomy is performed. However, even proven peritoneal penetration is not always indicative of organ injury. Some studies report that up to 30% of patients with proven peritoneal penetration do not have significant intra-abdominal injuries and that these patients may be managed with close observation alone.[5]

The increased use of laparoscopy for the evaluation of peritoneal penetration in anterior abdominal stab wounds is a reflection of its widespread availability and advances in laparoscopic technologies. In one study of 40 laparoscopies performed for penetrating abdominal stab wounds, half of the study patients had laparoscopies that were negative for peritoneal penetration and were able to avoid an unnecessary celiotomy.[8] Of the 22 patients with peritoneal penetration on laparoscopy, 3 had minor isolated liver injuries that did not require further intervention, 4 had injuries to the left diaphragm that were repaired laparoscopically, and the remaining 15 patients required celiotomy for open repair of intra-abdominal injuries. In total, the use of laparoscopy avoided unnecessary celiotomy in 66% of patients with penetrating abdominal injury. One benefit of this less invasive approach is the shorter length of hospital stay. For those with negative laparoscopy, the length of stay was 2.2 ± 1.1 days compared to 4.0 ± 1.7 days for those patients who underwent open exploration. These findings are similar to those of older studies[9] that also report negative laparoscopy rates of 50% and significantly shorter hospital stays following laparoscopy.

Laparoscopy has been used successfully in the evaluation of penetrating injuries to the left thoracoabdominal area. It has been shown that these injuries carry an 18% to 35% incidence of contemporaneous injury to the diaphragm.[10,11] Before the availability of laparoscopy, routine open exploration was the gold standard to avoid missed diaphragmatic injuries. In the early 1990s, studies proved that laparoscopy could be used to avoid the 30% to 65% negative celiotomy rate associated with routine celiotomy for thoracoabdominal injuries.[10,11] One important advantage of laparoscopy in these types of injuries is that it permits both the diagnosis and the repair of diaphragmatic injuries. The disadvantages of the laparoscopic approach are that it is invasive, costly, and it is inadequate for the evaluation of hollow viscus injuries. In addition, laparoscopy requires general anesthesia and carries with it the small, but significant risk of iatrogenic injury during trocar placement.

Helical CT has long been used for the evaluation of hemodynamically stable patients with blunt abdominal trauma. With its increasing availability, speed, and sensitivity, CT is emerging as a useful tool in the evaluation of penetrating abdominal trauma. Although several studies conclude that CT scan can accurately detect bowel injury, peritoneal penetration, and need for operative intervention, these studies are limited in that they are nonrandomized, retrospective reviews, and not limited to penetrating anterior abdominal wounds.[12,13] One potential application of CT scan in penetrating trauma is that it may be a useful adjunct in the evaluation of patients with reassuring abdominal examinations to allow for early discharge of patients with benign physical findings and negative CT scans.

EVALUATION OF GUNSHOT WOUNDS TO THE ABDOMEN

Although selective nonoperative management is practiced extensively for abdominal stab wounds, routine celiotomy is still considered the standard of care for anterior abdominal gunshot wounds in the combat theater and in many trauma centers. One argument for routine exploration is that gunshot wounds carry with them a higher incidence of intra-abdominal organ injury than stab wounds, ranging from 30% to 70%.[1]

One large retrospective review by Velmahos et al. of 1,405 patients with anterior abdominal gunshot wounds from a single institution reported the results of their nonoperative management strategy. Of these patients, 484 (34%) were initially selected for nonoperative treatment based on stable vitals signs and benign abdominal examinations. Within the nonoperative group, 65 patients (5%) required delayed celiotomy, and of these patients, 17 (26%) had negative celiotomies. The average time to delayed operative management was 6 hours from admission and there were no deaths among the patients treated nonoperatively. In all, 30% of patients with anterior abdominal gunshot wounds were successfully managed without operative exploration.[14] This is similar to the successful nonoperative management rate seen in studies of anterior abdominal stab wounds.

BLUNT ABDOMINAL TRAUMA

Blunt trauma is the most common mechanism of injury seen in the United States, and is most frequently caused by motor vehicle collision, motorcycle accidents, falls, assaults, and pedestrians struck. Colon and small bowel injuries are found in 1.2% and 0.3% of blunt trauma patients respectively.[15] Delay in diagnosis of >8 hours has been shown to increase morbidity and mortality directly attributable to the missed bowel injury. Mortality and complication rates were found to increase in parallel with time to operative intervention.[16]

Blunt traumatic bowel injuries are notoriously difficult to diagnose. Abdominal pain and peritonitis may take up to 6 to 8 hours to develop. One multi-institutional analysis demonstrated that 13% of patients with perforating small bowel injuries had normal abdominal CT scans preoperatively.[16] As nonoperative management of solid organ injuries becomes the standard of care, there is an increased risk of delayed diagnosis of blunt small bowel injuries.

In a review of the Pennsylvania trauma registry, Nance et al. showed a predictive relationship between solid and hollow viscus injuries in blunt abdominal trauma patients. The authors reviewed 3,089 patients who suffered a solid organ injury and found that 9.6% also had a hollow viscus injury. They further examined the number of solid organs injured and the percent of these patients who suffered hollow viscus injury. Among the 79% of patients with a single solid organ injury there were 7.3% patients with a hollow viscus injury. Of the patients with two solid organs injured, 15.4% also had a hollow viscus injury. Finally, in those patients with three or more solid organs injured, 34.4% also suffered a concomitant hollow viscus injury. The authors advocate a higher index of suspicion and early operative intervention for patients who suffer blunt abdominal trauma and have multiple solid organ injuries.[17]

Stable blunt abdominal trauma patients should initially undergo an oral and intravenous contrast-enhanced CT scan. If the CT scan is completely normal and the patient has no other injuries, the patient may be discharged from the hospital. Patients with one suspicious finding may either be admitted to undergo serial abdominal exams, have a repeat delayed CT scan, or a diagnostic peritoneal lavage (DPL) may be performed. If the DPL is negative, the patient should be observed. If the DPL is positive, an exploratory celiotomy is indicated. In patients who have multiple findings suspicious for bowel injury, operative exploration should be performed.[18]

When examining a stable blunt trauma patient, external signs of bowel injury should be noted. The seat-belt sign (ecchymosis to the anterior abdominal wall secondary to compressive force of the lap belt) is associated with a more than doubled relative risk of bowel injury (see Fig. 1).[19] Chance fractures (flexion-distraction

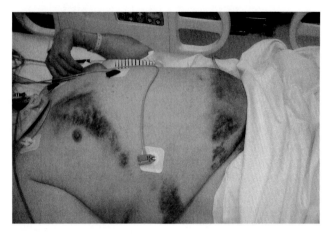

Figure 1 Ecchymosis across the anterior chest and abdomen of a patient using a three-point safety restraint. This physical examination finding is known as a *seat-belt* sign, and is associated with flexion-distraction fractures of the spine and blunt small bowel injury following motor vehicle collision. Photo courtesy of Bruce Ham, MD (Oregon Health and Science University).

fractures of the spine) are also associated with seat-belt use and should raise suspicion for a bowel injury.[20] Abdominal tenderness on physical examination may be associated with intra-abdominal organ injury. Often the examination is unreliable due to intoxication, head injury, intubation, or distracting injuries. When reliable, serial abdominal examinations may be used to guide therapy.

The focused assessment with sonography for trauma (FAST) examination looks for free intraperitoneal fluid in four areas: the Morrison pouch (the hepatorenal space), the splenorenal recess, the pouch of Douglas (inferior portion of the intraperitoneal cavity), and the pericardium. FAST has a sensitivity of 42% to 63%, specificity of 98% to 100%, a positive predictive value of 67% to 100%, a negative predictive value of 93% to 98%, and an accuracy of 92% to 98%.[21,22] Advantages of FAST examination include its rapidity, its noninvasive nature, its availability in the trauma bay, the absence of radiation exposure, and its low cost. Limitations of the test include interobserver variability and the inability to detect small volumes of fluid.

DPL is a rapid, inexpensive test to examine intraperitoneal contents. DPL may be performed with either an open or closed technique. With the closed technique, a needle is inserted two finger breadths below the umbilicus after infiltration with local anesthetic. A Seldinger technique is used to insert a guidewire. The needle is withdrawn and the peritoneal lavage catheter is inserted over the guidewire. If the initial aspiration is negative, 1 L of fluid is instilled and then drained by gravity. In patients with pelvic fractures, DPL must be performed above the umbilicus and with the open technique. To perform an open DPL, local anesthetic is infiltrated in the skin in the infra- or supraumbilical region. An incision is made through the skin and subcutaneous tissue. The fascia is incised and a purse-string suture is placed in the peritoneum. The peritoneum is opened and the catheter is inserted into the peritoneal cavity. Fluid is then instilled and returned as with the closed technique (see Fig. 2).

DPL is considered positive for intra-abdominal injury by the following criteria: aspiration of 10 mL or more of

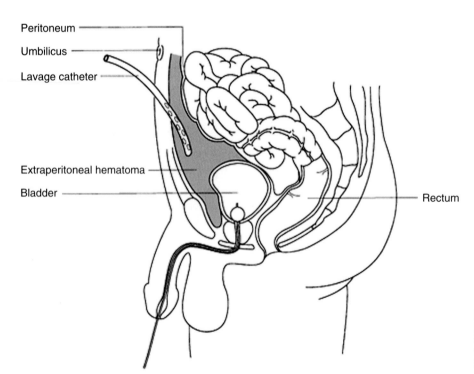

Peritoneum

Umbilicus

Lavage catheter

Extraperitoneal hematoma

Bladder

Rectum

Figure 2 Diagnostic peritoneal lavage (DPL). In the absence of pelvic fractures, the DPL catheter is inserted in the infraumbilical position and directed into the pelvis.

gross blood, red blood cell count >100,000 per mm³, white blood cell count >500 cells per mm³, alkaline phosphatase level >10 IU per L, amylase level >20 IU per L, or aspiration of bile, bacteria, or food fibers. A clear contraindication for DPL includes the need for exploratory celiotomy, and relative contraindications are pregnancy, obesity, and prior exploratory celiotomy. The accuracy of DPL, as reported in the Eastern Association for the Surgery of Trauma (EAST) guidelines, is 92% to 98% for intraperitoneal hemorrhage. Its usefulness for the detection of hollow viscus injury is disputed.[23] DPL may be most accurate in patients with intraperitoneal fluid in the absence of solid organ injury or in patients with a solid organ injury with significant abdominal pain that are being managed nonoperatively.[24] Complications of DPL are associated with misplaced catheters and have an incidence of 1%. An open technique may decrease the rate of misplacement. DPL results may be falsely positive if the patient has a pelvic fracture, or if there is bleeding from the anterior abdominal wall.

CT scan is recommended by EAST for the evaluation of hemodynamically stable patients with equivocal findings on physical examination, multiple other injuries, or neurologic injury. Disadvantages of CT are its high cost and the need to transport patients to the radiology suite. Patients with a negative CT scan should be admitted for observation and serial abdominal examinations.[23] CT scan diagnosis of bowel injury has a sensitivity of 64% to 88%, a specificity of 97% to 99%, and an accuracy of 82% to 99%.[18,25] Mesenteric infiltration (stranding) and free intraperitoneal fluid are the most frequent CT signs seen in bowel trauma.[25]

MANAGEMENT OF SMALL BOWEL INJURIES

Once the initial evaluation and resuscitation of the injured patient is complete, those with suspected or recognized small bowel injury should undergo immediate operative exploration. Under most circumstances, the abdomen should be explored through a midline incision. The incision should be extensive enough to permit evaluation of the entire abdominal cavity. In rare instances, patients with stab wounds may be explored through an extension of an existing abdominal wall defect.

Patients with extensive ongoing hemorrhage should be packed. Bleeding vessels in the mesentery should be individually ligated. Care should be taken to avoid mass ligation of the mesentery that may produce unnecessary bowel ischemia. Once initial control of significant hemorrhage is achieved, contamination from spilled gastrointestinal contents is addressed. Contamination from bowel perforation may be temporarily controlled with Babcock clamps, skin staples, or Vicryl sutures without causing additional injury to the bowel.

Intraoperative evaluation of the small bowel is performed in a systematic manner. The bowel is thoroughly examined from the ligament of Treitz to the ileocecal valve, and bowel perforations are controlled as they are encountered. Definitive repair is delayed until the entire length of bowel is inspected and all injuries are accounted for.

Treatment of individual small bowel injuries is based on the severity of injury. Small bowel injuries are graded by a scale developed by the American Association for the Surgery of Trauma (AAST) (see Table 1).[26] Grade I injuries

TABLE 1

AMERICAN ASSOCIATION FOR THE SURGERY OF TRAUMA (AAST) ORGAN INJURY SCALE (1990) FOR THE SMALL INTESTINE, COLON, AND RECTUM

Injured Structure	AAST Grade	Characteristic of Injury
Small bowel	I	Contusion or hematoma without devascularization; partial-thickness laceration
	II	Small (<50% circumference) laceration
	III	Large (>50% circumference) laceration
	IV	Transection
	V	Transection with devascularization or segmental tissue loss
Colon	I	Contusion or hematoma; partial-thickness laceration
	II	Small (<50% circumference) laceration
	III	Large (>50% circumference) laceration
	IV	Transection
	V	Transection with tissue loss; devascularized segment
Rectum	I	Contusion or hematoma; partial-thickness laceration
	II	Small (<50% circumference) laceration
	III	Large (>50% circumference) laceration
	IV	Full-thickness laceration with perineal extension
	V	Devascularized segment

are small, partial-thickness wounds that are managed by reapproximating the seromuscular layers with interrupted sutures. Full-thickness wounds that involve <50% of the bowel circumference, or grade II injuries, are repaired with limited debridement and primary closure. A transverse closure ensures a widely patent lumen and minimizes narrowing. Grade III injuries are full-thickness wounds that involve >50% of the circumference, without complete transection of the bowel. These may be repaired primarily if luminal narrowing can be avoided; otherwise, resection and anastomosis should be performed. Primary repair is performed as a two-layer closure with a running absorbable suture as the inner layer and interrupted silk sutures for the outer layer. Alternatively, a single-layer closure with running or interrupted sutures may also be performed.

Complete bowel transections and transections with segmental tissue loss are grade IV and V injuries, respectively. These more extensive small bowel injuries can be associated with devascularization. These injuries are typically managed by resection and anastomosis, the extent of which is determined by intestinal viability. Bowel perfusion is assessed first by inspection of the intestinal segment for color and the presence or absence of peristalsis. In addition, a Doppler probe may be employed on the antimesenteric border of the bowel to assess arterial flow. If an extensive proximal vascular injury leaves a large segment of intestine with questionable viability, temporary abdominal closure with planned second-look should be performed. In this setting, anastomosis is delayed for 24 to 48 hours when bowel perfusion can be reassessed.

Small bowel anastomoses may be hand sewn in one or two layers. Alternatively, stapled techniques may also be employed. There is conflicting data regarding the safety of stapled anastomoses in trauma patients with small bowel injuries. One retrospective study comparing stapled and hand-sewn anastomoses reported a significantly higher rate of intra-abdominal abscess and anastomotic leak requiring operative intervention in the stapled group.[27] However, this study did not distinguish between small bowel and colon injuries. Another retrospective study limited to small bowel injuries demonstrated no difference in the complication rates between sutured and stapled anastomoses.[28]

Because of the protected location of the duodenum and its close proximity to other vital organs, duodenal injuries often occur in the multiple-wounded trauma patient. Difficulty in diagnosis of duodenal injury results in delay of operative management and increased mortality. In one study of 163 small bowel injuries, management of duodenal injuries showed the greatest variability in the type of repair performed. Most blunt duodenal injuries were managed with a complex repair, such as pyloric exclusion, duodenal diverticulization, or pancreaticoduodenectomy. In contrast, the vast majority of duodenal stab wounds were successfully closed primarily. Gunshot wounds to the duodenum were repaired by either complex or primary techniques in equal numbers.[29]

MANAGEMENT OF COLON INJURIES

Treatment of colon injuries has evolved over the last century from mandatory colostomy to primary repair when safe and feasible. Management of colon injuries can be simplified by categorizing them as destructive or nondestructive. Nondestructive lesions are defined as wounds involving <50% of the bowel wall and do not involve devascularization. Destructive lesions are wounds that completely transect the colon or involve tissue loss and devascularized segments. With current management strategies, morbidity following colon injuries ranges from 20% to 35%, and mortality ranges from 3% to 15%.

Nondestructive lesions are the most common type of colonic injury. For partial-thickness wounds, inverting seromuscular sutures are sufficient. Full-thickness wounds may be treated by primary repair in either one or two layers. A recent review by Fabian et al. examined the prospective and retrospective studies comparing primary repair versus colostomy in patients with nondestructive colon lesions. Suture line failure rate occurred in 1.6% of patients who underwent primary repair. The incidence of intra-abdominal abscess was higher in the colostomy group as compared to the primary repair group (12% vs. 4.9%). The overall complication rate was 14% in primary repair group and 30% in the colostomy group. Mortality rates were equivalent at 0.1% in each group. There is good evidence to support the use of primary repair for nondestructive colon wounds.[30]

Patients with destructive wounds can also undergo primary repair safely. However, in these patients, other risk factors for complications must be considered. These risk factors include shock, delayed surgery, transfusion requirement >6 units, underlying comorbid conditions, or a penetrating abdominal trauma index (PATI) >25.[31,32] Patients who do not have any risk factors should be treated with resection and primary repair. In patients who do have risk factors, fecal diversion should be performed.

Fecal diversion may be accomplished by either a loop colostomy or an end colostomy based on surgeon preference. A loop colostomy may be formed using the injured colon segment, or the injured colon may be resected and a divided colostomy with mucous fistula may be formed. If the patient's condition permits, a primary repair may be performed with a diverting loop colostomy or ileostomy. Loop stomas are preferred because they are easier to close and result in less blood loss than end stomas. Loop ileostomies are less bulky, produce less odor, and are easier to fit with stoma appliances, when compared to loop colostomies.[33] Colostomy closure is typically performed after 3 to 6 months. However, some surgeons prefer early closure at 6 to 12 weeks. Colostomy takedown has an overall complication rate of 10% to 50%.

Studies have examined the morbidity associated with both colostomy creation and colostomy closure. One series of 75 patients reports a complication rate of 32% for colostomy creation compared to 5% for colostomy closure. The mean time to colostomy closure was 103 days (range 36 to 902 days). Fear of high morbidity associated with colostomy closure should not influence surgical decision making in colon injuries.[34]

Trunkey et al. surveyed practicing trauma surgeons about current management strategies for traumatic colon injuries. Of the 342 surveys completed, 98% of trauma surgeons would consider performing primary repair for traumatic colon injuries. Thirty percent said that they would never perform a diverting colostomy. Most respondents (54%) would perform a diverting colostomy for high-velocity gunshot wounds to the colon. Resection and anastomosis was preferred by 55% of surgeons when the isolated colon injury was a contusion with possible devascularization, laceration >50% of diameter, or transection. Surgeons who managed five or fewer colon injuries a year were significantly more likely to perform a diverting colostomy when compared to their counterparts who managed six or more of these injuries. This survey demonstrates that most trauma surgeons are practicing evidence-based management which supports the use of primary anastomosis in the repair of traumatic colon injuries.[35]

With current management strategies, morbidity following colon injuries ranges from 20% to 35%, and mortality ranges from 3% to 15%. Postoperative complications from colon repair include abscess formation (10%), fistula (1% to 3%), and stoma complications. Stomal complications are related to necrosis, stenosis, obstruction, or prolapse which together make up 5%.[36]

MANAGEMENT OF RECTAL INJURIES

Digital rectal examination should be performed on all patients in the trauma bay. The presence of blood should lead one to suspect rectal injury and investigate further with proctoscopy. Rectal injuries may be classified anatomically as intraperitoneal or extraperitoneal and then treated accordingly. Intraperitoneal injuries include injuries to the anterior and lateral upper two thirds of the rectum, and are treated in the same manner as the colonic injuries. The lower one third and the entire posterior rectum are not enveloped by serosa and are therefore extraperitoneal.

When treating extraperitoneal rectal injuries, the surgeon must decide how easily he or she can access the injury. Injuries that are easily accessible are repaired primarily followed by proximal fecal diversion. Inaccessible injuries are not explored, but are treated with proximal fecal diversion and presacral drainage (see Fig. 3).

To perform presacral drainage, a curvilinear incision is made in the skin between the coccyx and anus. Blunt dissection is then used to access the presacral space. Penrose drains are placed into the presacral space and gradually withdrawn on postoperative days 5 to 7. Complications following rectal injuries include sepsis, pelvic abscess,

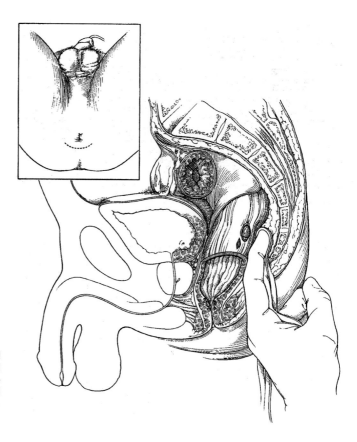

Figure 3 Presacral drainage is used to treat extraperitoneal rectal injuries. Blunt dissection is used to enter the presacral space where open drainage is achieved by way of Penrose drains. Weinberg JA, Fabian TC. Injuries to the Stomach, Small Bowel, Colon, and Rectum. In Souba WW, Fink MJ, Jurkovich GJ, et al. Trauma and Thermal Injury. New York: WebMD Inc, 2005.

urinary or rectal fistulas, rectal incontinence, stricture, loss of sexual function, and urinary incontinence.

REFERENCES

1. Demetriades D, Velmahos G, Cornwell E, et al. Selective nonoperative management of gunshot wounds of the anterior abdomen. *Arch Surg*. 1997;132(2):178–183.
2. Renz BM, Feliciano DV. Unnecessary laparotomies for trauma: A prospective study of morbidity. *J Trauma*. 1995;38(3):350–356.
3. Renz BM, Feliciano DV. The length of hospital stay after an unnecessary laparotomy for trauma: A prospective study. *J Trauma*. 1996;40(2):187–190.
4. Como JJ, Bokhari F, Chiu WC, et al. Eastern Association for the Surgery of Trauma, Practice Management Guideline Committee. *Practice management guidelines for the nonoperative management of penetrating abdominal trauma*. http://www.east.org/tpg/nonoppene.pdf. Accessed 2007.
5. Demetriades D, Rabinowitz B. Indications for operation in abdominal stab wounds: A prospective study of 651 patients. *Ann Surg*. 1987;205:129–132.
6. Shorr RM, Gottlieb MM, Webb K, et al. Selective management of abdominal stab wounds: Importance of the physical examination. *Arch Surg*. 1988;123:1141–1145.
7. Nagy K, Roberts R, Joseph K, et al. Evisceration after abdominal stab wounds: Is laparotomy required? *J Trauma*. 1999;47:622–626.
8. Simon RJ, Rabin J, Kuhls D. Impact of increased use of laparoscopy on negative laparotomy rates after penetrating trauma. *J Trauma*. 2002;53(2):297–302.
9. Fabian TC, Croce MA, Stewart RM, et al. A prospective analysis of diagnostic laparoscopy in trauma. *Ann Surg*. 1993;217(5):557–565.
10. Merlotti GJ, Dillon BC, Lange DA, et al. Peritoneal lavage in penetrating thoracoabdominal trauma. *J Trauma*. 1988;28:17.
11. Madden MR, Paull DE, Finkelstein JL, et al. Occult diaphragmatic injury from stab wounds to the lower chest and abdomen. *J Trauma*. 1989;29:292–298.
12. Salim A, Sangthong B, Martin M, et al. Use of computed tomography in anterior abdominal stab wounds. *Arch Surg*. 2006;141:745–752.
13. Shanmuganathan K, Mirvis SE, Chiu WC, et al. Penetrating torso trauma: Triple-contrast helical CT in peritoneal violation and organ injury: A prospective study in 200 patients. *Radiology*. 2004;231:775–784.
14. Velmahos GC, Demetriades D, Toutouzas KG, et al. Selective nonoperative management in 1,856 patients with abdominal gunshot wounds: Should routine laparotomy still be the standard of care? *Ann Surg*. 2001;234(3):395–403.
15. Watts DD, Fakhry SM. Incidence of hollow viscus injury in blunt trauma: An analysis from 275,557 trauma admissions from the EAST multi-institutional group. *J Trauma*. 2003;54:289–294.
16. Fakhry SM, Brownstein M, Oller D, et al. Relatively short diagnostic delays (<8hrs) produce morbidity and mortality in blunt small bowel injury: An analysis of time to operative intervention in 198 patients from a multicenter experience. *J Trauma*. 2000;48:408–415.
17. Nance ML, Peden GW, Schwab CW, et al. Solid viscus injury predicts major hollow viscus injury in blunt abdominal trauma. *J Trauma*. 1997;43:618–623.
18. Malhotra AK, Fabian TC, Croce MA, et al. Blunt bowel and mesenteric injuries: The role of screening computed tomography. *J Trauma*. 2000;48:991–1000.
19. Fakhry SM, Watts DD, Luchette FA. Current diagnostic approaches lack sensitivity in the diagnosis of perforated blunt small bowel injury: Analysis from 275,557 trauma admissions from the EAST multi-institutional HVI trial. *J Trauma*. 2003;54:295–306.
20. Weinberg, JA, Fabian TC. Injuries to the stomach, small bowel, colon, and rectum. *ACS surgery: principles and practice*, Web MD; 2005.
21. Miller MT, Pasquale MD, Cox J, et al. Not so fast. *J Trauma*. 2003;54:52–59.
22. Ollerton JE, Sugrue M, Wyllie P, et al. Prospective study to evaluate the influence of FAST on trauma patient management. *J Trauma*. 2006;60:785–791.
23. Hoff WS, Holevar M, Valenziano CP, et al. *Practice management guidelines for the evaluation of blunt abdominal trauma*. East practice management guidelines work group; 2001:1–27.
24. Otomo Y, Henmi H, Yamamoto Y, et al. New diagnostic peritoneal lavage crigeria for diagnosis of intestinal injury. *J Trauma*. 1998;44:991–998.
25. Gutela ST, Federle MP, Huang LF, et al. Performance of CT in detection of bowel injury. *Am J Radiol*. 2001;176:129–135.
26. Moore EE, Cogbill TH, Malagoni MA, et al. Organ injury scaling II: Pancreas, duodenum, small bowel, colon, and rectum. *J Trauma*. 1990;30:1427–1429.
27. Brundage SI, Jurkovich GJ, Hoyt DB, et al. Stapled versus sutured gastrointestinal anastomosis in the trauma patient: A multicenter trial. *J Trauma*. 2001;51:1054.
28. Witzke JD, Kraatz JJ, Morken JM, et al. Stapled versus hand-sewn anastomosis in patients with small bowel injury: A changing perspective. *J Trauma*. 2000;49:600–666.
29. Donohue JH, Crass RA, Trunkey DD. The management of duodenal and other small intestinal trauma. *World J Surg*. 1985;9:904–913.
30. Maxwell RA, Fabian TC. Current management of colon trauma. *World J Surg*. 2003;27:632–639.
31. Stewart RM, Fabian TC, Croce MA, et al. Is resection with primary anastomosis following destructive colon wounds always safe? *Am J Surg*. 1994;168:316–319.
32. Cornwell EE, Velhamos GC, Berne TV, et al. The fate of colonic suture lines in high-risk trauma patients. *J Am Coll Surg*. 1998;187:58–63.
33. Cleary RK, Pmerantz RA, Lampman RM. Colon and rectal injuries. *Dis Colon Rectum*. 2006;49:1203–1222.
34. Crass RA, Salbi F, Trunkey DD. Colostomy after colon injury: A low morbidity procedure. *J Trauma*. 1987;27:1237–1239.
35. Eshraghi N, Mullins RJ, Trunkey DD, et al. Surveyed opinion of American trauma surgeons in management of colon injuries. *J Trauma*. 1998;44:93–97.
36. Burch JM, Francoise RJ, Moore EE. Trauma. In: Brunicardi FC, ed. *Schwartz's principles of surgery*, 8th ed. New York: McGraw-Hill, 2005; 172.

Abdominal Vascular Injury

43

Brandon H. Tieu   **Minhao Zhou**   **Donald D. Trunkey**

Abdominal vascular injuries are highly lethal and a difficult challenge even for the most experienced trauma surgeons.[1] Patients can arrive in a stable condition with a contained hematoma, or in extremis and coagulopathic state with uncontrolled hemorrhage.[2,3] Hemorrhagic shock continues to be the second leading cause of mortality following trauma, but is the leading cause of preventable death.[4] It is important that early surgical control of bleeding is established as resuscitation and correction of coagulopathy are occurring. These injuries are relatively uncommon and are a result of penetrating injury in 88% to 95% of cases and blunt injury in 5% to 10%.[5-8] Accessing the retroperitoneal vessels can be difficult and iatrogenic injury can occur with rapid dissection through hematomas resulting in further blood loss. Owing to the location of the abdominal vasculature, associated injuries are the rule rather than the exception, with an estimated two to four associated intra-abdominal injuries that occur with visceral blood vessel trauma.[6,7] The presence of associated injuries increases the difficulty and time of management of abdominal vascular trauma even in damage control procedures. Even after initial control of exsanguinating hemorrhage, patients can still succumb to multisystem organ failure resulting in delayed mortality. Successful management of these injuries requires expedient surgical intervention, thorough knowledge of the anatomy and surgical precision to minimize iatrogenic injuries, and maximize the patient's chance of survival.

INCIDENCE

Historically, abdominal vascular injuries are more commonly seen in urban trauma settings than in the combat theater. Asensio et al. reported on 302 patients with abdominal vascular injuries over a 72-month period at a busy Level I trauma center that admits 7,000 to 7,500 cases per year.[1] A 30-year review of 5,760 cardiovascular injuries from another busy urban trauma center found 1,947 (33.8%) abdominal vascular injuries.[9] Goaley et al. reports that the Emory University Trauma service at Grady Memorial Hospital in Atlanta consistently treats 30 or more patients per year with abdominal vascular injuries.[5]

Compare this to reports during military conflict. In a review of 2,471 arterial injuries from World War II by Debakey and Simeone,[10] they found that only 49 (2%) of those were abdominal arterial injuries. Rich et al. reported that of 1,000 arterial injuries from the Vietnam War, only 29 (2.9%) involved the abdominal vessels.[11] In a recent publication from Clouse et al. reporting 301 vascular injuries from the Balad Vascular Registry in Iraq, only 18 (6%) were abdominal vascular injuries.[12]

DIAGNOSIS

Diagnosing abdominal vascular injuries starts with an astute awareness based on the mechanism of trauma that an injury may have occurred. Penetrating injuries in the midline should raise the suspicion for an injury to the aorta, inferior vena cava (IVC), or their respective branches.[13]

Patient presentation following abdominal vascular injuries is dependent on whether there is active exsanguination or if the bleeding is contained. If the hematoma is contained within the retroperitoneum or base of the mesentery, patients can either be hemodynamically stable or hypotensive but respond to intravenous (IV) fluid resuscitation. For those who have uncontrolled hemorrhage into the abdomen or retroperitoneum, they will present with severe hypotension or in cardiopulmonary arrest with losses of 40% to 50% of their blood volume.[6] The abdominal examination may reveal slight abdominal discomfort or acute peritonitis and a distended and rigid abdomen.

Baseline laboratory values that should be drawn include a complete blood count, an arterial blood gas, and coagulation studies. Rarely will these tests help with the diagnosis of an abdominal vascular injury but repeating them can help monitor resuscitation efforts as interventions are carried out. If the patient is in severe shock and in immediate need of surgical intervention then laboratory investigations should not delay transfer to the operating room (OR).

A plain radiograph of the abdomen can be quickly obtained in the trauma bay and may detect the presence, location, and trajectory of a penetrating missile. A computed tomography (CT) scan may show other associated injuries in a hemodynamically stable patient, but rarely are imaging studies helpful or required for diagnosis of abdominal vascular injury. The focused assessment with sonography for trauma (FAST) examination can be highly sensitive and specific for detecting hemoperitoneum in hypotensive patients following blunt abdominal trauma when performed by trauma team members,[14] but its reliability for penetrating trauma has yet to be determined.[6]

INITIAL RESUSCITATION

All trauma patients should be evaluated according to Advance Trauma Life Support protocols. For those with suspected abdominal vascular injury, after establishing a secure airway, assure adequate venous access with at least two large-bore IV lines, and start volume replacement with lactated Ringers solution. For those who do not respond to the initial 2 L of crystalloid solution, blood transfusions should be initiated. An attempt should be made to maintain a systolic blood pressure of 80 mm Hg until vascular control has been achieved. A Foley catheter should be placed after ruling out urethral injury to monitor resuscitation and test for hematuria, which could be a result of renal injury. Maneuvers to maintain normothermia should be instituted such as warming of the trauma bay, heated blankets, removal of wet clothing, and warmed IV fluids. Hypothermia can augment the development of coagulopathy and along with acidosis can result in the "lethal triad" of hypothermia, acidosis, and coagulopathy. For severely injured patients with coagulopathy, early use of fresh frozen plasma should be considered.[15,16]

Patients with penetrating injuries to the abdomen and present in extremis may need an emergency department (ED) thoracotomy. These patients present in

cardiopulmonary arrest or are in severe shock that is unresponsive to resuscitation.[6] ED thoracotomy allows for open cardiopulmonary massage and aortic cross-clamping to maintain cerebral and coronary arterial blood flow.[17] This technique limits intra-abdominal arterial bleeding but does not affect hemorrhage from venous injuries. Morbidity from thoracotomy itself includes an additional site for bleeding, another body cavity where heat can be lost, ischemia distal to the cross-clamp, and predisposes the patient to reperfusion injuries. Survival after ED thoracotomy range from 0% to 19.6% and for OR thoracotomy up to 10%.[1,18-20] Most of those patients who live longer than 24 hours after ED thoracotomy should have good neurologic recovery.[21]

OPERATIVE MANAGEMENT

The patient should have a standard trauma sterile preparation and draping from the neck to the mid thigh

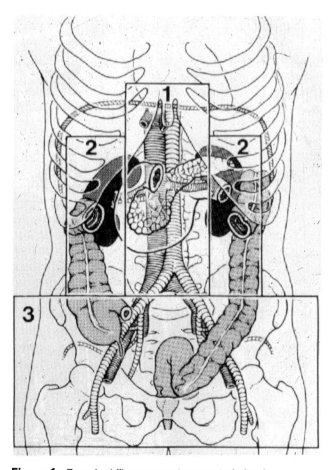

Figure 1 Zone 1 midline retroperitoneum includes the supramesocolic suprarenal aorta, celiac axis, proximal superior mesenteric artery, proximal renal artery, superior mesenteric vein, inframesocolic infrarenal aorta, and infrahepatic vena cava; zone 2 upper lateral retroperitoneum includes the renal artery and vein; zone 3 pelvic retroperitoneum includes the common, external and internal iliac arteries and veins. (Image from Dr. Trunkey's slides.)

and down to the operating table laterally to cover the entire torso. Assure that adequate amounts of all blood products are available. The OR should be warmed, heating blankets kept on the operating table, and warm air covers placed over the patient's legs, head, and upper extremities. Warmed fluids should be administered if needed and the temperature of the ventilator cascade increased to 42°C.[6] Prophylactic antibiotics should be given before surgery.

A standard midline incision should be made from the xyphoid process to the pubis. Immediate control of obvious life-threatening hemorrhage should be achieved, followed by control of gross spillage into the abdominal cavity. For solid organ hemorrhage, abdominal packs can be used to control bleeding. Direct digital pressure, sponge sticks, and formal proximal and distal control can be used for vascular hemorrhage. All four quadrants can be quickly packed for continued surface bleeding or if the bleeding cannot be immediately identified before embarking on a thorough inspection of the abdominal cavity and retroperitoneum. Feliciano et al. described a systematic approach to the management of vascular injuries that consists of classifying the location of the retroperitoneal hematoma in zones (see Fig. 1).[22]

AORTIC INJURIES

The aorta is located in zone I, midline retroperitoneum, and an aortic injury should be suspected in all penetrating trauma to this area. Injuries to the aorta can be divided into either supramesocolic or inframesocolic. Zone I retroperitoneal supramesocolic hematoma or hemorrhage can be an injury to the suprarenal aorta, the celiac axis, the proximal superior mesenteric artery (SMA), or proximal renal artery. Supramesocolic vascular injuries generally carry a higher mortality rate (65% to 90%) than inframesocolic injuries (55% to 66%) due to its difficult anatomic location.[1,23–26] If active hemorrhage is encountered, temporary control can be achieved by packing with laparotomy pads or manually compressing the aorta at the aortic hiatus with your fingers, an aortic root compressor, or placement of an aortic clamp.[25,27] Placement of a clamp at this location can be difficult and will require some dissection. Rapid exposure of the supraceliac abdominal aorta is achieved by dividing the lesser omentum, retracting the stomach and esophagus to the left, and manually dissecting the area just below the aortic hiatus of the diaphragm.[28] The left crus of the diaphragm may require transection to facilitate the

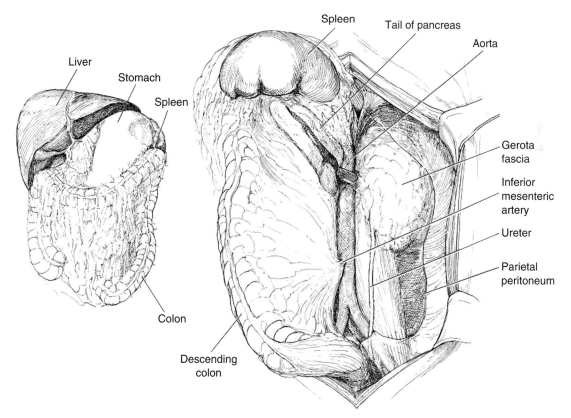

Figure 2 Left medial visceral rotation is performed to provide exposure of the entire length of the abdominal aorta, the left renal vasculature, the origins of the mesenteric arteries, and the common iliac bifurcation. (Figure from Thal ER, O'Keeffe T. Operative exposure of abdominal injuries and closure of the abdomen. In: Souba WW, Fink MP, Jurkovich GJ, et al. eds. *ACS surgery: principles and practice*. Chicago: WebMD Professional Publishing; 2006.)

exposure. Control of the suprarenal abdominal aorta is difficult due the anteriorly located celiac axis and SMA. Once hemorrhage is controlled, a left medial visceral rotation can completely expose the abdominal aorta (see Fig. 2). This is performed by incising the avascular line of Toldt of the left colon from the splenocolic flexure to the level of the distal sigmoid colon. The splenorenal ligament is also mobilized with a combination of sharp and blunt dissection. The left-sided viscera including the left colon, spleen, stomach, tail, and body of the pancreas are rotated using blunt dissection medially (Lim maneuver). For better access to the origin of the left renal artery, the left kidney can be mobilized and included in the medial rotation (Mattox maneuver). This exposes the entire length of the aorta including the aortic hiatus, the origin of the celiac axis, the origin of the SMA, the left iliac system, and the origin of the right common iliac artery. If the hemorrhage or hematoma is located in zone I inframesocolic area, rapid exposure can be achieved by retracting the transverse colon and mesocolon cephalad, eviscerating the small bowel to the right, and opening the midline retroperitoneum until the left renal vein is exposed (see Fig. 3). A proximal aortic cross-clamp can be placed inferior to the renal vessels to gain proximal control. For distal control, division of the midline retroperitoneum can be continued down to the aortic bifurcation taking care to avoid the origin of the inferior mesenteric artery (IMA) on the left. If the presence of a large retroperitoneal hematoma is distorting the entire inframesocolic area, the vascular defect is most likely located under the highest point of the hematoma (Mt. Everest phenomenon).[25] Once proximal and distal vascular control is achieved, surgical repair can proceed. Small injuries to the aorta should be adequately debrided

and repaired primarily with 3-0 or 4-0 vascular suture. For larger defects where primary repair will significantly narrow the lumen of the aorta, patch aortoplasty is indicated. For more extensive injuries where a large portion of the aorta needs to be resected, an interposition graft with 12 or 14 mm polytetrafluoroethylene (PTFE) or Darcon graft can be used. The graft is sewn in with 3-0 or 4-0 vascular suture, both ends of the aorta are flushed before the distal anastomosis is completed, and the distal aortic cross-clamp is removed before the final knot is tied to eliminate air from the system. Contamination from perforated viscous of the stomach, small bowel, and/or colon must be controlled and care must be taken to prevent graft infection. Vigorous intraoperative irrigation, proper graft coverage, and appropriate use of perioperative antibiotics can all be employed to decrease the incidence of graft infection, which is fairly rare in otherwise young healthy trauma patients.[25] The retroperitoneum should always be used to cover the repair with absorbable sutures in a watertight manner when feasible. Additional maneuvers for tissue coverage of the aortic graft include mobilizing the gastrocolic omentum, placing it into the lesser sac superiorly, and then bringing it down over the infrarenal aorta through a hole in the left transverse mesocolon. The gastrocolic omentum can also be mobilized away from the right side of the colon and brought into the left lateral gutter just below the ligament of Treitz to cover the graft. The omental pedicle is sutured in place to cover the graft and suture line to help prevent aortoenteric fistula.[29,30]

Cross-clamping the abdominal aorta in a hemodynamically unstable patient can cause profound ischemia to the lower extremities. The anesthesiologist should be notified when the proximal aortic cross-clamp is removed slowly

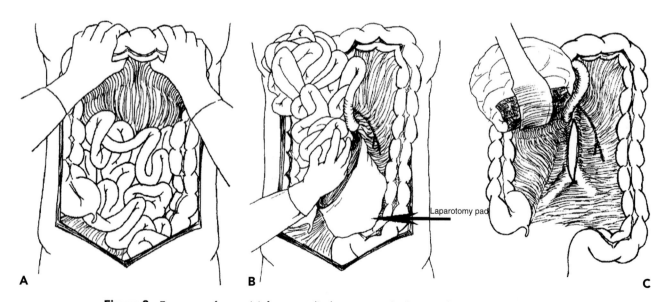

Figure 3 Exposure of zone I inframesocolic hematoma. **A:** Retract the transverse colon and mesocolon cephalad. **B:** Eviscerate the small bowel to the right. **C:** Open the midline retroperitoneum. (Figure from Master VA, McAninch JW. Operative management of renal injuries: Parenchymal and vascular. *Urol Clin North Am.* 2006;33:21–31, v–vi.)

A   **B**   **C**

while fluids and IV bicarbonate are rapidly infused to reverse washout acidosis from the previously ischemic lower extremities. Ischemia and reperfusion injury places the patient at very high risk for lower extremity compartment syndrome. Lower extremity compartment pressures should be measured (>30 mm Hg is high) and bilateral below-the-knee two-incision four-compartment fasciotomies should not be delayed.

INFERIOR VENA CAVA INJURIES

The vast majority of IVC injuries are due to penetrating trauma, with gunshot wounds being the most prevalent. If the injury is due to blunt trauma, it usually involves the retrohepatic or intrapericardial sections of the IVC due to rapid deceleration and shearing injury. Regardless of the mechanism of injury, IVC trauma carries approximately 50% mortality. The worse prognosis occurs in patients who arrive with hemodynamic instability or injuries involving the suprarenal or retrohepatic vena cava.[31,32]

The IVC has numerous tributaries including the right gonadal vein, right adrenal vein, renal veins, four to five pairs of lumbar veins, and hepatic and phrenic veins. Owing to this extensive collateral network, it is difficult to obtain complete proximal and distal control of the IVC.[31]

The venous circulation is a low-pressure system. More than half the number of patients who present will have a contained hematoma.[31] In patients with a stable midline nonpulsatile hematoma, controversy surrounds whether this needs to be explored. As many as 40% of patients may die from exsanguination after disruption of the hematoma secondary to surgical exploration.[33] Indications for exploration include concurrent injuries to the pancreas, duodenum, kidney, ureter, colon, or an associated arterial injury. Nonpulsatile hematomas due to injuries to the retrohepatic vena cava are probably best left unexplored because of the high risk and low probability of associated retroperitoneal injuries in that area. If active bleeding from the IVC is encountered, initial control can be obtained with manual compression of the bleeding point with a tightly rolled gauze pack until a more definitive exposure and control can be achieved.

Exposure of the suprahepatic IVC can be difficult. Upon entering the abdomen and gaining initial control of hemorrhage with packs, a diagnostic maneuver that can be useful is to gently retract the dome of the right lobe of the liver caudad. If a gush of blood is encountered, this usually implies an injury to the right or left hepatic vein. If there appears to be a large retroperitoneal hematoma when mobilizing the right lobe of the liver, it may become obvious that there is a retrohepatic cava injury. If the surgeon suspects that a hepatic vein has been injured, packs should be replaced and a sternotomy performed. This will allow control of the intrapericardial portion of the IVC with a Rummel tourniquet (Haeney technique).[34]

This, in combination with the Pringle maneuver, allows the surgeon approximately 30 minutes to repair the injured vessel.

The diaphragm can be split in the midline in a vertical manner to reveal the upper portion of the subdiaphragmatic cava and the hepatic veins. These can be repaired primarily or if one is completely avulsed, an appropriate lobectomy should be carried out. The best approach for blunt injuries to the retrohepatic cava is from the right side with medial rotation of the liver to the midline. This will often expose segmental veins coming from segment one directly into the cava that have been lacerated or the cava has a linear laceration reflecting that these veins have been detached from the anterior surface. For penetrating injuries to the retrohepatic cava and in rare instances it may be necessary to do a left hepatic lobectomy to gain access to the cava. This is preferred to a right hepatic lobectomy because the right lobe constitutes >60% of the liver mass. Intracaval shunts have also been described as well as the venoveno bypass.[35] However, we have found that the Haeney technique, as described in the preceding text, is preferable in most instances. Isolation of the liver blood supply using the Haeney technique can only be used for brief periods of time (up to 30 minutes) because the patient is in hypovolemic shock and the liver is already hypoxic.

To gain wide exposure of the infrahepatic vena cava, a right medial visceral rotation (Cattell-Braasch maneuver) can be performed (see Fig. 4). This involves incising the avascular line of Toldt of the right colon from the hepatic flexure down to the cecum. The colon is then retracted medially with blunt dissection. Additional exposure can be achieved by extending the inferior margin of the peritoneal incision to the root of the mesentery and performing a Kocher maneuver with medial rotation of the duodenum and the head of the pancreas. This maneuver provides wide exposure to the infrahepatic IVC and any associated aortic or renovascular injury inferior to the origin of the SMA.[36,37] The confluence of the common iliac veins to form the IVC is located posterior to the right common iliac artery. Access to this portion of the IVC can be achieved by division of the right common iliac artery, with subsequent reanastomosis after repair of the IVC.[38]

Proximal and distal control of the IVC with vascular clamps is often difficult due to extensive collaterals mentioned in the preceding text. Some useful techniques to facilitate control of the IVC in the face of hemorrhage are the use of balloon catheters inserted through the laceration and inflating it in the lumen of the IVC. Another technique is immediate tamponade of the wound with a tightly rolled pack, followed by the slow rolling of the pack down the wound from one end, exposing small portions of the injury while the remainder is still compressed. As the wound edges are exposed, Babcock clamps are applied sequentially until the entire wound has been coapted.[31] Care must be taken when occluding the entire IVC because this disrupts a large

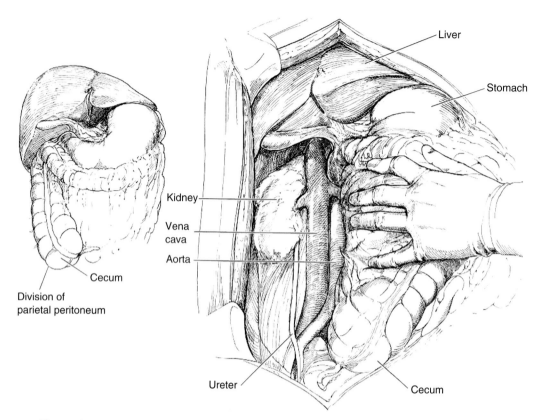

Figure 4 Right medial visceral rotation for exposure of the inferior vena cava, and the right renovascular pedicle. (Figure from Thal ER, O'Keeffe T. Operative exposure of abdominal injuries and closure of the abdomen. In: Souba WW, Fink MP, Jurkovich GJ, et al. eds. *ACS surgery: principles and practice*. Chicago: WebMD Professional Publishing; 2006.)

portion of the venous return to the right atrium and is poorly tolerated in severely hypovolemic patients.

Anterior caval injuries can usually be repaired primarily with a transverse continuous 4-0 or 5-0 vascular suture. Quick access to posterior caval injuries is difficult and can be achieved by opening the anterior wall or extending the anterior injury. If significant narrowing will result with primary repair (<50%), patch repair with saphenous or hypogastric vein can be performed. Revision of a narrowed infrarenal IVC repair should not be attempted in any patient who is hemodynamically unstable. The operating surgeon must remember that the first priority is stopping the hemorrhage and damage control. In fact, if the patient is in profound shock and has multiple vascular injuries, ligation of the infrarenal IVC is an acceptable method of management. Postoperative thrombosis and occlusion of the surgically repaired infrarenal IVC is not uncommon especially if the repair is narrow. This is usually very well tolerated and no further intervention is necessary.[31] Ligation of the suprarenal vena cava is less well tolerated because of the significant risks of renal failure. If the patient is in profound shock, it is reasonable to ligate the suprarenal IVC with planned reoperation and repair once the patient is properly resuscitated in the intensive care unit (ICU).

As with injuries to the aorta, injuries to the IVC can also compromise the lower extremities. Lower extremity compartment syndrome can develop especially if the IVC is ligated and should be managed with below-the-knee two-incision four-compartment fasciotomies. Postoperative lower extremity edema is common and is managed with elastic compression wraps, leg elevation, and sequential compression devices. Full-length custom-made compression support hose should be provided if lower extremity edema persists.

CELIAC AXIS INJURY

Injuries to the celiac axis are rare with only case reports and small case series ($n \leq 13$) reported in the literature. In a recent review from a large urban trauma center of 2,357 patients requiring a trauma laparotomy, the incidence of celiac axis injury was reported at 0.01%.[39] Mortality from this injury depends on associated injuries but approaches upward of 50%. The celiac axis gives off three main branches, common hepatic, left gastric, and splenic artery and is consistent in 90% of the population with the remainder 10% having some combination of two main branches.[6] There is extensive collateral circulation between the celiac axis and the SMA mainly through the superior and inferior pancreaticoduodenal arteries, gastroduodenal artery, and their rich anastomotic network surrounding the head of the pancreas.

Injuries to the celiac axis are located in zone I and can have hematoma formation at either the supramesocolic or inframesocolic location. Rapid exposure to this area can be achieved by left medial visceral rotation described previously. Injury to the celiac axis is usually treated with ligation for hemodynamically unstable patients with minimal complications because of the extensive collateral circulation. There have been no reported cases of ischemic bowel secondary to celiac axis ligation when there is an intact SMA. Only one case of an ischemic gallbladder has been reported to be due to traumatic celiac axis ligation.[40] Primary repair with 4-0 or 5-0 vascular suture can be attempted in stable patients without any other pressing associated injuries to address.

PORTA HEPATIS INJURIES

Injuries to the porta hepatis can present with hematoma or hemorrhage and can be due to injury of the portal vein and/or hepatic artery with a concomitant injury to the common bile duct. Initial control of hemorrhage can be achieved with direct digital pressure until a Pringle maneuver can be applied by placing a vascular clamp or vessel loop around the hepatoduodenal ligament. A Pringle maneuver should also be done before exploring a hematoma within this area. If the injury has occurred in the central portion of the porta, then a distal clamp can be applied just proximal to where these vessels enter the liver. After gaining adequate proximal and distal control, the structures within the hepatoduodenal ligament can be carefully dissected out for possible repair.

Injuries to the hepatic artery can be difficult to repair because of its small size. Although attempts at repair can be performed on occasion, ligation of the hepatic artery can be tolerated because of the vast collateral blood supply to the liver.[37] Ligation does increase the risk of liver necrosis if an associated hepatic injury is present.[5] If the right hepatic artery is ligated than a cholecystectomy should be performed.[5] If possible, the proper hepatic artery should be repaired.

Injuries to the portal vein can be highly lethal due to the size of the vessel and its posterior location within the hepatoduodenal ligament. Exposure of the anterior portion of the vein can be accomplished with mobilizing the common bile duct superiorly and to the left. An extensive Kocher maneuver is performed to allow for visualization of the posterior aspect of the vein down to the superior border of the pancreas. If hemorrhage is noted to be coming from behind the pancreas, then compression of the superior mesenteric vein (SMV) is performed to allow the pancreatic neck to be divided to expose the junction of the SMV

and splenic vein. Repair of the portal vein can be done with running 4-0 or 5-0 vascular suture. Extensive repair of the portal vein can be performed with an end-to-end anastomosis, PTFE interposition graft, portosystemic shunt, or splenic vein transposition but should not be attempted in patients with severe shock.[37] Ligation of the portal vein is more appropriate in patients in extremis. Following portal vein ligation, large volumes of crystalloid are required to reverse the transient peripheral hypovolemia that results from splanchnic hypervolemia.

Injury to the retrohepatic IVC has been briefly mentioned in this chapter. Nonruptured hematomas may be managed with perihepatic packing for 24 to 48 hours to minimize expansion and potential rupture. Obvious hemorrhage from behind the liver can be controlled with compression of the liver to compress the suspected injury to the IVC and a Pringle maneuver should be performed. The hepatic lobe nearest to the area of suspected injury to the cava is mobilized and lifted to expose the IVC.[41] Injury to the IVC or hepatic vein can be grasped and a curved vascular clamp is applied. Placement of a large-sized chest tube or endotracheal tube as an atriocaval shunt through the atrial appendage can be done if direct control of the injury is not successful.[42] The anesthesiologist should be made aware of the potential large volume of blood loss that will occur with exposure of the injury. This will allow for early transfusion of blood products and volume replacement to occur as control and repair are attempted. If control is obtained then repair can be performed with running 4-0 or 5-0 vascular suture.

SUPERIOR MESENTERIC ARTERY AND VEIN INJURIES

SMA injuries as with celiac axis injuries are also rare with an incidence of <1%.[43] Most series in the literature report a prevalence of penetrating trauma. However, in a 2001 large multicenter retrospective review, the incidence of blunt versus penetrating mechanisms of injury was approximately equal.[44] Interestingly, the mechanism of injury did not predict survival.

Approach to injuries to the SMA should be divided into zones and ischemic grade described by Fullen[45] (see Table 1). The hematoma or bleeding can be located in any retroperitoneal zone but most commonly in zone I with equal distribution in the supramesocolic and inframesocolic area.[44] Operative exposure to the SMA depends on the zone of injury. Fullen zone I injuries usually present as a supramesocolic hematoma and exposure can be achieved with left medial visceral rotation. Exposure of inframesocolic hematoma can be approached directly with an extensive Kocher maneuver or with the Catell-Braash maneuver. An alternative approach to Fullen zone I or II injuries is through the neck of the pancreas by transecting the avascular plane above

TABLE 1

THE FULLEN ANATOMIC CLASSIFICATION OF SUPERIOR MESENTERIC ARTERY INJURY BY ZONE AND GRADE

Zone	Segment of Superior Mesenteric Artery	Grade	Ischemic Category	Bowel Segments Affected
I	Trunk proximal to the first major branch inferior pancreaticoduodenal	1	Maximal	Jejunum, ileum, right colon
II	Trunk between inferior pancreaticoduodenal and middle colic	2	Moderate	Major segment, small bowel, right colon, or both
III	Trunk distal to middle colic	3	Minimal	Minor segment or segments, small bowel or right colon
IV	Segmental branches, jejunal, ileal or colic	4	None	No ischemic bowel

the mesenteric vessels. This approach is useful if direct pressure is required to the root of the mesentery to control bleeding, making lateral mobilization of the viscera for medial rotation difficult or impossible. After surgical repair of the vessels, the distal stump of the head of the pancreas can be oversewn in two layers, and the tail of the pancreas can either be resected (usually not necessary) or a pancreaticojejunostomy performed.

The SMA is the principal blood supply of the distal duodenum to the proximal two thirds of the colon with some collateral circulation from the celiac axis. In rare circumstances in young otherwise healthy trauma patients, ligation of the proximal SMA may be tolerated. In most of the patients, repair is necessary to prevent intestinal ischemia especially in the face of severe vasoconstriction due to exsanguinating hemorrhage. Injuries to Fullen zone I, II, or III should be repaired primarily if possible. Fullen zone IV injuries can be safely ligated, however, if there are multiple injuries in zone IV, ischemia is more likely and can be highly variable. If primary repair significantly narrows the artery, patch options include prosthetic PTFE or vein patch from the saphenous vein. Vein patch is recommended in a contaminated field from perforated viscus. The SMA, like the subclavian artery, has reduced elastic tissue and repair should be tensionfree. For complex injuries to the SMA that precludes primary or patch repair, an interposition or bypass graft is required. If the proximal anastomosis is to the aorta, it should be to the distal infrarenal aorta. For patients undergoing damage-control laparotomy, a temporary shunt can be inserted to maintain flow during resuscitation with planned delayed repair. Injuries to the IMA are usually ligated. Second-look laparotomy should be performed if there is concern for bowel ischemia, which can be a delayed presentation.

The most common associated vascular injury when the SMA is injured is the SMV.[44,46] Exposure to the SMV is the same as the SMA described in the preceding text. Primary venorrhaphy is preferred if rapid repair can be achieved. Complex repairs, however, are not recommended and ligation is the treatment of choice and is very well tolerated.[6,37,46] Ligation of the SMV can lead to immediate discoloration and swelling of the bowel. Temporary closure with planned second look is recommended if bowel ischemia is of significant concern. Vigorous postoperative fluid resuscitation is required to reverse the peripheral hypovolemia that can result from splanchnic hypervolemia with ligation of the SMV.[37,46] Injuries to the inferior mesenteric vein (IMV) are treated with ligation.

RENAL VASCULAR INJURY

Renovascular injuries are uncommon following trauma. In a review of the National Trauma Data Bank and >945,000 blunt trauma admissions, only 517 patients (0.05%) had injuries to the renal artery and of those only 29 had an associated renal vein injury.[47] In a multicenter report from six trauma centers over a 16-year period, only 55 patients were found to have renovascular injury.[48]

The decision to perform immediate nephrectomy depends on the clinical condition of the patient, long preoperative ischemia time, presence of associated injuries, and the presence of a normal contralateral kidney on palpation. For contained perirenal hematomas, associated intra-abdominal injuries should be addressed before renal exploration. This allows Gerota fascia to apply a tamponade effect on the hematoma.[49] However, if the patient undergoing laparotomy for blunt trauma is stable and the hematoma is contained then it need not be explored.[5] Revascularization following injury has been associated with a 14% to 40% renal salvage rate and can be associated with late complications including impaired renal function and delayed hypertension.[49,50] Recommended revascularization of a unilateral injury is advocated only within 5 hours of the injury.[50] Select patients with blunt and penetrating trauma who have sustained minor renal vascular injuries can be managed nonoperatively[47,51] and with less late complications.[47]

Management for renal artery thrombosis has been controversial with options including immediate revascularization, prophylactic nephrectomy, observation[47], or endovascular repair.[52] Angiographic and endovascular

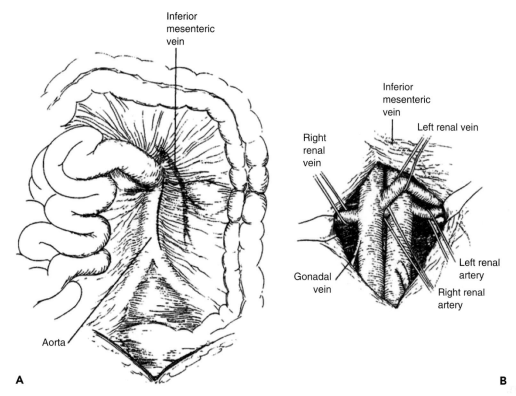

Figure 5 Operative exposure of the proximal renal vasculature. (Figure from Master VA, McAninch JW. Operative management of renal injuries: Parenchymal and vascular. *Urol Clin North Am.* 2006;33:21–31, v–vi.)

repair of renal vascular injuries has been successfully performed and can be considered in select patients with intimal tears, dissection, or thrombosis.[52]

Operative management for proximal control of the renal vasculature can be obtained through the midline of the retroperitoneum at the base of the mesentery (see Fig. 5). A longitudinal incision is made over the aorta extending from the SMA to the IMA. Dissection is carried out on the artery and the crossing left renal vein is identified and encircled with a vessel loop. The remaining renal vessels are then identified and controlled with vessel loops before perirenal hematomas are explored. The renal vessels can be occluded if there is massive hemorrhage from the parenchyma. Vascular occlusion should be limited to 30 to 60 minutes to minimize warm ischemic injury.[49,53] If active hemorrhage is present from Gerota fascia or from the retroperitoneum over the aorta then an incision lateral to the injured kidney should be made and the kidney should be elevated into the abdomen (Mattox maneuver). A vascular clamp is then placed across the hilar vessels of the kidney to control hemorrhage until a decision is made to repair the damaged vessels or perform a nephrectomy.

Partial penetrating injuries to the main renal artery can be repaired primarily following vascular control with 5-0 vascular sutures or by resection and an end-to-end tensionfree anastomosis.[54] Segmental arterial injury can

be safely ligated.[49] Blunt injuries to the renal artery resulting in thrombosis of a potentially viable kidney can undergo thrombectomy, debridement of the damaged arterial segment, and repair with anastomosis if the kidney is to be salvaged.[49] If a tensionfree anastomosis cannot be created, then an interposition graft can be considered but is usually reserved for patients with only one kidney.

Intimal tears following deceleration injury and noted on angiography can be managed by observation and anticoagulation, if flow to the kidney is preserved with repeat renal isotope scan or renal vascular ultrasonography. Alternatively, an endovascular stent may be placed which will then require a period of anticoagulation afterward.[55]

Major renal vein injury may require ligation for control with subsequent need for nephrectomy either at the initial surgery or at a subsequent one following damage control surgery. For partial renal vein injuries, once proximal and distal control of the vessel is obtained, then primary repair with a 5-0 vascular suture can be performed. Injuries to the segmental renal veins can be safely ligated because of the extensive collateral renal venous circulation.[49]

ILIAC ARTERY AND VEIN INJURY

The iliac arteries and veins lie in the lateral pelvis and are relatively protected by the bony pelvis and their posterior

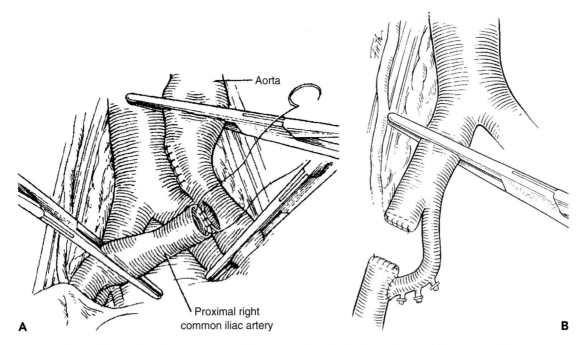

Figure 6   **A:** Contralateral common iliac transposition. **B:** Ipsilateral internal iliac transposition. (Figure from Lee JT, Bongard FS. Iliac vessel injuries. *Surg Clin North Am.* 2002;82:21–48, xix.)

location. Blunt injuries to the pelvis from motor vehicle crashes or direct blows to the pelvis result in vasculature injury by direct compression of the vessels over the bony pelvis or shearing forces created by sudden increase in intraluminal pressure from external compressive forces.[56] On physical examination of these patients, they may or may not have palpable femoral or distal lower extremity pulses. The absence of the pulses should raise the suspicion of arterial injury in patients with pelvic trauma. Angiography, CT angiography, or magnetic resonance angiography can be used to evaluate for vascular injuries in patients with blunt pelvic injuries. In addition to its diagnostic value, embolization of arterial bleeding can also be done with angiography.[5]

Penetrating injuries to pelvic vessels require surgical intervention. Hemorrhage can be controlled initially with compression while formal proximal and distal vascular control is obtained. After midline laparotomy the bowel is eviscerated to expose the bifurcation of the aorta. Incise the peritoneum overlying the bifurcation to gain proximal control of the iliac arteries and veins. Distal control of the external iliac artery and vein can be achieved where they emerge from the pelvis just proximal to the inguinal ligament. Continued back-bleeding from the internal iliac vessels can be controlled with vessel loops. If a complex vascular injury has occurred in a patient with severe shock then the vessel can be resected and a temporary intraluminal shunt (Argyle, Pruitt-Inahara) can be inserted to maintain flow while the patient is resuscitated in the ICU.[57] If bilateral iliac vascular injury is noted, then total pelvic vascular isolation can be performed. To do

this, the IVC and abdominal aorta are cross clamped above the bifurcation, and external iliac vessels are also cross clamped.[57] Standard repair of vessels after control of hemorrhage include lateral arteriography, end-to-end anastomosis, and resection and insertion of a saphenous vein or PTFE graft.[58] Contralateral common iliac and ipsilateral internal iliac transposition has been described to provide flow to the injured external iliac artery (see Fig. 6).[59] Primary arterial repair and especially synthetic grafts should not be placed in the presence of a large amount of enteric or fecal contamination. This may result in postoperative infection and abscess formation that can lead to a leak or blowout of the repair. An alternative to primary repair in this situation would be to divide the artery and close the proximal and distal ends with a double running row of 4-0 vascular suture and bury the ends in the retroperitoneum or omental pedicle.[5] An extra anatomic femofemoral bypass can be performed if the patient is stable to reestablish flow to injured extremity. If the patient is unstable, a four-compartment fasciotomy should be performed on the injured side with bypass planned within 6 hours of resuscitation in the ICU.

Injuries to the common or external iliac veins can also be initially controlled with direct compression. They can be repaired with 4-0 or 5-0 vascular suture or ligation for severe exsanguinating hemorrhage. If significant narrowing or occlusion is present following venorrhaphy then the patient needs postoperative anticoagulation to prevent thrombus formation or its propagation. Lower extremity elevation with support hose following venous ligation will limit the development of edema.[60]

ENDOVASCULAR OPTIONS FOR ABDOMINAL VASCULAR INJURIES

There have been many advances in endovascular technology and other minimally invasive techniques in the last decade. Current data in the literature regarding endovascular management of abdominal vascular trauma are still limited to small case series and case reports. Endovascular management is contraindicated in patients who are hemodynamically unstable, have other associated abdominal injuries requiring exploration, and have evidence of lower limb ischemia.[61] The vast majority of abdominal vascular injuries are due to penetrating trauma and this is a relative contraindication to endovascular repair because of other associated visceral injuries requiring surgical exploration. There has been one case report of endovascular repair of acute hemorrhage from an abdominal aorta injury due to a gunshot wound.[62] There was delayed hemorrhage two weeks after primary repair in a patient with multiple bowel perforations, significant stool contamination, and open abdomen. The patient's clinical condition prevented surgical intervention and underwent successful endovascular repair.[62] This case illustrates the potential of endovascular repair when surgical options are severely limited. A recently published larger trial ($n = 62$) evaluated the use of a covered stent in vascular injuries.[63] Most injuries were in the iliac arteries with 91.3% successful initial repair rate, 76.4% primary patency rate, and 74.3% of patients avoiding surgery after a 1-year follow-up.[63] Although this study was limited by the fact that 78% of the injuries were iatrogenic and the use of a historic control, it illustrates the potential of endovascular repair.

Endovascular repair is mostly relegated to blunt mechanisms of injury with intimal disruption. Blunt trauma is the most common mechanism of renal artery injury and there are several case reports of successful endovascular repair.[55,64,65] These first reported cases of successful endovascular repair of the abdominal aorta were performed in France in 1997.[66] Since then, there have been multiple case reports of successful stent repair of blunt abdominal aorta injuries and blunt and iatrogenic IVC injuries.[66–71] The long-term outcomes of these repairs are unknown. Bleeding vessels from severe blunt pelvic trauma can be embolized, which is a valuable tool in trauma and well documented in the literature.[61]

SUMMARY

Although trauma to major abdominal vessels is uncommon, they can be devastating injuries that carry high morbidity and mortality. Most of these injuries are due to penetrating trauma. Abdominal vascular trauma generally occurs with other associated injuries, which can increase the complexity and time of surgical intervention. Successful treatment of these injuries depends on a high suspicion of an injury and early control of uncontrolled bleeding. This requires a thorough knowledge of anatomy and exposure techniques to allow for quick and adequate control of the injured vessel. Patients arriving in extremis may require emergency room thoracotomy to gain proximal control of the aorta. Damage control laparotomy should be considered in coagulopathic patients after exsanguinating hemorrhage has been addressed.

REFERENCES

1. Asensio JA, Chahwan S, Hanpeter D, et al. Operative management and outcome of 302 abdominal vascular injuries. *Am J Surg.* 2000;180:528–533; discussion 533–524.
2. Brohi K, Singh J, Heron M, et al. Acute traumatic coagulopathy. *J Trauma.* 2003;54:1127–1130.
3. MacLeod JB, Lynn M, McKenney MG, et al. Early coagulopathy predicts mortality in trauma. *J Trauma.* 2003;55:39–44.
4. Kauvar DS, Lefering R, Wade CE. Impact of hemorrhage on trauma outcome: An overview of epidemiology, clinical presentations, and therapeutic considerations. *J Trauma.* 2006;60:S3–11.
5. Goaley TJ, Dente CJ, Feliciano DV. Torso vascular trauma at an urban level I trauma center. *Perspect Vasc Surg Endovasc Ther.* 2006;18:102–112.
6. Asensio JA, Forno W, Roldan G, et al. Visceral vascular injuries. *Surg Clin North Am.* 2002;82:1–20, xix.
7. Asensio JA, Petrone P, Karsidag T, et al. Abdominal vascular injuries: A continuing challenge. *Ulus Travma Derg.* 2002;8:189–197.
8. Asensio JA, Soto SN, Forno W, et al. Abdominal vascular injuries: The trauma surgeon's challenge. *Surg Today.* 2001;31:949–957.
9. Mattox KL, Feliciano DV, Burch J, et al. Five thousand seven hundred sixty cardiovascular injuries in 4459 patients. Epidemiologic evolution 1958 to 1987. *Ann Surg.* 1989;209:698–705; discussion 706–697.
10. Debakey ME, Simone FA. Battle injuries of the arteries in World War II: An analysis of 2471 cases. *Ann Surg.* 1946;123:534–579.
11. Rich NM, Baugh JH, Hughes CW. Acute arterial injuries in Vietnam: 1,000 cases. *J Trauma.* 1970;10:359–369.
12. Clouse WD, Rasmussen TE, Peck MA, et al. In-theater management of vascular injury: 2 years of the Balad vascular registry. *J Am Coll Surg.* 2007;204:625–632.
13. Mullins RJ, Huckfeldt R, Trunkey DD. Abdominal vascular injuries. *Surg Clin North Am.* 1996;76:813–832.
14. Rozycki GS, Ballard RB, Feliciano DV, et al. Surgeon-performed ultrasound for the assessment of truncal injuries: Lessons learned from 1540 patients. *Ann Surg.* 1998;228:557–567.
15. Gonzalez EA, Moore FA, Holcomb JB, et al. Fresh frozen plasma should be given earlier to patients requiring massive transfusion. *J Trauma.* 2007;62:112–119.
16. Holcomb JB, Jenkins D, Rhee P, et al. Damage control resuscitation: Directly addressing the early coagulopathy of trauma. *J Trauma.* 2007;62:307–310.
17. Feliciano DV, Bitondo CG, Cruse PA, et al. Liberal use of emergency center thoracotomy. *Am J Surg.* 1986;152:654–659.
18. Baker CC, Thomas AN, Trunkey DD. The role of emergency room thoracotomy in trauma. *J Trauma.* 1980;20:848–855.
19. Frame SB, Timberlake GA, Rush DS, et al. Penetrating injuries of the abdominal aorta. *Am Surg.* 1990;56:651–654.
20. Rhee PM, Acosta J, Bridgeman A, et al. Survival after emergency department thoracotomy: Review of published data from the past 25 years. *J Am Coll Surg.* 2000;190:288–298.
21. Baker CC, Caronna JJ, Trunkey DD. Neurologic outcome after emergency room thoracotomy for trauma. *Am J Surg.* 1980;139:677–681.
22. Ivatury R, Cayten CG, eds. *The textbook of penetrating trauma.* Baltimore: Williams & Wilkins; 1996.
23. Accola KD, Feliciano DV, Mattox KL, et al. Management of injuries to the suprarenal aorta. *Am J Surg.* 1987;154:613–618.

24. Davis TP, Feliciano DV, Rozycki GS, et al. Results with abdominal vascular trauma in the modern era. *Am Surg.* 2001;67:565–570; discussion 570–561.

25. Feliciano DV. Injuries to the great vessels of the abdomen. In: Souba WW, Fink MP, Jurkovich GJ, et al. eds. *ACS surgery: principles and practice.* Chicago: WebMD Professional Publishing; 2004:1–12.

26. Tyburski JG, Wilson RF, Dente C, et al. Factors affecting mortality rates in patients with abdominal vascular injuries. *J Trauma.* 2001;50:1020–1026.

27. Asensio JA, Forno W, Roldan G, et al. Abdominal vascular injuries: Injuries to the aorta. *Surg Clin North Am.* 2001;81:1395–1416, xiii–xxiv.

28. Veith FJ, Gupta S, Daly V. Technique for occluding the surpaceliac aorta through the abdomen. *Surg Gynecol Obstet.* 1980;151:426–428.

29. Bunt TJ, Doerhoff CR, Haynes JL. Retrocolic omental pedicle flap for routine plication of abdominal aortic grafts. *Surg Gynecol Obstet.* 1984;158:591–592.

30. Nothmann A, Tung TC, Simon B. Aortoduodenal fistula in the acute trauma setting: Case report. *J Trauma.* 2002;53:106–108.

31. Buckman RF, Pathak AS, Badellino MM, et al. Injuries of the inferior vena cava. *Surg Clin North Am.* 2001;81:1431–1447.

32. Wiencek RG, Wilson RF. Abdominal venous injuries. *J Trauma.* 1986;26:771–778.

33. Duke JH Jr, Jones RC, Shires GT. Management of injuries to the inferior vena cava. *Am J Surg.* 1965;110:759–763.

34. Heaney JP, Stanton WK, Halbert DS, et al. An improved technic for vascular isolation of the liver: Experimental study and case reports. *Ann Surg.* 1966;163:237–241.

35. Buckman RF Jr, Miraliakbari R, Badellino MM. Juxtahepatic venous injuries: A critical review of reported management strategies. *J Trauma.* 2000;48:978–984.

36. Cattell RB, Braasch JW. A technique for the exposure of the third and fourth portions of the duodenum. *Surg Gynecol Obstet.* 1960;111:378–379.

37. Feliciano DV. Injuries to the great vessels of the abdomen. In: Souba WW, Fink MP, Jurkovich GJ, et al. eds. *ACS surgery: principles and practice.* Chicago: WebMD Professional Publishing; 2004.

38. Salam AA, Stewart MT. New approach to wounds of the aortic bifurcation and inferior vena cava. *Surgery.* 1985;98:105–108.

39. Asensio JA, Petrone P, Kimbrell B, et al. Lessons learned in the management of thirteen celiac axis injuries. *South Med J.* 2005;98:462–466.

40. Kavic SM, Atweh N, Ivy ME, et al. Celiac axis ligation after gunshot wound to the abdomen: Case report and literature review. *J Trauma.* 2001;50:738–739.

41. Feliciano DV, Mattox KL, Jordan GL Jr, et al. Management of 1000 consecutive cases of hepatic trauma (1979–1984). *Ann Surg.* 1986;204:438–445.

42. Burch JM, Feliciano DV, Mattox KL. The atriocaval shunt. Facts and fiction. *Ann Surg.* 1988;207:555–568.

43. Asensio JA, Berne JD, Chahwan S, et al. Traumatic injury to the superior mesenteric artery. *Am J Surg.* 1999;178:235–239.

44. Asensio JA, Britt LD, Borzotta A, et al. Multiinstitutional experience with the management of superior mesenteric artery injuries. *J Am Coll Surg.* 2001;193:354–365.discussion 365–356.

45. Fullen WD, Hunt J, Altemeier WA. The clinical spectrum of penetrating injury to the superior mesenteric arterial circulation. *J Trauma.* 1972;12:656–664.

46. Asensio JA, Petrone P, Garcia-Nunez L, et al. Superior mesenteric venous injuries: To ligate or to repair remains the question. *J Trauma.* 2007;62:668–675; discussion 675.

47. Sangthong B, Demetriades D, Martin M, et al. Management and hospital outcomes of blunt renal artery injuries: Analysis of 517 patients from the National Trauma Data Bank. *J Am Coll Surg.* 2006;203:612–617.

48. Knudson MM, Harrison PB, Hoyt DB, et al. Outcome after major renovascular injuries: A western trauma association multicenter report. *J Trauma.* 2000;49:1116–1122.

49. Master VA, McAninch JW. Operative management of renal injuries: Parenchymal and vascular. *Urol Clin North Am.* 2006;33:21–31, vi.

50. Santucci RA, Fisher MB. The literature increasingly supports expectant (conservative) management of renal trauma—a systematic review. *J Trauma.* 2005;59:493–503.

51. Carroll PR, McAninch JW, Klosterman P, et al. Renovascular trauma: Risk assessment, surgical management, and outcome. *J Trauma.* 1990;30:547–552; discussion 553–544.

52. Breyer BN, Master VA, Marder SR, et al. Endovascular management of trauma related renal artery thrombosis. *J Trauma.* 2006.

53. Flye MW, Anderson RW, Fish JC, et al. Successful surgical treatment of anuria caused by renal artery occlusion. *Ann Surg.* 1982;195:346–353.

54. Brown MF, Graham JM, Mattox KL, et al. Renovascular trauma. *Am J Surg.* 1980;140:802–805.

55. Villas PA, Cohen G, Putnam SG III, et al. Wallstent placement in a renal artery after blunt abdominal trauma. *J Trauma.* 1999;46:1137–1139.

56. Baker WE, Wassermann J. Unsuspected vascular trauma: Blunt arterial injuries. *Emerg Med Clin North Am.* 2004;22:1081–1098.

57. Lee JT, Bongard FS. Iliac vessel injuries. *Surg Clin North Am.* 2002;82:21–48, xix.

58. Landreneau RJ, Lewis DM, Snyder WH. Complex iliac arterial trauma: Autologous or prosthetic vascular repair? *Surgery.* 1993;114:9–12.

59. Landreneau RJ, Mitchum P, Fry WJ. Iliac arterial transposition. *Arch Surg.* 1989;124:978–981.

60. Mullins RJ, Lucas CE, Ledgerwood AM. The natural history following venous ligation for civilian injuries. *J Trauma.* 1980;20:737–743.

61. Starnes BW, Arthurs ZM. Endovascular management of vascular trauma. *Perspect Vasc Surg Endovasc Ther.* 2006;18:114–129.

62. Yeh MW, Horn JK, Schecter WP, et al. Endovascular repair of an actively hemorrhaging gunshot injury to the abdominal aorta. *J Vasc Surg.* 2005;42:1007–1009.

63. White R, Krajcer Z, Johnson M, et al. Results of a multicenter trial for the treatment of traumatic vascular injury with a covered stent. *J Trauma.* 2006;60:1189–1195; discussion 1195–1186.

64. Lee JT, White RA. Endovascular management of blunt traumatic renal artery dissection. *J Endovasc Ther.* 2002;9:354–358.

65. Whigham CJ Jr, Bodenhamer JR, Miller JK. Use of the Palmaz stent in primary treatment of renal artery intimal injury secondary to blunt trauma. *J Vasc Interv Radiol.* 1995;6:175–178.

66. Vernhet H, Marty-Ane CH, Lesnik A, et al. Dissection of the abdominal aorta in blunt trauma: Management by percutaneous stent placement. *Cardiovasc Intervent Radiol.* 1997;20:473–476.

67. Castelli P, Caronno R, Piffaretti G, et al. Emergency endovascular repair for traumatic injury of the inferior vena cava. *Eur J Cardiothorac Surg.* 2005;28:906–908.

68. de Naeyer G, Degrieck I. Emergent infrahepatic vena cava stenting for life-threatening perforation. *J Vasc Surg.* 2005;41:552–554.

69. Erzurum VZ, Shoup M, Borge M, et al. Inferior vena cava endograft to control surgically inaccessible hemorrhage. *J Vasc Surg.* 2003;38:1437–1439.

70. Fontaine AB, Nicholls SC, Borsa JJ, et al. Seat belt aorta: Endovascular management with a stent-graft. *J Endovasc Ther.* 2001;8:83–86.

71. Teruya TH, Bianchi C, Abou-Zamzam AM, et al. Endovascular treatment of a blunt traumatic abdominal aortic injury with a commercially available stent graft. *Ann Vasc Surg.* 2005;19:474–478.

Genitourinary Injury

44

James J. Thomas   *Richard A. Santucci*
Allen F. Morey

Although rarely lethal in nature, genitourinary tract injuries may be associated with significant morbidity. Prompt recognition and treatment are imperative to reduce complications and improve outcomes. Hematuria is a common but imperfect indicator of urinary tract injury. Because of ongoing treatment requirements for nonurologic associated injuries, radiographic evaluation of the urogenital tract must be efficient and appropriately conducted, while erroneous or unhelpful negative studies must be avoided. Although minor injuries can be safely observed, maximal urinary drainage and/or immediate reconstruction are often appropriate means of management in more severe injuries. Prompt surgical reconstruction of most genital injuries usually leads to adequate and acceptable cosmetic and functional results. In this chapter, we review the contemporary evaluation and treatment of genitourinary injuries in the trauma patient.

RENAL INJURIES

Evaluation

Presentation
Blunt rapid deceleration injuries are the most common etiology for renal trauma. Although blunt renal injuries tend to be minor in nature, some may be associated with damage to the renal vessels, renal artery thrombosis, or renal pedicle avulsion. Major renal injuries are often associated with multiple associated nonurologic injuries in the setting of rapid deceleration or penetrating trauma.

Hematuria is the best indicator of urinary system injury, although the degree of hematuria and the severity of the renal injury may not correlate. Microscopic hematuria seems to herald the presence of renal injury more commonly when shock is present,[1–3] and less so when

it is not. Microscopy is not necessarily required to evaluate hematuria, as the dipstick method is rapid and has a sensitivity and specificity for detection of microhematuria of more than 97%.[4]

Indications for Renal Imaging
The indications for radiographic evaluation after blunt trauma are gross hematuria, microscopic hematuria with shock, and major deceleration injury in the presence of significant nonurologic-associated injuries.[3,5,6] Blunt trauma patients with isolated microhematuria do not in general require immediate imaging. Penetrating injuries with any degree of hematuria should be imaged.

Pediatric patients sustaining blunt abdominal trauma are at greater risk for renal injury than adults because children have less perirenal fat to protect and stabilize the kidney.[1] Shock may be a less useful criterion in children to determine if imaging studies should be performed.[7] Children with insignificant microhematuria (<50 red blood cell [RBC] per high power field [HPF]) after blunt trauma are a low-yield group and usually do not require urgent renal imaging.[7]

Imaging Studies
Computed tomography (CT) is the gold standard for the radiographic assessment of stable patients with renal trauma and should be performed whenever possible in cases where renal injury is suspected.[5,8,9] CT will accurately determine the location and depth of renal lacerations, the presence and amount of urinary or vascular contrast extravasation, as well as preexisting renal abnormalities. The American Association for the Surgery of Trauma (AAST) organ injury severity scale is the preferred classification scheme for grading of renal injuries, classified by abdominal CT or direct renal exploration (see Table 1).[6]

TABLE 1

AMERICAN ASSOCIATION FOR THE SURGERY OF TRAUMA (AAST) ORGAN INJURY SEVERITY SCALE FOR THE KIDNEY

Grade	Description of Injury
1	Contusion or nonexpanding subcapsular hematoma No laceration
2	Nonexpanding perirenal hematoma Cortical laceration <1 cm deep without extravasation
3	Cortical laceration >1 cm without urinary extravasation
4	Laceration: through corticomedullary junction into collecting system *or* Vascular: segmental renal artery or vein injury with contained hematoma, or partial vessel laceration or vessel thrombosis
5	Laceration: shattered kidney *or* Vascular: renal pedicle or avulsion

(Adapted from Moore EE, Shackford SR, Pachter HL, et al. Organ injury scaling: spleen, liver, and kidney. *J Trauma.* 1989;29(12): 1664–1666.; Nicolaisen GS, McAninch JW, Marshall GA, et al. Renal trauma: Re-evaluation of the indications for radiographic assessment. *J Urol.* 1985;133(2):183–187.)

Failure of the kidney to opacify after contrast administration is a hallmark of renal pedicle injury. Central parahilar hematoma is suggestive of renal pedicle injury, even if the renal parenchyma is well enhanced. In all cases of suspected renal trauma evaluated with spiral CT, additional delayed scans should be performed 10 to 15 minutes after contrast injection to evaluate the integrity of the collecting system.[10]

Unstable patients selected for immediate surgical intervention (and therefore unable to have a CT scan) should undergo one-shot intravenous pyelogram (IVP) in the operating suite if they need evaluation of renal or ureteral injury. The technique consists of a bolus intravenous injection of 2 mL per kg radiographic contrast followed by a single plain film taken after 10 minutes. The study is safe, efficient, and of high quality in most cases.[11] It provides important information concerning the injured kidney, and confirms a normal functioning kidney on the contralateral side. Although ultrasonography is a popular imaging modality in the initial evaluation of abdominal trauma, its role in staging renal trauma is not well established at this time.[12]

Treatment

Nonoperative Management

The kidney has remarkable healing properties, and nonoperative management has therefore become the treatment of choice for the vast majority of non–life-threatening renal injuries. Nonoperative management results in an excellent long-term outcome in most cases. All grade 1 and 2, and most grade 3 renal injuries can be managed nonoperatively. Exploration of grade 4 and 5 renal injuries often results in nephrectomy; recent data indicates that many of these patients can be managed safely with an expectant approach.[13,14]

Patients with suspected penetrating renal injury who are otherwise stable should undergo radiographic staging, whenever possible, to define the injury. Renal gunshot injuries require exploration only if they involve the hilum or are accompanied by signs of continued bleeding, ureteral injuries, or renal pelvis lacerations.[15] Stab wounds and low-velocity gunshot wounds may often be managed conservatively with an acceptably good outcome.[16] Tissue damage from high-velocity gunshot injuries may be more extensive.

The site of penetration by stab wound has an important influence on management—if posterior to the anterior axillary line, most (88%)[17] may be managed nonoperatively.[18,19] A systematic approach based on clinical, laboratory, and radiologic evaluation may minimize negative exploration after renal stabbing, without increasing morbidity from missed injury. Expectant management of renal stab wounds can be attempted on the hemodynamically stable patient, especially if ureteral and renal pelvis injuries can be ruled out. Ultimately, 98% of blunt renal injuries can be managed nonoperatively.

Grade IV and V injuries more often require surgical exploration, but even many of these can be managed without renal surgery if carefully staged and selected. Patients with high-grade injuries selected for nonoperative management should be closely monitored for persistent bleeding with repeat vital signs and serial hematocrits. If significant urinary extravasation persists beyond 48 hours, prompt urologic consultation with retrograde placement of an internal ureteral "double J" stent (and a urethral catheter to prevent urinary reflux) will often prevent prolonged urinary extravasation and improve perirenal urinoma formation, sepsis, and ileus.[20] Follow-up abdominal CT scans are reserved for high-grade injuries and symptomatic patients only (dropping hematocrit, flank pain, fever, etc.). Should renal bleeding persist, or delayed bleeding occur, angiographic studies with embolization of bleeding vessels will often obviate surgical intervention. It is popularly believed that attempts to repair a bleeding kidney in the days after injury when inflammation is maximal (say 3 to 30 days) will inevitably result in nephrectomy, so it seems prudent to attempt expedient angioembolization if possible.

Angiographic Techniques

Angiography is helpful in defining the exact location and degree of vascular injuries and is useful when planning selective embolization. Arteriography with selective renal embolization for hemorrhage control is a reasonable alternative to laparotomy, provided no other indication for immediate surgery exists.[21] The rate of successful hemostasis by embolization is reportedly identical in blunt and penetrating injuries.[22,23]

Operative Management: Indications

The only absolute indication for renal exploration is life-threatening hemodynamic instability due to renal hemorrhage, irrespective of the mode of injury.[24] Another strong indication for renal exploration is an expanding or pulsatile perirenal hematoma identified at exploratory laparotomy (this finding heralds a grade 5 vascular injury and is quite rare). Relative indications for surgery include suspected renal pelvis injury or persistent bleeding (≥3 units per 24 hours). It has been recognized that most injuries that have urinary extravasation and devitalized kidney fragments heal with nonoperative treatment.[25]

Renal Reconstruction

Renal reconstruction (renorrhaphy) by debriding, over-sewing, and covering the defect is feasible in most cases (see Table 2), but partial nephrectomy may be required when large amounts of tissue are damaged, especially at the pole of the kidney. Obtaining early vascular control before opening the Gerota fascia can decrease renal loss caused by bleeding during attempted renal repair (see Fig. 1).[26] In a series of 133 renal units in which early vessel isolation and control before opening the Gerota fascia was achieved, McAninch et al.[24] reported a very high renal salvage rate of 89%. Early vascular control does not increase postoperative azotemia or mortality.

Renovascular Injuries

Renovascular injuries are associated with extensive associated trauma and increased perioperative and postoperative mortality and morbidity. Prompt nephrectomy is usually the treatment of choice except in those very rare cases in which there is a solitary kidney or the patient has sustained bilateral vessel injuries (see Fig. 2).[17] Attempts at surgical repair of renal artery thrombosis largely fail, and certainly

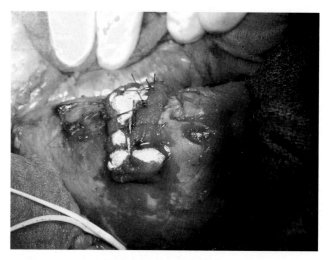

Figure 1 Repair of midpole renal laceration with multiple capsule sutures tied over Gelfoam bolster.

after 8 hours the kidney cannot be salvaged. Many patients with renal vascular injury are critically injured, with numerous associated organ injuries, low body temperature, and poor coagulation; the advisability of major vascular repair over a nephrectomy is limited in the unstable patient if a normal contralateral kidney is present. Damage control with placement of packs and planned return for corrective surgery within 24 hours is another reasonable alternative option.[27] Because the kidney is a paired organ it is sometimes sacrificed with alacrity in patients who would not truly be in danger from an attempted repair. In a recent series of 1,360 adult patients with renal lacerations 23% underwent surgery, and an appalling 64% of these got a nephrectomy.[28] This harmful practice must be avoided.

Complications

Early complications of renal injury include bleeding, infection, perinephric abscess, sepsis, urinary fistula, hypertension, urinary extravasation, and urinoma. Delayed complications include bleeding, hydronephrosis, calculus formation, chronic pyelonephritis, hypertension, arteriovenous fistula, and pseudoaneurysm, although these are all less common. Urinary extravasation can usually be managed expectantly as most resolve spontaneously. In cases where there is persistent leakage with fever and/or sepsis, ureteral stent placement or percutaneous drainage is usually feasible and curative.

URETERAL INJURIES

Evaluation

Presentation

Unlike renal injuries, nearly all ureteral injuries occur as a result of penetrating or iatrogenic trauma. And unlike renal

---

TABLE 2

PRINCIPLES OF RENAL RECONSTRUCTION AFTER TRAUMA

Consider preliminary vascular control—occlude vessels with Rommel tourniquet if major injury

Complete renal exposure

Judicious debridement of nonviable tissue

Hemostasis by individual suture ligation of bleeding vessels (4-0 chromic on RB-1 needle)

Watertight closure of the collecting system (either by suturing or by closing overlying parenchyma)

Coverage or approximation of the parenchymal defect

Consider use of hemostatic agent such as fibrin sealant over repair

Perirenal drain separated from repair, placed through dependant incision

RB, round body.

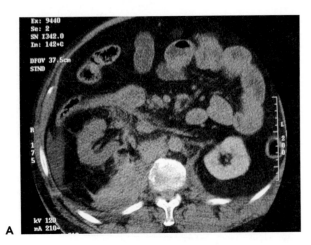
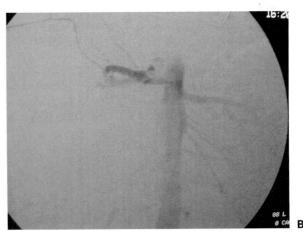

Figure 2 **A:** Computed tomography (CT) showing poor contrast uptake into right renal artery, concerning for renal artery thrombus. **B:** Confirmatory angiogram shows abrupt cutoff of right renal artery consistent with thrombus.

injuries, the presence of hematuria is not a reliable indicator of ureteral injury. Many (25% to 45%) cases of ureteral injury will not have even microscopic hematuria,[29,30] so a high index of suspicion is required.

The rare entity of ureteropelvic junction (UPJ) disruption consequent to rapid deceleration injury is associated with an unusual pattern of either medial or "circumrenal" contrast extravasation seen on CT.[31] Children are felt to be more susceptible because of their hyperextensible vertebral column.[32]

Diagnosis

Wound location is felt to be the best indicator of ureteral injury, and direct exploration is the best means of detecting its presence. Intraoperative detection requires a high degree of suspicion. The trajectory of the knife/missile must be carefully examined and ureteral exploration undertaken in all cases of potential injury. Intravenous infusion or direct ureteral injection of indigo carmine will often produce a pool of colored urine, which may guide intraoperative detection of ureteral injury.

Liberal use of preoperative diagnostic tools such as CT is helpful, whenever possible. Vigilance for delayed presentation of ureteral injuries will also allow detection of injuries missed on presentation. Fever, leukocytosis, and local peritoneal irritation are the most common signs of missed ureteral injury and should always prompt CT examination.

Computed Tomography

Ureteral injuries often manifest in the absence of contrast in the ureter on delayed images. This underscores the absolute necessity of tracing both ureters throughout their entire course on trauma CT scans.[33] Delayed images must be obtained 5 to 20 minutes after contrast injection.[34] Medial extravasation of contrast or nonopacification of the ipsilateral ureter on CT remains the most reliable finding, especially in UPJ avulsion (see Fig. 3). A late

finding of ureteral injury is a urinoma surrounding the ureter. A postcontrast kidney ureter and bladder (KUB) can supplement the CT images, which is created by getting a plain abdominal film after the CT with contrast is complete.

Retrograde Pyelography

Retrograde pyelography is used to delineate the level and extent of ureteral injury seen on CT scan or IVP, or if further clinical information is needed. At the same time, if appropriate, a retrograde ureteral stent can be attempted.

Treatment

Primary Repair

Repair of the ureter must be meticulous, and urologic consultation should be promptly sought to prevent adverse

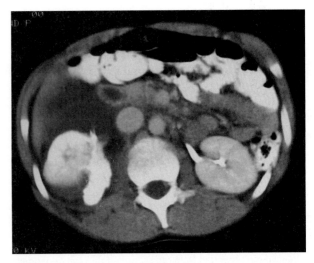

Figure 3 Delayed computed tomography (CT) scan with contrast showing medical extravasation of the right kidney, consistent with upper ureter or renal pelvis injury.

medicolegal consequences. Ureteral blood supply is tenuous and the sequelae of imperfect repair include urine leakage, abscess, fistula, and refractory ureteral stricture, requiring additional surgical procedures and/or nephrectomy.

Primary repair is recommended in most ureteral injuries. Principles of primary ureteroureterostomy involve limited debridement followed by creation of a spatulated, watertight closure using optical magnification, with interrupted or running 5-0 or 6-0 absorbable monofilament such as Maxon (polyglyconate).[29] An internal stent and retroperitoneal drain are placed in most cases. This technique is used primarily for injuries of the upper two thirds of the ureter.

Ureteroneocystotomy

Ureteroneocystotomy is used to repair ureteral injuries in the distal one third of the ureter. A tensionfree repair must be achieved—sometimes the ureteral stump can be reimplanted directly into the bladder. Other times, the bladder must be brought up to the ureter using either psoas hitch or Boari procedure, although complex reconstructions are often best reserved for a delayed setting (see Fig. 4). In trauma cases, we favor a simple refluxing, nontunneled anastomosis to decrease the chance of postoperative stenosis. Use of a stent or feeding tube across the anastomosis is advisable initially.

Damage Control

In unstable patients, delayed ureteral reconstruction may be preferred under more controlled conditions several months later. Immediate management in such cases should include ligation of the ureter just proximal to the injured area with concurrent placement of a long, 90-cm single-J ureteral stent up to the kidney, with the distal end brought out to the skin. Alternatively, planned percutaneous nephrostomy may be performed postoperatively after simple ureteral

ligation. Long silk ties are used to aid the dissection of the ureteral stump during the second-stage repair.

Ureteral Contusion

Minor ureteral contusions can be treated with stent placement. Caution must be exercised, however, as minor-appearing ureteral contusions may stricture later, or break down secondary to unappreciated microvascular damage to the ureter. When in doubt, the injured portion of the ureter should be debrided and ureteroureterostomy used to repair the injury.

GENITAL INJURIES

Penile Fracture

Penile fracture is the disruption of the tunica albuginea with rupture of the corpus cavernosum and is a surgical emergency. Fracture typically occurs during vigorous sexual intercourse. When the erect penis bends abnormally, the abrupt increase in intracavernosal pressure exceeds the tensile strength of the tunica albuginea, and a transverse laceration of the proximal shaft usually results.

The diagnosis of penile fracture is often straightforward and can be made reliably by history and physical examination alone. Patients usually describe a cracking or popping sound as the tunica tears, followed by pain, rapid detumescence, and discoloration and swelling of the penile shaft. If the Buck fascia remains intact, the penile hematoma remains contained between the skin and tunica, resulting in a typical "eggplant" deformity. If the Buck fascia is disrupted, hematoma can extend to the scrotum, perineum, and suprapubic regions. The mass effect of the hematoma often pushes the penis away from the tear. Because fear and/or embarrassment are commonly associated, patient presentation to the emergency department or

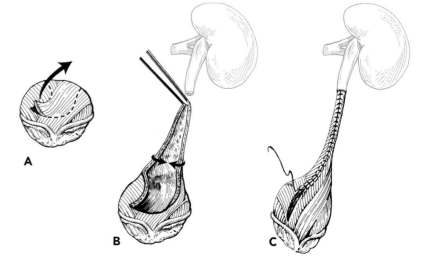

Figure 4 Boari bladder flap is used for lower ureteral reconstruction after extensive injury. The bladder is first completely mobilized anteriorly and laterally, then pexed to the psoas muscle tendon. After an anterior bladder wall flap is mobilized to the ureter, a tensionfree, stented anastomosis is performed.

clinic is sometimes significantly delayed. The typical history and clinical presentation of a fractured penis usually make adjunctive imaging studies unnecessary, but magnetic resonance imaging is reasonable in the evaluation of patients without the typical presentation and physical findings of penile fracture. Roughly 10% of penile fractures are associated with urethral lacerations, which are associated with gross hematuria, blood at the meatus, or inability to void, although the absence of these findings does not definitively rule out urethral injury.[35,36] Given that urethral injury occurs not infrequently, and that urethrography is a simple and reliable study, clinicians should have a low threshold for urethral evaluation in all cases of penile fracture.

Immediate exploration through a distal circumcising incision is appropriate in most cases, thereby providing exposure to all three penile compartments. Closure of the tunical defect with interrupted 2-0 or 3-0 absorbable sutures is recommended, while deep corporal vascular ligation or excessive debridement of the delicate underlying erectile tissue must be avoided. Partial urethral injuries should be oversewn using fine absorbable suture over a urethral catheter. Complete urethral injuries should be debrided, mobilized, and repaired in a tensionfree manner over a catheter. Broad-spectrum antibiotics and 1 month of sexual abstinence are recommended.

Immediate surgical reconstruction results in a faster recovery, decreased morbidity, lower complication rates, and a lower incidence of long-term penile curvature.[37,38] Conservative management of penile fracture results in penile curvature in >10% of patients, abscess or debilitating plaques in 30%, and significantly longer hospitalization times and recovery.[37,39]

Gunshot and Penetrating Wounds

Most penetrating wounds to the genitalia are due to gunshots and most require surgical exploration. Urethral injuries have been reported in 15% to 50% of penile gunshot wounds.[40] Retrograde urethrography should be strongly considered in any patient with penetrating injury to the penis, especially those with high-velocity missile injuries, blood at the meatus, difficulty voiding, or when bullet trajectory was near the urethra;[41] alternatively, intraoperative retrograde urethral injection of methylene blue or indigo carmine may identify the site of injury and the adequacy of closure.

Treatment principles include immediate exploration, copious irrigation, excision of foreign matter, antibiotic prophylaxis, and surgical closure. Excellent cosmetic and functional outcomes can be expected with immediate reconstruction.

Urethral injuries should be closed primarily utilizing standard urethroplasty principles (tensionfree, watertight repair using fine, absorbable sutures and optical magnification, performed over a small catheter); excellent results

have been reported.[35] Patients with urethral injury in the presence of extensive tissue damage and blast effect from high-velocity weapons or close-range shotgun blasts usually require staged repairs and urinary diversion.[42]

Animal and Human Bites

The morbidity of animal bites is directly related to the severity of the initial wound. Most victims are male children and dog bites are the most common injury.[43] Infectious complications are unusual because treatment is sought early, in contrast to most human bite victims who seek medical attention after a substantial delay, and are therefore more likely to present with gross infection.

Initial management of dog bites includes copious irrigation, debridement, and immediate primary closure, along with prophylactic broad-spectrum antibiotics.[44] Tetanus and rabies immunizations should be used as appropriate. Because of the risk of polymicrobial infection, empiric treatment with broad-spectrum antibiotics such as cefazolin or cephalexin is recommended. Wolf et al.[44] advised the additional use of penicillin V (500 mg four times daily) to provide additional coverage against *Pasteurella multocida*, present in 20% to 25% of dog-bite wounds. Alternatively, chloramphenicol alone (50 mg per kg daily for 10 days) is a readily available, inexpensive option which has proved effective in developing countries.[43] Human bites produce potentially contaminated wounds that often should not be closed primarily. Empiric antibiotic administration is warranted in the same manner as with dog bites, even though the bacteriology of the wounds is not identical.

Amputation

Traumatic amputation of the penis, although rare, is usually the result of genital self-mutilation. Sixty-five percent to 87% of patients performing genital self-mutilation are psychotic.[45] Psychiatric consultation should be sought in all such cases. Patients should be transferred to a facility with microsurgical capabilities; however, if unavailable, macroscopic anastomosis of the urethra and corporal bodies can be performed with good erectile results, albeit with less sensation and greater skin loss. Reconstruction of the urethra and reanastomosis of the corpora cavernosum with microsurgical repair of penile vessels and nerves achieves remarkably good results. The severed portion should be rinsed in saline solution, wrapped in saline-soaked gauze and sealed in a sterile plastic bag. The bag should then be placed into an outer bag with ice or slush.[46] Thermal injury to the amputated segment can occur if it is in direct contact with ice for a prolonged period. Successful reimplantation is possible after 16 hours of cold ischemia or 6 hours of warm ischemia.[46] If the severed part is not available, the penile stump should be formalized by closing the corpora and spatulating the urethral neomeatus, similar to a partial penectomy procedure for malignancy.

TABLE 3
STEP-BY-STEP APPROACH TO PENILE REATTACHMENT

Two-layer urethral closure over a catheter with 5-0 absorbable suture
Minimal dissection along the neurovascular bundle to identify severed vessels and nerves
Closure of the tunica albuginea with 3-0 absorbable suture
Microscopic anastomosis of the dorsal artery with 11-0 nylon
Microscopic dorsal vein repair with 9-0 nylon
Microscopic epineural repair of dorsal nerve with 10-0 nylon
Suprapubic cystostomy

Microvascular reconstruction of the dorsal arteries, vein, and nerves is the preferred method of repair for the amputated penis (see Table 3). Adequate erectile function is possible with both microvascular reanastomosis and macroscopic replantation. However, complications such as urethral strictures, skin loss, and sensory abnormalities are all much higher without microvascular repair. Penile skin loss, often complete, is a significant problem following macroscopic repair. One effective strategy is to denude the phallus of all skin and bury it in the scrotum, leaving the glans exposed, with separation of the structures after 2 months.[47]

Strangulation Injuries

Any child with unexplained penile swelling, erythema, or difficulty voiding should be examined closely for a hidden strangulating hair or string. Adults may place objects around the shaft as a means of sexual pleasure or to prolong an erection. Emergent treatment requires decompression of the constricted penis to allow for blood flow and micturition. Depending on the constricting device, significant physician resourcefulness may be required. String, hair, rubber bands, and plastic constricting devices can be incised, while metal objects might take more aggressive tools. Initial attempts to remove a solid constricting device causing penile strangulation involve lubricating the shaft and foreign body and attempted direct removal. A string or latex tourniquet can be wrapped around the distal shaft to decrease swelling and improve the odds of removing the device with lubrication. If the constricting object cannot be severed or removed, a string technique should be considered.[48] A thick silk suture or umbilical tape is passed proximally under the strangulation object and wound tightly around the penis distally toward the glans. The tag of suture or tape proximal to the ring is grasped; unwinding from the proximal end will push the object distally. Glandular puncture with a needle or blade will allow escape of dark trapped blood and improve the odds of removing the object with the string method. If there is any delay in decompression and the patient is unable to void and is uncomfortable or distended, a suprapubic bladder catheter should be placed.

Testicular Injuries

Presentation
Although the testis is relatively protected by the mobility of the scrotum, reflex cremasteric muscle contraction, and its tough fibrous tunica albuginea, blunt injury (usually the result of assault, sports-related events and motor vehicle accidents) can result in rupture of the tunica albuginea, contusion, hematoma, dislocation, or torsion of the testis. Testis injury results from blunt trauma in approximately 75% of cases.[49] Penetrating injuries due to firearms, explosions, and impalement injuries comprise the remainder. Rupture of the testis must be considered in all cases of blunt scrotal trauma. Most patients complain of exquisite scrotal pain and nausea. Swelling and ecchymosis are variable and the degree of hematoma does not correlate with the severity of testis injury; absence does not entirely rule out testis rupture, and contusion without fracture can present with significant bleeding. Scrotal hemorrhage and hematocele, along with tenderness to palpation often limit a complete physical examination. Penetrating injuries mandate careful examination of surrounding structures, especially the femoral vessels.

Imaging
Ultrasonography can be helpful to assess the integrity and vascularity of the testis. Ultrasonography is rapid, readily available, and noninvasive. Ultrasonographic findings suggestive of testis fracture include inhomogeneity of the testicular parenchymal texture and disruption of the tunica albuginea (see Fig. 5).[50] A normal or equivocal ultrasonographic study should not delay surgical exploration when physical examination findings are suggestive of testicular damage; definitive diagnosis is often made in the operating room.

Differential diagnosis of testis fracture includes hematocele without rupture, torsion of the testis or an appendage, reactive hydrocele, hematoma of the epididymis or spermatic cord, and intratesticular hematoma. Five percent of spermatic cord torsions are believed to be precipitated by trauma; torsion should be considered in all cases of significant scrotal pain without signs or symptoms of major scrotal trauma.[51]

Management
Early exploration and repair of testis injury is associated with increased testis salvage, reduced convalescence and disability, faster return to normal activities, and preservation of fertility and hormonal function.[35] Minor scrotal injuries without testis damage can be managed with ice, elevation, analgesics, and irrigation and closure in some circumstances.

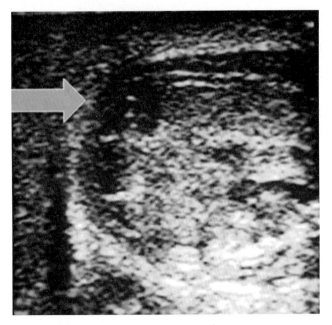

Figure 5 Ultrasonographic examination demonstrates hypoechoic intratesticular areas consistent with testicular rupture sustained by blunt trauma. Scrotal exploration revealed large hematocele and exposed seminiferous tubules.

The objectives of surgical exploration and repair are testis salvage, prevention of infection, control of bleeding, and reduced convalescence. Scrotal incision is preferable in most cases. The tunica albuginea should be closed with small absorbable sutures after removing necrotic and extruded seminiferous tubules. Even small defects in the tunica albuginea should be closed, because progressive swelling and intratesticular pressure can continue to extrude seminiferous tubules.

Every attempt to salvage the testis should be performed; loss of capsule tissue may require removal of additional parenchyma to allow closure of the remaining tunica albuginea (see Fig. 6). Significant intratesticular hematomas should be explored and drained even in the absence of testis rupture to prevent progressive pressure necrosis and atrophy, delayed exploration, and orchiectomy. Significant hematoceles should also be explored, regardless of imaging studies, because up to 80% are due to testis rupture.[35]

Penetrating scrotal injuries should be surgically explored to inspect for arterial and vasal injury. The vas deferens is injured in 7% to 9% of scrotal gunshot wounds. The injured vas should be ligated with nonabsorbable suture and delayed reconstruction performed if necessary. Approximately 30% of gunshot wounds injure both testes; consider exploring the contralateral testis depending on physical examination and the path of the projectile.

Complications

Nonoperative management of testis rupture is frequently complicated by infection, atrophy, necrosis, and delayed orchiectomy. Testis salvage rates exceed 90% with exploration and repair within 3 days of injury, versus orchiectomy rates three- to eightfold higher with conservative management and delayed surgery.[35] Testis salvage rates with conservative management are as low as 33%, with delayed orchiectomy rates between 21% and 55%. Approximately 45% of patients initially managed conservatively will ultimately undergo surgical exploration for pain, infection, and persistent hematoma, resulting in 21% to 22% of all conservatively managed men undergoing eventual orchiectomy.[52] Convalescence and time of return to normal activities are significantly reduced following early surgical repair.

Genital Skin Loss

Necrotizing gangrene due to polymicrobial infection in the genital area, or Fournier gangrene, is the most common cause of extensive genital skin loss. Loss is iatrogenic, caused

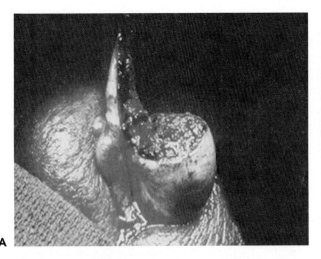

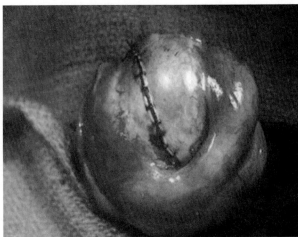

Figure 6 **A:** Seminiferous tubules debrided. **B:** Tunica albuginea reconstructed.

by the necessity for acute debridement of necrotic genital skin when the patient is seen initially. Although both cellulitis and Fournier gangrene are commonly associated with significant genital edema and erythema, the presence of skin ischemia is the hallmark of the latter. Scrotal ultrasonography and CT may both reveal subcutaneous air, a helpful indicator of necrotizing infection.

Penile skin loss can result from traction by mechanical devices, such as farm or industrial machinery, or by suction devices, such as vacuum cleaners. Because the penile tissue is a loose areolar tissue, it is often torn free without damage to the underlying structures. Significant scrotal skin loss resulting from penetrating trauma is uncommon.

Management

In cases of Fournier gangrene, multiple debridements are required over several weeks until active infection is controlled. Significant skin loss must be treated with wet-to-dry dressings until primary coverage is planned. Inspection atleast daily by the surgical team is mandatory. Suprapubic urinary diversion should be strongly considered for extensive injuries to simplify wound care and prevent urethral complications related to prolonged catheterization.

Genital burns are largely treated like other burns, with early resection of burn eschar and coverage with split-thickness skin grafts when possible. Partial-thickness skin loss or genital burns may be treated with silver sulfadiazine cream.

BLADDER INJURIES

Evaluation

Presentation

The urinary bladder is generally protected from external trauma because of its deep location in the bony pelvis. Most blunt bladder injuries are the result of rapid deceleration motor vehicle crashes, but also occur with falls, crush injuries, assault, and blows to the lower abdomen. Although disruption of the bony pelvis tends to tear the bladder at its fascial attachments, bony fragments can also directly lacerate the organ. Bladder laceration may also arise from penetrating trauma or various iatrogenic surgical complications, and may occur spontaneously in patients with altered sensorium, such as those who are intoxicated or have neuropathic disease.

Bladder injuries that occur with blunt external trauma are rarely isolated injuries; 80% to 94% of patients have significant associated nonurologic injuries.[53] Mortality in these multiply injured patients is primarily related to nonurologic injuries and ranges from 8% to 44%.[53] The most common associated injury is pelvic fracture, associated with 83% to 95% of bladder injuries.[54–56] Conversely, bladder injury has been reported to occur in only 5% to 10% of pelvic fractures.[56] Sudden force applied to a full bladder may result in a rapid rise in intravesical pressures and lead to rupture without pelvic fracture.

Bladder rupture does not occur as an isolated event in normal individuals. Most conscious patients have pronounced nonspecific symptoms such as suprapubic or abdominal pain and the inability to void. Associated abdominal and pelvic injuries may mask or confuse bladder symptoms. Physical signs include suprapubic tenderness, lower abdominal bruising, muscle guarding and rigidity, and diminished bowel sounds. Immediate catheterization should be performed because the most reliable sign of bladder injury is gross hematuria, which is present in 93% to 100% of cases.[57] If blood is noted at the meatus or the catheter does not pass easily, retrograde urethrography should be performed immediately because concomitant bladder and urethra injuries occur in 10% to 29% of patients.[56]

Imaging

Imaging of the bladder should be performed based on suspicion, examination, and the presence of hematuria or pelvic fracture. The absolute indication for immediate cystography after blunt external trauma is the presence of gross hematuria associated with pelvic fracture. Relative indications for cystography after blunt trauma include gross hematuria without a pelvic fracture, microhematuria with pelvic fracture, and isolated microscopic hematuria.[55] The diagnosis of bladder rupture is extremely low in these atypical groups (e.g., 0.6% in patients with pelvic fracture and microhematuria), but the index of suspicion should be raised by the presence of associated clinical indicators of bladder injury (see Table 4). Conversely, penetrating injuries of the buttock, pelvis, or lower abdomen with any degree of hematuria warrant cystography.

Retrograde or stress cystography is approximately 100% accurate for bladder injury, if performed appropriately. The bladder should be filled in cooperative and conscious patients to a sense of discomfort, otherwise to 350 mL. A three-film technique is recommended including precontrast image, full bladder anteroposterior (AP) film, and drainage

---

TABLE 4

CLINICAL INDICATORS OF BLADDER INJURY

Pelvic fracture with gross hematuria
Suprapubic pain or tenderness
Free intraperitoneal fluid on CT or ultrasonography
Inability to void, low urine output
Clots in urine
Signs of perineal or genital trauma
Unresponsive, intoxicated, altered sensorium
Preexisting bladder disease or urologic surgery
Abdominal distention or ileus

CT, computed tomography.

film. Posterior extravasation of contrast can be missed without a drainage film. Significant bladder distention is required to visualize small tears.

Dense, flame-shaped collections of contrast in the pelvis is characteristic of extraperitoneal extravasation. Depending on fascial integrity, contrast may extend beyond the confines of the pelvis and be visualized in the retroperitoneum, scrotum, phallus, thigh, and anterior abdominal wall. The amount of extravasation is not always proportional to the extent of bladder injury. Intraperitoneal extravasation is identified when contrast outlines loops of bowel.

CT cystography is as accurate and reliable as plain film cystography to evaluate suspected bladder injury as long as the bladder is filled in retrograde manner using contrast diluted to 2% to 4% (6:1 with saline) to a volume of 350 to 400 mL.[58] Drainage films are not required after CT cystography because the retrovesical space can be well visualized. Contrast dilution is mandatory because undiluted contrast material is so dense that the CT quality is compromised. Conventional abdominal CT imaging of the trauma patient may show findings suggestive of bladder injury, but is not considered to be adequate for bladder evaluation alone.[59]

Treatment

Management

The usual treatment for uncomplicated extraperitoneal bladder ruptures, when conditions are ideal, is conservative management with urethral catheter drainage alone. A large-bore Foley catheter (22 Fr) should be used to ensure adequate drainage. Cystography is recommended before catheter removal 14 days after injury to assess for persistent extravasation, in which case the catheter is maintained longer. Antimicrobial agents are instituted on the day of injury and continued until 3 days after the urinary catheter is removed.

Blunt extraperitoneal injuries with complicating features warrant immediate open repair to prevent complications such as fistula, abscess, or prolonged leak (see Table 5).

TABLE 5
INDICATIONS FOR IMMEDIATE REPAIR OF BLADDER INJURY

Intraperitoneal injury from external trauma
Penetrating or iatrogenic nonurologic injury
Inadequate bladder drainage/clots in urine
Bladder neck injury
Rectal or vaginal injury
Open pelvic fracture
Pelvic fracture requiring open reduction internal fixation
Selected stable patients undergoing laparotomy for other reasons
Bone fragments projecting into bladder

If a stable patient is undergoing exploratory laparotomy for other associated injuries, it is prudent to repair the extraperitoneal rupture; the anterior bladder wall is entered and the tear is closed intravesically with a single layer of absorbable suture. The perivesical pelvic hematoma should not be disturbed. When internal fixation of pelvic fractures is performed, concomitant bladder repair is recommended because urinary leakage from the injured bladder onto the orthopedic fixative hardware is prevented, thereby reducing the risk of hardware infection.

All penetrating or intraperitoneal injuries resulting from external trauma should be managed by immediate surgical repair. These injuries are often larger than suggested on cystography, are unlikely to heal spontaneously, and continued leak of urine causes a chemical peritonitis. When exploring bladder injuries, the ureteral orifices should be inspected for clear efflux, or ureteral integrity should be ensured utilizing intravenous indigo carmine or methylene blue, or retrograde passage of a ureteral catheter. Any injury in close proximity to or involving the ureteral orifice or intramural ureter should be stented or reimplanted. A perivesical drain should be employed. In patients with intraperitoneal rupture, antimicrobials are administered for 3 days, in the perioperative period only. If the bladder has been repaired, a cystogram is obtained 7 to 10 days after surgery.[54] When concurrent rectal or vaginal injuries exist, the organ walls should be separated, overlapping suture lines avoided, and every attempt made to interpose viable tissue in between the repaired structures. Fibrin sealant injected over the bladder wall closure may help reduce complications when intervening tissue is unavailable.[60]

Complications

The prompt diagnosis and appropriate management of bladder injuries allow for excellent results and minimal morbidity. Serious complications are usually associated with delayed diagnosis or treatment due to either a misdiagnosis or delayed presentation or complex injuries resulting from devastating pelvic trauma. Unrecognized bladder injuries may manifest as acidosis, azotemia, fever and sepsis, low urine output, peritonitis, ileus, urinary ascites, or respiratory difficulties. Unrecognized bladder neck, vaginal and rectal injury associated with the bladder rupture can result in incontinence, fistula, stricture, and a difficult delayed major reconstruction. Severe pelvic fractures may cause a transient or permanent neurologic injury and result in voiding difficulties despite an adequate bladder repair.

URETHRAL INJURIES

Posterior Urethra

Pelvic Fracture

Urethral disruption injuries typically occur in conjunction with multisystem trauma from vehicular accidents, falls, or industrial accidents. "Straddle fractures" involving all four pubic rami, open fractures, and those resulting in both vertical and rotational pelvic instability are associated with the highest risk of urologic injury.[61,62] The bulbomembranous junction is more vulnerable to injury during pelvic fracture.[63] In children, injuries are more likely to extend proximally to the bladder neck because of the rudimentary nature of the prostate.

Presentation

Urethral disruption is heralded by the triad of blood at the meatus, inability to urinate, and palpably full bladder. Urethral disruption is often first detected when a urethral catheter cannot be placed by the emergency department trauma team or when it is misplaced into pelvic hematoma. Pelvic hematoma often obscures the prostatic contour, resulting in a misdiagnosis of impalpable prostate. The digital rectal examination has poor sensitivity for the diagnosis of spinal cord, bowel, rectal, bony pelvis, and urethral injuries. Females with urethral injuries present with vulvar edema and blood at the vaginal introitus, thereby indicating the need for careful vaginal examination in all female pelvic fracture patients.[64]

Imaging

When blood at the urethral meatus is discovered, an immediate retrograde urethrogram should be performed to rule out urethral injury (see Fig. 7). A small-bore urethral catheter (16 Fr) is placed unlubricated 1 cm into the fossa navicularis, and the balloon is filled with 1 cm of water to achieve a snug fit. Alternatively, a Brodney clamp or rolled gauze bandage can be used to provide penile traction. Patients should be placed in an oblique or lateral decubitus position, and it is preferable to perform the study under fluorography when available; 25 mL of contrast is injected gently through a 60-mL catheter-tip syringe, and the film is taken during injection. Direct inspection by urethroscopy is suggested *in lieu* of urethrography in females with suspected urethral injury.[64,65]

Treatment

Management

Immediate suprapubic tube placement remains the standard of care. This is best accomplished through a small infraumbilical incision, which allows inspection and repair of the bladder and proper placement of a large-bore catheter at the bladder dome. Trochar suprapubic tube placement is reasonable when the bladder is distended and no other indications for surgery exist. However, over the long term, these smaller "punch" suprapubic tubes are more likely to become obstructed with debris or to fracture, requiring replacement.

Although orthopedists frequently suggest that a suprapubic tube not be placed if anterior pubic hardware is used in pelvic fracture repair due to concern that the suprapubic tube will lead to hardware infection, Koraitim et al.[65] have found that this complication is extremely rare, and that cystostomy can be safely used. However, the catheter should be placed high in the bladder and tunneled through the skin as high as possible on the lower abdominal midline to keep the tube away from the plated symphysis; this will also facilitate prostatic apex identification at the time of reconstruction.

An attempt at primary realignment of the distraction with a urethral catheter is reasonable in stable patients, either acutely or within several days of injury. We prefer a simple technique consisting of passage of a coude catheter antegrade by cystotomy, then tying it to another which can be drawn back into the bladder.

Incomplete urethral tears are best treated by stenting with a urethral catheter. Borrelli and Brandes[66] have not seen any evidence that a gentle attempt to place a urethral catheter can convert an incomplete into a complete transection. Caution is warranted because misplacement outside the bladder is distinctly possible; assurance of adequate positioning is imperative. In no case is traction used after urethral catheter placement; it is unnecessary and may cause incontinence.

Complex Injuries

In cases of female urethral disruption related to pelvic fracture, most authorities suggest immediate primary repair, or at least urethral realignment over a catheter, to avoid subsequent urethrovaginal fistulae or urethral obliteration.[64] Concomitant vaginal lacerations must also be closed acutely to prevent vaginal stenosis. Delayed reconstruction is problematic, because the female urethra is too short (~4 cm) to be amenable to anastomotic repair when it becomes embedded in scar.

Associated rectal injuries require open exploration, repair, irrigation, and placement of drains. Immediate suture reconstruction of posterior urethral disruption

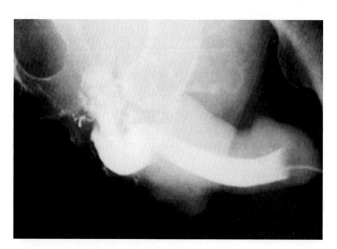

Figure 7 Retrograde urethrogram in pelvic fracture patient shows complete disruption of posterior urethra.

injuries is not recommended because of its association with unsatisfactory outcomes such as impotence and incontinence, stricture formation, and operative blood loss.

Anterior Urethra

In contrast to posterior urethral distraction, anterior injuries are most often isolated. Most occur after straddle injury and involve the bulbar urethra, which is susceptible to compressive injury due to its fixed location beneath the pubis. A smaller percentage is the result of direct penetrating injury to the penis.

As with posterior urethral injury, a high index of suspicion must be maintained in all patients with blunt or penetrating trauma in the urogenital region, and urethrography should be performed in any case of suspected urethral injury.[67] Clinical signs of anterior urethral injuries include blood at the meatus, perineal hematoma, gross hematuria, and urinary retention. In severe trauma, the Buck fascia may be disrupted, resulting in blood and urinary extravasation into the scrotum. The primary morbidity of straddle injury is urethral stricture, which may become symptomatic up to 10 years later.[68]

Anterior urethral injuries are divided on the basis of radiographic findings into contusion, incomplete disruption, or complete disruption. Contusions and incomplete injuries can be treated with urethral catheter diversion alone. Initial suprapubic cystostomy is the treatment of choice for major straddle injuries involving the urethra.

Primary surgical repair is recommended for low-velocity urethral gunshot injuries; catheter alignment alone is associated with a far worse stricture rate.[67] Debridement of the corpus spongiosum after trauma should be limited because corporal blood supply is usually robust, enabling spontaneous healing of most contused areas. Initial suprapubic urinary diversion is recommended after high-velocity gunshot wounds to the urethra, followed by delayed reconstruction.

REFERENCES

1. Nicolaisen GS, McAninch JW, Marshall GA, et al. Renal trauma: Re-evaluation of the indications for radiographic assessment. *J Urol*. 1985;133(2):183–187.
2. Mee SL, McAninch JW, Robinson AL, et al. Radiographic assessment of renal trauma: A 10-year prospective study of patient selection. *J Urol*. 1989;141(5):1095–1098.
3. Miller KS, McAninch JW. Radiographic assessment of renal trauma: Our 15-year experience. *J Urol*. 1995;154(2 Pt 1):352–355.
4. Chandhoke PS, McAninch JW. Detection and significance of microscopic hematuria in patients with blunt renal trauma. *J Urol*. 1988;140(1):16–18.
5. Steinberg DL, Jeffrey RB, Federle MP, et al. The computerized tomography appearance of renal pedicle injury. *J Urol*. 1984;132(6):1163–1164.
6. Moore EE, Shackford SR, Pachter HL, et al. Organ injury scaling: Spleen, liver, and kidney. *J Trauma*. 1989;29(12):1664–1666.
7. Morey AF, Bruce JE, McAninch JW. Efficacy of radiographic imaging in pediatric blunt renal trauma. *J Urol*. 1996;156:2014–2018.
8. Bretan PN Jr, McAninch JW, Federle MP, et al. Computerized tomographic staging of renal trauma: 85 Consecutive cases. *J Urol*. 1986;136(3):561–565.
9. Federle MP, Brown TR, McAninch JW. Penetrating renal trauma: CT Evaluation. *J Comput Assist Tomogr*. 1987;11(6):1026–1030.
10. Brown SL, Hoffman DM, Spirnak JP. Limitations of routine spiral computerized tomography in the evaluation of blunt renal trauma. *J Urol*. 1998;160:1979–1981.
11. Morey AF, McAninch JW, Tiller B, et al. Single-shot intraoperative IVP for immediate evaluation of renal trauma. *J Urol*. 1999;161:1088–1092.
12. McGahan JP, Richards JR, Jones CD, et al. Use of ultrasonography in the patient with acute renal trauma. *J Ultrasound Med*. 1999;18(3):207–213; quiz 215–206.
13. Santucci RA, McAninch JM. Grade IV renal injuries: Evaluation, treatment, and outcome. *World J Surg*. 2001;25(12):1565–1572.
14. Hammer CC, Santucci RA. Effect of an institutional policy of nonoperative treatment of grades I to IV renal injuries. *J Urol*. 2003;169(5):1751–1753.
15. Velmahos GC, Demetriades D, Cornwell EE III, et al. Selective management of renal gunshot wounds. *Br J Surg*. 1998;85(8):1121–1124.
16. Baniel J, Schein M. The management of penetrating trauma to the urinary tract. *J Am Coll Surg*. 1994;178(4):417–425.
17. Santucci RA, Wessells H, Bartsch G, et al. Evaluation and management of renal injuries: Consensus statement of the renal trauma subcommittee. *BJU Int*. 2004;93(7):937–954.
18. Bernath AS, Schutte H, Fernandez RR, et al. Stab wounds of the kidney: Conservative management in flank penetration. *J Urol*. 1983;129(3):468–470.
19. Armenakas NA, Duckett CP, McAninch JW. Indications for nonoperative management of renal stab wounds. *J Urol*. 1999;161(3):768–771.
20. Alsikafi NF, McAninch JW, Elliott SP, et al. Nonoperative management outcomes of isolated urinary extravasation following renal lacerations due to external trauma. *J Urol*. 2006;176:2494–2497.
21. Hagiwara A, Sakaki S, Goto H, et al. The role of interventional radiology in the management of blunt renal injury: A practical protocol. *J Trauma*. 2001;51(3):526–531.
22. Velmahos GC, Chahwan S, Falabella A, et al. Angiographic embolization for intraperitoneal and retroperitoneal injuries. *World J Surg*. 2000;24(5):539–545.
23. Sofocleous CT, Hinrichs C, Hubbi B, et al. Angiographic findings and embolotherapy in renal arterial trauma. *Cardiovasc Intervent Radiol*. 2005;28(1):39–47.
24. McAninch JW, Carroll PR, Klosterman PW, et al. Renal reconstruction after injury. *J Urol*. 1991;145(5):932–937.
25. Matthews LA, Smith EM, Spirnak JP. Nonoperative treatment of major blunt renal lacerations with urinary extravasation. *J Urol*. 1997;157(6):2056–2058.
26. Atala A, Miller FB, Richardson JD, et al. Preliminary vascular control for renal trauma. *Surg Gynecol Obstet*. 1991;172(5):386–390.
27. Coburn M. Damage control surgery for urologic trauma: An evolving management strategy [abstract #53]. *J Urol*. 2002;16(4, Suppl):13.
28. Wessells H, Suh D, Porter JR, et al. Renal injury and operative management in the United States: Results of a population-based study. *J Trauma*. 2003;54(3):423–430.
29. Presti JC Jr, Carroll PR, McAninch JW. Ureteral and renal pelvic injuries from external trauma: Diagnosis and management. *J Trauma*. 1989;29(3):370–374.
30. Brandes SB, Chelsky MJ, Buckman RF, et al. Ureteral injuries from penetrating trauma. *J Trauma*. 1994;36(6):766–769.
31. Kenney PJ, Panicek DM, Witanowski LS. Computed tomography of ureteral disruption. *J Comput Assist Tomogr*. 1987;11(3):480–484.
32. Boone TB, Gilling PJ, Husmann DA. Ureteropelvic junction disruption following blunt abdominal trauma. *J Urol*. 1993;150(1):33–36.
33. Townsend M, DeFalco AJ. Absence of ureteral opacification below ureteral disruption: A sentinel CT finding. *AJR Am J Roentgenol*. 1995;164(1):253–254.

34. Mulligan JM, Cagiannos I, Collins JP, et al. Ureteropelvic junction disruption secondary to blunt trauma: Excretory phase imaging (delayed films) should help prevent a missed diagnosis. *J Urol.* 1998;159(1):67–70.
35. Morey AF, Metro MJ, Carney KJ, et al. Consensus on genitourinary trauma. *BJU Int.* 2004;94:507–515.
36. Mydlo JH. Surgeon experience with penile fracture. *J Urol.* 2001;166:526–529.
37. Muentener M, Suter S, Hauri D, et al. Long-term experience with surgical and conservative treatment of penile fracture. *J Urol.* 2004;172:576–579.
38. El-Taher AM, Aboul-Ella HA, Sayed MA, et al. Management of penile fracture. *J Trauma.* 2004;56:1138–1140.
39. Orvis BR, McAninch JW. Penile rupture. *Urol Clin North Am.* 1989;16:369–375.
40. Goldman HB, Dmochowski RR, Cox CE. Penetrating trauma to the penis. *J Urol.* 1996;155:551–553.
41. Miles BJ, Poffenberger RJ, Farah RN, et al. Management of penile gunshot wounds. *Urology.* 1990;36:318–321.
42. Bandi G, Santucci RA. Controversies in the management of male external genitourinary trauma. *J Trauma.* 2004;56:1362–1370.
43. Gomes CM, Ribeiro-Filho L, Giron AM, et al. Genital trauma due to animal bites. *J Urol.* 2001;165:80–83.
44. Wolf JS, Turzan C, Cattolica EV, et al. Dog bites to the male genitalia: Characteristics, management and compairosn with human bites. *J Urol.* 1993;149:286–289.
45. Aboseif S, Gomez R, McAninch JW. Genital self-mutilation. *J Urol.* 1993;150:1143–1146.
46. Jezior JR, Brady JD, Schlossberg SM. Management of penile amputation injuries. *World J Surg.* 2001;25:1602–1609.
47. Bhanganada K, Chayavatana T, Pongnumkul C, et al. Surgical management of an epidemic of penile amputations in Siam. *Am J Surg.* 1983;146:376–382.
48. Noh J, Kang TW, Heo T, et al. Penile strangulation treated with the modified string method. *Urology.* 2004;64:591.
49. McAninch JW, Kahn RI, Jeffrey RB, et al. Major traumatic and septic genital injuries. *J Trauma.* 1984;24:291–298.
50. Micallef M, Ahman I, Ramesh N, et al. Ultrasound features of blunt testicular injury. *Injury.* 2001;32:23–26.
51. Lrhorfi H, Manunta A, Rodriguez A, et al. Trauma induced testicular torsion. *J Urol.* 2002;168:2548.
52. Del Villar RG, Ireland GW, Cass AS. Early exploration following trauma to the testicle. *J Trauma.* 1973;13:600–601.
53. Cass AS, Luxenberg M. Features of 164 bladder ruptures. *J Urol.* 1987;138:743–745.
54. Corriere JN, Sandler CM. Management of extraperitoneal bladder rupture. *Urol Clin North Am.* 1989;16:275–277.
55. Morey AF, Iverson AJ, Swan A, et al. Bladder rupture after blunt trauma: Guidelines for diagnostic imaging. *J Trauma.* 2001;51:683–686.
56. Cass AS. Diagnostic studies in bladder rupture. *Urol Clin North Am.* 1989;16:267–273.
57. Gomez RG, Ceballos L, Coburn M, et al. Consensus statement on bladder injuries. *BJU Int.* 2004;94:27–32.
58. Morey AF, Carroll PR. Evaluation and management of adult bladder trauma. *Contemp Urol.* 1997;9(7):13–22.
59. Mee SL, McAninch JW, Federle MP. Computerized tomography in bladder rupture: Diagnostic limitations. *J Urol.* 1987;137:207–209.
60. Evans LA, Ferguson KH, Foley JP, et al. Fibrin sealant for the management of genitourinary injuries, fistulas, and surgical complications. *J Urol.* 2003;169:1360–1362.
61. Brandes SB, Borelli J. Pelvic fracture and associated urologic injuries. *World J Surg.* 2001;25:1578–1587.
62. Koraitim MM. Pelvic fracture urethral injuries: The unresolved controversy. *J Urol.* 1999;161:1433–1441.
63. Mundy AR. Urethroplasty for posterior urethral strictures. *Br J Urol.* 1996;78:243–247.
64. Perry MO, Husmann DA. Urethral injuries in female subjects following pelvic fractures. *J Urol.* 1992;147:139–143.
65. Koraitim MM, Marzouk ME, Atta MA, et al. Risk factors and mechanism of urethral injury in pelvic fractures. *Br J Urol.* 1996;77:876–880.
66. Borrelli J, Brandes SB. Pelvic fractures: Assessment and management for the urologist. *AUA Update Series.* 2004;23(11):82–86.
67. Mundy AR. The role of delayed primary repair in the acute management of pelvic fracture injuries of the urethra. *Br J Urol.* 1991;68:273–276.
68. Husmann DA, Boone TB, Wilson WT. Management of low velocity gunshot wounds to the anterior urethra: The role of primary repair versus urinary diversion alone. *J Urol.* 1993;150:70–72.

FURTHER READINGS

Kane CJ, Nash P, McAninch JW. Ultrasonographic appearance of necrotizing gangrene: Aid in early diagnosis. *Urology.* 1996;48:142–144.
Park S, McAninch JW. Straddle injuries to the bulbar urethra: Management and outcomes in 78 patients. *J Urol.* 2004;171:722–725.

Management of the Difficult Abdomen and Damage Control Surgery

45

Jay S. Jenoff   *Patrick Kim*

Massive hemorrhage remains the second leading cause of injury-related, prehospital mortality, surpassed only by central nervous system injury.[1] Early trauma mortality is most frequently due to uncontrolled bleeding.[2] The evolution of care of the most severely injured patients has led to a step-wise approach of stabilization, resuscitation, and delayed definitive repair.[3] Patient evaluation and treatment at both the prehospital scene as well as in the emergency department have been shortened in these patients. This population, identified as suffering the "lethal triad" of ongoing acidosis, hypothermia, and coagulopathy, are being expedited both into and out of the operating room (OR). This process, termed *damage control surgery* by Rotondo et al., addresses immediately life-threatening hemorrhage and contamination at initial contact. This is followed by aggressive correction of metabolic derangement, with specific attention to the "triad" mentioned in the preceding text.

As the principles of trauma surgery have developed, damage control techniques have been applied to truncal injury in both the thoracic as well as the abdominal cavities. Vascular compromise in the extremities has also been addressed in this manner, with operative management aimed at early reperfusion followed by delayed, definitive repair. This chapter will describe the techniques and

sequence of the damage control, as named by Rotondo and Schwab in 1993, along with the resulting sequelae of this process.[4]

Traditionally, the phrase *damage control* is a naval term describing efforts to preserve a ship with extensive penetrating damage to its hull. The aim is to keep the vessel afloat and maintain overall mission integrity. Techniques would involve procedures to occlude gaps in the ship's body, the closing of compartmentalized watertight doors to limit the spread of damage, and local extinguishing of fires. Such procedures would keep the ship righted, buying time for definitive repair.[5]

In the care of the trauma patient, similar principles are applied. Early identification of appropriate patients allows limitation of pre-OR (prehospital scene, emergency department) resuscitation, expediting the patient to laparotomy. The initial goals are limited to control of hemorrhage through temporary intra-abdominal packing and large-vessel ligation, along with containment of contamination. This process is abbreviated to return the patient to the intensive care unit (ICU) setting for aggressive resuscitation aimed at rapid return to physiologic and metabolic normalcy. On successful resuscitation, the patient is returned to the OR for definitive repair of their injuries. If feasible, abdominal wall closure is performed at this time. For some, this may be done in a delayed manner, involving planned hernia repair up to a year from initial injury. Overall, this approach provides a strategy to combat the physiologic and metabolic mortality, which often follows successful technical intervention in the trauma patient.

HISTORY

Damage control techniques date back to the early 20th century.[6] In 1908, Pringle described intra-abdominal packing for hepatic hemorrhage.[7] Halsted went on to expand on this concept, placing protective rubber sheets between the packs and the liver parenchyma.[8] As the science of surgery progressed over the next few decades, these techniques were largely abandoned, with primary repair of injuries becoming the mainstay of treatment. This dominated surgical technique from the end of World War II and continued for the next 30 years.[9]

Interest in abbreviated laparotomy reemerged in 1976 when Lucas and Ledgerwood published a prospective study of hepatic packing at the Detroit General Hospital.[10] This was followed by Calne et al. who reported a similar experience in 1979.[11] In 1981, Feliciano et al. described a population exhibiting acidosis, hypothermia, and coagulopathy, and published a 90% survival rate in ten of these patients who underwent intra-abdominal packing for liver trauma.[12] In 1983, Stone et al. broadened and organized the process of damage control surgery. These techniques were not limited to hepatic trauma. The initial laparotomy was limited and coagulopathy corrected. On return of hemodynamic stability, operative intervention for definitive repair was pursued. Of note, 11 of 17 patients believed to possess lethal coagulopathy went on to survive their injuries.[13]

This approach to the traumatically injured patient would continue to grow over the next decade, and in 1993 Rotondo and Schwab coined the phrase "damage control." In detail, they standardized the three stages on which damage control surgery is based presently. Their initial study showed a 58% overall survival, which increased to 77% in selected population (major vascular injury with two or more visceral injuries).[4] The three stages were described as mentioned in the subsequent text.

Damage control stage one (DC I)—early laparotomy with control of hemorrhage and contamination followed by temporary abdominal closure.
Damage control stage two (DC II)—ICU resuscitation aimed at hemodynamic stabilization and correction of metabolic derangement.
Damage control stage three (DC III)—return to the OR for definitive repair with or without abdominal wall closure.

Johnson and Schwab defined a fourth stage, damage control Ground Zero (DC 0), in 2001. This stage begins in the prehospital setting and is aimed at identifying the select population that will benefit from damage control techniques, leading to limitation of preoperative resuscitation times.[14]

INDICATIONS FOR DAMAGE CONTROL

Over the last century, the indications for damage control have grown in number. Proper selection of appropriate patients is necessary, because just as failure to apply damage control principles may increase mortality, overuse will surely increase morbidity.

Rotondo et al. defined what they termed a maximal injury subset of patients who would benefit from damage control. These patients had a major vascular injury, two or more visceral injuries, and profound shock. Survival was 77% in these patients compared to 11% in those undergoing laparotomy with primary repair at initial surgery. In 1997, Rotondo and Zonies expanded on this by defining "key" factors in selecting the correct population for damage control.[15]

Moore et al. published their criteria for damage control in 1998. Their indications were similar and take into account available resources at the time of resuscitation.[16]

THE PHYSIOLOGY BEHIND DAMAGE CONTROL

With the improvement of transfusion services in trauma centers, blood banks developed the ability to rapidly provide the resources to meet massive transfusion requirements. However, patients ultimately succumbed to metabolic failure after bleeding was controlled and contamination eliminated. This "triad of death," metabolic acidosis, hypothermia, and coagulopathy, created an ongoing physiologic derangement with one entity augmenting the other two.[17] It is what Kashuk termed the bloody vicious cycle. It is these metabolic abnormalities that are the primary goal of the damage control two (DC II) phase of resuscitation.[18] The physiology of these processes is described in the subsequent text.

Acidosis

Hypovolemic shock leads to tissue ischemia and conversion from aerobic to anaerobic metabolism. Lactate, the end product, leads to a profound metabolic acidosis. This state leads to uncoupling of β-adrenergic receptors leading to catecholamine resistance. The resultant depressed cardiac output, hypotension, and ventricular arrhythmias exacerbate the shock state and further lactic acid production. Concomitantly, acidosis worsens the existing coagulopathy.[19]

Abramson et al. correlated lactate clearance with postinjury mortality. Survival was 100% when the body was able to clear lactate with 24 hours, whereas it fell to 14% if clearance took 48 hours or greater.[20] Rapid correction of metabolic acidosis is pursued during the damage control sequence. Control of hemorrhage in DC I and aggressive restoration of euvolemia in DC II are mainstays of therapy. Although controversial, adjunctive measures such as pulmonary artery catheter placement with measurement of continuous cardiac output and mixed venous oxygen saturation are often employed. They allow optimization of fluid resuscitation and pharmacologic therapy to maximize oxygen delivery to tissues.

Hypothermia

Hypothermia, defined as a core body temperature $<35^\circ C$, is present in two thirds of trauma patients admitted to a Level I trauma center.[21] At $32^\circ C$, mortality is 100% in the trauma population. Cushman et al. found a 40-fold higher incidence of death in patients with a core temperature $<35^\circ C$.[22]

Hypothermia in trauma patients stems from many etiologies. Environmental exposure at the prehospital scene, in the trauma bay, and in the OR is a common cause. Hypovolemic shock and the resultant decrease in oxygen delivery and consumption impair the ability of the body to generate heat. Compounding this are intoxication and pharmacologic intervention such as neuromuscular blocking agents administered with anesthesia. Room temperature resuscitation fluids and cooled blood products can quickly lower body temperature. Efforts to reverse these processes and prevent further cooling include warming the environment, limiting exposure to only that which is necessary, and active warming strategies (intravenous [IV] fluid/blood product warmers, Bair Hugger/Arctic Sun warming devices, cavitary irrigation), and should be employed as indicated. In extreme circumstances, continuous venovenous hemodialysis and even cardiopulmonary bypass may be employed for rapid warming in the most severe of circumstances.

The physiologic detriment due to hypothermia is a result of impaired myocardial contractility, arrhythmias, and a leftward shift of the oxygen–hemoglobin dissociation curve. Coagulopathy is also worsened by hypothermia. This may not be reflected in coagulation studies, as the blood samples are heated to $37^\circ C$ before evaluation, often giving falsely corrected values.

Coagulopathy

The coagulopathy observed in the severely injured patient can be attributed to several etiologies. Dilution of clotting factors can result from aggressive yet necessary resuscitation. Consumption of existing clotting factors can lead to both bleeding and clotting diatheses. Metabolic acidosis and hypothermia worsen coagulopathy, as previously stated. Quantitatively, massive transfusion leads to dilutional coagulopathy. After transfusion of one blood volume, there is a reduction in circulating platelets of approximately 60%. After 1.5 times replacement of blood volume, dilutional thrombocytopenia becomes the most common disorder of coagulation.[23] Qualitatively, platelet function is also impaired in the injured patient. Hypothermia reduces thromboxane B_2 production. Also, inositol triphosphate (IP_3), a regulatory mechanism for the GPIIb-IIIa platelet adherence sites, is temperature dependent.[24]

In the trauma patient, injury can lead to massive clotting factor activation and malfunction of the fibrinolytic system. Activation and congestion of the microvasculature with fibrin clotting can lead to further ischemia and acidosis. Conversely, such events may lead to consumption and depletion of necessary clotting factors in an actively exsanguinating patient.[25] Specific injury patterns, most notably head injury and pulmonary injury, often lead to this dysfunction of the coagulation cascade, worsening this problem.[26,27]

THE DAMAGE CONTROL SEQUENCE

Damage Control Ground Zero

Damage control ground zero begins in the prehospital setting, and continues through evaluation and resuscitation in the trauma bay. The goal of this stage is rapid assessment of injury patterns to provide early identification of patients who would appropriately benefit from a damage control approach. Doing so should lead first responders to limit time spent at the scene, and allow for advance notice of the trauma team that will be receiving this patient. This prehospital notification allows the resuscitating team ample time to optimize preparation of personnel and other necessary resources. Necessary steps such as rapid sequence intubation (RSI), chest tube placement, large-bore IV access, and indicated radiographic studies (chest and pelvic radiographs), as well as mobilization of blood bank resources can be expedited before surgery.

Damage Control Stage I

Initial Preparation

DC I involves a limited laparotomy aimed at the control of hemorrhage, limitation contamination, and temporary abdominal closure. Major hemorrhage is addressed with vascular ligation and intra-abdominal packing. Intraluminal vascular shunts are used to reestablish perfusion and avoid end-organ ischemia. Visceral injuries are resected without reanastomosis, with no attempt being made at definitive repair, limiting operative time.

Similar to the trauma bay, preparation is essential to the DC I stage. Warming of the OR, anesthesia circuit, fluids, and blood products to correct/prevent hypothermia is essential. OR personnel including anesthesia, nursing, and perfusion staff should be in place. A standard laparotomy set, chest instruments (including a sternal saw), and a vascular tray should be opened as the patient reaches the room.

The patient is positioned supine and prepped from the chin to below the knees, and to the OR table bilaterally. Electrocardiogram (ECG) leads, warming pads, and other monitoring equipment should be placed as posterior as possible so as to facilitate access to the entire anterior and lateral chest and abdomen. Both arms should be abducted on armboards at 90 degrees for access by the anesthesia staff.

Incision, Exploration, and Hemostasis

Abdominal exploration should commence with a vertical, midline incision from xiphoid process to pubic symphysis. In the reoperative abdomen, a bilateral subcostal incision may be considered. For suspected pelvic fracture with concomitant hematoma, the inferior portion of the midline may be left closed to maintain intra-abdominal pressure for tamponade effect. On entering the abdomen, a stepwise, organized exploration should take place. The bowel is eviscerated, a handheld abdominal wall retractor is employed, and all four quadrants are packed with laparotomy pads. While packing, the surgeon is afforded the opportunity to assess injury and prioritize repair. Once the abdomen is packed, a self-retaining retractor may be placed. If the patient has hemodynamic instability after abdominal packing or continued blood loss, proximal control of the supraceliac aorta may be obtained at the diaphragmatic hiatus. This will allow the anesthesia staff time to catch up with resuscitation as well as improve perfusion to the myocardium and brain.[28]

After major bleeding is controlled, the process of pack removal begins in the quadrant furthest from the presumed injury. Simple repair of arterial and venous injuries may be performed, with more complex reconstructions being delayed until the DC III stage. Intraluminal shunts should be placed at this time to maintain end-organ perfusion.[29,30]

Injury to solid organs should be addressed with simple repair or packing. More complex repairs will only prolong operative time, potentially exacerbating ongoing acidosis, hypothermia, and coagulopathy. Hepatic bleeding is treated with packing of the superior and inferior surfaces of the liver, obliterating the hepatodiaphragmatic recess and Morrison pouch. Division and ligation of the falciform ligament on initial laparotomy helps facilitate mobilization of the liver and prevents avulsion injury during packing. Continued bleeding may be controlled with the Pringle maneuver. Deeper parenchymal injuries may require finger fracture of the parenchyma with oversewing of visible vessels, as described by Pachter.[31] Following damage control of liver injuries, patients should undergo angiography and embolization during the DC II stage of

resuscitation. Careful coordination with the interventional radiology (IR) staff allows this to be accomplished on leaving the OR, before transport to the ICU.[32] Injury to other solid organs such as the spleen and kidneys may be handled in various ways. If simple repair is possible, it may be attempted. Care should be taken to avoid complex renorrhaphy and splenorrhaphy. Such efforts, although well described, will only delay correction of metabolic insufficiency. In such cases, resection may be the best option for survival.

Control of Contamination

Once bleeding has been controlled, hollow viscus injuries should be addressed. Spillage of succus entericus from the small bowel and stool from the large bowel should be promptly limited. Simple injuries may be repaired primarily. More extensively damaged bowel should be excluded with either circumferential umbilical tape or surgical staplers, with reanastomosis or diversion reserved for the DC III phase. Bowel viability and suitability for anastomosis is determined at the second-look laparotomy. Other injuries, such as pancreaticobiliary tract injuries, are treated with wide local drainage. Bladder injuries are treated by primary repair plus bladder drainage if intraperitoneal, and bladder drainage alone if extraperitoneal.

Temporary Abdominal Closure

No attempt should be made at definitive abdominal closure at the end of DC I laparotomy. Massive resuscitation and reperfusion injury will lead to intestinal wall edema and ongoing capillary leakage. Planned reoperation and risk of abdominal hypertension and subsequent abdominal compartment syndrome necessitate a loose closure. Skin-only closure allows for visceral protection and prevents further heat and fluid losses. This may be accomplished with a large, running, nonabsorbable suture. Historically, closure with sequential towel clamps was employed. However, with the frequent use of angiography following DC I, these metallic objects obscure necessary radiographic imaging; therefore, this quick and effective technique has been largely abandoned.

Often, by the end of even an abbreviated laparotomy, bowel edema is pronounced enough to preclude any abdominal closure. Silo-type devices such as the Bogota bag and Esmark dressings have been used. More recently, nonadherent dressings composed of Ioban (3M) encased towels, closed-suction drains, and occlusive dressing have been used. Commercial devices, such as the Vacuum-Assisted Closure (Hill-Rom), are also available.

Damage Control Stage II

The mainstay of DC II is resuscitation in the ICU. Although hemorrhage has been controlled and contamination limited, metabolic derangement leading to physiologic failure must be aggressively corrected. Preparation of the ICU environment should begin before the patient leaves the OR. Similar to the OR, environmental temperature, resuscitation fluids, and ventilator circuits should be warmed. Necessary personnel should be present and be well informed of the patient's injuries, operative course, and immediate needs upon arrival. Resources from the pharmacy and blood bank should be present, as well as monitoring and supportive devices. Importantly, DC II is often initiated in the IR suite before formal arrival in the ICU. Under these circumstances, it is essential to take the ICU to the patient, providing the same level of preparation and care at IR.

Paramount to DC II is the correction of acidosis, hypothermia, and coagulopathy. Acidosis is addressed by maximizing oxygen delivery. Arterial pressure monitoring with or without placement of a pulmonary artery catheter is used for goal-directed resuscitation. Of note, clearance of lactic acid within 24 hours of injury has been shown to correlate with improved survival.[33] Core rewarming, through active and passive, internal and external means is essential. Warming blankets, warm IV fluids, and heated ventilator circuits may act more as passive rewarming devices, doing more to prevent further heat loss than to actually improve body temperature by transferred energy. Active measures such as cavity lavage, continuous venovenous hemodialysis, and extracorporeal bypass allow rapid improvement in body temperature in appropriate patients.[34]

Despite operative intervention, the severely injured trauma patient will have continued blood loss unless ongoing coagulopathy is corrected. The administration of thawed or fresh-frozen plasma (FFP) should be instituted early. Fibrinogen levels should be assessed, with administration of cryoprecipitate if necessary. Platelet count should also be corrected. Clinical evaluation should complement laboratory evaluation, as specimens are evaluated at 37°C, causing this objective data to be misleading. Finally, without correction of ongoing acidosis and hypothermia, the patient will remain coagulopathic.

Tertiary Survey

The DC II stage of resuscitation allows for the performance of a tertiary survey. This allows repeated evaluation of the trauma patient, seeking out injuries not elucidated at the initial resuscitation. Plain radiographs may be obtained at the bedside in the ICU. If hemodynamically stable, the patient may undergo computed tomography as necessary.

Reoperation

Return to the OR should occur within 24 to 36 hours of initial surgery. Although the primary goal is transition to the DC III stage and definitive repair, many patients will require earlier "unplanned" reoperation before this. Several causes necessitate an earlier second-look than initially planned. The first is a missed injury at initial laparotomy, presenting as lack of physiologic "capture" during DC II. Continued bleeding despite corrected acidosis, core temperature, and coagulopathy portends a missed vascular injury and continued "surgical" bleeding. A missed visceral injury or inadequate drainage may present with ongoing shock despite resuscitation.[4]

The second common cause of early reoperation is the abdominal compartment syndrome. In 1863, Marey described the spectrum of symptoms accompanying intra-abdominal hypertension (IAH). These symptoms included a distended abdomen, hypoventilation with elevated peak airway pressures, decreased urine output, increased systemic vascular resistance (SVR), and decreased cardiac output.[35] Despite distensible, temporary abdominal closure techniques, IAH and the abdominal compartment syndrome may occur.[36] Ertel et al. described a 6% incidence of abdominal compartment syndrome following damage control laparotomy.[37] Measurement of peak airway pressures in ventilated patients, and bladder pressures through urinary catheters allows monitoring for such an entity.[38] However, the most important monitoring device is a high index of suspicion by the clinician at the bedside.

Damage Control Stage III

The goals of DC III are aimed at definitive repair of vascular, solid organ, and hollow viscus injuries. The critical decision lies in the determination of the timing of transition to this stage. The physiologic and metabolic values addressed in DC II should be corrected, with a normal lactate, core temperature, and coagulation profile. The patient should also be hemodynamically stable. This usually occurs within 24 to 36 hours of admission to the ICU.

In the OR, the patient is prepped and draped to allow for the planned procedure. The packs are removed by irrigation with copious amounts of fluid and gentle removal is employed to avoid damage from too vigorously removing packs that have adhered to internal structures. If repeat bleeding occurs, the packs may need to be replaced. A complete abdominal exploration should be performed, with attention to prior areas of repair. Intraluminal shunts should be removed and vascular injuries repaired. Bowel continuity is restored by primary anastomoses if feasible, and laterally placed diverting stomas where necessary. Repairs may be covered with greater omentum if available. Finally, feeding tubes are placed as indicated.

Abdominal closure should be attempted at this point. As in elective abdominal surgery, closure without tension is paramount. The fascial edges should be approximated to evaluate the mobility of the anterior abdominal wall. Persistent bowel and retroperitoneal edema may render definitive closure difficult or inadvisable at this time. Peak airway pressures should be closely monitored, with an elevation of >10 cm H_2O an indication to replace the temporary closure. Diuresis, if feasible, will help to reduce edema, promoting abdominal wall closure. An aggressive approach should be sought, as the complication rate rises significantly after the damage control has been open for 8 days or more.[39]

For many patients, fascial closure may take a prolonged period of time, and the surgeon is faced with the decision regarding options for bowel coverage. The first is closing the skin alone, with the fascia left open. This allows for coverage of the bowel, with a planned ventral hernia that may be fixed several months later. In some patients, even skin closure creates too much tension, and alternative means must be employed. Vicryl (polyglycolic) mesh may be used to cover the abdominal wall defect, being sewn to the fascial edges. Local wound care with saline-soaked gauze allows the bowel to form granulation tissue, which will ultimately cover the bowel and be amenable to skin grafting. This process takes 2 to 3 weeks, leaving an abdominal wall defect that can be fixed in 6 to 12 months. Several other methods of abdominal wall closure are in practice. A multidisciplinary approach, including the involvement of a plastic and reconstructive surgeon and wound care professionals, is often helpful.

The Sequelae of Damage Control Surgery

The endpoint of damage control surgery is patient survival. With this comes the possibility of several known complications. A thorough knowledge of these potential morbidities should guide the surgeon in caring for the severely injured patient. These include wound infection, intra-abdominal sepsis, bile leak, dehiscence, abdominal compartment syndrome, abdominal wall necrosis, enteroatmospheric fistulae, and multisystem organ failure as well as others.[40] Miller et al. found a significant increase in complication rate when abdominal wall closure was delayed 8 days or more post-DC I, with an overall morbidity associated with the open abdomen of 25%.[39] These complications should not be seen as a failure, but rather a preferable alternative to mortality. It should, however, underscore the importance of proper patient selection before embarking on the damage control pathway. Overall, with aggressive management and exquisite attention to detail, the surgeon should strive to prevent the preventable and promptly recognize and treat that which cannot be prevented.

REFERENCES

1. MacKenzie EJ, Fowler CJ. Epidemiology. In: Mattox KL, Feliciano DV, Moore EE, eds. *Trauma*, 4th ed. New York: McGraw-Hill; 2000:21–39.
2. Sauaia A, Moore FA, Moore EE, et al. Epidemiology of trauma deaths: A reassessment. *J Trauma*. 1995;38:185–193.
3. Feliciano DV, Moore EE, Mattox KL. *Trauma*, 4th ed. New York: McGraw-Hill; 2000:907–931.
4. Rotondo MF, Schwab CW, McGonigal MD, et al. Damage control: An approach for improved survival in exsanguinating penetrating abdominal injury. *J Trauma*. 1993;35:373–383.
5. Gaynor F. *The new military and naval dictionary*. New York: Philosophical Library Publishers; 1951.
6. Richardson JD, Franklin GA, Lukan JK, et al. Evolution in the management of hepatic trauma: A 25-year perspective. *Ann Surg*. 2000;232:324–330.
7. Pringle J. Notes on the arrest of hepatic hemorrhage due to trauma. *Ann Surg*. 1908;48:541–549.
8. Halsted W. Ligature and suture material: The employment of fine silk in preference to catgut and the advantages of transfixing tissues and vessels in controlling hemorrhage-also an account of the introduction of gloves, gutta-percha tissue and silver foil. *JAMA*. 1913;LX:1119–1126.
9. Sharp K, LoCicero R. Abdominal packing for surgically uncontrollable hemorrhage. *Ann Surg*. 1992;215:467–474.
10. Lucas C, Ledgerwood A. Prospective evaluation of hemostatic techniques for liver injuries. *J Trauma*. 1976;16:442–451.
11. Calne R, McMaster P, Pentlow B. The treatment of major liver trauma by primary packing with transfer of the patient for definitive treatment. *Br J Trauma*. 1978;66:338–339.
12. Feliciano D, Mattox K, Jordan G. Intra-abdominal packing for control of hepatic hemorrhage: A reappraisal. *J Trauma*. 1981;21:285–290.
13. Stone H, Strom P, Mullins R. Management of the major coagulopathy with onset during laparotomy. *Ann Surg*. 1983;197:532–535.
14. Johnson JW, Gracias VH, Schwab CW, et al. Evolution in damage control for exsanguinating penetrating abdominal injury. *J Trauma*. 2001;51:261–271.
15. Rotondo MF, Zonies DH. The damage control sequence and underlying logic. *Surg Clin North Am*. 1997;77:779–782.
16. Moore EE, Burch JM, Franciose RJ, et al. Staged physiologic restoration and damage control surgery. *World J Surg*. 1998;22(12):1184–1190.
17. Burch JM, Denton JR, Noble RD. Physiologic rational for abbreviated laparotomy. *Surg Clin North Am*. 1997;77:779–782.
18. Kashuk JL, Moore EE, Millikan JS, et al. Major abdominal vascular trauma: A unified approach. *J Trauma*. 1982;22:672–679.
19. Ferrara A, MacArthur J, Wright H, et al. Hypothermia and acidosis worsen coagulopathy in the patient requiring massive transfusion. *Am J Surg*. 1990;169:515–518.
20. Abramson D, Scalea T, Hitchcock R, et al. Lactate clearance and survival following injury. *J Trauma*. 1993;35:584–588.
21. Jurkovich GJ, Greiser WB, Luterman A, et al. Hypothermia in trauma victims: An ominous predictor of survival. *J Trauma*. 1987;27:1019–1024.
22. Cushman JG, Feliciano DV, Renz BM, et al. Iliac vessel injury: Operative physiology related to outcome. *J Trauma*. 1997;42:1033–1040.
23. Lynn M, Jeroukhimov I, Klein Y, et al. Updates in the management of severe coagulopathy in trauma patients. *Intensive Care Med*. 2002;28:s241–s247.
24. McGowan E, Detwiler T. Modified platelet response to thrombin. Evidence for two types of receptor or coupling mechanism. *J Biol Chem*. 1986;261:739–746.
25. Gentilello LM, Pierson DJ. Trauma critical care. *Am J Respir Crit Care Med*. 2001;163:604–607.
26. Goodnight SH, Kenoyer G, Rapaport SI, et al. Defibrination after brain tissue destruction: A serious complication of head injury. *N Engl J Med*. 1974;290:1043–1047.
27. Kearney T, Bennt L, Grode M, et al. Coagulopathy and catecholamines in severe head injury. *J Trauma*. 1992;32:608–611.
28. Garcia-Rinaldi R, Defore WW, Mattox KL Jr, et al. Unimpaired renal, myocardial, and neurologic function after cross clamping of the thoracic aorta. *Surg Gynecol Obstet*. 1976;143:249–252.
29. Reilly PM, Rotondo MF, Carpenter JP, et al. Temporary vascular continuity during damage control: Intraluminal shunting for proximal superior mesenteric artery injury. *J Trauma*. 1995;39:757–760.
30. Johansen KH, Hedges G. Successful limb reperfusion by temporary arterial shunt during a 950-mile air transfer. *J Trauma*. 1989;29:1289–1291.
31. Pachter HL, Spencer FC, Hofstetter SR, et al. Significant trends in the treatment of hepatic trauma. Experience with 411 injuries. *Ann Surg*. 1992;215:492–500.
32. Kushimoto S, Arai M, Aiboshi J, et al. The role of interventional radiology in patients requiring damage control laparotomy. *J Trauma*. 2003;54:171–176.
33. Abramson D, Scalea TM, Hitchcock R, et al. Lactate clearance and survival following injury. *J Trauma*. 1993;35:584–589.

34. Gentilello LM, Cobean RA, Offner PJ, et al. Continuous arteriovenous rewarming: Rapid reversal of hypothermia in critically ill patients. *J Trauma.* 1992;32:316–325.

35. Ivatury RR, Sugerman HJ. Abdominal compartment syndrome: A century later, isn't it time to pay attention? *Crit Care Med.* 2000;28:2137–2138.

36. Gracias VH, Braslow B, Johnson J, et al. Abdominal compartment syndrome in the open abdomen. *Arch Surg.* 2002;137:1298–1300.

37. Ertel W, Oberholzer A, Platz A, et al. Incidence and clinical pattern of the abdominal compartment syndrome after "damage control" laparotomy in 311 patients with severe abdominal and/or pelvic trauma. *Crit Care Med.* 2000;28:1747–1753.

38. Kron IL, Harman PK, Nolan SP. The measurement of intra-abdominal pressure as a criterion for exploration. *Ann Surg.* 1984;199:28–30.

39. Miller RS, Morris JA Jr, Diaz JJ Jr, et al. Complications after 344 damage-control open celiotomies. *J Trauma.* 2005;59(6):1365–1374.

40. Shapiro MB, Jenkins DH, Schwab CW, et al. Damage control: Collective review. *J Trauma.* 2000;49:969–978.

Diagnosis and Management of Extremity Vascular Injuries

46

C. Kristian Enestvedt   *David Cho*   *Donald D. Trunkey*

INTRODUCTION

Extremity vascular injuries continue to pose clinical challenges to trauma and vascular surgeons. More than three fourths of all vascular trauma occurs in the extremity.[1–5] Although most clinically significant peripheral vascular injuries result from penetrating trauma, the contribution to this cohort from blunt trauma may be higher depending on the injury mechanism and setting.[2,4–14] The accumulated experience with vascular trauma has seen considerable contributions from surgeons in combat settings, where most injuries result from penetrating trauma. Historically, many arterial injuries were managed with simple ligation followed by amputation. Current management yields high rates of successful vascular repair and significantly improved limb salvage rates compared to vessel ligation. In addition, the development of endovascular techniques will impact the future of surgical management for vascular trauma.

Patient Evaluation

The evaluation of trauma victims with vascular injury should follow the basic protocols of Advanced Trauma Life Support (ATLS). A thorough, focused vascular examination is paramount when an arterial injury is suspected. Palpation of the arterial pulse at all levels in the affected limb(s) should begin distally and move proximally, with note made of the quality, strength, and rate at each level.

Throughout the examination, the injured limb should be compared to the contralateral limb. Occasionally, hard signs of arterial disruption will be encountered such as active arterial hemorrhage, expanding hematoma, limb ischemia, thrill, bruit, or absent pulses (see Table 1). Of these, pulse deficit is reportedly the most common.[15] Although compression techniques—including placement

---

TABLE 1

HARD AND SOFT SIGNS OF VASCULAR INJURY

Hard signs
- Arterial bleeding
- Ongoing hemorrhage with shock
- Pulsatile hematoma
- Limb ischemia
- Bruit or thrill
- Loss or absence of distal pulses

Soft signs
- Nonexpanding hematoma
- Injury to nerve associated with vessel
- Wound or injury tract <1 cm from major vessel
- Decreased ABI
- Knee dislocation
- History of massive bleeding now stopped

ABI, Ankle Brachial Index.

of tourniquets—can be used as temporizing measures for active arterial hemorrhage in the trauma bay, further management should be performed in the operating room. Radiographic or ultrasonographic assessment of a limb with an absent pulse, however, is obligatory if other issues do not require immediate attention in the multiply injured patient.

Evaluation of the affected extremity with a handheld Doppler ultrasound should be performed routinely in all patients with nonpalpable pulses. It is important to make note of the phase pattern of the waveforms. Absent Doppler signals warrant further imaging—either with angiography, duplex ultrasonography, or computed tomography with angiogram (CTA). Every Doppler examination, whether normal or abnormal, should be followed by the Ankle Brachial Index (ABI) measurement. An ABI >1.0 is considered normal. Any measurement <0.9 warrants further evaluation, usually with angiography. Again, it is important to compare findings between limbs.

Combined with ABI, the physical examination (PE) has proved to be an accurate measure of arterial injury.[8,15–19] A high negative predictive value has been well documented when the PE is used as a screening test in the trauma setting, with fewer than 1.5% of occult vascular injuries ultimately requiring operative intervention.[16] The robust sensitivity of screening with PE and ABI has been validated by multiple authors for both penetrating and blunt injury. Gonzalez et al.[15] examined the utility of PE for the evaluation of penetrating extremity trauma in 406 patients with 489 vascular injuries. The authors demonstrated a sensitivity of 92% and a specificity of 95%. Their screening protocol included PE for hard signs of vascular injury, assessment of injury trajectory, and Doppler ultrasound. Those patients without hard signs were observed and those with hard signs were either taken directly to the operating room or for angiography. There were four missed injuries, for a negative predictive value of 99%. Miranda et al.[20] reported a positive predictive value of 94.3% and a negative predictive value of 100% for PE in a retrospective review of their institution's protocol for managing posterior knee dislocations. Thirty-five patients with knee dislocations were either taken emergently to the operating room (8 patients, 23%) because of hard signs of vascular injury, or they were observed with serial examinations (27 patients, 77%). In the latter group, no vascular injuries were diagnosed during hospitalization, nor at a mean follow-up of 13 months (12 patients). Long-term studies have also validated the nonoperative management of occult vascular injuries. In a longitudinal study of patients with penetrating extremity trauma, Dennis et al.,[16] demonstrated that PE alone can be safely used to triage this patient population. The mean follow-up for patients in the group who underwent evaluation only with PE was 5.4 years, and none of the patients surveyed required vascular intervention and none reported symptoms related to vascular insufficiency.

Pathophysiology

The arterial wall is composed of three anatomic layers—the intima, media, and adventia—and vascular injury can affect one or all vessel layers. Blunt force trauma seen with crush injury can lead to vessel contusion. Hematoma formation occurs between the intima and media or the media and adventia and cause compression and partial or complete vessel occlusion. Disruption between the intima and media can also lead to an intimal flap with subsequent dissection and thrombosis. Whenever the intimal layer is disrupted, the highly thrombogenic internal elastic lamina is exposed. When the inner two layers are disrupted but the adventitia is intact, a pseudoaneurysm forms outside the vessel lumen (see Fig. 1). Stretch injury to the vessel causes disruption between the layers due to shearing forces. These injuries often occur in the setting of posterior knee dislocation with resulting occlusion of the popliteal artery. Vessel lacerations or complete transections are typically the result of penetrating injury from missiles or other projectiles, and less commonly from fractured bone (see Fig. 4). Arteriovenous fistulae (AVFs) commonly result when concomitant arterial and venous injuries occur in close proximity (see Figs. 2 and 6).

Etiology, Injury Mechanism, and Location

The etiology of vascular trauma often depends on both the setting in which injuries are reported and the particular vessel injured. For instance, in the civilian setting at an urban trauma center, penetrating injury accounted for 81% of approximately 360 vascular injuries at the Ben Taub General Hospital in Houston, Texas, from 1981 to 1985.[2] Likewise,

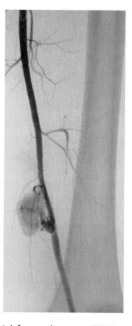

Figure 1 Superficial femoral artery (SFA) pseudoaneurysm following gunshot wound the thigh.

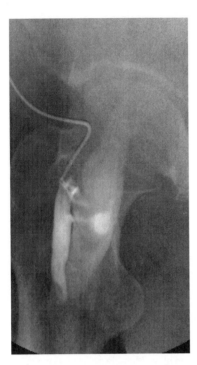

Figure 2 Common femoral artery (CFA) →femoral vein arteri-ovenous fistulae (AVF) following penetrating injury to upper thigh.

Vessel	Number of Injuries	Percentage
CFA	55	8.3
Profunda femoral	34	5.1
SFA	238	35.9
Above knee popliteal	129	19.5
Below knee popliteal	86	13.0
Combined above/below knee popliteal	22	3.3
Crural	99	14.9

TABLE 2

LOCATION OF VESSEL INJURY IN LOWER EXTREMITY, 550 PATIENTS IN 663 COMBINED VASCULAR INJURIES

CFA, common femoral artery; SFA, superficial femoral artery. (Adapted from Hafez HM, Woolgar J, Robbs JV. Lower extremity arterial injury: Results of 550 cases and review of risk factors associated with limb loss. *J Vasc Surg.* 2001;33(6):1212–1219.)

recent wartime experience demonstrates that approximately 94% of battlefield vascular injuries (of which 78% were extremity injuries) were the result of penetrating trauma.[1] In contrast, injury to the popliteal artery is the result of blunt mechanisms in most reported cases.[12,21,22] In their review of the National Trauma Data Bank to evaluate outcomes from popliteal artery injury, Mullenix et al.[22] noted that 61% of the injuries were the result of blunt mechanisms, with only 39% occurring from penetrating injury. Likewise, Hossny et al.[12] reported that of 39 popliteal artery injuries occurring over a 9-year period, 31 (79%) were the result of blunt trauma.

Penetrating injury most often occurs from gunshot or stab wounds in the civilian setting, and from fragment wounds in combat settings.[1,8,11] Surgeons in combat settings also routinely encounter blast injury from improvised explosive devices (IEDs).[1] Blunt injury most often results from motor vehicle collisions (MVCs), falls, and crush injury in both civilian and battlefield environments.

Lower extremity vascular injuries are defined as those occurring below the inguinal ligament. The most commonly injured vessel is the femoral artery.[6,11] Injuries to the common femoral artery (CFA), profunda femoris, superficial femoral artery (SFA), and popliteal artery both above and below the knee represent the bulk of clinically significant vascular trauma requiring revascularization procedures or surgical exploration (see Table 2). Because there is more redundancy in the blood supply to the calf and foot, with anterior tibial, posterior tibial, and peroneal arteries all supplying this distribution, one or sometimes two of these vessels can be disrupted without loss of distal perfusion and limb ischemia. The one *caveat* to this point is that significant bleeding from any of these vessels or their branches can lead to elevated compartment pressures in the calf and subsequent compartment syndrome. Trauma and vascular surgeons should maintain a high index of suspicion for the compartment syndrome and intervene with fasciotomy as necessary, as discussed later in this chapter.

Vascular injury to the upper extremity is relatively common, representing 30% to 40% of vascular injuries in urban civilian settings.[23,24] For the purposes of this discussion, the vessels of the upper extremity are defined as coursing from the axilla to the wrist. Injuries to the subclavian vessels are commonly reported together with those of the axillary vessels, and surgical management and associated injuries are similar.[10,25,26] Therefore, axillosubclavian vessel injuries are discussed here as well. The most commonly injured vessel in the upper extremity is the brachial artery with an incidence of approximately 50%, followed by the radial and ulnar arteries (~25% each), with the least common being the axillary and subclavian arteries (~3% to 5%).[23,24] The most common mechanism for vascular injury in the upper extremity is penetrating trauma.[10,23-25]

Iatrogenic injuries account for an increasing number of peripheral vascular lesions.[27] The rise in these injuries has come with the growth of percutaneous therapies for coronary and peripheral arterial disease processes. Although many of these injuries can be managed by noninvasive methods (compression and/or fibrin injection under ultrasonographic guidance, endovascular stent grafts, etc.), some require more extensive management. Although a full discussion of the incidence, etiology, prevention, and management of these injuries is beyond the scope of this chapter, they remain an important diagnostic and treatment challenge for vascular surgeons.

Imaging Techniques

Angiography

Contrast angiography (CA) is considered the gold standard for the evaluation of arterial injury. Proposed for the diagnostic evaluation of extremity vascular trauma as early as the 1960s, arteriography has seen significant advances mostly in the realm of catheter-based therapy (discussed later in this chapter).[28,29] As a purely diagnostic modality, angiography has sensitivities of 92% to 96%, specificity above 96%, and 98% reported diagnostic accuracy.[30–34] Indications for angiography are mostly based on the clinical findings of the evaluating surgeon and include those mentioned in the preceding text. Some authors use emergency room angiography to quickly triage patients with soft signs of vascular injury.[8,35,36] Owing to the potential for multiple lesions within the same vessel or extremity, intraoperative angiography should always be an important part of the surgeon's armamentarium. This procedure can be performed both before and after repair of identified lesions. In the latter case, after repairing an injured vessel that demonstrated hard signs of injury it may be necessary to perform intraoperative angiography to rule out concomitant distal injury (see Figs. 3 and 4).

Although several scoring systems have been developed to better select patients for CA, such as those with penetrating injury proximity to major vascular structures or relative to injury mechanism, they have not proven to be effective and are not an appropriate substitute for a high index of suspicion following a thorough examination.[37–39] For instance, it was historically believed that posterior knee dislocations always warranted angiographic investigation because of a high rate of popliteal artery injury. However, because of the low incidence (<16%) of vessel damage in this patient cohort with very few of these injuries of clinical significance, angiogram is only indicated on a selective basis—that is, where PE findings are abnormal.[38,40] This is also true for penetrating injury proximity to vascular structures, which is a poor indicator for positive angiography.[39]

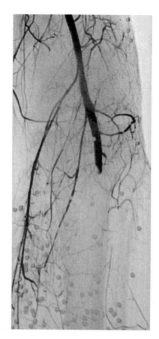

Figure 4 Popliteal artery injury in patient in preceding figure following shotgun blast. Multiple pellets lodged in lower extremity.

Duplex

Duplex ultrasonography can also play a crucial role in evaluating patients with vascular injuries. Although duplex is somewhat limited by operator dependence, several studies have shown that it is a valuable diagnostic tool. In a study of 198 patients with 319 potential injuries, Bynoe et al.[41] reported a sensitivity of 95%, a specificity of 99%, and an overall accuracy of 98%. In centers without computed tomography (CT) or angiography readily available, or in-theater forward combat hospitals, ultrasonography may be an invaluable imaging option.

Computed Tomography with Angiogram

Most investigations of the utility of CTA in evaluating vascular injury have focused on either injuries to the neck vessels or those in the lower extremity. For the

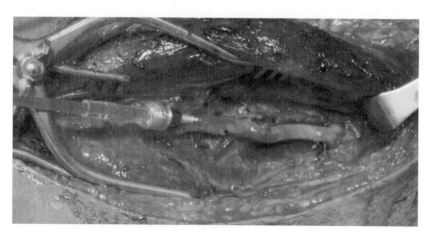

Figure 3 Intraoperative angiography in patient with multiple vascular injuries to a single limb following gunshot wound.

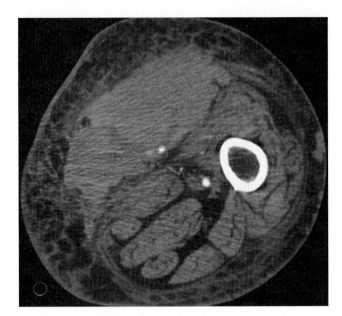

Figure 5 Large thigh hematoma with contrast extravastion from branch of superficial femoral artery (SFA).

purposes of this chapter, the discussion will be centered on the latter. With the advent of improved CT scans, particularly the multidetector contrast-enhanced spiral scanners, detection of vascular injuries has vastly improved. In fact, CTA is becoming a viable alternative to angiography for the detection of arterial injury, particularly in those patients without hard signs. Lesions that can routinely be diagnosed include intimal dissections, pseudoaneurysms, AVFs, thromboses and/or occlusions, hematomas, and laceration with active bleeding as evidenced by contrast extravasation (see Figs. 5 and 6). Occasionally, CTA may be nondiagnostic due to significant artifact from bullet fragments or other foreign bodies.[42] Reported sensitivities range from 90% to 100%, with specificities of 98% to 100% (see Table 3). However, some of the recent

reports lack comparison to a gold standard (operative exploration or CA) and most are limited by inadequate or short-term follow-up. The sensitivity of CTA in detecting small, although clinically significant lesions such as intimal flaps—particularly those around the knee—is unknown. Large, prospective studies are needed to validate the use of CTA as a substitute for angiography.

Magnetic Resonance Angiography

Magnetic resonance imaging (MRI) or magnetic resonance angiography (MRA) is used less frequently in the acute setting. Metal implants such as cerebral aneurysm clips and cardiac pacemakers preclude the use of MRI, and it may be difficult to ascertain whether patients have such devices in the acute setting. Many orthopaedic fixation devices are also contraindications for MRI. Additionally, MRI typically takes longer and requires more cooperation from the patient than does CT, which makes it less favorable to use with acutely injured or combative patients. It may also be less effective than CT, as one group of authors showed in a randomized controlled trial that it was not as accurate as CTA in evaluating nontraumatic limb ischemia.[47] The ability to discriminate infrapopliteal lesions is limited, and MRA is not as accurate as CA in identifying clinically significant distal lesions in the lower extremity.[48] Despite these drawbacks, MRA can provide highly detailed images in the hemodynamically stable patient. In the event that angiography is indicated, but the patient's renal insufficiency precludes the use of iodinated contrast, MRA may be a good option.

Management

Temporizing Methods

If brisk arterial bleeding is encountered in the primary survey of a trauma patient, digital or manual compression is typically the first method employed for hemorrhage control. In the event of a penetrating injury associated

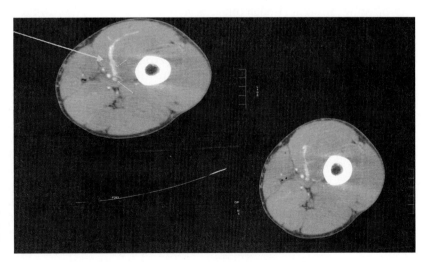

Figure 6 Contrast extravasation (*large arrow*) from superficial femoral artery (SFA) injury with arteriovenous fistulae (AVF) (note contrast filling vein, *small arrows*).

TABLE 3

THE UTILITY OF COMPUTED TOMOGRAPHY WITH ANGIOGRAM (CTA) IN IDENTIFYING PERIPHERAL ARTERIAL INJURY

Author	Year	Number of CT Scans	Sensitivity (%)	Specificity (%)	Missed Injuries	Mean Follow-up (months)
Soto et al.[43]	1999	45	90	100	NR	NR
Soto et al.[44]	2001	139	95.1	98.7	NR	NR
Busquets et al.[45]	2004	95	100	NR	0	8
Inaba et al.[46]	2006	62	100	100	0	1.5

NR, not reported.

with brisk bleeding, a Foley catheter can be inserted into the wound tract and inflated to provide compression and partial occlusion. Depending on the setting, tourniquets may be employed for temporary vascular occlusion. These devices are often appropriate in the setting of traumatic amputation or when triaging patients who are in shock at sites a considerable distance from definitive care. It should be noted that tourniquets worsen the ischemic insult, and prophylactic fasciotomy is often routinely used for limbs with prolonged ischemia times. Blindly applying vascular clamps is not advised, as this can cause damage to both the vessel and associated structures.

Ligation

Although obviously suboptimal for restoring tissue oxygenation to the affected limb, vessel ligation may be a necessary life-saving option in certain settings. Battlefield or forward theater triage units may perform such maneuvers when definitive vascular surgical repair is not available. This may also be true in the civilian setting where a patient in hemorrhagic shock requires immediate attention to control bleeding before transfer to a Level I trauma center. If vessel ligation is required, it is always advisable to tag the distal end of the vessel and tie it off as well. There are several reasons for this practice. First, significant back-bleeding can occur through collateral vessels and lead to continued shock. Second, when significant blast injury with major tissue disruption occurs, the vessel ends may be more readily identifiable early in the injury evolution. Additionally, muscular arteries have a tendency to contract, requiring extensive dissection during future attempts at repair. It is therefore advisable to make both ends of the ligated vessel readily identifiable for the treating surgeon.

Simple ligation can typically be performed for small distal branches such as tibial arteries in the leg or the radial artery in the forearm without untoward consequences.[9,49–51] This strategy requires at least one open vessel below the knee or elbow and no evidence of distal ischemia.[49] In fact, this operative strategy has been advocated as more cost effective with outcomes equivalent to repair.[51]

Intravascular Shunt

Temporary intravascular shunts (TIVSs) have been one of the mainstays of trauma surgery for decades.[52,53] Providing critical limb perfusion in the case of significant vascular disruption, intravascular shunts are typically used in proximal locations where injury to a major vessel leads to tissue ischemia due to the absence of adequate collateral circulation. This is particularly true at the CFA, SFA and popliteal artery in the lower extremity, and at the subclavian and axillary arteries in the upper extremity (see Fig. 7). Shunts tend to have lower patency rates in smaller, distal vessels.[54] Most authors do not advocate prolonged shunting, although case reports have demonstrated shunt patency up to 24 hours.[55] Temporary shunts can be invaluable temporizing measures before transfer to a more specialized center for definitive management or before reduction and repair of associated orthopaedic injury.

There are some important principles to keep in mind when employing temporary shunts. First, the tubing must be noncompressible so that it does not collapse when secured proximally and distally within the artery. Commercially available Sundt and Argyle carotid shunts are good options. In the event that these devices are not readily available, sterile, rigid plastic tubing such as intravenous tubing often works well, as do endotracheal suction catheters. Second, the shunt should be sized accordingly, with a diameter slightly smaller than the injured artery. Too large a catheter may cause further intimal damage if it is forcibly passed into the vessel. Likewise, if the catheter is too small, distal flow will be further compromised. Rummel tourniquets with umbilical tape—which is relatively atraumatic to vessel architecture—are a favored technique to secure the shunt within the damaged vessel (Fig. 7). Shunt patency is most dependent on duration of *in situ* shunting, and systemic heparinization is not required.[56,57] Thrombectomy is often necessary, and most authors advocate local intraluminal heparin.[52–55,57–59] Outcomes with TIVS are typically good, with significantly fewer complications in shunted versus nonshunted limbs and high limb-salvage rates.[12,57,59]

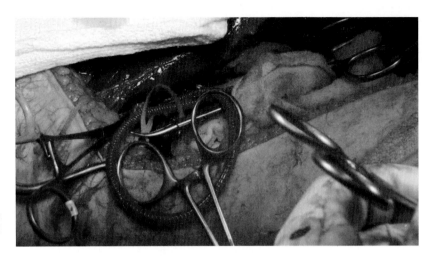

Figure 7 Superficial femoral artery (SFA) shunt in a patient who suffered a gunshot wound (GSW) to the femoral artery.

Operative Management—Lower Extremity

Exposure for injured vessels in the lower extremity follows the principles used in elective revascularization procedures. Preoperative or intraoperative angiography can help pinpoint the specific location of vessel injury and can also help delineate multiple vascular injuries to a single extremity (Fig. 1). Because limb-salvage rates are poor when reoperation is required, definitive repair should be attempted at the first operative intervention unless patient instability dictates otherwise.[11,60] Incisions are located longitudinally over the affected area. The one exception to this rule is in the case of CFA injury, where an oblique incision made above the inguinal ligament allows for dissection of the external iliac artery to establish proximal control. Alternatively, a longitudinal incision in the groin may be carried superiorly, dividing the inguinal ligament to gain similar exposure. As in elective vascular procedures, obtaining proximal and distal control is paramount. If this cannot be accomplished by controlling the vessel with vascular clamps, a Fogarty balloon may be passed through the vessel defect and inflated for vessel occlusion. Temporary control can also be established with finger

compression or lateral suture. In some instances, the latter may be all that is required to definitively repair a vessel injury, so long as there is not an associated intimal dissection and the repair does not significantly narrow the vessel. Alternatively, a portion of the vessel may be left *in situ* and a vein patch used to repair the injured portion. This technique works well when the patch angioplasty is appropriately sized. A large, bulging patch may lead to turbulent flow, thrombosis, and embolism.

In the event that a complete transection is encountered or the vessel has been lacerated leaving a ragged wound, the vessel edges should first be debrided. Primary end-to-end anastomosis may be performed by reapproximation of the vessel so long as a tension free repair can be accomplished. The affected extremity should not be maintained in a flexed position during anastomosis, as undue tension and stretch will occur when the limb is subsequently extended.

If an interposition graft is to be used, harvesting the contralateral saphenous vein or using another autogenous graft is the preferred technique (see Fig. 8).[61,62] Preoperative planning should always include prepping both lower extremities for potential vein harvest. Interposition vein

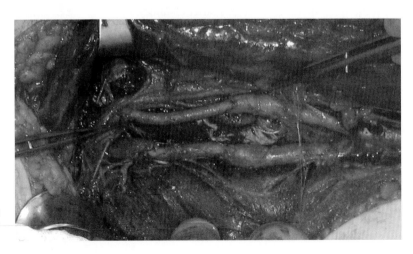

Figure 8 Repaired femoral artery and vein with interposition reversed saphenous vein graft following gunshot wound (GSW).

TABLE 4

OUTCOME BASED ON TYPE OF VASCULAR REPAIR IN 550 PATIENTS AS MEASURED BY REQUIREMENT FOR AMPUTATION

Procedure	Number of Injuries	Amputations (Number)	OR for Amputation (95% CI)	p Value
Ligation	64	11	1.1 (0.5–2.1)	0.5
Suture repair	109	9	0.45 (0.22–0.93)	0.01
Vein graft	317	40	0.7 (0.4–1.1)	0.08
Prosthetic graft	58	11	1.4 (0.7–2.9)	0.2
Vein tied	92	14	0.9 (0.5–1.7)	0.5
Fasciotomy	258	46	1.2 (0.7–1.9)	0.22
Reexplored	19	7	3.1 (1.2–8.4)	0.02
Failed revascularization	32	14	5.2 (2.4–11.0)	<0.001

OR, odds ratio.
(Adapted from Hafez HM, Woolgar J, Robbs JV. Lower extremity arterial injury: Results of 550 cases and review of risk factors associated with limb loss. *J Vasc Surg.* 2001;33(6):1212–1219.)

grafts have excellent limb salvage and long-term patency rates.[63–65] As in elective revascularization procedures, the vein graft should be reversed. Although there are no large trauma series comparing conduits other than saphenous vein, experience in nontraumatic revascularization validates the superiority of other autogenous grafts (such as upper extremity vein grafts) over prosthetics.[66] Synthetic interposition grafts traditionally have lower patency rates than autogenous grafts. However, they may be necessary options when a long conduit is needed or the patient does not have suitable vein for harvest.

For the multiply injured patient with concomitant orthopaedic and vascular injuries, any long bone fractures should be permanently fixated only after definitive vascular repair. Again, intravascular shunts can restore critical blood flow to an ischemic limb while orthopaedic injuries are being managed with temporizing measures. An appropriate management plan should be coordinated between orthopaedic, vascular, trauma, and plastic surgeons as necessary for complex extremity injuries.

Mortality from lower extremity arterial injury is low, with survival well above 90% in large series.[6] Outcomes for limb salvage in lower extremity arterial injury are outlined in Table 4. Best results are obtained with interposition vein grafts, while ligation, the need for reexploration, and failed revascularization portend worse outcomes and higher amputation rates.[11] Failed limb salvage in recent combat experience, where amputation rates of roughly 7% are reported, are classically higher than in civilian trauma.[1] Other reported predictors of poor limb salvage include combined venous and arterial injury, multiple associated fractures, concomitant nerve injury, blunt mechanism, and infection (see Table 5).[2,6,8,11,22,67] Functional outcomes are often suboptimal, and particularly high rates of disability are reported in this patient population.[68]

Operative Management—Upper Extremity

The patient should be placed in the supine position. For subclavian and axillary injuries, the arm should be abducted to not more than 30 degrees, as excessive abduction can distort the anatomy.[10] The chest and any areas of possible autogenous vein harvest such as the lower extremities should be included in the surgical field. In the forearm, brachial artery injuries should be repaired within 12 hours due to a high rate of compromise of function after this period.[50]

Exposure of the subclavian and proximal axillary vessels begins with an incision at the sternoclavicular junction, extending over the medial clavicle, and curving downward over the deltopectoral groove. Exposure of the aortic arch or root of the subclavian artery can be achieved with the addition of a median sternotomy. For distal axillary

TABLE 5

PREDICTORS FOR LIMB SALVAGE

Poor Outcome/Low Limb Salvage Rates	Good Outcome/High Limb Salvage Rates
■ Ligation	■ Vein graft
■ Failed Revascularization	■ Successful revascularization
■ Need for reoperation	■ Lateral suture repair
■ Combined arterial and venous injury	■ Single vessel injury
■ Multiple associated fractures	■ Short-segment vessel injury
■ Multiple fractures/soft tissue loss/mangled extremity	■ No associated fractures
■ Concomitant nerve injury	■ Absence of nerve injury
■ Blunt mechanism	■ Penetrating mechanism
■ Infection	

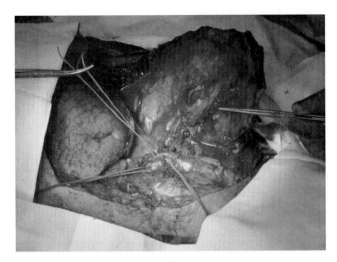

Figure 9 Trap door incision to expose injured subclavian vein.

injuries, the incision begins at the middle of the clavicle and curves over the deltopectoral groove. Traditionally, the "trap door" incision has been advocated for left subclavian artery injuries (see Fig. 9). However, some authors have reported excellent exposure of either left or right side with the clavicular incision and addition of the median sternotomy if needed.[10,26] The "trap door" incision can be associated with severe bleeding because of the division of muscle, as well as additional postoperative pain and respiratory compromise. The medial portion of the clavicle should be resected or divided and retracted for subclavian injuries. When a sternotomy is required, the anterior scalene must be divided or retracted, taking care to avoid the phrenic nerve. Exposure of the brachial artery and forearm vessels should be through longitudinal incisions so that the option of increased exposure exists, if needed. Care should be taken when crossing joints and when in proximity to the median nerve.

Debridement is followed by primary repair when possible with an end-to-end anastomosis. This is usually more feasible with the brachial and forearm arteries than the more proximal vessels.[10,50] In the subclavian and axillary positions, it has been suggested that prosthetic and autogenous grafts are equivalent, but one 13-year series of 38 patients reported a 21% infection rate, although these authors did not use prosthetic graft.[10,26,50] This suggests that autogenous vein grafts should be used when time and anatomic considerations permit. In the arm and forearm, however, prosthetic graft is contraindicated. Other than the risk of infection, prosthetic grafts consistently perform poorly when compared to autogenous graft in terms of patency.[50] Fogarty catheters should be passed in the arm and forearm to clear the vessels of distal thrombus. Spasm is also more of a concern distally than proximally, and can be managed with topical lidocaine, papaverine, direct stretch by infusion of saline, or excision. If both forearm arteries are injured and only one can be repaired, the larger

ulnar artery should be reconstructed.[50] Generally, ligation can be performed as a lifesaving maneuver if the patient is in extremis.

Transected nerves, when found, should be tagged for reexploration at a later surgery. It has also been recommended that without preoperative documentation of the status of the brachial plexus, it should not be explored until a later date.[10] Again, a fasciotomy should be performed if a compartment syndrome is suspected. In the forearm, a carpal tunnel release is performed in conjunction with fasciotomy. Systemic anticoagulation is generally not feasible due to significant bleeding, but local instillation of heparin saline is commonly practiced.[69]

Mortality due to vascular injury in the upper extremity is variable depending on the location of the injury, with axillary and subclavian injuries being highly lethal (up to 60%), whereas mortality from forearm vessel injuries is usually due to associated injuries.[10,50] Morbidity is variably and sparsely reported in the literature, owing in part to the difficulty in obtaining follow-up in this population. It is related in large part to the degree of associated injury, particularly injury to the brachial plexus in the proximal upper extremity, and median nerve in the forearm.

Amputation rates, where published, range from 2.6% to 18.8%.[14,25,70] In their 13-year review of 38 patients with injuries to the subclavian and axillary arteries, Aksoy et al. reported a 31.5% rate of permanent neurologic deficit and one case (2.6%) of permanent brachial plexus deficit in surviving patients.[25] Their wound infection and early postoperative thrombosis rates were 21% and 2.6% respectively. At 7 months their patency rate was 84.6%, which represents 11 of 13 patients out of the original 38 for which follow-up was available.

Endovascular Management

Background

Utilization of endovascular techniques in the treatment of peripheral vascular disease, the military conflict in Iraq, and growing experience with endovascular management of truncal and cervical injury have generated substantial interest in the endovascular management of vascular injury to the extremities.[71–75] Advances in radiologic capability and device technology have made a variety of injuries amenable to endovascular repair.[74,76] However, use of endovascular techniques to treat vascular injury of the extremity has to date been restricted to case reports and small series. Although prospective, randomized studies are needed to validate the endovascular management of extremity vascular injuries, current reports confirm the safety and feasibility of these techniques.

A number of advantages of endovascular methods over traditional open techniques can be directly applied from the accumulated experience in treating nontraumatic vascular lesions (see Table 6).[71,73,75,77–79] For example, Xenos et al. reported a threefold decrease in blood loss and a

TABLE 6

ADVANTAGES/DISADVANTAGES OF ENDOVASCULAR REPAIR

Advantage	Disadvantage
■ Distant access	■ Specialized personnel and equipment required
■ Decreased potential injury to surrounding structures (e.g., nerves, soft tissue)	■ Contrast load
■ Avoids dissection in distorted tissue	■ Does not allow evaluation of surrounding tissues
■ Minimizes dissection in contaminated field	■ Does not correlate with degree of blood loss
■ Does not require general anesthesia	■ Need for anticoagulation is undefined
■ Decreased procedure time	
■ Decreased blood loss	
■ Minimally invasive temporizing measure	

TABLE 7

INCLUSION/EXCLUSION CRITERIA FOR ENDOVASCULAR REPAIR OF PERIPHERAL ARTERY TRAUMA

Indicated	Contraindicated
Lesion specific	
■ Short segment or focal lesion	■ Long segment lesion
■ Pseudoaneurysm	■ Total vessel transection
■ Arteriovenous fistula	■ Area of significant compression or flexion/extension (e.g., third portion of axillary artery, popliteal artery)
■ Intimal flap	
■ Proximal to axillary or popliteal artery	■ Distal to axillary or popliteal arteries
■ Adequate proximal/distal fixation points	■ Inadequate proximal/distal fixation points
Patient/setting specific	
■ Hard signs absent	■ Hard signs present
■ Full endovascular capability	■ No endovascular capability
■ Hemodynamic stability	■ Hemodynamically unstable
■ Cannot tolerate general anesthesia	■ Temporizing "bridge" to definitive repair

60-minute decrease in procedure time in seven patients with axillosubclavian injury repaired with covered stents when compared to five patients who underwent traditional open repair.[79] There were no significant differences in 1-year patency between groups. One caution amidst the enthusiasm and increased applicability of endovascular therapies is that the supportive data, although encouraging, is lacking in well-documented, consistent long-term follow up.[71–73,76,77,79–81]

Indications/Contraindications

The management of vascular injury, whether by the open or endovascular approach, is always guided by the basic tenets of timely intervention, adequate exposure, proximal and distal control, careful assessment of associated injuries, and avoidance of prosthetic material within a contaminated field.[69,75] Table 7 summarizes these recommendations. There are no clearly defined indications for endovascular repair of vascular injury to the extremity. Most authors adhere to the principle of direct open exploration for "hard" signs of vascular injury, whereas "soft" signs warrant adjunct diagnostic modalities depending on the clinical situation and the judgment of the treating clinician.[78,82] Traditional treatment strategies for utilizing these adjunct measures are presented elsewhere in this chapter. It is within this well-established framework that endovascular management is incorporated.

Lesion type is another consideration to this approach. As previously noted, total transection or bleeding associated with hemodynamic instability is best treated by an open procedure. Additionally, nonfocal (>5 cm) lesions are likely to have poor success rates based on the nontrauma experience.[73,78] Pseudoaneurysms and AVFs appear to be the most widely reported types of lesions treated by endovascular techniques, with intimal flaps and dissections being increasingly reported (see Figs. 1 and 2). White et al. reported 26 of 62 (42%) cases of endovascular treatment of pseudoaneurysm or AVF in the extremity, with 1-year exclusion of the lesion of 90% for subclavian and 62% for femoral locations.[81] Primary patency at 1 year was 86% for subclavian and femoral lesions combined. There is currently little evidence to support the use of endovascular techniques in smaller, more peripheral vessels of either the upper or lower extremity, in light of the poor patency rates in the nontrauma experience.[73,78] Isolated case reports exist, but no conclusions as to their applicability can be made until a larger experience has accumulated. Therefore, there is currently little role for these techniques in vessels distal to the axillary or the popliteal arteries.

The around-the-clock availability of an interventional radiologist or vascular surgeon experienced in endovascular techniques is critical, as well as a support team facile in these techniques in the settting of vascular trauma. A suite or operating room with full endovascular capability as well as a full complement of guidewires, sheaths, coils, stents, and stent grafts is another necessity. The possibility of converting to a formal open procedure must always be entertained, and a seamless transition should be anticipated when managing extremity injury by an endovascular approach.

Upper Extremity

The location of the injury can suggest the type of management. For example, endovascular techniques may confer the greatest advantage in the axillosubclavian region.[74] Subclavian and axillary arterial injuries are uncommon, comprising 5% to 10% of arterial trauma in civilians, and have been associated with mortality as high as 30% to 60%.[26,76,79] It has been reported that 23% to 60% of patients who sustain this injury die before reaching the emergency department.[26] Open surgical exposure in this area is highly morbid, and can include a thoracotomy, clavicular resection, and sternotomy. The brachial plexus and phrenic nerve are in close proximity and have a high potential for injury, particularly in the context of soft tissue injury and distortion of tissue planes. Danetz et al. performed a retrospective review of 46 patients with axillosubclavian injuries with the aim of establishing the feasibility of endovascular repair specifically in trauma patients.[71] They determined that 43% of patients who maintained vital signs in the emergency department had lesions amenable to endovascular repair using a stent or stent graft. These authors defined feasibility as a hemodynamically stable patient with (a) a focal arterial laceration, (b) intimal flap, (c) first order branch avulsions or lacerations, (d) AVF, or (e) pseudoaneurysm with adequate proximal and distal fixation points. They also noted that including the use of proximal balloon tamponade until definitive repair can be performed would increase the proportion of patients in which endovascular techniques are feasible. Xenos et al. reported a series of 23 patients with axillary or subclavian injury. Of these, 12 patients (52%) with lesions amenable to vascular repair, of which 7, or 58% of amenable lesions, ultimately underwent endovascular repair, depending on surgeon preference. They reported no statistical difference between groups regarding 1-year patency.[79] Castelli et al. reported a series of seven patients who underwent either stent graft (five) or stent (two) placement for injuries in this location with no operative complications and 100% patency rate at 22 months of follow-up.[76]

Lower Extremity

Femoral injuries are also amenable to endovascular therapy, although it is currently considered an experimental modality. However, because femoral injuries comprise up to 70% of arterial injuries, the frequency of lesions potentially treatable with endoluminal methods is high, and use of these procedures is likely to increase.[83] Currently, the utility of embolization for refractory bleeding from the deep femoral artery is accepted practice.[78,84] Covered stents have been used successfully to treat pseudoaneurysms and AVFs in this region, although cumulative case numbers are small.[74,77,78,85,86] Parodi et al.[8] reported 4 cases of stent graft deployment in the femoral position in a series of 29 cases of posttraumatic pseudoaneurysms and AVFs.[77] Also included in the authors' review were 17 total cases of stent deployment in the extremity. The index procedure in the femoral position was successful in 100% of cases, while 16 of 17 (94%) were successful for all extremity positions. Although early results are promising, one additional caution

with regard to the lower extremity is that limb salvage rates are not well reported.

Endovascular Techniques

A number of devices and techniques are available to the endovascular surgeon. A full discussion of the technical aspects is beyond the scope of this chapter, but a brief introduction in regards to the management of vascular injury of the extremity is presented here.

Balloons have been used for temporary occlusion of massive bleeding as a damage control measure until a definitive open or endovascular repair can be performed.[74,75,78] They have also been successfully used to "tack down" intimal flaps.[73]

A variety of materials are available to embolize bleeding vessels, including coils, polymeric biomaterials, synthetic microspheres, and liquid adhesives.[75] The guiding principle is to precisely introduce thrombogenic material over a focal length while avoiding distal embolization or end-tissue ischemia. Although well established in the treatment of cerebrovascular or pelvic bleeding, it has been suggested that embolization has little role in the extremity other than exclusion of small pseudoaneurysms and AVFs, in collateral vessels of the elbow and knee, or in deep muscular branches of the leg which may be otherwise difficult to reach.[74,78,84]

Metallic stents were originally designed to expand the lumen of atherosclerotic vessels, but their use has been increasingly reported in trauma, primarily in the case of intimal dissection.[75,76] Stents are either self-expanding or balloon expandable, with the former being advantageous in vessels that curve or move, and the latter being useful in vessels that are straight or calcified.[78] Stent grafts are nonporous materials supported by a metallic stent that are designed to span a defect in a vessel wall and exclude the lesion. Corresponding to the most commonly reported type of lesion managed by endovascular means (pseudoaneurysm or AVF), the stent graft is the most frequently used device for treating these lesions.[71,73,74,78,79,81,86]

Regardless of device used, the basic technical principles are similar. After angiographic characterization of the lesion, including size, type (dissection, AVF, transection, etc), proximity to branches, and vessel size, a guidewire is introduced through a distant access site. Once the area of interest is approached, the device is delivered across the lesion. In the case of a stent or stent graft, a 10% to 20% oversize is recommended to ensure a proper seal.[78] Heparin can be delivered locally but the role of systemic peri- and postprocedural anticoagulation is unclear.[69,85] Typically, systemic heparinization is not required postoperatively.

Outcomes for Endovascular Repair

Data regarding complications must be reviewed with caution for two primary reasons. First, follow-up is

TABLE 8

COMPLICATIONS RELATED TO ENDOVASCULAR REPAIR OF VASCULAR INJURY OF THE EXTREMITY

Access site hematoma
Access site infection
Pseudoaneurysm
Endoleak
Stenosis/occlusion
Neointimal hyperplasia
Limb claudication or ischemia
Distal embolization
Graft infection
Inadvertent branch occlusion
Limb loss

historically poor in trauma patients. Second, because endovascular repair of arterial injury is an emerging field, long-term data are not available. However, many of the complications seen are those inherent to any vascular repair (see Table 8). Early follow-up appears to be promising. Overall, rates of adverse events range from 6.5% to 17% in most reports, while follow-up ranges from 6 weeks to 4 years, with three authors reporting follow-up >20 months.[76,77,80,81,86] By comparison, historical data from large series of traditional repairs report overall complication rates between 9% and 30%.[87] These include large series of battlefield casualties from the Vietnam and Korean conflicts as well as civilian series.

White et al.[81] reported their experience with 62 repairs in the iliac, subclavian, or femoral arteries after 6 months. The authors noted a 14.5% early (<30 days) adverse event rate and a 6.5% late (>30 days) adverse event rate. These events included pseudoaneurysm, access site infection, graft thrombosis, and stenosis. Seven endoleaks (11%) were also reported. They found a decrease in perioperative complications (57.7% vs. 21.2%), equivalent late complication rate (6% vs. 12%), decreased post procedure mortality (27.3% vs. 9.1%), and decreased all-cause late mortality (33.9% vs. 15.2%) when endovascular repair was compared to open procedures. Further, they commented that the complications that occur with endovascular repair (e.g., stenosis and occlusion) are generally less morbid than those seen in open repair (e.g., disseminated intravascular coagulation, sexual dysfunction, and nerve injury) and are more amenable to repair with further minimally invasive techniques.

Although a lack of well-designed prospective trials prevent definitive conclusions from being drawn, there continues to be rapid growth in the utilization of endoluminal surgery for arterial trauma. Enthusiasm for minimally invasive techniques must be tempered with a solid foundation in the traditional principles guiding the management of vascular injury. Good candidates are generally hemodynamically stable and without hard signs of vascular injury. Advantages appear to be greatest with axillary and subclavian injuries, where historical mortality is high and exposure is difficult and morbid. Other uses include embolization of difficult to reach deep muscular arteries and temporary balloon tamponade as an adjunct to definitive treatment for a patient in extremis. Pseudoaneurysms and AVFs are the lesions most amenable to treatment. As experience grows, the range of treatable lesions and the role of endovascular therapy are likely to expand. Larger, well-designed trials are needed to bolster this growing experience and provide sound practice guidelines.

Further Considerations

The Compartment Syndrome and Fasciotomy

A high index of suspicion for the development of the compartment syndrome must be entertained in the patient with vascular injury to the extremity. This condition arises in an extremity when increased compartmental pressures exceed capillary perfusion pressure.[88] In the setting of limited perfusion, hypoxia leads to the generation of free radicals which subsequently initiate a cycle of cellular injury, swelling leading to increased pressure, a further decline in perfusion, and progressive injury. Ultimately, cell death and limb loss occur. Multiorgan failure and death may result from the inflammatory cascade that is set into motion by the compartment syndrome.

Diagnosing the compartment syndrome continues to be a difficult clinical challenge. Although the underlying pathophysiologic sequence is generally well accepted, the timing of its evolution and the pressures needed to cause compartment syndrome are not well understood.[88,89] It is exceedingly difficult to differentiate intracompartmental hypertension and compartment syndrome based on the gradient that exists between the two. A wide range of presenting signs and symptoms is frequently encountered, from mild edema and pain on passive stretch to a cold, insensate, pulseless extremity. Patients at risk for the compartment syndrome also often have severe, multiple injuries which necessitate the need for more than one intervention simultaneously. Aggressive fluid resuscitation in these patients can often precipitate the development of compartment syndrome, either from the dislodgement of clot from injured vessels or from reperfusion injury and capillary leak in an already ischemic limb.

Ultimately, the diagnosis of compartment syndrome is clinical, based on a high index of suspicion. Classic findings such as pulselessness or paresthesias are often late findings. The mechanism of injury itself should lead to its early consideration, and includes most vascular injuries. Other types of injuries that may predispose to the compartment syndrome are combined venous and arterial injuries and crush injuries.[72,88] The most common sign on PE is pain on passive stretch of the extremity, although this finding may be obscured in patients with a depressed level of consciousness or distracting injuries. A swollen, tense compartment—particularly in the setting of pulse variation between affected and unaffected limbs—are other hallmarks that should raise suspicion. If the diagnosis is uncertain, compartment pressures may be measured, and several handheld devices are available. A compartment pressure above 30 mm Hg or within 10 to 20 mm Hg of diastolic blood pressure is worrisome. It should be emphasized that measurement of compartment pressures or ancillary testing should not delay decompression when indicated, nor should it be a substitute for repeated PE. This has proved to be particularly salient in the combat setting, where extremity injury approaches 70% of all injuries and compartment pressures are not measured as a matter of protocol.[7,72,74] Similarly, in a review of combined orthopaedic and vascular injuries in a large, inner-city Level I trauma center in the United States, McHenry et al.[72] performed 12 fasciotomies in 27 patients (44%) without measuring compartment pressures. The authors reported no cases of delayed fasciotomy for unrecognized compartment syndrome.

Numerous incisions have been described, and the most commonly performed are discussed here. There are three compartments in the thigh: the anterior, lateral, and posterior. Fasciotomy of the thigh involves a single incision on the lateral thigh, exposure and division of the fascia lata, retraction of the vastus lateralis, and identification and incision of the lateral intermuscular septum.[90] The leg has four compartments: the anterior, lateral, superficial, and deep posterior. Decompression is most commonly and most definitively achieved by the two-incision technique, the first incision centered between the anterior and lateral compartments and the second positioned 1 to 2 cm posterior to the posteromedial aspect of the tibia.[69] The forearm has three compartments: the superficial, deep flexor, and the extensor. Some references acknowledge four compartments, considering the mobile wad of Henry, consisting of the brachioradialis and the extensor carpi radialis longus and brevis muscles as a separate compartment.[91] Regardless, the treatment is the same. Decompression should begin with a volar fasciotomy, which begins medial to the biceps tendon, crosses the elbow obliquely, continues in a curvilinear manner along the brachioradialis muscle, crosses the wrist at an angle, and extends along the thenar crease. A carpal tunnel release is sometimes performed at the same time. If this does not adequately decompress the forearm, a dorsal fasciotomy may be performed, which begins just distal to the lateral epicondyle and extends down the middle of the dorsal aspect of the forearm to the wrist.[69]

Closure can be achieved by a variety of methods. Most commonly, a split-thickness skin graft is employed. Primary or delayed primary closure, closure by secondary intent, and, rarely, various soft tissue flaps have all been successfully utilized.[69,88,89]

Complications primarily include incomplete fasciotomy and infection. Sequelae of prolonged tissue ischemia in this setting include limb loss, nerve injury, and rhabdomyolysis. Most complications are the result of either a delay in presentation, diagnosis, or intervention. Williams et al.[88] reported an approximately fourfold increase (28% vs. 7.3%) in infectious complications in patients undergoing fasciotomy after 12 hours from injury as compared to those undergoing fasciotomy before 12 hours. It must also be noted that McHenry et al.[31] found an almost doubling in hospital stay in patients who required fasciotomy versus those who did not (18 vs. 10 days). Again, it is clear that none of these concerns should delay timely and complete decompression.

The role of prophylactic fasciotomy is difficult to define for a number of reasons. The diagnosis of compartment syndrome itself is not reliably predicted by a set range of circumstances, locations, or mechanisms of injury. Next, the timing and indications for therapeutic fasciotomy itself are often unclear. Data are limited and marked by a lack of consensus. Traditional teaching dictates ischemia time >6 hours as an indication for fasciotomy. However, one review noted only a difference in infectious complications when comparing fasciotomies performed greater than or less than 12 hours from injury.[88] Abouezzi et al.,[92] in an 8-year review of 45 fasciotomies performed for 163 vascular injuries, noted only popliteal vessel location as significantly associated with the need for fasciotomy. They noted no difference in frequency of fasciotomy for combined arterial and venous injury. Further, they described seven delayed fasciotomies, but define delay only as after the index surgery. However, this was a review in which multi- or univariate analysis was not undertaken. In contrast, another recent review found an increase in fasciotomy with combined arterial and venous injury.[72] On the other end of the spectrum, in the combat theater in Iraq and Afghanistan, fasciotomy is performed if the measurement of compartment pressures is even contemplated.[7] Granted, this is a markedly different set of circumstances than seen in civilian trauma, with a far greater incidence of massive tissue loss and high energy and blast mechanisms of injury. However, Williams et al.[88] also report their experience with fasciotomy without the measurement of compartment pressures in their civilian series. In addition, fasciotomy is another surgical procedure and is subject to its own attendant risks such as infection, increased hospital stay, and the need for multiple surgeries to provide coverage of the defect if primary closure is not achieved.

Prophylactic fasciotomy is therefore a concept fraught with controversy. Several different indications exist as outlined in the preceding text, but have not been supported by sound data. Prolonged ischemia, popliteal vessel injury, and combined arterial and venous injury are reasonable circumstances in which to consider prophylactic fasciotomy, but their incorporation into formulaic treatment practices should be avoided.

Venous Injury

The management of venous injury or combined arterial and venous injury has undergone a substantial change in management over the last 4 decades. Before the Vietnam conflict, venous injuries were routinely ligated. However, with improved limb salvage rates in patients who had venous repairs reported by combat surgeons during this era, ligation fell out of favor until the early 1980s.[93] The natural history of venous ligation rarely leads to clinically significant or incapacitating edema. Although a majority of repaired lower extremity veins thrombose early in the postoperative period, these clots rarely propagate.[94,95] When followed over time, it appears that many thrombosed vessels recanalize. Serial examinations with duplex or venography reveal that as many as 78% of vein repairs are patent at 30 days, with lesion location highly predictive for patency.[95,96] The rates for limb salvage are equivalent with either venous ligation or repair, leading most authors to recommend venous repair if it can be accomplished expeditiously and with minimal dissection in a hemodynamically stable patient.[6,94,97] Retrospective analysis suggests that combined venous and arterial injury portends a worse prognosis for limb salvage than single vessel injury.[6] Vein lacerations repaired with patch angioplasty have the highest patency rates, followed by lateral suture and interposition grafts.[96] Complex spiral interpositions frequently thrombose and have the lowest reported patency rates.[94,95] Repairs with reversed vein interposition typically employ the greater saphenous vein, which has a narrower diameter than the femoral vein and likely contributes to the high incidence of thrombosis (Fig. 8).

MANGLED EXTREMITIES: AN EDITORIAL COMMENT

In a perfect world, it should be possible for a general or orthopaedic surgeon to assess a patient with a mangled extremity and to make a perfect decision as to whether to do prompt amputation or to attempt reconstruction. Unfortunately, the literature does not help us that much in making these decisions, and most of the literature that addresses the mangled extremity focuses on the lower extremity. These fractures have been classified as 3C and are invariably open.[98,99] Some have vascular injuries, and some do not. Some are insensate, and some are not.

In a recent study by Swiontkowski et al. of 569 patients with severe leg injuries who underwent reconstruction or amputation, the sickness impact profile (SIP) showed no difference in outcomes between these two groups.[100] Their study did show that there was a poorer score for the SIP if the

patient was rehospitalized or had a major complication, a lower educational level, non–white race, poverty, lack of private health insurance, poor social support network, low self-efficiency, smoking, and involvement in disability-compensation litigation. Interestingly, patients who underwent reconstruction were more likely to be rehospitalized than those who underwent amputation. Return to work between the two groups was similar. The fact the groups were similar reflects the surgeons made good decisions.

Many scoring systems have been developed to predict those patients who should undergo immediate amputation and those who should have reconstruction. My own bias is reflected by Bonanni, Rhodes, and Lucke, who state that predictive scoring is an exercise in futility.[101] In their study, they could not show reliable sensitivity or specificity using the mangled extremity syndrome index (MESI), predictive salvage index (PSI), mangled extremity severity score (MESS), or the limb salvage index (LSI). Surgical judgment based on experience is still the gold standard.

There are few areas in trauma care where there is so much controversy as to whether amputations for mangled extremities should be done early or delayed. The most common reasons for delayed amputation are loss of wound cover in ununited fractures, infection in a nonunion fracture, an insensate limb, recurrent ulcerations, a dystrophic limb, sympathetic dystrophy, and phantom pain to name a few. Some surgeons have argued that functional recovery is faster and less costly following amputation than with multiple procedures for salvage and reconstruction. In addition to the study by Bosse listed earlier, there is a study by Pozo et al., who studied 35 patients who had amputation following the failure of treatment for severe lower limb trauma.[102] Seven of the amputations were for ischemia within 1 month of the injury; 13 were between 1 month and 1 year for infection, complicating loss of limb cover or ununited fractures; and 15 were later than 1 year after injury mainly for infected nonunion. This latter group had an average of 12 surgeries and 50 months of treatment, including 8 months in hospital. Factors that contributed to salvage failure were vascular injuries, nerve damage, bone damage, muscle damage, skin cover, and sepsis. Overall, these authors concluded that if one attempts lower limb reconstruction, they should be assessed very early on by two specialists, one in trauma surgery and the other in plastic surgery, as to whether or not futility is inevitable. Obviously, this requires experience, and persistent attempts at salvage can be extremely difficult.

Another study that might influence surgeons as to salvage versus amputation comes from Case Western Reserve, where they followed up 34 patients, of whom 16 had a successful limb salvage procedure, and 18 had an immediate below knee amputation (BKA). The patients who had a successful limb salvage procedure took significantly more time to achieve full weight bearing, were less willing or able to work, and had higher hospital charges than the patients who had been managed with an early BKA. Furthermore, those patients who had limb salvage considered themselves severely disabled, and they had more problems than the amputation group with the performance of occupational and recreational activities. These quality of life evaluations, however, must be put into the perspective that Swiontkowski et al.[100] have already outlined.

A final study for consideration is one by Roessler et al.[103] They reviewed 80 patients for a 4-year period and asked the question when to amputate. They concluded that neurologic, bone, and tissue status did influence the decision regarding immediate amputation, but had little to do with delayed loss of limb or life. Somewhat surprisingly, they found that the circulation as determined by the presence or absence of a palpable or Doppler-detected pulse was critical. They concluded that in cases in which salvage is attempted, amputation should be performed at 24 hours if the patient's condition, including a markedly positive fluid balance, indicates systemic compromise. They also made the observation that in the absence of a distal pulse on presentation, the eventual amputation rate is high.

Donald D. Trunkey, MD

REFERENCES

1. Clouse WD, Rasmussen TE, Peck MA, et al. In-theater management of vascular injury: 2 years of the Balad Vascular Registry. *J Am Coll Surg.* 2007;204(4):625–632.
2. Feliciano DV, Herskowitz K, O'Gorman RB, et al. Management of vascular injuries in the lower extremities. *J Trauma.* 1988;28(3):319–328.
3. Fox CJ, Gillespie DL, O'Donnell SD, et al. Contemporary management of wartime vascular trauma. *J Vasc Surg.* 2005;41(4):638–644.
4. Oller DW, Rutledge R, Clancy T, et al. Vascular injuries in a rural state: A review of 978 patients from a state trauma registry. *J Trauma.* 1992;32(6):740–745; discussion 5–6.
5. Peck MA, Clouse WD, Cox MW, et al. The complete management of extremity vascular injury in a local population: A wartime report from the 332nd Expeditionary Medical Group/Air Force Theater Hospital, Balad Air Base, Iraq. *J Vasc Surg.* 2007; 45(6):1197–1205.
6. Asensio JA, Kuncir EJ, Garcia-Nunez LM, et al. Femoral vessel injuries: Analysis of factors predictive of outcomes. *J Am Coll Surg.* 2006;203(4):512–520.
7. Beekley AC, Starnes BW, Sebesta JA. Lessons learned from modern military surgery. *Surg Clin North Am.* 2007;87(1):157–184, vii.
8. Bowley DM, Degiannis E, Goosen J, et al. Penetrating vascular trauma in Johannesburg, South Africa. *Surg Clin North Am.* 2002;82(1):221–235.
9. Cakir O, Subasi M, Erdem K, et al. Treatment of vascular injuries associated with limb fractures. *Ann R Coll Surg Engl.* 2005;87(5):348–352.
10. Demetriades D, Asensio JA. Subclavian and axillary vascular injuries. *Surg Clin North Am.* 2001;81(6):1357–1373, xiii.
11. Hafez HM, Woolgar J, Robbs JV. Lower extremity arterial injury: Results of 550 cases and review of risk factors associated with limb loss. *J Vasc Surg.* 2001;33(6):1212–1219.
12. Hossny A. Blunt popliteal artery injury with complete lower limb ischemia: Is routine use of temporary intraluminal arterial shunt justified? *J Vasc Surg.* 2004;40(1):61–66.
13. Melton SM, Croce MA, Patton JH Jr, et al. Popliteal artery trauma. Systemic anticoagulation and intraoperative thrombolysis improves limb salvage. *Ann Surg.* 1997;225(5):518–527; discussion 27–29.
14. Rozycki GS, Tremblay LN, Feliciano DV, et al. Blunt vascular trauma in the extremity: Diagnosis, management, and outcome. *J Trauma.* 2003;55(5):814–824.
15. Gonzalez RP, Falimirski ME. The utility of physical examination in proximity penetrating extremity trauma. *Am Surg.* 1999;65(8):784–789.
16. Dennis JW, Frykberg ER, Veldenz HC, et al. Validation of nonoperative management of occult vascular injuries and accuracy of physical examination alone in penetrating extremity trauma: 5- to 10-year follow-up. *J Trauma.* 1998;44(2):243–252; discussion 2–3.
17. Frykberg ER, Dennis JW, Bishop K, et al. The reliability of physical examination in the evaluation of penetrating extremity trauma for vascular injury: Results at one year. *J Trauma.* 1991;31(4):502–511.
18. Mills WJ, Barei DP, McNair P. The value of the ankle-brachial index for diagnosing arterial injury after knee dislocation: A prospective study. *J Trauma.* 2004;56(6):1261–1265.
19. Stannard JP, Sheils TM, Lopez-Ben RR, et al. Vascular injuries in knee dislocations: The role of physical examination in determining the need for arteriography. *J Bone Joint Surg Am.* 2004;86-A(5):910–915.
20. Miranda FE, Dennis JW, Veldenz HC, et al. Confirmation of the safety and accuracy of physical examination in the evaluation of knee dislocation for injury of the popliteal artery: A prospective study. *J Trauma.* 2002;52(2):247–251; discussion 51–52.
21. Huynh TT, Pham M, Griffin LW, et al. Management of distal femoral and popliteal arterial injuries: An update. *Am J Surg.* 2006;192(6):773–778.
22. Mullenix PS, Steele SR, Andersen CA, et al. Limb salvage and outcomes among patients with traumatic popliteal vascular injury: An analysis of the National Trauma Data Bank. *J Vasc Surg.* 2006;44(1):94–100.
23. Bongard F, Dubrow T, Klein S. Vascular injuries in the urban battleground: Experience at a metropolitan trauma center. *Ann Vasc Surg.* 1990;4(5):415–418.
24. Myers SI, Harward TR, Maher DP, et al. Complex upper extremity vascular trauma in an urban population. *J Vasc Surg.* 1990;12(3):305–309.
25. Aksoy M, Tunca F, Yanar H, et al. Traumatic injuries to the subclavian and axillary arteries: A 13-year review. *Surg Today.* 2005;35(7):561–565.
26. Demetriades D, Chahwan S, Gomez H, et al. Penetrating injuries to the subclavian and axillary vessels. *J Am Coll Surg.* 1999;188(3):290–295.
27. Giswold ME, Landry GJ, Taylor LM, et al. Iatrogenic arterial injury is an increasingly important cause of arterial trauma. *Am J Surg.* 2004;187(5):590–592; discussion 2–3.
28. Lumpkin MB, Logan WD, Couves CM, et al. Arteriography an an aid in the diagnosis and localization of acute arterial injuries. *Ann Surg.* 1958;147(3):353–358.
29. Wholey MH, Bocher J. Angiography in musculoskeletal trauma. *Surg Gynecol Obstet.* 1967;125(4):730–736.
30. Rees R, Bonneval M, Batson R, et al. Angiography in extremity trauma: A prospective study. *Am Surg.* 1978;44(10):661–663.
31. Snyder WH III, Thal ER, Bridges RA, et al. The validity of normal arteriography in penetrating trauma. *Arch Surg.* 1978;113(4):424–426.
32. Menzoian JO, Doyle JE, LoGerfo FW, et al. Evaluation and management of vascular injuries of the extremities. *Arch Surg.* 1983;118(1):93–95.
33. Sirinek KR, Gaskill HV III, Dittman WI, et al. Exclusion angiography for patients with possible vascular injuries of the extremities–a better use of trauma center resources. *Surgery.* 1983;94(4):598–603.
34. Geuder JW, Hobson RW II, Padberg FT Jr, et al. The role of contrast arteriography in suspected arterial injuries of the extremities. *Am Surg.* 1985;51(2):89–93.
35. MacFarlane C, Boffard KD, Saadia R, et al. Emergency room arteriography: A useful technique in the assessment of peripheral vascular injuries. *J R Coll Surg Edinb.* 1989;34(6):310–313.
36. O'Gorman RB, Feliciano DV, Bitondo CG, et al. Emergency center arteriography in the evaluation of suspected peripheral vascular injuries. *Arch Surg.* 1984;119(5):568–573.

37. Reid JD, Weigelt JA, Thal ER, et al. Assessment of proximity of a wound to major vascular structures as an indication for arteriography. *Arch Surg.* 1988;123(8):942–946.

38. Hollis JD, Daley BJ. 10-year review of knee dislocations: Is arteriography always necessary? *J Trauma.* 2005;59(3):672–675; discussion 5–6.

39. Francis H III, Thal ER, Weigelt JA, et al. Vascular proximity: Is it a valid indication for arteriography in asymptomatic patients? *J Trauma.* 1991;31(4):512–514.

40. Kendall RW, Taylor DC, Salvian AJ, et al. The role of arteriography in assessing vascular injuries associated with dislocations of the knee. *J Trauma.* 1993;35(6):875–878.

41. Bynoe RP, Miles WS, Bell RM, et al. Noninvasive diagnosis of vascular trauma by duplex ultrasonography. *J Vasc Surg.* 1991;14(3):346–352.

42. Miller-Thomas MM, West OC, Cohen AM. Diagnosing traumatic arterial injury in the extremities with CT angiography: Pearls and pitfalls. *Radiographics.* 2005;25(Suppl 1):S133–S142.

43. Soto JA, Munera F, Cardoso N, et al. Diagnostic performance of helical CT angiography in trauma to large arteries of the extremities. *J Comput Assist Tomogr.* 1999;23(2):188–196.

44. Soto JA, Munera F, Morales C, et al. Focal arterial injuries of the proximal extremities: Helical CT arteriography as the initial method of diagnosis. *Radiology.* 2001;218(1):188–194.

45. Busquets AR, Acosta JA, Colon E, et al. Helical computed tomographic angiography for the diagnosis of traumatic arterial injuries of the extremities. *J Trauma.* 2004;56(3):625–628.

46. Inaba K, Potzman J, Munera F, et al. Multi-slice CT angiography for arterial evaluation in the injured lower extremity. *J Trauma.* 2006;60(3):502–506; discussion 6–7.

47. Ouwendijk R, de Vries M, Pattynama PM, et al. Imaging peripheral arterial disease: A randomized controlled trial comparing contrast-enhanced MR angiography and multi-detector row CT angiography. *Radiology.* 2005;236(3):1094–1103.

48. Hingorani A, Ascher E, Markevich N, et al. A comparison of magnetic resonance angiography, contrast arteriography, and duplex arteriography for patients undergoing lower extremity revascularization. *Ann Vasc Surg.* 2004;18(3):294–301.

49. Ballard JL, Bunt TJ, Malone JM. Management of small artery vascular trauma. *Am J Surg.* 1992;164(4):316–319.

50. Fields CE, Latifi R, Ivatury RR. Brachial and forearm vessel injuries. *Surg Clin North Am.* 2002;82(1):105–114.

51. Johnson M, Ford M, Johansen K. Radial or ulnar artery laceration. Repair or ligate? *Arch Surg.* 1993;128(9):971–974; discussion 4–5.

52. Johansen K, Bandyk D, Thiele B, et al. Temporary intraluminal shunts: Resolution of a management dilemma in complex vascular injuries. *J Trauma.* 1982;22(5):395–402.

53. Khalil IM, Livingston DH. Intravascular shunts in complex lower limb trauma. *J Vasc Surg.* 1986;4(6):582–587.

54. Rasmussen TE, Clouse WD, Jenkins DH, et al. The use of temporary vascular shunts as a damage control adjunct in the management of wartime vascular injury. *J Trauma.* 2006;61(1):8–12; discussion 5.

55. Nalbandian MM, Maldonado TS, Cushman J, et al. Successful limb reperfusion using prolonged intravascular shunting in a case of an unstable trauma patient–a case report. *Vasc Endovascular Surg.* 2004;38(4):375–379.

56. Granchi T, Schmittling Z, Vasquez J, et al. Prolonged use of intraluminal arterial shunts without systemic anticoagulation. *Am J Surg.* 2000;180(6):493–496; discussion 6–7.

57. Reber PU, Patel AG, Sapio NL, et al. Selective use of temporary intravascular shunts in coincident vascular and orthopedic upper and lower limb trauma. *J Trauma.* 1999;47(1):72–76.

58. Nunley JA, Koman LA, Urbaniak JR. Arterial shunting as an adjunct to major limb revascularization. *Ann Surg.* 1981;193(3):271–273.

59. Sriussadaporn S, Pak-art R. Temporary intravascular shunt in complex extremity vascular injuries. *J Trauma.* 2002;52(6):1129–1133.

60. Leguerrier A, Lebeau G, Leveque JM, et al. Vascular injuries of the limbs. Evaluation of 106 lesions in 76 patients. *J Chir (Paris).* 1986;123(2):108–116.

61. McCready RA, Logan NM, Daugherty ME, et al. Long-term results with autogenous tissue repair of traumatic extremity vascular injuries. *Ann Surg.* 1987;206(6):804–808.

62. Thomas JH, Pierce GE, Iliopoulos JI, et al. Vascular graft selection. *Surg Clin North Am.* 1988;68(4):865–874.

63. Bastounis E, Pikoulis E, Leppaniemi AK, et al. Revascularization of the limbs using vein grafts after vascular injuries. *Injury.* 1998;29(2):105–108.

64. Keen RR, Meyer JP, Durham JR, et al. Autogenous vein graft repair of injured extremity arteries: Early and late results with 134 consecutive patients. *J Vasc Surg.* 1991;13(5):664–668.

65. Pasch AR, Bishara RA, Lim LT, et al. Optimal limb salvage in penetrating civilian vascular trauma. *J Vasc Surg.* 1986;3(2):189–195.

66. Faries PL, Logerfo FW, Arora S, et al. A comparative study of alternative conduits for lower extremity revascularization: All-autogenous conduit versus prosthetic grafts. *J Vasc Surg.* 2000;32(6):1080–1090.

67. Lin CH, Wei FC, Levin LS, et al. The functional outcome of lower-extremity fractures with vascular injury. *J Trauma.* 1997;43(3):480–485.

68. Busse JW, Jacobs CL, Swiontkowski MF, et al. Complex limb salvage or early amputation for severe lower-limb injury: A meta-analysis of observational studies. *J Orthop Trauma.* 2007;21(1):70–76.

69. Vogel T, Jurkovich G. Injuries to the peripheral blood vessels. In: Fink M, Jurkovich G, Kaiser L, et al. eds. *ACS surgery: principles and practice 2007.* New York: WebMD; 2007.

70. Shanmugam V, Velu RB, Subramaniyan SR, et al. Management of upper limb arterial injury without angiography–Chennai experience. *Injury.* 2004;35(1):61–64.

71. Danetz JS, Cassano AD, Stoner MC, et al. Feasibility of endovascular repair in penetrating axillosubclavian injuries: A retrospective review. *J Vasc Surg.* 2005;41(2):246–254.

72. McHenry TP, Holcomb JB, Aoki N, et al. Fractures with major vascular injuries from gunshot wounds: Implications of surgical sequence. *J Trauma.* 2002;53(4):717–721.

73. Lonn L, Delle M, Karlstrom L, et al. Should blunt arterial trauma to the extremities be treated with endovascular techniques? *J Trauma.* 2005;59(5):1224–1227.

74. Starnes BW, Arthurs ZM. Endovascular management of vascular trauma. *Perspect Vasc Surg Endovasc Ther.* 2006;18(2):114–129.

75. Weiss VJ, Chaikof EL. Endovascular treatment of vascular injuries. *Surg Clin North Am.* 1999;79(3):653–665.

76. Castelli P, Caronno R, Piffaretti G, et al. Endovascular repair of traumatic injuries of the subclavian and axillary arteries. *Injury.* 2005;36(6):778–782.

77. Parodi JC, Schonholz C, Ferreira LM, et al. Endovascular stent-graft treatment of traumatic arterial lesions. *Ann Vasc Surg.* 1999;13(2):121–129.

78. Risberg B, Lonn L. Management of vascular injuries using endovascular techniques. *Eur J Surg.* 2000;166(3):196–201.

79. Xenos ES, Freeman M, Stevens S, et al. Covered stents for injuries of subclavian and axillary arteries. *J Vasc Surg.* 2003;38(3):451–454.

80. Brandt MM, Kazanjian S, Wahl WL. The utility of endovascular stents in the treatment of blunt arterial injuries. *J Trauma.* 2001;51(5):901–905.

81. White R, Krajcer Z, Johnson M, et al. Results of a multicenter trial for the treatment of traumatic vascular injury with a covered stent. *J Trauma.* 2006;60(6):1189–1195; discussion 95–96.

82. Britt LD, Weireter LJ, Cole FJ. Newer diagnostic modalities for vascular injuries: The way we were, the way we are. *Surg Clin North Am.* 2001;81(6):1263–1279, xii.

83. Carrillo EH, Spain DA, Miller FB, et al. Femoral vessel injuries. *Surg Clin North Am.* 2002;82(1):49–65.

84. Henry SM, Tornetta P III, Scalea TM, Damage control for devastating pelvic and extremity injuries. *Surg Clin North Am.* 1997;77(4):879–895.

85. McArthur CS, Marin ML. Endovascular therapy for the treatment of arterial trauma. *Mt Sinai J Med.* 2004;71(1):4–11.

86. Thalhammer C, Kirchherr AS, Uhlich F, et al. Postcatheterization pseudoaneurysms and arteriovenous fistulas: Repair with percutaneous implantation of endovascular covered stents. *Radiology.* 2000;214(1):127–131.

87. Rich NM. Complications of vascular injury management. *Surg Clin North Am.* 2002;82(1):143–174, xxi.

88. Williams AB, Luchette FA, Papaconstantinou HT, et al. The effect of early versus late fasciotomy in the management of extremity trauma. *Surgery.* 1997;122(4):861–866.

89. Dente CJ, Feliciano DV, Rozycki GS, et al. A review of upper extremity fasciotomies in a level I trauma center. *Am Surg.* 2004;70(12):1088–1093.

90. Azar F. Traumatic disorders. In: Canale ST, ed. *Campbell's operative orthopaedics,* 10th ed. Philadelphia: Mosby; 2003.

91. Jobe MT. Compartment syndromes and volkmann contractures. In: Canale ST, ed. *Campbell's operative orthopaedics,* 10th ed. Philadelphia: Mosby; 2003.

92. Abouezzi Z, Nassoura Z, Ivatury RR, et al. A critical reappraisal of indications for fasciotomy after extremity vascular trauma. *Arch Surg.* 1998;133(5):547–551.

93. Mullins RJ, Lucas CE, Ledgerwood AM. The natural history following venous ligation for civilian injuries. *J Trauma.* 1980;20(9):737–743.

94. Meyer J, Walsh J, Schuler J, et al. The early fate of venous repair after civilian vascular trauma. A clinical, hemodynamic, and venographic assessment. *Ann Surg.* 1987;206(4):458–464.

95. Pappas PJ, Haser PB, Teehan EP, et al. Outcome of complex venous reconstructions in patients with trauma. *J Vasc Surg.* 1997;25(2):398–404.

96. Kuralay E, Demirkilic U, Ozal E, et al. A quantitative approach to lower extremity vein repair. *J Vasc Surg.* 2002;36(6):1213–1218.

97. Bermudez KM, Knudson MM, Nelken NA, et al. Long-term results of lower-extremity venous injuries. *Arch Surg.* 1997;132(9):963–967; discussion 7–8.

Editorial Comment

98. Hansen ST Jr. The type-IIIC tibial fracture: Salvage or amputation. *J Bone joint Surg Am.* 1987;69:799–800.

99. Gustilo RB, Mendoza RM, Williams DN. Problems in the management of type III (severe) open fractures: A new classification of type III open fractures. *J Trauma.* 1984;24:742–746.

100. Swiontkowski MF, MacKenzie EJ, Bosse MJ, et al. Factors influencing the decision to amputate or reconstruct after high-energy lower extremity trauma. *J Trauma.* 2002;52:641–649.

101. Bonanni F, Rhodes M, Lucke JF. The futility of predictive scoring of mangled lower extremities. *J Trauma.* 1993;34:99–104.

102. Pozo JL, Powell B, Hutton PAN, et al. The timing of amputation for lower limb trauma. *J Bone Joint Surg Br.* 1990;72B:288–292.

103. Roessler MS, Wisner DH, Holcroft JW. The mangled extremity: When to amputate? *Arch Surg.* 1991;126:1243–1249.

104. Lange RH. Limb reconstruction versus amputation decision making in massive lower extremity trauma. *Clin Orthop.* 1989;243:92–99.

105. Johansen K, Daines M, Howey T, et al. Objective criteria accurately predict amputation following lower extremity trauma. *J Trauma.* 1990;30:568–573.

106. Matsen SL, Malchow D, Matsen FA III. Correlations with patients' perspectives of the result of lower-extremity amputation. *J Bone Joint Surg Am.* 2000;82:1089–1095.

107. Dagum AB, Best AK, Schemitsch EH, et al. Salvage after severe lower-extremity trauma: Are the outcomes worth the means? *Plast Reconstr Surg* 1999;103:1212–1220.

108. Bondurant FJ, Cotler HB, Buckle R, et al. The medical and economic impact of severely injured lower extremities. *J Trauma.* 1988;23:1270–1273.

109. Butcher JL, MacKenzie EJ, Cushing B, et al. Long-term outcomes after lower extremity trauma. *J Trauma.* 1996;41:4–9.

110. Georgiadis GM, Behrens FF, Joyce MJ, et al. Open tibial plateau fractures with severe soft-tissue loss. Limb salvage compared with below-the-knee amputation. *J Bone Joint Surg Am.* 1993;75A:1431–1442.

111. MacKenzie EJ, Burgess AR, McAndrew MP, et al. Patient oriented functional outcome after unilateral lower extremity fracture. *J Trauma.* 1993;7:393–401.

112. Fairhurst MJ. The function of below-knee amputee versus the patient with salvaged grade III tibial fracture. *Clin Orthop.* 1994;301:227–232.

113. Caudle RJ, Stern PF. Severe open fractures of the tibia. *J Bone joint Surg Am.* 1987;69:801–807.

114. Pierce RO Jr, Kernek CB, Ambrose TA II. The plight of the traumatic amputee. *Orthopedics.* 1993;16:793–797.

Fractures of the Upper Extremity

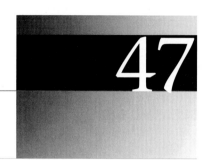

David A. Volgas   *Rena L. Stewart*

Fractures of the upper extremity occur in approximately one third of all multitrauma patients. These injuries will have a profound impact on the patient's recovery because they often preclude the use of crutches and even wheelchairs. Injuries to the upper extremity associated with blunt trauma are indicative of injury to deeper structures such as lung and heart. The trauma surgeon must look past the obvious deformity or blood and focus on the deeper structures which may endanger the patient's life. In general, fractures of the upper extremity heal within 6 to 8 weeks. The section will describe the various types of upper extremity fractures, the operative indications, and general approach to the management of these injuries.

FRACTURES OF THE SCAPULAR BODY

The scapula is a flat bone that lies approximately 30 degrees to the chest wall posteriorly. It is quite mobile under normal circumstances. It is very thin, in most places only 1 mm thick. It is covered by the origin of the rotator cuff muscles anteriorly and posteriorly. Also, the medial border serves as the insertion of the rhomboids and levator scapula and more inferiorly of the serratus muscles. Fractures can be adequately imaged by standard radiography and it is rare that a computed tomography (CT) scan is needed.

Scapula fractures occur as a result of direct penetrating trauma such as a gunshot wound or, more commonly, as a result of blunt trauma to the chest wall and shoulder. Because they are generally treated nonoperatively, their greatest importance is that they are a harbinger of significant thoracic trauma. The presence of a scapula fracture should lead the surgeon to consider other diagnoses

such as pulmonary contusion, multiple rib fractures, pneumothorax, or cardiac contusion.

Treatment typically consists of sling immobilization for comfort as well as early range of motion exercises. On rare occasions, fragments of the scapula can be oriented at right angles to their normal position and may cause skin breakdown or lung penetration. They may prompt the orthopaedic surgeon to perform an open reduction or excision of the offending fragment.

SCAPULOTHORACIC DISSOCIATION

Scapulothoracic injuries are rare but serious injuries which indicate tremendously high-energy trauma.[1] They are generally caused by a traction injury to the upper extremity and involve the near-amputation of the shoulder girdle from the torso. They can be life threatening when the injury causes disruption of the subclavian vein or artery.[2,3] Morbidity is universal even with prompt recognition and treatment. Vascular injury occurs in >80%,[3] while permanent neurologic injury occurs in 94%. There is a 10% mortality associated with these injuries primarily due to hemorrhagic shock. The diagnosis may be delayed when the injury is a closed injury. The telltale radiographic sign of lateralization of the scapula may be overlooked if there is a low index of suspicion.

A vascular surgeon or an experienced trauma surgeon should be called immediately if scapulothoracic dissociation is suspected.[4] Repair is difficult, because of the traction nature of the vascular injury. There is often a wide zone of injury to the artery and there may be persistent vasospasm. Additionally, the vein may be torn from its origin or in the axilla. A wide approach, which may include a supraclavicular approach, may be required. The clavicle may be divided with a saw to permit better visualization of the vessels as they travel laterally.

GLENOID FRACTURE

Glenoid fractures are uncommon fractures of the scapula. They are generally caused by direct blunt trauma to the chest wall and may therefore be a sign of more significant injury to the lungs. In isolation, glenoid fractures can often be managed nonoperatively, but when displaced >2 mm, they may require operative treatment. Operative treatment can safely be delayed 10 to 14 days to allow recovery from the associated lung injury. The surgical approach is normally posterior, with the patient in a lateral decubitus position for 2 to 4 hours, depending on the experience of the surgeon.

CLAVICLE FRACTURES

The clavicle is an "S" shaped bone which articulates the sternum medially (the sternoclavicular joint) and the acromion laterally (the acromioclavicular or A-C joint). The function of the clavicle is to both suspend the shoulder and to act as a strut to keep the shoulder at an appropriate distance away from the body. Clavicle fractures are the most common fracture in the human body, comprising 3% to 10% of all fractures.[5] They are seen most frequently in young, active individuals and result from force applied to the upper extremity and transmitted to the thorax or, infrequently, a direct blow to the clavicle.[6,7] Although only a small percentage of clavicle fractures are "open" or "compound" injuries, the open clavicle fracture should alert the trauma surgeon to the possibility of concomitant life-threatening injury. The largest review of this topic revealed that open clavicle fractures are associated with head injury in 65% of cases, pulmonary injury in 75%, spine fractures in 35%, and facial trauma in 55%.[8] Like all

open fractures, open fractures of the clavicle are surgical emergencies.

In the past, clavicle fractures were thought to be a benign injury and were treated almost exclusively nonoperatively. This treatment strategy was based on early reports that showed that virtually all clavicles "healed" with nonunion rates of <1%.[9] However, surgeons are now rethinking the treatment of these common injuries as new data comes to light regarding functional outcomes and union rates. An understanding of this paradigm shift is important for the general surgeon treating trauma patients. The traumatologist is frequently the only surgeon caring for a patient with a clavicle fracture, because orthopaedic consultation has traditionally been rare for closed clavicle fractures. New evidence suggests that referral to an orthopaedic surgeon for evaluation of most clavicle fractures is extremely important.

There are two significant problems with nonoperative treatment of clavicle fractures, particularly fractures which are significantly displaced (usually shortened). The first factor is that careful review of existing literature reveals a much higher rate of nonunion than previously thought. In a systematic review of all English literature, the Evidence-Based Orthopaedic Trauma Working Group revealed that the nonunion rate is actually 6% for all fractures and rises to 15% for displaced fractures, more than 10 times the rate previously thought.[10] The second factor encouraging more frequent operative management is that patients are much less satisfied with the outcomes of nonoperative management than previously believed.[7,11–14] A study of "healed" fractures revealed that at >4 years after the fracture, 50% of patients were partially or totally dissatisfied with their outcome and 40% had been unable to return to their previous work.[15] This poor functional outcome for patients is related to the fact that displaced clavicle fractures heal in a shortened position and cause significant changes in the biomechanical functioning of the shoulder (see Fig. 1).

Evaluation of clavicle fractures should include careful examination of the neurologic and vascular status of the upper extremity and also of the skin overlying the

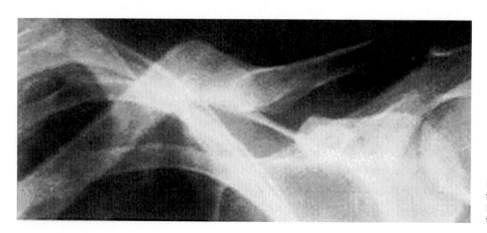

Figure 1 A "healed" clavicle fracture after nonoperative treatment. Note the significant shortening of the clavicle.

clavicle to look for "skin tenting." While almost all clavicle fractures will cause swelling and some stretching of the skin over the displaced fragments, true skin tenting is rare and represents a serious condition requiring urgent orthopaedic consultation. If the skin is blanched or necrotic, an orthopaedic surgeon should be summoned without delay. In the past, treatment with a figure-of-eight brace was thought to pull clavicle fractures back into a better position and thereby remove the pressure on the skin. Studies have shown that this is not the case and fracture position is unchanged with the use of a figure-of-eight brace (compared to a simple sling).[16] This type of brace is also extremely uncomfortable and results in high rates of patient dissatisfaction. Therefore, treatment with figure-of-eight brace has largely been abandoned. Nonoperative management now consists of treatment in a sling for a short period of time (not more than 2 weeks) followed by early range of motion exercises.

Operative management has recently been shown in a randomized controlled trial to yield superior results for displaced clavicle fractures.[17] Therefore, referral to an orthopaedic surgeon is appropriate for virtually all clavicle fractures, with the possible exception of nondisplaced fractures. Although no consensus exists on the definition on a "displaced fracture," there is agreement that any fracture that has shortened >1 cm and/or displaced more than the width of the clavicle should be evaluated by an orthopaedic surgeon (see Fig. 2A). Several methods of operative fixation of clavicle fractures exist including plates and screws (most common) (see Fig. 2B) and screws or pins placed in the central medullary cavity of the bone.[17-21]

SHOULDER DISLOCATION

Shoulder dislocations are common and are often seen as a result of a sports-related injury. They may also occur during falls (especially in the elderly), after high-energy impacts, or after seizures. The most common dislocation is anteroinferior. Rarely, a posterior dislocation may occur and it is most often seen after seizures or electric shock. The rarest dislocation is a straight inferior dislocation, termed *luxatio erecta*, because the patient presents with the arm fully raised, as if raising the hand in class.

Treatment is normally simple and most emergency department physicians are comfortable with the reduction. After conscious sedation, a sheet is looped around the torso under the arm of the affected side. An assistant is asked to provide countertraction by simply pulling on the sheet from the other side of the patient, whereas the surgeon grasps the arm with the elbow in extension and the arm abducted approximately 30 degrees. Moderate traction and adequate sedation will usually accomplish the reduction. Pain relief is immediate after reduction. Alternatively, a 10-lb weight can be tied to the arm while the patient is lying prone on a gurney or table with the arm hanging down. After approximately 10 to 15 minutes, with adequate sedation, the shoulder will spontaneously reduce.

If the shoulder cannot be reduced, an orthopaedic surgeon should be contacted. Postreduction treatment depends on the patient's age. Young patients have a much higher redislocation rate than older patients. Because of this, many orthopaedic surgeons recommend operative treatment to reinforce the anterior capsule acutely, but others prefer to give 6 weeks of physical therapy and only consider surgical treatment if the patient dislocates a second time. A shoulder immobilizer or sling is used until the patient can follow up with an orthopaedic surgeon.

Complications of shoulder dislocation include redislocation, axillary nerve injury, and musculoskeletal nerve injury. Vascular injuries are rare, but may occur.[22-25] Most commonly venous thrombosis may occur, more commonly with luxatio erecta. Pseudoaneurysm of the axillary or brachial artery has also been reported.

THE "FLOATING SHOULDER"

The *floating shoulder* is a term used to describe ipsilateral fractures of the clavicle and glenoid neck. This injury is uncommon and treatment is controversial. Some surgeons advocate repair of one of the fractures to restore the shoulder girdle,[26] whereas others advocate nonoperative treatment for both fractures.[27] The consensus appears to be that operative fixation is reserved for fractures with marked displacement.[26,28,29]

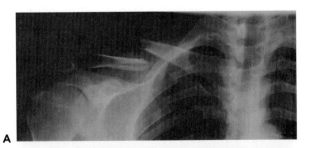

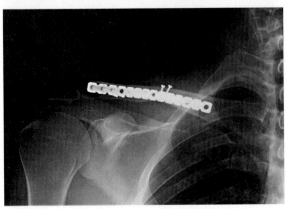

Figure 2 **A:** A displaced clavicle fracture. Referral to an orthopaedic surgeon is appropriate. **B:** Fixation of a displaced clavicle fracture using plate and screws.

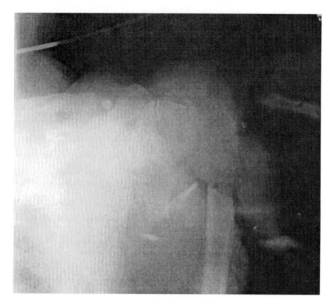

Figure 3   A comminuted proximal humerus fracture.

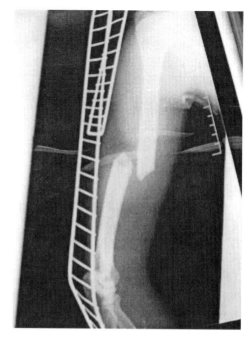

Figure 4   Midshaft humerus fracture at the level of the spiral groove where the radial nerve passes close to bone.

PROXIMAL HUMERUS FRACTURES

Fractures of the proximal humerus are very common, especially in the elderly. All elderly or postmenopausal patients should be screened for osteoporosis. These fractures may also occur as a result of high-energy blunt (see Fig. 3) or penetrating trauma. Many of these fractures may be definitively treated nonoperatively; however, fractures which involve the shoulder joint or significant displacement will often require surgical intervention. In the acute setting, a sling is generally all that is required unless the joint cannot be reduced or there is an open fracture.

Nerve injuries can occur and usually involve the axillary nerve. This may be detected by examining the shoulder for decreased sensation over the lateral deltoid ("shoulder patch" distribution) or by palpating the deltoid muscle and asking the patient to contract the muscle. Arterial injuries (axillary or brachial artery) are reported, but rare.

MIDSHAFT HUMERUS FRACTURES

Fractures of the shaft of the humerus are common. They may be caused by blunt or penetrating trauma. They may be associated with other upper extremity injuries. Anatomically, the fractures often occur at the level of the spiral groove, which courses posteriorly approximately at the middle of the arm. The radial nerve travels against bone along this groove and is often injured by the fracture (see Fig. 4). Nerve injuries occur in approximately 12% of cases, but complete recovery of function is the rule.[30] Arterial injuries are uncommon with blunt injures, but do occur with penetrating injuries.

Isolated fractures of the humerus may be successfully treated nonoperatively in a clamshell splint (Sarmiento brace). Indications for operative management include the following:

- Multiple extremity fractures where the patient may need early use of the arm to assist with ambulation or transfer
- Morbidly obese patients
- Open fracture
- Markedly comminuted or segmental fractures
- Fractures with neurologic deficit which develops after an attempted reduction

Operative treatment may be performed with a plate and screws or an intramedullary nail at the surgeon's preference. Nonunion rates are low for nonoperatively treated fractures. Operatively treated fractures carry about the same rate of nonunions, 5%.

SIMPLE ELBOW DISLOCATIONS

Because elbow motion is complex (allowing both flexion/extension and rotation of the forearm), the anatomy is also complex. The elbow consists of a hinged joint formed by the distal humerus and the "C" shaped olecranon portion of the ulna. Of particular interest in high-energy trauma is the coronoid process of the olecranon, which is a frequently missed site of fracture leading to recurrent dislocation. The remainder of the elbow joint is made up of the radial head, which rotates against the proximal ulna to allow rotation of the forearm (see Fig. 5).

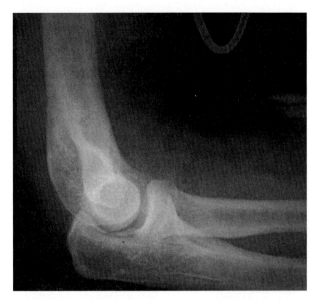

Figure 5 A lateral x-ray view of the normal elbow. Note the coronoid process at the anterior tip of the olecranon.

After the shoulder, dislocations of the elbow are the second most common dislocation in the upper extremity. Dislocations are classified as simple (dislocations without accompanying fracture) and complex (dislocations combined with fractures). The rate of complications for combined fracture-dislocations is higher than for simple dislocations.[31-35]

Treatment should consist of immediate reduction of the elbow if an orthopaedic surgeon is not readily available. This is normally accomplished quite easily with sedation of the patient and the simple maneuver of gentle longitudinal

traction on the arm, followed by flexion of the elbow. Once reduced, it is essential to obtain good quality radiographs to confirm that the joint is reduced and to look for other elbow injuries such as fractures that may be difficult to see when the elbow is dislocated. The patient should then undergo a detailed neurologic and vascular examination followed by splinting with the elbow at 90 degrees of flexion. Most simple dislocations are stable and after a brief period of splint immobilization (7 to 10 days) range of motion can begin. Immobilization for >3 weeks results in poorer outcome, therefore, follow-up with an orthopaedic surgeon should occur before this time (Josefsson,[32]).

COMPLEX ELBOW DISLOCATIONS, CORONOID FRACTURES, AND FRACTURES OF THE RADIAL HEAD

Dislocations of the elbow can be associated with fractures of the radial head or the coronoid process of the olecranon or both (the so-called terrible triad).[36-38] These "complex dislocations" are far less stable than simple dislocations, more difficult to treat, and have inferior outcomes. These injuries require surgical repair by an experienced orthopaedist and therefore prompt referral is necessary[38-40] (see Fig. 6A and B). Disaster can result from delays during which patients with complex dislocations can redislocate while in a splint.

FRACTURES OF THE OLECRANON

Olecranon fractures, like all injuries about the elbow, must begin early range of motion within 10 days of

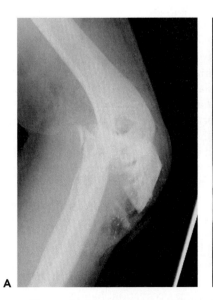

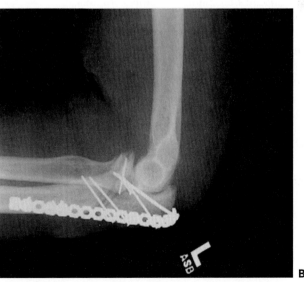

A   B

Figure 6 **A:** Complex open fracture/dislocation of the elbow including fracture of the olecranon, radial head and coronoid. This pattern is unstable and requires prompt orthopaedic consultation. **B:** Complex fracture/dislocation following surgical fixation of the olecranon, radial head and coronoid. Note the concentric reduction of the elbow joint.

the injury to achieve optimal functional results. The vast majority of olecranon fractures are displaced and therefore require surgical fixation to anatomically restore the joint surface and to provide sufficient stability for early motion.[41]

FRACTURES OF THE FOREARM

Fractures of the radius and ulna are common with >500,000 per year.[42] Falls are the most common mechanism of injury, with patients younger than 15 years accounting for 25% of these injuries.[42] In the forearm, the radius and ulna form a functional unit with the radius rotating about the ulna both proximally and distally to create forearm rotational movement. With the exception of isolated fractures of the ulna resulting from a direct blow (the "night-stick" fracture), injury of only one component of the forearm complex is rare. Therefore, when evaluating forearm fractures careful attention must be paid to the proximal and distal radioulnar joint to identify concomitant dislocations.

There are four major patterns of forearm fractures: fractures of the shaft of the radius and ulna (most common), isolated ulna fractures, fractures of the ulna combined with dislocation of the radial head (Monteggia fractures), and fractures of the radius combined with dislocation of the distal radioulnar joint at the wrist (Galeazzi fractures).

Evaluation of forearm fracture should include a careful neurologic examination, with particular attention to the function of the posterior interosseous nerve (PIN) branch of the radial nerve when the radial head is dislocated. High-energy trauma poses the risk of compartment syndrome and the patient should be carefully examined for this.[43] The forearm must be examined circumferentially for open fracture wounds. X-rays should be obtained of the forearm and also the elbow and/or wrist if there is suspicion of a proximal or distal radioulnar dislocation associated with the fracture.

Initial management should include splinting of the entire arm, which immobilizes both the wrist and the elbow. In adults, operative fixation of forearm fractures is indicated in virtually all cases so as to restore the complex biomechanics of the forearm.[44–47] For closed fractures, this surgery can be delayed for several days. Fractures combined with proximal or distal dislocations (Monteggia and Galeazzi fractures) are unstable and the joints will not remain reduced even with splinting. Therefore, these injuries require prompt surgical management. All open fractures require emergent surgical management. The cornerstone of surgical fixation of forearm fractures is with plates and screws, which allows for the anatomic restoration of the forearm biomechanics and early range of motion (see Fig. 7A and B).

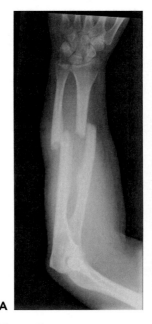
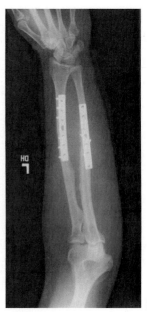

Figure 7 **A:** Fracture of the radius and ulna, the so-called both bone forearm fracture. **B:** Surgical stabilization of the both bone forearm fracture with plate and screws.

WRIST FRACTURES

Fractures of the distal radius and ulna (see Fig. 8) are among the most common fractures encountered in trauma, with approximately 2,000,000 occurring in 2004. They are often a result of a fall, but are also commonly associated with motor vehicle collisions. When encountered in elderly patients, they may be the initial sign of osteoporosis. Like fractures of the hip, proximal humerus, or spine in the elderly population, wrist fractures should prompt an osteoporosis workup.[48]

Many closed fractures are managed initially in the emergency department with closed reduction and casting or splinting. Conscious sedation is normally used for anesthesia. The reduction maneuver is typically to recreate the fracture, then pull longitudinal traction and finally to correct the dorsal angulation. Fractures which are minimally displaced initially will often be definitively managed with a cast. In highly comminuted fractures or in osteoporotic fractures, the closed reduction will often be lost over time.

If the fracture cannot be adequately reduced or is at high risk of losing the reduction, operative treatment is recommended. There are a variety of operative interventions and the choice of a particular procedure is largely a result of surgeon preference.[49] Surgeons will choose a particular method of operative treatment based on patient-related factors such as occupation, handedness, osteoporosis, comorbidities, and age. The first goal of treatment is to restore the normal anatomy to enable the highest function. The

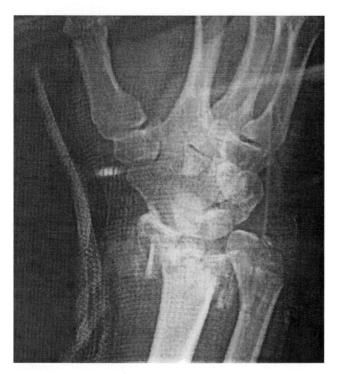

Figure 8   A highly comminuted distal radius fracture.

or excision may be used depending on the fracture pattern and size of the ulnar fragment.

Distal radius fractures are commonly closed, but open fractures can occur. When they occur, urgent irrigation and debridement are required. Nerve injuries often occur and usually involve the median nerve as it passes through the carpal tunnel. Decreased sensation in the thumb, index finger, and middle finger is a sign of a median nerve injury. The nerve should be decompressed as soon as practical to avoid permanent damage to the nerve and loss of thumb function. Loss of reduction is rare after plate fixation, but common when other methods of treatment are used. Nonunion and malunion occur, especially in comminuted fractures. Arterial injuries to the radial or ulnar nerve are uncommon. The ulnar artery is normally the dominant arterial supply to the hand. If the Allen test is abnormal, the diagnosis of vascular injury (spasm or laceration) is confirmed. As long as one of the two vessels is intact, the hand will be viable and the injured vessel can safely be ligated, although ligation of the ulnar artery may lead to some cold intolerance.

COMPARTMENT SYNDROME IN THE UPPER EXTREMITY

The pathophysiology of compartment syndrome is that of acute muscular and neural ischemia caused by elevated intramuscular pressure. This is caused either by muscle swelling or, less commonly, by external compression. Compartment syndrome in the upper extremity is much less well studied than in the lower extremity. However, many of the same risk factors apply and all are common in trauma patients. A variety of conditions may produce compartment syndrome including fractures, crush injuries, vascular injury, prolonged compression of the limb (such as entrapment), and penetrating trauma. The most important factor in making the correct diagnosis is a high index of suspicion. In any patient with a painful swollen limb, the diagnosis of compartment syndrome should be considered. It is also important to remember that the presence of an open fracture does not eliminate the risk of compartment syndrome but rather indicates an *increased* risk. In one study, 9% of open fracture patients also had compartment syndrome.[53] The diagnosis is made even more challenging in patients who are intubated, sedated, intoxicated, or otherwise unable to provide a reliable clinical examination.

The older teaching that the diagnosis of compartment syndrome should be based on the "5 'P's" (pain, pallor, pulselessness, paraesthesia, and paralysis) is no longer valid. All of these symptoms except pain are late findings and usually indicate that irreversible damage to muscle and nerve has already occurred. Therefore, the diagnosis should be made before these symptoms occur. "Pain out of proportion to the injury" is frequently described as a

second goal is to provide early rigid fixation to allow for early range of motion treatment and thereby prevent stiffness, which is common after wrist fractures.

External fixation may be used either for intraoperative traction to allow better reduction of the fracture and provide some stability while the plate is applied, or as definitive fixation in older patients, or where there is significant destruction of the joint. Percutaneous pinning is sometimes used to augment a reduction which is suspected of being too unstable to be treating in a cast, but not so unstable as to require a plate.[50]

Plate osteosynthesis is used for many intra-articular fractures or fractures which are unstable because of comminution. Reduction of the articular surface to <2 mm of displacement is considered standard of care in young patients.[51] In addition to articular displacement, attention must be paid to restoring radial height, ulnar inclination, and volar tilt. Failure to achieve adequate reduction will lead to loss of motion, early arthritis, and pain. Volar plates are currently favored so as to avoid the problems encountered with dorsal plates, joint stiffness, pain, and tendon rupture.[52] Techniques continue to change rapidly in response to the development of new plates, which attempt to gain better fixation by anatomically directing screws into good bone and locking the screws to the plate to avoid toggle of the screws within the plate. Fixation that is strong enough to allow early full range of motion is the goal for plate fixation. The ulnar fracture is repaired if it remains displaced after reduction of the radius. Wires, plates, suture, reliable symptom but this is difficult to quantify in the face of severe and multiple injuries. More helpful is "pain on passive stretch." This test is performed by having the examiner passively flex the fingers (to examine the extensor muscles of the forearm) and then extend the fingers (to examine the flexor compartment forearm muscles). This is a completely passive stretch, the patient does not move the fingers actively, and any fractures present must be stabilized while the test is performed. This test should be performed on all awake patients who are at any risk for compartment syndrome. If increased pressure exists within the muscle compartments, this test will be exquisitely painful.

The diagnosis of compartment syndrome can be made on clinical findings alone. For example, a patient whose arm has been severely crushed for an extended period of time beneath an overturned car who then develops severe swelling, pain, and severe pain on passive stretch clearly has a compartment syndrome. In such a patient, no further time should be wasted performing further tests before the patient is taken urgently to the operating room. In cases that are less clear, a suspicious clinical picture can be confirmed by measurement of the compartment pressure. This can be done with a portable compartment pressure monitor or by using a large bore needle connected to a central venous pressure (CVP) or arterial pressure monitor. In patients who are intubated or sedated, a catheter can be left in place for continuous monitoring. It is important to measure the pressure at several sites within the arm and forearm. The safest "threshold" for diagnosing compartment syndrome is the perfusion pressure or "δ P." This is calculated as

$$\delta P = \text{diastolic blood pressure} - \text{compartment pressure}$$

Prompt fasciotomy should be performed when the δ P (perfusion pressure) is <30 mm Hg (McQueen, 1996). Fasciotomy of the upper extremity should release all of the compartments completely, including release of the carpal tunnel and lacertus fibrosis at the elbow. Fasciotomies should be left open and closed or covered at a later time. Consultation with an orthopaedic or hand surgeon is very appropriate.

It is essential to remember that irreversible muscle and nerve damage occurs at 6 hours of ischemic time. Therefore, the diagnosis and timely treatment of compartment syndrome should be considered "limb saving" surgery. A high index of suspicion must be accompanied by prompt transfer of the trauma patient to the operating room if compartment syndrome is to be treated successfully. In rare cases where a patient is too unstable to be moved to the operating room, fasciotomies can be performed at the bedside.

REFERENCES

1. Estrada LS, Alonso J, Rue LW III. Continuum between scapulothoracic dissociation and traumatic forequarter amputation: A review of the literature. *Am Surg.* 2001;67(9):868–872.
2. Clements RH, Reisser JR. Scapulothoracic dissociation: A devastating injury. *J Trauma.* 1996;40(1):146–149.
3. Damschen DD, Cogbill TH, Siegel MJ. Scapulothoracic dissociation caused by blunt trauma. *J Trauma.* 1997;42(3):537–540.
4. Katsamouris AN, Kafetzakis A, Kostas T, et al. The initial management of scapulothoracic dissociation: Challenging task for the vascular surgeon. *Eur J Vasc Endovasc Surg.* 2002;24(6):547–549.
5. Nordqvist A, Petersson C. The incidence of fractures of the clavicle. *Clin Orthop Relat Res.* 1994;300:127–132.
6. Crenshaw AH. Fractures of the shoulder girdle, arm and forearm. In: Crenshaw AH, ed. *Campbell's operative orthopaedics*, 8th ed. St. Louis: Mosby–Year Book; 1992:989–1053.
7. Robinson CM, Cairns DA. Primary nonoperative treatment of displaced lateral fractures of the clavicle. *J Bone Joint Surg.* 2004; 86–A:778–782.
8. Taitsman LA, Nork SE, Coles CP, et al. Open clavicle fractures and associated injuries. *J Orthop Trauma.* 2006;20:396–399.
9. Neer CS II. Nonunion of the clavicle. *JAMA.* 1960;172:1006–1011.
10. Zlowodzki M, Zelle BA, Cole PA, et al. Treatment of the acute midshaft clavicle fractures; systematic review of 2144 fractures. *On behalf of the evidence-based orthopaedic trauma working group.* *J Orthop Trauma.* 2005;19(7):504–507.
11. Hill JM, McGuire MH, Crosby LA. Closed treatment of displaced middle-third fractures of the clavicle gives poor results. *J Bone Joint Surg.* 1997;79–B:537–539.
12. Lazrides S, Zafiropulos G. Conservative treatment of fractures at the middle third of the clavicle: The relevance of shortening and clinical outcomes. *J Shoulder Elbow Surg.* 2006;15(2):191–194.
13. Nordqvist A, Redlund-Johnell I, von Scheele A, et al. Shortening of clavicle fracture: Incidence and clinical significance, a 5-year follow-up of 85 patients. *Acta Orthop Scand.* 1997;68(4):349–351.
14. Nordqvist A, Petersson CJ, Redlund-Johnell I. Mid-clavicle fractures in adults: End results study after conservative treatment. *J Orthop Trauma.* 1998;12(8):572–576.
15. McKee MD, Pedersen EM, Jones C, et al. Deficits following nonoperative treatment of displaced midshaft clavicular fractures. *J Bone Joint Surg.* 2006;88:35–40.
16. Anderson K, Jensen PO, Lauritzen J. Treatment of clavicular fractures. Figure-of-eight bandage versus a simple sling. *Acta Orthop Scand.* 1987;58:71–74.
17. Canadian Orthopaedic Trauma Society. Nonoperative treatment compared with plate fixation of displaced midshaft clavicular fractures. *J Bone Joint Surg.* 2007;89(1):1–10.
18. Chuang T, Ho W, Hsieh P, et al. Closed reduction and internal fixation for acute midshaft clavicular fractures using cannulated screws. *J Trauma.* 2006;60(6):1315–1321.
19. Denard PJ, Koval KJ, Cantu RV, et al. Management of midshaft clavicle fractures in adults. *Am J Orthop.* 2005;527–536.
20. Haidar SG, Krishnan KM, Deshmukh SC. Hook plate fixation for type II fractures of the lateral end of the clavicle. *J Shoulder Elbow Surg.* 2006;15(4):419–423.
21. Jackson WFM, Bayne G, Gregg-Smith SJ. Fractures of the lateral third of the clavicle: An anatomic approach to treatment. *J Trauma.* 2006;61:222–225.
22. Maweja S, Sakalihasan N, Van Damme H, et al. Axillary artery injury secondary to anterior shoulder dislocation: Report of two cases. *Acta Chir Belg.* 2002;102(3):187–191.
23. Popescu D, Fernandez-Valencia JA, Combalia A. Axillary arterial thrombosis secondary to anterior shoulder dislocation. *Acta Orthop Belg.* 2006;72(5):637–640.
24. Stahnke M, Duddy MJ. Endovascular repair of a traumatic axillary pseudoaneurysm following anterior shoulder dislocation. *Cardiovasc Intervent Radiol.* 2006;29(2):298–301.
25. Tsutsumi K, Saito H, Ohkura M. Traumatic pseudoaneurysm of the subclavian artery following anterior dislocation of the shoulder: A report of a surgical case. *Ann Thorac Cardiovasc Surg.* 2006; 12(1):74–76.
26. Owens BD, Goss TP. The floating shoulder. *J Bone Joint Surg Br.* 2006;88(11):1419–1424.
27. Edwards G, Whittle AP, Wood GW II. Nonoperative treatment of ipsilateral fractures of the scapula and clavicle. *J Bone Joint Surg Am.* 2000;82(6):774–780.

28. Egol KA, Connor PM, Karanuakar MA, et al. The floating shoulder: Clinical and functional results. *J Bone Joint Surg Am.* 2001;83–A(8): 1188–1194.

29. Pasapula C, Mandalia V, Aslam N. The floating shoulder. *Acta Orthop Belg.* 2004;70(5):393–400.

30. Shao YC, Harwood P, Grotz MR, et al. Radial nerve palsy associated with fractures of the shaft of the humerus: A systematic review. *J Bone Joint Surg Br.* 2005;87(12):1647–1652.

31. Hildebrand KA, Patterson SD, King GJ. Acute elbow dislocations: Simple and complex. *Orthop Clin North Am.* 1999;30(1):63–79.

32. Josefsson PO, Johnell O, Gentz CF. Long term sequealae of simple dislocation of the elbow. *J Bone Joint Surg Am.* 1984;66: 927–930.

33. McKee MD, Jupiter JB. Trauma to the adult elbow and fractures of the distal humerus. In: Browner B, Jupiter JB, Levine A, et al. eds. *Skeletal trauma,* Vol. 2. Philadelphia: WB Saunders; 2001: 1455–1522.

34. Ring D, Jupiter JB. Fracture dislocation of the elbow: Current concepts review. *J Bone Joint Surg Am.* 1998;80(14):566–580.

35. Schmeling GJ. Elbow and forearm: Adult trauma. In: Koval KJ, ed. *Orthopaedic knowledge update 7.* Rosemont: American Academy of Orthopaedic Surgeons; 2002:307–316.

36. Cook RE, McKee MD. Techniques to tame the terrible triad: Unstable fracture dislocations of the elbow. *Op Tech Orthop.* 2003;13(2): 130–137.

37. Frankle MA, Koval KJ, Sanders RW, et al. Radial head fractures with dislocations treated by immediate stabilization and early motion. *J Shoulder Elbow Surg.* 1999;8:355–356.

38. Ring D, Jupiter JB, Zilberfarb J. Posterior dislocation of the elbow with fractures of the radial head and coronoid. *J Bone Joint Surg Am.* 2002;84–A:547–551.

39. Pugh DM, Wild LM, Schemitsch EH, et al. Standard surgical protocol to treat elbow dislocations with radial head and coronoid fractures. *J Bone Joint Surg Am.* 2004;86–A:1122–1130.

40. King GJW, Evans DC, Kellam JF. Open reduction and internal fixation of radial head fractures. *J Orthop Trauma.* 1991;5(1): 21–28.

41. Bailey CS, MacDermid J, Patterson SD, et al. Outcome of the plate fixation of olecranon fractures. *J Orthop Trauma.* 2001;15: 542–548.

42. Chung KC, Spilson SV. The frequency and epidemiology of hand and forearm fractures in the United States: Abstract. *J Hand Surg [Am].* 2001;26:908–915.

43. McQueen MM, Gaston P, Court-Brown CM. Acute compartment syndrome: Who is at risk? *J Bone Joint Surg Br.* 2000;82: 200–203.

44. Chapman MW, Gordon JE, Zissimos AG. Compression-plate fixations of acute fractures of the diaphysis of the radius and ulna. *J Bone Joint Surg Am.* 1989;71:159–169.

45. Moed BR, Kellam FJ, Foster JR, et al. Immediate Internal fixation of open fractures of the diaphysis of the forearm. *J Bone Joint Surg Am.* 1986;68:1008–1017.

46. Burwell HN, Charnley AD. Treatment of forearm fractures in adults with particular reference to plate fixation. *J Bone Joint Surg Br.* 1964;46:404–425.

47. Yasutomi T, Nakatsuchi Y, Koike H, et al. Mechanism of limitation of pronation/supination of the forearm in geometric models of deformities of the forearm bones. *Clin Biomech (Bristol, Avon).* 2002;17:456–463.

48. Court-Brown CM, Caesar B. Epidemiology of adult fractures: A review. *Injury.* 2006;37(8):691–697.

49. Simic PM, Weiland AJ. Fractures of the distal aspect of the radius: Changes in treatment over the past two decades. *Instr Course Lect.* 2003;52:185–195.

50. Rosati M, Bertagnini S, Digrandi G, et al. Percutaneous pinning for fractures of the distal radius. *Acta Orthop Belg.* 2006;72(2): 138–146.

51. Knirk JL, Jupiter JB. Intra-articular fractures of the distal end of the radius in young adults. *J Bone Joint Surg Am.* 1986;68(5): 647–659.

52. Tavakolian JD, Jupiter JB. Dorsal plating for distal radius fractures. *Hand Clin.* 2005;21(3):341–346.

53. Blick SS, Brumback RJ, Poka A, et al. Compartment syndrome in open tibial fractures. *J Bone Joint Surg Am.* 1986;68(9):1348–1353.

Hand Injuries

48

Allan Durkin   David Halpern   Richard D. Klein

The human hand is a marriage of form and function. It allows us to interact and react to our environment with efficiency and accuracy. Because of its vulnerable position, it is commonly injured at both work and play. Hand injuries are, for the most part, nonlethal, but they have potential for significant morbidity due to loss of function. This morbidity can largely be avoided by timely, appropriate management of these injuries. This chapter will review the fundamentals of hand anatomy and physiology, as well as the management principles for common injuries.

ANATOMY AND PHYSIOLOGY

The human hand is a symphony of bones, muscles, nerves, and tendons, and each of these components is critical for efficient function.

Bony Anatomy

The hand consists of five fingers—thumb, index, long, ring, and small fingers. Each digit holds two major neurovascular bundles on its ulnar and radial aspects. In these bundles lie the proper digital arteries, veins, and nerves. The bony platform of each finger consists of three nonsesamoid phalanx bones with the exception of the thumb, which harbors only two. The phalangeal bones of the hand articulate with five metacarpal bones, which connect the fingers to the base of the hand. The base of the hand consists of eight carpal bones. Traveling radial to ulnar, proximal to distal, the eight carpal bones are the: (i) scaphoid (ii) lunate, (iii) triquetrum, (iv) pisiform, (v) trapezium, (vi) trapezoid, (vii) capitate, and (viii) hamate bones (see Fig. 1). The carpal bones articulate with the radius and ulnar bones, and are supported laterally by a triangular shaped fibrocartilaginous complex, and anteriorly by a complex of ligaments extending from the distal radius into the base

of the hand. An important bony structure is the Guyon canal. This bony conduit lies between the pisiform and the hook of the hamate bone. It provides an access route for the ulnar artery and nerve at the base of the hypothenar eminence.

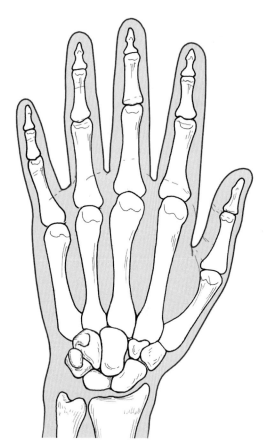

Figure 1 Bony structure of the hand. The eight carpal bones from proximal to distal, radial to ulnar are (i) scaphoid, lunate, triquetrum, and pisiform (proximal row) and (ii) trapezium, trapezoid, capitate, and hamate.

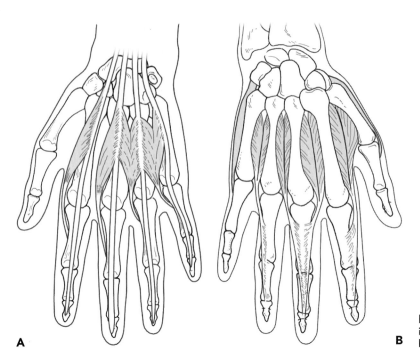

A

B

Figure 2 **A:** Intrinsic muscles of the hand—interosseous muscles. **B:** Intrinsic muscles of the hand—lumbrical muscles.

Muscle Anatomy

The hand is acted upon by both intrinsic and extrinsic muscles, the extrinsic muscles having the muscle belly within the forearm. The intrinsic muscles are the: (i) thenar, (ii) hypothenar, (iii) lumbrical, and (iv) the palmar and dorsal interossei muscle groups (see Fig. 2). There are three thenar muscles: (i) opponens pollicis, (ii) flexor pollicis brevis (deep and superficial heads), and (iii) abductor pollicis brevis. These three muscles are innervated by the median nerve. There are three hypothenar muscles: (i) abductor digiti minimi, (ii) flexor digiti minimi, and (iii) the opponens digiti minimi. These three muscles are innervated by the ulnar nerve. There are four lumbricals, two of which are innervated by the median nerve on the radial side of the hand, and two of which are innervated by the ulnar nerve on the ulnar side of the hand. These muscles originate from the flexor digitorum profundus as it courses from the wrist toward the distal phalanx. Cumulatively, these muscles provide flexion at the metacarpophalangeal joint, as well as extension at the interphalangeal joint.

The interosseous muscles are innervated exclusively by the ulnar nerve. They are divided into two groups—the dorsal and palmar interossei. The dorsal interossei consists of four muscles, and provides abduction of the index, middle, and ring fingers. The palmar interossei consists of three muscles, and allows adduction of the small, index, and ring fingers toward the middle finger.

The extrinsic muscles of the hand impact on both wrist and digit motion. They are subclassified into anterior (flexor) (see Fig. 3) and posterior (extensor) compartment groups (see Fig. 4), with the intrinsic muscles having their muscle belly within the hand itself. The anterior

compartment is conventionally divided into three separate muscle groups: (i) superficial, (ii) middle, and (iii) deep. With the exception of the palmaris longus tendon, all tendons of these muscles traverse the wrist deep to the flexor retinaculum. The superficial flexor muscles are the flexor carpi radialis, flexor carpi ulnaris, and palmaris longus. These muscles are innervated by the median nerve, with the exception of the flexor carpi ulnaris, which is innervated by the ulnar nerve. The middle flexors consist of the flexor digitorum superficialis, which is also innervated by the median nerve. This muscle terminates in four separate tendons, which themselves bifurcate at the middle phalanx of the medial four fingers (all except the thumb). At the middle phalanx, the tendon inserts into the medial and lateral surface of the bone. The chiasm generated by the split in the distal superficialis tendon creates a small conduit, through which the flexor digitorum profundus tendons travel to insert on the distal phalanx. The deep flexor muscles are the flexor digitorum profundus, the flexor pollicis longus, and the pronator teres. The flexor digitorum profundus is innervated by the median nerve on the radial side and the ulnar nerve on the ulnar side, whereas the flexor pollicis longus and pronator teres are innervated by the anterior interosseous branch of the median nerve.

The extensor (posterior) compartment is classified by function and is categorized as: (i) hand motion at level of wrist, (ii) finger motion, and (iii) thumb motion. All muscle tendons enter the hand deep to the extensor retinaculum. Hand motion at the wrist is generated by three muscles: (i) extensor carpi radialis longus, (ii) extensor carpi radialis brevis, and (iii) extensor carpi ulnaris. The extensor carpi radialis longus is innervated by the radial nerve, whereas

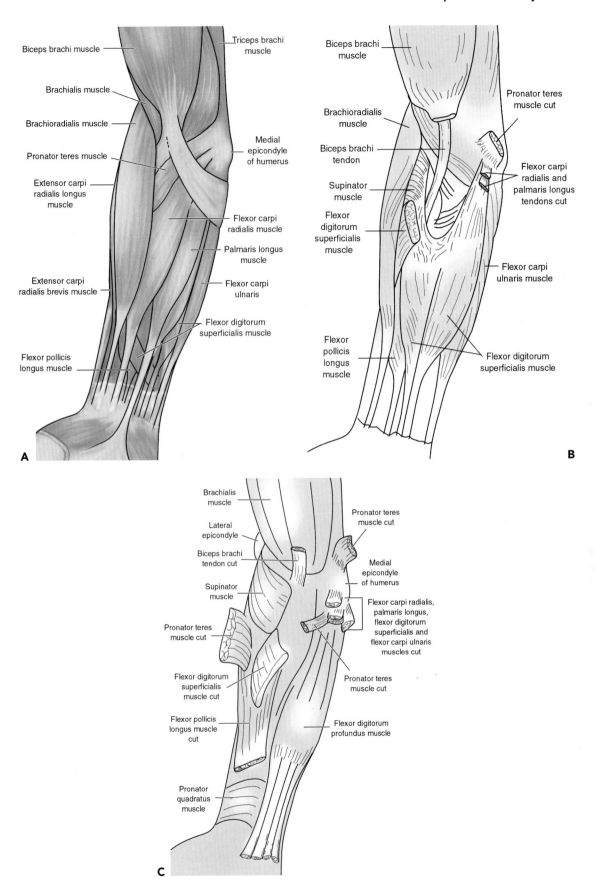

Figure 3   A: Superficial extrinsic flexors of the hand. **B:** Intermediate extrinsic flexors of the hand. **C:** Deep extrinsic flexors of the hand.

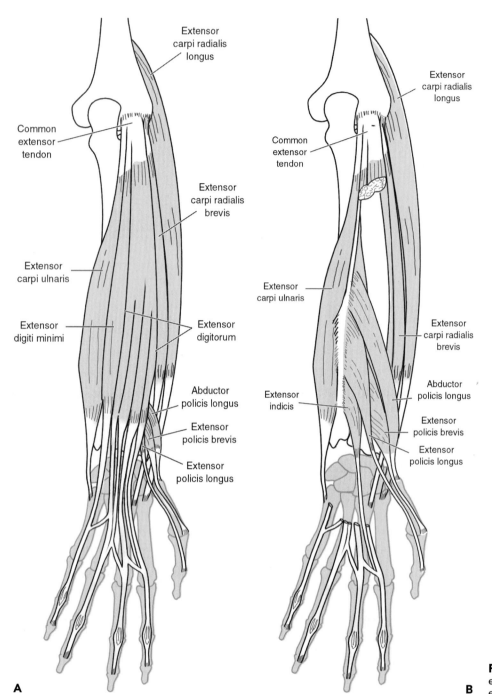

Extensor
carpi radialis
longus

Common
extensor
tendon

Extensor
carpi radialis
brevis

Extensor
carpi ulnaris

Extensor
digiti minimi

Extensor
digitorum

Abductor
policis longus

Extensor
policis brevis

Extensor
policis longus

Extensor
carpi radialis
longus

Common
extensor
tendon

Extensor
carpi ulnaris

Extensor
indicis

Extensor
carpi radialis
brevis

Abductor
policis longus

Extensor
policis brevis

Extensor
policis longus

A

B

Figure 4 **A:** Superficial extrinsic extensors of the hand. **B:** Deep extrinsic extensors of the hand.

the two remaining muscles are innervated by the posterior interosseous branch of the radial nerve. Finger motion is generated by three muscles: (i) extensor indicis, (ii) extensor digitorum profundus, and (iii) the extensor digiti minimi. These three muscles are exclusively innervated by the posterior interosseous branch of the radial nerve. Thumb motion is generated by three muscles: (i) extensor pollicis brevis, (ii) abductor pollicis longus, and (iii) the extensor pollicis longus. These three muscles are also innervated by the posterior interosseous nerve. The anterior interosseous nerve is a branch of the median nerve, whereas the posterior

interosseous nerves correspond to the deep branch of the radial nerve.

Vascular

The radial and ulnar arteries provide two major conduits for arterial inflow to the hand. (see Fig. 5) These arteries form two separate arterial arcades—the superficial and deep palmar arches. The superficial arch is primarily supplied by the ulnar artery, whereas the deep arch is primarily supplied by the radial artery. These arches supply the common digital

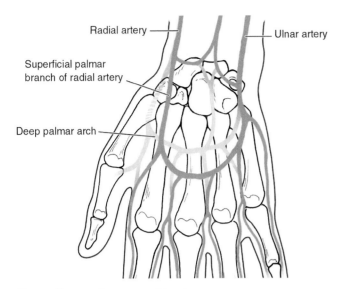

Radial artery

Ulnar artery

Superficial palmar branch of radial artery

Deep palmar arch

Figure 5 Vascular system of hand.

arteries and the princeps pollicis artery to the thumb. These common digital arteries and the princeps pollicis artery then bifurcate and extend medially and laterally along the long axis of each digit, thereby becoming the proper digital arteries. Loss of one digital bundle will not compromise digital vascular inflow resulting in clinically evident ischemia.

PHYSICAL EXAMINATION

Injuries to the human hand are rarely life threatening. However, patients who have sustained injury to their hand commonly present with other injuries. It is crucial for the surgeon to not lose sight of this, and concentrate on an obvious hand injury, and undertriage simultaneous injury.

After completing standardized primary and secondary trauma surveys, and assuring that all life-threatening injuries have been addressed, an accurate history regarding the injury should be taken. Of note, the physician should determine early on as to whether the patient injured his/her dominant or nondominant hand. The physician should attempt to define the mechanism of injury (i.e., crush, laceration, burn, etc.), and its perceived effect by the patient. An attempt to define the exact position and orientation of the hand at the time of injury should be made. By so doing, significant clues toward injured internal structures can be determined. Next, define how the patient feels his/her hand. Do they have normal sensation and movement? If not, how does it differ? Again, an adequate catalog of these characteristics offers insight regarding internal damage. The magnitude of injury should also be addressed. Injury from engine-powered machinery will produce a deeper injury pattern in most cases than hand-powered machinery. The time of injury should be accurately recorded, as well as the time evaluated. This time interval can be critical, especially

if ischemia is involved. The patient should be asked about any prior hand injuries. Finally, an accurate determination of pertinent medical comorbidities should be undertaken.

The examination of the hand begins with inspection. First, observe the hand in its resting position, and then examine the hand for active function by having the patient put wrist and digits separately through as full range of motion as possible. If the injury is severe and if immediate surgery is indicated, probing the wound in the emergency room may injure and contaminate the tissues needlessly. In these cases, leave the wound sterilely dressed until the patient is anesthetized in the operating room, otherwise gently palpate the hand to evaluate tender or swollen areas.

The hand receives both the radial and ulnar arteries, with the radial artery traveling laterally, and the ulnar artery traveling medially. Both vessels should be inspected for laceration/transaction. Injuries to these vessels are usually obvious. In the absence of arterial hemorrhage, however, both structures should be palpated, and pulsatile flow should be present.

With the hand in neutral (aka beer-can) position, evaluate for any obvious abnormalities in the position of the hand. For example, if a single digit shows evidence of flexion while at rest, the possibility of an extensor tendon injury must be entertained. Conversely, extension of a digit or phalanx could indicate a flexor tendon injury. There are numerous surface anatomic features, which can be utilized by the physician to define injury. On the flexor surface of the hand, the wrist harbors two separate skin creases (see Fig. 6). At the proximal crease, both the radial and ulnar arteries can be palpated. The distal crease corresponds to the proximal aspect of the flexor retinaculum, which lies superior to the median nerve, and the synovial sheaths of the flexor carpi radialis, flexor pollicis longus, flexor digitorum profundus, and flexor digitorum superficialis. Notably, the tendon of the palmaris longus lies superficial to the flexor retinaculum, and extends to this skin crease. If the patient flexes thumb to ring finger, the palmaris longus tendon will become prominent in 90% of patients.

With this crease in view, ask the patient to individually move each metacarpophalangeal joint. This evaluates the tendons of the flexor digitorum superficialis, which terminates on the middle phalanx. Next, the patient should move each distal phalanx while the physician blocks motion at the middle phalanx. This evaluates the tendons for the flexor digitorum profundus, which also traverse the flexor retinaculum. Finally, the hand should be clenched into a fist, and flexed at the wrist. In this position, the tendons of the palmaris longus, flexor carpi radialis, and flexor carpi ulnaris can be palpated volarly.

The pisiform bone is also palpable immediately distal to the distal wrist crease. This bone, along with the hook of the hamate bone, forms the start of the Guyon canal. The ulnar artery and nerve travel within this canal, and injury to either of these structures is very possible in this

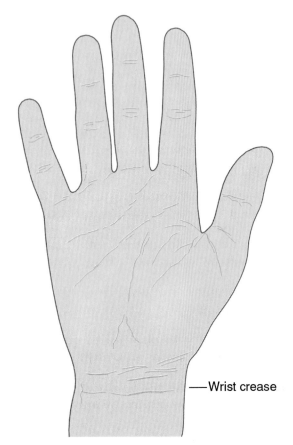

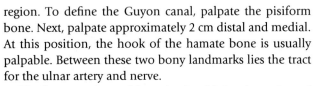

—Wrist crease

Figure 6   Palmar creases.

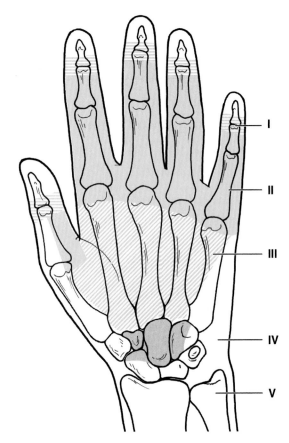

Figure 7   Flexor tendon zones.

region. To define the Guyon canal, palpate the pisiform bone. Next, palpate approximately 2 cm distal and medial. At this position, the hook of the hamate bone is usually palpable. Between these two bony landmarks lies the tract for the ulnar artery and nerve.

The flexor tendons of the wrist should then be evaluated (see Fig. 7). With the wrist in supine position, ask the patient to oppose his thumb and short finger. This will expose the palmaris longus tendon. The flexor tendons lie on the ulnar side of this structure. Next, ask the patient to flex each digit at the proximal interphalangeal (PIP) joint while palpating the wrist on the ulnar side of the palmaris longus tendon. Next, the distal interphalangeal (DIP) joint should be flexed. Again, all tendons lie on the ulnar side of the palmaris longus, but the middle, ring, and small fingers will all flex in unison given that they have a common muscle belly. During these examinations, abnormalities in motion should be evaluated.

There are 12 extensor tendons (see Fig. 8). Each tendon can be palpated during motion to confirm position and function. The examiner will commonly have difficulty separating the extensor pollicis brevis from the abductor pollicis brevis, because the extensor pollicis brevis is much narrower, and in close proximity to the abductor pollicis longus, which is itself prominent. Distinction is made by

palpation of the base of the first metacarpal beyond the attachment of the abductor pollicis longus.

After completing the history and physical examination, plain radiographs should be taken of the injured hand. Most commonly, three views of the hand should be obtained—posterior-anterior (PA), medial, and lateral views. The presence of significant fracture or dislocation at the wrist mandates specialty consultation.

INJURIES

Burns

The mnemonic "RBC" has been utilized to classify hand burns as first, second, and third degree: R = red, first degree; B = blister, second degree; and charred = C, third degree. First-degree burns usually present with erythema and a few small blisters, as these injuries only involve the superficial epidermal structures. First-degree burns are cleansed with soap and water, and dressed with a nonadherent petroleum-based dressing. Conversely, second-degree burns extend into the deeper aspect of the dermis, and can ultimately evolve into full-thickness injury, especially within the context of infection. Second-degree burns present with deep erythema and

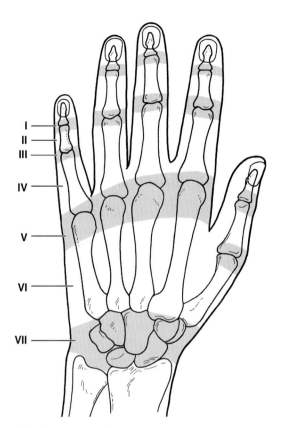

Figure 8 Extensor tendon zones.

Nonthermal burns are also commonly encountered in the emergency department. The therapeutic foundation of treating chemical burns is copious irrigation with sterile water. Patients who are conscious and lucid should be interviewed and specifically asked about the offending chemical agent. Alkaline burns should undergo sterile water lavage, followed by treatment with dilute acetic acid. In patients with acidic burns, dilute sodium bicarbonate should be administered following sterile water irrigation. A notable exception is injuries from hydrofluoric acid. Burns caused by hydrofluoric acid should be flushed with cold water, treated with benzalkonium chloride, and subcutaneously injected with 10% calcium gluconate until subjective pain resolves. Alternatively, for superficial hydrofluoric acid burns, 10% calcium gluconate can be applied topically utilizing sterile KY jelly as a delivery matrix.

Electrical burns can be caused by either an electrical spark and its inherent heat or by an actual electrical current, which passes through the patient. It is absolutely critical that this distinction be made during the patient's initial presentation as management of thermal and electrical burns differs. Patients who have a thermal injury due to an electrical spark should undergo local management of their injury. However, patients who sustain an electrical current injury have significant systemic issues that cannot be ignored. Exposure to 500 V or greater can generate both local and distant tissue damage remote from the point of entry. When biological organisms are exposed to an electrical current, the body acts essentially as a resistor, and will absorb voltage as the current passes from its entry to its exit point. This mandates a head to toe examination by the physician to define the current exit point. The electrical current commonly produces significant soft tissue loss at the entry, exit, and transit sites. Furthermore, patients should undergo electrocardiogram (ECG) evaluation for evidence of cardiac dysrhythmia. If any abnormalities are noted on ECG, cardiac telemetry monitoring is indicated. Tissue necrosis will require debridement and secondary reconstruction. However, debridement of necrotic wounds should be delayed for 24 hours, even if patients present with necrotic wounds. Large electrical injuries will often extend in the first 24 hours, and immediate debridement of wounds will often necessitate further operative debridement as the injury evolves.

Extreme thermal conditions due to very hot and cold temperatures may also cause severe burns. First-degree frostbite is a superficial injury and the patient is best served by local wound care until healing occurs. Treatment with petrolatum-based dressings usually suffices. Second-degree frostbite refers to a partial-thickness loss of dermis, and like its burn counterpart, is well served by topical antimicrobials with petrolatum-based dressings. Third-degree frostbite involves loss of the dermis and requires excision and grafting. Fourth-degree frostbite involves a full-thickness dermal injury as well as injury to the deeper tissue. Many of these injuries will ultimately require amputation.

require vigilant surveillance or consultation with a burn specialist. These wounds should be protected with a nonadherent petroleum-based dressing, and application of 1% silver sulfadiazine is indicated. Notably, early referral to a hand physical therapist is crucial with these injuries because immobility can foster a robust scarring response, which can ultimately limit overall function.

A third-degree burn represents a complete-thickness dermal injury. The skin will appear dry and contracted with a pathologic hue ranging from charred, to light yellow, to brown. The viability of these wounds can often be determined by physical examination. However, in undetermined cases, administration of 2 mL of 10% fluorescein intravenously and subsequent observation with a Wood lamp can be employed to evaluate tissue viability. Patients with third-degree burns should be admitted to the hospital, and scheduled to undergo debridement and skin graft closure. Furthermore, these wounds must be inspected for circulation, especially in cases involving a circumferential injury. If any evidence of vascular compromise is present, emergency escharotomy to restore distal circulation is indicated. A fourth-degree burn is one which involves deep vital structures of the digit or hand, such as tendons. Amputation is often advisable, but sometimes portions of the functionally useless digits can be salvaged as flap substrate for wound closure.

Tendon Injuries

There are 12 extrinsic flexor tendons in the hand and wrist. Injuries to these structures are classified on the basis of anatomic location of the flexor insult. The hand is divided into five separate zones, as follows:

Zone 1—distal phalanx of thumb and digits: insertion of flexor digitorum profundus

Zone 2—proximal to Zone 1 to the distal palmar crease

Zone 3—distal carpal ligament to distal palmar crease

Zone 4—carpal tunnel

Zone 5—forearm tendons

All flexor tendon injuries, once identified, should be explored and repaired in an operating room under regional or general anesthesia. The rationale for this approach is twofold: (i) maximization of flexor repair outcome and (ii) the opportunity to explore the region for concomitant injury. Flexor tendon injuries in all zones, especially laceration injuries, are frequently associated with injuries to nearby neural structures, and this injury association should be recognized preoperatively, and utilized intraoperatively to address additional problems within the zone of injury. Initial care consists of copious wound irrigation, followed by loose closure of overlying soft tissue, splinting, and administration of antibiotics. When confronted with a tendinous injury, subspecialty consultation with a hand specialist is indicated.

Following surgery, favorable results are often observed with repair in zones I, III, IV, and V; however, the functional results are much less certain in zone II. The patient should be informed that intense hand therapy is always indicated following a flexor tendon repair and that recovery is slow. Furthermore, the patient should be aware that a great deal of hard workis necessary to achieve favorable outcomes. Postoperative attention to protect the healing tendon must be considered while still allowing for some motion to prevent irreversible adhesions. The necessity for a second revisional surgery is not unusual, and is usually undertaken to alleviate traumatic adhesions in patients who sustained a flexor tendon injury.

Extensor Injuries

Extensor tendon injuries are in actuality more common than flexor injury, most likely due to reduced anatomic protection on the posterior surface of the hand as compared to anterior. These tendons are separated into eight separate zones, which were initially described by Vater.

Zone I—Distal phalanx

This zone encompasses extensor tendon insertion onto the distal phalanx. Disruption of this articulation results in a flexed position of the distal phalanx, referred to as *Mallet finger*. These injuries are further classified into six subtypes:

1. Type I—Closed injury. Treated most commonly with splinting for 6 weeks, followed by mobilization

2. Type II—Open laceration. Treated with tendon reapproximation and wound closure.

3. Type III—Open laceration with soft tissue and tendon loss. Immediate treatment consists of wound washout with soft tissue coverage. Future tendon reconstruction indicated.

4. Type IVa—Epiphyseal plate laceration in children. Treatment is closed reduction with splinting.

5. Type IVb—Hyperflexion with <50% articular surface fracture. Splinting for 6 weeks.

6. Type IVc—Hyperextension injury with >50% articular surface fracture. Treatment involves K-wire open fixation of joint, followed by splinting time for 6 weeks.

Zone II—Middle phalanx

Injuries are more commonly from crushing or shearing force, rather than lacerations. Injuries that involve <50% of tendon diameter should undergo splinting for 6 weeks, followed by physical therapy. If >50% of the tendon is injured, primary repair with postoperative splinting is indicated.

Zone III—Proximal interphalangeal joint

Injury in this region commonly results in what is known as a Boutonniere deformity, with unopposed flexion at the PIP, and hyperextension at the DIP. Initial therapy consists of splinting the PIP joint in extension, and reevaluation of the injury in 72 hours. If on reexamination, the patient is unable to extend the PIP, a zone III extensor tendon injury can be conclusively diagnosed. Therapy consists of splinting for 6 weeks. Surgical reduction is indicated only with concomitant fracture, or with failure of medical management after 6 weeks.

Zone IV—Proximal phalanx

Injuries to this region are commonly diagnosed by inspection. Extensor tendon injury tends to be partial in nature in this region, and in the presence of normal extensor function, operative repair is not indicated. If, however, a complete tendon laceration is present, open repair is indicated, with 6 weeks of splinting in extension. Partial lacerations are traditionally treated with splinting in extension for 3 to 4 weeks, but many authors advocate early mobilization with partial tears.

Zone V—Metacarpophalangeal joint

Most injuries to this region of the hand are open in nature, and laceration of the extensor tendon is common in this region. Open repair of injuries in this region is indicated.

Zone VI—Dorsal hand

Injuries to this region are difficult to diagnose because partial tears to extensor tendons can be effectively hidden by associated tendons during examination. These injuries commonly require exploration subsequent to injury management. Injuries to this area should be evaluated by hand specialists.

Zone VII—Wrist

Tendon laceration to this region requires operative exploration and repair.

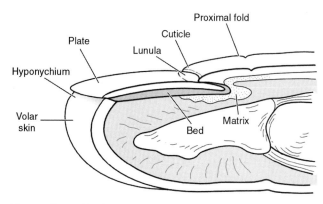

Figure 9 Nail bed anatomy.

Zone VIII—Dorsal forearm

Most deep injuries to this region involve multiple extensor tendons. Operative exploration of this region is advocated for best functional outcomes.

Nail Bed

The nail bed lies on the dorsal surface of the distal phalanx. In this position, it is commonly the first anatomic structure to interact with our environment. This position frequently places the nail bed within harm's way, and expectedly, injury to the nail bed is a common presenting complaint in the emergency department. Unfortunately, many of these injuries are not taken seriously at presentation, and are mismanaged. Improper management of these injuries commonly results in chronic finger deformities.

The nail itself is a complex structure that begins at the nail fold (see Fig. 9). The nail fold refers to the skin which overlaps the nail root. The nail bed refers to the dermis underneath the nail body. The germinal matrix, which is responsible for approximately 90% of all nail growth, begins here underneath the nail fold and nail root. It extends out into the lunula, which is the whitish "moon" structure found distal to the nail fold, underneath the nail body. Distal to the lunula, the sterile matrix is found. This structure extends from the distal tip of the lunula to the end of the nail bed. The eponychium is a transparent structure that is bound to the skin of the nail fold, and covers the nail root. It serves as a barrier against infection for the germinal matrix. Notably, the eponychium is commonly mistaken for the nail cuticle. However, the nail cuticle itself consists of sloughed epithelial cells from the skin of the nail fold, and

overgrowth of the eponychium. Hence, the eponychium and nail cuticle are related, but separate structures.

The most commonly encountered nail bed injuries are: (i) lacerations, (ii) crush, and (iii) avulsion injuries. Regardless of mechanism of injury, the following are a number of management principles regarding nail bed injuries, which should be adhered to.

1. Remove damaged portions of nail body for improved examination of nail bed
2. Minimize debridement of the nail bed
3. Operative stabilization of distal phalanx, if indicated
4. Prompt repair of nail bed and/or any associated skin lacerations
5. Lost sterile matrix should be replaced with a sterile matrix graft
6. Replace nail body with native nail. If unable to use native nail body, use biomaterial substitute (silastic, etc.)

CONCLUSION

This chapter offers a brief overview of hand anatomy, examination of the hand, and an overview of commonly seen injuries. Management of these injuries, however, is rarely brief. Despite appropriate diagnosis and successful management, optimal outcome in patients with injured hands is ultimately dependent on the patient's willingness and motivation to undergo rehabilitation. Most hand injuries require some degree of immobilization, which implicitly generates stiffness of the hand joints, and atrophy of hand musculature. For optimal function to return, all patients with significant hand injuries requiring immobilization should be evaluated by hand occupational therapy after their acute management has concluded. Failure to involve appropriate hand therapists will in many cases obviate even the most effective surgical management.

SUGGESTED READINGS

Brown RE. Acute nail bed injuries. *Hand Clin.* 2002;18:2.
Idler RS. Anatomy and biomechanics of the digital flexor tendons. *Hand Clin.* 1985;1:3.
Kaplan EB. Anatomy, injuries and treatment of the extensor apparatus of the hand and the digits. *Clin Orthop.* 1995;13:24.
Lister G. *The hand: diagnosis and indications.* Churchill Livingstone; 1977.
Strickland JW. Flexor tendon injuries I: Foundations of treatment. *J Am Acad Orthop Surg.* 1995;3:44.
Strickland JW. Flexor tendon injuries II: Operative technique. *J Am Acad Orthop Surg.* 1995;3:55.

Special Interdisciplinary Problem: Pelvic Fracture

49

H. Claude Sagi

INTRODUCTION AND ANATOMY

Pelvic fractures are serious injuries associated with a diverse assortment of morbidities and mortality rates ranging from 10% to 50%. Life-threatening associated nonpelvic injuries are common due to the enormous forces that are required to disrupt the pelvic ring.

Figure 1 shows the three bones that combine to form the pelvic ring—the two innominate bones (which arise from the fusion of the embyronic pubic, ilium, and ischium) and the midline sacrum (the caudal segment of the axial skeleton). The acetabulum (hip socket) is located at the center of the fusion site where the three embryonic innominate bones come together on each side.

The pelvic bones unite anteriorly in the midline through the articulation between the pubic bones and the symphyseal ligaments. Posteriorly, the sacrum is situated between the right and left iliac portions of the innominate bones forming the bilateral sacroiliac (SI) joints, which are secured by the SI (which have dorsal and ventral components behind and in front of the SI joints), sacrotuberous (ST), and sacrospinous (SSp) ligaments. Because of the inherent bony structural instability of the symphysis and SI joints, the integrity of the pelvic ring depends completely on the integrity of these ligaments. In addition to supplying structural support for the pelvic ring, these ligaments provide support for the many vascular, neural, and visceral structures contained in the pelvis. This critical set of functions of the pelvic ligaments explains the association between traumatic ligament disruption and increased short- and long-term pelvic fracture morbidity.

The major trunks of the iliac arterial system pass near the SI joints ventrally (see Fig. 2), and disruption of these ligaments increases the risk of significant arterial injury and hemorrhage, which usually involves the anterior and posterior divisions of the internal iliac arteries. We have observed two instances of injury to the main trunks of the internal and external iliac arteries from femoral

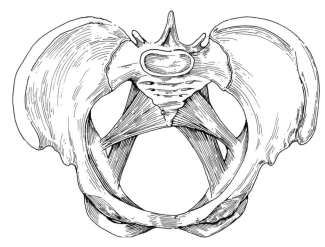

Figure 1 Anatomy of the pelvis analogous to the inlet view seen on radiographic views. Shown are the bony elements and the sacrotuberous ligaments.

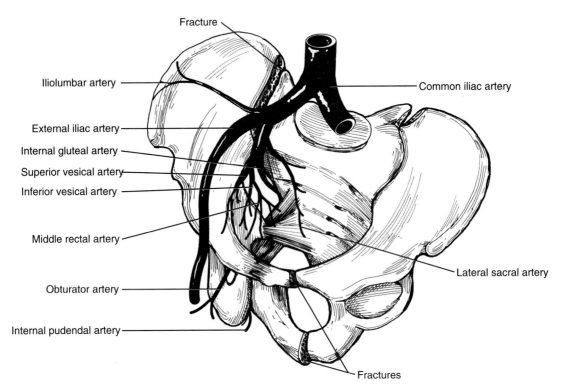

Figure 2 Association of pelvic vasculature to the disrupted sacroiliac joint.

head protrusion into the pelvis associated with acetabular fractures.

The bladder and urethra are located immediately posterior to the pubic symphysis and the rectum is immediately anterior to the sacrum. Because of the intimate association of these pelvic visceral structures to the bony pelvis, visceral injury is common. Major force transfer is required to produce pelvic fracture. Because of this, associated major nonpelvic injuries are commonly encountered. Indeed, clinical research by Demetriades et al.,[1] Poole and Ward[2] and Cydulka et al,[3] have documented that associated neurologic, thoracic, and abdominal visceral injuries are more predictive than the pelvic fracture in determining mortality and functional outcome.

The pubic symphysis is the weakest link in the pelvic ring, supplying only 15% of the inherent pelvic stability.[4] The SI joints are the strongest in the body, relying primarily on the posterior SI ligamentous attachments in resisting vertical and anterior-posterior (AP) displacement. Being a ring structure, disruption and displacement in one area implies (biomechanically) that there must be disruption (fracture or dislocation) and displacement in another area of the ring.

EPIDEMIOLOGY OF PELVIC FRACTURES

Traumatic pelvic fractures result from (in descending order) motorcycle crashes, auto-pedestrian collisions, falls, and motor vehicle crashes.[5,6] Crush injuries may also result in pelvic fractures (see Table 1). As the incidence of high-velocity motor vehicle collision (MVC) increases, so does the incidence of pelvic fracture. Side impact with lateral impact and damage and vehicle incompatibility (small vs. large vehicles) are the main risk factors for pelvic fracture morbidity and mortality.[7–9]

PREHOSPITAL INTERVENTION

Information gleaned from witnesses at the scene in addition to that from prehospital care professionals regarding patient presentation and examination may raise the suspicion for these injuries. Uniform prehospital transport protocols are helpful and should be followed. Appropriate

---

TABLE 1

INJURY PATTERNS ASSOCIATED WITH PELVIC FRACTURE

Motorcycle crash
Vehicle–pedestrian collision
Side impact motor vehicle collision
Fall >15 ft
Motor vehicle crash

immobilization, airway protection, and initial circulatory support with expedient transport to a definitive care facility are the main goals. Application of the pneumatic antishock garment in the field is an option to stabilize the pelvic fracture; however, this device can lead to other problems (as noted in the subsequent text) and many prehospital care systems no longer carry the military antishock trouser (MAST) device.

INITIAL ASSESSMENT

The multiply injured patient is at risk for thoracic, intra-abdominal, soft tissue, pelvic, and extremity hemorrhage. Once the primary survey is completed with a secure airway and oxygenation, sources of hemorrhage must be identified and controlled. Radiographic studies of the chest, abdomen, and pelvis can help identify these sources. The focused abdominal ultrasonographicy (focused assessment sonography for trauma [FAST]) can detect abdominal hemorrhage, and, when positive in a hemodynamically unstable patient, is an indication for laparotomy.[10] Diagnostic peritoneal lavage (DPL) is also helpful, but should be performed above the umbilicus in a patient with known or suspected pelvic hemorrhage to avoid false-positive results. The sequence of assessments outlined in the Advanced Trauma Life Support course is helpful for organizing an approach to managing potentially unstable trauma patients. However, this sequence is not helpful in determining hemodynamic instability for individual patients. Individual hemodynamic measurements are snapshots in time and by themselves are not helpful. Hemodynamic trends are helpful and the time required, in the trauma resuscitation area, to make a decision as to hemodynamic stability is a worthwhile investment.

EARLY DETECTION AND MANAGEMENT OF ASSOCIATED INJURIES

As a result of the considerable energy imparted to the pelvis to cause fractures and dislocations, associated injuries are common. Reports by Biffl and Demetriades[1,10] indicate that the most common injuries associated with pelvic fractures in descending order are chest injury in up to 63%, long bone fractures in 50%, brain and abdominal injury (spleen, liver, bladder, and urethra) in 40%, and spine fractures in 25%. Demetriades' study, for example, observed that intestinal injury alone can be found in 4% to 14% of patients with pelvic fractures. An early decision for exploration of the chest or abdomen when thoracic or abdominal bleeding and/or intestinal injury are suspected is central to lowering mortality in multiply injured patients with pelvic fractures.

The secondary survey focuses on identifying other injuries, particularly those that may be contributing to ongoing blood loss. Once thoracic and abdominal

---

TABLE 2

ELEMENTS OF THE CLINICAL EXAMINATION FOR SIGNS OF PELVIC FRACTURE

Does the patient have pelvic pain?
Are there neurologic deficits involving sciatic, femoral, or obturator nerve?
Are there contusions, ecchymoses, or abrasions at or near the bony prominences of the pelvis?
Are there ecchymoses of the scrotum or perineum?
Is there blood at the urethral meatus?
Is there blood in or around the rectum and is the prostate normal?
Are there open wounds of the groin, buttock, or perineum?
Is there a leg length difference or is the resting position of one leg different from the other?
Is there pain or abnormal pelvic motion on compression of the anterior iliac spines, lateral compression of the iliac crests, rotation of the lower extremity, or hip flexion-extension?

---

hemorrhage have been ruled out, persistent blood loss is assumed to be pelvic in origin until proved otherwise. Clinical findings that are highly suggestive of a pelvic fracture are listed in Table 2. Clinical findings of patients at high risk for ongoing bleeding are listed in Table 3. The clinical examination should assess for gross instability of the pelvis.

Observation of the patient may reveal scrotal/labial or flank and perineal ecchymosis, and blood from the rectum, vagina, or urethra. Additionally, rectal and vaginal examinations are mandatory to rule out mucosal tears that communicate with the fracture, indicating an open and contaminated injury. An abnormally high prostate position in males on rectal examination is suggestive of a urethral tear.

AP and lateral compression (LC) on the iliac wings may elicit pain or frank rotational instability or there may even be a palpable gap or separation of the symphysis. External rotation and shortening of the lower extremity may indicate an "open-book" type injury and/or vertical

---

TABLE 3

CLINICAL FEATURES INDICATING INCREASED RISK FOR PELVIC FRACTURE BLEEDING

Prehospital hypotension
Admission base deficit >5
Persistent tachycardia in face of normal oxygenation and adequate pain control
Recurrent hypotension during resuscitation
Requirement for >6 units blood during first 24 hr

TABLE 4

MYOTOMES OF THE LOWER EXTREMITY AND THE ASSOCIATED MOTOR FUNCTION

- L1/2: Hip flexors
- L3/4: Quadriceps/knee extension
- L4/5: Ankle and toe dorsiflexion
- S1: Ankle flexion
- S2/3: Toe plantar flexion

TABLE 5

TILE CLASSIFICATION OF PELVIC FRACTURE

Type A: Pelvic ring stable

(a) A1: Fractures not involving the ring (i.e., avulsions, iliac wing or crest fractures)

(b) A2: Stable minimally displaced fractures of the pelvic ring

Type B: Pelvic ring rotationally unstable, vertically stable

(a) B1: Open book

(b) B2: Lateral compression, ipsilateral

(c) B3: Lateral compression, contralateral or bucket-handle type injury

Type C: Pelvic ring rotationally and vertically unstable

(a) C1: Unilateral

(b) C2: Bilateral

(c) C3: Associated with acetabular fracture

shear (VS) injury. Gonzales et al.[11] documented that clinical examination in conscious patients who could comply with the physical examination yielded a 90% sensitivity for the diagnosis of pelvic fracture The addition of the AP pelvic radiograph will permit accurate identification and initial classification of the pelvic fracture.

An accurate neurologic examination is often difficult to obtain secondary to variable patient cooperation. However, a rapid examination of a few major areas is important because the sciatic nerve and branches of the sacral plexus lie in close proximity to common fracture sites. Rectal examination for tone and bulbocavernosus reflex is easy to perform and can be accomplished in the obtunded or noncompliant patient to rule out cauda equina syndrome. The bulbocavernosus reflex in the female is elicited by gently tugging on the Foley catheter. Perianal sensation and voluntary sphincter contraction are much more difficult to examine in the acute trauma injury setting. Peripheral nerve examination is possible for distal motor groups at the ankle and foot, but proximal muscle weakness is difficult to examine secondary to pain. See Table 4 for muscle groups and functional tests for motor nerves passing through the pelvis to the lower extremity.

Patients who respond to volume expansion and are stable over a 15- to 30-minute period of observation may be safely moved to receive further diagnostic studies. The trauma team leader must decide which diagnostic maneuver is the most appropriate given the clinical picture and initial screening studies.

Computed tomographic (CT) scanning is useful in gauging the amount of pelvic hemorrhage that has occurred, in addition to helping guide treatment of the pelvic fracture itself. Blackmore et al.[12] observed a direct relationship between the volume of pelvic hematoma seen on CT scan and patient transfusion requirements. CT may be done especially when a contrast blush is seen, which indicates significant ongoing pelvic hemorrhage and the need for pelvic therapeutic angiography.[12]

CLASSIFICATION OF PELVIC FRACTURES

Classification of pelvic fractures and dislocations requires adequate plain radiography (AP, inlet, and outlet x-rays) and thin-cut (3 mm) CT scan imaging. If possible, the AP pelvis is obtained before bladder catheterization and cystography to avoid obscuring landmarks. Several classification schemes are currently employed, but all have evolved from the early work performed by Pennal[13] and Tile[14] (see Table 5). The most widely used classification scheme is that of Young and Burgess,[15] which focuses on the mechanism of injury (see Table 6). The classification system put forth by the Orthopaedic Trauma Association (OTA) and Association for the Study of Internal Fixation (AO-ASIF) group is more comprehensive and serves primarily to provide a widely accepted and standardized classification system for data collection and reporting.[16]

TABLE 6

YOUNG AND BURGESS PELVIC FRACTURE CLASSIFICATION

Lateral compression (LC): Anterior injury = rami fractures

(a) LC I: Sacral fracture on side of impact

(b) LC II: Crescent fracture on side of impact

(c) LC III: Type I or II injury on side of impact with contralateral open-book injury

Antero posterior compression (APC): Anterior injury = symphysis diastasis/rami fractures

(a) APC I: Minor opening of symphysis and sacroiliac (SI) joint anteriorly

(b) APC II: Opening of anterior SI, intact posterior SI ligaments

(c) APC III: Complete disruption of SI joint

Vertical shear (VS) type: Vertical displacement of hemipelvis with symphysis diastasis or rami fractures anteriorly, iliac wing, sacral facture, or SI dislocation posteriorly.

Combination (CM) type: Any combination of above injuries

CM, combined mechanism.

Treatment is based on accurate assessment of the resultant injury and instability pattern. It is important to remember two points: First, that the posterior pelvic ring injury defines ultimate stability. Second, although in an intact pelvis the anterior ring (symphysis) supplies only 10% to 15% of the total stability, in an unstable pelvis where there is complete disruption of the posterior ring, stabilization of the anterior ring contributes significantly to the strength of the reconstruction and maintenance of reduction. Possible posterior ring injuries are iliac wing fractures, SI dislocations, and sacral fractures. Possible anterior ring injuries are rami fractures and symphyseal disruptions. Pelvic injuries can include any combination of anterior and posterior injuries, unilateral or bilateral.

LC fractures are the most commonly encountered. At the time of impact, the hemipelvis on the side of impact is pushed (internally rotated) into the contralateral pelvis. This usually involves rami fractures anteriorly with a sacral impaction iliac wing fracture. This type of injury is rotationally unstable, but usually vertically stable (see Fig. 3).

Anterior-posterior compression (APC) injuries result in the commonly termed *open-book* pelvis. The impact causes external rotation of one or both hemipelvises, with the fulcrum or point of rotation being the SI joints. The first point of failure is the symphysis pubis. Because increasing external rotation is applied, ST, SSp, and anterior SI ligaments fail under tension. Anterior SI ligament disruption is present when there is more than 2.5 cm of diastasis of the symphysis. With further external rotation, the posterior SI ligaments ultimately fail as well. When this stage is reached, all of the supporting ligaments of the pelvic ring are disrupted in addition to the pelvic floor and perineal musculature (see Fig. 4)

VS injuries are the most unstable and usually encompass some form of rotational injury as well. In these cases, a cranially directed force shears the hemipelvis causing

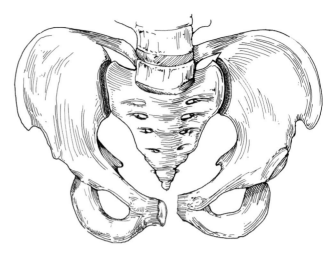

Figure 4   Open-book pelvic fracture.

severe skeletal, muscular, and ligamentous disruption. The iliac crest of the injured hemipelvis is seen to be riding cephalad compared to the contralateral side, often with a fracture of the ipsilateral transverse process of L5 (see Fig. 5). Significant urogenital, vascular, and neurologic injuries are accompanied by the APC and VS injuries due to the stretch and traction placed on these structures as the injuring forces are applied.

DIAGNOSIS OF PELVIC FRACTURE BLEEDING

Bleeding and vascular injury, however, are the most commonly associated problem with pelvic fractures. Huittinen and Slatis,[17] in a classic contribution to the field of pelvic fracture care, showed with postmortem angiography that pelvic fracture hemorrhage results most frequently from

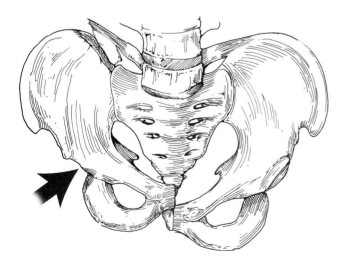

Figure 3   Lateral compression pelvic fracture.

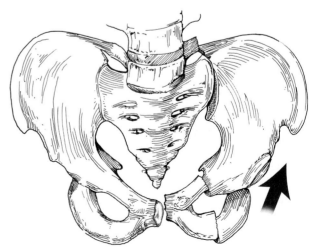

Figure 5   Vertical shear pelvic fracture.

the venous structures and bleeding bone edges. This hemorrhage stops in most patients secondary to tamponade from increasing tissue pressure in the pelvic retroperitoneal space. However, in patients who died of pelvic fracture hemorrhage, single or multiple arterial lacerations were more likely to be present. Arterial bleeding can overcome the tamponade effect of the retroperitoneal tissues leading to shock; this is the most common cause of death related to the pelvic fracture itself. Arterial bleeding usually arises from branches of the internal iliac system, with the superior gluteal and pudendal arteries being the most commonly identified source.

As outlined in the preceding text, bleeding and hemorrhage from pelvic fracture alone is and should be a diagnosis of exclusion. Once resuscitation is under way and a search for thoracic and abdominal bleeding has been completed, further analysis of the fracture pattern can be performed to see if this may be the cause of ongoing blood loss. However, the radiographic representation of the fracture alone is inadequate in determining the risk of ongoing hemorrhage because only the current degree of displacement is visible and not that which occurred at the time of impact. Metz et al.[18] documented an equal number of arterial bleeding sites seen on angiography in patients with APC and LC injury patterns. The take-home message is that severe bleeding can occur in all fracture patterns and the whole clinical picture should dictate clinical strategy rather than just the radiograph.

Supporting this assertion is a report by Miller et al.,[19] which observed that patients could be chosen for pelvic angiography based on the recurrence of hypotension within 2 hours of an initially successful resuscitation. They discovered that active arterial bleeding occurred in 73% of patients selected by these means. Details of our preferences and treatment strategies are shown in the accompanying algorithm and discussed in the following section (see Fig. 6).

If pelvic fracture bleeding is suspected, patients get blood transfusions as needed. Four to six units of blood may be given before venous bleeding subsides. If the patient is still requiring transfusion after this point is reached, specific therapy for the bleeding is chosen on the basis of the criteria discussed in the subsequent text. CT scans of the pelvis may allow quantification of the volume of blood loss and may disclose a contrast "blush" indicating active arterial bleeding.

TREATMENT OF PELVIC FRACTURE HEMORRHAGE—PERSISTENT CONTROVERSIES

Fortunately, most bleeding from pelvic fracture arises from torn small- and medium-sized veins and edges of fractured bone. These sites will usually stop by natural hemostatic mechanisms if patient cardiovascular function, blood volume, and coagulation status are kept within

acceptable limits. We transfuse all patients who do not immediately stabilize after being administered 2,000 mL of balanced salt solution. If a patient requires more than 4 units of blood transfusion, support of coagulation with fresh frozen plasma infusion is begun. Platelets are given to keep the platelet count above 100,000 per mm^3. For those patients who have persistent bleeding, controversy has continued concerning the desirability of efforts to reduce pelvic volume and stabilize bone edges versus the use of selective angiography and embolization or emergent surgical exploration with packing. There is a large body of evidence to suggest that closure of symphysis pubis separations with reduction of pelvic volume improves the prospect of tamponade of pelvic bleeding. Holding bone edges so that motion is minimized is intuitively appealing as a means of stopping hemorrhage. The time-honored tenet of fracture care—"splint them where they lie"—is an example of the long-held conviction that immobilization of fractures controls bleeding around fracture sites and improves pain control.

Reports of the efficacy of the pneumatic antishock garment supported this concept for the management of bleeding due to pelvic fracture.[20,21] This device served three potential functions: first, it returned blood from the lower extremities to the central vascular system; second, it could close, at least partially, open-book type injuries; and third, it stabilized the pelvis. Brotman et al.[22] discussed the shortcomings and failures of the pneumatic antishock garment, particularly the fact that the garment had to be partially or completely removed to allow access to the abdomen in patients who required abdominal exploration as well as reports of compartment syndrome and skin necrosis following the use of the device hindered acceptance of this approach.

The adoption of aggressive fracture fixation strategies pioneered by European trauma surgeons accelerated interest in early application of external fixation for control of bleeding, and several experienced orthopaedic trauma surgeons support the use of early external fixation as a means of controlling pelvic bleeding. Although some assert that external fixation is superior to angiography for control of bleeding, no head-to-head comparison has been done.

Two basic types of external skeletal fixation are currently employed: anterior frames (which are applied percutaneously to the iliac bones either above the acetabulum or into the iliac crest), and the pelvic clamps (which are applied to the posterior iliac fossae at the iliac groove).[23] Both devices can be positioned so that access to the abdomen is possible. Anterior frames function by internally rotating and restoring alignment to an externally rotated pelvis (an open book), but only if the posterior ring is intact. Pelvic clamps apply an internal vector that translates the hemipelvis medially and therefore does not rely on an intact posterior ring. Ertel et al.[24] reported use of the C-clamp in patients with severe pelvic bleeding and noted that laparotomy with pelvic packing was occasionally

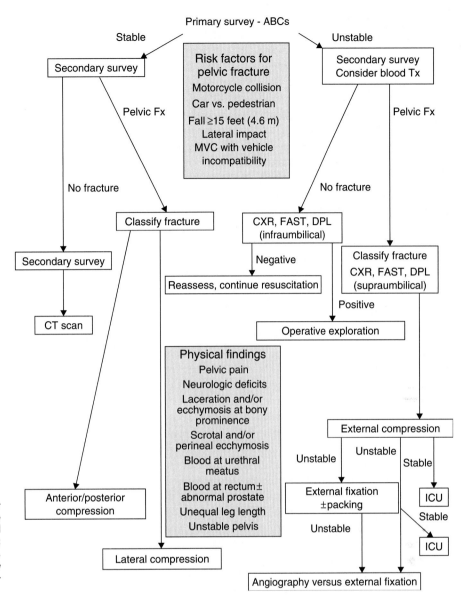

Figure 6 Treatment strategies for pelvic fracture. MVC, motor vehicle crash; CXR, chest x-ray; FAST, focused assessment with sonography for trauma; DPL, diagnostic peritoneal lavage; CT, computed tomography; ICU, intensive care unit; ABC, airway breathing circulation.

needed when the C-clamp failed to control bleeding. Their overall mortality due to bleeding was 25%. This approach is also supported in a report by Gansslen et al.[25]

Potential drawbacks to the use of external fixation are the need for expert orthopaedic support, which must be readily available soon after the patient arrives at the definitive care facility. Specific training is needed for successful application of external fixation devices. Indeed, there have been reports of pelvic visceral injury following application of external fixation devices.[26,27] Some orthopaedic surgeons feel strongly that application in the operating room (rather than in the resuscitation area) using sterile technique and image intensifier control is necessary for safe placement of external fixators. Because of these concerns and the availability of other devices for pelvic compression, application of external fixators for persistent hemodynamic instability in the resuscitation area has not been universally accepted.

The application of a folded bedsheet anchored anteriorly by towel clips can reduce pelvic volume and can be applied safely and quickly in the emergency room (ER) by caregivers who are not trained orthopaedic surgeons. The bedsheet is applied in a straight transverse manner with the primary force vector being delivered to the greater trochanters. Recently, Bottlang et al.[28] reported an adjustable fabric device for pelvic compression, which is now commercially available (T-Pod Bio-cybernetics International, La Verne, California).

One potential hazard of applying external compression devices is overcorrection of the fracture. This is particularly true in fractures where the posterior ring is completely unstable. Compression of the ilium with overcorrection can result in injury to the neurovascular and pelvic visceral structures. Therefore, in conscious, responsive patients, careful assessment of neurovascular status is essential before and after the application of any pelvic fixation device in addition to follow-up radiographs. Another complication of external compression devices such as sheets or pelvic binders is the development of pressure ulceration and full-thickness skin necrosis and slough. These devices are often employed in critically ill patients who will spend many days in the intensive care unit (ICU). If the binder is successful in controlling pelvic hemorrhage and is left in place for more than 48 hours because of fear of recurrent bleeding, the potential for major skin and soft tissue problems is significant.[29]

For patients who have persistent hemodynamic instability despite pelvic compression, appropriate resuscitation, and exclusion of thoracic, abdominal, and extremity hemorrhage, expeditious clinical decisions are necessary. The two options at this point are angiographic embolization of presumed pelvic arterial bleeding versus open exploration and packing. The lack of readily available experts in angiography obviously limits any radiologic approach. Experienced trauma surgeons have reported instances of death during angiography in desperately ill patients who are actively bleeding. Rather than take a desperately ill, unstable patient to the angiography suite, laparotomy with pelvic packing before angiography is preferable.

The choice of angiography versus external fixation or pelvic compression is made on the basis of a careful assessment of the fracture pattern and resources available at each hospital and agreement, in advance, as to which specialists will participate in the management of pelvic fracture with hemorrhage. Commitment to immediate availability is critical from all specialists involved. If the fracture pattern is not amenable to compression, then angiography should be sought. If it is amenable to compression, then at least a trial of sheet wrapping or pelvic binder is indicated. These basic tenets are well outlined in the practice management guidelines promulgated by the Eastern Association for the Surgery of Trauma.[30]

Transfemoral angiography offers the opportunity to identify bleeding points and stop bleeding using selective embolization. Concern has been expressed, especially by Hak,[31] that many patients who undergo angiography do not have active bleeding sites visualized. With improved patient selection, as noted in the subsequent text, the number of positive studies has progressively increased. In some cases of multiple bilateral bleeding points, filling of the internal iliac vessels bilaterally with embolic material has been utilized. Necrosis of pelvic viscera such as the rectum is a risk of bilateral internal iliac occlusion. Sexual dysfunction, a feared long-term complication of bilateral internal iliac occlusion, has not been regularly observed.[32] There is, apparently, a small chance of tissue necrosis in patients who have undergone definitive pelvic fixation following angiography through large "extensile exposure" incisions. So far, these reports have been single case experiences. Patients older than 60 years are more likely to have arterial bleeding in conjunction with pelvic

fracture, and increasing mortality risk as age rises has been well documented.[33,34] The demonstration of bleeding sites is common when angiography is used in these patients perhaps because of aging of the vessels and atherosclerosis. Despite successful angiography, mortality remains significant in this group at 11% to 15%.[35] Similar findings were reported by Velmahos et al.[36] They observed a higher frequency of positive angiograms in patients older than 55 years. Recurrent bleeding after embolization was seen in 6% of their patients after "successful" embolization.

It is clear that successful management of pelvic fracture bleeding is best accomplished by a multidisciplinary team approach with choices as the strategy made on the basis of availability of local resources and clearly agreed upon protocols for management.

DIAGNOSIS AND MANAGEMENT OF GENITOURINARY INJURIES IN PATIENTS WITH PELVIC FRACTURE

Injuries to the bladder and urethra are common with pelvic fractures with an incidence as high as 15% to 20%.[37–39] Because of the significant force required to rupture a hollow viscus within the pelvis, mortality can be as high 22% to 34% when pelvic fractures are accompanied by a bladder rupture.[40] Bladder injuries tend to cluster in those patients with lateral compression mechanism, whereas urethral injury is seen with both anterior compression and lateral compression mechanisms.

The clinical finding most consistently observed after bladder injury is gross hematuria which is present in 95% of patients. The remaining 5% of patients will have microscopic hematuria. Patients with gross hematuria and pelvic fracture are evaluated carefully for urethral injury or bladder rupture, as discussed in the subsequent text. The presence of a pelvic fracture, particularly combined with penile and scrotal ecchymosis, should raise suspicion for a bladder and/or urethral injury. When bladder injury is suspected, contrast cystography is performed in stable patients following placement of a Foley catheter. Stable patients who are to undergo CT scanning can have CT cystography as described in the report by Peng et al.[41] Properly performed CT cystography is as accurate as conventional cystography. Extraperitoneal bladder injury is treated, usually, with Foley catheter drainage. Intraperitoneal bladder rupture is treated with exploration and suture closure. Suprapubic catheterization is not usually necessary, but when indicated, placement of the catheter must take into account the potential for contamination of anterior internal fixation.

The classic findings of abnormal position of the prostate, inability to void, and blood at the urethral meatus are seen in a minority of patients. Lowe[42] documented that the appearance of these symptoms and signs is a function of

STEPS IN PERFORMING RETROGRADE CONTRAST URETHROGRAPHY (RUG)

Carefully insert bladder catheter
Cease insertion immediately for any resistance to passage
  or drainage of thick blood or thick bloody urine
Withdraw catheter until 4 cm of catheter is in penile urethra
Inflate catheter balloon with 3 mL saline
Inject 15–20 mL of water soluble contrast

the interval between injury and evaluation. Patients seen early after injury are unlikely to manifest clear-cut clinical evidence of bladder or urethra injury. A high index of suspicion is necessary.

Clinical examination and pelvic x-rays are obtained and, on the basis of these, a decision to attempt bladder catheterization is made. When pelvic fracture is present, catheterization should be attempted by a clinician experienced in passing catheters in patients with urethral injury. Unless there is easy and unobstructed passage of the catheter into the bladder, efforts at passing the catheter are stopped and a contrast urethrogram is obtained by inflating the Foley catheter balloon in the penile urethra with 2 to 3 mL of saline and instilling 10 to 15 mL of water-soluble contrast material and obtaining an oblique film of the pelvis. Table 7 lists the steps in performing retrograde contrast urethrography (RUG). The grading scale for urethral injury, as promulgated by the American Association for the Surgery of Trauma, is shown in Table 8.

Failure to pass contrast into the bladder indicates urethral disruption. Extravasation of contrast into the surrounding soft tissues may be observed. Cephalad displacement of the bladder by the pelvic hematoma with

GRADING SYSTEM FOR URETHRAL INJURIES AS PROMULGATED BY THE EASTERN ASSOCIATION FOR THE SURGERY OF TRAUMA

Grade	Designation	Clinical Findings
1	Contusion	Blood at meatus, retrograde contrast urethrography (RUG) normal
2	Stretch injury	Elongation of urethra, no extravasation
3	Partial disruption	Extravasation, contrast in bladder
4	Complete disruption	Extravasation, no contrast in bladder, <2 cm separation

passage of the contrast into the bladder is the finding typical of stretch injury to the urethra with continuity maintained. Endoscopic placement of a transurethral bladder drainage catheter is indicated, where possible, to facilitate management and later repair. When transurethral catheterization of the bladder is not possible, open or ultrasound-guided percutaneous suprapubic cystography are indicated.

Despite the short length of the urethra in women, anterior compression fractures and VS injuries associated with perineal injury cause urethral tears in women. Blood around the urethral orifice and lacerations of the vaginal introitus suggest an elevated risk of this injury. Most urethral injuries in women are amenable to treatment with Foley catheter drainage.

Open, frequent, and frank communication among the specialists providing care for the patient with pelvic fracture is necessary to make certain that the choices and sequencing of interventions lead to an optimal outcome.

OPEN PELVIC FRACTURES

Open pelvic fractures occur when there is communication between a fracture fragment and the skin or a pelvic visceral cavity. These injuries are observed in 4% to 5% of patients with pelvic fracture[43]. The incidences of pelvic infection including soft tissue infection and osteomyelitis as well as high mortality and long-term disability are raised in patients with open pelvic fracture as documented in the reports by Brenneman et al.[44] and Raffa et al.[45] Skin lacerations communicating with pelvic fracture sites may be found along the course of the iliac crest, in the groin, and in the perineum and should raise the suspicion of rectal or vaginal injury. During the acute evaluation of genitourinary injury in the patient with a pelvic fracture, a careful digital rectal and, if appropriate, vaginal examination is mandatory. Palpable vaginal lacerations indicate open pelvic fracture. Occasionally, rectal lacerations can also be palpated but, in most of them, the most consistent finding indicating rectal injury in the patient with pelvic fracture is the finding of blood in the rectal lumen.

Vaginal speculum examination and proctoscopic examination are postponed until it is safe to place the patient in lithotomy or lateral decubitus position. Speculum and sigmoidoscopic examinations, when they may be safely done, supplement the careful digital vaginal and rectal examination. Pelvic and anal sphincter muscle damage may accompany perineal lacerations. Evaluation for fecal continence is not an emergency diagnostic procedure for patients with pelvic fracture. Damage to the anal sphincter with a perineal laceration suggests the need for diverting colostomy. Fecal diversion is done selectively based on the position of the laceration (perineal lacerations will usually require and groin lacerations may sometimes require diversion). When fecal soilage of an open wound is possible, diversion is performed to reduce the chance of pelvic wound infection. Five patients with perineal lacerations in Brenneman's series did not undergo fecal diversion and all suffered serious infectious complications.

Plans for definitive repair of the pelvic fracture need to be understood before the decision to perform fecal diversion is made so that best placement of the ostomy can be assured. If colostomy is to be performed, it should be done within the first 6 to 8 hours of injury to reduce the incidence of sepsis and death.[46]

Wounds of the perineum, anorectum, and vagina are managed using open techniques with repeated dressing changes/irrigations using general anesthesia as necessary. These wounds are usually allowed to heal by secondary intention to maintain an open tract to the fracture site. Our bias is that maintaining an open tract offers some protection against infection but data to support this bias are not available. Similarly, there is no convincing evidence that antibiotic treatment, either systemically, by topical application, or by irrigation lowers pelvic infection rate or osteomyelitis. Groin and iliac crest wounds are managed selectively. Some of these are amenable to early closure if contamination and tissue damage are not severe.

PRINCIPLES OF FIXATION FOR PELVIC FRACTURES

Basic Tenets

1. With complete instability of the posterior ring (i.e., the posterior SI ligaments are disrupted), anterior fixation alone is inadequate.

2. With complete instability of the posterior ring and vertical instability, any posterior fixation should be supplemented with some form of anterior stabilization.
3. With partial instability of the pelvic ring (i.e., the posterior SI ligaments are intact), anterior fixation alone is adequate and full weight bearing may be permitted.

Anterior Pelvic Ring Injuries

Symphysis Diastasis

The options for stabilizing symphyseal disruptions include anterior external fixators or internal fixation with plate and screws. Available data from biomechanical studies have shown that there is no significant difference between external or internal fixation of the pelvis for controlling the symphysis.[47,48] In addition, there is significant improvement in pelvic stability when posterior fixation is augmented with some form of anterior fixation in VS injury patterns.[49] Figure 7A shows an open-book pelvic fracture complicated by ongoing bleeding. After angiographic control of the bleeding, fixation with a combined anterior and posterior approach was accomplished (see Fig. 7B). Earlier clinical studies have shown no difference between two-hole plates and multihole plates; however, newer data suggests that two-hole plates may have a higher reoperation rate and incidence of pelvic malreduction.

Pros and Cons of External Fixation

Pros

- Can be used just as easily with rami fractures as symphysis disruption
- Can be applied in the ER, ICU, or OR

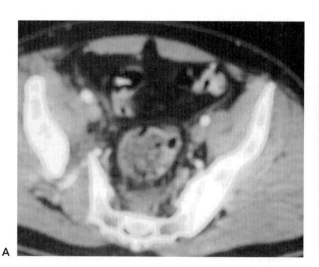
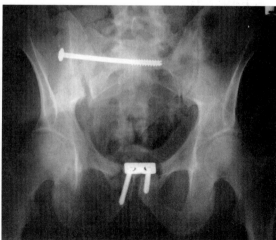

Figure 7   **A:** Open-book pelvic fracture with complete posterior disruption and instability. Contrast blush indicates continuing pelvic hemorrhage, which was controlled angiographically. **B:** Open-book pelvic fracture stabilized with combined anterior and posterior fixation.

- Can be used when contamination from abdominal and genitourinary injuries complicates the clinical picture
- Can be removed in the clinic or office setting

Cons

- External device that interferes with positioning, sitting, and clothing
- Pin-site care and infection can be problematic, particularly with obese patients
- More difficult to obtain and maintain an anatomic reduction of the anterior pelvic ring

Pros and Cons of Internal Fixation

Pros

- No interference with positioning, sitting, or clothing
- No problems with pin-site care

Cons

- Cannot be used with abdominal or pelvic contamination
- If hardware removal is required (not infrequently) then formal reoperation is necessary
- Can potentially interfere with relaxation of the pelvic ring in females delivering the fetus

Rami Fractures

Options are essentially the same; however, internal fixation with plating does not carry the same long-term obstetrical or hardware failure sequelae. The retrograde medullary ramus screw is a novel technique that allows percutaneous application of internal fixation of the ramus fracture; however, a closed percutaneous reduction must be possible.

Posterior Pelvic Ring Injuries

Iliac Wing Fractures

Iliac wing fractures can be fixed with the patient prone using a posterior approach with an incision along the crest and elevation of the gluteal musculature from the outer table of the ilium, or supine using an anterior approach with the lateral window of the ilioinguinal or Smith-Peterson exposures of the inner table. Depending on the fracture pattern and the patient's condition and/or associated injuries, one approach may offer advantages over the other. As a general rule, the anterior approach is better tolerated by the patient and associated with less blood loss. However, if the iliac wing fracture is very posterior, then exposure of both sides of the fracture and application of fixation may be difficult.

Usually, a single pelvic reconstruction plate or lag screw along the crest supplemented with a second reconstruction plate or lag screw at the level of the pelvic brim or sciatic buttress will suffice in neutralizing deforming forces until healing occurs (see Figs. 8A and B).

Sacroiliac Joint Dislocations

Again, the SI joint can be approached from either anterior or posterior as described in the preceding text, but it is often easier to reduce the SI joint and apply reduction clamps from posterior. Attention must be paid to closing the anterior aspect of the SI joint, which can be difficult from the posterior approach. Fixation options include iliosacral screws, anterior SI plating, and posterior transiliac plating or compression rods; however, biomechanical studies have not shown any significant differences between these techniques.[40,51–54]

Pros and Cons of Iliosacral Screw Fixation

Pros

- Can be applied percutaneously if closed reduction is possible
- Can be applied in either the prone or supine position
- Can be applied in situations of severe soft tissue damage where open procedure would be compromised

Cons

- Experienced surgeons and excellent intraoperative fluoroscopic quality with clear imaging are a must[55,56]

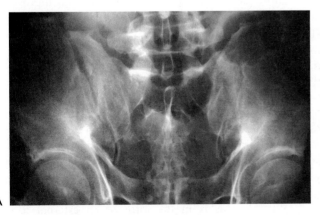
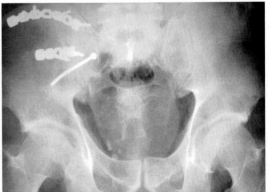

A   B

Figure 8   **A:** Iliac wing fracture before internal fixation. **B:** Iliac wing fracture after stabilization.

Pros and Cons of Anterior Sacroiliac Plating

Pros

- Particularly useful if additional ipsilateral anterior pelvic/acetabular procedures are performed

Cons

- Requires dissection and placement of fixation onto the sacral ala, which places the L5 nerve root at risk

Pros and Cons of Transiliac Bars or Plates

Pros

- Crosses the normal contralateral SI joint

Cons

- In thin patients, fixation can be prominent and bothersome occasionally causing skin breakdown

Crescent Fractures (Sacroiliac Joint Fracture-Dislocations)

This injury involves a fracture of the iliac wing posteriorly that starts at the crest and exits into the SI joint. A variable-sized fragment of posterior crest containing the posterior superior iliac spine (PSIS) remains attached to the sacral ala through the posterior SI ligaments. This constant fragment can be used as an aid to reduction as it is located anatomically. Standard fixation involves a superiorly placed reconstruction plate along the crest with supplemental lag screws from the posterior inferior iliac spine (PIIS) into the sciatic buttress just above the greater notch. As the constant fragment becomes smaller, this injury approaches an SI dislocation, and consideration must be given to supplemental SI screws or plates.

Sacral Fractures

The topic of sacral fractures encompasses a whole discussion. Suffice it to say that these injuries, depending on fracture pattern, can be regarded as pelvic ring injuries or spinal injures. In addition, sacral fractures often involve some form of neurologic deficit, either unilateral peripheral nerve root (as in the case of VS injuries) or cauda equina lesions (as in the case of transverse fractures that involve the central spinal canal). Occasionally, the L5/S1 joint is disrupted and the stability of the lumbosacral junction is compromised. All of these issues need to be taken into consideration when treating sacral fractures. Figure 9 illustrates a CT image of a sacral fracture causing neural as well as skeletal damage.

Fixation largely depends on what is disrupted, that is, the pelvic ring, the lumbosacral junction, or both. Some sacral fractures that arise from lateral compression injuries result in impaction of the ala and may be inherently stable, not requiring any fixation. Other fractures that are unstable will incorporate some form of posterior fixation as outlined in the preceding text.

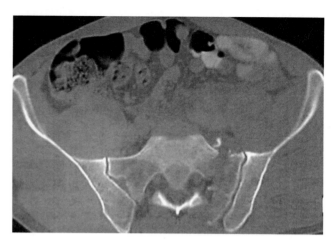

Figure 9   Sacral fracture creating posterior instability.

OUTCOME STUDIES FOR PELVIC FRACTURES

Stabilization of unstable pelvic injuries has only recently evolved to include early internal fixation and restoration of anatomic relations. Before the 1980s, very little was understood regarding the biomechanics and contributions to stability of the various pelvic bony and ligamentous structures. As recently as the 1970s, many pelvic ring disruptions were treated with nonoperative techniques; generally skeletal traction and pelvic slings to prevent excessive cephalad migration of the hemipelvis. However, many clinicians have documented the high incidence of poor functional outcome and chronic pain in patients with vertically unstable pelvic fractures treated nonoperatively.[14,57,58] The results of these and other studies provided the impetus to pursue operative means to achieve and maintain anatomic reduction.

Operative stabilization began with anteriorly placed external fixators alone, which were found to be nearly totally ineffective at controlling vertical and posterior displacement of the posterior aspect of the ring 59. Clinical outcome studies with the use of external fixators subsequently found that results were not improved over nonoperative management[60,61] and in fact, traction and pelvic sling alone may have been more successful at treating this unstable injury.

Improved short-term patient outcome with early stabilization of the pelvic fracture and mobilization of the patient[62,63] as well as numerous reports citing improved outcome with anatomic reduction of the posterior ring continued to provide the impetus to develop more rigid and stable posterior fixation constructs.

Supplemental fixation of the anterior aspect of the pelvic ring has been shown to provide further biomechanical stability in the case of the vertically unstable hemipelvis. Whether this is in the form of an external fixator or symphyseal plate seems to be of little significance; however, more orthopaedic trauma surgeons are moving toward routine use of symphyseal plates that can be placed at the time of exploratory laparotomy, and do not give rise to the attendant pin-site complications seen with external fixators.

Early outcome studies support the position that the long-term functional results are improved if reduction with <1 cm of combined displacement of the posterior ring is obtained, especially with pure dislocations of the SI complex. Fractures of the posterior ring tend to do better, presumably because bone healing can restore initial strength and stability, SI dislocations rely purely on ligamentous healing and scar formation and these patients tend to fare worse in terms of short-term and long-term problems with pain and ambulation when compared to patients with other fracture patterns.

However, despite seemingly anatomic reductions (or near anatomic) more recent clinical outcome studies have shown that with modern fixation techniques, a substantial proportion of patients continues to have poor outcomes with chronic posterior pelvic pain.[64-67] This is likely related to the following multiple confounding factors:

1. Trauma patients often have a borderline socioeconomic status with poor social and financial support groups
2. Extensive soft tissue damage and associated long bone and extremity fractures
3. Associated neurologic, visceral, and urogenital injuries with dyspareunia, sexual dysfunction, and incontinence
4. Prolonged recovery and rehabilitation time with loss of job, home, and family

Outcome studies after fixation of pelvic injuries are difficult to interpret because of poor follow-up, heterogeneity of the injury pattern, associated visceral and neurologic injury, and the lack of a reliable outcome measure for pelvic ring injuries. Debate continues regarding the definition of adequate reduction of the pelvic ring and how malreduction affects functional outcome, if at all. Recent clinical outcome studies have shown that with current fixation techniques, a substantial proportion of patients continue to have poor outcomes with chronic posterior pelvic pain despite seemingly anatomic reductions and healing, with <50% returning to previous level of function and work status.[47,63,65,68]

REFERENCES

1. Demetriades D, Karaiskakis M, Toutouzas K, et al. Pelvic fractures: Epidemiology and predictors of associated abdominal injuries and outcomes. *J Am Coll Surg.* 2002;195:1–10.
2. Poole GV, Ward EF. Causes of mortality in patients with pelvic fractures. *Orthopedics.* 1994;17:691–696.
3. Cydulka RK, Parreira JG, Coimbra R, et al. The role of associated injuries on outcome of blunt trauma patients sustaining pelvic fractures. *Injury.* 2000;31:677–682.
4. Hearn TC, Tile M. The effects of ligament sectioning and internal fixation of bending stiffness of the pelvic ring. *In Proceedings of the 13th International Conference on Biomechanics.* Perth, Australia; December 1991.
5. Dalal SA, Burgess AR, Siegel JH, et al. Pelvic fracture in multiple trauma: Classification by mechanism is the key to pattern of organ injury, resuscitative requirements, and outcome. *J Trauma.* 1989;29(7):981–1002.
6. Rowe SA, Sochor MS, Staples KS, et al. Pelvic ring fractures: Implications of vehicle design, crash type, and occupant characteristics. *Surgery.* 2004;136:842–847.
7. Adams JE, Davis GG, Alexander CB, et al. Pelvic trauma in rapidly fatal motor vehicle accidents. *J Orthop Trauma.* 2003;17:406–410.
8. Inaba K, Sharkey PW, Stephen DJ, et al. The increasing incidence of severe pelvic injury in motor vehicle collisions. *Injury.* 2004;35:759–765.
9. Biffl WL, Smith WR, Moore EE, et al. Evolution of a multidisciplinary clinical pathway for the management of unstable patients with pelvic fractures. *Ann Surg.* 2001;233:843–850.
10. Blackmore CC, Jurkovich GJ, Linnau KF, et al. Assessment of volume of hemorrhage and outcome from pelvic fracture. *Arch Surg.* 2003;138:504–509.
11. Pennal GF, Tile M, Waddell JP, et al. Pelvic disruption: Assessment and classification. *Clin Orthop.* 1980;151:12–22.
12. Gonzalez RP, Fried PQ, Bukhalo M. The utility of clinical examination in screening for pelvic fractures in blunt trauma. *J Am Coll Surg.* 2002;194:121–125.
13. Tile M. Pelvic fractures: Should they be fixed? *J Bone Joint Surg.* 1988;70–B:1–12.
14. Young JWR, Burgess AR, Brumback RJ, et al. Pelvic fractures: Value of plain radiography in early assessment and management. *Radiology.* 1986;160:445–451.
15. Orthopaedic Trauma Association. OTA classification of fractures. *J Orthop Trauma.* 1996;10(Suppl):66–75.
16. Huittinen V-M, Slatis P. Postmortem angiography and dissection of the hypogastric artery in pelvic fractures. *Surgery.* 1973;73:454–462.
17. Metz CM, Hak DJ, Goulet JA, et al. Pelvic fracture patterns and their corresponding sources of hemorrhage. *Orthop Clin North Am.* 2004;35:431–437.
18. Miller PR, Moore PS, Mansell E, et al. External fixation or arteriogram in bleeding pelvic fracture: Initial therapy guided by markers of arterial hemorrhage. *J Trauma.* 2003;54:437–443.
19. Mattox KL, Bickell W, Pepe PE, et al. Prospective randomized evaluation of antishock MAST in post-traumatic hypotension. *J Trauma.* 1986;26:779–786.
20. Flint LM, Brown A, Richardson JD, et al. Definitive control of hemorrhage in pelvic crush injuries. *Ann Surg.* 1979;189:709–716.
21. Brotman S, Browner BD, Cox EF. MAS trousers improperly applied causing a compartment syndrome in the lower extremity. *J Trauma.* 1982;22:598–599.
22. Pohlemann T. Pelvic emergency clamps: Anatomic landmarks for a safe primary application. *J Orthop Trauma.* 2004;18:102–105.
23. Ertel W, Keel M, Eid K, et al. Control of severe hemorrhage using C-clamp and pelvic packing in multiply injured patients with pelvic ring disruption. *J Orthop Trauma.* 2001;15:468–474.
24. Gansslen A, Giannoudis P, Pape HC. Hemorrhage in pelvic fracture: Who needs angiography? *Curr Opin Crit Care.* 2003;9:515–523.
25. Bartlett CS, Ali A, Helfet DL. Bladder incarceration in a traumatic symphysis pubis diastasis treated with external fixation: A case report and review of the literature. *J Orthop Trauma.* 1998;12:64–67.
26. Geracci JJ, Morey AF. Bladder entrapment after external fixation of traumatic pubic diastasis: Importance of follow-up computed tomography in establishing prompt diagnosis. *Mil Med.* 2000;165:492–493.
27. Bottlang M. Noninvasive reduction of open-book pelvic fractures by circumferential compression. *J Orthop Trauma.* 2002;16:367–373.
28. Ghanayem AJ. Emergent treatment of pelvic fractures. Comparison of methods of stabilization. *Clin Orthop.* 1995;318:75–80.
29. Pasquale M, Fabia TC. Eastern Association for the Surgery of Trauma. Practice management guidelines for hemorrhage in pelvic fracture. *J Trauma.* 1998;44(6):941–956.
30. Hak DJ. The role of pelvic angiography in evaluation and management of pelvic trauma. *Orthop Clin North Am.* 2004;35:439–443.

31. Ramirez JI, Velmahos GC, Best CR, et al. Male sexual function after bilateral iliac artery embolization for pelvic fracture. *J Trauma.* 2004;56:734–739.

32. O'Brien DP, Luchette FA, Pereira SJ, et al. Pelvic fracture in the elderly is associated with increased mortality. *Surgery.* 2002;132:710–714.

33. Kimbrell BJ, Velmahos GC, Chan LS, et al. Angiographic embolization for pelvic fractures in older patients. *Arch Surg.* 2004;139:728–733.

34. Velmahos GC, Toutouzas KG, Vassiliu P, et al. A prospective study on the safety and efficacy of angiographic embolization for pelvic and visceral injuries. *J Trauma.* 2002;53:303–308.

35. Fallon B, Wendt JC, Hawtrey CE. Urological injury and assessment in patients with fractured pelvis. *J Urol.* 1984;131:712–714.

36. Peng MY, Parisky YR, Cornwell EE, et al. CT cystography versus conventional cystography in evaluation of bladder injury. *AJR Am J Roentgenol.* 1999;173:1269–1272.

37. Rothenberger DA, Velasco R, Strate R, et al. Open pelvic fracture: A lethal injury. *J Trauma.* 1978;18:184–187.

38. Brenneman FD, Katyal D, Boulanger BR, et al. Long term outcome in open pelvic fractures. *J Trauma.* 1997;42:773–777.

39. Richardson JD, Harty J, Amin M, et al. Open pelvic fractures. *J Trauma.* 1982;22:533–538.

40. Stocks GW, Gabel GT, Noble PC, et al. Anterior and posterior internal fixation of vertical shear fractures of the pelvis. *J Orthop Res.* 1991;9:237–245.

41. Webb LX, Gristina AG, Wilson JR Jr, et al. Two-hole plate fixation for traumatic symphysis pubis diastasis. *J Trauma.* 1988;28(6):813–817.

42. Sagi HC, Ordway NT, DiPasquale T. Biomechanical analysis of fixation for vertically unstable sacro-iliac dislocations with ilio-sacral screws and symphyseal plating. *J Orthop Trauma.* 2004;18(3):135–139.

43. Matta JM, Saucedo T. Internal fixation of pelvic ring fractures. *Clin Orthop.* 1989;242:83–97.

44. Comstock CP, van der Meulen MCH, Goodman SB. Biomechanical comparison of posterior internal fixation techniques for unstable pelvic fractures. *J Orthop Trauma.* 1996;10(8):517–522.

45. Gorczyca JT, Varga E, Woodside T, et al. The strength of ilio-sacral lag screws and trans-iliac bars in the fixation of vertically unstable pelvic injuries with sacral fractures. *Injury.* 1996;27(8):561–564.

46. Simonian PT, Routt ML. Biomechanics of pelvic fixation. *Orthop Clin North Am.* 1997;28(3):351–367.

47. Routt ML, Simonian PT, Mills WJ. Iliosacral screw fixation: Early complications of the percutaneous technique. *J Orthop Trauma.* 1997;11(8):584–589.

48. Routt ML, Simonian PT, Agnew SG, et al. Radiographic recognition of the sacral alar slope for optimal placement of iliosacral screws: A cadaveric and clinical study. *J Orthop Trauma.* 1996;10(3):171–177.

49. Routt ML, Nork SE, Mills WJ. High energy pelvic ring disruptions. *Orthop Clin North Am.* 2002;33:59–72.

50. Holdsworth F. Dislocation and fracture dislocation of the pelvis. *J Bone Joint Surg.* 1948;30B:461–466.

51. Slatis P, Huittenen V-M. Double vertical fractures of the pelvis: A report on 163 patients. *Acta Chir Scand.* 1972;138:799–807.

52. Semba R, Yasukawa K, Gustilo R. Critical analysis of results of 53 Malgaigne fractures of the pelvis. *J Trauma.* 1983;23:535–537.

53. Cole JD, Blum DA, Ansel LJ. Outcome after fixation of unstable posterior pelvic ring injuries. *Clin Orthop.* 1996;329:160–179.

54. Kregor PJ, Routt ML. Unstable pelvic ring disruptions in unstable patients. *Injury.* 1999;30(Suppl 2):SB19–SB28.

55. Goldstein A, Phillips T, Sclafani SJ, et al. Early open reduction and internal fixation of the disrupted pelvic ring. *J Trauma.* 1986;26(4):325–333.

56. Latenser BA, Gentilello LM, Tarver AA, et al. Improved outcome with early fixation of skeletally unstable pelvic fractures. *J Trauma.* 1991;31(1):28–31.

57. Tornetta P, Matta JM III. Outcome of operatively treated unstable posterior pelvic ring disruptions. *Clin Orthop.* 1996;329:186–193.

58. Dujardin FH, Hossenbaccus M, Duparc F, et al. Long-term functional prognosis of posterior injuries in high-energy pelvic disruption. *J Orthop Trauma.* 1998;12(3):145–150.

59. Nepola JV, Trenhaile SW, Miranda MA, et al. Vertical shear injuries: Is there a relationship between residual displacement and functional outcome? *J Trauma.* 1999;46(6):1024–1030.

60. Van den Bosch EW, Van der Kleyn R, Hogervorst M, et al. Functional outcome of internal fixation for pelvic ring fractures. *J Trauma.* 1999;47(2):365–371.

61. Copeland CE, Bosse MJ, McCarthy ML, et al. Effect of trauma and pelvic fracture on female genitourinary, sexual, and reproductive function. *J Orthop Trauma.* 1997;11(2):73–81.

62. Lowe MA, Mason JT, Luna GK, et al. Risk factors for urethral injury in men with traumatic pelvic fractures. *J Urol.* 1988;140:506–507.

63. Yinger K, Scalise J, Olsen SA, et al. Biomechanical comparison of posterior pelvic ring fixation. *J Orthop Trauma.* 2003;17(7):481–487.

64. Cass AS, Godec CJ. Urethral injury due to external trauma. *Urology.* 1978;11:607–611.

65. Palmer JK, Benson GS, Corriere JN. Diagnosis and initial management of urological injuries associated with 200 consecutive pelvic fractures. *J Urol.* 1983;130:712–714.

66. Kellam J. The role of external fixation in pelvic disruptions. *Clin Orthop.* 1989;241:66–82.

67. Cass AS. The multiply injured patient with bladder trauma. *J Trauma.* 1984;24:731–734.

68. Raffa J, Christensen NM. Compound fractures of the pelvis. *Am J Surg.* 1976;132:282–286.

FURTHER READINGS

Oliver CW, Twaddle B, Agel J, et al. Outcome after pelvic ring fractures: Evaluation using the medical outcomes short-form SF-36 *Injury.* 1996;27(9):635–641.

Pohlemann T, Gansslen A, Schellwald O, et al. Outcome after pelvic ring injuries. *Injury.* 1996;27(Suppl 2):SB31–SB38.

Fractures of the Lower Extremity

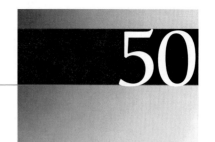

50

James P. Stannard   *Justin N. Duke*   *Jorge E. Alonso*

Lower extremity fractures are often severe injuries that may lead to long-term disability in patients who are involved in trauma. Most orthopaedic traumatologists spend their careers focusing on pelvic and lower extremity trauma. However, understanding these injuries is vitally important to general surgery traumatologists as well. As the "captain of a ship," it is critical for traumatologists to understand how lower extremity trauma frequently has a major systemic impact. This chapter will initially focus on the management of lower extremity trauma patients when they present to the trauma room. Following that, we will discuss the concepts of damage control orthopaedics, open fractures, gunshot wounds, dislocations, geriatric patients, and heterotopic ossification. Finally, we will briefly discuss various lower extremity skeletal injuries and their appropriate management.

Severe lower extremity trauma is increasingly common as a result of our increasingly mobile society, high-speed driving, and the influence of alcohol, drugs, and firearms. As we become more mobile, the speed and thereby the achieved kinetic energy at which we can injure ourselves keeps pace with the engineering design changes intended to prevent these same injuries. The combination of improved automotive safety features and continued trauma system improvements have led to more patients' surviving their injuries. It is important to understand the systemic impact of high-energy lower extremity injuries on multiply injured patients, in order to decrease their morbidity and increase the potential function following rehabilitation.

INITIAL PRESENTATION AND PHYSICAL EXAMINATION

Once the *Airway*, *Breathing*, and *Circulation* (ABCs) of resuscitation have been initiated and the extremity examinations are completed, it is time to pay special attention to many details. The history provided by the patient, emergency medical services (EMSs), or other witnesses can be very significant in evaluating the nature and severity of the patient's skeletal injury. Here, because we are concerned with the lower extremity, facts such as potential environmental contamination become very important. Quantitating the energies associated with the injury can be very useful (see Fig. 1). For example, a young individual who sustains a relatively low-energy accident, such as a fall from standing, with a femoral neck fracture raises our suspicion for an underlying pathologic process. Although this information may seem appropriate for the nonacute treatment phase of care, it illustrates the importance of history when available. The presence of any crush injury is particularly important, especially if there was a prolonged extraction time at the scene of the accident. Rhabdomyelisis and compartment syndrome become much more likely with a crush injury than with other mechanisms of trauma.

The initial survey of the lower extremity should be concerned with gross deformity, skeletal stability, soft tissue assessment, and the neurovascular status of each limb (see Fig. 2). With an awake and alert patient, these conditions

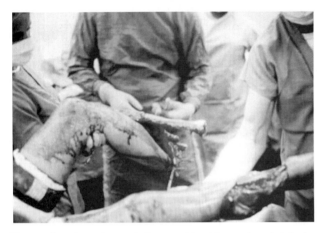

Figure 1 Bilateral mangled extremities. The patients' right leg was able to be salvaged.

baseline neurologic and vascular examination possible. The quality of this examination may dictate the subsequent treatment course of the lower extremity over the initial 48- to 72-hour resuscitation period.

Many patients will present with fractures that demonstrate obvious deformity during the secondary survey. Radiographs should be obtained for the area of interest and the joint proximal and distal to the fracture. Unstable long bone should be temporarily stabilized using traction or splinting while a definitive plan for treatment is formulated. Stabilization is important not only for pain control but also to minimize hemorrhage and secondary soft tissue injury, as well as to maintain soft tissues properly.

may be relatively easy to assess, but are more challenging and important in the obtunded and/or mechanically ventilated patient. If at all possible, the orthopaedic service should be consulted as early as possible, preferably during the initial assessment of the patient. This will allow a much more complete extremity neurovascular examination and involve orthopaedic surgery in the overall clinical decisions early in the course of care. Unfortunately, the realities of the care of trauma patients will dictate that patients often require airway management with intubation before evaluation by orthopaedics. Consequently, it is essential that the general surgery trauma team obtain the best

DAMAGE CONTROL ORTHOPAEDICS

The topic of damage control orthopaedics is currently in evolution and somewhat controversial. It is well established that many patients benefit from early definite stabilization of long bone fractures of the lower extremities. However, the observation that some patients develop systemic complications following skeletal stabilization has led the concept of damage control orthopaedics.[1,2] This approach is based on the observation that some patients with multiple systemic injuries may not tolerate, and in fact may be harmed by undergoing early definitive treatment of their fractures. The scenario most frequently studied is that of the polytrauma patient with a femoral fracture[3] (see Fig. 3). It has been established that early fixation

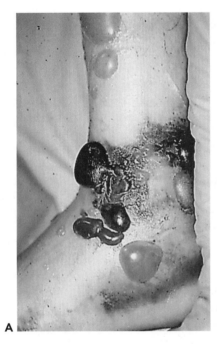
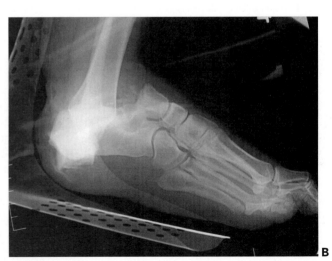

Figure 2 Talar dislocation with impressive blistering of the overlying skin. This patient will need to wait before surgery can be attempted, although the dislocation needs closed reduction as soon as possible.

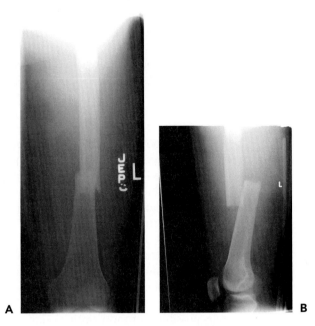

Figure 3 **A:** Anterior-posterior (AP) view of transverse femur fracture. **B:** Lateral view of transverse femur fracture.

reduces many risks of pulmonary complication for many patients; however, the type of fixation is a point of contention. There is concern that a subset of patients, often those with severe thoracic injuries or lung contusions, may not respond well to intramedullary nailing in the acute phase of their resuscitation. The second hit theory states that during the initial treatment course, polytrauma patients develop elevated levels of inflammatory markers and cytokines as part of their systemic response to trauma. Some investigators have expressed concern that performing invasive orthopaedic procedures during the immediate posttrauma period can be associated with an exaggerated inflammatory response that can overwhelm the body and can lead to multiorgan system failure, sepsis, and death. The greatest elevation in the level of inflammatory markers seems to be associated with reamed intramedullary nailing of the femur, although new methods of reaming while irrigating and suctioning moderate these risks.[4,5] Consequently, research is under way as to the specifics of this second hit theory, and it remains highly controversial regarding which patients will benefit from early intramedullary stabilization, and those who would benefit from minimizing the initial orthopaedic surgical procedures and cultivating a damage control approach.

Patients who have sustained particularly severe multi-system trauma may benefit from minimizing the initial orthopaedic procedures. If a patient is hemodynamically tenuous or has sustained a severe chest or brain injury, a temporizing procedure such as external fixation may be the wisest initial treatment. Advantages of external fixation include that it can be applied very quickly and with minimal blood loss[6] and that it can be performed concurrently while another surgical team performs a procedure on another site of the body. Disadvantages include the poor long-term results if the external fixation is used as definitive fixation, and the cost and risk of pin tract infections if the fixator is intended for only temporary stabilization.[7]

It is important that the primary trauma surgery team realizes that many external fixators are placed only for temporary stabilization of the fracture. Communication with the orthopaedic service should be maintained because external fixators require diligence to insure that the pin sites are kept clean, and that it does not stay in place too long. Ideally, the patient will be able to tolerate definitive fixation within the first 3 to 4 days of their admission, as the risk of complications with the exchange of external fixations for nails or plates increases the longer they stay in place. One potential exception involves open fractures with severe soft tissue injury. They may need to be spanned for a longer period of time until the wound and soft tissues have recovered enough to allow definitive fixation and coverage.

OPEN FRACTURES

Open fracture is one category of skeletal injury that requires prompt attention to optimize clinical outcome (see Fig. 4). Most North American orthopaedic surgeons employ the Gustilo and Anderson classification system to grade the severity of open fractures (see Table 1).[8]

The introduction of negative pressure wound therapy (NPWT) devices (vaccum-assisted closure [VAC], Kenetic Concepts, Inc., San Antonio, TX) has remarkably improved our ability to cover open fractures that have significant soft tissue destruction without resorting to large free tissue transfers.[9–12] The VAC is often placed at the end of the initial debridement, and then changed with each subsequent debridement (see Fig. 5). NPWT is thought to work through three mechanisms. First, it increases

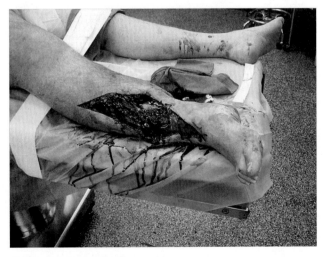

Figure 4 A grade III open tibia.

TABLE 1

GUSTILO AND ANDERSON SYSTEM OF OPEN FRACTURE CLASSIFICATION

Type of Fracture	Description
Type I	Injuries involving simple fracture patterns and a skin incision <1 cm long, without gross contamination
Type II	Open fractures having a skin laceration longer than 1 cm, with a mild to moderate degree of soft tissue damage and contamination
Type III	High-energy injuries with a severe soft tissue injury; further divided into three categories
Subtype IIIA	Fractures having adequate soft tissue available for coverage
Subtype IIIB	Fractures having inadequate soft tissue available to cover the bone
Subtype IIIC	Fractures having inadequate soft tissue available to cover the bone, plus an arterial injury that requires vascular repair

blood flow and angiogenesis.[13] Second, it is thought to improve the wound by removing excess fluid.[14] This mechanism is very important in some injury patterns such as compartment syndrome and burns, but less important with other skeletal injuries. The third proposed mechanism of NPWT action involves mechanical stimulation of cell cytoskeletons leading to the production of substances and proteins associated with wound healing.[15,16] An additional benefit of using NPWT in the operating room is that the wound is sealed off from the outside environment by the VAC dressing. This can be particularly helpful in patients who are in the intensive care unit environment where resistant organisms are more commonly encountered.[17,18]

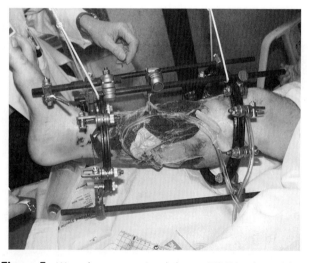

Figure 5 Wound vaccum-assisted closure (VAC) in place with an external fixator.

The use of NPWT may be associated with more rapid wound closure and a lower rate of infection in selected orthopaedic trauma patients.

The initial treatment of open fracture should begin as soon as possible. Of course, life-threatening injuries always take precedence over limb-threatening injuries. However, once the trauma team has successfully addressed the initial ABCs and the patient is stable, the open fracture must be a priority. There are some important principles that should be kept in mind during the treatment of patients with open fractures: (i) limit the evaluation of the open wound to a single look; (ii) initiate antibiotics early; and (iii) initiate surgical irrigation and debridement expeditiously[19–22] (see Fig. 6). The first principle is that the open fracture wound should be viewed once, and then kept covered. It will be very helpful if a digital photo can be taken when the wound is initially evaluated, so that subsequent caregivers can look at the photo rather than repetitively exposing the wound. The second principle is that antibiotic therapy should be initiated as soon as possible. For most open wounds this will include cefazolin 1 g every 8 hours, with the addition of an amiglycoside if the fracture is type II or III. If the wound is contaminated with soil or other sources of organic infection (i.e., ditch water or farm accidents) then penicillin or metronidazole should be added to the regimen. Alternatively, a broad-spectrum antibiotic plus penicillin, if there is organic contamination, can be employed. The rapidity of the initiation of appropriate antibiotic coverage is associated with decreasing the likelihood of the patient developing an infection or osteomyelitis.[18,19] The tetanus status of the patient must also be determined; and without proof of tetanus vaccination status, patients should receive both toxoid of 0.5 mL and immunoglobulin of 250 U if they are older than 10 years. Following initial inspection, the wound should be covered with a sterile dressing, radiographs obtained, and a reduction attempted with splinting. The patient should be taken expeditiously to the operating room for a formal debridement and irrigation procedure and surgical stabilization of the fracture. If the patient is too unstable to be taken to the operating room quickly, a limited debridement and irrigation procedure should be undertaken in the intensive care unit. This procedure is performed using a sterile field, limited debridement, and pulsatile irrigation with at least 8 L of sterile saline (see Fig. 7). It is more controversial whether a cleansing procedure should be undertaken in the emergency room if a delay is anticipated in getting the patient to the operating room. Debridement should clearly not be performed in the emergency room or trauma bay, but a gentle washing with removal or gross contaminants is permissible. Sterile saline may be used with a "water can" cap that allows gentle irrigation, and one can add Betadine to the solution until the fluid is the color of iced tea. Any visible bone fragments should not be removed outside the operating room. There is no clear data to support or condemn a single gentle cleansing in the

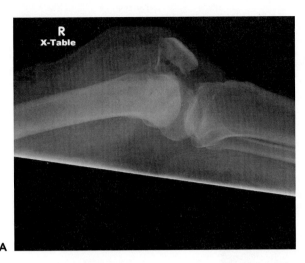
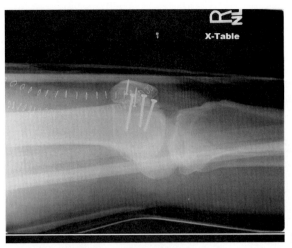

Figure 6 **A:** Penetrating trauma from a meat slicer that resulted in an open fracture. The patient was taken to the operating room urgently for irrigation and fixation. **B:** Postoperative films of the patient who suffered an open wound caused by an industrial meat slicer. Notice the staple lines that correspond to the slice made in the anterior thigh.

emergency room. If such a procedure is performed, it is very important to understand that it is not a substitute for formal intraoperative debridement and irrigation.

GUNSHOT WOUNDS INVOLVING A FRACTURE

Fractures to the lower extremities caused by firearms require special consideration. As with all fractures, the mechanism can be very important to guiding the treatment

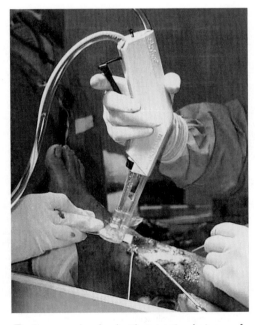

Figure 7 An example of pulsatile irrigation being performed in the operating room.

of these fractures (see Fig. 8). Knowing whether the projectile came from a handgun, hunting or assault rifle, or shotgun, and from what range the injury occurred will aid in treatment. A close range injury is usually associated with higher energy than a bullet fired from a distance. More importantly, knowing the caliber and specifics of the ammunition can be of help. High-energy gunshot wounds create fargreater soft tissue damage in the zone of injury surrounding the fracture. These wounds require great vigilance and frequent trips to the operating room in order to avoid complications such as osteomyelitis, nonunion, or compartment syndrome. Treatment should be based on a thorough physical and neurovascular examination and supplemented by radiographs.

The gunshot is a clinical challenge due to the contaminated nature of the wound. The skin, clothing, and other foreign material must be debrided from the wound and are potential sources of infection. Soft tissue damage is caused not only by the fracture of the bone and resultant instability but also by the shock wave of the projectile passing through the tissue. The ballistic zone of injury is far greater with a high-energy gunshot wound than with a low-energy injury. The patient depicted in Fig. 8 sustained a gunshot wound to the lower extremity that was suspicious of vascular injury due to decreased capillary refill. Appropriate evaluation requires vascular studies to determine the extent of damage, to include Duplex ultrasonography, computed tomography (CT) angiography, and intraoperative and formal angiography (see Fig. 9).

OPEN JOINTS

Any laceration in the immediate vicinity of a joint must be considered to be an open joint until proved otherwise.

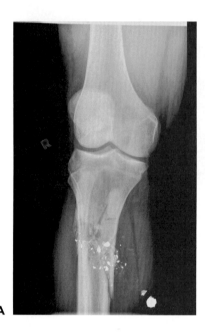

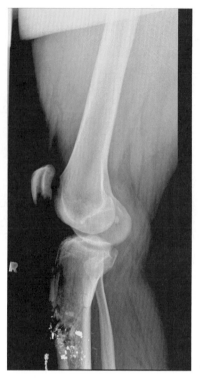

Figure 8   A and B: Gunshot wound to proximal tibia, anterior-posterior (AP), and lateral.

The reason for this high level of suspicion is due to the adverse consequences of subsequent joint infection if this diagnosis is overlooked. A septic joint is an excruciatingly painful condition that represents a surgical emergency. In an infected joint, the bacteria can replicate at alarming rates, resulting in severe and often irrevocable damage to the articular cartilage of the joint. The net result of a missed or untreated septic joint is early and often severe degenerative arthritis with subsequent permanent disability or systemic sepsis and death.

The joint under suspicion should be challenged with an injection of sterile saline, with the volume used depending on the joint involved. Usually 60 mL is adequate for challenging a knee, and lower volumes being adequate for

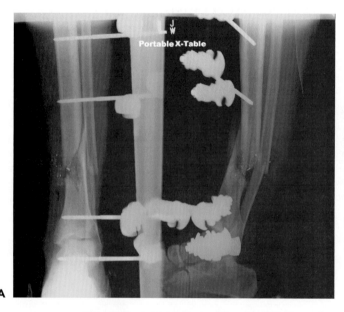

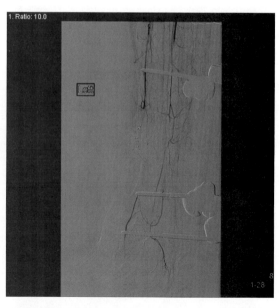

Figure 9   A: Gunshot wound to the tibia. Treated as type IIIC due to contamination and suspicion of vascular injury. **B:** CT angiogram of patient. Notice vascular insufficiency distal to the injury. This patient was placed in an external fixator, but the vascular team was unable to repair the injury.

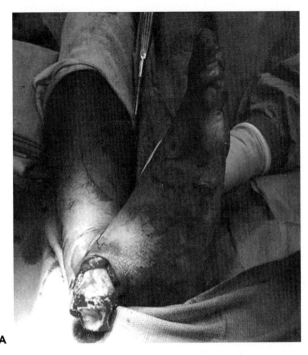

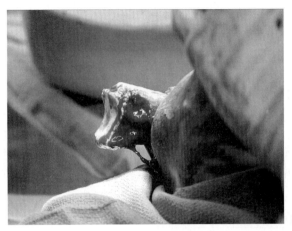

A   B

Figure 10 An open fracture with dislocation. Notice the exposed articular cartilage of the distal tibia.

most other joints. Strict care should be taken to adhere to sterile technique so that an iatrogenic septic joint does not occur. Once it has been established that there is an open joint, surgical debridement and irrigation is urgent. If the patient is stable and adequately resuscitated, there should be little delay in getting to the operating room. The longer the surgical team delays debriding and irrigating the joint, the greater the chance of damage to the articular cartilage (see Fig. 10). It is also important to rapidly initiate systemic antibiotics as an adjunct to the surgical treatment of the open joint.

DISLOCATIONS

As with most conditions, the severity of dislocations can vary widely depending on the severity of the trauma. The potential long-term consequences of dislocation are remarkably different depending on the joint involved. Dislocations of the hip, knee, and ankle are all injuries associated with a high risk of complications. Dislocations of the hip are particularly important to recognize and treat early. There is a high risk of severe damage to the femoral head from osteonecrosis due to an interruption in the vascular supply. Knee dislocations are addressed in another chapter. They are complex injuries that must be recognized rapidly in order to exclude the possibility of a popliteal artery injury. Current trends favor physical examination with or without supplemental ankle brachial indices to exclude vascular injuries following knee dislocations. This

protocol is now well established in the literature.[23–29] The risks associated with ankle and foot dislocations are primarily associated with skin necrosis in the region of the dislocation (see Fig. 11). The skin around the foot and ankle has a tenuous blood supply and does not tolerate

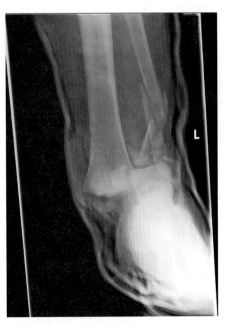

Figure 11 Anterior-posterior (AP) ankle film of complete talardislocation. Notice the plaster splint in place, indicating that closed reduction was attempted. This dislocation was only reducible by open reduction that was urgently carried out.

the deformity of a dislocation well. These three types of lower extremity dislocations require urgent or emergent reduction of the joint.

In most situations, closed reduction should be attempted as soon as possible. The initial attempt is normally done under conscious sedation. If reduction is not achieved with one or two good efforts, then the patient should be taken to the operating room for a reduction under general anesthesia. As noted previously, the longer a dislocated joint remains unreduced, the greater the risk of permanent morbidity due to vascular or soft tissue injury. Many trauma patients are young, and the options for reconstruction of a hip that has developed severe posttraumatic arthritis secondary to osteonecrosis are quite limited, and less than ideal. Dislocations of the femoral head are usually posterior, but can occasionally be anterior. Anterior dislocations are usually associated with higher energy trauma and often additional fractures are associated with hip dislocations.

GERIATRIC LOWER EXTREMITY TRAUMA

As the US population ages, the number of elderly patients involved in high-energy traumas and sustaining lower extremity fractures is increasing.[30–32] This demographic also suggests that a significant number of patients with periprosthetic fractures will be encountered. These periprosthetic fractures require more careful and detailed preoperative planning when compared to standard fractures, and often a total joint surgeon may be essential to successfully treat these complex injuries.

Another major concern regarding geriatric patients with fractures is their associated medical comorbidities. Additionally, the status of their soft tissues and their bone quality can remarkably influence the surgical plan. A detailed medical history from a reliable source can be beneficial in assisting the orthopaedic team to form a treatment plan. Because some patients will have poor quality soft tissue, it is important to be particularly gentle when applying dressings and splints. Care should be taken not to further jeopardize already friable tissue. Any splints or casts should be well padded and must be frequently inspected to avoid pressure ulcers. It is important to point out that many surgical treatments of the lower extremity can be undertaken with the use of regional or spinal anesthesia, thereby reducing the risks of endotracheal intubation and general anesthetics in this population.

HETEROTOPIC OSSIFICATIONS

The topic of heterotopic ossifications warrants brief mention. Certain injuries such as high-energy fractures with severe comminution, gunshot wounds, and closed head injury are prone to produce heterotopic ossification. Heterotopic ossification is the formation of bone outside the original periosteum. These formations can limit the range of motion of a joint, cause significant pain, or even completely immobilize the joint. It is important for the trauma team to be aware of the risk of this complication. Common injuries associated with debilitating heterotopic ossification are hip or acetabulum fractures or dislocations. Also, patients who require a posterior pelvic (Kocher Langenbeck) surgical approach are at high risk. Femoral head injuries are also commonly associated with lower extremity heterotopic ossification. High-risk patients should be considered for prophylactic treatment with either a single low-dose treatment of radiation therapy or a 6-week course of indomethacin. Failure to prevent this complication can leave a polytrauma patient with permanent impairment despite recovery from their other injuries.

FRACTURES OF THE ACETABULUM

The hip socket, which comprises the femoral head and the acetabulum, can be subjected to fractures that can range from nonoperative fractures to life-threatening injuries. In patients who have sustained high-energy trauma, the screening anterior-posterior (AP) pelvis film should be carefully evaluated for fractures of the acetabulum. Iliac oblique and obturator oblique views should also be obtained to evaluate the posterior and anterior column respectively once the patient has been stabilized.

The most common form of acetabular fracture is the posterior wall fracture. This pattern is frequently seen when an occupant in a motor vehicle strikes the dashboard with their knee and the force is transmitted proximally. This injury can be associated with distal femur fractures, patella fractures, and hip or knee dislocations. The classification of acetabulum fractures is lengthy and beyond the scope of this chapter. If there is evidence suggestive of a fracture, the patient should have a CT scan with fine (usually 2 mm) cuts through the acetabulum. The CT scan is excellent at showing whether there are bony fragments in the joint, which will necessitate early intervention to preserve the articular surface. It is also critical for documenting marginal impaction of the bone, which the orthopaedic surgeon must address if it is present. The results of the CT scan are necessary to determine the need for skeletal traction as well as how quickly the patient requires surgical stabilization. Many acetabular fractures are also associated with hip dislocations. Fracture dislocations should be treated by first promptly reducing the hip, and then obtaining CT scans and other studies to look for associated injuries (see Fig. 12). It is very difficult to assess extent of the acetabular fractures by CT scan with the hip dislocated. The femoral head may be reducible, but if unstable, can repeatedly dislocate. In this situation, femoral traction can be used to maintain the femoral head in place until surgery. Skeletal traction can also be performed to maintain tissue length, and to allow delayed reconstruction of the

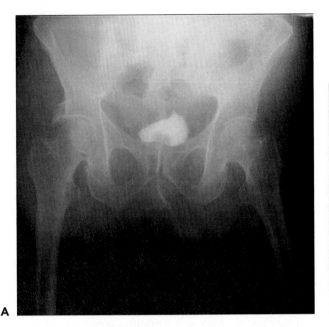

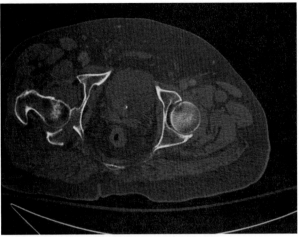

A   B

Figure 12 A: Anterior-posterior (AP) pelvis of a 73-year-old man involved in a motor vehicle collision (MVC). **B:** Computed tomography (CT) shows patient. Notice the posterior wall fragment. This hip was grossly unstable and required open reduction internal fixation. The femoral head was evaluated for associated injury.

acetabulum safely while other injuries are addressed if needed.

In general, if bony debris is present in the joint, if the joint is unstable, or if there is displacement or fracture of the weight-bearing surface of the acetabulum, surgery will be indicated and the patient should be prepared for such procedures. Open reduction and internal fixation of the acetabulum can result in significant blood loss; therefore, it is necessary that patient's hemodynamic status be optimized before surgery.

FEMORAL HEAD

Femoral head fractures are most commonly associated with hip dislocations. It is important to understand the blood supply to the femoral head because dislocations that are not reduced within 6 to 8 hours have an increased risk of developing osteonecrosis.[33] The foveal artery that branches from the obturator artery runs inside the ligamentum teres and is often compromised with displacement of the femoral head from the acetabulum. Though this artery provides only a minor amount of the blood supply in adults, it is very important in pediatric patients. The vast majority of blood flow to the femoral head is supplied by the medial femoral circumflex artery and its branches. Reducing the dislocation helps reduce distortion and damage to this critical artery.

Some small fractures of the femoral head that do not involve the weight-bearing surface may be treated closed, but most fractures involving the weight-bearing surface will require surgery. The complications of femoral head fracture

include posttraumatic arthritis and avascular necrosis of the femoral head. These complications can be reduced with early anatomic reduction and fixation of the fracture.

FEMORAL NECK

Femoral neck fractures seen in the young trauma population are the result of very high-energy trauma such as automobile accidents or a fall from a significant height. This fracture is a completely different injury than low-energy hip fractures in geriatric patients. Displaced high-energy femoral neck fractures in young patients are an urgent priority. This injury, like hip dislocations, may interrupt the blood supply to the femoral head. The anatomic reduction and stable fixation of these fractures should be of very high priority in young patients who are not good candidates for total hip arthroplasty. Clearly, life-threatening injuries should take priority over these injuries. However, the timing of fixation of femoral neck fractures in young patients is nearly as important as reducing lower extremity dislocations. Particular attention should be paid to nondisplaced femoral neck fractures in young patients. They should be given a high priority for stabilization to prevent the fracture from displacing and thereby threatening the blood supply to the head of the femur.

Isolated fractures of the femoral neck will most likely be seen in the elderly population because of low-energy impact, such as a fall from standing, or falling out of bed. An AP view of the pelvis along with AP and lateral views of the proximal femur will aid in evaluation. A careful history can help illuminate risk factors that lead to the fracture, and possibly uncover other associated conditions that need attention such as vertigo or pathologic fractures. A recent history of groin or hip pain could indicate a pathologic fracture, and this may alter the treatment plan.

Factors such as general health, medical comorbidities, ambulation status, and expectation of outcomes should be taken into account while treating an elderly patient. The more osteoporotic their bone stock, the more complicated fixation can become. In many instances, hip arthroplasty is the preferred treatment. There are also indications for nonoperative treatments; however, these indications are usually for the nonambulators with minimal pain or for those who would not tolerate the procedure well.

TROCANTERIC REGION OF THE FEMUR

The trochanteric region lies immediately distal to the neck of the femur. There are two distinct fracture patterns that occur in this area—intertrochanteric and subtrochanteric. Like the fractures of the femoral neck, intertrochanteric fractures most frequently occur in elderly patients who have experienced a low-energy injury. On presentation they usually have a shortened and externally rotated limb that is painful to range of motion (see Fig. 13). Intertrochanteric fractures may also present in the young population but will be associated with high-energy trauma. Most intertrochanteric fractures will require surgery when the patient is medically stable and great care must be exercised in establishing the rotational alignment of the femur. However, unlike fractures of the femoral neck, intertrochanteric fractures rarely

threaten the blood supply of the femoral head. Consequently, intertrochanteric fractures in young patients do not require the same sense of urgency that is necessary with femoral neck fractures.[34] Fixation can range from hip screws to plating, and cephalograde intramedullary nailing with locking screws. Isolated fractures of the greater trochanter can be seen in the elderly population, and if there is minimal displacement the treatment can be nonoperative. For the young patient or the active elderly patient with a displaced greater trochanter, fracture fixation of the fragment is recommended using tension band techniques. Isolated lesser trochanteric fracture should raise suspicion for the possibility of a pathologic fracture and further workup is warranted.

Fractures in the subtrochanteric region can also be of a pathologic nature, but more commonly will be the result of high-energy trauma. Fractures of the subtrochanteric region are defined as fractures between the lesser trochanter and 5 cm distal to the lesser trochanter. This region of the femur bears the highest forces and is very strong. It requires remarkable trauma to cause a subtrochanteric fracture, particularly in young patients. Great care should be taken to evaluate these patients for other injuries. These fractures are also often very challenging to reduce, and are much more prone to nonunion than other regions of the femur. Femur fractures, particularly in the subtrochanteric region, may be associated with significant bleeding. Stabilization, either temporary or definitively, can help with maintenance of hemodynamic stability.

FEMORAL SHAFT

Fractures of the femoral shaft are usually the result of high-energy trauma, unless the patient has weakened bone stock as a result of a pathologic condition. Patients will usually present with obvious deformity of the femur and with the leg in a field traction splint. Great care should be taken to insure that a patient is not to be left in a field traction splint for an extended period of time. These splints are excellent for transport and temporary stabilization; however, severe soft tissue and nerve damage may result from a splint that is not removed in a timely manner at the treatment center. After removal of the splint and assessment of the stability of the limb, radiographs should be obtained of the entire femur. At a minimum, this includes AP and lateral of the entire bone. It may be desirable to obtain oblique views if there is a unique fracture pattern that requires further evaluation. Many femur fractures will result in limb shortening and require traction for both patient comfort and for maintaining the tissues out to length. A traction pin should be placed from medial to lateral in the distal femur or from lateral to medial in the proximal tibia. Reducing the fracture with traction can help alleviate pain, aid reduction during the definitive surgical procedure, and reduce the amount of hemorrhage into the compartments of the leg.

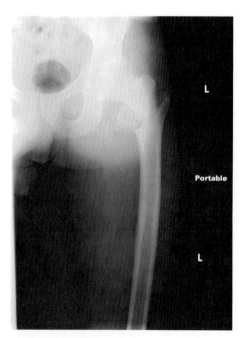

Figure 13   Intertrochanteric fracture.

The femur is surrounded by some of the largest muscle groups in the body, and is therefore subject to great deforming forces. The large volume of the compartments make compartment syndrome less likely than in some other areas such as the tibia where the swelling is not tolerated as well. However, compartment syndrome can still occur and frequent neurovascular examinations are warranted to insure that it is not worsening. A more detailed discussion of this topic is covered elsewhere in this text. As noted in the preceding text, the large compartments of the leg make it possible for a patient to lose considerable amounts of blood into the perifemoral space. It is common to lose more than a liter of blood into this area. For patients who are hemodynamically unstable, femur fractures, particularly if bilateral, should command the attention of the trauma team who must identify these injuries early and effect appropriate stabilization.

Femur fractures are one of the primary areas of controversy regarding damage control orthopaedics. There is no debate regarding whether a femur fracture needs stabilization. The debate centers on the appropriate timing of skeletal surgery in multitrauma patients with femur fractures. The second hit model suggests that some patients do not respond well to reamed nailing of the femur in the presence of a systemic inflammatory response, as may be seen in the polytrauma patient. Temporary stabilization with an external fixator is one potential solution in patients who are too sick to undergo intramedullary nailing. Recently, a reamer has been developed that aspirates the reamings from the medullary canal, remarkably decreasing embolization to the lungs. Animal studies have been favorable with Reamer Irrigator Aspirator (Synthes, Paoli, PA), and the device is currently in use in many trauma centers. Thee use of this device may improve the safety of intramedullary nailing in multitrauma patients with femur fractures.

SUPRACONDYLAR

Fractures of the distal (or supracondylar) femur can be quite complex due to the mechanics of the knee joint itself. The initial examination should scrutinize the neurovascular structures that pass behind the knee, and swift action must be taken if there is evidence of vascular compromise. If a fracture is seen on initial radiographs, complete knee films consisting of an AP, lateral, and two 45-degree obliques should be obtained. If the fracture involves the articular surface and the patient can tolerate the examination, a CT scan should be performed to reveal the articular status. When knee instability is present on physical examination, a magnetic resonance imaging (MRI) of the knee can also facilitate diagnosis of an associated knee dislocation and aid in preoperative planning. Most fractures will require internal fixation, and those fractures that have involvement of the articular surface will require meticulous reduction

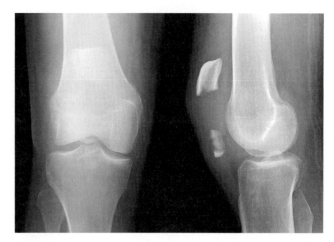

Figure 14 Anterior-posterior (AP) and lateral view of patella fracture.

and fixation to avoid the long-term complications of posttraumatic arthritis.

PATELLA

The patella, one of the most unique bones of the body, should be considered together with the extensor mechanism of the knee. The evaluation of the injured extensor mechanism involves active extension of the knee. If this is not possible, then radiographs are indicated (see Fig. 14). AP, lateral, and sunrise views should be obtained and evaluated. One potential pitfall to avoid is the presence of a two-part or bipartite patella that may be mistaken for a fracture. Radiographic clues include smooth edges of the two bones and the finding that the condition exists in the contralateral patella for approximately 50% of the time.

There are a variety of fracture patterns of the patella. The patterns that lend themselves to nonoperative treatment are those in which the extensor mechanism is intact and there is minimal displacement of the fragments, and minimal disruption of the articular surface. Extensor mechanism disruptions may also present as avulsion fractures of the patella. This injury occurs when the force pulling on the tendon exceeds the strength of the bone attachment. These fractures may appear as part of bone pulled away from the proximal or distal ends of the patella. The quadriceps tendon and patella tendon are also subjected to rupture or tear, which also interrupts the extensor mechanism. This injury requires surgical repair to restore function to the lower extremity.

TIBIAL PLATEAU

Injury to the tibial plateau can vary widely depending on the energy of the trauma and the quality of the patient's bone. These two factors impart an almost binary classification of injury based on the mechanism of injury. The initial assessment of the tibia should involve a thorough neurovascular assessment of the limb and a diligent assessment of the soft tissue covering the fracture. Should there be any suspicious laceration near the knee, the wound should be challenged to insure that the injury does not include an open joint. If the joint is open, urgent operative debridement and irrigation are necessary. A thorough history of the mechanism of injury can be very helpful in the assessment of the soft tissue, and when and whether surgical intervention may proceed.

Initially, AP and lateral radiographs of the injured knee should be obtained. If articular disruption is evident, a CT scan may be indicated to assess the severity of the articular damage of the tibia. It has long been recognized

that medial tibial plateau fractures are frequently associated with ligament injuries. Recent data has demonstrated that ligament and other soft tissue injuries in the knee occur in the vast majority of patients with tibial plateau injury. To fully evaluate the knee following tibial plateau fractures, some authors advocate MRI rather than CT scans.[35–40] The MRI can provide adequate detail of the bony injury while also providing detail regarding the ligaments, menisci, and articular cartilage of the knee. There are additional specialized radiographs, such as traction views, that the treating physician may obtain if other methods have failed to provide adequate information, or if the fracture pattern is such that the essential radiographic information in not clear.

Low-energy trauma to the lateral plateau rarely presents an urgent situation. These types of fractures can often

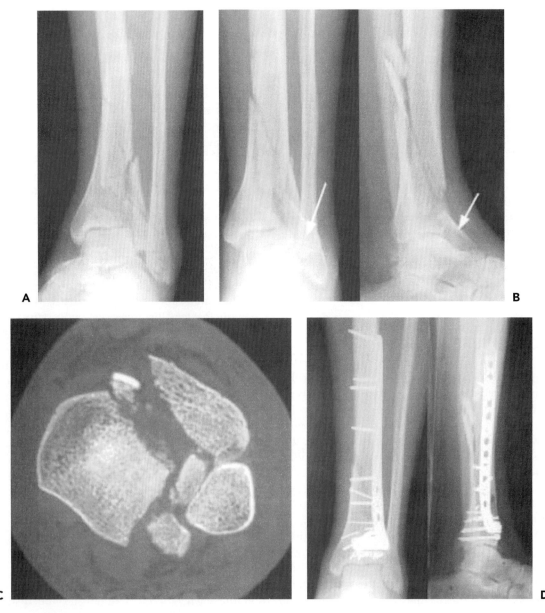

Figure 15 Images of a plafond fracture.

be treated nonoperatively with casting and subsequent application of a knee brace, provided the fracture is limited to the lateral plateau, the knee is stable, and the articular surface is not significantly displaced.

High-energy tibial plateau fractures are severe injuries. In addition to the knee injuries discussed in the preceding text, these fractures are commonly associated with soft tissue injuries such as severe contusions, crush injuries, or open fractures. Infection is a frequent problem following tibial plateau injuries. There is a current trend toward delaying surgery for 3 to 10 days to allow the soft tissues to recover before performing surgical fixation. A well-established link between high-energy tibial plateau fractures and compartment syndrome is recognized.[41] It is important that both the trauma and orthopaedic teams keep this association in mind and examine the leg frequently in the initial 24 to 72 hours following injury.

TIBIAL SHAFT AND FIBULA FRACTURES

Fractures of the tibia are frequently associated with high-energy trauma. The presentation can vary from an open, contaminated, vascular compromised limb at high risk of amputation to simple closed fractures that can be treated with reduction and casting. The initial evaluation of the tibia should focus on the neurovascular status of the limb, the condition of the soft tissue, and the status of the compartments of the leg. Compartment syndrome must always be considered with any tibia fracture. The soft tissues of the lower leg are also some of the least forgiving in the body due to the scant muscular coverage of the tibia anteriorly.

Open tibia fractures present problems that can tax the limits of modern orthopaedic intervention. If a vascular injury is present it must be addressed immediately. Leg length and skeletal stability should be established with external fixation before the vascular repair if time allows, so that the vascular repair is not later damaged when definitive skeletal fixation occurs. Preferably, both surgical teams are present intraoperatively to expedite the management of these complex injuries. Because the tissues of the tibia are unforgiving, great care must be given to the location of the external fixation pin sites if utilized for either temporary or definitive fixation. Appropriate care for the pin sites is essential to prevent infections that may limit future surgical options. Should there be a considerable soft tissue injury, the external fixator should be placed with future surgical approaches in mind.

Isolated fractures of the fibula are not common, but can occur in the instance of a lateral blow to the leg. If there is no tibial involvement, isolated fibula fractures can frequently be treated without surgery. Usually the fibula is fractured in tandem with the tibia, but its stabilization is often not essential to fixation of the leg if the tibia is repaired. The fibula will generally heal on its own, or will form an asymptomatic nonunion.

A complicated distal tibia injury that involves the articular surface is called a *plafond* or *pilon fracture* (see Fig. 15). This injury requires evaluation by CT in most cases to fully appreciate the extent of articular damage and to formulate a surgical plan for fixation. Injury to the soft tissues further complicates treatment, and tissue preservation must be a priority. If there is significant swelling, compartments must be assessed and an external fixator might be indicated to stabilize the fracture until the swelling subsides and the tissues are ready for surgery. This protocol of early spanning external fixation with planned delay of definitive internal fixation is the one currently used in major trauma centers.

ANKLE FRACTURES

Ankle fractures can range from those that present with pain on ambulation to an open ankle fracture dislocation. If the ankle is grossly dislocated, an attempt to reduce it should be undertaken as quickly as possible. The radiographs of interest are AP, lateral, and mortise views of the ankle. Physical examination should take special note of the skin overlying the fracture and assess for fracture blisters, abrasions, and any suspicious signs for an open joint. The integrity of the tibial or fibula syndesmosis should be evaluated by compressing the leg approximately 2 in. above

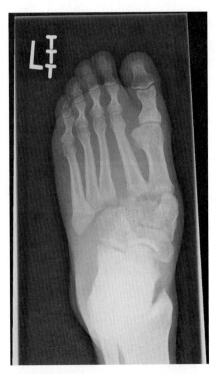

Figure 16 Anterior-posterior (AP) foot film showing Lisfranc fracture dislocation.

the malleolus to see if there is severe tenderness, indicating a possible syndesmotic disruption.

CALCANEUS FRACTURES

The calcaneus is most frequently fractured in falls from a height or motor vehicle collisions (MVCs). Consequently, there should be a high suspicion for other injuries. It is well documented that bilateral calcaneus fractures are associated with vertebral fractures, open injuries, and compartment syndrome of the foot.[42] In diabetic patients and those with poor bone stock, the presentation of the fractures can be different and so can their treatment. Because the calcaneus has a large volume of cancellous bone surrounded by a relatively thin shell of cortical bone, internal fixation can be problematic. The soft tissue surrounding the calcaneus has skin with a somewhat tenuous blood supply, and very little muscle or other soft tissue. As a result, the risks of soft tissue breakdown and infection are significant, particularly in patients with microvascular disease, such as chronic nicotine abuse, and diabetes.

Radiographs that should be obtained include an ankle series, an AP of the foot, lateral foot, and a Harris axial view. Should there be articular involvement, a CT scan is warranted. As with ankle fractures, the status of the soft tissues can compromise therapy and calcaneus fractures frequently exhibit significant swelling and fracture blisters. Most surgeons delay definitive fixation for 7 to 14 days to allow the soft tissues to recover from the initial trauma.

TALUS FRACTURES

The talus is responsible for the force transmission of the entire weight of the body. For this reason, its role in a functional limb is great. Unfortunately, most injuries to the talus will interfere with long-term function. By recognizing these fractures early and by treating them urgently, many of the complications of osteonecrosis and posttraumatic arthritis can be minimized.

When evaluating a talus fracture, ankle (AP, lateral, and mortise) and foot (AP, lateral, and oblique) radiographs should be obtained. Also, a Canale view may be helpful

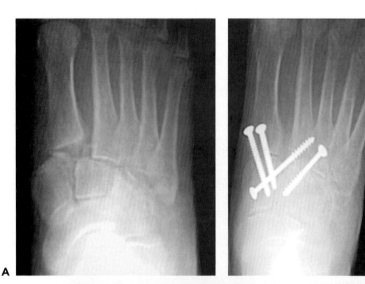

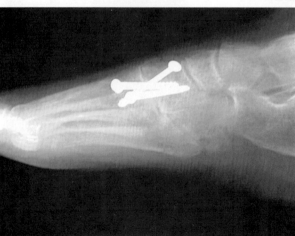

Figure 17 A–C: Pre- and postimages of a typical Lisfranc fracture.

in evaluating the talar neck. CT scans will occasionally be necessary to appreciate all the details of the fracture. The talus is susceptible to osteonecrosis because of its tenuous blood supply. The likelihood of osteonecrosis is relative to the degree of fracture displacement. The talus is also subject to various dislocations with its neighboring bones, but the most serious example is a complete dislocation that occurs with massive twisting forces on the foot. Prompt reduction is essential for the possibility of a favorable outcome. If the talus is not reducible, then open reduction should proceed as soon as possible (Fig. 11).

FRACTURES OF THE MIDFOOT

Fractures of the midfoot are often caused by direct trauma to the foot. Radiographs should include AP, lateral, and oblique views of the foot. Should there be moderate comminution and/or articular involvement, a CT scan is also indicated. As with other fractures, assessment of any open injuries, open joints, or compartment syndrome must be considered. Lisfranc fracture dislocations are severe injuries involving the midfoot (see Fig. 16). It is important to recognize the injury and reduce and stabilize it (see Fig. 17). Occasionally, the radiographs may appear relatively normal despite remarkable pain and swelling. In this scenario, a Lisfranc fracture should be suspected and stress radiographs should be obtained.

FRACTURES OF THE FOREFOOT

A direct blow most commonly causes injury to the metatarsals and phalanges. When fractures of the forefoot are suspected, a foot series including AP, lateral, and oblique should be obtained. Frequently, fractures that are either nondisplaced or adequately reduced can undergo closed management. Surgery is primarily needed when there is articular involvement, or gross instability if the fracture does not lend itself to closed treatment.

CONCLUSION

The myriad of fractures and their complexity in the lower extremity can be overwhelming. The prompt recognition of the nature of these injuries and taking appropriate action can minimize acute and long-term morbidity of patients. Lower extremity skeletal trauma can have a significant impact on the patient's overall condition and long-term outcome. The timing of surgical intervention and the need for damage control orthopaedic techniques must be determined for the individual patient. It is critical that the trauma team and the orthopaedic team work closely together in providing care to these severely injured patients.

REFERENCES

1. Pape HC, Giannoudis P, Krettek C. The timing of fracture treatment in polytrauma patients: Relevance of damage control orthopedic surgery. *Am J Surg.* 2002;183:622–629.
2. Hildebrand F, Giannoudis P, Krettek C, et al. Damage control: Extremities. *Injury.* 2004;35:678–689.
3. Nowotarski PJ, Turen CH, Brumback RJ, et al. Conversion of external fixation to intramedullary nailing for fractures of the shaft of the femur in multiply injured patients. *J Bone Joint Surg Am.* 2000;82:781–788.
4. Joist A, Schult M, Ortmann C, et al. Rinsing-suction reamer attenuates intramedullary pressure increase and fat intravasation in a sheep model. *J Trauma.* 2004;57:146–151.
5. Schult M, Kuchle R, Hofmann A, et al. Pathophysiological advantages of rinsing-suction-reaming (RSR) in a pig model for intramedullary nailing. *J Orthop Res.* 2006;24:1186–1192.
6. Scalea TM, Boswell SA, Scott JD, et al. External fixation as a bridge to intramedullary nailing for patients with multiple injuries and with femur fractures: Damage control orthopedics. *J Trauma.* 2000;48:613–621.
7. Harwood PJ, Giannoudis PV, Probst C, et al. The risk of local infective complications after damage control procedures for femoral shaft fracture. *J Orthop Trauma.* 2006;20:181–189.
8. Gustilo RB, Anderson JT. Prevention of infection in the treatment of one thousand and twenty-five open fractures of long bones: Retrospective and prospective analyses. *J Bone Joint Surg.* 1976;58(4):453–458.
9. Mehbod AA, Ogilvie JW, Pinto MR, et al. Postoperative deep wound infections in adults after spinal fusion: Management with vacuum-assisted wound closure. *J Spinal Disord Tech.* 2005;18(1):14–17.
10. Argenta LC, Morykwas MJ. Vacuum-assisted closure: A new method for wound control and treatment: Clinical experience. *Ann Plast Surg.* 1997;38(6):563–577.
11. Gustafsson R, Johnsson P, Algotsson L, et al. Vacuum-assisted closure therapy guided by C-reactive protein level in patients with deep sternal wound infection. *J Thorac Cardiovasc Surg.* 2002;123(5):210–215.
12. Fabian TS, Kaufman HJ, Lett ED, et al. The evaluation of subatmospheric pressure and hyperbaric oxygen in ischemic full-thickness wound healing. *Am Surg.* 2000;66(12):1136–1143.
13. Chen SZ, Li J, Li XY, et al. Effects of vacuum-assisted closure on wound microcirculation: An experimental study. *Asian J Surg.* 2005;28(3):211–217.
14. Webb LX. New techniques in wound management: Vacuum-assisted wound closure. *J Am Acad Orthop Surg.* 2002;10(5):303–311.
15. Morykwas MJ, Argenta LC, Shelton-Brown EI, et al. Vacuum-assisted closure: A new method for wound control and treatment: Animal studies and basic foundation. *Ann Plast Surg.* 1997;38(6):553–562.
16. Morykwas MJ, Faler BJ, Pearce DJ, et al. Effects of varying levels of subatmospheric pressure on the rate of granulation tissue formation in experimental wounds in swine. *Ann Plast Surg.* 2001;47(5):547–551.
17. Wongwarawat MD, Schnall SB, Holtom PD, et al. Negative pressure dressings as an alternative technique for the treatment of infected wounds. *Clin Orthop.* 2003;414:45–48.
18. Genecov DG, Schneider AM, Morykwas MJ, et al. A controlled sub-atmospheric pressure dressing increases the rate of skin graft donor site reepithelialization. *Ann Plast Surg.* 1998;40(3):219–225.
19. Patzakis MJ, Wilkins J. Factors influencing infection rate in open fracture wounds. *Clin Orthop Relat Res.* 1989;243:36–40.
20. Zalavras CG, Patzakis MJ, Holtom PD, et al. Management of open fractures. *Infect Dis Clin North Am.* 2005;19(4):915–929.
21. Webb LX, Bosse MJ, Renan CC. Analysis of surgeon-controlled variables in the treatment of the limb-threatening Type-III open tibial diaphyseal fractures. *J Bone Joint Surg Am.* 2007;89:923–928.
22. Harley BJ, Beaupre LA, Jones CA, et al. The effect of time to definitive treatment on the rate of nonunion and infection in open fractures. *J Orthop Trauma.* 2002;16(7):484–490.

23. Stannard JP, Sheils TM, Lopez-Ben RR, et al. Vascular injuries in knee dislocations following blunt trauma: Evaluating the role of physical examination to determining the need for arteriography. *J Bone Joint Surg.* 2004;86-A:910–915.

24. Abou-Sayed H, Berger DL. Blunt lower-extremity trauma and popliteal artery injuries. *Arch Surg.* 2002;137:585–589.

25. Martinez D, Sweatman K, Thompson EC. Popliteal artery injury associated with knee dislocations. *Am Surg.* 2001;67:165–167.

26. Dennis JW, Jagger C, Butcher JL, et al. Reassessing the role of arteriograms in the management of posterior knee dislocations. *J Trauma.* 1993;35(5):692–697.

27. Kendall RW, Taylor DC, Salvian AJ, et al. The role of arteriography in assessing vascular injuries associated with dislocations of the knee. *J Trauma.* 1993;35(6):875–878.

28. Treiman GS, Yellin AF, Weaver FA, et al. Examination of the patient with a knee dislocation: The case for selective arteriography. *Arch Surg.* 1992;127:1056–1063.

29. Miranda FE, Dennis JW, Veldenz HC, et al. Confirmation of the safety and accuracy of physical examination in the evaluation of knee dislocation for injury of the popliteal artery: A prospective study. *J Trauma.* 2002;52(2):247–252.

30. Koval KJ, Meek R, Schemitsch E, et al. Geriatric trauma: Young ideas. *J Bone Joint Surg.* 2003;85-A(7):1380–1387.

31. Mears DC. Surgical treatment of acetabular fractures in elderly patients with osteoporotic bone. *J Am Acad Orthop Surg.* 1999;7(2):128–141.

32. Heyburn G, Beringer T, Elliott J, et al. Orthogeriatric care in patients with fractures of the proximal femur. *Clin Orthop Relat Res.* 2004;425:35–43.

33. Hougaard K, Thomsen PB. Traumatic posterior dislocation of the hip—orognostic factors influencing the incidence of avascular necrosis of the femoral head. *Arch Orthop Trauma Surg.* 1986;105(1):32–35.

34. Sims SH. Subtrochanteric femur fractures. In: Stannard JP, Schmidt AH, Kregor PJ, eds. *Surgical treatment of orthopaedic trauma*, 1st ed. New York: Thieme; 2007:589–610.

35. Barrow BA, Fajman WA, Parker LM, et al. Tibial plateau fractures: Evaluation with MR imaging. *Radiographics.* 1994;14(3):553–559.

36. Brophy DP, O'Malley M, Lui D, et al. MR imaging of tibial plateau fractures. *Clin Radiol.* 1996;51(12):873–878.

37. Holt MD, Williams LA, Dent CM. MRI in the management of tibial plateau fractures. *Injury.* 1995;26(9):595–599.

38. Kode L, Lieberman JM, Motta AO, et al. Evaluation of tibial plateau fractures: Efficacy of MR imaging compared with CT. *AJR Am J Roentgenol.* 1994;163(1):141–147.

39. Shepherd L, Abdollahi K, Lee J, et al. The prevalence of soft tissue injuries in nonoperative tibial plateau fractures as determined by magnetic resonance imaging. *J Orthop Trauma.* 2002;16(9):628–631.

40. Yacoubian SV, Nevins RT, Sallis JG, et al. Impact of MRI on treatment plan and fracture classification of tibial plateau fractures. *J Orthop Trauma.* 2002;16(9):632–637.

41. Stannard JP, Martin SL. Tibial plateau fractures. In: Stannard JP, Schmidt AH, Kregor PJ, eds. *Surgical treatment of orthopaedic trauma*, 1st ed. New York: Thieme; 2007:713–741.

42. Weber TG, Brokaw DS, Scharfenberger A, Broderick JS. Foot fractures. In: Stannard JP, Schmidt AH, Kregor PJ, eds. *Surgical treatment of orthopaedic trauma*, 1st ed. New York: Thieme; 2007:815–851.

51

Special Interdisciplinary Problem: Knee Dislocation

Troy Caron   *H. Claude Sagi*

The number of patients who present to the emergency department with a knee dislocation is estimated to be <0.02% of all orthopaedic injuries.[1] There are many instances where a dislocated knee has spontaneously reduced before the patient arrives at the treating facility, but this number is unknown. Patients presenting with a multiligamentous knee injury but not a frank dislocation should be treated as having sustained a knee dislocation that spontaneously reduced.

On initial presentation, the patient with a dislocated knee should be treated like any other patient in the trauma setting. Once the patient is stabilized and the primary survey parameters have been addressed, attention should then be directed toward the secondary survey and the status of the extremities. If a knee dislocation is identified or suspected based on position or ligamentous instability, the knee should be reduced and the limb aligned and stabilized as soon as possible. Careful attention to subtle asymmetry in neurologic or vascular examination findings before and following reduction is key.

Only when the knee is reduced and the neurovascular status of the patient is confirmed to be normal can definitive treatment and stabilization for knee instability be considered. Many different combinations of structures in the knee can be damaged with a knee dislocation. These structures include the anterior cruciate ligament (ACL), posterior cruciate ligament (PCL), medial collateral ligament (MCL), lateral collateral ligament (LCL), posterolateral corner (PLC), menisci, articular cartilage, and bone.

Clinical examination, x-rays, and magnetic resonance imaging (MRI) must be obtained for definitive diagnosis of the damaged structures. The treatment options and timing for repair will depend on stability of the patients, what structures have been damaged, and other injuries that the extremity has sustained. The ultimate goal is to restore stability and painfree functional mobility.

CLASSIFICATION

Like all deformity in orthopaedic surgery, dislocations are described by what direction the distal fragment (the tibia) moves in relation to the proximal fragment (the femur). These include anterior, posterior, medial, lateral, and rotatory dislocations.[2] Posterior dislocations, the result of a force causing the tibia to be driven anteriorly, are the most common representing more than 70% of the dislocations and likely result from a hyperextension mechanism (see Fig. 1). Studies have shown that when the knee is hyperextended greater than 30 degrees the knee will dislocate.[3]

The next most common dislocation is the posterior dislocation (see Fig. 2). Posterior knee dislocations result from a direct force striking the anterior tibia, driving it posteriorly. This occurs most commonly with motor vehicle collisions or sports-related injuries when the knee strikes the dashboard or an oncoming opponent.

Medial and lateral dislocations (see Fig. 3) are much less common. These occur when a force is directed from

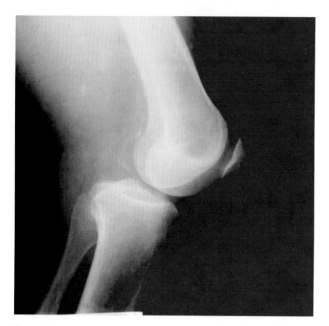

Figure 1   Posterior dislocation.

the side causing a varus (toward the midline) or valgus (away from the midline) stress across the knee. Neurologic injury is more likely to occur in lateral knee dislocations as a result of tethering of the peroneal nerve at the fibular head and neck.[4] Rotatory dislocations are far less common (see Fig. 4). Rapid twisting or torsion results in rotatory dislocation with or without neurovascular injury. It is almost always accompanied by protrusion of the medial femoral condyle through the medial retinaculum and capsule. With enough twisting, invagination of the MCL into the joint results in incarceration and trapping (buttonholing effect) of the medial femoral condyle and

an irreducible knee dislocation.[5-9] The invagination of the joint capsule and prominence of the femoral condyle medially produce a dimple in the skin at the joint line which can clinically help distinguish this kind of injury from other dislocations.[10]

The condition of the static (ligamentous, bony, meniscal, and cartilaginous structures) and the dynamic (muscles) stabilizers determine the stability of the knee. The ligamentous structures include the ACL, PCL, MCL, LCL, and PLC. The PLC is made up of the iliotibial band, popliteus complex, the middle third of the lateral capsular ligament, the fabellofibular ligament, the arcuate ligament, the posterior horn of the lateral meniscus, the lateral coronary ligament, and the posterolateral portion of the joint capsule. In order for the knee to dislocate many of these structures must be disrupted.

Typically, for anterior or posterior dislocations, both ACLs and PCLs are disrupted. However, there are many reports in the literature in which only one of the cruciates is torn.[4,11-13] The ACL is always disrupted with an anterior dislocation and the PCL with a posterior dislocation. When a valgus stress is applied the MCL will be disrupted. When a varus stress is applied the LCL will be disrupted.

Other more comprehensive classification schemes exist describing the combinations of ligamentous injury rather than the direction of displacement. However, they relate more to the planning of ligamentous reconstruction and are beyond the scope of this chapter.

Fractures of the femoral condyles and tibial plateau need to be recognized because they can significantly influence knee stability in the face of intact ligamentous structures. Injury to articular and/or meniscal cartilage also occurs; however, these injuries have less impact on stability and are more important for the subsequent development of posttraumatic osteoarthritis.

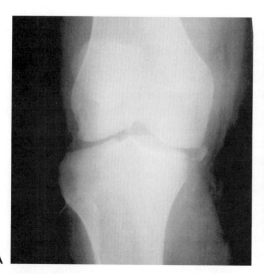
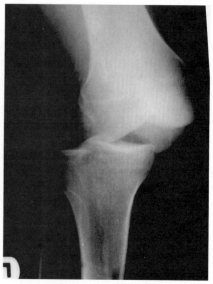

Figure 2   **A:** Lateral dislocation with associated medial capsule avulsion. **B:** Lateral dislocation.

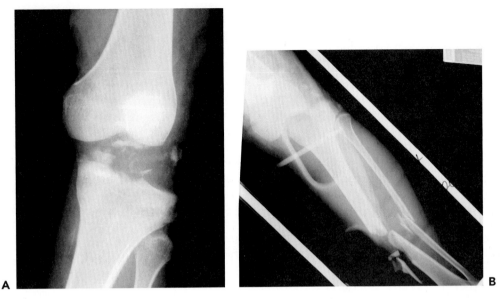

Figure 3 **A:** Posterolateral dislocation. **B:** Posterolateral dislocation. This x-ray also shows the importance of getting views of the femur and tibia.

EVALUATION AND ACUTE MANAGEMENT

Once a knee dislocation is identified it should be reduced as soon as possible; however, a quick neurovascular examination should precede the reduction maneuver. The posterior tibial artery and dorsalis pedis artery should be palpated. If the pulses cannot be palpated secondary to vasospasm, hypotension, edema, or soft tissue defects, then Doppler examination should be performed to ensure adequate perfusion to the distal extremity. The sensorimotor status of the deep and superficial peroneal nerves and tibial nerve should be evaluated and documented. Nerve damage occurs with an incidence of 16% to 35% of all knee dislocations.[14–17] The peroneal nerve innervates ankle and toe dorsiflexors,

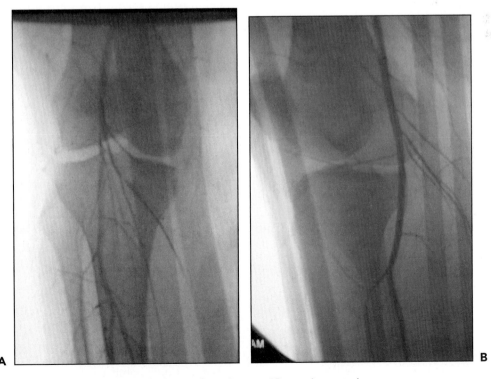

Figure 4 **A:** Normal AP and **(B)** Lateral arteriogram. AP, anterior-posterior.

whereas the tibial nerve innervates ankle and toe plantar flexors.

After the neurovascular status is confirmed and documented, reduction can be performed under conscious sedation if the patient's status permits. This can be successfully accomplished in most of the patients with gentle longitudinal traction and a force is directed opposite the direction of dislocation by an assistant. In grossly unstable knees, particularly in an unconscious or sedated/relaxed patient, care must be taken to avoid excessive force and overdistraction of the joint and neurovascular structures.

Radiographic evaluation of the knee should be performed to identify the type of dislocation and any fractures about the femur and tibia. However, if a dislocation is identified, neurovascular examination and reduction/immobilization should be performed before any radiographic examination to avoid unnecessary prolonged kinking, traction, or pressure on the neurovascular structures.

The paramount concern in a patient with a knee dislocation is the vascular status of the extremity. Therefore, following reduction the pulses should be palpated for symmetry and an Ankle Brachial Index (ABI) should be performed to rule out occult vascular injury in the case of palpable pulses. An ABI is performed by placing a blood pressure cuff about the calf and using the Doppler to detect the pulse at the ankle or foot. The systolic pressure is recorded when a Doppler-able pulse returns. This is repeated on the ipsilateral upper extremity, and the ratio of the ankle systolic pressure to the brachial systolic pressure is calculated. Normally, the ABI should be >1, with anything below 0.9 highly suggestive of an occult vascular injury (i.e., an intimal tear or flap).[18]

If the knee is irreducible and the pulse is absent or asymmetric with an abnormal ABI, then emergent operative reduction should be undertaken followed by repetition of ABI. If the ABI or physical examination suggests a vascular injury despite anatomic reduction, then contrast arteriography is recommended to investigate vascular structures.

The incidence of an associated popliteal artery injury ranges from 7% to 80%.[2,19-23] If a vascular injury has not been addressed within the first 6 to 8 hours, the amputation rate has been reported to be as high as 86%.[2] Because of the high incidence of associated vascular injury and its catastrophic sequelae, many sources in the past have recommended arteriography for *all* patients with knee dislocations.[21-23] However, more recent publications by Stannard and Mills have shown the reliability of both the physical examination and ABI in treating the patient with a knee dislocation. Provided the patient was admitted for close observation and the physical examination or ABI remained within normal limits, no vascular complications were encountered. The complication rate of arteriography ranges from 2% to 3% for allergic reactions, vasculitis, thrombosis, and renal failure; however, in the patient with

an abnormal physical examination or ABI this does not outweigh the potential benefits.[24-26] If any abnormality is noted on arteriography other than vasospasm, vascular consultation is required.

If the pulses are normal and an ABI of >0.9 is found, further evaluation of the ligamentous structures can be attempted using physical examination to assess damage. In the acute setting it can be difficult to perform these tests on an alert patient because of discomfort. The examination is based on stress-testing the stability of the ligamentous structures:

ACL: The Lachman test is done with the patient's knee held at 20 to 30 degrees of flexion. The patient's femur is stabilized with one hand while the other hand attempts to translate the tibia anteriorly. The degree of laxity and the firmness of the endpoint are compared to the contralateral knee. This is the most sensitive clinical examination for testing the ACL.[27]

PCL: The posterior drawer test is used to assess the PCL. This is done by flexing the patient's knee up to 90 degrees. A posteriorly directed force is then applied to the proximal tibia. The degree of laxity and the endpoint should be assessed and compared to the contralateral side. This is the most sensitive test for the PCL.

MCL: The MCL is assessed with the knee at 30 degrees of flexion with a valgus stress applied to the knee. If the knee is stressed in full extension, the ACL and PCL help to stabilize against a valgus stress and may give a false-negative examination. At 30 degrees of flexion, these ligaments no longer help stabilize against the valgus stress. If the medial joint space opens then the MCL is likely incompetent.

LCL: The LCL is tested at 30 degrees of flexion for the same reason as the MCL. A varus stress is applied to the knee. If the lateral joint space opens then the LCL is likely incompetent.

PLC: The PLC is assessed using the posterior drawer test at both 30 degrees and 90 degrees of flexion. If there is increased laxity at 30 degrees when compared to 90 degrees, a PLC injury should be considered. The dial test is also used to test the PLC. The tibia is externally rotated at 30 degrees of knee flexion and at 90 degrees of flexion. If there is increased rotation at 30 degrees but not 90 degrees then there is an isolated PLC injury. If there is laxity at both 30 degrees and 90 degrees then there is a PLC injury and a PCL tear.[28]

After the physical examination is completed, the patient should be placed in a long leg splint or a knee immobilizer. Radiographs should be repeated once the knee is immobilized in order to ensure that the knee joint remains reduced in the splint. If the knee joint does not remain reduced in the splint then the patient should be taken to the operating room for application of a spanning external fixator to maintain a concentric reduction and prevent posterior subluxation.

After satisfactory perfusion is assured and the knee joint is reduced and stabilized, MRI should be performed to assess the extent of soft tissue or ligamentous injury.[29,30] MRI has been found to be 85% to 100% accurate in predicting the extent of soft tissue injury.[31]

The patient should subsequently be admitted for 24-hour observation and frequent (every 2 hours) neurovascular monitoring for compartment syndrome and changes in vascular status.

Timing of definitive stabilization is the source of much debate in the orthopaedic community. Whereas some orthopaedic surgeons advocate early physical therapy and reestablishment of range of motion and delayed ligamentous repair or reconstruction at around 6 weeks, others recommend early reconstruction.[32-35] Opinion also differs as to whether all structures or only certain key stabilizers need to be reconstructed, these issues will be discussed to some degree later in the chapter. Emergent or urgent operative intervention is indicated only in those patients presenting with a vascular injury, compartment syndrome, an irreducible dislocation, or an open wound communicating with the knee joint.

Neurologic injuries rarely involve complete transection of the nerve and result primarily from stretch neuropraxia or axonotmesis. If a neurologic deficit is identified, the patient is observed for a period of 6 to 12 weeks. If no recovery is noted electromyography and nerve conduction studies can be performed. Fibrillation and denervation potentials in the muscle may be a sign of complete transection and if there is a conduction block at the level of the knee then the nerve should be explored and repaired if necessary.

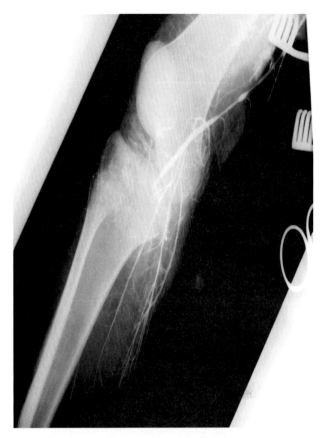

Figure 5   Arteriogram with obstruction in popliteal space.

COMPLICATIONS

Vascular Injury

Identifying a vascular injury in a patient with a dislocated knee is crucial for the viability of the limb. With passing time, the chance for successful vascular repair decreases; therefore, this injury must be considered with every knee dislocation or suspected knee dislocation. The rate of popliteal artery injury reported in the literature ranges from 7% to 80%; the amputation rate for delayed vascular repair (>8 hours of warm ischemia time) is as high as 86%.[2,19,20,36] Reasons for the high amputation rate relate to failure of reperfusion, compartment syndrome, and neuromuscular necrosis. During World War II, ligation of the popliteal artery was associated with a 73% amputation rate. Amputation decreased to 32% during the Korean War with attempts at popliteal repair.[20] If repair of the popliteal artery is accomplished within 6 hours of warm ischemia time, the amputation rate is further decreased to 8.3%.[37]

Anatomically, the popliteal artery is fixed at the adductor hiatus proximally and the fibrous arch of the soleus distally. During dislocation of the knee, the popliteal artery is stretched between these two points resulting in arterial injury (see Figs. 5 and 6). In a cadaveric study,

Kennedy noted that rupture of the popliteal artery occurred with greater than 50 degrees of hyperextension.[3] Vascular injury can range from a complete tear that requires surgical intervention to an intimal lesion that can be observed. Intimal lesions (tears and flaps) can form pseudoaneurysms, thrombose, or conversely have no adverse effect.[38]

The key to not missing an arterial injury in a patient with a knee dislocation is to do the appropriate physical examination and perform arteriography when appropriate. The physical examination should include palpation of the dorsal pedal pulse as well as the posterior tibial pulse. An ABI should also be documented because an arterial injury may be present in 5% to 15% of those patients with a seemingly normal pulse on palpation.[32,33,39-41] The positive predictive value of detecting an arterial injury with palpation of pulses ranges from 79% to 90%, the specificity ranges from 91% to 99%, and the positive predictive value ranges from 75% to 99%.[20,41] Therefore, a normal pulse does not obviate an arterial injury. Conversely, an abnormal pulse does not necessarily indicate an arterial injury. Several factors can account for this discrepancy ranging from vasospasm and hypotension in the trauma patient to the palpatory skills of the examiner. This underscores the importance of the ABI. When the ABI is found to be <0.9,

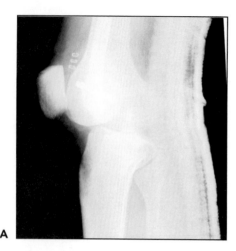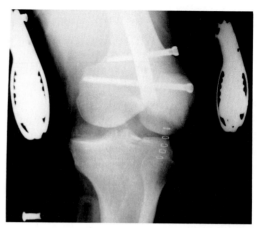

Figure 6 **A:** Persistent subluxation of the knee joint after application of a posterior splint. **B:** Persistent subluxation of the knee joint after application of a hinged brace.

the sensitivity for major arterial injury is 95% to 100%, and the specificity is 97% to 100%.[18,42]

Duplex ultrasonography has been proposed as a safer and cheaper alternative to arteriography with comparable accuracy (98%).[34] However, this test may be difficult to obtain in the trauma patient because of pain, splintage, and the distorted anatomy of the dislocated knee.[43] Magnetic resonance contrast angiography using gadolinium has been examined as a less invasive alternative with fewer complications. In a small study it was found to be equivalent to angiography but because of little support for it in the literature, angiography remains the standard.[29]

In the setting of a knee dislocation with a normal pulse, arteriography has detected occult vascular injury in 23% of patients; with an abnormal pulse the yield is 79%.[44] Complications with arteriography occur at a rate of 2% to 3%.[24–26,34] and are listed in Table 1.

The reported incidence of false-positive results that may lead to unnecessary surgery has ranged from 2.4% to 7%.[20] Many of the reports in the literature discuss the positive findings on arteriogram despite having a normal physical examination. Most of these findings are actually intimal tears or lesions that may require close clinical follow-up but not surgical treatment.[38,40,44–49] A prior animal model has shown that an intimal flap or tear without hemodynamically significant stenosis (i.e., <50% luminal narrowing) has only a 3% rate of developing thrombosis.[50] These controlled laboratory findings have been confirmed in the clinical environment and the current recommendation for patients diagnosed with a noncritical intimal tear is observation for 48 to 72 hours with serial clinical examinations.[48]

Therefore, arteriography is not recommended or necessary for all knee dislocations. The risks and costs of this study do not always outweigh the clinical benefits. Selective arteriography is indicated if a prehospital abnormal examination suggested arterial injury, ABI is <0.9, no pulse is palpable, or an abnormal pulse is present when compared to the contralateral side.[39,43,51–54]

When it is decided that vascular repair will be necessary, both the orthopaedic and vascular surgeon should discuss the future plans for the patient. This includes the location of incisions, type of temporary stabilization, and timing of definitive fixation.

Nerve Injury

Apart from the peroneal nerve at the fibular head and neck, the nerves in the popliteal space are not tethered like the popliteal artery. Nerve injuries therefore are less common than arterial injuries. The incidence of peroneal nerve injury with knee dislocations ranges from 14% to 35%, and is more common with the posterolateral dislocation.[14,17]

Nerve injuries can range from neuropraxia to complete transection, although as mentioned previously, complete transection is rare. Typically, the injury is caused by the

TABLE 1

COMPLICATIONS ASSOCIATED WITH ARTERIOGRAPHY

Reactions to contrast media
Vasovagal response to arterial puncture
Local hemorrhage
Vein and nerve injury
Subintimal injection of contrast material
Vasculitis
Arterial thromboembolism
Problems related to catheters/guide wires
Intravascular injection of foreign substances
Renal impairment
Arteriovenous fistula
Puncture site hemorrhage

peroneal nerve stretching across the posterior aspect of the lateral femoral condyle leading to axonotmesis over a broad area. Recovery of neurologic function is unpredictable with most studies reporting no recovery in more than 50% of injuries. The superficial peroneal nerve is usually the first to recover and can extend up to 18 months. Because these injuries are typically traction injuries with a large zone of injury, primary repair of the nerve is impossible and nerve grafting over a large distances has a poor prognosis.[14–17]

The patient with a peroneal nerve injury typically presents with a foot drop. These patients should be placed in an ankle-foot orthosis (AFO) to help keep the foot in a plantigrade position and prevent the development of equinus contractures. The AFO can remain in place until the nerve recovers, or until surgical treatment (usually some form of tendon transfer) is performed. In many cases, the AFO can be the definitive treatment.

TREATMENT

The current recommendations for definitive treatment of a knee dislocation are repair or reconstruction of the collateral ligaments, the cruciate ligaments, and the PLC. The goal is to restore stability in order to give the patient a painless, stable, and functional extremity.[55–62] Typically, the dislocation is stabilized to allow the inflammatory process to decrease and then allow gentle range of motion in the hope of decreasing the risk of arthrofibrosis that occur after the definitive reconstruction procedure. It has been found that patients with an Injury Severity Score of >26 treated with acute reconstruction are at high risk for the development of heterotopic ossification and severe joint stiffness.[63]

The acute setting treatment can include a posterior splint, knee immobilizer, external fixator, cross pinning, or olecranization of the patella.[64] Typically, an external fixator is used when splintage does not maintain an anatomic reduction; however, cross pinning or olecranization of the patella are other good options for temporary stabilization (see Figs. 7 and 8).

OUTCOME

Outcome after knee dislocation is variable with inconsistent reports in the literature. As recently as the last 2 decades, knee dislocations have been treated with many different algorithms ranging from nonoperative to multiligament reconstruction either acutely or in a delayed manner. Factors that must be considered when interpreting the results and outcome studies include which ligaments were reconstructed, length of time between injury and definitive surgical repair, and any neurovascular injury or associated fractures.

Outcome studies evaluate range of motion, pain, return to work, instability, and posttraumatic arthritis. The recovery of range of motion for operatively treated cases has varied from 106 to 130 degrees. Almost half of all patients develop some degree of flexion contracture with approximately 20% of contractures greater than 5 degrees.[65,66]

Chronic pain is variable between studies because of the subjective nature of this parameter. The most important factors that contribute to chronic pain are instability, articular injury, and posttraumatic arthritis. Many patients are unable to return to the same job that they had before the injury. Most patients do go back to work but only

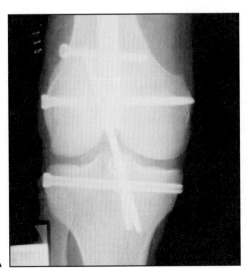
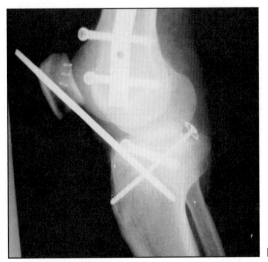

Figure 7 A: Olecronization of the patella—the posterior cruciate ligament (PCL) was reconstructed and the tibial plateau was fixed. Clinically the knee was still unstable. **B:** Lateral projection of the knee.

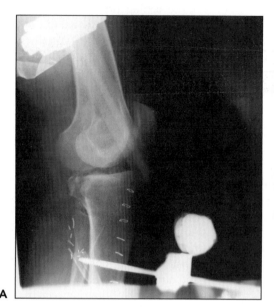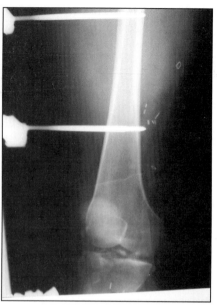

Figure 8   Knee dislocation requiring spanning external fixation for maintenance of reduction.

approximately half return to their previous job and level of function.[65,67]

REFERENCES

1. Rihn JA. The acutely dislocated knee: Evaluation and Management. *J Am Acad Orthop Surg.* 2004;12:334–346.
2. Green NE, Allen BL. Vascular injuries associated with dislocation of the knee. *J Bone Joint Surg Am.* 1977;59:236–239.
3. Kennedy JC. Complete dislocation of the knee joint. *J Bone Joint Surg Am.* 1963;45:889–904.
4. Brautigan B, Johnson D. The dislocated knee. The epidemiology of knee dislocations. *Clin Sports Med.* 2000;19:387–397.
5. Kontakis G, Christoforakis J, Katonis P, et al. Irreducible knee dislocation due to interposition of the vastus medialis associated with neurovascular injury. *Orthopedics.* 2003;26:645–646.
6. Siegmeth A, Menth-Chiari WA, Amsuess H. A rare case of irreducible knee dislocation in a seventy-three-year old male. *J Orthop Trauma.* 2000;14:70–72.
7. Huang FS, Simonian P, Chansky HA. Irreducible posterolateral dislocation of the knee. *Arthroscopy.* 2000;16:323–327.
8. Silverberg DA, Acus R. Irreducible posterolateral knee dislocation associated with interposition of the vastus medialis. *Am J Sports Med.* 2004;32:1313–1316.
9. Baxamusa T, Galloway M. Irreducible knee dislocations secondary to interposed menisci. *Am J Orthop.* 2001;30:141–143.
10. Reckling FW, Peltier LF. Acute knee dislocations and their complications. *Clin Orthop Relat Res.* 2004;422:135–141.
11. Bratt HD, Newman AP. Complete dislocation of the knee without disruption of both cruciate ligaments. *J Trauma.* 1993;34:383–389.
12. Toritsuka Y, Horibe S, Hiro-oka A. Knee dislocation following anterior cruciate ligament disruption without any other ligament tears. *Arthroscopy.* 1999;15:522–526.
13. Cooper D, Speer K, Wickiewicz T, et al. Complete knee dislocation without posterior cruciate ligament disruption. *Clin Orthop.* 1992;284:228–233.
14. Hegyes MS, Richardson MW, Miller MD. Knee dislocation: Complications of nonoperative and operative management. *Clin Sports Med.* 2000;19:519–543.
15. White J. The results of traction injuries to the common peroneal nerve. *J Bone Joint Surg Br.* 1968;50:346.
16. Wood MB. Peroneal nerve repair. Surgical results. *Clin Orthop.* 1991;267:206–210.
17. Niall DM, Nutton RW, Keating JF. Palsy of the common peroneal nerve after traumatic knee dislocation. *J Bone Joint Surg Br.* 2005;87:664–667.
18. Mills W, Barei D, McNair P. The value of the ankle – brachial index for diagnosing arterial injury after knee dislocation: A prospective study. *J Trauma.* 2004;56:1261–1265.
19. Kendall RW, Taylor DC, Salvian AJ. The role of arteriography in assessing vascular injuries associated with dislocations of the knee. *J Trauma.* 1993;35:875–878.
20. Stannard JP, Sheils TM, Lopez-Ben RR, et al. Vascular injuries in knee dislocations: The role of physical examination in determining the need for arteriography. *J Bone Joint Surg Am.* 2004;86:910–915.
21. Alberty RE, Goodfried G, Boyden AM. Popliteal artery injury with fratural dislocation of the knee. *Am J Surg.* 1981;142:36–40.
22. Cone JB. Vascular injury associated with fracture-dislocation of the lower extremity. *Clin Orthop.* 1989;243:30–35.
23. Kremchek TE, Welling RE, Kremchek EJ. Traumatic dislocation of the knee. *Orthop Rev.* 1989;18:1051–1057.
24. AbuRahma AF, Robinson PA, Boland JP, et al. Complications of arteriography in a recent series of 707 cases: Factors affecting outcome. *Ann Vasc Surg.* 1993;7:122–129.
25. Hessel SJ, Adams DF, Abams HL. Complications of angiography. *Radiology.* 1981;138:273–281.
26. Nunn DB. Complications of peripheral arteriography. *Am Surg.* 1978;44:664–669.
27. Donaldson WF, Warren RF, Wickiewicz T. A comparison of acute anterior cruciate ligament examinations. *Am J Sports Med.* 1992;10:100–102.
28. Covey DC. Injuries of the posterolateral corner of the knee. *J Bone Joint Surg Am.* 2001;83:106–118.
29. Potter H, Weinstein M, Allen A, et al. Magnetic resonance imaging of the multiple – ligament injured knee. *J Orthop Trauma.* 2002;16:330–339.
30. Tsiagadigui JG, Sabri F, Sintzoff S, et al. Magnetic resonance imaging for irreducible posterolateral knee dislocation. *J Orthop Trauma.* 1997;11:457–460.
31. Twaddle BC, Hunter JC, Chapman JR, et al. MRI in acute knee dislocation. *J Bone Joint Surg Br.* 1996;78:573–579.
32. Lohmann M, Lauridsen K, Vedel P. Arterial lesions in major knee trauma: Pedal pulse a false sign of security? *Arch Orthop Trauma Surg.* 1990;109:238–239.

33. McCutchan JD, Gillham NR. Injury to the popliteal artery associated with dislocation of the knee: Palpable distal pulses do not negate the requirement for arteriography. *Injury.* 1989;20: 307–310.

34. Bynoe RP, Miles WS, Bell RM. Noninvasive diagnosis of vascular trauma by duplex ultrasonography. *J Vasc Surg.* 1991;14: 346–352.

35. Fanelli GC. Treatment of combined anterior cruciate ligament-posterior cruciate ligament-lateral side injuries of the knee. *Clin Sports Med.* 2000;19:493–502.

36. Miller HH, Welch CS. Quantitative studies on the time factor in arterial injurys. *Ann Surg.* 1949;130:538.

37. Wolma FJ. Arterial injurys of the legs associated with fractures and dislocations. *Am J Surg.* 1980;140:186.

38. Winkelaar G, Taylor DC. Vascular trauma associated with fractures and dislocations. *Semin Vasc Surg.* 1998;11:261–273.

39. Gable DR, Allen JW, Richardson JD. Blunt popliteal artery injury: Is physical exam alone enough for evaluation? *J Trauma.* 1997;43:541–544.

40. McCoy GF, Hannon DG, Barr RJ, et al. Vascular injury associated with low – velocity dislocations of the knee. *J Bone Joint Surg Br.* 1987;69:285–287.

41. Barnes C, Pietrobon R, Higgins L. Does the pulse examination in patients with traumatic knee dislocation predict a surgcial arterial injury? A Meta-analysis. *J Trauma.* 2002;53:1109–1114.

42. Johnson K, Lynch K, Paun M, et al. Non-invasive vascular test reliably exclude occult arterial trauma in injured extremities. *J Trauma.* 1991;31:515–519.

43. Miranda F, Dennis J, Veldenz H, et al. Confirmation of the safety and accuracy of physical examination in the evaluation of knee dislocation for injury of the popliteal artery: A prospective study. *J Trauma.* 2002;52:247–252.

44. Trieman GS, Yellin AF, Weaver FA. Evaluation of the patient with a knee dislocation: The case for selective arteriography. *Arch Surg.* 1992;127:1056–1063.

45. Kaufman SL, Martin LG. Arterial injuries associated with complete dislocation of the knee. *Radiology.* 1992;184:153–155.

46. Varnell RM, Coldwell DM, Sangeorzan BJ, et al. Arterial injury complicating knee disruption. *Am Surg.* 1989;55:699–704.

47. Wascher DC, Dvirnak PC, DeCoster TA. Knee dislocation: Initial assessment and implication for treatment. *J Orthop Trauma.* 1997;11:525–529.

48. Wascher DC. High velocity knee dislocation with vascular injury. Treatment principles. *Clin Sports Med.* 2000;19:457–477.

49. Applebaum R, Yellin AE, Weaver FA, et al. Role of routine arteriography in blunt lower extremity trauma. *Am J Surg.* 1990;160: 221–225.

50. Sawchuck AP, Eldrup-Jorgenssen J, Tober C, et al. The natural history of intimal flaps in a canine model. *Arch Surg.* 1990; 125:1614–1616.

51. Melton MM, Croce MA, Patton JH, et al. Popliteal artery trauma. *Ann Surg.* 1997;225:518–529.

52. Rose SC, Moore EE. Trauma angiography: The use of clinical findings to improve patient selection and case preparation. *J Trauma.* 1988;28:240–245.

53. Bryan T, Merritt P, Hack B. Popliteal arterial injuries associated with fractures or dislocations about the knee as a result of blunt trauma. *Orthop Rev.* 1991;20:525–530.

54. Klineberg E, Crites B, Flinn W, et al. The role of arteriography in assessing popliteal artery injury in knee dislocations. *J Trauma.* 2004;56:786–790.

55. Ricter M, Bosch U, Wipperman B, et al. Comparison of surgical repair or reconstruction of the cruciate ligaments versus nonsurgical treatment in patients with traumatic knee dislocations. *Am J Sports Med.* 2002;30:718–727.

56. Fanelli GC, Giannotti BF, Edson CJ. Arthroscoically assisted combined anterior and posterior cruciate ligament reconstruction. *Arthroscopy.* 1996;12:5–14.

57. Cole BJ, Harner CD. The multiligament injured knee. *Clin Sports Med.* 1999;18:241–262.

58. Good L, Johnson RJ. The dislocated knee. *J Am Acad Orthop Surg.* 1995;3:284–292.

59. Schenck RC, Hunter RE, Ostrum RF, et al. The dislocated knee. *Instr Course Lect.* 1994;43:127–136.

60. Roman PD, Hopson CN, Zenni E. Traumatic dislocation of the knee: A report of 30 cases and literature review. *Orthop Rev.* 1987;16:917–924.

61. Shapiro MS, Freedman EL. Allograft reconstruction of the anterior and posterior cruciate ligaments after traumatic knee dislocation. *Am J Sports Med.* 1995;23:580–587.

62. Harner C, Waltrip R, Bennett C, et al. Surgical management of knee dislocations. *J Bone Joint Surg.* 2004;86:262–273.

63. Mills W, Tejwani N. Heterotopic ossification after knee dislocation: The predictive value of the injury severity score. *J Orthop Trauma.* 2003;17:338–345.

64. Rungee JL, Fay MJ, Deberdino TM. Olecranization of the patella. *Orthopedics.* 1995;18:27–34.

65. Almekinders LC, Dedmond BT. The dislocated knee: Outcomes of the operatively treated knee dislocation. *Clin Sports Med.* 2000;19:503–518.

66. Demond BT, Almekinders LC. Operative versus nonoperative treatment of knee dislocations: A meta-analysis. *Am J Knee Surg.* 2001;14:33–38.

67. Mariani PP, Santoriello P, Iannone S, et al. Comparison of surgical treatments for knee dislocation. *Am J Knee Surg.* 1999;12: 214–221.

SUGGESTED READINGS

Covey D. Injuries of the posterolateral corner of the knee. *J Bone Joint Surg Am.* 2001;83:106–118.

Wilson T, Talwalker J, Johnson D. Lateral patella dislocation associated with an irreducible posterolateral knee dislocation: Literature review. *Orthopedics.* 2005;28:459–461.

Wong CH, Tan JL, Chang HC, et al. Knee dislocations – a retrospective study comparing operative versus closed immobilization treatment outcomes. *Knee Surg Sports Traumatol Arthrosc.* 2004;12:540–544.

Anesthesia for Trauma Surgery

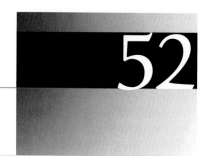

Christopher R. Turner

Anesthesia for trauma is unique in its requirement for a rapid assessment of a dynamically changing clinical situation while engaging in ongoing resuscitation and initiating and maintaining an anesthetic. Anesthetic priorities must be triaged quickly, therapy initiated rapidly, and monitoring established speedily while constantly assessing the changing condition of the patient and staying on guard for sudden clinical events from hidden injuries or surgical manipulation. This chapter is intended to outline the issues facing the anesthesia team for a number of trauma scenarios and to emphasize the communication and team approach necessary to bring about a successful trauma anesthetic and hospital course.

PREPARING FOR TRAUMA

The trauma anesthetic begins long before the patient's injury. One or more operating rooms (ORs) must be immediately available for the trauma-to-come. These rooms should either be rapidly warmed (upon notification of a trauma) or prewarmed, should be immediately adjacent to the emergency department (ED), trauma burns intensive care unit (TBICU), interventional radiology, and the required sterile gear, and staffed by experienced personnel well known to the rest of the trauma team.

Trauma rooms should be set up with the basic gear to begin an anesthetic. The anesthesia machine should be on and the checkout completed, physiologic monitors should be on with electrodes attached, a variety of airway equipment ready to use, intravenous (IV) setups immediately available, in addition to having suction and drugs ready. The drugs that must be ready include sedative hypnotics

(often etomidate or ketamine is preferable to the standard propofol or sodium thiopental) and succinylcholine as well as a nondepolarizing muscle relaxant (often rocuronium), lidocaine, and basic vasopressors such as ephedrine, phenylephrine, and epinephrine. In addition, scopolamine should be stocked to be given for amnesia if the patient is unable to tolerate any anesthetic, insulin and D50 should be available for treatment of hypo- or hyperglycemia, and mannitol and furosemide in stock for treatment of intracranial hypertension. Other vasopressors such as dopamine and norepinephrine should also be available, as well as vasopressin and hydrocortisone. Narcotics should be checked out ahead of time to the anesthesia trauma team and either be carried on their persons in the hospital during call or kept in a locked location immediately available to the trauma ORs. Multiple sizes of catheters—IV, arterial, central venous, introducer sheath—and pulmonary artery catheters (PACs) should all be in the room, along with the gowns, gloves, and sterile drapes for inserting these catheters if time permits. High-volume fluid warmers should be in the room or immediately outside, and it is usually preferable to prestage bagged kits of the required disposables for the warmers along with instructions (with pictures) of the setup steps. These can be left indefinitely if not opened but minimize the time required to set up the fluid warmer in a crisis. Crash carts must be immediately available to the trauma OR and checked daily.

Unfortunately we must address the issue of OR security. After hours trauma ORs must be locked, must be within a secured operating suite, or must be under constant observation according to Centers for Medicare and Medicaid Services (CMS) regulations.[1] This is primarily to allow prepared drugs to be left on top of the anesthesia carts rather than locked up in the cart itself. Unfortunately, a properly set up trauma OR is also a magnet for other hospital personnel who need gear and may elect to scavenge it from the OR, thereby making their life easier but potentially compromising the care of the acutely injured patient. Proper room security can help avoid this situation.

Aside from the trauma OR setup, there are several other preparations that can be made, which help smooth the anesthetic care of the trauma patient. Of primary importance is a rapid and reliable communication system, which integrates the anesthesiology team into the hospital trauma response. It is not practical for the trauma team to find a phone or computer, look up an anesthesia pager number, transmit an informative message, and await a response all the while engaging in the ED stabilization of a critical patient. A designated anesthesia walkie-talkie or cell phone should be linked to the trauma system's announcement of patient acquisition, arrival, and immediate disposition. In addition, this device should allow the trauma team to transmit anesthesia-specific information rapidly and with prompt acknowledgement of receipt. This is particularly critical if an anesthesiologist is not part of the ED trauma response team in your institution.

Another preparation that can pay big dividends is mobile airway equipment in the form of an airway bag, tackle box, or "airway cart." When responding to an airway crisis in the ED, radiology suite, or TBICU, a well-equipped airway box can be a lifesaver. The contents of the airway box will depend on the favored airway interventions in your institution but may include a variety of blades for direct laryngoscopy (DL), assistive stylets such as the gum elastic bougie, laryngeal mask airways (LMAs) and/or intubating LMAs, a portable flexible fiber optic bronchoscope, a portable rigid fiber optic laryngoscope such as a Bullard, and percutaneous cricothyrotomy kits. The immediate availability of a variety of airway devices that are familiar to all department personnel can keep an unpleasant airway situation from deteriorating into frank disaster.

The last preparation that should be undertaken is the establishment of a protocol for massive transfusion between the blood bank, the trauma service, and the anesthesia service. When a trauma patient requires massive transfusion, it is helpful for everyone to have agreed in advance how rapidly blood will be available, what kind of blood will be released under what circumstances, and when and how rapidly factors and platelets will accompany the packed cells. This helps to avoid arguments during resuscitation over product availability and allows providers to focus on the patient instead.[2]

PREOPERATIVE HISTORY

The hallmark of the typical anesthetic is a careful preoperative evaluation, which thoroughly explores the patient's history and current condition, thereby leading to a carefully considered anesthetic plan with appropriately chosen monitoring and carefully titrated anesthetic dosing. In the trauma situation this often goes out the window; under the worst of circumstances you may receive a page that the patient is already in the OR! Therefore, the trauma preoperative evaluation must focus on the essential areas of immediate relevance to the performance of a limited anesthetic, is often obtained from an emergency medical technician (EMT), ED nurse, or surgical resident, and is usually incomplete. Laboratory or radiologic studies or professional consultations, which under other circumstances might be essential, may have to be deferred to the intraoperative or postoperative period. Even basic necessities such as IV access may have to be performed in the OR in concert with surgical preparation and/or activity.

Time for a history can often be obtained by meeting the patient in the ED trauma bay. Even if the patient is unconscious and undergoing multiple procedures, it is often possible to get the relevant history by listening to the ED "chatter" and asking targeted questions. This also places the anesthesia team in a position to assist with airway or access procedures as needed. Alternatively, with the increasing importance of interventional radiology in the treatment of the trauma patient with abdominal or pelvic bleeding, it may be possible for a member of the anesthesia crew to be present in angiography to assist with patient management if necessary and to obtain a more complete history with the benefit of a little breathing room.

A useful mnemonic for the emergency history is "AAMPLE": (A = allergies, A = age, M = medications, P = past medical history, L = last meal, E = events up to the trauma). However, even this much history is often unknown or known imperfectly. Allergies are useful to know for obvious reasons, but are often completely unknown and in the event that resuscitation is proceeding poorly, anaphylaxis should be kept as part of the differential diagnosis. Age is important in broad ranges. Although adolescent and young adult males are most likely to be involved in trauma, physiologically they are most able to tolerate it.[3] The very young and the very old are most susceptible to trauma and its associated complications. Questions about medications should focus on those of immediate relevance to the anesthetic—cardiovascular medications (β-blockers, calcium channel blockers, and particularly angiotensin-converting enzyme [ACE] inhibitors), pulmonary medications (bronchodilators), neurologic medications (anticonvulsants, antipsychotics, and antidepressants), analgesics, and recreational drugs (alcohol and other depressants, opiates, and sympathomimetics such as cocaine and methamphetamine). Past medical history likewise focuses on areas of immediate relevance to the anesthetic and may often, to some extent, be inferred from the medication list if known. A history of coronary artery disease or congestive heart failure, neurologic disease,[4] asthma or chronic obstructive pulmonary disease (COPD), renal disease, diabetes, psychiatric disorder, or recreational drug abuse will immediately impact the conduct of the anesthetic, the physiologic targets for therapy, and postoperative management. Events leading to the trauma help to focus attention on the most life-threatening conditions, while also triggering a targeted search for possible associated injuries.

It is often important to know the general details of the out-of-hospital management: What was the time of injury, what was the mechanism of injury, what injuries were noted at the scene and what was the patient's neurologic status, and what treatment was given at the scene and en route? Most important in many cases is what airway management occurred: Did the patient need to be intubated, if so was the attempt successful, and if not what was used as a rescue airway?

It is also useful to know the results of any diagnostic studies done as part of the trauma workup. Did the focused abdominal sonography for trauma (FAST) show abdominal or pelvic fluid? What were the results of the chest and abdominal plain films? Were any bone studies done? Was angiography performed and what were the results? Were any bleeding vessels embolized? Was head, neck, thoracic, or abdominal computed tomography (CT) or magnetic resonance imaging (MRI) done; if so, are the results available and what were they?

PERIOPERATIVE TREATMENT

Anesthetic management of the trauma patient focuses on the immediate and most life-threatening priorities. Generally these are (i) intravascular volume, access, and resuscitation; (ii) airway management; (iii) establishing necessary monitoring; and (iv) provision of whatever anesthetic the patient will tolerate. These priorities are somewhat fluid and must often be done simultaneously. The presence of a trauma anesthesia team contributes materially to successful outcomes. By dividing up the responsibilities for airway management, access, fluid management, monitor placement, drug administration, record keeping, and overall direction among multiple people, each team member can successfully focus on discrete tasks. Note that the "anesthetic" portion of the anesthetic is low on the list of priorities. The time-honored axiom that the trauma patient must "earn" the anesthetic is due to the cardiovascular collapse sometimes seen with even small doses of anesthetics.

RESUSCITATION AND ACCESS

Usually, but not always, this process has started before arrival in the OR; either in the field or in the ED. A minimum standard should be two free-flowing short large bore (16 or 14 gauge) peripheral IVs, and more as necessary. Short peripheral lines in general have higher flow rates and are preferred for acute resuscitation.[5,6] Sometimes

peripheral IVs have been started but may be antecubital and/or of inadequate caliber. Small antecubital catheters can be changed over a wire to a "rapid infusion catheter (RIC)" or short single lumen central venous pressure (CVP) catheter, but the existing antecubital must be at least 20 gauge for this to work, and the vein has to be large enough to accept the larger catheter. The saphenous vein is often large, readily accessible, and provides a direct route to the inferior vena cava (IVC); minor problems such as long-term infection rate offset by ease of access and remoteness from surgical sites. However, use caution in the potential presence of venous bleeding below the diaphragm or you may merely contribute your resuscitation fluid to the ongoing hemorrhage. Central venous catheters are started more rapidly than a peripheral cut down and should be obtained if peripheral catheters cannot be quickly started, or after the initial resuscitation to obtain secure IV access and to facilitate operative and postoperative management. Massive transfusion may require multiple introducer sheaths in the central circulation.

At this point, there is no outcome data to support the choice of a particular fluid to be used in the initial resuscitation. There is likewise no data to support the use of colloid over crystalloid in the initial resuscitation of a trauma patient.[7,8] The particular crystalloid used does not appear to be very important. There is no outcome data to support the use of one crystalloid over another; therefore, the choice of crystalloid will depend upon secondary indicators. Lactated Ringers (LR) is the most common fluid used in anesthesia and OR resuscitation. It is balanced and buffered and can be given in large volumes with little effect on acid–base status but is slightly hypoosmolar, at least transiently decreases serum osmolarity,[9] and is incompatible with blood transfusion. Normal saline (NS) is readily available, slightly hyperosmolar, and compatible with transfusions and medications; however, it is associated with a hyperchloremic acidosis when given rapidly.[10] Hypertonic saline has been studied for decades but there is no clearly established role for it that changes outcome,[8] with the possible exception of patients with head trauma. Other solutions are available such as Normosol, which is also balanced, is isoosmolar, and is buffered with acetate. These types of solutions may prove to be better for volume resuscitation; however, there is again no outcome data to support this notion.

Like hypertonic saline, colloids have been extensively studied in resuscitation for decades, and as yet there is no clinically established role for them. Colloids studies include human albumin and various synthetic colloids such as dextran and hydroxyethyl starch. Although colloids are more efficient at expanding intravascular volume, increase indices of tissue perfusion, and may decrease peripheral edema, they have also been associated with brain and lung edema and the synthetic colloids have a significant incidence of anaphylactic reaction.[8] They are also substantially more expensive than crystalloids and in the case of albumin, sometimes in short supply. In summary, although colloids are often mixed with crystalloids during trauma resuscitation, there is at present no clear justification for their use or expense.

None of the crystalloid or colloid solutions provide what is often most needed in the trauma patient—oxygen carrying capacity. In the continued absence of a non–human blood oxygen carrier, only red blood cells (RBCs) can augment oxygen uptake and delivery. A requirement for transfusion is associated with increased mortality from trauma, but it is not clear whether this is due to adverse effects of transfusion or due to the greater acuity of trauma patients who require transfusion.[11] Indications for transfusion will depend on the patient and the situation, but include evidence of end-organ ischemia, increasing base deficit (lactic acidosis), a hematocrit measurement below which it is dangerous for the patient (approximately 20 to 25 in young previously healthy patients to 30 or higher for older patients with systemic diseases), or ongoing hemorrhage.

The specific kind of RBC will depend on the urgency of the transfusion. When time permits (usually about an hour), transfusion should be performed with blood that has been typed and crossed. This procedure performs a blood typing (including Rh), performs a minor cross match testing donor plasma against the recipient's RBCs as well as a major cross match of donor RBC against recipient plasma, and tests for antibodies against Kell, Kidd, and Duffy antigens. This testing decreases the chance of any transfusion reaction to approximately 1:50,000. If time is short, typed and screened blood can be administered, which omits the major and minor cross matches and has approximately a 1:10,000 incidence of allergic or nonallergic transfusion reaction. Unfortunately, this only saves a few minutes of processing time, hence it is generally not recommended to use type and screen over type and cross. Type-specific blood, on the other hand, only tests for ABO and Rh type and can be available in 10 minutes. Type-specific blood carries a 1:1,000 incidence of transfusion reaction and therefore should be avoided except when necessary. If there is no time to wait, then prestaged universal donor (O−) blood should be available in the ORs for immediate transfusion requirements. If more than four units of O− blood are used, then transfusion should be continued with O− blood to avoid graft versus host type reactions. O+ blood can also be used unless the patient is a woman of child-bearing age.

Cell salvage techniques may be life saving during massive hemorrhage. Blood can be suctioned from the field, and the red cells washed, concentrated, and retransfused. While the washed red cells do not contain any clotting factors and can contain traces of anticoagulant, nevertheless blood can often be processed faster than it can be obtained from the blood bank, and by recycling hemorrhaged blood transfusion requirements can be decreased.

There is some evidence that supports modest improvements in outcome if patients are allowed to have lower than normal blood pressure and intravascular volume up to the time that major hemorrhage is controlled.[12] Although this has been controversial, there is general agreement that once major hemorrhage has been controlled resuscitation should be aggressive but not excessive. End points for resuscitation will be addressed in the section on later stages of the anesthetic.

THE TRAUMA AIRWAY

Often concurrently with resuscitation for the anesthesiologist comes the necessity of airway management. A definitive airway may have been placed before arrival in the OR; otherwise rapid decisions must be made regarding airway management.

There must be a very low threshold for endotracheal intubation: Airways rarely improve during trauma treatment and the airway that is manageable now may be unobtainable later. If the airway has been secured already, either in the field or in the ED, the anesthesiologist must verify that the existing airway is secure, properly placed, and appropriate for further hospital care. An endotracheal tube (ETT) placed in the field may be esophageal (with the patient spontaneously ventilating around it), may be endobronchial, or may be of inadequate size for the anesthetic or for subsequent critical care.

Most trauma anesthetics will be general anesthetics, necessitating a secure, properly placed ETT. Regional anesthetics or monitored anesthesia care (MAC) cases will be the minority and reserved for more minor trauma and surgery. Although these anesthetics have the wonderful attributes of facilitating neurologic examination and potentially avoiding airway management, in practice the intoxication or lack of cooperation on the part of the patient, the extent of the surgery, presence (or possibility) of coagulopathy, or hemodynamic instability usually prevent the use of awake anesthetic techniques. The airway is best secured early and electively; attempting to avoid a difficult intubation in the trauma patient invites disaster later when the airway worsens or the surgery takes a turn for the worse. If an awake anesthetic is chosen to avoid immediate airway management, there must be several options planned and prepared to quickly manage the airway later should that become necessary.

Airway assessment is done in the usual manner except that the patient may not be cooperative with the airway examination. Particular attention is paid to signs of airway trauma: external trauma to the neck, swelling (symmetric or asymmetric), coughing, or breathing through secretions or blood, or stridor. As always, the anterior neck is examined for the feasibility of a surgical airway should that be necessary. A high index of suspicion is necessary for airway injuries, as airway injuries may be markedly greater than suspected based on the external examination.

Endotracheal Intubation

In the event that the patient arrives without a secured airway, there are several considerations that are unique to the trauma airway. The first is the risk of aspiration; trauma patients should be considered to have full stomachs and to be at increased risk for aspiration.[13] Gastric emptying slows or stops at the time of trauma, so unless the patient last ate 8 hours before the trauma the patient may have retained gastric contents. Multiple attempts at mask ventilation often inflate the stomach and compromise ventilation and oxygenation as well as further increase the risk of vomiting and aspiration. While cooperative patients may be able to take PO nonparticulate antacids, other interventions to reduce gastric volume or acidity are likely to be ineffective in the time available in an emergency situation.

A rapid-sequence induction with cricoid pressure is the most common intervention used in the face of a full stomach, but this may not be the best approach if the patient has facial or airway injuries, a difficult airway, or has a potential cervical spine injury. In addition, the airway may be even more difficult than it was initially due to swelling and/or bleeding due to trauma, repeated airway instrumentation, or resuscitation. Trauma patients tend to desaturate very quickly, even when preoxygenated, and trauma patients in general and head trauma patients in particular will not tolerate periods of hypoxia and hypotension that would be tolerated by healthier individuals.[14]

When the patient is cooperative, an awake fiber optic intubation can deal with most of these issues with the greatest safety; otherwise, an awake intubation by DL (with or without muscle relaxants) or a sedated spontaneously ventilating fiber optic intubation may be the wisest choice. The oral route in general is preferred to the nasal route due to the lower incidence of complications,[15] the lower incidence of sinusitis for prolonged intubations, and because of the potential for intracranial passage of a tube in the presence of skull base trauma. Patients should only be anesthetized and relaxed for intubation when there is great confidence that intubation will be successful, that mask ventilation can be performed if it is not, and that the patient will not experience cardiovascular collapse from the anesthetics.

In the event that intubation techniques are unsuccessful and the patient acutely desaturates, the accepted emergency airway now is cricothyrotomy because it can be done more quickly than a formal tracheotomy. This should be converted to a formal tracheotomy as early as possible due to the high incidence of glottic injuries seen when cricothyrotomies remain in place more than 24 hours.

Airway Trauma

The airway itself can be involved in the trauma; the presence of head or thoracic trauma increases the likelihood of trauma to the airway. Severe laryngeal or tracheal disruption is often fatal at the scene. If the patient survives to reach the anesthesiologist airway trauma, limited mouth opening, oral or pharyngeal debris, edema, bleeding, secretions, or the creation of false passages all increase the difficulty of airway management. Airway trauma distal to the glottic opening can create false passages which may quickly form subcutaneous emphysema, pneumomediastinum, or pneumothorax leading to inability to ventilate and disaster. If there is a possibility of airway trauma, and the patient is at all cooperative or can be made cooperative pharmacologically, the airway is best managed awake and spontaneously ventilating while guiding the ETT with a flexible fiber optic scope, with careful attention paid to the anatomy both above and below the vocal cords inspecting for signs of trauma.

The Potentially Unstable Cervical Spine

Another unique consideration in the trauma patient is the potential for cervical spinal instability and/or cord injury. It is very common for the trauma patient to present for surgery in a cervical collar with the cervical spine uncleared. Often the necessary radiographic studies have been done but not read. While every trauma anesthesiologist should have a basic understanding of reading C-spine films and should be able to identify obvious fractures and dislocations, nevertheless it is not uncommon to face an airway that must be secured with a neck of unknown stability. In this setting, the hallmark of the intubation is that it must be done in a neutral position, and subsequently immobilization must be maintained for the protection and preservation of the spinal cord in order to prevent secondary injury.

If the patient is awake and cooperative, an elective awake intubation over a fiber optic bronchoscope is the gold standard. This has been shown to generate relatively little cervical motion, allows the patient to protect himself or herself from cervical injury, and last but not least allows a postintubation neurologic examination to demonstrate that the function of the cervical cord is intact and unaffected by the intubation.

If the patient is not cooperative, either from intoxication or from hemodynamic or neurologic instability, then it is generally better to do the intubation asleep. Again, however, this must be done in a neutral position and must be performed with an awareness of the risk of aspiration. In a patient whose cervical cord is intact or who has a cord injury of <24 to 48 hours' duration, succinylcholine may be used to relax the patient for intubation, and *may* permit a return to spontaneous ventilation in the event that intubation is unsuccessful. Cricoid pressure (the Sellick maneuver) is generally a good idea except in those situations where there is cervical instability in the segments directly under the cricoid ring. Placement of a second hand supporting the neck for two-handed cricoid pressure may reduce movement of an unstable cervical spine. Mask ventilation, if provided at pressures that will not insufflate the stomach, may dramatically improve the time to desaturation but mask ventilation can cause motion at unstable cervical segments equal to that seen with DL.[16]

There is no outcome data to support the particular choice of one technique of neutral intubation over another, and precious little experimental data. Intubation may be attempted with DL with manual in-line stabilization (the most common choice), asleep fiber optic, rigid fiber optic such as a Bullard or Wu-scope, lightwand, or optical lightwands such as the Bonfils. The choice of technique should be the one that the anesthesiologist has the greatest familiarity and facility with, with the *caveat* that only the DL and the lightwand are potentially useful in the setting of airway blood—all of the optical techniques will fail when the optics are covered with blood. However, if one technique proves difficult the anesthesiologist should switch to another before the struggles are enough to alter the neutral position or cause airway injury. Again, cricothyrotomy or tracheostomy should be done early in the progression toward airway disaster in an attempt to absolutely minimize the duration of hypoxia. Likewise, the airway is more important than the C-spine: while C-spine injury must be a part of the thought process, hypoxia definitely injures while an unstable C-spine only might injure.

Managing the Rescue Airway

If the field crew or the ED were unable to place an ETT, the patient may come to you with an unsecured airway, an oropharyngeal airway (such as a Combitube), an LMA, with an ETT placed through an intubating LMA, or with a surgical airway. It is the anesthesiologist's responsibility to transform a temporizing airway into a standard ETT or to recommend tracheostomy.

Of primary interest is whether a rescue airway offers a method for accessing the trachea when it is changed over to a standard ETT. If the temporizing airway can be removed over a tube changer, it offers a greater likelihood that changing the airway will be successful because the tube changer offers a visual and mechanical guide to the placement of the definitive airway. If the rescue airway does not permit the placement of a tube changer or facilitation of a laryngoscopy with the airway in place, then the existing airway must be sacrificed in order to attempt to place the definitive one. This moves a formal surgical airway considerably higher on the decision tree: it may prove wise to perform a surgical airway in the presence of the rescue airway (particularly if the patient is likely to eventually need a tracheotomy anyway), or to move more quickly to a surgical airway in the event that placing the definitive airway proves problematic.

MONITORING

If time allows it is useful to establish the monitoring for the resuscitation and anesthetic before initiating treatment so that the results of therapy can be followed, but unlike the typical anesthetic establishing monitoring must sometimes take a secondary role to therapeutic interventions. Again, it is useful to have multiple personnel participating in the anesthetic so that the leader can focus on the big picture while others are simultaneously performing resuscitation, airway management, and initiating monitoring.

If resuscitation or airway management delays the initiation of monitoring, it is important to establish monitoring at the earliest opportunity so that the resuscitation can be titrated and neither insufficient nor excessive. Basic monitors for resuscitation are generally standard monitors, a Foley catheter, orogastric tube, and an arterial line. The standard monitors are pulse oximetry (for oxygenation, cardiac rate and rhythm, and peripheral perfusion), electrocardiogram (ECG) (monitoring both for preexisting myocardial injury and for ischemia during resuscitation), blood pressure (organ perfusion), end-tidal (Et) CO_2 (adequacy of ventilation and cardiac output), temperature, and airway pressures and spirometry (monitoring for pulmonary injury and edema). It is usually wise to establish an arterial line while the patient has a blood pressure, particularly if cardiovascular collapse is a possibility later in the anesthetic. The arterial line is helpful because multiple laboratory draws are usually necessary, the blood pressure often changes more rapidly than a noninvasive blood pressure can keep up with, it is less susceptible to interference from the surgeons bumping or leaning against it, and it provides an excellent assessment of the volume responsiveness of hypotension to fluid therapy by systolic pressure variation (SPV).

SPV is the cyclic change in systolic blood pressure (SBP) secondary to positive pressure ventilation. During normal mechanical inspiration, systolic pressure may slightly increase (↑up) but will then decrease (↓down) as the inspiratory phase progresses. Systolic pressure will subsequently return to baseline during the expiratory phase. These systolic pressure changes are very reproducible with positive pressure ventilation under normal circumstances. The difference between the greatest or least systolic pressure during inspiration and the baseline systolic pressure during apnea is the ↑up SPV or ↓down SPV, respectively. SPV (specifically ↓down) has been increasingly used as a monitor of intravascular volume and has been shown to be useful in hemorrhagic shock in dogs and pigs.[17] SPV normally is approximately 5 mm Hg, with values >10 mm Hg consistent with hypovolemia and >15 mm Hg consistent with severe hypovolemia.

Temperature monitoring is particularly important in the trauma patient and must be established early. The trauma setting, the cold transport, ED, and ORs, exposure of the patient for triage and treatment, and the suppression of hypothalamic temperature control by anesthetics[18] all contribute to the high incidence of hypothermia in the trauma patient. Rapid warming is essential as hypothermia increases perioperative hemorrhage due to both inhibition of platelet function[19] as well as inhibition of the enzymes of the clotting cascades. Hypothermia is an indicator of poor prognosis if not rapidly reversed.[20] Because the full exposure and preparation of the trauma patient renders ineffective air warming systems, the most effective method of warming the trauma patient is treatment in a (very) warm environment.[21]

Central venous and pulmonary artery pressure monitoring, cardiac output monitoring, and/or a transesophageal echocardiography (TEE) are generally reserved for later in the resuscitation when the patient has received what appears to be appropriate resuscitation and still remains hypotensive, thereby necessitating the differentiation of the cause of the hypotension. A CVP catheter may also be of utility later in the patient's intensive care unit (ICU) course as secure IV access for fluids, medications, laboratory draws, and nutrition.

ANESTHESIA

If the patient's condition permits, an anesthetic can be established in part or whole before airway management. Again, follow the axiom of making the patient "earn" the anesthetic, other than muscle relaxation. Recall of intraoperative events is higher during trauma anesthetics precisely because patients often do not tolerate a sufficiently deep anesthetic to prevent awareness.[22] Most anesthetic regimens not only cause cardiovascular depression and vasodilation but also interfere with the compensatory mechanisms that respond to hypotension. If the patient will not tolerate any anesthetic at all, IV scopolamine may be used to help prevent recall at a dose of 0.4 mg IV for a typical adult as long as the surgeons are warned that the fixed and dilated pupils they will see in the ICU will not be indicative of the state of the patient's brain.

If the patient will tolerate anesthesia, then a steady progression should move gradually up the scale of cardiac depression and vasodilation: start with narcotics (particularly the "cleaner" synthetic opiates such as fentanyl), move to relatively nondepressing sedative hypnotics (etomidate or ketamine), progress to low-dose volatile anesthetics or (perhaps) nitrous oxide, and only if the patient has proved that he or she will tolerate these doses, the anesthetic progress to agents with more cardiac depression and/or vasodilation effects such as thiopental, propofol, midazolam, or a higher-dose volatile anesthetic. Nitrous oxide is a questionable choice in this setting; while it has the advantage of relatively little cardiac depression, it limits the FIO_2 that can be administered and can greatly expand

a pneumocephalus, pneumomediastinum, or pneumothorax. Once it has been established that the patient will tolerate the anesthetic, maintenance is retained as for any anesthetic with a greater likelihood of having to decrease the anesthetic again should changing clinical situations warrant it. Consideration should be given to administration of β-blockers to patients with thoracic injury and/or blunt myocardial injury with elevated troponin levels.[23]

LATER STAGES OF THE ANESTHETIC

It is critically important during the anesthetic to maintain constant two-way communication with the surgical team. The team must be kept abreast of how the patient is doing including the status of volume resuscitation, the patient's vital signs, and the level of anesthesia. Conversely, they need to keep the anesthesia team informed as to where they are in the procedure, when they have controlled major hemorrhage, when they expect further hemorrhage, and what their expectations are for postoperative care/course. By coordinating the resuscitation and anesthetic with surgical events, the patient is more likely to do well.

Intraoperative complications will depend on the clinical scenario, but many manifest as persistent hypotension. Hypotension before adequate volume resuscitation can be treated with vasopressors as a temporizing measure. Vasopressin[24] and hydrocortisone[25] can be used to treat hypotension refractory to the common vasopressors in trauma patients. However, if the hypotension does not respond to relatively small doses of these agents it is inappropriate to continue to treat hypotension with vasopressors without establishing its cause. Common etiologies include ongoing (perhaps occult) bleeding, pneumothorax or tamponade, neurogenic shock, embolus, or direct myocardial injury. These must be sorted out quickly, and if the intraoperative survey does not reveal a cause, then a TEE examination performed by a competent echocardiographer can often establish the reason for persistent hypotension. If this is not available, then placement of a PAC and measurement of filling pressures, cardiac output, and vascular resistance are advisable.

Once more than the patient's total blood volume has been lost (and transfused), several other considerations come in to play. Hyperkalemia can result from large transfusions particularly when given rapidly. Dilution and consumption may necessitate the replacement of platelets, clotting factors, (fresh frozen plasma [FFP] and/or cryoprecipitate), and calcium. Replacing these are ideally guided by laboratory studies, but often in the acute setting anesthesiologist must transfuse these products based on the clinical scenario and tissue (not vessel) bleeding.[26] There is some evidence that preemptive treatment may ultimately reduce the total amount of factors required.[27] Keep in mind that coagulation studies performed at 37°C may be normal in a patient who is coagulopathic due to hypothermia. In cases of severe coagulopathy, recombinant factor VIIa has been shown to improve measures of coagulopathy, but may worsen outcome and is extremely expensive.[28,29]

Persistent lactic acidosis (as manifested by the base deficit on arterial blood gas [ABG] analysis) is another potential intraoperative complication and a marker for poorer outcomes.[30] Increasing base deficit is a sign of hypoperfusion and need for further resuscitation (volume or red cells or both), but sometimes once the patient is volume replete the base deficit, although not rising, persists or falls very slowly. In such cases, it is generally better to accept the base deficit rather than continuing to treat it with further aggressive volume and transfusion. If the patient's pH is below 7.20 (a somewhat arbitrary value but one below which plasma enzymes begin to malfunction), it may be wise to increase it with sodium bicarbonate, but if the pH is >7.20 and stable or rising it is often better to follow the base deficit and allow it to resolve on its own.

As discussed earlier, it may be appropriate to accept lower blood pressures and perhaps lower intravascular volume during the initial resuscitation period. However, once the major hemorrhage has been controlled you should be more aggressive restoring intravascular volume and blood pressure. Adequate intravascular volume is probably more important than blood pressure *per se*. Overresuscitation is probably associated with a poorer outcome[31] but persistent hypoperfusion leads to permanent organ injury.

With some good luck the team will reach a point after the start of the anesthetic where they "hit their stride." Resuscitation will be keeping up with ongoing blood loss, essential monitors will have been established, the patient will be receiving more than minimal anesthetic agents, and the patient will be warm or at least getting warmer. At this point, it is appropriate to reconsider both the current situation and plans for future intraoperative and postoperative care.

The end points for resuscitation and transfusion therapy and targets for the anesthetic are individualized for each patient but involve blood pressure and heart rate within normal limits, SPV <10 mm Hg, urine output of at least 0.5 mL per kg (preferably higher), good peripheral pulses, acceptable oxygen saturation, a hematocrit not lower than the patient can safely tolerate (and higher than that if ongoing bleeding is expected), relatively normal or normalizing acid–base status with a stable or improving base deficit, near normal electrolytes, and an acceptable anesthetic depth likely to prevent recall. These endpoints are empirically derived; there is currently no evidence that titration to any particular parameter improves outcome.[32]

At the end of the anesthetic, should the patient be extubated? This decision must consider several unusual factors: (i) Is the patient likely to return to the OR soon? (ii) Will ongoing resuscitation or hemodynamic support be needed? (iii) How difficult was the airway to manage in the first place, and how much worse is it now?

What are the effects on the airway of injury, burn, or edema from the resuscitation? Was the patient's cervical spine unstable or uncleared? (iv) How important is a postoperative neurologic examination? (v) Was the patient intoxicated or combative at the start of the resuscitation, is he or she likely to still be intoxicated or combative, or is there the likelihood of withdrawal from some substance postoperatively?

Often it is better to leave the patient intubated and transport to the ICU for further stabilization. In that case the transport must be done with full monitoring, with agents and equipment along for emergencies, sometimes with resuscitation ongoing, usually with assisted ventilation ongoing, and if tolerated with sedation (aside from muscle relaxation) in progress.

If the patient is maintained in the ICU postoperatively, the anesthesiologist may continue to provide care and support, either as a member of the critical care team or as an airway consultant for longer-term issues. Unfortunately, common is the patient who makes it through the initial treatment in relatively good shape but has an untoward event in the ICU, and often these events are related to the airway. Neurologic and respiratory status may wax and wane post trauma, necessitating airway intervention where none was needed before. The anesthesiologist may be consulted for advice or presence during the extubation of a patient with a difficult airway—this is a laudable practice that should be encouraged. Often extubation can be made safer by the use of adjunct devices such as Cook airway exchange catheters. Alternatively, the anesthesiologist can counsel to proceed to a formal tracheostomy for patients deemed too risky to extubate or who will need ventilatory support for some time to come. The elective tracheostomy is always preferable to the emergency one.

SOME SPECIAL SITUATIONS IN TRAUMA ANESTHESIA

Pediatrics

Pediatrics represents a special situation for the trauma anesthesiologist. Differences between pediatric and adult anesthetics are not the focus of this chapter but include airway anatomy and management, head and cervical spine anatomy, circulation, and the responses to shock.[33] As mentioned in the preceding text, young children have a relatively higher mortality from trauma. The younger the patient and the worse the injury the more necessary is treatment at a pediatric trauma centers, but any hospital in the trauma system may be called upon to provide the assessment and treatment of a pediatric trauma patient. In any case, the overall priorities for the pediatric trauma anesthetic are the same as those for adults: resuscitation and airway management followed by monitoring and then by provision of an anesthetic.

A pediatric patient's relatively small size means less margin for error, more difficult IV access, and greater force over smaller area protected less by an immature skeleton, thereby making more likely multisystem injury. Rapid rewarming is even more essential for pediatric trauma patients than for adults because hypothermia develops more rapidly due to their relatively greater surface area and they have a more limited ability to maintain core temperature.

Children with multiple injuries can maintain normal blood pressure until 25% to 35% of their estimated blood volume (EBV) is lost; nevertheless they often present in shock. Hemorrhage is often underestimated in pediatric patients.[34] Younger children have high sympathetic tone and infants are critically dependent on heart rate for their blood pressure: Bradycardia manifests early as hypotension because they have limited ability to augment stroke volume. If access is not obtained quickly it can be peripherally gained through cut downs, central lines, or intraosseous access. Intraosseous access is relatively easily done with a low complication rate but requires specialized needles and some training to perform.[35]

Two aspects of pediatric trauma airway management should be mentioned. The first is that due to their smaller airway diameter, a given amount of airway edema will result in greater airway compromise. The second is that the patient's age may make awake fiber optic intubation techniques unusable. Monitoring and anesthesia should progress in the same general manner as for adults with the *caveat* that younger children may be even more susceptible to the cardiovascular depression associated with many anesthetic regimens.

Burns and Burn Debridement

Anesthesia for burn debridement is based on the same principles and priorities as for trauma anesthesia—resuscitation, airway, monitoring, and then anesthetizing. It is not uncommon for burn injuries to coexist with other injuries, and pediatric patients are frequent victims of burn injuries; therefore, some of the earlier discussions will apply here as well.

Once again, IV access and resuscitation take center stage.[36] In place of or in addition to hemorrhage, there is now massive fluid loss from burned skin and tachypnea. Surface area of burn is more important in determining volume loss than is depth of burn. Once the protective epidermal layer is lost, volume loss occurs at a tremendous pace and hypovolemia is a primary cause of mortality in the first 24 hours. IV access in these patients is often difficult due to intravascular volume depletion and also access must be obtained through burn or scar. Again, central venous lines and/or peripheral cut downs should be performed early in the resuscitation if needed. A Foley catheter is required for all significant burn patients, and the patients must be kept warm by any means necessary. Capillary membrane disruption allows massive amounts of leak to form peripheral edema—the classic "Michelin Man." Renal blood flow (RBF) diminishes and the tubules are burdened by the toxic products of breakdown of muscle and burned tissue as well as the diminished RBF. Alkalinization of the urine with IV sodium bicarbonate may be useful in helping to clear these renally toxic products.

The Parkland and modified Brooke formulas both attempt to quantify the massive volumes that may be required to resuscitate burn patients. These represent starting points and should be increased or decreased as the clinical scenario dictates. The use of colloid in the first day after a burn may be associated with increased edema.[36] Data from a guinea pig model suggested markedly better survival for animals resuscitated with Ringers acetate as opposed to LR or NS[37] but this has not been repeated in humans.

The airway should be secured early in the burn patient with at least an 8.0 ETT, particularly if there is any possibility of airway or respiratory tract burn. Warning signs predicting future airway compromise include a smoky or enclosed fire, facial, neck, or nares burns, hoarseness, stridor, cough with carbonaceous sputum, or tachypnea. An airway that is manageable now may not be in the near future after edema sets in, and surgical airways are more difficult and carry increased mortality in the setting of airway burns. Intubation helps protect against airway obstruction and facilitates mechanical ventilation and pulmonary toilet-copious secretions that are common in pulmonary burn injury. When intubating the patient, pay particular attention to the state of the airway, looking for evidence of burn, chemical injury, or smoke irritation. After intubation, it is wise to perform fiber optic bronchoscopy, looking for injury below the vocal cords, soot, secretions, or hemorrhage. Subglottic injury is uncommon except with steam burns but can still occur and should be diagnosed early.

Pulmonary edema may form during the volume resuscitation needed for treating burns and injuries and often progresses to adult respiratory distress syndrome (ARDS). Positive pressure ventilation and positive end-expiratory pressure (PEEP) are often required in burn patients, even some with relatively small areas of burn. High FIO_2 is usually required to compensate for the higher metabolic rate associated with burn injury. Bronchospasm and pulmonary edema should be treated in the usual manner.

Particularly in the setting of burns from enclosed fires, be aware of the possibility of carbon monoxide (CO)[38] or cyanide poisoning from smoke inhalation. CO poisoning can be recognized by bright red skin, headache, nausea, restlessness, and confusion, and CO can be measured using cooximetry. CO has a 210-fold increased affinity for hemoglobin over oxygen; at 100% O_2 the halftime for CO-Hgb dissociation is 40 to 60 hours. Because central nervous system (CNS) binding is increased compared to blood, 100% O_2 therapy should continue as long as neurologic symptoms persist. CO in addition to smoke inhalation increases mortality. Cyanide poisoning must be approached with a high index of suspicion in the setting of smoky fires involving textiles or upholstery because there is still no readily available rapid test for cyanide exposure. The manifestations of cyanide toxicity under anesthesia are nonspecific and include acidosis, seizures, hypertension, tachycardia, and arrhythmias up to and including cardiac arrest. If cyanide toxicity is suspected it should be treated with high FIO_2, supportive measures, and if necessary a cyanide binding agent such as sodium thiosulfate.[38,39]

Monitoring should be more intense than for an equivalent nonburn case particularly in the presence of inhalation injury, >40% body surface area burn, or extremes of age. Despite the need for massive volume resuscitation, normovolemia is the goal and over-resuscitation increases mortality. ECG monitoring may require the use of needle electrodes, as standard electrodes may not stick to the burned area. Temperature monitoring is critical as hypothermia is life threatening, but oftentimes these patients are hypermetabolic and hyperthermic. $EtCO_2$ is essential because the hyperdynamic state generates more CO_2 than normal and hyperventilation may be required. An arterial line is essential for blood pressure and SPV monitoring and recurring blood gas and electrolyte analysis—pay particular attention to sodium (as a measure of relative free water load), potassium (from rapid transfusion or injured tissue), and calcium (which can be markedly decreased in the face of transfusions). Urine output is likewise essential, and for the trauma patient, CVP, PAC, and TEE monitoring are usually reserved for later in the resuscitation in the face of a confusing clinical picture.

The anesthetic agents used for burn surgery are not vitally important. The biggest issue in the choice of anesthetic agents is that these patients often come for repeated procedures and therefore develop tolerance and accumulate anesthetic agents. Succinylcholine should be avoided after the first day of a burn because extrajunctional acetylcholine (ACH) receptors proliferate and increase the risk of hyperkalemia in this setting. This may also make them resistant to nondepolarizing relaxants and may require a 50% to 100% increase in the intubating dose of a nondepolarizer. The anesthetic should be heavy on analgesia because these injuries and surgeries are intensely painful and these patients are often receiving high doses of opioids with resulting tolerance. Ketamine is a time-honored drug for its lack of respiratory depression or accumulation and its potent analgesia. Dexmedetomidine appears to be increasing in popularity for similar reasons.

These patients may present for excisions and debridement and/or skin grafts. Expect to see massive blood loss that is difficult to estimate, anticipate the complications of massive transfusion (including hypocalcemia and coagulopathy), and do whatever it takes to keep the patients normothermic. Patients will often be placed in multiple positions during the procedures. In general, the surgery should be terminated or staged *before* the patient becomes

coagulopathic (more than one blood volume lost) or hypothermic (below 35°C).

These patients may also require escharotomy for compartment syndrome of the extremities (for perfusion), thorax or abdomen (for hemodynamics or ventilation), or of the face or neck (for airway support). These are usually straightforward unless the eschar involves the airway. In this case, an ETT is usually present by the time an eschar forms, but dislodgement of the ETT can be fatal because it may be impossible to replace and surgical salvage of the airway is doubtful.

Head Trauma

The anesthetic management of head injury has changed markedly over the last decade. The standard therapy of mannitol and hyperventilation to prevent cerebral edema for every head injury has been replaced by a new emphasis on maintenance of cerebral perfusion pressure (CPP) of at least 70 mm Hg,[40] maintaining oxygenation and assiduous avoidance of hypoxia. Because intracranial pressure (ICP) is a major determinant of CPP, the threshold for ICP monitoring is lowered, particularly if the patient is unlikely to be awakened postoperatively for whatever reason. Sustained increases in ICP above 20 mm Hg are associated with poorer outcomes.[41] Hyperventilation, mannitol, furosemide, and hypertonic saline are now used selectively to treat elevated ICP as opposed to the universal treatment done in the past. Cerebrospinal fluid (CSF) drainage is a useful intervention to control ICP, which will often be preferred by the neurosurgical service in view of its preservation of cerebral blood flow, and many of the methods for ICP monitoring such as ventriculostomy also allow CSF drainage to control ICP. In situations where cerebral edema and ICP increases are resistant to therapy, barbiturate coma (not propofol due to its association with acidosis after prolonged infusion)[42] or craniectomy may control ICP long enough for the brain swelling to diminish, but these are last-ditch efforts and often associated with a grim prognosis.

This is one situation in trauma where the choice of resuscitation fluid may make a significant difference. It is recognized that there is little that can be done about the edema formed by injured brain but that the maintenance of cerebral perfusion and serum osmolarity can help prevent the formation of edema in normal brain. As mentioned earlier, LR is hypoosmolar and contributes the equivalent of approximately 200 mL of free water to the resuscitation. If resuscitation is extensive, this free water may be sufficient enough to decrease serum osmolarity to cause edema in normal brain, thereby worsening intracranial dynamics. In this case, maintenance of serum osmolarity with NS, Normosol, or hypertonic saline may prove to be beneficial.[40]

Although patients with traumatic brain injury and mild hypothermia on admission tend to have better outcomes, induced hypothermia as a therapy has not been clearly shown to be of benefit in this setting and is probably not worthwhile given the other complications attendant to hypothermia.[43] On the other hand, hyperthermia is clearly associated with worsened neurologic outcome, perhaps in part through its effects on ICP[44] and so should be assiduously avoided.

On occasion head injury can cause neurogenic shock. This is the result of the sudden loss of sympathetic nervous system signals to the smooth muscle in vessel walls, resulting in fixed vasodilated vasculature with hypotension, bradycardia, and hypothermia. The anesthetic management of neurogenic shock will be discussed in the following section.

Spinal Injury

Issues concerning C-spine injury and airway management have been addressed already in the airway section. Here we will discuss other anesthetic issues raised by spinal injuries. It is important to differentiate spinal injury from spinal cord injury: Generally, bony injuries are most important in the degree that they have caused or might cause either primary or secondary spinal cord injury through vascular compromise and ischemia. Prevention of secondary injury is the hallmark of anesthesia care for spinal cord injury; therefore, maintenance of neutral position of the spine is of paramount importance throughout the perioperative period. In addition, maintenance of cord perfusion and oxygen delivery is vital because spinal cord injury is exacerbated by hypotension, hypoxia, stress response, or hyperthermia. Even with impeccable care, the natural history of these injuries waxes and wanes due to edema and inflammatory changes.

The level and completeness of a spinal cord injury influence the difficulty posed for an anesthetic. Incomplete injuries may preserve some sensory, motor, or autonomic function below the level of the injury, thereby potentially necessitating an anesthetic that will not only block pain sensation from below the lesion but also perhaps provide some vasomotor tone and/or inhibition of mass reflexes. While low (lumbar or low thoracic) lesions pose difficulties for the patient in terms of respiratory function due to loss of abdominal assistance to ventilation, for the anesthesiologist, once the increased vascular capacitance below the level of the lesion has been accounted for (and succinylcholine avoided after the first 24 hours), these injuries generally do not pose undue difficulties for management. Midlevel lesions (mid to high thoracic) begin to pose more potential for postoperative respiratory compromise and a greater likelihood of coexisting thoracic injuries. Weeks later in the patient's course, these lesions may also produce episodes of autonomic hyperreflexia. High (high thoracic or cervical) lesions may generate immediately life-threatening compromise to all parameters of respiratory function, potential phrenic nerve involvement, increased aspiration risk, and the potential for sinus arrest due to unopposed

vagal activity, as well as the airway issues that have been addressed earlier.

In a manner analogous to head trauma management, maintenance of cord perfusion involves at least a normal blood pressure (cord perfusion pressure) with somewhat higher pressure if cord edema is thought to be present by MRI or neurologic examination, normal oxygen saturation and normal acid–base and blood gas parameters, and normocarbia because spinal cord blood supply, like cerebral blood supply, vasoconstricts in the presence of hypocarbia. Mannitol may be of some use in reducing spinal cord edema. Although newer data suggests that the early enthusiasm over reducing spinal cord deficits was overstated, if methylprednisolone has been started by the trauma service, it should be continued through the perioperative period.

Neurogenic (spinal) shock due to spinal cord trauma is the result of massive dysfunction of the spinal cord below the level of the lesion. Generally, the lesion must be above the splanchnic innervation (midthoracic) for spinal shock to be a clinical problem. Sympathetic denervation results in a dilated, fixed capacitance with decreased cardiac return, bradycardia, lost orthostatic and pressor reflexes, and decreased contractility. Thermoregulation is also lost. Spinal shock lasts hours to weeks, but less than the period of flaccid paralysis.

The general approach to treating spinal shock is aggressive volume resuscitation until the CVP begins to rise or SPV to fall, at which time the resuscitation is dramatically slowed. The fixed dilated intravascular capacitance needs to be filled, but over-resuscitation will dump crystalloid into the lungs. Have a low threshold for PAC monitoring to assist in balancing fluid resuscitation and left-sided filling, cardiac output, and systemic vascular resistance (SVR) in the face of a confusing clinical picture.[45]

Thoracic

Thoracic trauma is often immediately life threatening because of the structures contained within the thorax. Thoracic trauma can lead to unilateral or bilateral pneumothorax or hemothorax, injury to the lower airways, blunt cardiac injury, injury to the great vessels, and direct pulmonary or thoracic cage trauma. Many thoracic injuries which survive to reach the hospital are relatively straightforward after chest tube placement, but some will require emergency thoracotomy for hemorrhage control. Major thoracic injuries can not only pose difficulties in pulmonary or cardiac management but may also be associated with thoracic-level spinal cord injuries.

CONCLUSION

Although the patient suffering traumatic injury poses substantial challenges to the anesthesia team, proper preparation before the anesthetic, knowledge of the clinical situation, setting appropriate priorities during the anesthetic, and maintaining good communication with the trauma team will markedly enhance the chances for a positive outcome.

REFERENCES

1. Center for Medicare and Medicaid Services. Medicare and medicaid programs; hospital conditions of participation: Requirements for history and physical examinations; authentication of verbal orders; securing medications; and postanesthesia evaluations. *Fed Registr*. 2005;70(57):15266–15274.
2. Malone D, Hess J, Fingerhut A. Massive transfusion practices around the globe and a suggestion for a common massive transfusion protocol. *J Trauma*. 2006;60:S91–S96.
3. Oreskovich MR, Howard JD, Copass MK, et al. Geriatric trauma: Injury patterns and outcome. *J Trauma*. 1984;24:565.
4. Rembert F. State of health at time of injury. In: Giesecke AH, ed. *Anesthesia for surgery and trauma*. Philadelphia: FA Davis Co; 1976.
5. Millihan J, Cain TL, Hansbrough J. Rapid volume replacement for hypovolemic shock: A comparison of techniques and equipment. *J Trauma*. 1984;26:428.
6. Chen I, Huang Y, Lin W. Flow-rate measurements and models for colloid and crystalloid flows in central and peripheral venouse line infusion systems. *IEEE Trans Biomed Eng*. 2002;49(12): 1632–1638.
7. Boldt J. Fluid choice for resuscitation of the trauma patient: A review of the physiological, pharmacological, and clinical evidence. *Can J Anaesth*. 2004;51(5):500–513.
8. Rizoli S. Crystalloids and colloids in trauma resuscitation: A brief overview of the current debate. *J Trauma*. 2003;54(5):S82–S88.
9. Williams E, Hildebrand K, McCormick S, et al. The effect of intravenous lactated Ringer's solution versus 0.9% sodium chloride solution on serum osmolality in human volunteers. *Anesth Analg*. 1999;18:999–1003.
10. Scheingraber S, Rehm M, Sehmisch C, et al. Rapid saline infusion produces hyperchloremic acidosis in patients undergoing gynecologic surgery. *Anesthesiology*. 1999;90(5):1265–1270.
11. Eastridge B, Malone D, Holcomb J. Early predictors of transfusion and mortality after injury: A review of the data-based literature. *J Trauma*. 2006;60:S20–S25.
12. Bickell W, Wall M, Pepe P. Immediate versus delayed fluid resuscitation for hypotensive patients with penetrating torso injuries. *N Engl J Med*. 1994;331(17):1105–1109.
13. Olsson G, Hallen B, Hambreaus-Jonson K. Aspiration during anaesthesia: A computer aided study of 185358 anaesthetics. *Acta Anaesthesiol Scand*. 1986;30:84–92.
14. Hukkelhoven C, Steyerberg E, Habbema J, et al. Predicting outcome after traumatic brain injury: Development and validation of a prognostic score based on admission characteristics. *J Neurotrauma*. 2005;22(10):1025–1039.
15. Dronen S, Merigian K, Hedges J, et al. A comparison of blind nasotracheal and succinylcholine-assisted intubation in the poisoned patient. *Ann Emerg Med*. 1987;16:650–652.
16. Donaldson W, Towers J, Doctor A, et al. A methodology to evaluate motion of the unstable spine during intubation techniques. *Spine*. 1993;18:2020–2023.
17. Preisman S, Pfeiffer U, Lieberman N, et al. New monitors of intravascular volume: A comparison of arterial pressure waveform analysis and the intrathoracic blood volume. *Intensive Care Med*. 1997;23(6):651–657.
18. Sessler D. Mild perioperative hypothermia. *N Engl J Med*. 1997; 336(24):1730–1737.
19. Michaelson ASMH, Bernard MR, Kestin AS, et al. Reversible inhibiton of human platelet activation by hypothermia in vivo and in vitro. *Thromb Hemost*. 1994;71:633–640.
20. Wang H, Callaway C, Peitzman A, et al. Admission hypothermia and outcome after major trauma. *Crit Care Med*. 2005; 33(6):1296–1301.
21. Morris R. Operating room temperature and the anesthetized, paralyzed patient. *Arch Surg*. 1971;102:95–97.
22. Bogetz M, Katz J. Recall of surgery for major trauma. *Anesthesiology*. 1984;61:6–9.
23. Martin M, Mullenix P, Rhee P, et al. Troponin increases in the critically injured patient: Mechanical trauma or physiologic stress? *J Trauma*. 2005;59(5):1086–1091.
24. Haas T, Voelckel W, Wiedermann F, et al. Successful resuscitation of a traumatic cardiac arrest victim in hemorrhagic shock with vasopressin: A case report and brief overview of the literature. *J Trauma*. 2004;57(1):177–179.
25. Hoen S, Mazoit J, Asehnoune K, et al. Hydrocortisone increases the sensitivity to alpha-1 adrenoceptor stimulation in humans following hemorrhagic shock. *Crit Care Med*. 2005;33(12): 2737–2743.
26. Hess J, Lawson J. The coagulopathy of trauma versus disseminated intravascular coagulation. *J Trauma*. 2006;60:S12–S19.
27. Ketchum L, Hess J, Hippala S. Indications for early fresh frozen plasma, cryoprecipitate, and platelet transfusion in trauma. *J Trauma*. 2006;60:S51–S58.
28. Dutton R, McCann M, Hyder M, et al. Factor VIIa for correction of traumatic coagulopathy. *J Trauma*. 2004;57(4):709–718.
29. Lynn M, Jeroukhimov I, Klein Y, et al. Updates in the management of severe coagulopathy in trauma patients. *Intensive Care Med*. 2002;28(Suppl 1):S241–S247.
30. Krishna G, Sleigh J, Rahman H. Physiological predictors of death in exsanguinating trauma patients undergoing conventional surgery. *Aust N Z J Surg*. 1998;68(12):826–829.
31. Revell M, Greaves I, Porter K. Endpoints for fluid resuscitation in hemorrhagic shock. *J Trauma*. 2003;54:S63–S67.
32. Wade C, Holcomb J. Endpoints in clinical trials of fluid resuscitation of patients with traumatic injuries. *Transfusion*. 2005;45: 4S–8S.
33. Feldman D, Reich N, Foster J. Pediatric anesthesia and postoperative analgesia. *Pediatr Clin North Am*. 1998;45(6):1525–1537.
34. Dykes EH. Paediatric trauma. *Br J Anaesth*. 1999;83(1):130–138.
35. Ross AK. Pediatric trauma. Anesthesia management. *Anesthesiol Clin North America*. 2001;19(2):309–337.
36. MacLennan N, Heimbach D, Cullen B. Anesthesia for major thermal injury. *Anesthesiology*. 1998;89(3):749–770.
37. Conahan S, Dupre A, Giaimo M, et al. Resuscitation fluid composition and myocardial performance during burn shock. *Circ Shock*. 1987;23:37–49.
38. Lee-Chiong T. Smoke inhalation injury. *Postgrad Med*. 1999; 105(2):55–64.
39. Barillo D, Good R, Esch V. Cyanide poisoning in victims of fire: Analysis of 364 cases and review of the literature. *J Burn Care Rehab*. 1994;15(1):46–57.
40. Ghajar J. Traumatic brain injury. *Lancet*. 2000;356:923–929.
41. Prough D, Lang J. Therapy of patients with head injuries: Key parameters for management. *J Trauma*. 1997;42(5S):10S–18S.
42. Burow B, Johnson M, Packer D. Metabolic acidosis associated with propofol in the absence of other causative factors. *Anesthesiology*. 2004;101:239–241.
43. Tisherman S. Hypothermia and injury. *Curr Opin Crit Care*. 2004; 10(6):512–519.
44. Rossi S, Zanier E, Mauri I, et al. Brain temperature, body core temperature, and intracranial pressure in acute cerebral damage. *J Neurol Neurosurg Psychiatry*. 2001;71(4):448–455.
45. Cobby T, Hardman J, Baxendale B. Anaesthetic managment of the severely injured patient: Spinal injury. *Br J Hosp Med*. 1997; 58(5):198–201.

Special Considerations in Trauma in Children

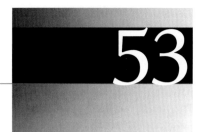

Thane A. Blinman   Michael L. Nance

There is no greater health concern in the pediatric population than trauma. Trauma is the leading cause of death among children between 1 and 18 years of age, greater than all other causes combined.[1] Injury-related death is responsible for approximately 30% of all years of potential life lost.[1] For every one injury-related death in the pediatric population, there are 12 children hospitalized for injury and more than 60 treated for an injury in an emergency department (ED) (see Fig. 1).[1] Despite well-intentioned safety laws and apparently better safety products, the problem persists.

Care of the injured child differs in important ways from routine care of the injured adult. In addition to the anatomic differences, injury patterns and physiologic responses diverge for adult and pediatric trauma patients. The biomechanics of pediatric patients differ from adults in discreet ways, as follows:

- Decreased mineralization of bone means that bone offers less protection to structures in the central nervous system (CNS), thorax, and abdomen.
- Decreased muscle strength per unit volume means not only diminished protection of the cervical spine and abdomen, but decreased Starling effect in the heart.
- Increased surface area relative to body mass means dramatically increased vulnerability to radiative and evaporative loss of heat and fluid.

Not only are the patterns of injury different than in adults (e.g., pulmonary contusion in the absence of rib fracture) but the physiologic responses to hemorrhage and resuscitative interventions differ substantially from those exhibited by adults (e.g., increased heart rate [HR] instead of preload-recruitable stroke work in order to maximize delivery). Failure to consider these differences can lead to treatment that is incorrect either in terms of therapeutic choice (e.g., early splenectomy for spleen laceration) or of degree (e.g., over- or under-resuscitation of the child in shock or traumatic brain injury [TBI]). In addition, the largely nonoperative nature of pediatric trauma has lulled some into believing that no injured children need surgical consultation, a myth easily dispelled by the case logs of any major children's trauma center.[2,3]

The objective of this chapter is to describe clinically important differences in the care of the injured child with emphasis on resuscitation and surgical care of specific injuries. Orthopaedic injuries, burns, and exposures are excluded.

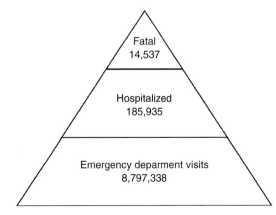

Figure 1 Injury pyramid demonstrating fatal injuries, injuries requiring hospitalization and injuries resulting in an emergency department visit for children aged 0 to 18 years, 2004. (Data from National Center for Injury Prevention and Control. Available at: http://www.cdc.gov/ncipc/wisqars/; Accessed May 4, 2007.)

TRAUMA SYSTEMS

Trauma centers were developed to provide the best care to the injured patient. By concentrating resources in identified institutions, and by directing the most severely injured patients to these centers, outcomes were optimized.[4] The American College of Surgeons (ACS) has established guidelines to accredit hospitals as trauma centers. Similar guidelines were established to verify pediatric trauma centers as well. Most states have adopted these (or locally modified) ACS guidelines as a foundation for a trauma system. Despite the existence of pediatric resource centers for trauma, more than three fourths of pediatric trauma care occurs outside of such centers.[5] Of concern, the overall survival of the younger (age younger than 10 years) and most injured (Injury Severity Score [ISS] greater than 15) patients treated in a freestanding pediatric hospital was improved compared to adult hospitals and non–freestanding pediatric hospitals.[6] Pediatric trauma centers have also shown improved outcomes compared to nonpediatric trauma centers for specific injury types including head and spleen injuries.[7,8] However, the fact remains that given the limitations of geography or availability of resources, most injured children will be treated outside of pediatric trauma centers. Therefore, it is imperative that all practitioners treating pediatric patients (up to 25% of typical trauma center volume) are comfortable with and equipped to provide care for the injured child. The basic equipment recommended by the American Academy of Pediatrics and American College of Emergency Physicians to care for injured children was found in only 5.5% of hospitals in the United States.[9] Equipment essential for treatment of the pediatric trauma patient is listed in Table 1.

PREHOSPITAL CARE

There is evidence that paramedics deliver good prehospital care to children as well as to adults.[10] Although properly sized equipment is often absent on a standard rescue ambulance, paramedics appear to improvise and adapt existing equipment well to protect the injured child. Response times and extrication methods are independent of patient age, of course. Heavy use of helicopter evacuation and transport (in patients who tend to have less severe injuries) is perhaps evidence that emergency medical service (EMS) providers prefer to err on the side of caution.[11]

Nevertheless, prehospital providers struggle with some important aspects of pediatric care, especially the pediatric airway, intravenous (IV) access, and C-spine immobilization. Recent evidence indicates that airway management short of endotracheal intubation (in particular, oral airway and bag-valve-mask ventilation) is superior to unsuccessful attempts at field intubation, especially in a child with traumatic brain injury (TBI).[12,13] Meanwhile, complications are seen in as many as half of prehospital intubations and attempts, with unrecognized esophageal intubations alarmingly common. Current recommendations are to avoid attempts at endotracheal intubation in the field and to transport using oral airway and bag-valve-mask ventilation with chin-lift/jaw-thrust unless these maneuvers are demonstrably inadequate. An exception may be the pediatric patient requiring prolonged transport in whom a stable airway is preferable. EMS staff who must intubate a child should clearly understand the anatomic differences of the pediatric airway (see subsequent text).

IV access in the pediatric patient is frequently challenging. A high percentage of pediatric trauma patients arrive in the ED with *no* IV access. Intraosseus (IO) catheters seem underused, despite their demonstrated effectiveness in children. The thin sternum of a child makes this location contraindicated; practitioners should preferentially use the tibia if an IO is used. The risk of infection remains, and definitive IV access including central venous access should be established as soon as feasible in the hospital setting.

C-spine precautions are often misapplied or not employed. Pediatric patients whose C-spines are immobilized often suffer from one of three errors: incorrectly sized C-collar (almost always so large that it slips over the chin, simultaneously obstructing the airway and providing no C-spine protection); absent C-collar (usually with the possibly effective but inadequately tested work-around of a rolled towel and tape); inadequate padding beneath the thoracic spine to compensate for the prominent occiput of the child (which produces flexion at the neck instead of neutral positioning).

Other prehospital issues, such as "hypotensive resuscitation" or the use of intentional hypothermia have been inadequately studied in the pediatric population to make thoughtful recommendations.

ACUTE CARE

Primary Survey

Early hospital care of the pediatric trauma patient parallels standard Advanced Trauma Life Support (ATLS) protocols, and the usual rubric of primary survey (*A*irway, *B*reathing, *C*irculation, *D*isability, and *E*xposure [ABCDE]), secondary survey, and tertiary survey provides a good structure for discussion, with emphasis on clinically important anatomic and physiologic differences.

Airway

Safe control of the airway is paramount in pediatric trauma resuscitation. Success here prevents secondary injury from hypoxia, but success depends upon a clear understanding of the indications for intubation, an organized clinical approach, and facility with anatomic differences of the airway of a child.

TABLE 1

GUIDELINES FOR EQUIPMENT AND SUPPLIES FOR USE IN PEDIATRIC PATIENTS IN THE EMERGENCY DEPARTMENT (ED)[a]

Monitoring equipment
- Cardiorespiratory monitor with strip recorder
- Defibrillator with pediatric and adult paddles (4.5 and 8 cm) or corresponding adhesive pads
- Pediatric and adult monitor electrodes
- Pulse oximeter with sensors and probe sizes for children
- Thermometer or rectal probe
- Sphygmomanometer
- Doppler blood pressure device
- Blood pressure cuffs (neonatal, infant, child, and adult arm and thigh cuffs)
- Method to monitor endotracheal tube and placement[b]
- Stethoscope

Airway management
- Portable oxygen regulator and canisters
- Clear oxygen masks (standard and nonrebreathing—neonatal, infant, child, and adult)
- Oropharyngeal airways (sizes 0–5)
- Nasopharyngeal airways (12F through 30F)
- Bag-valve-mask resuscitator, self-inflating (450- and 1,000-mL sizes)
- Nasal cannulae (child and adult)
- Endotracheal tubes: uncuffed (2.5, 3.0, 3.5, 4.0, 4.5, 5.0, 5.5, and 6.0 mm) and cuffed (6.5, 7.0. 7.5, 8.0, and 9.0 mm)
- Stylets (infant, pediatric, and adult)
- Laryngoscope handle (pediatric and adult)
- Laryngoscope blades: straight or Miller (0, 1, 2, and 3) arid Macintosh (2 and 3)
- Magill forceps (pediatric and adult)
- Nasogastric/feeding tubes (5F through 18F)
- Suction catheters—flexible (6F, 8F, 10F, 14F, and 16F)
- Yankauer suction tip
- Bulb syringe
- Chest tubes (8F through 40F) [c]
- Laryngeal mask airway (sizes 1, 1.5, 2, 2.5, 3, 4, and 5)

Vascular access
- Butterfly needles (19–25 gauge)
- Catheter-over-needle devices (14–24 gauge)
- Rate limiting infusion device and tubing[c,d]
- Intraosseous needles (may be satisfied by standard bore needle aspiration needles)
- Arm boards[d]
- Intravenous fluid and blood warmers[c]
- Umbilical vein catheters[c,e] (size 5F feeding tube may be used)
- Seldinger technique vascular access kit[c]

Miscellaneous
- Infant and standard scales
- Infant formula and oral rehydrating solutions[c]
- Heating source (may be met by infrared lamps or overhead warmer)[c]
- Towel rolls, blanket rolls, or equivalent
- Pediatric restraining devices
- Resuscitation board
- Sterile linen[f]
- Length-based resuscitation tape or precalculated drug or equipment list based on weight

Specialized pediatric trays
- Tube thoracotomy with water seal drainage capability[c]
- Lumbar puncture
- Pediatric urinary catheters
- Obstetric pack
- Newborn kit[c]
- Umbilical vessel cannulation supplies[c]
- Venous cutdown[c]
- Needle cricothyrotomy tray
- Surgical airway kit (may include a tracheostomy tray or a surgical cricothyrotomy tray)[c]

(continued)

TABLE 1
(CONTINUED)

Fracture management
- Cervical immobilization equipment[c,b]
- Extremity splints[c]
- Femur splints[c]

Medical photography capability

[a]Adapted from Middleton KR, Burt CW. Committee on Pediatric Equipment and Supplies for Emergency Departments, National Emergency Medical Services for Children Resource Alliance. *Adv Data.* 2006;28(367):1–16; United States, 2002–03.
[b]Many types of cervical immobilization devices are available, including wedges and collars. The type of device chosen depends on local preferences and policies and procedures. Chosen device should be stocked in sizes to fit infants, children, adolescents, and adults. Use of sandbags to meet this requirement is discouraged, because they may cause injury if the patient has to be turned.
[c]Equipment that is essential but may be shared with the nursery, pediatric ward, or other inpatient service and is readily available to the ED.
[d]Equipment or supplies that are desirable but not essential.
[e]Ensure availability of pediatric sizes within the hospital.
[f]Available within hospital for burn care.
[g] Suitable for hypothermic and hyperthermia measurements with temperature capability from 25°C to 44 °C.
[h]May be satisfied by a disposable CO_2 detector of appropriate size for infants and children. For children 5 years or older who are >20 kg in body weight, an esophageal detection bulb or syringe may be used additionally.
[i]To regulate rate and volume.
(Adapted from Care of Children in the Emergency Department: Guidelines for preparedness. *Pediatrics.* 2001;107:777–781.)

All trauma centers should have an established protocol for pediatric intubation, a pediatric intubation cart stocked with appropriate sizes of tubes and laryngoscopes, and a guide (such as a Broselow tape) that facilitates choice of tubes and dosing of key medications.

Every institution should maintain a rapid sequence intubation protocol (see Fig. 2). Any unstable child should be intubated by the *most experienced person present*; unstable trauma patients cannot tolerate multiple unskilled attempts.

The pediatric airway differs from the adult in (at least) six discreet ways, as follows (see Fig. 3):

1. Shorter trachea (even relative to body size)
2. Anteriorly displaced epiglottis
3. Prominent occiput
4. High larynx
5. Proportionately large tongue and smaller mouth
6. Narrowed at the cricoid cartilage

These differences mean that a different strategy for intubation of the child is required. In particular, the short trachea necessitates caution to avoid a mainstem intubation. One strategy is to carefully observe the double lines on the endotracheal tube (ETT), when these have just passed the cords, the tube is likely in good position. Careful auscultation using the axilla and observation of the chest rise can confirm good tube position. The anterior epiglottis can be compensated for by less aggressive head tilt (to be avoided in any case if the C-spine is not clear), opting instead for a gentle "sniffing position." Meanwhile, an assistant can direct the epiglottis into a more favorable

position with careful cricoid pressure, even maneuvering the larynx left or right slightly as needed. The prominent occiput can be obviated by gentle padding behind the shoulders (not the neck). The small mouth and large tongue are handled by having reliable suction at the ready, using a

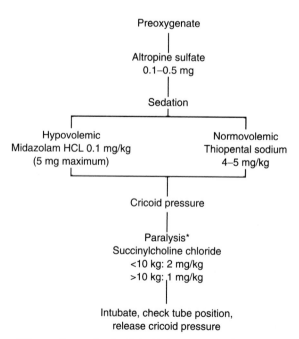

Figure 2   Algorithm for rapid sequence induction of the pediatric trauma patient. (From American College of Surgeons, 1997.)

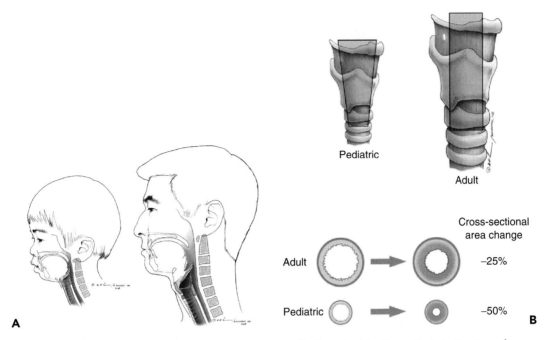

Figure 3 A: Anatomic differences between the pediatric and adult airway. **B:** Anterior view of airway demonstrating narrowing at the level of the cricoid cartilage in the pediatric airway and proportionately greater impact on airway diameter due to edema (Courtesy Brian Denham, MD).

correctly sized laryngoscope (especially the narrower Miller blade), and having the assistant pull gentle traction at the side of the mouth. Finally, the typical narrowing of the cricoid cartilage has traditionally translated into use of uncuffed tubes for children in order to avoid subglottic stenosis from balloon pressure injury, and while some have recently questioned this practice in the intensive care unit (ICU) setting, it remains true that a correctly sized (a classic heuristic is to choose a tube with the same external diameter as the pinky finger) uncuffed tube is easier to place. Finally, all of these anatomic differences mean that esophageal intubation is common but easily detected with use of end-tidal CO_2 devices now widely available.

Indications for intubation include the following:

- Inability to spontaneously protect the airway (e.g., Glasgow Coma Scale [GCS] <8, overdose, drugs, facial trauma)
- Inability to ventilate (e.g., flail chest)
- Inability to oxygenate (e.g., pulmonary contusion, smoke inhalation, and cardiac instability)

Breathing
Several factors can inhibit breathing in infants and children in ways not seen in adults. Aside from the airway considerations listed in the preceding text, clinicians should remember that infants are obligate nose-breathers; tubes, debris, and blood in the nose impede air movement in these patients. Calculations for minute ventilation are somewhat different as well. Children require higher respiratory rates and lower tidal volumes, especially during

bag-valve-mask ventilation. Bradypnea/respiratory arrest is the most common cause of cardiac arrest in babies. The clinician should give rapid (approximately 30 to 40 bpm) breaths using a pressure valve, taking care to not exceed peak inspiratory pressures greater than 25 to 30 mm Hg. Higher pressures are unlikely to improve tidal volume but more likely to inflict barotrauma/volutrauma. In addition, because gastric distension is one of the chief causes of respiratory embarrassment in the younger pediatric trauma patient, the overflow ventilation at higher pressures is more likely to diminish tidal volumes. Early recognition and tube decompression of a distended stomach in a crying, injured child can prevent unnecessary ventilation failure.

Circulation
The total circulating blood volume of the child can be surprisingly small. For young children, blood volume is approximately 80 mL per kg; therefore a 5-kg baby has just 400 mL of total blood volume, and has sustained a 40% hemorrhage (class IV shock) with a loss of only 160 mL (just over 5 oz). Similarly a 25-kg child with a total blood volume of $80 \times 25 = 2,000$ mL can quietly lose 25% of his blood volume in little time from a scalp wound that bleeds just 0.5 L in an hour, or 8.3 mL per minute. The small starting volumes can fool the complacent clinician who ignores these seemingly small but persistent sources of blood loss in the resuscitation suite. Pediatric patients have a remarkable ability to compensate for blood loss, however. The initial response to hypovolemia (i.e., hemorrhage) is tachycardia. In the active trauma resuscitation area, it would not be surprising to see tachycardia in a frightened, injured

child. Distinguishing the source of the tachycardia can be challenging. Often, the pediatric patient will maintain a normal blood pressure until 40% or more of the estimated blood volume has been lost. Hypotension in the pediatric patient is always concerning.

Control of the circulation begins with good venous access. According to ATLS protocol, two attempts should be made to place large-bore IV cannulas in the upper extremities. If this is unsuccessful, an IO line can be placed in the tibia. Large volumes can be readily infused through IO lines, and they can be used for the usual blood products and IV medications. However, they should be regarded as temporary and infection prone; rarely should a child leave the trauma bay with IO catheters in place.

In children, the elements governing oxygen delivery as defined by the oxygen delivery (D_{O_2}) equation are the same as adults. However, the relative contribution of each of these to oxygen delivery differs importantly in children. Oxygen delivery depends on blood oxygen content multiplied by cardiac output (CO). This section considers only CO, which is governed not by one equation, but by two simultaneous equations:[14]

$$CO = HR \times SV = HR \times EF \times EDV$$

and

$$CO = (MAP - CVP)/SVR$$

So the elements of CO are:

HR (heart rate)
SV (stroke volume)
EDV (end diastolic volume, i.e., "preload")
EF (ejection fraction, i.e., "contractility")
MAP (mean arterial pressure)
SVR (systemic vascular resistance, i.e., "afterload")

The mainstay of resuscitation in adult trauma patients has been to maintain circulating volume, and to take advantage of preload (EDV) recruitable increases in CO. In other words, aggressive volume resuscitation in an otherwise healthy adult trauma patient could be shown to boost CO and oxygen delivery as far as EDV could be pushed upward. Although enthusiasm for "supraphysiologic" D_{O_2} (appropriately) has waned, it is largely true that large volumes can be administered to young adults with little negative effect.

The same is not true for babies and children. Starling's law of the heart does not function over nearly the same range of preload, and children rely more on scaling up HR in order to increase CO. Rather than responding to increased stretch with increased stroke work, the pediatric heart will more quickly yield to edema (which increases wall stiffness) and begin to fail. Consequently, clinicians must use more caution in children to avoid not only under-resuscitation but over-resuscitation. Frequently, children in shock require earlier use of pharmacologic agents to alter

SVR/afterload or EF/contractility rather than the aggressive fluid volume resuscitation that succeeds in adults and teens.

This has implications for choice of resuscitation fluid as well. Recommendations for the sick pediatric trauma patient include limiting crystalloid volume resuscitation (and the importance of using warm fluids is even more pronounced in children; see section "Exposure" in the subsequent text) to just two boluses of 20 mL per kg, then switching to O(−) packed red blood cells (PRBCs) for ongoing hemodynamic instability. In this way, circulating volume is more likely to approach "euvolemia" using a fluid that also increases oxygen carrying capacity, thereby maximizing D_{O_2}.

As always, children benefit from "just right" interventions, for example, specific treatments continued just until clinical endpoints are achieved. Endpoints for resuscitation include the following:

- Normalization of HR (to age-appropriate levels)
- Increasing pulse pressure
- Improved skin color and extremity warmth
- Clearing sensorium (as measured by GCS)
- Increasing MAP
- Production of urine (2 mL/kg/hour in infants, 1 mL/kg/hour in adolescents)

Disability

A modified GCS has been validated in children (see Table 2).[15] As in adults, a GCS of 8 or less is an indication for intubation. Importantly, a low GCS is also an independent risk factor for other major injury. Unlike

TABLE 2

GLASGOW COMA SCALE REVISED FOR USE IN PEDIATRIC POPULATION

Best Response	Pediatric GCS	Score
Eye	No eye opening	1
	Eye opening to pain	2
	Eye opening to speech	3
	Eyes open spontaneously	4
Verbal	No vocal response	1
	Inconsolable, agitated	2
	Inconsistently consolable, moaning	3
	Cries, but is consolable, inappropriate interactions	4
	Smiles, oriented to sounds, follows objects, interacts	5
Motor	No motor response	1
	Extension to pain	2
	Flexion to pain	3
	Withdrawal from pain	4
	Localizing to pain	5
	Obeys commands	6

GCS, Glasgow Coma Scale.

adults, children are more likely to have seizures associated with injury and therefore to have transient altered mental status from postictal states. The routine use of prophylactic antiseizure medication, however, has not been shown to be efficacious.[16] In addition, children seem to suffer more mental status degradation from shock and therefore better recovery from resuscitation.

Children are more prone to severe TBI. The head makes up a larger fraction of body mass than in adults and is less well supported by the neck, and the brain is less protected by the bony skull. More importantly, children suffer disproportionately more from transient deficiencies in cerebral oxygen delivery, either from hypoxia or hypotension. Even brief episodes of either measurably increase the risk of death and disability in severe TBI.

Exposure

"Exposure" in the pediatric trauma patient should be understood to mean the following:

- Unobstructed visualization and palpation of the entire body
- Determination of exposure to toxins (CO, acid, petroleum distillates, etc.)
- *Protection from* exposure in the trauma bay in particular, protection from hypothermia

While complete exposure and thorough examination of the injured child is crucial, so is protecting the child from hypothermia in the trauma bay, computed tomography (CT) scanner, and operating room (OR). After the traditional "strip and flip," early effort to covering the child with warm blankets as much as possible greatly protects against iatrogenic heat loss. Covering or bundling can also decrease anxiety in the awake child. Meanwhile, a warm ambient temperature in the trauma bay, overhead warming lights and/or underbody warmers, and warm fluids should be employed to prevent hypothermia. Efforts should also be made to remove all trauma patients, but especially children, from hard spine boards expeditiously (when clinically appropriate). It is demonstrable that remaining on a hard board causes pain in <30 minutes, and can cause skin injury within an hour.[17]

Secondary Survey

During the head-to-toe secondary survey, a number of other measures should be considered:

Chest X-ray (CXR): The ordinary anterior-posterior chest x-ray (AP-CXR) is a rich source of information and is fast. It is a good practice to have a plate positioned on the table before the child arrives, and to shoot the film during the primary survey. Often, problems with airway or breathing (mainstem intubation, pneumothorax, gastric distension, etc.) are identified or confirmed by the film.

Electrocardiogram Monitoring, Pulse Oximetry: They are routinely used, as in adults.

Placement of Central Venous Catheter: This should be considered for any unstable child. However, central lines in children can be challenging to those who lack experience. Landmarks are subtly different, the hardware smaller, and the mechanical response of the needle and wire in the vein misleading. If there are two large-bore peripheral IV catheters, central access can be delayed until later in the resuscitation or in the OR or ICU.

Placement of Bladder Catheter: During inspection of the perineum, the rectal examination is commonly omitted in children because the anal aperture is very small compared to most examiners' fingers, and the information gained from the examination is limited. Similarly, the classic "pelvic rock" is to be avoided, or performed at most once, and gently. If visual, gentle physical examination of the perineum and urethral meatus show no evidence of injury, a size-appropriate bladder catheter can be placed. Resistance or blood indicates the need for urethrogram, especially in the setting of pelvic fracture demonstrated by x-ray.

Placement of Nasogastric (NG): The NG tube is useful to decrease the risk of aspiration of gastric contents, to administer oral contrast, and to diminish abdominal respiratory compromise from gastric distention. Gastric distension can be profound in a crying, aerophagic child, or in a child undergoing bag-valve-mask respiration. In this case, the ventilatory compromise can produce hypoventilation severe enough to lead to cardiac arrest. NG tubes are contraindicated in cases of basilar skull fracture or midface instability; an orogastric (OG) tube can be substituted in this case. Common sense indicates that gastric tubes are not to be inflicted on every patient arriving in the trauma bay.

Laboratory Studies: Recent literature indicates that *few* laboratory studies (e.g., liver function tests [LFTs], metabolic panel) are useful for directing care. Little effort should be made at attempting blood draws in injured children, except for complete blood count (CBC) and a type and cross.[18] An arterial blood gas may add some information in the critically injured child because the admission base deficit reflects injury severity and predicts mortality. Mortality increases in children with a base deficit <–8 mEq per L, and is strong evidence of potentially lethal injuries or uncompensated shock.[19] In patients with significant head injury, thrombin and partial thromboplastin times should be drawn to help determine the need for correction of coagulation abnormalities.

Re-evaluation: Resuscitation is a dynamic process. The practitioner must frequently reassess the physiologic response to resuscitation to ensure goals have been achieved. At the same time, the trauma team leader should anticipate a plan and destination for the child (e.g., CT scanner, pediatric intensive care unit [PICU], OR, or transfer to a higher level of care (e.g., pediatric trauma center). It is the trauma team leader's principal responsibility to drive the patient toward execution of a treatment plan efficiently.

DIAGNOSTIC PROCEDURES

Unstable patients with an obvious source of ongoing hemorrhage (e.g., hard signs of arterial injury, hemothorax, etc.) need to go directly to the OR. The primary decision to be made once ABCs are secured is operative approach and incision. But these circumstances are uncommon in the pediatric patient, and the surgeon frequently benefits from this additional information. Several diagnostic tools are available to help with this diagnostic process.

Plain X-rays

Plain films are useful screening tools, but are probably less helpful overall than in adults because of the variable sizes and extent of ossification of bony structures. The anterior-posterior chest film, ideally taken immediately on patient arrival, is probably the most helpful. The AP-CXR may reveal pneumothorax/hemothorax, pneumoperitoneum, foreign objects, widened mediastinum, and misplaced tubes (especially ETTs).

Other films may not be as useful. Pelvic x-rays are both less sensitive and less specific for fractures in children. C-spine films generally show bony deformity, but should be considered screening tools only: Positive findings always require further definition (usually with CT and/or magnetic resonance imaging [MRI]), but even negative results should be viewed with suspicion in a child with a suggestive mechanism of injury or tenderness on physical examination. Injuries to the spinal cord without bony injury are much more common in children.

Ultrasonograph/Focused Abdominal Sonography for Trauma

Most centers report that Focused Abdominal Sonography for Trauma (FAST) is reliable in discerning the following:

- The presence or absence of fluid in the abdominal cavity
- The presence or absence of fluid in the thorax
- The presence of fluid in the pericardium (where it is the test of choice for tamponade)

FAST does not, however, give one important piece of information—the actual source of fluid in the abdomen. In experienced hands, FAST is reported to be useful to exclude the abdomen as a source of bleeding in the unstable child. However, it is critical to validate physician-performed diagnostic accuracy before employing FAST as a basis for operative decisions.[20]

Computed Tomography Scanning

CT scanning has become the workhorse of trauma diagnostic information. Although there are reports of measurable, albeit very small, lifetime increases in neoplastic risk from CT radiation, these worries should be discounted in the face of immediate injury.[21,22] Rather, scanning protocols that employ weight-specific radiation dosing should be utilized. The rapid scan acquisition and processing made possible by multislice scanners and modern software mean few children need to be restrained or sedated in the scanner.

IV contrast is contraindicated in initial head scans. For abdominal CT scans, IV contrast is required to optimally visualize the solid organs, and in particular, to determine active extravasation: a "blush" from a liver, spleen, or kidney signifies arterial bleeding that may not be suitable for nonoperative protocols. For most injuries, CT angiography has supplanted more invasive methods of detecting injury to thoracic and carotid vessels, and can even exclude some extremity vascular injuries.[23] Meanwhile, oral contrast is often omitted during initial abdominal CT scans because administration of contrast takes time, typically elicits vomiting in children, and usually does not have time to travel to the distal bowel. Oral contrast may, however, help identify proximal injuries such as duodenal hematomas. CT scanning reliably detects bony injuries, but children can sustain severe injuries to brain, spinal cord, lung, and genitourinary (GU) tract without fractures because of the decreased mineralization and stiffness of the bony structures protecting these organs. In particular, CT is poor at detecting spinal cord injuries without radiologic abnormality (SCIWORA); MRI is the modality of choice here, but only in the stabilized patient. Currently, MRI has no role in the acute workup.

Diagnostic Peritoneal Lavage

Diagnostic peritoneal lavage (DPL) is rarely used in children now as the information it provides is similar (fluid or no fluid) to that gleaned from other sources (e.g., FAST). It can give some information about source of fluid that FAST cannot (e.g., presence of vegetable fibers implies viscus injury). However, DPL is more difficult to perform (particularly in an awake child), takes more time than other tests, evaluates only the peritoneum, not the retroperitoneum, and has greater associated risk (e.g., bleeding, perforation, or infection).

Nevertheless, it is still conceivable that DPL could be useful in detecting hemorrhage in a trauma patient when FAST or CT was unavailable. DPL is performed as in adults, with the following few differences:

1. Decompress the bladder and stomach.
2. Use a *supraumbilical* incision to avoid the high-riding pediatric bladder, and use the open or seldinger technique to direct a catheter toward the pelvis.
3. Gross blood is a positive result. If no blood is seen, instill 10 mL per kg (up to 1 L) of warmed Ringers lactate solution and allow it to drain. As in adults, with microscopic analysis, a positive test is given by: >100,000 RBC per mm^3, >500 WBC per mm^3, bile, urine, or food material.

Emergency Department Thoracotomy

Emergency department thoracotomy (EDT) has a poor track record in all trauma patients, but in children it has been particularly unhelpful. As early as 1987, it was apparent that in pediatric blunt trauma, EDT had no influence on survival.[24] Later, it was demonstrated that if pediatric patients had no signs of life (SOL) in the field, they never survived, even with EDT. Worse, there have been no *neurologically intact* survivors among pediatric blunt trauma patients who presented to the trauma bay without SOL.[25] Even those with limited SOL on presentation had a survival of only 23.5% with the risk of fatality after cardiopulmonary resuscitation (CPR) increased for children with a systolic blood pressure below 60 mm Hg on arrival. Although children with penetrating injury had better survival, for all survivors of traumatic arrest, 64% had at least one impairment in the functional activities of daily living.[26] These findings and other data have consistently demonstrated that the potential for survival in pediatric trauma arrest is quite poor, contrary to the popular perception of extraordinary resilience in the pediatric patient. EDT may have value only in cases where arrest occurs in the trauma bay, regardless of mechanism.

Recommendations

Declare death for:

- CPR >20 minutes (in or out of hospital)
- Asystole
- Pulseless and HR <40
- EDT not indicated for blunt trauma victim with no SOL

Perform limited resuscitation for:

- Respiratory arrest
- Pulseless or HR <40
- Severe hypotension with arrest
- Intubation in the field
- EDT of limited value for penetrating with no SOL

Perform EDT for:

- Penetrating injury to chest with witnessed SOL and arrest
- Peripheral vascular injury with witnessed SOL

MANAGEMENT OF INJURIES

The management is similar for most injuries in pediatric and adult patients. Several types of injuries in children are worth additional comment, including the following:

- Traumatic brain injury (TBI)
- Blunt trauma to organs of the thoracic and abdominal cavities
- Cervical spine
- Penetrating trauma
- Nonaccidental trauma

Traumatic Brain Injury

Head injury is the leading cause of death and disability in injured children. Management goals for severe TBI are similar in children and adults and are directed at minimizing additional brain damage from secondary brain injury by hypoxia, hypotension, and elevated intracranial pressure (ICP). Consensus guidelines for the management of severe pediatric brain injury were issued by the trauma, neurosurgical, neurologic, and critical care societies.[27] Practical points for management of the pediatric brain injured patient include the following:

- Intubate for a GCS of 8 or less.
- Avoid routine use of mannitol or hyperventilation.
- Use ICP monitoring for GCS of 8 or less.
- It is not true that open fontanels or sutures prevent high ICP and therefore obviate pressure monitoring. Ventriculostomy offers some control of ICP in addition to monitoring and is preferred in severe TB Cerebral perfusion pressure (CPP) should be maintained above 40 mm Hg in children.
- ICP can be managed by drainage, neuromuscular blockade, sedation, or 3% saline at 0.1 to 1.0 mL/kg/hour. Serum osmolarity should maintained <320 mOsm per L. In the setting of acute deterioration or herniation, aggressive hyperventilation ($PaCO_2$ <30 mm Hg) and/or mannitol 0.25 to 1 g per kg can be attempted. Surgical treatment of ICP may allow ICP reduction by 9 to 74 mm Hg with decompressive craniectomy.
- Steroids have no proven role.
- Antiseizure prophylaxis is generally not recommended.[16]
- Even minor head injury can lead to measurable cognitive deficits that persist for months after the injury in children. Routine follow-up is strongly encouraged.
- There is a growing body of evidence supporting the efficacy of decompressive hemicraniectomy for selected pediatric trauma patients with refractory intracranial hypertension.[28,29] This therapy, while encouraging, should be applied on a case-by-case basis.

Blunt Trauma

Chest: Lung and Trachea, Esophagus, Great Vessels

The most common blunt chest trauma in children is pulmonary contusion. Pulmonary contusion may be seen without rib fracture, can progress ("blossom") over 48 hours after injury, and can precipitate acute respiratory distress syndrome (ARDS) in the uninjured lung. Suspicion should be increased in any case of spleen or liver laceration, especially grade III or higher. Other predictors of thoracic injury in children sustaining blunt torso trauma include low systolic blood pressure, elevated respiratory rate, abnormal results on thoracic examination, abnormal chest auscultation findings, femur fracture, and a GCS score <15.[30] The appearance of pulmonary contusion on CT does not correlate with mortality.[31]

Most pulmonary contusions are self-limited; however, on occasion they may be problematic. In the most extreme example, children (like adults) with severe posttraumatic ARDS can be treated successfully with extracorporeal support. Pulmonary hemorrhage occurs frequently, but is manageable.[32] Although children and adults differ in regard to injury mechanism, overall injury severity, and associated injuries, outcomes for thoracic trauma are quite similar in contradistinction to previous reports.[33] Contusions do not typically cause late pulmonary dysfunction.[34]

Great vessel injuries are rare in the pediatric population, but, if suspected, are most readily investigated with CT angiography. Traumatic aortic injuries are rare in children, with none noted in one institutional review.[35] The most common findings on plain films are a left apical cap, pulmonary contusion, aortic obscuration, and mediastinal widening. Helical CT and transesophageal echocardiography can be used in the diagnosis of traumatic aortic injuries in children. Associated injury is the most important mortality factor. Thoracic surgeries can be performed with minimal morbidity and without mortality in children with blunt thoracic trauma.[36] Cardiac contusions are the most common of these injuries encountered, but rarely have clinical significance.

Blunt trauma to the esophagus is quite rare and often identified late.[37] In the largest series, the most common cause was motor vehicular trauma. The cervical and upper thoracic esophagus was the site of perforation in 82%. In 78% of the cases, there were findings consistent with esophageal injury, but there was a delay in diagnosis attributed to a lack of specific symptom complex. Infectious complications were common (38%) especially when diagnosis was delayed and sepsis-related mortality can reach almost 10%.[38] On the other hand, early diagnosis allows management consisting only of wide drainage and antibiotics.

Diaphragmatic injury results from blunt and penetrating torso trauma, is uncommon, rarely occurs in isolation, and is associated with a high morbidity and mortality.[39,40] Given the large amount of energy required, blunt diaphragmatic injury most commonly occurs from falls and motor vehicle collisions.[41] Plain film findings suggested the diagnosis in most with CT and MRI as useful diagnostic adjuncts.[42] Isolated diaphragmatic injuries do occur in children more frequently than in adults. As in adults, diaphragmatic rupture prevails in the left side, and purposeful surgical diagnosis and early management determine the effectiveness of treatment. Management consists first of management of associated injuries; while incarceration and obstruction are risks of diaphragmatic rupture, usually associated closed head injury (CHI) is more pressing. If the patient is stable, laparoscopic or thoracoscopic repair is feasible. Whether approached open or endoscopically, from the chest or abdomen, repair is predicated on (a) reduction of abdominal viscera, and (b) creating a low tension closure using permanent, interrupted suture and

patch such as Surgisys or Goretex if needed. Avulsion of the costal origin of the diaphragm is a peculiar type of injury described in children. The intercostal muscle flap is a useful tool to bridge diaphragmatic defects.[43] Postoperative small bowel intussusception was the most frequent complication after repair.[41]

Solid Organ Injuries

The management of solid organ injuries (e.g., liver, spleen, and kidney) in the pediatric population has evolved over the last decade to a largely nonoperative approach. Guided by early studies demonstrating the safety and efficacy of this approach, contemporary studies have demonstrated success rates in excess of 90% for nonoperative management.[44-46] The intra-abdominal organs (e.g., liver and spleen), which in the adult are protected by the thoracic cage, are larger proportionately in the child and extend beyond the costal margin. Because of increased compliance of the ribs, more energy is transmitted to the underlying structures. Also, the abdominal wall musculature is less well developed and affords relatively less protection to the internal organs. For these reasons, abdominal injuries are common in the pediatric patient. Although the patterns for peak time to operative intervention vary for the specific organs injured and injury severity, most children with a solid organ injury requiring surgery will need operative intervention within 24 hours of admission.[46]

Liver

Liver laceration after blunt trauma is the second most common abdominal injury in pediatric trauma, but the most common intra-abdominal injury leading to death. Injuries are graded according to the same organ injury scale used in adults. As in adults, the right (and larger) lobe is injured more frequently, with the dual blood supply and high vascularity responsible for potential for significant hemorrhage. Fortunately, liver lacerations in children rarely need to be explored, with >90% amenable to nonoperative management. However, they can go undetected if suspicion is low, and subsequent failure to manage these can lead to complications such as biloma, uncontrolled hemorrhage, or even ascites severe enough to produce abdominal compartment syndrome.

Common symptoms of liver injury in the setting of trauma include right upper quadrant (RUQ) pain, abdominal distension, and right shoulder pain. Elevated transaminases suggest liver injury but are not sensitive or specific, and do not predict severity.[18,47] Liver laceration is most commonly diagnosed by CT scan, with IV contrast. Injury pathways are frequently utilized for liver and other solid organ injuries to optimize care. Such a pathway was proposed and validated by the American Pediatric Surgical Association (see Table 3).[48,49] Patients responding appropriately are monitored in the ICU for 24 hours with a goal of keeping Hb >8. Controversy continues regarding the transfusion threshold in this patient population. It is

TABLE 3

AMERICAN PEDIATRIC SURGICAL ASSOCIATION GUIDELINES FOR MANAGEMENT OF ISOLATED LIVER OR SPLEEN INJURIES IN THE PEDIATRIC PATIENT

	CT Grade			
	I	II	III	IV
ICU days	None	None	None	1
Hospital stay	2	3	4	5
Predischarge imaging	None	None	None	None
Postdischarge imaging	None	None	None	None
Activity restriction (wk)[a]	3	4	5	6

[a]Return to full-contact, competitive sports (i.e. football, wrestling, hockey, lacrosse, and mountain climbing) should be at the discretion of the individual pediatric trauma surgeon. The proposed guidelines for return to unrestricted activity include "normal" age-appropriate activities.
Stylianos S. Evidence-based guidelines for resource utilization in children with isolated spleen or liver injury. The APSA Trauma Committee. *J Pediatr Surg.* 2000;35:164–167.

generally accepted that if transfusion requirements exceed 40 mL per kg, intervention is indicated.

Nevertheless, some children will require exploration. More options exist for control of exsanguinating liver trauma than previously. Adult trauma experience has demonstrated the utility of damage control techniques, particularly the staged celiotomy, and this has been proved of use in the pediatric patient as well.[50] New surgical glues, especially FloSeal, can dramatically improve hemostasis. When confronting an exsanguinating liver laceration, the initial focus as in the adult should be on control of hemorrhage, not definitive control or repair of injuries. Packing of the abdomen with lap pads is highly effective at staunching hepatic parenchymal bleeding for pediatric patients as well. A cold, coagulopathic patient can have a temporary abdominal closure and return for unpacking and definitive repair or resection once physiologically improved, typically 12 to 24 hours later. Meanwhile, interventional radiology techniques have kept pace allowing selective embolization of bleeding sources, obviating the need for celiotomy in highly selected cases or complimentary liver packing and damage control in operative cases.

The clinician should be aware of other organs commonly injured in patients with proven liver laceration. In addition to injuries to other solid organs, pulmonary contusion of the right lower lobe (RLL) is common, and can complicate care.

Spleen

The spleen is the most commonly injured abdominal organ. Splenic trauma is suspected in any blunt trauma to the lower chest or upper abdomen. Patients often exhibit left upper quadrant (LUQ) pain and tenderness, abdominal distension, tachycardia, and the Kehr sign (referred pain to the left shoulder from diaphragmatic irritation). In addition, as with liver trauma, rib fractures are rare but pulmonary contusions are not. Pleuropulmonary involvement (i.e., effusion, contusion) was observed in almost half the number of patients with blunt splenic trauma. Pleuropulmonary involvement occurred either early as a result of direct chest trauma or was delayed.[51] Diagnosis and grading by CT scanning is fast and reliable. Grading in children is the same as for adults (see Chapter 41).

Management of splenic trauma in children is the prototype for nonoperative strategy in abdominal trauma. More than 90% of splenic injuries can be managed by observation, fluid resuscitation, and judicious use of transfusion. Indeed, most children with splenic injuries require no surgery and no transfusion. Nonoperative treatment has produced a fourfold decrease in blood transfusions in children with splenic injury over the last decade.[52]

As with liver injury, most centers employ an algorithmic approach to splenic lacerations. In general, grade III and higher injuries are slotted into the solid organ injury pathway. Importantly, nonoperative management should not be confused with "benign neglect." Success of nonoperative management and preservation of functioning spleen is higher in pediatric trauma centers than adult facilities, with few missed injuries and rare delayed complications (such as splenic rupture), suggesting that algorithm-guided expert attention is indeed effective.

Indications for intervention include refractory bleeding (>40 mL per kg transfused), peritonitis suggesting a hollow organ injury, or abdominal compartment syndrome. Selective embolization of arterial branches by interventional radiology can preserve functioning spleen, although evaluation of splenic function is difficult and these patients may require vaccination even without operative splenectomy. If operating for another indication and a splenic injury is encountered, partial resection, repair, and FloSeal can all be attempted. If these are ineffective, splenectomy proceeds as with adults, with surgical stapling the most reliable method of dividing the hilum. Although associated with higher grades of injury, the CT scan with contrast blush does not mandate embolization or surgical intervention in children with blunt splenic trauma. Severe splenic injuries with a "blush sign" on the initial CT scan may be successfully treated nonoperatively according to a defined treatment protocol based on physiologic response to injury rather than radiologic features of the injury.[53]

If all measures are unsuccessful in preserving a functioning spleen, vaccination reduces the risk of overwhelming postsplenectomy infection (OPSI). Although OPSI is estimated to be rare (0.23% to 0.42% per year), it can be lethal. The risk for OPSI has been reported to be fivefold higher in pediatric than in the adult patients.[54]

Current recommendations include education, immuno-prophylaxis, and chemoprophylaxis for patients following splenectomy.[55] Despite strong scientific data to demonstrate the efficacy of postsplenectomy vaccination, it has been our practice to provide vaccination against infection with encapsulated organisms, in particular *Streptococcus pneumoniae* (the most common agent of OPSI), *Hemophilus influenzae*, and *Neisseiria meningitides* after splenectomy for trauma in the pediatric patient. In addition, our patients, regardless of vaccination status, are maintained on oral penicillin until they are 18 years old.

Follow-up routine imaging of solid organ injuries is no longer recommended in the absence of clinical symptoms suggestive of an intra-abdominal process.

Kidney

The kidney is the third most commonly injured solid organ in blunt trauma, with football placing kidneys at the highest risk.[56] The injury scale as described by the American Association for Surgery of Trauma (AAST) is used in children as well (see Chapter 44).[57] Although ultrasonography and urinalysis may be helpful in screening for injury, exact classification is afforded only by CT scan.[58] Despite their hollow component, the kidneys are amenable to nonoperative management strategies. Success with nonoperative management was noted in 94.7% of children with a 98.9% renal salvage rate.[59] In higher grade injuries (grade III and above), delayed extravasation of contrast was seen on occasion. For such injuries, follow-up CT scan at 48 to 72 hours postinjury is recommended. Even in the face of significant extravasation, patients are likely to respond to closed techniques (e.g., ureteral stenting, percutaneous nephrostomy) obviating the need for laparotomy and possible renal loss.[60] Selective embolization by an experienced interventional radiologist of bleeding renal lacerations of higher grade is certainly possible in children, even with abnormal renal anatomy such as horseshoe kidney.[61]

Bladder

Most bladder injuries result from blunt trauma, with penetrating injuries (as well as some iatrogenic injuries) reported less commonly.[62,63] Children have a higher risk of bladder injury in blunt trauma than adults because the bladder is less well protected by the bony pelvis. The full bladder in an infant or small child protrudes high above the pubic symphysis, at times easily extending to (or even above) the umbilicus. Any lower abdominal blunt trauma (such as a lap-belt injury) can lead to rupture of the bladder.

Evidence of bladder damage comes from urethral blood, abdominal pain, a suggestive mechanism, and presence of fluid on imaging studies. The diagnosis is confirmed by conventional cystogram, or CT cystogram by delayed contrast images on CT. CT cystogram is the most accurate.

Isolated extraperitoneal bladder perforation can be managed with Foley catheter drainage for 7 days, antibiotics,

and pain control. Intraperitoneal bladder injury is managed by laparotomy and primary repair. A layered method using absorbable monofilament is most commonly used. Female urethral and bladder neck injury occurs with pelvic fracture, presents with gross hematuria and/or blood at the introitus, and requires operative repair for avulsions and longitudinal lacerations. These patients are at risk for significant sexual and lower urinary tract dysfunction and may require pediatric urologic follow up.[64]

Pancreas

Pancreatic injuries are comparatively relatively rare, but present challenging management issues. The "handlebar injury" typifies the pancreatic injury pattern.[65,66] Here, a child is struck in the upper midabdomen with the end of a bicycle handlebar during a crash. As a result, the sharp blow transects the pancreas, usually in the tail or distal body. The pancreas sustains the only injury, aside from the telltale round hematoma seen in the lower epigastrium.

The child who presents immediately after injury may be deceptively asymptomatic and well appearing, with tachycardia the first evidence of deeper injury. Later, the child will develop anorexia and nausea, abdominal pain (often both epigastric and right lower quadrant [RLQ]). Fever and peritonitis may follow within the first 48 hours. CT scan with IV contrast timed to highlight the pancreas reveals the injury.[67] Patients requiring delayed surgical intervention after an unsuccessful period of observation or a subsequent operation due to undetected pancreatic duct injury demonstrated a higher rate of pancreas-specific mortality and morbidity.[68] In other cases, children present days after the injury with nausea and epigastric pain. Here, CT or ultrasonography may reveal a pancreatic pseudocyst.

Treatment of pancreatic injuries depends on (a) the severity of injury and (b) the timing of presentation (see Table 4). Minor injuries (no evidence of major duct disruption) to the pancreas discovered early may require no treatment. If uncertainty remains about whether a ductal injury has occurred, endoscopic retrograde cholangiopancreatography (ERCP) allows definitive delineation of the duct anatomy and the potential stent placement even in young children.

Unrecognized (either through test sensitivity or late presentation) duct injuries may progress to pseudocyst formation over the weeks following injury. Small pseudocysts with mild or no symptoms may resolve without treatment.[69] Large, symptomatic pseudocysts require drainage (see subsequent text).

Controversy surrounds the treatment of obvious ductal disruption with total or near transection of the pancreas. As nonoperative treatment of various organ injuries in children became more common (even dogmatic), advocates reported many such successful cases for severe pancreatic injuries in children. However, others have noted that these children often had long hospital courses, with weeks of bowel rest and multiple drainage procedures for

TABLE 4		

TABLE 4
MANAGEMENT OF PANCREATIC INJURIES

	Minor	Severe (Transection)
Early (first 24 hr)	No treatment	Resection
Late (pseudocyst)	Observation, serial US	Drainage

US, ultrasound.

treatment of pseudocysts.[70] The evidence now suggests that early surgical intervention dramatically shortens hospital stays and decreases complications.

In general, complete, or near complete pancreatic transection is managed with spleen-preserving distal pancreatectomy (if physiologically stable in the OR). Recently, several groups, including our own have completed the procedure laparoscopically with excellent results.[71] Regardless of operative approach, however, the goals of the procedure are to perform the following:

- Remove the injured portion of the pancreas
- Close the duct
- Preserve the spleen

Method of duct closure seems to matter little; good results have been reported with stapling, suturing, and Roux-en-Y anastomosis. It should be noted that staplers are not scaled to children, and casual use of the stapler may be technically more challenging (placing the splenic vessels at particular risk) and may lead to a greater pancreatic resection than needed.[70]

Long-term functional results of distal pancreatectomy should be excellent. Pancreatic exocrine insufficiency is rare, and there are no reported cases of diabetes or other endocrine dysfunction (as expected given that the bulk of the Islet cell mass is concentrated in the head).

Duodenum and Small Intestine

Intestinal injuries comprise up to 15% of intra-abdominal injuries in children.[72] While the duodenum is most commonly injured after blunt trauma in children, small bowel injuries such as mesenteric avulsion, enterotomy, and even transections are well described.[73] Overall, intestinal injuries in children are rare, but still carry a high mortality risk (>25%).[74] Although the high energy transfer required to produce these injuries doubtless contributes to this risk, the difficulty in diagnosing these injuries also produces delays in treatment. Too often, small bowel injuries are suspected hours or even days after the original trauma, when peritonitis is clinically apparent. Diagnosis and treatment of duodenal and small bowel injuries differ.

Duodenal injuries present with similar mechanisms to pancreatic injuries (both frequently coexist): a single, epigastric blow from a handlebar, fist, or other blunt trauma producing an obstructing duodenal hematoma much more commonly than perforation. Patients look well initially, but usually develop increased pain and bilious emesis as the hematoma occludes the duodenal lumen. Diagnosis is confirmed by CT (or upper gastrointestinal [UGI]). Rarely do these injuries require surgical intervention. Instead, NG decompression and total parenteral nutrition (TPN) support nearly always allows resolution without late sequelae within 1 to 2 weeks. Occasionally, patients require more time, and the surgeon is advised to wait; patience is rewarded in the management of these injuries, with well over 90% able to be managed nonoperatively.[75] In cases where repair is required (such as perforation, or failure of conservative treatment), primary repair (simple hematoma evacuation, or primary closure) is usually possible. In larger injuries, pyloric exclusion or gastrojejunostomy may occasionally be required.

In contrast, small bowel perforations and transections must be repaired. Any blunt trauma to the abdomen may injure the small bowel, but the classic is the lap-belt injury, often associated with the child "submarining" beneath the belt during a frontal impact, and producing a horizontal stripe of abdominal wall ecchymosis ("seat-belt sign"). Unfortunately, diagnosis is difficult because free air is absent frequently, and even CT has low sensitivity to these injuries. This insensitivity is theoretically worsened by the use of noncontrast scanning; however, even with contrast, rarely is the contrast given time to reach a jejunal or ileal injury, and sensitivity degrades as the contrast travels distally. Still, the diagnosis may be suspected in a patient with a suspicious mechanism, focal, tenderness, and unexplained fluid on the CT scan. Even with this evidence, the diagnosis is rarely definitive, and options available include to wait and watch, to explore, or to perform DPL. Fortunately, definitive diagnosis with neither delay nor undue patient harm can be obtained with exploratory laparoscopy (see subsequent text on minimally invasive methods). Injuries detected can be repaired laparoscopically or pulled to an expanded trocar site incision (usually the umbilicus) for repair extracorporeally. Even without traumatic enterotomy, blunt trauma may spur development of small bowel–small bowel intussusception, manifesting days after the injury.[76]

Penetrating Trauma

Penetrating injuries are responsible for more than 10% of admissions at most major pediatric trauma centers, with firearm injuries accounting for almost 7% of all patients treated in these centers. According to the 2005 annual pediatric report of the National Trauma Data Bank (NTDB), penetrating mechanisms accounted for approximately 8.5% of all injuries (but more than 20% of deaths) in those younger than 19 years.[77] The rate of firearm injuries increases dramatically with age in the pediatric population (from 2/100,000 at age 6 years to 6/100,000 by age 12 years to 103/100,000 by age 18 years).[78] Firearm injuries had the longest average lengths of hospital stay of all injury mechanisms. Of great concern, the lethality of penetrating injuries (gunshot wound [GSW], stab) was threefold greater than that of blunt injury mechanisms (e.g., motor vehicle related, pedestrian injury, falls).[77] The mortality risk is higher in younger children compared to adolescents, due perhaps to the closer relationship of vital structures and the smaller frame in the younger ages.[79,80] As with their adult counterparts, a thorough understanding of the management principles for penetrating injuries is necessary for practitioners involved in the care of the pediatric trauma patient.

Most firearm injuries in children are due to handguns.[81] Shotgun wounds typically account for as many as 20% of firearm-related injuries in children and adolescents. The lethality of long guns, related to projectile dispersion and higher kinetic energy, may be of even greater concern in the small child than in the adult.[80,82] In addition, an estimated 30,000 air rifle injuries occur annually in the United States. Because air rifles can produce muzzle velocities greater than many low-velocity handguns and rifles, even these small projectiles can deliver dangerous and deep injury.[83] Although the injuries sustained by most children with an air rifle injury are minor, all mandate a thorough evaluation and high index of suspicion for visceral injury.

Fatal Penetrating Injuries

Gunshot injuries to the head are by far the most lethal. Pediatric patients with a GSW to the head were more than three times as likely to die (61% vs. 18%) compared to those involving all other body regions.[84] Patients presenting with a GCS <8, unilateral dilated pupil, and transventricular or bihemispheric trajectories were associated with mortality rates of 70% to 98%.[85] In addition, patients with an infratentorial trajectory had improved outcomes compared with those sustaining a transtentorial injury.[86]

Patients with a GSW to the head quite frequently are nonsalvageable. However, those patients with nonintracranial firearm injuries will survive in 75% to 80% of cases. A study of patients with non-intracranial but fatal GSWs demonstrated injuries to the thorax were most common, but approximately 50% had injuries to multiple body regions (see Table 5).[87] The most common injuries identified included lung, major vascular and hemopneumothorax. The frequency of organ injuries in all pediatric patients with GSWs to the thorax or abdomen are provided in Tables 6 and 7.

Although routine use of FAST in the blunt injured child has not been embraced, FAST provides a noninvasive means of establishing priorities in children with multiple torso wounds.[88] FAST also provides a means of evaluating the patient for evidence of pericardial fluid, hemothorax, or hemodynamically significant intraperitoneal fluid in the pediatric patient in extremis.

TABLE 5

ORGANS INJURED IN CHILDREN WITH A FATAL, NONINTRACRANIAL FIREARM INJURY

Organ	Frequency (%)
Lung	56.5
Any major vascular	54.6
Hemopneumothorax	49.2
Heart	44.6
Liver	28.8
Thoracic major vascular	26.6
Bowel	26
Abdominal major vascular	24.9
Diaphragm	22
Kidney	11.3
Spleen	9.6
Esophagus	9.6
Larynx/trachea	5.6
Pancreas	4.5
Spinal cord	4
Tracheobronchial	2.3
Ureter/bladder	2.3

(Adapted from Nance ML, Branas CC, Stafford PW, et al. Nonintracranial fatal firearm injuries in children: Implications for treatment. *J Trauma*. 2003;55(4):631–635.)

The management of organ-specific penetrating injuries in the pediatric population is similar to that in the adult population. The treating surgeon must not underestimate the significance of any blood loss in the small child and the propensity toward hypothermia with an open body cavity.

TABLE 6

FREQUENCY OF INTRATHORACIC ORGANS INJURED IN CHILDREN WITH PENETRATING TRAUMA

Organ	Frequency (%)
Pneumo/hemothorax	64
Pneumothorax	23
Pneumohemothorax	24
Hemothorax	18
Lung	29
Contusion	14
Laceration	10
Diaphragm	15
Heart	13
Major vessel	10
Esophagus	1

(Adapted from Cooper A, Barlow B, DiScala C, et al. Mortality and truncal injury: The pediatric perspective. *J Pediatr Surg*. 1994;29(1): 33–38.)

TABLE 7

FREQUENCY OF INTRA-ABDOMINAL ORGANS INJURED IN CHILDREN WITH PENETRATING TRAUMA

Organ	Frequency (%)
Gastrointestinal tract	70
Stomach	13
Duodenum	4
Jejunum/ileum	24
Colon/rectum	27
Liver	27
Major vessel	19
Kidney	10
Spleen	9
Genitourinary tract	8
Pancreas	6

(Adapted from Cooper A, Barlow B, DiScala C, et al. Mortality and truncal injury: The pediatric perspective. *J Pediatr Surg.* 1994;29(1): 33–38.)

The indications for emergency room thoracotomy (ERT) in the child with a penetrating injury are of some debate. An ERT may be indicated in the child with loss of documented vital signs (in the ER or en route) but is of limited value in the patient with no documented SOL. ERT may be useful in cases of suspected cardiac tamponade from penetrating chest trauma.

Data regarding the use of damage control laparotomy in the pediatric population is limited to anecdotal reports; however, damage control would appear justified in the pediatric patient meeting the traditional adult criteria of severe injury, hypothermia, coagulopathy, acidosis, and early blood transfusion.

Abuse

Treatment of the abused child represents one of the most challenging aspects of pediatric medicine and trauma care. In addition to the complex medical issues, there are frequently daunting social and ethical problems that compound the care. The United States has one of the highest reported rates of child maltreatment in the industrialized world, accounting for as many as 17% of all injury deaths in the pediatric population.[89] In 2004, an estimated 3,503,000 investigations were initiated into suspected child abuse and neglect. Of these, approximately 872,000 cases of abuse or neglect were substantiated, including 1,490 child fatalities.[90] The recognition of death as due to inflicted injury, however, is often underappreciated. The underascertainment of child abuse homicides may be as high as 50% to 61% using traditional International Classification of Diseases-9 (ICD-9) coding strategies, making child abuse deaths likely a much greater problem than is generally recognized.[91,92] In the nonfatally injured child, it has been suggested that child abuse may be responsible for as many as 10% of all visits to the ED.[93] In a review of the National Pediatric Trauma Registry, more than 10% of children younger than 5 years entered into the dataset had inflicted injuries.[94] In large urban pediatric trauma centers, 1.4% of all admissions (all ages) were due to child abuse.[93] Because of the unacceptably high incidence of child physical abuse, health care professionals must be ever observant and questioning. Nonaccidental injuries are commonly seen in trauma centers and children's hospitals, often presenting as head injury, burns, abdominal trauma, or fractures without adequate explanation.

Nonaccidental injuries in children should be suspected based on findings from the history and physical examination. Red flags for abuse are listed in Table 8.

Shaken Impact Syndrome

Abusive head trauma has the highest incidence in children younger than 1 year and is the site most likely to have a fatal outcome. The risk of a child suffering nonaccidental head injury by age 1 year is 1 in 4,065. These brain injuries occur almost exclusively in young infants (median age 2.2 months).[95] The rapid deceleration and acceleration as a mechanism to produce a pattern of intracranial and retinal hemorrhages without external evidence of impact was proposed in the 1970s. The exact pathophysiology of the brain injury in shaken impact syndrome is unclear; however, it is likely a combination of mechanical forces, hemorrhage, hypoxia, and possibly seizures.[96] Accidental subdural hematoma (SDH) is rare in small children. Subdural and subarachnoid hemorrhages are the most common intracranial findings associated with

TABLE 8

HISTORY AND PHYSICAL EXAMINATION FINDINGS CONCERNING FOR CHILD ABUSE

History

1. Delay in seeking medical advice
2. Repeated episodes of trauma treated in different emergency departments
3. Inappropriate response (e.g., hypervigilance, withdrawal) to extent of injury
4. History differs or changes between parents or care providers

Physical examination

1. Multiple subdural hematomas (particularly if of varying age)
2. Retinal hemorrhage
3. Perioral injuries
4. Physical findings out of proportion to reported mechanism of injury (e.g., visceral injury minor trauma)
5. Genital or perianal trauma
6. Evidence of old injuries (bruises, scars)
7. Healing fractures
8. Long bone fractures in nonambulatory patients
9. Patterned marks or burns (cigarette burn, belt mark)
10. Scald burns without associated splash or spill areas

inflicted head injuries. Although subdural hemorrhage with evidence of impact as well as a history of fall or motor vehicle accident (MVA) is not suggestive of abuse, diffuse subdural bleeding (associated with shearing of bridging veins) is certainly suspicious. Retinal hemorrhages are identified in 80% of children with nonaccidental head trauma. The combination of retinal hemorrhages and SDH is highly suggestive of nonaccidental cranial trauma.[97]

Management of these head injuries follows the principles of all TBIs as described earlier. However, complete skeletal survey and/or bone scan should be included to identify other injuries. Nonaccidental head trauma is the predominant cause of SDH and epidural hematoma (EDH). The presentation for an infant with an SDH or EDH can be variable and nonspecific, but must be considered in any child who is unwell.[98] Overall, the spectrum and degree of severity of neurologic abnormalities in survivors of nonaccidental head trauma is extremely variable, with most of these children being moderate or severely abnormal.[99]

MRI is the best modality for demonstrating the presence and extent of diffuse axonal injuries.[100] MRI is also useful to establish timing (acute, subacute, and chronic) of intracranial bleeds to support or contradict the reported mechanism. Furthermore, MRI appears to accurately delineate hypoxic-ischemic injury which is more suggestive of inflicted trauma, likely a result of delay in seeking care.[101]

Fractures

Owing to the compliant nature of the pediatric skeletal system, the forces required to cause a fracture can be quite substantial. Any skeletal injury may be produced by abuse. However, some fractures (especially in infants) should always raise suspicion: mid-shaft long bone fractures, rib fractures (especially ribs fractured in two places or posterior fractures), scapular fractures, spinous process fractures, and sternal fractures. A suspicious history often accompanies these injuries, examples including implausible stories (1-month-old infants "rolling" from a couch) or inconsistent mechanisms like falling from a bed (a mechanism which almost never produces serious injury). Occasionally, multiple fractures of different ages will be explained as being associated with metabolic disorders, especially osteogenesis imperfecta. However, abuse is considerably more common in the population than osteogenesis imperfecta. Although osteogenesis imperfecta and other conditions should be considered, clinicians should not hesitate to report suspected child abuse and institute protective measures until diagnostic workup is complete. When multiple or suspicious fractures are detected, a complete skeletal survey should be performed on any child younger than 2 years.[102] In one report, 24% of skeletal surveys were positive, with a mean of 2.5 fractures per child (range 0 to 9). The age of positive cases ranged from 2 weeks to 36 months with the majority (82%) younger than 12 months of age.[103]

Infants younger than 1 year of age with fractures have a high prevalence of abuse. The risk of abuse as cause for the fracture is greater in those aged younger than 4 months. Infants with nonaccidental fractures have a high risk of further abuse even with intervention.[104] In the infant, it has been demonstrated that 82% of rib fractures are due to child abuse compared with 7.7% from accidental injury, 7.7% from bone fragility, and 2.6% from birth trauma.[105] Rib fractures have a 95% positive predictive value of nonaccidental trauma in children younger than 3 years and are the only skeletal manifestation of inflicted injury in 29% of cases.[106]

Burns

Most burns in children are accidental, with children younger than 5 years particularly susceptible to scald injuries from reaching for containers of hot liquid. However, other burns fall under the "nonaccidental" category whether the result of malice or neglect. Patterns of nonaccidental burns that are highly suspicious usually result from immersion injuries, such as a "stocking feet" injury with or without perineal involvement. Craniofacial immersion injury is infrequent. Instead, bilateral lower extremity burns are the most common, and are typically the result of inflicted tap water immersions. Meanwhile, buttock/perineal immersions are more common with abuse than accident.[107] Generally, a splash pattern is more consistent with accidental injury.

Burning by neglect is far more prevalent than abuse. Parental drug abuse, single parent families, delay in presentation, and a lack of first aid were statistically more prevalent in neglected children than in those with accidental burn injuries. Neglected children were also statistically more likely to have deeper burns and require skin grafting. Most (83%) children whose burns were deemed to be due to neglect had at least one previous contact with local child protection services, and 48.8% required foster care.[108]

Management of burn injuries is detailed elsewhere. The standard body surface area diagrams used to calculate burn percentage are provided in Fig. 4.

Abdominal Trauma

After head injury, nonaccidental trauma to the abdomen is the leading cause of death from abuse, with a fatality rate as high as 50%.[109] Abdominal injuries are the second leading cause of death (behind head injuries) in children with fatal physical abuse.[110] This fact may be due to the often extreme forces (e.g., punch or kick) imparted on the small torso of an abuse victim. Toddlers seem to be particularly vulnerable, suffering punches, kicks or impacts after being thrown against objects. Typically, as with other nonaccidental trauma, there will be an implausible story ("the dog jumped on him") offered by a caretaker. It is reasonable to include CT of the abdomen for any child

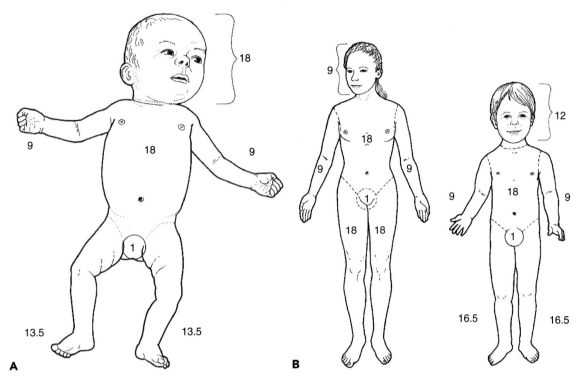

Figure 4   **A:** Body surface area diagram to estimate burn size in newborn. **B:** Body surface area comparison between adult and pediatric patient.

who exhibits other injury patterns consistent with abuse. The liver, duodenum, and small bowel are particularly vulnerable in nonaccidental abdominal trauma. Major abdominal injuries were identified in 0.5% of physically abused children, 45% of whom were fatally injured (Cooper 1988). Abdominal injuries were identified in 11.4% of abused children (vs. 6.8% of general pediatric trauma population) in a review of the National Pediatric Trauma registry that included more than 18,000 children younger than 5 years.[94]

Sexual Abuse

Sexual abuse can affect children of any age, race, gender, or socioeconomic background. The true prevalence is unknown, but is likely dramatically underreported due to the highly stigmatized nature of the event. Of all reported cases of abuse, approximately 10% were sexual abuse. Child sexual abuse includes any sexual activity (vaginal/anal intercourse, oral–genital contact, genital–genital contact, fondling and exposure to pornography or to adults engaging in sexual activity) involving a child who is unable to give consent.[111]

Evaluation of a child with suspected sexual abuse should be done by a well-organized, multidisciplinary team. The assessment should include a thorough history and physical examination as many children will have coexisting physical abuse. Rectal or vaginal perforations from sexual abuse may present as an acute abdomen. Appropriate forensic evidence

should be collected including photodocumentation of physical findings. Cultures should be sent for sexually transmitted diseases that may support or confirm the diagnosis of sexual abuse. Physical findings strongly suggestive of sexual abuse include hymenal laceration (acute or healed), ecchymosis of the hymen, or deep perianal lacerations.

An examination under anesthesia is often beneficial to allow a more thorough assessment of the injuries and minimize psychological trauma. Severe perineal trauma or rectal perforation may require intestinal diversion to heal. Long-term follow-up is necessary to help minimize the risk of adverse psychosocial sequelae.

MINIMALLY INVASIVE METHODS

Laparoscopy and thoracoscopy have been reported for management of pediatric trauma since 1995.[112] As minimally invasive methods (both equipment and expertise) have become more generally available, the use of minimally invasive surgery (MIS) for trauma has grown. There are a number of scenarios and requirements for excellent application of MIS methods in pediatric trauma. As a prerequisite, MIS for trauma is best used in a center with a brisk minimally invasive practice. Ease of access and familiarity with the equipment among both the nursing and physician staff is essential to prevent delay and enhance yield. Considerable experience to handle the nonstandard pathology and faster pace needed for trauma is required.

An excellent use of laparoscopy is for diagnosis of bowel injury.[113] For example, a small child with a seat-belt sign and fluid in the pelvis on CT scan, a tender abdomen, tachycardia, and no solid organ injury is at high risk for a small bowel injury, which is notoriously difficult to diagnose. As mentioned earlier, CT may not be adequately sensitive, and DPL presents a number of problems in the pediatric patient. In contrast, the patient mentioned earlier would benefit from exploratory laparoscopy and inspection of the bowel. Small perforations can be repaired endoscopically, and larger injuries can be mobilized and brought to a slightly enlarged umbilical incision (or other small incision) and repaired extracorporeally.[113] Other organs, even duodenum and pancreas, can be well visualized by experienced surgeons.[114] Conversion to laparotomy should not be delayed should the surgeon need better visualization or access for complex or technically difficult repairs.

Similarly, the thoracic cavity is well visualized thoracoscopically. Typically, low-velocity penetrating injuries, such as stab wounds that produce persistent high bloody output from a chest tube, can be evaluated and treated without resorting to a debilitating thoracotomy. Chest wall bleeders, pulmonary parenchymal tears, and diaphragmatic injuries are all candidates for thoracoscopic repair.

Naturally, a child for whom laparoscopy is being contemplated should meet some selection criteria. MIS is contraindicated for the following:

- Massive hemoperitoneum
- Any unstable patient
- Any patient unable to tolerate abdominal insufflation (or single lung ventilation for thoracoscopy)

REFERENCES

1. National Center for Injury Prevention and Control. Available at: http://www.cdc.gov/ncipc/wisqars/; Accessed May 4, 2007.
2. Green SM, Rothrock SG. Is pediatric trauma really a surgical disease? *Ann Emerg Med.* 2002;39(5):537–540.
3. Nance ML, Stafford PW. Pediatric trauma is a surgical disease. *Ann Emerg Med.* 2003;41(3):423–424; author reply 424–5.
4. MacKenzie EJ, Rivara FP, Jurkovich GJ, et al. A national evaluation of the effect of trauma-center care on mortality. *N Engl J Med.* 2006;354(4):366–378.
5. Segui-Gomez M, Chang DC, Paidas CN, et al. Pediatric trauma care: An overview of pediatric trauma systems and their practices in 18 US states. *J Pediatr Surg.* 2003;38(8):1162–1169.
6. Densmore JC, Limb HJ, Oldham KT, et al. Outcomes and delivery of care in pediatric injury. *J Pediatr Surg.* 2006;41:92–98.
7. Potoka DA, Schall LC, Gardner MJ, et al. Impact of pediatric trauma centers on mortality in a statewide system. *J Trauma.* 2000;49(2):237–245.
8. Mooney DP, Forbes PW. Variation in the management of pediatric splenic injuries in New England. *J Trauma.* 2004;56(2):328–333.
9. Middleton KR, Burt CW. Availability of pediatric services and equipment in emergency departments: United States, 2002–03. *Adv Data.* 2006;28(367):1–16.
10. Paul TR, Marias M, Pons PT, et al. Adult versus pediatric prehospital trauma care: Is there a difference? *J Trauma.* 1999;47(3):455–459.
11. Eckstein M, Jantos T, Kelly N, et al. Helicopter transport of pediatric trauma patients in an urban emergency medical services system: A critical analysis. *J Trauma.* 2002;53(2):340–344.
12. Bernard SA. Paramedic intubation of patients with severe head injury: A review of current Australian practice and recommendations for change. *Emerg Med Australas.* 2006;18(3):221–228.
13. DiRusso SM, Sullivan T, Risucci D, et al. Intubation of pediatric trauma patients in the field: Predictor of negative outcome despite risk stratification. *J Trauma.* 2005;59:84–91.
14. Blinman T, Maggard M. Rational manipulation of oxygen delivery. *J Surg Res.* 2000;92(1):120–141.
15. Kraus JF, Fife D, Conroy C. Pediatric brain injuries: The nature, clinical course, and early outcomes in a defined United States' population. *Pediatrics.* 1987;79(4):501–507.
16. Young KD, Okada PJ, Sokolove PE, et al. A randomized, double-blinded, placebo-controlled trial of phenytoin for the prevention of early posttraumatic seizures in children with moderate to severe blunt head injury. *Ann Emerg Med.* 2004;43(4):435–446.
17. Cordell WH, Hollingsworth JC, Olinger ML, et al. Pain and tissue-interface pressures during spine-board immobilization. *Ann Emerg Med.* 1995;26(1):31–36.
18. Capraro AJ, Mooney D, Waltzman ML. The use of routine laboratory studies as screening tools in pediatric abdominal trauma. *Pediatr Emerg Care.* 2006;22(7):480–484.
19. Kincaid EH, Chang MC, Letton RW, et al. Admission base deficit in pediatric trauma: A study using the National Trauma Data Bank. *J Trauma.* 2001;51(2):332–335.
20. Suthers SE, Albrecht R, Foley D, et al. Surgeon-directed ultrasound for trauma is a predictor of intra-abdominal injury in children. *Am Surg.* 2004;70(2):164–167; discussion 167–8.
21. Hall EJ. Lessons we have learned from our children: Cancer risks from diagnostic radiology. *Pediatr Radiol.* 2002;32(10):700–706.
22. Kim PK, Zhu X, Houseknecht E, et al. Total effective radiation dose from diagnostic radiology in pediatric trauma patients. *World J Surg.* 2005;29(12):1557–1662.
23. Inaba K, Potzman J, Munera F, et al. Multi-slice CT angiography for arterial evaluation in the injured lower extremity. *J Trauma.* 2006;60(3):502–506; discussion 506–7.
24. Beaver BL, Colombani PM, Buck JR, et al. Efficacy of emergency room thoracotomy in pediatric trauma. *J Pediatr Surg.* 1987;22(1):19–23.
25. Boyd M, Vanek VW, Bourguet CC. Emergency room resuscitative thoracotomy: When is it indicated? *J Trauma.* 1992;33(5):714–721.
26. Li G, Tang N, DiScala C, et al. Cardiopulmonary resuscitation in pediatric trauma patients: Survival and functional outcome. *J Trauma.* 1999;47(1):1–7.
27. Adelson PD, Bratton SL, Carney NA, et al. American Association for Surgery of Trauma; Child Neurology Society; International Society for Pediatric Neurosurgery; International Trauma Anesthesia and Critical Care Society; Society of Critical Care Medicine; World Federation of Pediatric Intensive and Critical Care Societies. Guidelines for the acute medical management of severe traumatic brain injury in infants, children, and adolescents. Chapter 6. Threshold for treatment of intracranial hypertension. *Pediatr Crit Care Med.* 2003;4(Suppl 3):S25–S27.
28. Taylor A, Butt W, Rosenfeld J, et al. A randomized trial of very early decompressive craniectomy in children with traumatic brain injury and sustained intracranial hypertension. *Childs Nerv Syst.* 2001;17(3):154–162.
29. Josan VA, Sgouros S. Early decompressive craniectomy may be effective in the treatment of refractory intracranial hypertension after traumatic brain injury. *Childs Nerv Syst.* 2006;22(10):1268–1274.
30. Holmes JF, Sokolove PE, Brant WE, et al. A clinical decision rule for identifying children with thoracic injuries after blunt torso trauma. *Ann Emerg Med.* 2002;39(5):492–499.
31. Kwon A, Sorrells DL Jr, Kurkchubasche AG, et al. Isolated computed tomography diagnosis of pulmonary contusion

does not correlate with increased morbidity. *J Pediatr Surg.* 2006;41(1):78–82; discussion 78–82.

32. Fortenberry JD, Meier AH, Pettignano R, et al. Extracorporeal life support for posttraumatic acute respiratory distress syndrome at a children's medical center. *J Pediatr Surg.* 2003;38(8):1221–1226.

33. Johannigman JA, Campbell RS, Davis K Jr, et al. Combined differential lung ventilation and inhaled nitric oxide therapy in the management of unilateral pulmonary contusion. *J Trauma.* 1997;42(1):108–111.

34. Haxhija E, Nores H, Scober P, et al. Lung contusion-lacerations after blunt thoracic trauma in children. *Pediatr Surg Int.* 2004;20(6):412–414.

35. Tiao GM, Griffith PM, Szmuszkovicz JR, et al. Cardiac and great vessel injuries in children after blunt trauma: An institutional review. *J Pediatr Surg.* 2000;35(11):1656–1660.

36. Balci AE, Kazez A, Eren S, et al. Blunt thoracic trauma in children: Review of 137 cases. *Eur J Cardiothorac Surg.* 2004;26(2):387–392.

37. Sartorelli KH, McBride WJ, Vane DW, et al. Perforation of the intrathoracic esophagus from blunt trauma in a child: Case report and review of the literature. *J Pediatr Surg.* 1999;34(3):495–497.

38. Beal SL, Pottmeyer EW, Spisso JM. Esophageal perforation following external blunt trauma. *J Trauma.* 1988;28(10):1425–1432.

39. Simpson J, Lobo DN, Shah AB, et al. Traumatic diaphragmatic rupture: Associated injuries and outcome. *Ann R Coll Surg Engl.* 2000;82(2):97–100.

40. Soundappan SV, Holland AJ, Cass DT, et al. Blunt traumatic diaphragmatic injuries in children. *Injury.* 2005;36(1):51–54.

41. Karnak I, Senocak ME, Tanyel FC, et al. Diaphragmatic injuries in childhood. *Surg Today.* 2001;31(1):5–11.

42. Koplewitz BZ, Ramos C, Manson DE, et al. Traumatic diaphragmatic injuries in infants and children: Imaging findings. *Pediatr Radiol.* 2000;30(7):471–479.

43. Shehata SM, Shabaan BS. Diaphragmatic injuries in children after blunt abdominal trauma. *J Pediatr Surg.* 2006;41(10):1727–1731.

44. Upadhyaya P, Simpson JS. Splenic trauma in children. *Surg Gynecol Obstet.* 1968;126(4):781–790.

45. Ein SH, Shandling B, Simpson JS, et al. Nonoperative management of traumatized spleen in children: How and why. *J Pediatr Surg.* 1978;13(2):117–119.

46. Nance ML, Holmes JH, Wiebe DJ. Timeline to operative intervention for solid organ injuries in children. *J Trauma.* 2006;61(6):1389–1392.

47. Keller MS, Coln CE. The utility of routine trauma laboratories in pediatric trauma resuscitations. *Am J Surg.* 2004;188(6):671–678.

48. Stylianos S. Evidence-based guidelines for resource utilization in children with isolated spleen or liver injury. The APSA Trauma Committee. *J Pediatr Surg.* 2000;35(2):164–167.

49. Stylianos S. Compliance with evidence-based guidelines in children with isolated spleen or liver injury: A prospective study. *J Pediatr Surg.* 2002;37(3):453–456.

50. Hamill J. Damage control surgery in children. *Injury.* 2004;35(7):708–712.

51. Gorenstein A, Witzling M, Haflell T, et al. Pleuro-pulmonary involvement in children with blunt splenic trauma. *J Paediatr Child Health.* 2003;39(4):282–285.

52. Kilic N, Gurpinar A, Kiristioglu I, et al. Ruptured spleen due to blunt trauma in children: Analysis of blood transfusion requirements. *Eur J Emerg Med.* 1999;6(2):135–139.

53. Lutz N, Mahboubi S, Nance ML, et al. The significance of contrast blush on computed tomography in children with splenic injuries. *J Pediatr Surg.* 2004;39(3):491–494.

54. Holdsworth RJ, Irvin AD, Cushierr A. Postsplenectomy sepsis and its mortality rate: Actual versus perceived risk. *Br J Surg.* 1991;78:1031–1038.

55. Brigden ML, Patullo AL. Prevention and management of overwhelming postsplenectomy infection – an update. *Crit Care Med.* 1999;27(4):836–842.

56. Wan J, Corvino TF, Greenfield SP, et al. Kidney and testicle injuries in team and individual sports: Data from the national pediatric trauma registry. *J Urol.* 2003;170(4 Pt 2):1528–1533; discussion 1531–2.

57. Kuan JK, Wright JL, Nathens AB, et al. American Association for the Surgery of Trauma Organ Injury Scale for kidney injuries predicts nephrectomy, dialysis, and death in patients with blunt injury and nephrectomy for penetrating injuries. *J Trauma.* 2006;60(2):351–356.

58. Wessel LM, Scholz S, Jester I, et al. Management of kidney injuries in children with blunt abdominal trauma. *J Pediatr Surg.* 2000;35(9):1326–1330.

59. Nance ML, Lutz N, Carr MC, et al. Blunt renal injuries in children can be managed nonoperatively: Outcome in a consecutive series of patients. *J Trauma.* 2004;57(3):474–478.

60. Philpott JM, Nance ML, Carr MC, et al. Ureteral stenting in the management of urinoma following severe blunt renal trauma in children. *J Pediatr Surg.* 2003;38(7):1096–1098.

61. Legg EA, Herbert FB, Goodacre B, et al. Super-selective arterial embolization for blunt trauma in the horseshoe kidney. *Urology.* 1998;51(2):320–321.

62. Shindel AW, Rollins M, Dillon PA, et al. Bladder injury from a shard of glass. *J Trauma.* 2006;61(6):1557.

63. Kim S, Linden B, Cendron M, et al. Pediatric anorectal impalement with bladder rupture: Case report and review of the literature. *J Pediatr Surg.* 2006;41(9):E1–E3.

64. Black PC, Miller EA, Porter JR, et al. Urethral and bladder neck injury associated with pelvic fracture in 25 female patients. *J Urol.* 2006;175(6):2140–2144.

65. Fraser GC. "Handlebar" injury of the pancreas. Report of a case complicated by pseudocyst formation with spontaneous internal rupture. *J Pediatr Surg.* 1969;4(2):216–219.

66. Arkovitz MS, Johnson N, Garcia VF. Pancreatic trauma in children: Mechanisms of injury. *J Trauma.* 1997;42(1):49–53.

67. Sivit CJ, Eichelberger MR, Taylor GA, et al. Blunt pancreatic trauma in children: CT diagnosis. *AJR Am J Roentgenol.* 1992;158(5):1097–1100.

68. Olah A, Issekutz A, Haulik L, et al. Pancreatic transection from blunt abdominal trauma: Early versus delayed diagnosis and surgical management. *Dig Surg.* 2003;20(5):408–414.

69. Holland AJ, Davey RB, Sparnon AL, et al. Traumatic pancreatitis: Long-term review of initial non-operative management in children. *J Paediatr Child Health.* 1999;35(1):78–81.

70. Stringer MD. Pancreatic trauma in children. *Br J Surg.* 2005;92(4):467–470.

71. Reynolds EM, Curnow AJ. Laparoscopic distal pancreatectomy for traumatic pancreatic transection. *J Pediatr Surg.* 2003;38(10):E7–E9.

72. Bruny JL, Bensard DD. Hollow viscous injury in the pediatric patient. *Semin Pediatr Surg.* 2004;13(2):112–118.

73. Sandiford NA, Sutcliffe RP, Khawaja HT. Jejunal transection after blunt abdominal trauma: A report of two cases. *Emerg Med J.* 2006;23(10):e55.

74. Ameh EA, Nmadu PT. Gastrointestinal injuries from blunt abdominal trauma in children. *East Afr Med J.* 2004;81(4):194–197.

75. Clendenon JN, Meyers RL, Nance ML, et al. Management of duodenal injuries in children. *J Pediatr Surg.* 2004;39(6):964–968.

76. Erichsen D, Sellstrom H, Andersson H. Small bowel intussusception after blunt abdominal trauma in a 6-year-old boy: Case report and review of 6 cases reported in the literature. *J Pediatr Surg.* 2006;41(11):1930–1932.

77. National Trauma Data Bank. *National Trauma Data Bank report 2005.* Accessed through URL http://www.facs.org/trauma/ntdb .html, 2005.

78. Agran PF, Winn D, Anderson C, et al. Rates of pediatric and adolescent injuries by year of age. *Pediatrics.* 2001;108:E45.

79. Holland AJ, Kirby R, Browne GT, et al. Penetrating injuries in children: Is there a message? *J Paediatr Child Health.* 2002;38:487–491.

80. Beaver BL, Moore VL, Peclet M, et al. Characteristics of pediatric firearm fatalities. *J Pediatr Surg.* 1990;25:97–100.

81. Nance ML, Denysenko L, Durbin DR, et al. The rural-urban continuum: Variability in statewide serious firearm

injuries in children and adolescents. *Arch Pediatr Adolesc Med.* 2002;156(8):781–785.

82. Nance ML, Sing RF, Branas CC, et al. Shotgun wounds in children: Not just accidents. *Arch Surg.* 1997;132(1):58–62.

83. McNeill AN, Annest JL. The ongoing hazard of BB and pellet gun related injures in the United States. *Ann Emerg Med.* 1995;26:187–194.

84. Beaman V, Annest JL, Mercy JA, et al. Lethality of firearm related injuries in the United States population. *Ann Emerg Med.* 2003;35(3):258–266.

85. Martin RS, Siqueria MG, Santos MT, et al. Prognostic factors and treatment of gunshot wounds to the head. *Surg Neurol.* 2003;60:98–104.

86. Nathoo N, Chite SH, Edwards PJ, et al. Civilian infra-tentorial gunshot injuries: Outcome analysis of 26 patients. *Surg Neurol.* 2002;58:225–233.

87. Nance ML, Branas CC, Stafford PW, et al. Nonintracranial fatal firearm injuries in children: Implications for treatment. *J Trauma.* 2003;55(4):631–635.

88. Asensio JA, Arroyo H, Veloz W Jr. Penetrating thoraco-abdominal injuries: Ongoing dilemma—which cavity and when? *World J Surg.* 2002;26:539–543.

89. UNICEF. *A league table of child maltreatment deaths in rich nations. Innocenti Report Card.* Florence: Innocenti Research Centre; 2003.

90. Administration for Child and Families. Available at: http://www.acf.hhs.gov/programs/cb/stats_research/index.htm#can. Accessed March 19, 2007.

91. Crume TL, DiGuiseppi C, Byers T, et al. Underascertainment of child maltreatment fatalities by death certificates, 1990–1998. *Pediatrics.* 2002;110:18.

92. Herman-Giddens ME, Brown G, Verbiest S, et al. Underascertainment of child abuse mortality in the United States. *JAMA.* 1999;281:463.

93. Chang DC, Knight V, Ziegfeld S, et al. The tip of the iceberg for child abuse: The critical roles of the pediatric trauma service and its registry. *J Trauma.* 2004;57:1189.

94. DiScala C, Sege R, Li G, et al. Child abuse and unintentional injuries: A 10-year retrospective. *Arch Pediatr Adolesc Med.* 2000;154:16.

95. Barlow KM, Minns RA. Annual incidence of shaken impact syndrome in young children. *Lancet.* 2000;356(9241):1571–1572.

96. Duhaime AC, Gennarelli TA, Thibault LE, et al. The shaken baby syndrome. A clinical, pathological, and biomechanical study. *J Neurosurg.* 1987;66(3):409–415.

97. Demaerel P, Casteels I, Wilms G. Cranial imaging in child abuse. *Eur Radiol.* 2002;12(4):849–857.

98. Hobbs C, Childs AM, Wynne J, et al. Subdural haematoma and effusion in infancy: An epidemiological study. *Arch Dis Child.* 2005;90(9):952–955.

99. Barlow K, Thompson E, Johnson D, et al. The neurological outcome of non-accidental head injury. *Pediatr Rehabil.* 2004;7(3):195–203.

100. Parizel PM, Van Goethem JW, Ozsarlak O, et al. New developments in the neuroradiological diagnosis of craniocerebral trauma. *Eur Radiol.* 2005;15(3):569–581.

101. Ichord R, Naim M, Pollock A, et al. Hypoxic-ischemic injury complicates traumatic brain injury in young children: The role of diffusion weighted imaging. *J Neurotrauma.* 2007;24(1):106–118.

102. Jenny C. Evaluating infants and young children with multiple fractures. *Pediatrics.* 2006;118(3):1299–1303.

103. Day F, Clegg S, McPhillips M, et al. A retrospective case series of skeletal surveys in children with suspected non-accidental injury. *J Clin Forensic Med.* 2006;13(2):55–59.

104. Skellern CY, Wood DO, Murphy A, et al. Non-accidental fractures in infants: Risk of further abuse. *J Paediatr Child Health.* 2000;36(6):590–592.

105. Bulloch B, Schubert JC, Brophy PD, et al. Cause and clinical characteristics of rib fractures in infants. *Pediatrics.* 2000;105:48.

106. Barsness KA, Cha E, Bensard DD, et al. The positive predictive value of rib fractures as an indicator of nonaccidental trauma in children. *J Trauma.* 2003;54:1107.

107. Daria S, Sugar NF, Feldman KW, et al. Into hot water head first: Distribution of intentional and unintentional immersion burns. *Pediatr Emerg Care.* 2004;20(5):302–310.

108. Chester DL, Jose RM, Aldlyami E, et al. Non-accidental burns in children – are we neglecting neglect? *Burns.* 2006;32(2):222–228.

109. Trokel M, DiScala C, Terrin NC, et al. Blunt abdominal injury in the young pediatric patient: Child abuse and patient outcomes. *Child Maltreat.* 2004;9:111.

110. O'Neill JA Jr, Meacham WF, Griffin JP, et al. Patterns of injury in the battered child syndrome. *J Trauma.* 1973;13:332.

111. Sapp MV, Vandeven AM. Update on childhood sexual abuse. *Curr Opin Pediatr.* 2005;17(2):258–264.

112. Chen MK, Schropp KP, Lobe TE. The use of minimal access surgery in pediatric trauma: A preliminary report. *J Laparoendosc Surg.* 1995;5(5):295–301.

113. Streck CJ, Lobe TE, Pietsch JB, et al. Laparoscopic repair of traumatic bowel injury in children. *J Pediatr Surg.* 2006;41(11):1864–1869.

114. Lebedyev A, Zmora O, et al. Laparoscopic distal pancreatectomy. *Surg Endosc.* 2004;18(10):1427–1430.

FURTHER READING

Cooper A, Floyd T, Barlow B, et al. Major blunt abdominal trauma due to child abuse. *J Trauma.* 1988;28:1483.

Trauma in Pregnancy

54

Mark R. Hemmila

Trauma is the leading cause of death for both pregnant and nonpregnant woman in their childbearing years.[1] Approximately 5% of all pregnancies are complicated by trauma.[2-4] Of woman aged between 12 and 51 who are listed in the National Trauma Databank, 1.5% were injured while pregnant. The rate of mortality for the pregnant mother is 1.4% and the rate of fetal demise in pregnant woman following traumatic injury is 6.1%.[4] The preponderance of trauma during pregnancy is due to a blunt mechanism of injury with penetrating trauma being relatively infrequent. Motor vehicle accidents account for more than 50% of all traumas during pregnancy and most fetal deaths (82%) from trauma are due to motor vehicle accidents.[5,6] The pregnant female is at risk for trauma from the following etiologies in descending order: motor vehicle accidents, domestic abuse and assault, falls, and burns.[5] Domestic assault is an important and often overlooked cause of trauma in pregnant patients.

Central to the management of traumatic injury of the pregnant patient is the fact that two separate, but linked patients are involved. A key principle is to treat the mother first because most medical measures which aid in the resuscitation of the mother will be helpful to the fetus. Assessment and patient management can be complicated by the anatomic and physiologic changes of pregnancy. These changes can mimic or camouflage injury and result in a patient who can be difficult to characterize. A multidisciplinary approach to the patient that includes specialists from trauma surgery, emergency medicine, obstetrics, nursing, and prehospital providers is strongly recommended. Ultimately, trauma management of the pregnant patient revolves around minimizing fetal loss and optimizing both the maternal and fetal outcome.

PHYSIOLOGY

Many changes occur to the anatomy and physiology of a pregnant woman throughout the gestational period. These changes influence the pattern of injury, assessment, and management of the pregnant trauma patient. A summary of these changes is provided in Table 1.

Reproductive Organs

The most obvious physical change during pregnancy is the gradual enlargement of the uterus (see Fig. 1). At 12 weeks' gestation, the uterus transitions from being a pelvic organ to becoming an intraabdominal organ by rising over the pelvic brim.[7] Around 20 weeks' gestation, the vertex of the gravid uterus can be palpated at the level of the umbilicus. At 36 weeks of gestation, the uterus has reached the costal margins and in the last few weeks of pregnancy the fundal height decreases as the fetal head drops back into the pelvis. Concomitant with uterine enlargement is the displacement of maternal abdominal organs laterally and cephalad. In the late stages of pregnancy, most of the gastrointestinal tract is located above the inferior costal margin. The diaphragm may be elevated with corresponding compression of the lungs and mediastinum. Uterine blood flow increases from 50 mL per minute at 10 weeks' gestation to 500 mL per minute in the term female, which is equivalent to 17% of the cardiac output.[8] Compensatory dilation of the uterine and pelvic veins will occur to handle this increased blood flow. This increase in vascularity can result in massive hemorrhage with pelvic injury.

Cardiovascular

By the end of the first trimester, the plasma volume increases by 40% to 50% and a smaller increase in red cell volume is also present (20% to 30%).[9] The result is the physiologic anemia of pregnancy and in late pregnancy a hematocrit of 31% to 34% is normal.[7] This hypervolemia is meant to compensate for the 1 to 1.5 L hemorrhage that occurs at childbirth. The pregnant patient also experiences a decrease in peripheral vascular resistance resulting in

TABLE 1

PHYSIOLOGIC CHANGES DURING PREGNANCY

Organ System	Normal	Pregnant
Reproductive organs		
Uterine location	Pelvis	Abdomen
Uterine blood flow (mL/min)	50	500–700
Cardiovascular		
Cardiac output (L/min)	5–6	↑ 30 %–40%
Heart rate (beats/min)	70–80	↑ 15–20 beats/min
Blood pressure (mm Hg)	110/70	↓ 10–15 mm Hg second trimester, normal at term
Respiratory		
Tidal volume (mL)	450	↑ 30%–50%
Respiratory rate (breaths/min)	12–16	↑ 15%
Functional residual capacity (mL)	1,800	↓ 25%
Oxygen consumption (mL/min)	250	↑ 20%
pH	7.34–7.44	7.41–7.46
PaO_2 (mm Hg)	95–100	↑ 105
$PaCO_2$ (mm Hg)	35–45	↓ 27–32
HCO_3 (mmol/L)	24–30	↓ 19–24
Diaphragm	Normal	Elevated up to 4 cm
Gastrointestinal		
Lower esophageal sphincter	Normal	Relaxed, predisposes to GERD and aspiration
Hepatobiliary	Normal	↑ Progesterone results in ↓ cholecystokinin, cholestasis and ↑ gallstone formation
Hematologic		
Blood volume (mL)	4,000	↑ 30%–50%
Plasma volume (mL)	2,400	↑ 3,700
White blood cell count (WBC/mm³)	4.5–10	↑ 5–12, can rise up to 20
Hematocrit (%)	36–46	↓ 31–34
Coagulation factors	Normal	↑ Factors I, VII, VIII, IX, X, ↓ Protein S
Musculoskeletal		
Ligaments	Normal	Soften

GERD, gastroesophageal reflux disease; WBC, white blood cells; ↑, increase; ↓, decrease.

supine hypotension, a decrease in blood pressure of 15% to 20%, and an increase in cardiac output by up to 40%. These changes nadir at 28 weeks' gestation and can mask signs of acute blood loss.[10-12] Gravid patients can experience traumatic hemorrhage of up to 2,000 mL without demonstrating clinical deterioration through the typical signs and symptoms of shock.

The amount of replacement fluid needed in a pregnant patient changes as the plasma volume increases. A third trimester patient can require 1.5 times the amount of intravenous fluid resuscitation to compensate for the same level of hemodynamic compromise in a nonpregnant patient.[13] The gravid uterus can lead to supine hypotension by direct compression of the inferior vena cava that diminishes venous return. This can be minimized by using a foam wedge or rolled blanket to displace the backboarded patient to a moderate left-lateral decubitus position during transport and resuscitation. This maneuver should be employed to improve blood flow in patients >20 weeks' gestation.

Respiratory

Progressive uterine enlargement results in elevation of the diaphragm as abdominal organs are displaced. A rise in the resting level of the diaphragm by as much as 4 cm occurs.[14] This results in a decreased residual volume, an increase in the diaphragmatic excursion, and results in larger tidal volumes. At 12 weeks of gestation, the functional reserve capacity decreases by 10% to 25%.[13] Consequently, apnea is poorly tolerated and supplemental oxygen should always be given to pregnant trauma patients. Mild hyperventilation leads to respiratory alkalosis and a shift in the oxyhemoglobin dissociation curve to the left, increasing the maternal affinity for hemoglobin to be bound to oxygen. A increase in the pH level leads to a

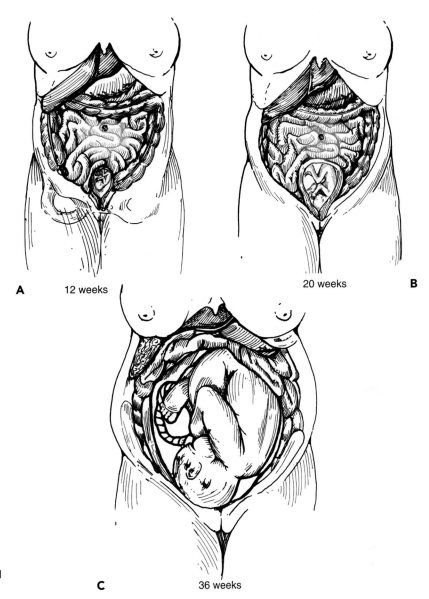

A 12 weeks

20 weeks B

C 36 weeks

Figure 1 **A–C:** Enlargement of the uterus and fundal height during pregnancy.

simultaneous rise in the level of 2,3 diphosphoglycerate, which shifts the oxyhemoglobin dissociation curve back to the right and facilitates the unloading of oxygen from maternal hemoglobin to fetal hemoglobin across the placenta.[15,16]

Gastrointestinal

Progressive enlargement of the uterus stretches out the abdominal wall and displaces the abdominal viscera. The response to peritoneal irritation is altered and the change in organ location can make the physical examination confusing and potentially unreliable. Compression of the gastrointestinal viscera cephalad, diminished motility, and hormone-mediated relaxation of the lower esophageal sphincter can predispose the gravid patient to

gastroesophageal reflux disease and increase the risk of aspiration.[17] A high level of the female hormone progesterone inhibits cholecystokinin production resulting in decreased gallbladder contractility. This leads to cholestasis and an increase in the susceptibility to gallstone development.[18]

Hematologic

Pregnancy increases the cellular synthesis of many procoagulant factors; however, most pregnant women have normal anticoagulant factor levels except for a decrease in protein S.[19] In total, pregnancy is a hypercoagulable state but bleeding time and clotting time are unchanged when measured. The risk of deep venous thrombosis and venous thromboembolism is markedly increased in pregnancy.[20] Platelets are more reactive and their destruction is enhanced. Most pregnant patients have an increased production of platelets within the bone marrow. The relative leukocytosis of pregnancy is well known and accounts for a slight rise in the overall white blood cell count. Blood volume increases and total red blood cell mass may be 30% higher in the pregnant patient despite a drop in the measured circulating hemoglobin per unit volume.

Musculoskeletal

Interosseus ligaments soften and relax during pregnancy. This results in increased mobility and laxity of joints such as the sacroiliac, and symphysis pubis in preparation for expansion of the birth canal. These changes in addition to uterine enlargement affect the pregnant female center of gravity and gait such that they are predisposed to falls.

PREGNANT PATIENT ASSESSMENT AND MANAGEMENT

Prehospital

The initial care of the patient is usually by prehospital personnel at the scene and in transport. To begin resuscitation and treatment of the patient, it is essential that prehospital providers be aware of the physiologic changes present in the pregnant patient. Provision of the Airway, Breathing, and Circulation (ABCs) of trauma care is paramount to both the mother and fetus. Awareness of airway management problems such as tissue edema in the oropharynx is essential. The relative hypervolemia of pregnancy may mask the signs and symptoms of blood loss and shock until an acute rapid decompensation occurs. Intravenous solutions should be administered in a liberal manner during transport to avoid sudden deterioration in a compensated, but injured patient. These patients should be transported with spine precautions on a backboard tilted to the left to avoid uterine compression of the vena cava.[21] In addition to the standard patient history, appropriate information regarding prenatal care, gestational age, and pregnancy complications should be obtained and relayed to the accepting trauma center when feasible.

Primary Survey

The conduct of the primary survey in the pregnant patient is the same as for the nonpregnant patient. The goal is to identify, triage, and treat life-threatening injuries by addressing ABC with the mother given treatment priority. Assessment and establishment of the maternal airway is critical and all pregnant patients should receive supplemental oxygen at a minimum. Late in gestation the oropharynx is swollen from tissue edema and endotracheal intubation of the gravid patient can be difficult; therefore, use of a

smaller than normal diameter endotracheal tube, such as a 6.5 mm ID or less, may be necessary.[22] Injury can stimulate a stress response release of catecholamines. Maternal catecholamine surges can lead to uterine–placental vasoconstriction that can compromise the delivery of oxygen to the fetal circulation.[23] Small differences in the maternal Pao_2 can markedly change the oxygen saturation of the fetal blood because of a leftward shift in the fetal oxyhemoglobin dissociation curve when compared to the maternal curve.[24] Aggressive crystalloid intravenous fluid resuscitation is recommended in the pregnant patient, even if evidence of hemodynamic compromise is not immediately apparent. Late in pregnancy, supine hypotension is present due to vena cava compression. This should be alleviated by placing the patient in a mild left lateral decubitus position using a wedge or rolled blankets placed under the transport backboard.

Secondary Survey

After the ABCs of the primary survey have been addressed, the secondary survey is performed. A brief, focused history should be obtained if the patient is not obtunded. Areas of importance include circumstances of the traumatic event, loss of consciousness, medical and obstetric history, time of last meal, medications, allergies, and a review of systems. A head-to-toe physical examination is carried out including a pelvic examination. Radiologic studies appropriate to the trauma evaluation should be ordered and usually include a chest and pelvic x-ray for the blunt trauma patient. A Foley catheter should be placed to monitor urine output and consideration should be given to placing a nasogastric tube given the pregnant patient's likelihood of vomiting and risk for aspiration. Fetal monitoring is initiated during the secondary survey.

Obstetric history includes date of last menstrual period, expected delivery date, status of the current pregnancy, history of fetal movement, history of pregnancy-related medical problems such as gestational diabetes, preeclampsia, congenital disorders, preterm labor, placental abruption, placental previa, and prior fetal outcomes. Gestational age can be estimated using fundal height measured by palpation on the physical examination. Fundal height at the umbilicus is consistent with 20 weeks fetal gestation.[24] Fetal viability is considered feasible approximately 24 to 26 weeks gestation, but can vary depending on the experience of the local neonatology support.[25] A pelvic and rectal examination should be performed by an experienced team member, and attention must be focused on evidence of vaginal discharge (blood or amniotic fluid), cervical effacement and dilation, fetal station, and umbilical cord prolapse. Obstetrical presence as part of the trauma team effort in the evaluation of the gravid patient is highly recommended.

Five conditions are associated with signaling an acute status of the pregnancy. These include vaginal bleeding, rupture of amniotic sac, presence of contractions, bulging perineum, and abnormal fetal heart rate and rhythm.[24] Vaginal bleeding before the onset of full-term labor is abnormal. It is potentially indicative of preterm labor, placental abruption, or placenta previa. Rupture of the amniotic sac can allow prolapse of the umbilical cord resulting in compression of the cord and potential compromise of the fetal circulation. Suspected amniotic fluid can be tested using Nitrazine paper, which will turn deep blue if the test is positive. Rupture of the amniotic sac is an obstetrical emergency because of the risk of infection and umbilical cord prolapse. Bulging of the perineum represents pressure from a presenting part of the fetus and delivery or spontaneous abortion may be in progress. The presence of strong contractions ascertained on the physical examination is associated with true labor and preparations should be made for delivery and resuscitation of the neonate.

Traumatic injury to the placenta can result in transplacental or fetomaternal hemorrhage. A small amount of fetal blood (0.01 mL) is capable of sensitizing an Rh-negative maternal trauma patient. The Kleihauer-Betke (KB) test is used to detect the presence of fetal cells in the maternal circulation. Because of its high sensitivity, the KB test by itself does not necessarily indicate pathologic fetal–maternal hemorrhage.[26] The KB test is recommended for injured Rh-negative patients in the second or third trimester to detect impending fetal exsanguination and determine risk of Rh isosensitization in these patients. If the initial test is positive, the KB test should be repeated in 24 hours to identify ongoing fetomaternal hemorrhage. Treatment of positive fetomaternal Rh exposure consists of an initial intravenous dose of 300 μg of Rh-immune globulin, with an additional dose of 300 μg for every 30 mL of fetomaternal transfusion as estimated by the KB test. Recent evidence suggests that the KB test accurately predicts the risk of preterm labor, and in a patient with a negative KB test fetal monitoring duration can be limited safely.[27] When used as a predictor of preterm labor, the KB test has benefit to all maternal trauma patients, regardless of Rh status. Therefore, a KB test should be performed on all pregnant patients >12 weeks of gestation.[28]

Fetal Assessment

Direct assessment of the fetus is limited following traumatic injury. Initial fetal evaluation is undertaken as part of the secondary survey and consists of uterine assessment, fundal height, recording of fetal heart tones with regard to rate and rhythm, and evaluation of fetal movement. Fetal heart rate monitoring is best accomplished with an external cardiotocographic device that records both fetal heart tones and uterine contractions. The normal fetal heart rate is between 120 and 160 beats per minute. Bradycardia (fetal heart rate <100 beats/minute) is associated with severe hypoxia and should be recognized as potential fetal

distress.[29] Late decelerations of fetal heart rate after uterine contractions can be related to uteroplacental insufficiency and may warrant monitoring or intervention following injury.

Separation of the placenta from the uterine wall is termed *placental abruption*. Following blunt trauma, major cases of placental abruption in which there is >50% separation are usually fatal to the fetus. Minor cases of placental abruption are not always initially detected, but may be manifested as early fetal distress picked up as decelerated heart rate associated with uterine contractions. These cases usually become evident within the first few hours of traumatic injury. All pregnant patients who are ≥20 weeks' gestation and who suffer trauma should receive cardiotocographic monitoring for a minimum of 4 hours and preferably 6 hours in the absence of signs, symptoms, or monitoring abnormalities.[28,29] A 24-hour course of monitoring is recommended for patients with frequent uterine activity (≥6 contractions/hour), a nonreassuring fetal heart rate pattern, abdominal or uterine pain, vaginal bleeding, serious maternal injury, or hypotension.[29]

Ultrasonography is a valuable tool in screening the trauma patient and is utilized in the focused abdominal sonography for trauma (FAST). The same device can be used to rapidly determine fetal viability based on fetal cardiac movement and fetal movement. The ultrasonographic examination can also determine fetal size and placental location. Placental abruption can sometimes be identified as a retroplacental lucency or echogenic structure in the amniotic fluid.[30] The combination of ultrasonographic examination and cardiotocographic monitoring is very sensitive at detecting all fetal or pregnancy associated complications of trauma.[31] These complications are usually manifested within 6 hours of admission. An ultrasonographic examination demonstrating oligohydramnios (<1 cm layer of amniotic fluid) is consistent with uteroplacental injury secondary to uterine rupture or rupture of the amniotic sac membrane.

DIAGNOSTIC CONSIDERATIONS

After the primary survey and stabilization of the patient, diagnostic modalities are used to determine the scope and extent of injuries to the mother and fetus. Laboratories pertinent to the trauma setting are obtained and all female patients of childbearing age should have a β-human chorionic gonadotropin (β-hCG) test performed.[32] Evaluation of the abdomen for hemoperitoneum can be performed by ultrasonography (FAST), diagnostic peritoneal lavage, or computed tomography (CT) scan. The FAST examination is preferred because it is noninvasive and does not utilize ionizing radiation. If a diagnostic peritoneal lavage is necessary, the open, supraumbilical technique should be used.

TABLE 2

UTERINE (FETAL) RADIATION DOSES FOR COMMON TRAUMA IMAGING STUDIES

Type of Examination	Radiation Dose	
	mGy	rads
Radiography		
Skull, any projection	0	0
Cervical spine, any projection	0	0
Chest AP	0.001	0.0001
Thoracic spine, AP, or lateral	0.001	0.0001
Abdomen, AP	0.79	0.079
Pelvis, AP	1.03	0.103
Pelvis, lateral	0.84	0.084
Lumbar spine, AP	0.90	0.090
Lumbar spine, lateral	0.28	0.028
GI/GU studies		
Cystogram	6.2	0.62
IVP	4.4	0.44
Computed tomography		
CT brain	0	0
CT chest	0.02	0.002
CT chest and abdomen	1.2	0.12
CT chest and abdomen, aorta	16.1	1.6
CT chest/abdomen/pelvis, aorta	45.3	4.5
CT PE protocol, including pelvis and LE for DVT	12.2	1.2
CT abdomen	1.2	0.12
CT abdomen and pelvis	16.2	1.6
CT pelvis	15	1.5
Fluoroscopy		
Abdomen or pelvis[a]	7/min	0.7/min

Doses provided are for the nongravid uterus in the average-sized mother. Fetal doses are approximated by uterine doses; however, accurate estimates are not available for later in gestation for a gravid uterus (late-term fetus).
[a]Estimated fetal dose with the fetus in the field of view (@ 8 kVp and 2 mA). Based on a measured exposure rate value of 2.5 R/min at tabletop of fluoroscopic unit.
AP, anterior-posterior; GI, gastro intestinal; GU, gastric ulcer; IVP, intravenous pyelogram; CT, computed tomography; PE, pulmonary embolus; LE, lower extremity; DVT, deep venous thrombosis.

Regarding radiologic studies, a study deemed necessary for maternal evaluation should not be withheld on the basis of its potential danger to the fetus. Unnecessary duplication of studies should be avoided and appropriate shielding/reduced radiation exposure protocols must be followed whenever possible. Radiologic exposure is measured using units of rad (radiation absorbed dose) or Gray (1 rad = 10 mGy). Dosages of common radiologic tests are listed in Table 2. Fetal radiation dosing without shielding is 30% of dose administered to the mother. No study has shown an increase in teratogenicity above baseline at fetal exposures below 10 rad to the fetus, and x-ray exposure below 10 rad represents an acceptable risk to the human embryo and fetus.[29]

Radiation risk can be divided into three categories: low, <10 mGy; intermediate, 10 to 250 mGy; high, >250 mGy.[33] Estimated doses are 2 mGy per exposure (radiographs), 5 mGy per slice (CT), and 10 mGy per minute of fluoroscopy, when the fetus is within the x-ray field. Fetal radiation exposure in the "low" category carries a minimal risk for random mutations. As an example, although the probability of an exposed conceptus developing a childhood cancer is tripled compared to that of a nonexposed pregnancy, no childhood cancer will occur in 99.9% of such "low" dose cases.[34] When radiation dose exceeds approximately 150 mGy ("intermediate" category), teratogenic mutations potentially attributable to x-rays are found. These mutations only occur between gestational ages of 2 to 15 weeks. Radiation-induced mutagenesis is many times more likely when the fetus dose is "high," which results in teratogenic or carcinogenic mutations at 2% to 3% greater than background rates. Once organogenesis is complete, the main increased risk is that of childhood cancer such as leukemia. Growth restriction, microcephaly, and mental retardation can occur with high dose radiation (>100 rad), well above the amounts used in medical imaging.[35,36] The fetus is most at risk for central nervous system effects between weeks 8 and 15 and the dose appears to be at least 20 to 40 rads.[36,37]

The American College of Obstetricians and Gynecologists' recommendations for diagnostic imaging in pregnant patients states that a 5 rad exposure to the fetus is not associated with any increased risk of fetal loss or birth defects.[38] The National Council on Radiation Protection has published that fetal risk is considered to be negligible at 5 rad or less when compared to the other risks of pregnancy, and the risk of malformations is significantly increased above control levels only at doses above 15 rad.[39] The Eastern Association for the Surgery of Trauma practice management guidelines state that exposure to <5 rad has not been associated with an increase in fetal anomalies or pregnancy loss and is considered safe at any point during gestation.[29] Consultation with a radiologist is recommended for calculation and monitoring of the estimated fetal dose when multiple diagnostic x-rays are necessary. The pregnant patient's abdomen should be shielded with a lead apron whenever possible to reduce fetal exposure to radiation.

OPERATIVE INDICATIONS AND TECHNIQUE

Blunt Trauma

Following diagnosis, the management of the pregnant patient with blunt traumatic injuries varies little from the nonpregnant scenario. Just as in nongravid patients, nonoperative management of solid organ injuries to the liver, spleen, or kidney in hemodynamically stable patients is the treatment of choice because it avoids the risk of general anesthesia and laparotomy in these patients. In an unstable patient or patient with peritonitis/hollow viscous injury, early surgery is the preferred option as hypotension and intraabdominal infection are harmful to the fetus and increase the risk of preterm delivery or fetal demise.[40] A standard midline laparotomy excision is employed and four-quadrant packing with subsequent exploration performed. The uterus should be left intact unless it has been directly injured or impairs exposure and treatment of maternal injuries. If labor ensues, vaginal delivery should be attempted unless it presents an increased risk to the mother or fetus. A cesarean section can prolong the operative time and drastically increase blood loss by 1 to 1.5 L. Indications for a cesarean section during a trauma laparotomy include (i) refractory maternal shock, viable fetus; (ii) threat to life from exsanguination; (iii) mechanical limitation of uterus to maternal treatment; (iv) risk of fetal distress exceeds the risks of prematurity; and (v) unstable thoracolumbar spinal injury.[30]

The fetus is usually well protected from blunt force injury by the pelvic bones (until engagement of the head during the third trimester), elasticity of the myometrium, and cushion effect of the amniotic fluid.[40] Direct fetal injury from blunt trauma is therefore rare but can occur and result in fractures to the extremities or skull, and intracerebral hemorrhage. Pelvic fracture is a common injury to the mother that may result in fetal death and has a rate of fetal demise as high as 25%.[24] Management of blunt injury to the pelvis is often difficult during pregnancy. Injury to engorged retroperitoneal blood vessels can easily result in severe hemorrhage and shock.[41] Bleeding from pelvic blood vessels should be managed with interventional angiography embolization; however, the radiation dose usually exceeds the amount considered to be safe during pregnancy. Appropriate dose estimation and counseling should occur in these patients following successful treatment.

Uterine rupture is rare, but can happen at the site of a previous cesarean section.[42,43] It presents as massive intraabdominal hemorrhage or more subtly as vaginal bleeding if the rupture is away from the major uterine blood vessels. Lacerations of the uterus are repaired primarily in one or two layers with a running locking stitch of large (1-0) absorbable suture. The decision as to whether to deliver the fetus is based on viability (gestational age) and fetal status. In cases where the fetus is nonviable (<24 to 26 weeks' gestation), it is possible to perform a primary repair of the uterus and allow the pregnancy to progress toward term. For severe injury and hemorrhage the option of hysterectomy is available, but infrequently needed and should only be performed as a last resort.

The placenta is not elastic, but the myometrium is.[44] In blunt trauma, a shearing effect can occur at the uterine placental interface due to this difference in tissue properties that results in separation and bleeding of the two tissues.[45] This is termed *placental abruption*. Placental abruption can occur in the absence of obvious abdominal injury.[44] It presents as vaginal bleeding, abdominal pain, presence of contractions, and unexplained hypotension.[30] Severe cases in which more than 50% of the placenta is separated almost uniformly result in fetal demise. Ultrasonographic examination alone is unfortunately not very sensitive at diagnosing placental abruption.[46] Cardiotocographic monitoring in conjunction with ultrasonography and careful examination for signs and symptoms such as vaginal bleeding, abdominal cramps, or leakage of amniotic fluid in the patient at risk for rapid deceleration injury is the recommended approach for diagnosis of major and minor episodes of placental abruption likely to result in fetal distress.

Penetrating Trauma

Because of its front and center location, the uterus in the later stage of pregnancy is a frequent target in penetrating trauma. Stab wounds that do not penetrate the thick uterine wall present little risk to the mother or fetus. Management is identical to that in the nonpregnant patient and based on the likelihood of intra-abdominal injury. Uterine lacerations are repaired primarily. Because the uterus acts a potential shield, death to the mother following abdominal gunshot wounds is low and only 20% to 30% have injuries beyond the uterus.[47] Gunshot wounds to the upper abdomen can result in a multitude of injuries to the mother late in pregnancy because considerable crowding of the visceral organs occurs as the uterus enlarges. Unfortunately, following an abdominal gunshot wound, 70% of the fetuses will sustain an injury and 40% to 65% will suffer demise depending on the severity of injury and gestational viability at the time of wounding.[47–49] Gunshot wounds with penetration into the abdominal cavity are managed with laparotomy. If a bullet has penetrated the uterus and the fetus is viable, a cesarean section should be performed and the neonatal injuries addressed by a surgeon if indicated. Pediatric surgical and neonatology assistance is recommended when available at the treating institution.

EMERGENT CESAREAN SECTION FOR TRAUMA

Performance of an emergency cesarean section at more than 25 weeks' gestation for appropriate indications following trauma is associated with 45% fetal survival and 72% maternal survival.[25] The absence of fetal heart tones ordinarily predicts mortality from an emergent cesarean section following traumatic injury to the mother. When fetal heart tones are present and the estimated gestational age is ≥26 weeks, emergent cesarean section following trauma results in a 75% infant survival.[25] However, the long-term morbidity of this procedure may be high. If an emergent cesarean section is deemed necessary, performance of the procedure in an operating room is preferable to the trauma resuscitation bay. Use of a midline incision is recommended to facilitate surgical exploration of the abdomen looking for injuries following delivery of the fetus.

The need for perimortem cesarean section is extremely rare. Because the procedure is an often futile and emotional event, it should only be considered in any moribund pregnant woman of ≥24 weeks' gestation.[29] Whenever possible, all efforts at cardiopulmonary resuscitation should be exhausted before proceeding with a perimortem cesarean section. Delivery must be accomplished within 20 minutes of maternal death, but ideally should begin within 4 minutes of maternal arrest.[3,29,30,50] The fetal neurologic outcome is directly related to the length of time after maternal death that delivery occurs.

Viability should be determined by assuring that the fundal height is several fingerbreaths above the umbilicus.[24,25] A midline incision is created from the xiphoid to the symphysis pubis through all layers of the abdominal wall. A vertical uterine incision is made, the fetus removed, umbilical cord double clamped and divided, and the infant handed to appropriate personnel to begin resuscitation. The placenta should be completely removed. Efforts at cardiopulmonary resuscitation should continue simultaneously with delivery as reports of maternal survival have occurred after the uterus is emptied resolving any supine hypotension from vena caval compression that is present.[43,51]

MATERNAL AND FETAL OUTCOMES

Trauma causes death in the fetus more often than in the mother. Independent risk factors for fetal demise include Injury Severity Score (ISS) >15; Abbreviated Injury Score ≥3 in the head, abdomen, thorax, or lower extremities; Glasgow Coma Scale score ≤8; increasing fluid requirements; maternal acidosis; and maternal hypoxia.[4,52] In patients with an ISS >15, the adjusted odds ratio for fetal mortality can be as high as 9.[4] The presence of abruptio placentae is associated with almost uniform fetal mortality.[53] In general, the measurement of maternal physiologic and laboratory parameters fails to accurately predict fetal outcome. The incidence of fetal death is increased in the following traumatic situations; maternal death, direct uteroplacental fetal injury, maternal shock, pelvic fracture, severe head injury, and hypoxia.[54,55] Injured pregnant patients with an ISS >8 demonstrate similar mortality, morbidity, and length of stay when matched to nonpregnant control patients.[55] Risk factors predictive of contractions or preterm labor include gestational age >35 weeks, assaults, and pedestrian collisions.[56]

Prenatal care is essential for optimal care of the unborn child. Good prenatal care involves education and screening for prevention of injury and identification of patients at risk. Episodes of domestic abuse can begin or escalate during pregnancy. Often the abuser is well known to the patient. Interpersonal violence is not a function of marital status, race, age, or economic standing. Significant percentages of

woman test positive for the presence of illegal drugs or alcohol when they are injured during pregnancy. Substance abuse is known to contribute to both intentional and unintentional injury in pregnant woman as well as placing the fetus at risk for low birth weight. Supplemental motor vehicle restraint systems such as lap belts and air bags are considered safe during pregnancy. Lap belt–associated injury can be reduced by educating woman as to proper seat belt position—low across and at the pelvic brim and not on top of the gravid uterus. The shoulder belt should lie to the side of the uterus, between the breasts and over the midportion of the clavicle.[3,24,57]

REFERENCES

1. Fildes J, Reed L, Jones N, et al. Trauma: The leading cause of maternal death. *J Trauma*. 1992;32:643–645.
2. Weiss HB. Pregnancy-associated injury hospitalizations in Pennsylvania, 1995. *Ann Emerg Med*. 1999;34:626–636.
3. Mattox KL, Goetzl L. Trauma in pregnancy. *Crit Care Med*. 2005; 33:S385–S389.
4. Ikossi DG, Lazar AA, Morabito D, et al. Profile of mothers at risk: An analysis of injury and pregnancy loss in 1,195 trauma patients. *J Am Coll Surg*. 2005;200:49–56.
5. Connolly AM, Katz VL, Bash KL, et al. Trauma and pregnancy. *Am J Perinatol*. 1997;14:331–336.
6. Weiss HB, Songer TJ, Fabio A. Fetal deaths related to maternal injury. *JAMA*. 2001;286:1863–1868.
7. Tsuei BJ. Assessment of the pregnant trauma patient. *Injury*. 2006; 37:367–373.
8. Gant NF, Worley RJ. Measures of uteroplacental blood flow in the human. In: Rosenfeld CR, ed. *The uterine circulation*. Ithaca: Perinatology Press; 1993:53–73.
9. Henderson SO, Mallon WK. Trauma in pregnancy. *Emerg Med Clin North Am*. 1998;16:209–228.
10. Wilson M, Morganti AA, Zervoudakis I, et al. Blood pressure, the renin-alsosterone system and sex steroids throughout normal pregnancy. *Am J Med*. 1980;68:97–104.
11. Lees MM, Taylor SH, Scott DB, et al. A study of cardiac output at rest throughout pregnancy. *J Obstet Gynaecol Br Commonw*. 1967;74: 319–328.
12. Mashini IS, Albazzaz SJ, Fadel HE, et al. Serial noninvasive evaluation of cardiovascular hemodynamics during pregnancy. *Am J Obstet Gynecol*. 1987;156:1208–1213.
13. Brooks DC, Parungo CP. The pregnant surgical patient. In: Souba WW, Fink MP, Jurkovich GJ, et al. eds. *ACS surgery principles and practice*. New York: WebMD; 2006:9.3.1–9.3.21.
14. Elkus R, Popovich J. Respiratory physiology in pregnancy. *Clin Chest Med*. 1992;13:555–565.
15. Cunningham FG, MacDonald PC. Maternal adaptions to pregnancy. In: Gant NF, et al. eds. *Williams Obstetrics*, 20th ed. Norwalk: Appleton & Lange; 1997:191–225.
16. Tsai CH, de Leeuw NK. Changes in 2,3 diphosphoglycerate during pregnancy and puerperium in normal woman and in beta-thalassemia heterozygous women. *Am J Obstet Gynecol*. 1982;142: 520–523.
17. Winbery SL, Blaho KE. Dyspepsia in pregnancy. *Obstet Gynecol Clin North Am*. 2001;28:333–350.
18. Braverman DZ, Johnson ML, Kern F Jr. Effects of pregnancy and contraceptive steroids on gallbladder function. *N Engl J Med*. 1980; 302:362–364.
19. Bremme K, Ostlund E, Almqvist I, et al. Enhanced thrombin generation and fibrinolytic activity in normal pregnancy and the puerperium. *Obstet Gynecol*. 1992;80:132–137.
20. Toglia MR, Weg JG. Venous thromboembolism during pregnancy. *N Engl J Med*. 1996;335:108–114.
21. Clark SL, Cotton DB, Pivarnik JM, et al. Positional change and central homodynamic profile during normal third trimester

pregnancy and post partum. *Am J Obstet Gynecol.* 1991;164: 883–887.

22. Munnur U, de Boisblanc B, Suresh MS. Airway problems in pregnancy. *Crit Care Med.* 2005;33:S259–S268.

23. Clark KE, Irion GL, Mack CE. Differential responses of uterine and umbilical vasculatures to angiotensin II and norepinephrine. *Am J Physiol.* 1990;259:H197–H203.

24. Knudson MM, Rozycki GS, Paquin MM. Reproductive system trauma. In: Moore EE, Feliciano DV, Mattox KL, eds. *Trauma,* 5th ed. New York: McGraw-Hill; 2004:851–874.

25. Morris JA, Rosenbower TJ, Jurkovich GJ, et al. Infant survival after cesarean section for trauma. *Ann Surg.* 1996;223:481–488.

26. Dhanraj D, Lambers D. The incidences of positive Kleihauer-Betke test in low-risk pregnancies and maternal trauma patients. *Am J Obstet Gynecol.* 2004;190:1461–1463.

27. Muench MV, Baschat AA, Reddy UM, et al. Kleihauer-Betke testing is important in all cases of maternal trauma. *J Trauma.* 2004; 57:1094–1098.

28. Pearlman MD, Tintinalli JE, Lorenz RP. A prospective controlled study of outcome after trauma during pregnancy. *Am J Obstet Gynecol.* 1990;162:1502–1510.

29. Barraco RD, Chiu WC, Clancy TV, et al. *Practice management guidelines for the diagnosis and management of injury in the pregnant patient: The EAST practice management guidelines work group.* Available at http://www.east.org/tpg/pregnancy.pdf. Accessed February 8, 2007.

30. Rozycki GS. Trauma in pregnancy. In: Mulholland MW, Lillemoe KD, Doherty GM, et al. eds. *Greenfield's surgery: scientific principles & practice,* 4th ed. Philadelphia: Lippincott Williams & Wilkins; 2006:484–493.

31. Towery R, English TP, Wisner D. Evaluation of pregnant women after blunt injury. *J Trauma.* 1993;35:731–735.

32. Bochicchio GV, Napolitano LM, Haan J, et al. Incidental pregnancy in trauma patients. *J Am Coll Surg.* 2001;192:566–569.

33. Upton AC. Radiobiologic effects of low doses: Implications for radiological protection. *Radiat Res.* 1977;71:51–74.

34. Mann FA, Nathens A, Langer SG, et al. Communicating with the family: The risks of medical radiation to conceptuses in victims of major blunt-force torso trauma. *J Trauma.* 2000;48:354–357.

35. Bohnen NI, Ragozzino MW, Kurland LT. Brief communication: Effects of diagnostic irradiation during pregnancy on head circumference at birth. *Int J Neurosci.* 1996;87:175–180.

36. Otake M, Schull WJ. Radiation-related brain damage and growth retardation among prenatally exposed atomic bomb survivors. *Int J Radiat Biol.* 1998;74:159–171.

37. Otake M, Schull WJ. In utero exposure to A-bomb radiation and mental retardation; a reassessment. *Br J Radiol.* 1984;57: 409–414.

38. American College of Obstetricians and Gynecologists Committee on Obstetric Practice. Committee opinion #299: Guidelines for diagnostic imaging during pregnancy. *Obstet Gynecol.* 2004;104: 647–651.

39. National Council on Radiation Protection and Measurements. *Medical radiation exposure of pregnant and potential pregnant women.* NRCP report no. 54. Bethesda: NCRP; 1977.

40. Petrone P, Asensio JA. Trauma in pregnancy: Assessment and treatment. *Scand J Surg.* 2006;95:4–10.

41. Lavin JP Jr, Polsky SS. Abdominal trauma during pregnancy. *Clin Perinatol.* 1983;10:423–438.

42. Shah AJ, Kilcline BA. Trauma in pregnancy. *Emerg Med Clin North Am.* 2003;21:615–629.

43. Pearlman MD, Tintinalli JE. Evaluation and treatment of the gravida and fetus following trauma and pregnancy. *Obstet Gynecol Clin North Am.* 1991;18:371–381.

44. Higgins SD, Garite TJ. Late abrupto placentae in trauma patients: Implications for monitoring. *Obstet Gynecol.* 1984;63: 10S–12S.

45. Crosby WM, Snyder RG, Snow CC, et al. Impact injuries in pregnancy I. Experimental studies. *Am J Obstet Gynecol.* 1968;101: 100–110.

46. Reis PM, Sander CM, Pearlman MD. Abruptio placentae after auto accidents: A case control study. *J Reprod Med.* 2000;45:6–10.

47. Patterson RM. Trauma in pregnancy. *Clin Obstet Gynecol.* 1984; 27:32–38.

48. Sandy EA, Koerner M. Self inflicted gunshot wound to the pregnant abdomen: Report of a case and review of the literature. *Am J Perinatol.* 1989;6:30–31.

49. Franger AL, Buchsbaum HJ, Peaceman AM. Abdominal gunshot wounds in pregnancy. *Am J Obstet Gynecol.* 1989;160: 1124–1128.

50. Rothenberger D, Quattlebaum FW, Perry JF Jr, et al. Blunt maternal trauma: A review of 103 cases. *J Trauma.* 1978;18:173–179.

51. DePace NL, Betesh JS, Kotler MN. "Postmortem" cesarean section with recovery of both mother and offspring. *JAMA.* 1982;248: 971–973.

52. Hoff WS, D'Amelio LF, Tinkoff GH, et al. Maternal predictors of fetal demise in trauma during pregnancy. *Surg Gynecol Obstet.* 1991; 172:175–180.

53. Ali J, Yeo A, Gana TJ, et al. Predictors of fetal mortality in pregnant trauma patients. *J Trauma.* 1997;42:782–785.

54. Kissinger DP, Rozycki GS, Morris JA Jr, et al. Trauma in pregnancy. Predicting pregnancy outcome. *Arch Surg.* 1991;126: 1079–1086.

55. Shah KH, Simons RK, Holbrook T, et al. Trauma in pregnancy: Maternal and fetal outcomes. *J Trauma.* 1998;45:83–86.

56. Curet MJ, Schermer CR, Demarest GB, et al. Predictors of outcome in trauma during pregnancy: Identification of patients who can be monitored for <6 hours. *J Trauma.* 2000;49:18–24.

57. Pearlman MD. Motor vehicle crashes, pregnancy loss and preterm labor. *Int J Gynaecol Obstet.* 1997;57:127–132.

Geriatric Trauma

55

Lawrence Lottenberg   *Darwin Noel Ang*

The geriatric population makes up 12.5% of the current population and could double in 30 years.[1-3] These patients are typically defined as individuals equal to or older than 65 years. A landmark study[4] recently completed in the state of Florida identified the elderly population (older than 65 years) comprising 24% of the state's population, more than twice the national average. The study also noted a 71% undertriage rate for motor vehicle crashes and approximately 90% undertriage rate for falls. Finally, it should be noted that while 70% of young patients are appropriately triaged to trauma centers, only 50% of the elderly find their way to designated trauma centers. The effects of aging are highly variable across an entire population, with many patients remaining healthy and vigorous until near the end of life.[5] Many elderly injured patients are at increased risk of mortality and morbidity because of diminished functional status (frailty syndrome) and the need for emergency care for their injuries. Both these factors have been associated with poorer outcomes.[6]

Trauma is the fifth leading cause of death for all ages and the seventh leading cause of death for those older than 65 years.[7] Falls are the most common cause of blunt trauma for the geriatric population. Many falls are from a standing height but falls from heights >10 ft are not uncommon, especially in the Southeast during times of storm preparation and damage. Motor vehicle collisions are the second most common cause of injuries in the elderly, while vehicle-pedestrian collisions are the third most common cause of injury to the elderly.[8] Interestingly, these three injury mechanisms are also known to be associated with large force transfer and, when present, they comprise the criteria for defining high-impact trauma with increased chance for serious injury (see Table 1). Finally, while penetrating trauma from suicide and homicide occurs less frequently in the geriatric population, its consequences are oftentimes more severe due to more comorbidity and less physiologic reserve than younger patients. The total cost to our health care system is approximately $3.2 billion annually in hospital charges, making care of the elderly injured patient an important topic to address.[9]

The goal of this chapter is to identify specific issues that are important in the management of the geriatric trauma patient and identify key features in the treatment of select organ system injuries. Because elderly patients frequently present with an array of comorbidities and physiologic patterns which are influenced by preexisting disease, the drugs used to treat those diseases, and the effects of the injuries incurred, the goal of trauma care for these patients is guided by efforts to gain early control of the injury so that complications may be minimized. When these treatment approaches are based on protocol-driven, evidence-based principles, improved outcomes can be realized.

IMPORTANT GERIATRIC-RELATED MEDICAL ISSUES

Polypharmacy

Elderly patients have more health issues and, as a result, take more medications for age-related comorbid problems. Therefore, polypharmacy is a unique medical issue to the geriatric trauma patient population and it is important to obtain this information during the initial hospital admission. Medications may have a direct impact on falls, bleeding, and mental status changes (see Table 2).

TABLE 1

CRITERIA FOR HIGH-IMPACT INJURIES

1. Collision ≥30 mph
2. Fall from 15 ft
3. Car striking a pedestrian

TABLE 2

ROLE OF DRUGS ON INJURY AND POSTINJURY PATHOPYSIOLOGY

Falls	Bleeding	Mental Status Changes
Antihypertensives	Coumadin	Alcohol
Antihistamines	Heparin products	Amphetamines
Antispsychotics	Antiplatelet	Antihistamines
Benzodiazepines		Antipsychotics
Muscle relaxants		Benzodiazepines
Narcotics		Cocaine
Vasodilators		Narcotics
Laxatives		

For the geriatric trauma patient, it is especially helpful to identify medications that will complicate or hinder their emergent medical or surgical management. One of the most dreaded surgical complications is bleeding while on anticoagulation. Multiple injury patients are at risk for coagulopathy due to shock, resuscitation with isotonic fluids, and infusion of multiple blood products. When this is compounded with the effects of systemic anticoagulation, the results can be lethal.

Surprisingly, age has not been proved to be an independent determining factor for bleeding complications from anticoagulation.[10] However, there is a clear association of increased use of anticoagulation with age and this results in a large increase in the number of patients at risk for increased bleeding when injury occurs in an anticoagulated patient. There is controversy regarding the utility of anticoagulation for nonrheumatic atrial fibrillation in older patients. While increases in quality-adjusted life years of survival have not been shown, the risk of bleeding due to warfarin therapy seems to be counterbalanced by a protective effect against stroke.[11,12] Most authors agree that careful management of the intensity of anticoagulation, keeping the international normalized ratio (INR) at or below 3.5 is essential to maximizing effectiveness while reducing complications. Low-intensity warfarin therapy (INR 2.0) is not associated with a reduced risk of bleeding.[13] Anticoagulation, especially when the INR exceeds 3.5, may place the elderly patient at a higher risk for bleeding as a result of trauma. The consequences of anticoagulation, especially in the patient with brain injury, seem to carry a higher percentage of mortality compared to patients not on anticoagulation.[14] This effect can be especially seen with cerebral hemorrhage and in patients older than 85 years.[15] Several studies suggest that mortality is greater from fall-related intracranial bleeding in patients on warfarin where the INR exceeds 2.5 by as much as 10-fold.

If an unstable geriatric patient is known to be taking warfarin or heparin products, immediate correction of their coagulopathy is required with fresh frozen plasma. Recent reports suggest the utility of activated factor VIIa to rapidly reverse the deleterious effects of warfarin and massive coagulopathy from over resuscitation.[16,17] Vitamin K is not considered as an adequate means of immediately reversing the effects of warfarin because of its time of effect. However, it is not unreasonable to administer if available for foreseeable long-term bleeding complications.[18]

Medications associated with increased risk of falls include antiarrhythmics, antihistamines, antihypertensives, antipsychotics, benzodiazepines, digoxin, laxatives, monoamine oxidase inhibitors, muscle relaxants, narcotics, tricyclics, selective seratonin reuptake inhibitors, and vasodilators.[3]

Prior Medical History

Advanced age is associated with an increased number of medical conditions. Several authors have shown through retrospective studies that preexisting medical conditions increase the mortality of the trauma patient between 2 and 8 times, and depending on the severity number of medical problems.[19-21] Medical conditions that are likely to complicate the geriatric patient's hospital course and affect mortality from significant trauma include previous history of myocardial infarction, significant chronic obstructive pulmonary disease (COPD), poorly controlled diabetes, bleeding disorders, previous history of deep vein thrombosis (DVT), Alzheimer dementia, adrenal insufficiency, and osteoporosis.

Some past medical problems have themselves been associated with organ-specific trauma. For example, cerebral atrophy has been associated with intracranial hemorrhages, osteoporosis with fractures, and COPD with pneumothoraces and ventilator-associated pneumonia. Appropriate precautions should be taken if these medical problems are already known, and attention to detail becomes especially important in recognizing these potential issues that may arise during the hospital admission.

Prior Surgical History

Previous surgery can be a complicating factor during a trauma laparotomy. Intra-abdominal adhesions can play a role in hollow viscous and solid organ injury by means of shear force and tear injuries. Oftentimes, adhesiolysis may become necessary during a damage control laparotomy taking valuable time away from obtaining hemostasis and the identification of major injuries. In addition, anatomy may be distorted due to previous resections and intestinal reconstruction.

In the chest, previous median sternotomy and thoracotomy will increase the level of difficulty in tube thoracostomy insertion and if needed, trauma-related thoracotomy or sternotomy. Extensive experience in reoperative surgery is necessary for successful outcomes.

ORGAN SYSTEM INJURIES

Brain and Spinal Cord

The prognosis and outcomes from traumatic brain injuries in the geriatric patient have been shown to be much worse than in younger patients. Some studies have reported that mortality rates are doubled for patients older than 55 years who have traumatic brain injuries compared to younger patients.[22] The Eastern Association for the Surgery of Trauma (EAST) practice management guideline for geriatric trauma recommends an initial course of aggressive treatment, followed by a reevaluation of the patient's neurologic status at 72 hours postadmission.[7] These recommendations are based on the data supporting admission Glasgow Coma Score (GCS) versus delayed GCS scoring. While the consensus is that a low-admission GCS confers a poorer prognosis, the actual score ranges from 7 to 11 with no consensus on a score to reliably predict outcomes. The data for delayed GCS scoring clearly shows high mortality percentages ranging from 90% to 100% for GCS scores between 8 and 9.[23,24]

Traumatic brain injuries with GCS <8 and computed tomography (CT) findings consistent with increased intracranial pressure (ICP) require invasive ICP monitoring. Once elevated ICPs are established, aggressive therapy to decrease this with hyperventilation, propofol, and mannitol should be expeditiously pursued. All these treatments have been shown to decrease ICP by different mechanisms. Hyperoxia, by increasing the fraction of inspired oxygen, has been shown to reduce cerebral lactate levels and possibly improve brain oxygen tension. Decompressive craniectomy is the last resort and is especially controversial among the geriatric population.

Spinal cord injuries are a significant source of morbidity and mortality in the elderly. Comparative studies have suggested that patients older than 65 years have approximately a fivefold increase in mortality after spinal cord injury compared to younger patients.[25] Mortality has also been reported to be higher in patients older than 50 years especially when the cord injury is severe. Patients older than 65 years are more likely to fracture their cervical spines by low-energy mechanisms compared to younger patients, causing these fractures to be often overlooked.[26]

The elderly are particularly susceptible to dens and second cervical vertebrae fractures on the basis of biomechanical changes from degenerative disease in the mid and lower cervical spine. Predictors of cervical spinal injuries include neurologic deficits, severe head injury, and high-energy mechanism of injury.[27] CT scan in this setting has been proved to be both effective and cost saving for initial diagnosis. Magnetic resonance imaging (MRI) has a role in planning later definitive management when prompt evaluation by a neurosurgical specialist has been done.

Acute management for geriatric spinal injuries include immobilization, adequate pain control, invasive monitoring with pulmonary artery (PA) catheter with correction of hypotension and bradycardia, and corticosteroids. Our institutional practice has been to administer methylprednisolone based on the National Acute Spinal Cord Injury Study ([NASCIS] I and II) trials in patients with known blunt injury to the spinal cord who present within 8 hours of injury despite the lack of convincing evidence that functional outcomes are improved.[28,29] Patients are given a 30 mg per kg bolus followed by a 5.4 mg/kg/hour infusion of steroid for 48 hours. Patients with transient neurologic deficit with negative radiologic studies should have flexion and extension cervical films before removal of the cervical collar. This is especially important in geriatric patients with known osteoporosis, cervical surgery, and degenerative disease of the cervical spine. The incidence of central cord syndrome is higher in the elderly population because of the aforementioned degenerative disease almost always present.

Thoracic Injuries

The elderly are especially prone to rib fractures, pulmonary contusions, hemothoraces, and pneumothoraces from blunt trauma. Chest trauma resulting in rib and vertebral fractures has been increasingly recognized as one of the most commonly seen injuries in the elderly, especially in motor vehicle collisions. There is some evidence to suggest that there is a linear relationship between age, number of rib fractures, and complications.[30]

The three most common blunt chest injuries of geriatric patients are rib fractures, flail chest, and sternum fractures.[31] The chest x-ray and physical examination play a key part in the early management of geriatric trauma patients with chest trauma because rapid identification of pneumothorax and decompression are essential in management. While younger patients can tolerate small to moderate pneumothoraces, older patients will deteriorate rapidly. A pneumothorax that does not appear on plain films and is present on CT scan only warrants mandatory intervention in the elderly patient because of limited ventilatory reserve.

Patients with more than six fractured ribs are especially at risk from these aforementioned complications.[32] Another study pointed to the fact that although elderly patients with rib fractures have less severe injuries, as measured by lower injury severity scores and higher GCSs, overall trauma mortality is higher than in younger patients with rib fractures[33] (see Table 3). After adjusting for severity, comorbidity, and multiple fractures, Bergeron et al. observed that patients older than 65 years had five times the odds of dying when compared to younger patients.[34]

Early intervention with tube thoracostomy and mechanical ventilation and adequate pain control are both important in the treatment of chest wall injuries in this population. Some centers are now advocating rib fracture stabilization for certain injuries. One group was able to show

TABLE 3

MORTALITY BY AGE AND NUMBER OF RIB FRACTURES

Age	Number of Rib Fractures				Total
	1–2	**3–4**	**5–6**	**7**	
	Percentage				
Younger than 65 y	6.1	7.6	16.2	23.3	11.4
Equal to or older than 65 y	12.3	11.2	28.1	37.8	20.1
Total	7.9	8.8	20.3	27.9	14.1
$p = 0.001$					

ventilator days decreased from 9.4 to 2.9 days with plating of fractures.[35] Proponents of rib fracture stabilization cite that failure to gain the benefits of pain control and chest wall stability may result in death from pneumonia, adult respiratory distress syndrome (ARDS), aspiration pneumonia, ventilator-associated pneumonia, and empyema.[36] Experience in American trauma centers with this technique has been limited.[37] Another recent study looked into a model controlling multiple known risk factors; age and Injury Severity score were the only two predictors of mortality in patients with rib fractures and multiple system injury. However, pneumonia was significantly associated with mortality in patients with isolated thoracic trauma.[38]

Acute pain management of patients with multiple rib fractures deserves attention, because lack of pain management leads to poor pulmonary effort with avoidable consequences. Multiple methods of analgesia exist. Systemic opioids, nonsteroidal anti-inflammatory drugs, regional anesthetics such as intercostal nerve block, epidural analgesia, intrathecal opioids, intrapleural analgesia, and thoracic paravertebral block all have strengths and weakness, and knowledge of the alternatives will result in improved outcomes.[39]

Abdomen

Intra-abdominal organ injury is the third most common injury pattern in the elderly.[40] These injuries carry a 4.7 greater risk of mortality compared to younger patients.[41] After addressing the airway, breathing, and circulation issues, a prompt evaluation of the abdomen is required. Physical examination is paramount; however, distracting injuries, especially bony injuries and traumatic brain injury sustained by the geriatric patient can obfuscate the diagnosis.

Focused assessment using sonography for trauma should be part of the diagnostic workup of every patient who demonstrates hemodynamic instability and/or a high suspicion for intra-abdominal injury of sufficient severity to warrant immediate surgery. In the hands of an experienced surgeon, the specificity of the abdominal ultrasonography can be as high as 95%.[42]

Injury to the liver is approached in a similar manner for all age groups of patients; nonoperative management should include angioembolization if there is an arterial blush on CT scan.

Perhaps one of the more controversial topics in geriatric trauma is the management of splenic injury. Previously, a dictum for the management of splenic injuries in individuals older than 55 years was splenectomy because nonoperative management led to unacceptable failure rates. In some studies this is as high as 91%.[43,44] These data came largely from single-institution retrospective studies. The strongest data to support early surgery for those older than 55 years comes from a multi-institution retrospective study looking at 1,488 adult patients from 27 trauma centers.[44] In this study, nonoperative management failed more commonly in elderly patients, with resultant increased mortality regardless of success or failure rates for nonoperative management of younger patients in the same institution.

There is support nonoperative management as an acceptable algorithm in the treatment of solid organ injury in the geriatric population. In the study by Cocanour,[45] the failure rates of nonoperative management were the same for younger and older patients; however, the mortality was higher in the older patient population. The authors point out though that the deaths of their older patients were due to other comorbid problems and not directly as a result of the splenic injury.

Overall, it is generally agreed that geriatric patients with injuries similar to young patients will have worse outcomes due to their multiple comorbidities and decreased physiologic reserve. This leads to the conclusion that a single-minded approach is probably hazardous in older patients with spleen injury. An open mind to the full constellation of the patient's injuries and comorbidities will dictate that all available modalities should be considered to select the optimum approach for each patient.

Musculoskeletal and Vascular

Orthopaedic management in the elderly should adhere to the same principles of any age with early fracture fixation when indicated and damage control with external fixation as necessary.

Approximately 60% of all individuals older than 65 years have some sort of atherosclerotic disease. When dealing with long bone fractures of both the upper and lower extremities, it is difficult to determine whether the pulse examination has been influenced by preexisting atherosclerotic disease. Ankle Brachial Index (ABI) is a method of screening but of late CT angiography has been shown to obviate the need for invasive arteriography. Endovascular stenting of injuries to the extremities is beginning to show promise. Careful attention to the symptoms and diagnosis of compartment syndrome either clinically or by compartment pressure measurement will prevent significant morbidity for elderly patients.

Pelvis

The lifetime risk for hip fractures in men older than 65 years is 5%.[46] The annual hospital admission for hip fractures exceeds 250,000 per year. This is a very serious problem in the geriatric population because the overall mortality has been reported to be sixfold higher compared to younger patients.[47] Geriatric patients who present with pelvic fractures generally have higher injury severity scores because the amount of force required to create pelvic fractures is also transmitted to the rest of the body. Some have suggested that there is also a predominant pattern of injury with lateral compression fracture occurring more commonly. Measures such as external fixation and external compression with a pelvic binder will not be consistently effective as a means of achieving hemostasis in these fractures.

Early detection is perhaps the most important aspect in the management of a pelvic fracture in the elderly. If the fracture is amenable to external stabilization with a pelvic binder, then this is followed by resuscitation, stabilization, and angioembolization. As a rule, older patients with pelvic fractures will have longer hospital stays, more morbidity associated with being immobile, and higher mortality. Aggressive management aimed toward hemostasis, early physical therapy, and attention to comorbid factors should all be factored in the successful treatment of pelvic fractures in this age-group.

HOSPITAL MANAGEMENT

Resuscitation

Ideally, geriatric patients should be triaged to Level 1 trauma centers because of their likelihood of sustaining more injury from both penetrating and blunt trauma.[48] Elderly trauma patients are undertriaged in the prehospital phase of care and the likelihood of appropriate triage diminishes as the distance from a trauma center and the injury site increases.[49] Endpoints of resuscitation have been a controversial topic among geriatric patients because of their potential to have decreased cardiac function from preexisting coronary, myocardial, or valvular disease. Rapid control of airway, removal of dentures, timely intubation, and appropriate early administration of blood products all become essential in the early management of the elderly trauma patient. Laboratory assessments must include blood urea nitrogen (BUN), creatinine, INR, proficiency testing (PT), and electrolytes in all of these critically injured patients. Central venous access and arterial line monitoring are both advantageous in the management of these patients.

Intensive Care

Once a geriatric patient requires intensive care admission, invasive hemodynamic monitoring has been the standard practice of many trauma centers. Available data have supported early intensive management and invasive monitoring in geriatric populations on the basis of preexisting conditions that may mask the true severity of injury sustained by the patient.[50] Scalea et al. were able to show that early invasive monitoring with a PA catheter and arterial line disclosed that nearly half of their geriatric trauma patients were in unsuspected cardiogenic shock.[51] By optimizing their patients to a cardiac index of >4 L/minute/m^2 or improving the oxygen consumption index to 170 mL/minute/m^2, they were able to improve survival.

All geriatric patients should be placed on DVT prophylaxis, which includes sequential compression devices and subcutaneous heparin products. It is now well accepted that low molecular weight heparin is superior to subcutaneous heparin in preventing DVT. One interesting study looked at the epidemiology of diagnosed pulmonary embolism and DVT in the elderly.[52] Both DVT and pulmonary emboli increase with age and the most significant increase appears to be after the age of 70. Routine screening for DVT and consideration for inferior vena cava (IVC) filters should be part of the assessment for all geriatric trauma patients.

β-blockade may be a useful adjunct for those patients with identifiable increased cardiovascular risk and arterial pressure and heart rate within acceptable ranges. Data is available that supports the protective effect of this intervention when it is applied to appropriate patient groups.[53] Tight glucose control is also essential in geriatric patients as both morbidity and mortality have been associated with glucose levels higher than 110.[54] Aggressive pulmonary toilet and early ambulation are equally important for better pulmonary function and in decreasing the risk of infection. Patients with underlying pulmonary disease or severe injuries from trauma are more likely to develop ventilator-associated pneumonia, which carries 38% mortality.[55] If the patient has a normal functioning gastrointestinal (GI) tract, then enteral feeds are preferred over total parenteral nutrition. Finally, the question of maintaining the hemoglobin above a certain level has remained

TABLE 4

REQUIRED INTENSIVE CARE UNIT (ICU) OPTIMIZATION FOR THE GERIATRIC PATIENT

ICU Requirements	Management
DVT/PE prophylaxis	Heparin (LMWH and UH), sequential compression devices, and IVC filter
Perioperative β-blockade	Scheduled metoprolol IV or PO
Glucose control	Insulin drip preferred over sliding scale
Pulmonary toilet regimen	Incentive spirometry, elevation HOB 30 degrees, and subglottic suction ET tubes
Early extubation	Protocol-driven ventilator wean and extubation
Invasive monitoring	Pulmonary artery catheter, arterial line, and noninvasive Doppler esophageal probe

DVT, deep vein thrombosis; PE, pulmonary embolism; LMWH, low molecular weight heparin; UH, unfractionated heparin; IVC, inferior vena cava; HOB, head of bed; ET, endotracheal tube.

controversial because several popular studies have shown that packed red blood cell transfusion has a correlation with increased morbidity or mortality or equivocal outcomes in critically ill patients.[56] Our practice has been to transfuse geriatric patients with significant cardiac or coronary artery disease that are symptomatic from anemia to a hemoglobin concentration above 10 mg per dL. The thought behind this is to improve oxygen delivery as well as to optimize cardiac output in a patient with cardiovascular compromise. For these patients, symptoms may manifest either in the form of refractory tachycardia or hypoxia. Table 4 summarizes important parameters that should be optimized as a major component of the critical care of the elderly injured patient.

Delirium is a particularly troublesome problem in the elderly injured patient. Rates of delirium diagnosed in hospitalized elderly patients may exceed 15% and this rate rises to 70% in critically ill geriatric patients. Patients have variable clinical presentations, which include agitation, hyperactivity, hypoactivity, or mixed forms. Patients with preinjury histories of alcohol abuse, poor nutrition, and diminished functional status are at increased risk. Prevention is a key to successful management. Early mobilization, avoidance of excessive use of narcotics and sedatives, and provision of adequate psychological support and sleep time are important preventive measures. If pharmacologic therapy is needed, haloperidol is preferred because of fewer sedative, anticholinergic, and hypotensive side effects.

Clinicians are increasingly recognizing the usefulness of assistance by a dedicated geriatrician consultant to assist in achieving improved outcomes for critically ill elderly patients.

DISCHARGE AND REHABILITATION

Once the geriatric patient begins recovery from trauma, the posthospital course becomes an important factor in long-term recovery. The phenomenon of deconditioning has been observed with increased frequency in elderly patients recovering from severe illness and injury.[57] Measures to ameliorate or reverse this condition include careful attention to nutrition and aggressive physical, occupational, and psychological therapy. Although some have suggested that patients requiring rehabilitation for trauma compared to those who were discharged to nursing homes showed no statistical differences in outcomes, this observation seems particularly counterintuitive.[58] However, discharge planning should begin with admission. Preinjury living arrangements need to be assessed. Patients in independent living facilities or living at home alone or with a spouse likely will not be able to return to their previous living situations without home health care or a short or long stay in a nursing home or rehabilitation facility. Participating in twice-weekly multidisciplinary sit-down rounds with physicians, nurses, physical therapists, physiatrists, occupational therapists, speech pathologists, dietitians, and social workers is essential in planning an appropriate outcome for the geriatric trauma patient. A recent study points out that patients who survive injuries experience residual impairments in functional capacity and quality of life for as long as 1 year after injury.[59]

SUMMARY

Trauma in the elderly represents a significant population-based group of patients with unique preexisting conditions and comorbidities. Management principles require prompt recognition of hemodynamic abnormality early in the course of treatment and must be protocol driven with evidence-based principles. Meticulous attention to detail will ensure optimal outcomes.

REFERENCES

1. Rzepka SG, Malangoni MA, Rimm AA. Geriatric trauma hospitalization in the United States: A population-based study. *J Clin Epidemiol.* 2001;54(6):627–633.
2. Spencer G. *Projections of the population of the United States by age, sex and race: 1988–2080,* Vol. 1018. Washington, DC: U.S. Bureau of the Census; 1989.
3. Miller KE, Zylstra RG, Standridge JB. The geriatric patient: A systematic approach to maintaining health. *Am Fam Physician.* 2000;61(4):1089–1104.
4. Durham R, Pracht E, Orban B, et al. Evaluation of a mature trauma system. *Ann Surg.* 2006;243(6):775–783; discussion 775–783.
5. Christmas C, Makary MA, Burton JR. Medical considerations in older surgical patients. *J Am Coll Surg.* 2006;203(5):746–751.
6. Turrentine FE, Wang H, Simpson VB, et al. Surgical risk factors, morbidity, and mortality in elderly patients. *J Am Coll Surg.* 2006;203(6):865–877.

7. Jacobs DG, Plaisie BR, Barie PS, et al. *Practice management guidelines for geriatric trauma.* 2001.
8. Mandavia DNK. Geriatric trauma. *Emerg Med Clin North Am.* 1998;16:257–274.
9. Mackenzie EJMJ, Smith GS, Fahey M. Acute hospital costs of trauma in the United States: Implications for regionalized systems of care. *J Trauma.* 1990;30:1096–1103.
10. Fihn SD, Callahan CM, Martin DC, et al. The National Consortium of Anticoagulation Clinics. The risk for and severity of bleeding complications in elderly patients treated with warfarin. *Ann Intern Med.* 1996;124(11):970–979.
11. Gage BF, Birman-Deych E, Kerzner R, et al. Incidence of intracranial hemorrhage in patients with atrial fibrillation who are prone to fall. *Am J Med.* 2005;118(6):612–617.
12. Desbiens NA. Deciding on anticoagulating the oldest old with atrial fibrillation: Insights from cost-effectiveness analysis. *J Am Geriatr Soc.* 2002;50(5):863–869.
13. Fang MC, Chang Y, Hylek EM, et al. Advanced age, anticoagulation intensity, and risk for intracranial hemorrhage among patients taking warfarin for atrial fibrillation. *Ann Intern Med.* 2004;141(10):745–752.
14. Franko J, Kish KJ, O'Connell BG, et al. Advanced age and preinjury warfarin anticoagulation increase the risk of mortality after head trauma. *J Trauma.* 2006;61(1):107–110.
15. Karni A, Holtzman R, Bass T, et al. Traumatic head injury in the anticoagulated elderly patient: A lethal combination. *Am Surg.* 2001;67(11):1098–1100.
16. Boffard KD, Riou B, Warren B, et al. Recombinant factor VIIa as adjunctive therapy for bleeding control in severely injured trauma patients: Two parallel randomized, placebo-controlled, double-blind clinical trials. *J Trauma.* 2005;59(1):8–15; discussion 15–18.
17. Harrison TD, Laskosky J, Jazaeri O, et al. "Low-dose" recombinant activated factor VII results in less blood and blood product use in traumatic hemorrhage. *J Trauma.* 2005;59(1):150–154.
18. Coimbra R, Hoyt DB, Anjaria DJ, et al. Reversal of anticoagulation in trauma: A North-American survey on clinical practices among trauma surgeons. *J Trauma.* 2005;59(2):375–382.
19. Milzman DP, Boulanger BR, Rodriguez A, et al. Pre-existing disease in trauma patients: A predictor of fate independent of age and injury severity score. *J Trauma.* 1992;32(2):236–243; discussion 234–243.
20. Charlson ME, Pompei P, Ales KL, et al. A new method of classifying prognostic comorbidity in longitudinal studies: Development and validation. *J Chronic Dis.* 1987;40(5):373–383.
21. Gubler KD, Davis R, Koepsell T, et al. Long-term survival of elderly trauma patients. *Arch Surg.* 1997;132(9):1010–1014.
22. Vollmer D. Age and outcome following traumatic coma: Why do older patients fare worse? *J Neurosurg.* 1991;75:S37–S49.
23. Kotwica Z, Jakubowski JK. Acute head injuries in the elderly. An analysis of 136 consecutive patients. *Acta Neurochir (Wien).* 1992;118(3–4):98–102.
24. Ross AM, Pitts LH, Kobayashi S. Prognosticators of outcome after major head injury in the elderly. *J Neurosci Nurs.* 1992;24(2):88–93.
25. Jackson AP, Haak MH, Khan N, et al. Cervical spine injuries in the elderly: Acute postoperative mortality. *Spine.* 2005;30(13):1524–1527.
26. Spivak JM, Weiss MA, Cotler JM, et al. Cervical spine injuries in patients 65 and older. *Spine.* 1994;19(20):2302–2306.
27. Bub LD, Blackmore CC, Mann FA, et al. Cervical spine fractures in patients 65 years and older: A clinical prediction rule for blunt trauma. *Radiology.* 2005;234(1):143–149.
28. Bracken MB, Shepard MJ, Collins WF, et al. A randomized, controlled trial of methylprednisolone or naloxone in the treatment of acute spinal-cord injury. Results of the Second National Acute Spinal Cord Injury Study. *N Engl J Med.* 1990;322(20):1405–1411.
29. Bracken MB, Shepard MJ, Holford TR, et al. Administration of methylprednisolone for 24 or 48 hours or tirilazad mesylate for 48 hours in the treatment of acute spinal cord injury. Results of the Third National Acute Spinal Cord Injury Randomized Controlled Trial. National Acute Spinal Cord Injury Study. *JAMA.* 1997;277(20):1597–1604.
30. Testerman GM. Adverse outcomes in younger rib fracture patients. *South Med J.* 2006;99(4):335–339.
31. Lee WY, Cameron PA, Bailey MJ. Road traffic injuries in the elderly. *Emerg Med J.* 2006;23(1):42–46.
32. Flagel BT, Luchette FA, Reed RL, et al. Half-a-dozen ribs: The breakpoint for mortality. *Surgery.* 2005;138(4):717–723; discussion 715–723.
33. Stawicki SP, Grossman MD, Hoey BA, et al. Rib fractures in the elderly: A marker of injury severity. *J Am Geriatr Soc.* 2004;52(5):805–808.
34. Bergeron E, Lavoie A, Clas D, et al. Elderly trauma patients with rib fractures are at greater risk of death and pneumonia. *J Trauma.* 2003;54(3):478–485.
35. Nirula R, Allen B, Layman R, et al. Rib fracture stabilization in patients sustaining blunt chest injury. *Am Surg.* 2006;72(4):307–309.
36. Ahmed Z, Mohyuddin Z. Management of flail chest injury: Internal fixation versus endotracheal intubation and ventilation. *J Thorac Cardiovasc Surg.* 1995;110(6):1676–1680.
37. Mayberry JC, Terhes JT, Ellis TJ, et al. Absorbable plates for rib fracture repair: Preliminary experience. *J Trauma.* 2003;55(5):835–839.
38. Brasel KJ, Guse CE, Layde P, et al. Rib fractures: Relationship with pneumonia and mortality. *Crit Care Med.* 2006;34(6):1642–1646.
39. Karmakar MK, Ho AM. Acute pain management of patients with multiple fractured ribs. *J Trauma.* 2003;54(3):615–625.
40. Oreskovich MR, Howard JD, Copass MK, et al. Geriatric trauma: Injury patterns and outcome. *J Trauma.* 1984;24(7):565–572.
41. Finelli FC, Jonsson J, Champion HR, et al. A case control study for major trauma in geriatric patients. *J Trauma.* 1989;29(5):541–548.
42. Rozycki GS, Ochsner MG, Jaffin JH, et al. Prospective evaluation of surgeons' use of ultrasound in the evaluation of trauma patients. *J Trauma.* 1993;34(4):516–526; discussion 517–526.
43. Smith JS Jr, Cooney RN, Mucha P Jr. Nonoperative management of the ruptured spleen: A revalidation of criteria. *Surgery.* 1996;120(4):745–750; discussion 741–750.
44. Harbrecht BG, Peitzman AB, Rivera L, et al. Contribution of age and gender to outcome of blunt splenic injury in adults: Multicenter study of the eastern association for the surgery of trauma. *J Trauma.* 2001;51(5):887–895.
45. Cocanour CS, Moore FA, Ware DN, et al. Age should not be a consideration for nonoperative management of blunt splenic injury. *J Trauma.* 2000;48(4):606–610; discussion 602–610.
46. Schwartz AV, Kelsey JL, Sidney S, et al. Characteristics of falls and risk of hip fracture in elderly men. *Osteoporos Int.* 1998;8(3):240–246.
47. Henry SM, Pollak AN, Jones AL, et al. Pelvic fracture in geriatric patients: A distinct clinical entity. *J Trauma.* 2002;53(1):15–20.
48. Lane P, Sorondo B, Kelly JJ. Geriatric trauma patients-are they receiving trauma center care? *Acad Emerg Med.* 2003;10(3):244–250.
49. Papa L, Langland-Orban B, Kallenborn C, et al. Assessing effectiveness of a mature trauma system: Association of trauma center presence with lower injury mortality rate. *J Trauma.* 2006;61(2):261–266; discussion 266–267.
50. Demetriades D, Karaiskakis M, Velmahos G, et al. Effect on outcome of early intensive management of geriatric trauma patients. *Br J Surg.* 2002;89(10):1319–1322.
51. Scalea TM, Simon HM, Duncan AO, et al. Geriatric blunt multiple trauma: Improved survival with early invasive monitoring. *J Trauma.* 1990;30(2):129–134; discussion 126–134.
52. Kniffin WD Jr, Baron JA, Barrett J, et al. The epidemiology of diagnosed pulmonary embolism and deep venous thrombosis in the elderly. *Arch Intern Med.* 1994;154(8):861–866.
53. Auerbach AD, Goldman L. Beta-blockers and reduction of cardiac events in noncardiac surgery: Scientific review. *JAMA.* 2002;287(11):1435–1444.
54. van den Berghe G, Wouters P, Weekers F, et al. Intensive insulin therapy in the critically ill patients. *N Engl J Med.* 2001;345(19):1359–1367.

55. Tejerina E, Frutos-Vivar F, Restrepo MI, et al. Incidence, risk factors, and outcome of ventilator-associated pneumonia. *J Crit Care.* 2006;21(1):56–65.

56. Vincent JL, Piagnerelli M. Transfusion in the intensive care unit. *Crit Care Med.* 2006;34(5 Suppl):S96–101.

57. Killewich LA. Strategies to minimize postoperative deconditioning in elderly surgical patients. *J Am Coll Surg.* 2006;203(5):735–745.

58. Kramer AM, Steiner JF, Schlenker RE, et al. Outcomes and costs after hip fracture and stroke. A comparison of rehabilitation settings. *JAMA.* 1997;277(5):396–404.

59. Sampalis JS, Liberman M, Davis L, et al. Functional status and quality of life in survivors of injury treated at tertiary trauma centers: What are we neglecting? *J Trauma.* 2006;60(4):806–813.

Burn Injury

56

Frederick W. Endorf   *Saman Arbabi*

Approximately 500,000 Americans suffer burn injuries each year, with approximately 40,000 requiring hospital admission for treatment of their burns. It is estimated that 4,000 people will die annually in the United States as a result of burns.[1] A proper understanding of the diagnosis and treatment of burn injuries is essential for trauma and critical care surgeons.

HISTORY

Burn care has undergone a remarkable evolution over the course of the last century. In the early 1900s, burn patients typically faced an extremely grim prognosis. If one third of the body surface area was involved, even with superficial burns, death was considered inevitable.[2] Great strides were made in understanding burn resuscitation following major disasters such as the 1930 Rialto Concert Hall,[3] 1942 Cocoanut Grove,[4] and 1947 Texas City fires.[5] The advent of early excision of the burn wound in the 1970s decreased burn wound sepsis and shortened hospital stays.[6,7] Subsequent improvements in critical care and wound management have decreased mortality to the point that survival is often expected. Long-term functional outcomes have instead become the goals of burn care. The American College of Surgeons (ACS), along with the American Burn Association (ABA), realizing that burn care is a specialized and constantly changing field, initiated a burn center verification process to ensure that high standards are met in the care of burn patients. Participating burn centers are verified every 3 years with the goal of providing reliable, excellent care to burn patients.[8] Burn care has evolved into a multidisciplinary effort that sets it apart from many other subspecialties, with attention to psychological and rehabilitation issues along with traditional medical and surgical care. The wide-ranging nature of this comprehensive care exceeds the scope of this chapter, and here we focus primarily on the surgical and critical care topics germane to the care of burn patients.

MECHANISMS OF BURN INJURY

Burns may be caused by any number of agents, but are most commonly grouped into thermal, electrical, and chemical burns. Thermal burns are the most common, including fire or flame burns, scalds, and contact burns. Of patients admitted to burn centers, 46% have fire or flame injuries, 32% scalds, and 8% contact burns from hot objects. Of the 4,000 burn-related deaths each year, approximately 3,500 are linked with residential fires, and often are a result of inhalation injury and carbon monoxide (CO) poisoning.[1] Electrical injuries are less common (4% of burn admissions)[1] but can be severe. Special considerations in the care of electrical injury include the potential for cardiac arrhythmias, extremity compartment syndromes, and rhabdomyolysis. An electrocardiogram (ECG) is recommended in all patients with electrical injury, but low-voltage injuries without ECG abnormalities or other injuries do not necessarily require hospital admission.[9] A high index of suspicion should be maintained for compartment syndrome with concurrent rhabdomyolysis, and fasciotomies should be performed as indicated by neurologic or vascular compromise. Examination of vision and hearing is also important, particularly in lightning injuries.[10] Chemical burns are also less common, but can also cause severe burns. Attention should be given to complete removal of the substance from the patient through copious irrigation of the affected area for at least 30 minutes. One must also look for metabolic insults caused by the offending agent, such as acidosis, hemolysis, and hemoglobinuria with formic acid or hypocalcemia with hydrofluoric acid.[11] Hydrofluoric acid is a common culprit due to its inclusion in industrial cleansers. Treatment is neutralization with calcium, through calcium gluconate in dimethyl sulfoxide applied directly to wounds, or subcutaneous or intravenous infiltration of calcium gluconate.[12,13] Intra-arterial infusion of calcium gluconate has been reported in facial hydrofluoric acid burns.[14]

BURN DEPTH

Traditionally, burn depth was classified using first, second, and third degrees. This system has gradually been replaced with the terms superficial, superficial partial thickness, deep partial thickness, and full thickness. Superficial burns are typically caused by ultraviolet light (i.e., "sunburn") or by very short flash burns. These burns are dry and red, blanch with pressure, are painful to touch, and heal in 3 to 6 days without scarring. Partial-thickness burns may be further divided into superficial and deep depending on the depth of dermis involved. Superficial partial-thickness burns are often caused by splash scalds or short flash burns. They will blister, and are red and weeping and blanch with pressure (see Fig. 1). These burns are painful to touch, air and temperature, and most will heal without surgery after 7 to 20 days. Scarring is uncommon, although pigment changes in the skin may be seen. Deep partial-thickness burns may be caused by scalds, flame burns, or oil or grease burns. These burns also blister, but can be wet or have a waxy dry texture, with a patchy red or white appearance. Deep partial-thickness burns are typically insensate. Surgery is usually required because these burns take more than 3 weeks to heal, and are especially prone to infection, hypertrophic scarring, and contractures if allowed to heal without excision and grafting. Full-thickness burns are white, gray, or black. They are insensate and do not blanch

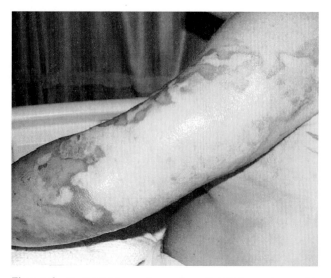

Figure 1 Partial-thickness burn: A partial-thickness burn with pink and moist burn area.

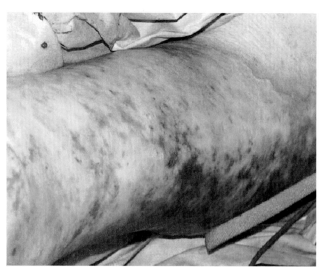

Figure 2 Full-thickness burn: A full-thickness burn with gray-white and dry burn area.

with pressure (see Fig. 2). Any full-thickness burns >2% of the total body surface area (TBSA) are not likely to heal, and even small full-thickness burns have severe risks of scarring and contractures.[15]

Assessment of burn depth is important because the vast majority of superficial partial-thickness burns will heal without surgery, but most deep partial-thickness burns require excision and skin grafting. Even the most adept burn surgeons can be fooled when predicting whether partial-thickness burns will heal, and several areas of research have been devoted to improving estimations of burn depth. Histologic diagnosis by full-thickness skin biopsy gives a consistently accurate measure of burn depth. Unfortunately, pathologic diagnosis is painful for the patient, slow, and subject to the availability of histopathologists.[16] Frozen section with immunofluorescence may be a faster method but has not made the transition to clinical use.[17] Ultrasonography has shown promise as a less painful modality that may help predict which partial-thickness burns may not heal.[18] Laser Doppler imaging has generated much interest for measuring skin perfusion and is used to predict burn depth and potential for healing.[19] Serial laser Doppler examinations have been reported to result in high specificity and positive predictive value when attempting to predict the healing of partial-thickness burns.[20] Other technologies have been useful in laboratory investigations of burn depth, but methods using techniques such as indocyanine green angiography[21] and optical coherence tomography[22] are not practical for routine clinical use. It is important to remember that burn wound depth is dynamic, and may convert from superficial partial-thickness to deep partial thickness as a result of wound infection and even under-resuscitation, according to animal studies.[23] Serial examinations of burns by an experienced surgeon are therefore mandatory throughout a patient's hospital course.

BURN SIZE

It is essential to make an accurate estimation of burn size to help determine resuscitation strategies and to give a preliminary indication of prognosis. Most formulas for resuscitation rely on the percent of body surface area burned (%TBSA). The "rule of nines" may give a quick estimation of burn size in the absence of other measuring tools (see Fig. 3). For adult patients, the anterior and posterior trunk each make up 18% of the TBSA, each lower extremity 18%, each upper extremity 9%, and the head 9%. The head in children may account for more of the total surface area. The patient's palmar surface of the hand usually approximates 1% of the TBSA, and may be used to estimate total burn size. A card of standardized size with corresponding nomograms for modified body surface area has been reported as useful for rapidly and accurately assessing burn size.[24] The Lund and Browder chart is a commonly used topographic diagram that is easy to use and accurate for estimating burn size.[25]

PROGNOSTIC INDICATORS

The classic equation for predicting mortality in burn patients in the past was simply that mortality equals patient age in years plus the %TBSA.[26] Continuing advancements in burn care have markedly decreased mortality overall, resulting in overestimation of mortality by this formula. Clearly, age, depth of burn injury, and %TBSA, along with inhalation injury, are still major contributors to mortality. One review of 1,665 burn patients led to a mortality formula with three risk factors: age older than 60 years, more than 40% TBSA burned, and presence of inhalation injury. This accurately stratifies patients into four groups based on 0, 1, 2, or 3 risk factors.[27] Mathematically adjusted functions based primarily on age also correlate with overall mortality in some series.[28] Attempts have been made to apply other existing scoring systems for critically ill patients to the burn population, but correlation with mortality is poor. Adding a burn size factor to existing scoring systems may improve their predictive value.[29] Female patients,

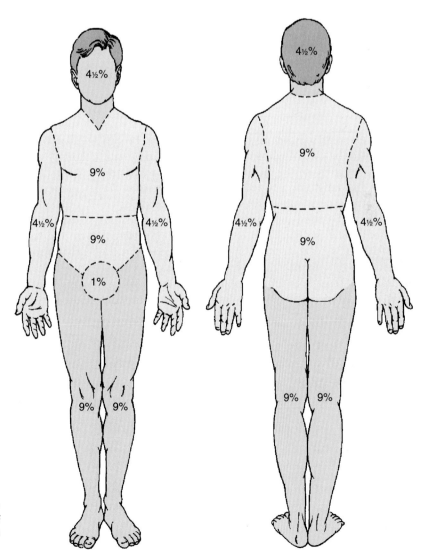

Figure 3 Rule of Nines: In "rule of nines," the adult body is divided into surface areas of fraction or multiples of 9%, which may give a quick estimation of the burn size.

especially in the 30- to 59-year-old age-group, may have a higher mortality than their male counterparts in the same age-group.[30]

RECOMMENDATIONS FOR BURN CENTER TRANSFER

In an attempt to optimize care for burn patients, the ABA and the ACS have encouraged the transfer of patients with severe burns to a verified burn center. The established guidelines for transfer include partial-thickness burns of more than 10% TBSA, and/or third-degree burns in any age-group. Patients with burns involving the face, hands, feet, genitalia, perineum, or joints should be transferred, as well as patients with electrical or chemical burns or the presence of inhalation injury. Other patients who should be referred to a burn center include those with complicated preexisting medical disorders or those who will require specialized care for social, emotional, or rehabilitative needs. This includes children in hospitals not equipped for pediatric care. Patients with associated trauma, where traumatic injuries are the primary immediate threat, must be evaluated and stabilized at an appropriate trauma center before transfer to a burn center.[31]

INITIAL MANAGEMENT OF BURN INJURIES

There are several immediate measures that must be undertaken in the care of burn patients, the most important of which is attention to the airway. The larynx typically protects the subglottic airway from direct burns, but the supraglottic airway may be exposed to heat. Swelling in this area can be rapid and cause lethal airway obstruction. Signs of inhalation injury may include facial burns, singeing of the eyebrows and nasal hair, or carbon deposits in the oropharynx or sputum. A history of explosion or confinement in a closed space during a fire may also be a harbinger of inhalation injury.[32] Known aspiration of hot liquid can precipitate a condition similar to epiglottitis and will require immediate intubation.[33] A carboxyhemoglobin level of more than 10% should also warrant closer investigation of the airway. The presence of these markers, or any other clinical suspicion of inhalation injury, should prompt elective endotracheal intubation. A patient being transferred to a burn center should be intubated before transfer.

A crucial step in the immediate care of burn patients is to stop the burning process. All clothing should be removed because many synthetic fabrics can melt into a residue that may cause ongoing burning of the patient. Dry chemical powders should be carefully brushed from the wound, and all chemical burns should be irrigated with large quantities of water for at least 20 to 30 minutes.[33] Expeditious placement of intravenous access is mandatory.

Two large-caliber peripheral intravenous lines should be placed through nonburned skin if possible, although burned skin should not deter appropriate intravenous placement. If peripheral access is difficult, central venous catheters may be necessary. Intraosseous lines should be considered in both pediatric and adult patients[34] with difficult venous access. Infusion of lactated Ringers solution should be started immediately. Discussion of resuscitation strategies will be covered later in this chapter, but regardless of formula used, unexpected hemodynamic lability during the initial evaluation may be an indication of other injuries and should prompt further investigation.

THE SECONDARY SURVEY AND ESCHAROTOMY

The secondary survey of the burned patient should include a thorough history and physical examination, with special attention paid to the burn size and depth. Evaluation of tissue perfusion is important, especially in circumferential extremity burns, in which performance of escharotomies may be necessary. Pain, numbness, delayed capillary refill, or loss of peripheral pulses may signal the need for escharotomy in the extremities. Circumferential abdominal eschar may lead to an abdominal compartment signaled by decreased urine output, hypotension, and increased airway pressures. Bedside escharotomies using simple electrocautery result in a visible release of underlying subcutaneous tissue and separation of the edges of the escharotomy line. Extra caution must be maintained to avoid injury in the areas of the upper arm (brachial artery), elbow (ulnar nerve), and knee (peroneal nerve). Thoracic escharotomies are done overlying the midline sternum and can be extended bilaterally in the subcostal areas. Lateral abdominal incisions release the abdomen and are easily extended to the lateral lower extremities if necessary. Extremity escharotomies are performed longitudinally on the medial and lateral aspects. Hand incisions extend to the thenar and hypothenar eminences, with digit escharotomies placed on the dorsolateral aspects of the fingers. Incomplete response of signs and symptoms after sufficiently generous escharotomies may signal the need for fasciotomies, which are typically performed in an operating room setting.[35]

Baseline laboratory studies should include a complete blood count (CBC), type and screen, carboxyhemoglobin, blood glucose, electrolytes, and pregnancy test in females of appropriate age. A chest x-ray may be indicated after endotracheal intubation or central line placement.[33] A nasogastric tube should be considered, and an indwelling urinary catheter is mandatory to monitor urine output as an endpoint of resuscitation. It is occasionally necessary to incise a severely burned foreskin to permit access to the urethral meatus.[36] Short-acting intravenous sedatives and narcotics should be used liberally for patient comfort. Initial coverage of the burns with clean linen helps keep the patient warm and relieves pain from air currents, and unroofing of blisters or debridement of the wound should be postponed until arrival at the location of definitive care. Prophylactic systemic antibiotics are not indicated in the treatment of acute burns.[33]

AIRWAY, BREATHING, AND VENTILATORY MANAGEMENT

Most patients with severe burn injury are intubated early for airway management and respiratory support. Pulmonary insufficiency and failure in severely burned patients are multifactorial.[37] The etiology can be differentiated into direct pulmonary and upper airway inhalation injury and indirect or secondary acute lung injury due to activation of the systemic inflammatory response.[37] Inhalation of hot air may cause upper airway, above vocal cords, burn that is particularly dangerous because swelling in this area can be rapid and cause lethal airway obstruction. In addition, inhalation of carbon particles, products of incomplete combustion, toxic gases, and organic acids can cause upper airway, lower airway, and alveolar injury. CO intoxication is a lethal complication of inhalation injury, which is covered at the end of this section. As already mentioned, any history of closed space fire should raise suspicion for inhalation injury. This is particularly important if there is history of prolonged exposure and confinement, such as being unconscious in a closed space fire. Early intubation before development of airway or pulmonary dysfunction is essential.

There is also secondary delayed pulmonary injury due to the systemic inflammatory response syndrome, sepsis, and pneumonia. In addition, ventilator-associated lung injury has been described as an important iatrogenic factor contributing to the secondary accentuation of pulmonary injury.[38] The reduced pulmonary compliance and chest wall rigidity of burn patients can lead to aggressive ventilator management and high airway pressures, exacerbating acute lung injury. Institution of low-tidal volume ventilation, allowing permissive hypercapnia was shown to reduce the development of ventilator-associated lung injury and significantly improve outcomes.[38] Additionally, use of alternate ventilation strategies such as high-frequency oscillatory and percussive ventilations may be beneficial in selected burn patients.[39] Although there is limited comparative data regarding these two strategies, it appears that high-frequency percussive ventilation is especially useful in inhalation injuries.[40]

Clinical suspicion of inhalation injury can be quickly confirmed by fiber optic bronchoscopy. Significant findings include erythema, carbonaceous deposits, edema, bronchorrhea, and friability, which infrequently progresses to frank hemorrhage. Mucosal sloughing can lead to endoluminal obliteration.[41] Adjunctive radiology is generally not helpful, although thoracic computed tomography (CT), ^{99}Technetium (^{99}Tc) scanning, and xenon scanning have been investigated for use in inhalation injury.[42]

Treatment of inhalation injury is still restricted primarily to supportive care. Inhaled β-agonists may ameliorate bronchospasm, and investigation continues regarding the use of other nebulized agents such as acetylcysteine and aerosolized heparin. These additional therapies have been shown to transiently improve pulmonary variables but have not impacted mortality.[25] Steroids have no benefit after inhalation injury, and may actually worsen outcomes.[43] Recombinant human antithrombin[44] and aerosolized tissue plasminogen activator[45] are effective in animal models of inhalation injury, but have not yet seen widespread clinical use. For patients with inhalation injuries that are refractory to treatment with conventional therapies, intrabronchial surfactant[46] or inhaled nitric oxide[47] may be useful in salvage situations.

An important and potentially lethal complication of inhalation injury is CO poisoning. It should be suspected in patients with inappropriate neurologic symptoms, and may be manifested by a "cherry red" appearance of the patient's skin. Pulse oximetry is inaccurate in patients with CO poisoning, so carboxyhemoglobin levels must be obtained by arterial blood gas. A carboxyhemoglobin level of 5% or less is considered normal, and levels above 10% may be associated with clinical symptoms such as headache, confusion, and disorientation. Prolonged exposure or high levels of carboxyhemoglobin may be associated with significant complications and death. Therapy with 100% oxygen is the gold standard for elimination of CO. The half-life of CO is approximately 250 minutes in room air but drops to 40 to 60 minutes with administration of 100% oxygen.[48] Hyperbaric oxygen therapy has been used in an attempt to improve neurologic outcomes in severe inhalation injury,[49] but "diving" of critically ill patients often presents logistic difficulties that have limited its use in burn patients.

RESUSCITATION

Burn trauma leads to a combination of hypovolemic and distributive shock on the basis of generalized microvascular injury and interstitial third-spacing through collagen and matrix degeneration.[37] Burn injury is marked by a dynamic and ongoing fluid shift that has led to the development of fluid resuscitation formulas based on percentage of TBSA burn and weight. Fluid resuscitation based on the Parkland burn formula is extensively used in burn centers and has helped minimize the occurrence of burn shock.[50] Most surgeons agree that the estimated need of a burn patient in the first 24 hours is 2 to 4 mL/kg/% body surface burn, half of which is given in the first 8 hours and the other half is given in subsequent 16 hours. Therefore, a 100 kg patient with 30% body surface area burn will require 6 to 12 L of fluid, commonly warm Ringers lactate, in the first 24 hours. However, a recent survey of 28 burn centers found that in 58% of patients actual fluid resuscitation exceeded the 4 mL per kg recommended by Baxter.[51] Over-resuscitation has been shown to correlate directly with rising intra-abdominal pressure and the development of abdominal compartment syndrome.[52] Apart from the well-described extremity compartment syndrome, orbital compartment syndrome requiring canthotomy in patients receiving supranormal resuscitation was recently described.[53] The current high-volume fluid regimens have shifted postburn resuscitation complications from renal failure to pulmonary edema with increased requirement for ventilatory support, the need for fasciotomies in unburned limbs, and the occurrence of the abdominal compartment syndrome.[54]

Warm crystalloid solutions such as lactated Ringers solution and normal saline are still first line fluid replacements in burn resuscitation.[37] Owing to reduced intravascular fluid retention, large volumes have to be infused, which accentuate tissue edema, and the development of tissue edema can lead to worsening outcomes.[55] Hypertonic saline (HTS) resuscitation (7.5% NaCl) has been promoted for its efficient intravascular volume resuscitation, rapid restoration of blood pressure and cardiac output with improved cerebral perfusion, and potential for expanding circulating volume by reabsorption of fluid from the interstitial space.[56] More recently, HTS has been studied as a fluid with significant modulation of systemic inflammatory response secondary to reperfusion injury, which may be beneficial in patients with shock.[57,58] In animal models of trauma and burn, use of HTS resuscitation has been associated with decreased edema and improved organ perfusion and outcomes.[59–61] Data on the effectiveness of HTS to prevent organ damage in the clinical setting are inconsistent.[62] Some of the studies in burn patients have demonstrated that HTS may decrease the fluid load, tissue edema, and complications such as abdominal compartment syndrome.[63–65] However, others have noted no benefit in fluid requirement and potentially increase the risk of renal failure.[66] It appears that the benefit of HTS is seen in early resuscitation,[67] and some researchers have recommended stopping HTS infusion when serum sodium concentration exceeds 160 mEq per L.[54,68] Currently, HTS is not routinely used in burn patients, and further research is required to better define potential benefits, the timing, and the optimal volume.

Theoretically, the use of colloids in resuscitation of hypovolemic patients may be associated with preservation of plasma osmotic pressure, more efficient plasma volume expansion, and decreased tissue and pulmonary edema.[37] However, clinical studies have not demonstrated a significant improvement in patient outcomes with colloid resuscitation.[56,69,70] In burn patients, treatment with albumin did not improve outcomes.[69]

A recent multicenter cohort analysis found an increased mortality in burn patients associated with blood transfusions.[71] Therefore, there is a push to decrease blood transfusion in burn patients. Recombinant human erythropoietin has been shown to be useful in treatment of chronic anemia, and theoretically may decrease the need for blood transfusion in the intensive care unit (ICU). However, in a prospective double-blinded randomized study of 40 severely burned patients, recombinant human erythropoietin did not prevent the development of postburn anemia or decrease transfusion requirements.[72]

NUTRITION AND METABOLIC RESPONSE

Severely burned patients have an impressive hyperdynamic response. A study in pediatric patients with >40% TBSA burn demonstrated that the resting metabolic rate is increased in the ranges between 160% and 200%.[73] This global hypermetabolism is associated with tachycardia, fever, muscle protein catabolism, and derangement in hepatic protein synthesis.[74,75] This response may be associated with significant complications such as immunodeficiency, impaired wound healing, sepsis, loss of lean body and muscle mass, cardiac ischemia, and potential death.[37] Primary treatment modalities include avoidance of infectious complications such as sepsis and early excision of full-thickness burns, which is associated with attenuation of hypermetabolism.[75–77] The use of early enteral feeding in burn patients may attenuate catabolic response after thermal injury.[78] Because there is significant increase in energy expenditure after burns, high-calorie nutritional support was thought to decrease muscle catabolism. However, aggressive high-calorie feeding with a combination of enteral and parenteral nutrition was associated with increased mortality.[79] Most authors recommend adequate calorie intake through enteral feeding and avoidance of overfeeding. The protein requirement is raised to 1.5 to 2.0 g/kg/day in treatment of severely burned patients.[77]

Management of elevated glucose levels should be part of the nutritional support in patients with thermal injury. In a study of 58 pediatric burn patients, there was a significant association between poor glucose control and complications such as increased bacteremia, reduced skin graft take, and increased mortality.[80] In another study, tight glucose control in severely burned patients appeared to be safe and associated with decreased risk of infection and improved survival.[81] Therefore, aggressive monitoring and treatment of hyperglycemia are recommended.

Immune Enhancing Agents

The immune-enhancing agents include arginine, glutamine, Omega 3 fatty acids, and antioxidants such as ascorbic acid (vitamin C) and α-tocopherol (vitamin E).[37] Most researchers agree that an indiscriminate use of a combination formula immunonutrition-diet in the critically ill patients is not beneficial.[82,83] Therefore, a more selective approach is proposed, and there is a need for more clinical studies. For instance, use of high doses of ascorbic acid in experimental burn sheep was associated with decreased edema and fluid requirement.[84] In a randomized trial of critically ill surgical patients, a combination of ascorbic acid and α-tocopherol reduced the incidence of organ failure and ICU length of stay.[85] Early use of high-dose antioxidant therapy in the injured patients appears to be beneficial; however, further clinical trials are required to confirm this potential effect and better define the timing and the required dose.[86,87]

Modulation of Endocrine and Hormonal Response

Burn injury is associated with increased levels of catecholamines.[37] In burn patients, β-blockers can blunt the catecholamine effect by attenuating hypermetabolism, decreasing oxygen demand and resting energy expenditure, and decreasing heart rate and cardiac oxygen demand.[77] β-blockers may also attenuate catecholamines-induced muscle catabolism and lipolysis.[88,89] Moreover, there is data to suggest that β-blockers can modify catecholamine-mediated defect in lymphocyte activation and improve immune response with decreased infectious complications.[90] In a randomized study of 25 children with severe burns, treatment with propranolol-attenuated hypermetabolism and reversed muscle-protein catabolism.[91] In a retrospective study of adult burn patients, use of β-blockers was associated with decreased mortality, wound infection rate, and wound healing time.[92] There are no large randomized studies looking at mortality and wound healing in burn patients. However, many burn units use β-blockers such as propranolol or metoprolol as the most effective catabolic treatment in burn patients.[37]

Burn injury is associated with increased levels of catabolic hormones, and use of anabolic steroids may attenuate hypermetabolism or blunt catabolic response after burn injury. Oxandrolone, a testosterone analog, is an anabolic hormone that is commonly used in burn patients. In a study of 14 severely burned children, oxandrolone improved muscle protein metabolism through enhanced protein synthesis efficiency.[93] In adult burn patients, oxandrolone significantly decreased weight loss and net nitrogen loss and increased donor site wound healing compared with placebo controls.[94] In a prospective randomized study of 81 patients, 10 mg oxandrolone every 12 hours was associated with decreased hospital stay.[95] Although there was no hepatic insufficiency, a significant increase in hepatic transaminases was observed.

OUTPATIENT MANAGEMENT OF BURN INJURIES

Patients with minor burns and no evidence of inhalation injury can potentially be managed as outpatients. The ABA classifies minor burns as <10% TBSA in an adult or <5% TBSA in children or the elderly, with <2% TBSA full-thickness burns for any patient.[31] However, some patients with minor burns may still need hospital admission. These are patients with circumferential injury, immunosuppressed patients, or patients with a high-voltage electrical injury and ECG abnormalities.[96] Also, any suspicion of child abuse in burned children mandates hospital admission. It has been reported that up to 11% of pediatric burns are not accidental, with children aged 13 to 24 months at highest risk.[97]

For those patients meeting requirements for outpatient burn care, their burn wounds must first be thoroughly cleaned. Pretreatment with narcotics may be necessary for the initial cleansing. Washing with mild soap and water is optimal, and disinfectant solutions are not recommended as they may interfere with healing.[98] Ruptured blisters should be debrided, and blisters that appear likely to rupture should be unroofed and washed, rather than aspirated.[99] Tetanus immunization should be updated if necessary in superficial partial-thickness burns or deeper. Superficial burns do not require topical antibiotics, but deeper burns require silver sulfadiazine cream (Silvadene) and covering with a sterile dressing. Contraindications to the use of Silvadene include facial burns, sulfa allergies, and pregnant or breast-feeding patients as well as newborns due to the risk of sulfonamide kernicterus.[100] Bacitracin is an alternative in these situations and is favored by some due to its lower cost.[101] Silver-impregnated dressings such as Acticoat (Westhaim Biomedical, Saskatchewan, Canada) or Aquacel-Ag (Convatec, Princeton, NJ) are costlier but have the advantage of less frequent dressing changes. Biologic wound membranes such as Porcine Xenograft (Brennan Medical, St. Paul, MN) or Biobrane (Dow-Hickham, Sugarland, TX) mimic physiologic wound closure, giving the underlying wound time to heal. Because these are typically occlusive dressings and are changed at longer intervals, it is essential that they only be used in very clean, superficial partial-thickness burns.[102] Patients managed as outpatients should be seen the day after injury to assess adequacy of pain control and wound management. Subsequent follow-up can be extended to once or twice weekly after that, unless concerns about patient or family competence with wound care mandate more frequent visits.[103] Long-term issues such as scar management and reconstruction are beyond the scope of this article, but suffice it to say that any concerns with inadequate healing should prompt referral to a surgeon experienced in the management of burn wounds.

SURGERY

When a burned patient has been adequately stabilized and fully resuscitated, attention may be turned to surgical treatment of their burn wounds. The traditional approach of expectant management of the wound until sloughing of the eschar was prone to high risks of wound sepsis and mortality. Though Janzekovic described early excision and skin grafting in 1970,[6] it took several years before this approach became widely accepted. As more studies continued to show improved survival and shorter stay, even for patients with large burns, this became the standard of care.[7,104–107] The extent of excision at this time was limited not only by available donor sites but also by intraoperative blood loss. Techniques such as tourniquets, epinephrine clysis,[108] and topical thrombin[25] have dramatically reduced intraoperative bleeding and transfusion needs.[109]

Newer studies consistently show that earlier wound excision decreases invasive wound infection, shortens time to definitive closure, and decreases overall hospital stay.[110] Earlier excision also plays a role in decreasing the profound inflammatory and hypermetabolic response seen in patients with large burns,[111] and in conjunction with early enteral nutrition can decrease catabolism of muscle protein.[112] Earlier, time to wound closure may also decrease the risk of heterotopic ossification.[113] All these findings have led surgeons to push for even earlier complete excision in extremely large burns. An approach using early near-total wound excision will typically require cadaveric allograft or synthetic skin substitutes given a shortage of donor sites.[25]

Tangential excision of the burn wound is the standard method for preserving viable dermis, which will have a whitish appearance with diffuse punctuate bleeding. Deep full-thickness burns may require excision to fascia to adequately remove all burned tissue. Debridement of difficult anatomic areas such as the face and hands may be accomplished with a pressurized water dissector.[114] Autografting of the patient's nonburned skin is the optimal method for wound coverage after burn excision. Split-thickness donor skin is harvested with a pneumatic dermatome, preferably from less conspicuous sites such as the thighs and back. Meshing of the donor skin allows for greater surface area coverage, and allows drainage and prevention of hematoma or seroma formation. However, nonmeshed skin should be used if possible in cosmetically sensitive areas. Staples and absorbable sutures have traditionally been used for graft fixation. A multicenter randomized trial showed that fibrin sealant may be superior to staples for securing autologous sheet grafts.[115] Reinforcement with vacuum-assisted closure devices has been shown to be helpful in decreasing graft loss and shortening hospital length of stay.[116,117] If immobilization of a body part is necessary to ensure graft adherence, the affected part should be immediately splinted in an antideformity position by an experienced therapist.[118]

Unfortunately, even the use of meshed grafts may not provide adequate donor skin for extremely large burns. This has led to investigation into potential skin substitutes. Hope of a permanent skin substitute comprising both epidermal and dermal layers is yet unfulfilled. Temporary biologic membranes such as cryopreserved split-thickness human allograft (cadaveric skin),[119] porcine xenograft,[120] and human amniotic membrane[121] allow for excellent temporary coverage but require excision at a later date followed by autografting for definitive coverage. Because of these limitations, efforts have been focused on developing permanent substitutes. Integra (Integra LifeSciences Corporation, Plainsboro, NJ) is the most widely used synthetic skin substitute in burn patients. Integra is a bilaminar structure consisting of a collagen-chondroitin 6-sulphate inner layer coated on one side with a silicone membrane that mimics epidermal function.[122] Integra use requires a two-stage procedure. After initial application, a 2- to 3-week period is required for the artificial dermis to become vascularized. During this period, the silastic coating prevents fluid loss and bacterial invasion. After the neodermis is established, the silastic may be removed and an epithelial autograft placed over the involved areas. Integra has been especially useful in large burns[123] and difficult areas such as the hands[124] and face.[125] The use of several sequential layers of Integra has been successfully used in treating complex wounds with volume loss, and in fourth-degree burns involving tendon or bone.[126] Alloderm (LifeCell, Woodlands, TX) is a similar dermal substitute consisting of processed and freeze-dried acellular human cadaveric dermis. This in combination with thin split-thickness skin grafts may be equivalent to thicker autografts alone.[127]

Despite their obvious contributions to burn surgery, the dermal substitutes are hampered by the persistent need for subsequent epidermal coverage. Cultured epithelial autografts, despite logistic difficulties such as poor handling and lengthy time for culture and harvest, are still used in clinical practice for extensive burns.[128] An exciting new development is a cultured skin substitute made up of a collagen-glycosaminoglycan substrate with autologous fibroblasts and keratinocytes. Studies using this new substitute in combination with Integra have resulted in good graft take, adequate cosmetic results, and less donor site use in large burns.[129,130] Larger partial-thickness burns are usually managed expectantly without surgical intervention. Particularly in the pediatric population, however, frequent dressing changes can be painful and may require longer inpatient therapy. Bioengineered skin substitutes such as TransCyte (Smith & Nephew) may hasten reepithelialization and decrease the overall number of dressing changes.[131]

There is a wide array of coverings available for donor sites, including calcium alginate dressings, hydrocolloids, transparent films, xenografts, xeroform and petrolatum gauze, Scarlet Red, and Biobrane.[132] Though it can be largely a matter of surgeon preference, optimal coverage of donor sites has been examined in several recent studies. One animal study showed that glycosaminoglycan hydrogels in combination with a transparent film accelerated donor site healing compared to a transparent film alone.[133] A β-glucan polymer was superior to calcium sodium alginate dressings in another prospective study of donor site dressings.[134] Silver-impregnated dressings, despite being effective for burn wounds, showed worse scarring of donor sites when compared to a hydrophilic polyurethane dressing.[135]

Long-term scar management and reconstruction, as well as physical therapy and rehabilitation, would each warrant their own reviews and will not be covered here. We simply recommend early involvement of a multidisciplinary team including physical and occupational therapists and surgeons experienced in burn reconstructive surgery.

FUTURE PROMISING THERAPIES

Severe burn injury is associated with increased risk of sepsis and systemic inflammatory response syndrome, which are correlated with a high risk of end-organ failure.[39,136–138] Therefore, many investigators have studied the benefit of immune-modulation in severely burned patients. The therapies discussed here are currently either experimental or are not yet proved to be beneficial in patients with thermal injury.

Recombinant Human Activated Protein C

Recombinant human activated protein C (activated drotrecogin alfa) is the first U.S. Food and Drug Administration (FDA)-approved agent for treatment of severe sepsis. *Post hoc* analyses of 532 possible surgical patients in the Protein C Worldwide Evaluation in Severe Sepsis (PROWESS) trial demonstrated a favorable benefit/risk profile in surgical patients.[139,140] Twenty-four patients in this group were defined as having a skin surgical procedure in the 30 days before the study. Increased risk of bleeding was similar to the medical patients, and there was no fatal bleeding in the surgical cohort. There was a 12-hour waiting period after a surgery before starting the treatment and patients with anticipated need for surgery within the ensuing 96-hour period were excluded. In a case presentation of 12 patients with soft tissue injury (8 patients with burn injury and 2 with toxic epidermal necrolysis) and sepsis, Brunsvold et al. concluded that recombinant human activated protein C is a potential treatment modality for patients with large soft tissue injury and severe sepsis.[141] The mortality rate was 50%, which compares to reported 3 months survival of 58.9% in the *post hoc* analysis of patients with severe sepsis in the PROWESS trial. Three patients had soft tissue/dermal bleeding, which stopped after early cessation of drotrecogin alfa. It should also be noted that since 90% of the drug is eliminated within 2 hours of discontinuation of infusion, stopping the treatment should rapidly stop drotrecogin alfa-induced bleeding.[139] Although there are no published trials in burn patients, on the basis of available information, those with severe sepsis who lack the exclusion criteria may be considered for recombinant activated protein C.

Topical Immunomodulation

Thermal injury induces dermal inflammatory and proapoptotic signaling. The burn wound is the inflammatory source triggering systemic inflammatory response through liberation of a plethora of potentially deleterious proinflammatory mediators and attraction/activation of neutrophils.[142–144] Studies using rodent models of thermal injury have demonstrated that controlling the source of inflammation at the dermis may attenuate systemic inflammatory response and acute lung injury.[145,146] In these studies, topical application of p38-mitogen–activated protein kinase-inhibitor to the burn wound decreased dermal inflammation, postburn skin apoptosis, and secondary pulmonary complications. Topical inflammatory modulation in severe burns is attractive because it can be readily used in patients who are already receiving topical antimicrobial agents, and it may avoid some of the systemic complications. However, currently there are no clinically approved topical immunomodulators for burn patients.

Plasma Exchange in Treatment of Burn Patients

Some authors have suggested plasma exchange in treatment of burn patients in shock who continue to require high-volume resuscitation and are not responsive to conventional therapy. The hypothesis is that this process will remove the systemic inflammatory mediators in the serum of burn patients and improve their outcomes. In therapeutic plasma exchange, patient plasma is removed and replaced with a colloid replacement solution such as 5% human serum albumin (most common) in saline or fresh frozen plasma.[147] A randomized trial of plasma exchange in treatment of burn shock in 22 patients demonstrated no significant difference in the total fluid requirement but there was an increase in mean urine output.[148] Further studies are required to study this potential therapy.

BURN PREVENTION

The ideal treatment for burns is prevention of the initial injury. Unfortunately, there is much room for improvement in the area of burn prevention. Several interventions have proved their worth in community-based interventions. A working smoke alarm reduces the risk of death from residential fire by at least 50%. Despite this, only 75% of US households have a functioning smoke alarm, and low-income households are at particular risk. The Centers for Disease Control and Prevention (CDC) instituted a program in which they installed 212,000 smoke alarms in

126,000 high-risk homes, with fire safety education and 6-month follow-up to ensure functioning alarms. They estimated that at least 610 lives were saved as a direct result of the program, with potential additional benefit through lateral teaching of friends and neighbors.[149] It is crucial that education on installation and use of alarms be included in any community intervention because mere distribution of free smoke alarms without any directed teaching does not incur the same benefit.[150] Other successful community interventions have included flame-retardant sleepwear for children[151] and regulation of hot water temperatures below 49°C.[152] One detailed scald prevention program used education, home inspections, and installation of antiscald devices. Though resource intensive, this program was associated with a decrease in scald admissions by more than 50% in the involved community over a 2-year period.[153]

SUMMARY

Burns continue to be a major source of injury throughout the world. Breakthroughs in critical care and wound management have led to dramatic decreases in mortality for even large burns, but much work remains. Even as progress continues on improving burn survival, the burn community is striving to better address the functional outcomes of patients with severe burns. The implementation of new technologies into the structure of multidisciplinary burn care makes this a dynamic and exciting field. It behooves all trauma, critical care, and acute care surgeons to become familiar with the basics of burn care and to stay abreast of new developments in this constantly evolving specialty.

REFERENCES

1. American Burn Association. *Burn incidence and treatment in the US: 2007 fact sheet.* Available at http://www.ameriburn.org/resources_factsheet.php. Accessed April 10, 2007.
2. Burke JF. Burn treatment's evolution in the 20th century. *J Am Coll Surg.* 2005;200:152–153.
3. Underhill FP. The significance of anydremia in extensive superficial burns. *JAMA.* 1930;95:852–857.
4. Saffle JR. The fire at Boston's Cocoanut Grove nightclub. *Am J Surg.* 1993;166:581–591.
5. Thompson JC. Gifts from surgical research. Contributions to patients and to surgeons. *J Am Coll Surg.* 2000;190:509–521.
6. Janzekovic Z. A new concept in the early excision and immediate grafting of burns. *J Trauma.* 1970;10(12):1103–1108.
7. Burke JF, Quinby WC Jr, Bondoc CC. Primary excision and prompt grafting as routine therapy for the treatment of thermal burns in children. *Surg Clin North Am.* 1976;56:477–494.
8. Supple KG, Fiala SM, Gamelli RL. Preparation for burn center verification. *J Burn Care Rehabil.* 1997;18:58–60.
9. Arnoldo B, Klein M, Gibran NS. Practice guidelines for the management of electrical injuries. *J Burn Care Res.* 2006;27(4):439–447.
10. Koumbourlis AC. Electrical Injuries. *Crit Care Med.* 2002;30(11): S424–S430.
11. Goodwin CW, Finkelstein JL, Madden MR. Burns. In: Schwartz SI, Shires TG, Spencer FC, eds. *Principles of surgery,* 6th ed. New York: McGraw-Hill; 1994.
12. Hatzifotis M, Williams A, Muller M, et al. Hydrofluoric acid burns. *Burns.* 2004;30(2):156–159.
13. Dunser MW, Ohlbauer M, Rieder J, et al. Critical care management of major hydrofluoric acid burns: A case report, review of the literature, and recommendations for therapy. *Burns.* 2004;30(4):391–398.
14. Nguyen LT, Mohr WJ III, Ahrenholz DH, et al. Treatment of hydrofluoric acid burn to the face by carotid artery infusion of calcium gluconate. *J Burn Care Rehabil.* 2004;25(5):421–424.
15. Morgan ED, Bledsoe SC, Barker J. Ambulatory management of burns. *Am Fam Physician.* 2000;62:2015–2026, 2029–2030, 2032.
16. Watts AM, Tyler MP, Perry ME, et al. Burn depth and its histological measurement. *Burns.* 2001;27(2):154–160.
17. Ho-Asjoe M, Chronnell CM, Frame JD, et al. Immunohistochemical analysis of burn depth. *J Burn Care Rehabil.* 1999;20(3):207–211.
18. Iraniha S, Cinat ME, VanderKam VM, et al. Determination of burn depth with noncontact ultrasonography. *J Burn Care Rehabil.* 2000;21(4):333–338.
19. Bray R, Forrester K, Leonard C, et al. Laser Doppler imaging of burn scars: A comparison of wavelength and scanning methods. *Burns.* 2003;29(3):199–206.
20. Mileski WJ, Atiles L, Purdue G, et al. Serial measurements increase the accuracy of laser Doppler assessment of burn wounds. *J Burn Care Rehabil.* 2003;24:187–191.
21. Kamolz LP, Andel H, Haslik W, et al. Indocyanine green video angiographies help to identify burns requiring operation. *Burns.* 2003;29(8):785–791.
22. Srinivas SM, de Boer JF, Park H, et al. Determination of burn depth by polarization-sensitive optical coherence tomography. *J Biomed Opt.* 2004;9(1):207–212.
23. Kim DE, Phillips TM, Jeng JC, et al. Microvascular assessment of burn depth conversion during varying resuscitation conditions. *J Burn Care Rehabil.* 2001;22(6):406–416.
24. Malic CC, Karoo RO, Austin O, et al. Resuscitation burn card – a useful tool for burn injury assessment. *Burns.* 2007;33:195–199.
25. Ramzy PI, Barret JP, Herndon DN. Thermal injury. *Crit Care Clin.* 1999;15(2):333–352.
26. Zawacki BE, Azen SP, Imbus SH, et al. Multifactorial probit analysis of mortality in burn patients. *Ann Surg.* 1979;189:1–5.
27. Ryan CM, Schoenfeld DA, Thorpe WP, et al. Objective estimates of the probability of death from burn injuries. *N Engl J Med.* 1998;338:362–366.
28. Moreau AR, Westfall PH, Cancio LC, et al. Development and validation of an age-risk score for mortality prediction after thermal injury. *J Trauma.* 2005;58(5):967–972.
29. O'Mara MS, Tran T, Palmieri TL, et al. Standard scoring systems correlate with survival in burn patients, but underestimate mortality. *Presented in Abstract form at the American Burn Association 2007 Annual Meeting.* San Diego; 2007. March 20–23.
30. O'Keefe GE, Hunt JL, Purdue GF. An evaluation of risk factors for mortality after burn trauma and the identification of gender-dependent differences in outcomes. *J Am Coll Surg.* 2001;192:153–160.
31. American College of Surgeons. *Resources for optimal care of the injured patient: 2007.* Chapter 14. Available at www.ameriburn.org/Chapter14.pdf. Accessed April 30, 2007.
32. American College of Surgeons Committee on Trauma. Injuries due to burns and cold. In: *Advanced trauma life support student manual,* 6th ed. Chicago: American College of Surgeons; 1997:273–288.
33. Sheridan RL. Recognition and management of hot liquid aspiration in children. *Ann Emerg Med.* 1996;27:89–91.
34. Frascone R, Kaye K, Dries D, et al. Successful placement of an adult sternal intraosseous line through burned skin. *J Burn Care Rehabil.* 2003;24(5):306–308.
35. Wolf SE, Herndon DN. Burns. In: Townsend CM, ed. *Sabiston textbook of surgery,* 17th ed. Philadelphia: WB Saunders; 2004:578.
36. Sheridan RL. Burns. *Crit Care Med.* 2002;30(11):S500–S514.
37. Ipaktchi K, Arbabi S. Advances in burn critical care. *Crit Care Med.* 2006;34(Suppl 9):S239–S244.

38. The Acute Respiratory Distress Syndrome Network. Ventilation with lower tidal volumes as compared with traditional tidal volumes for acute lung injury and the acute respiratory distress syndrome. *N Engl J Med.* 2000;342(18):1301–1308.

39. Cartotto R, Ellis S, Smith T. Use of high-frequency oscillatory ventilation in burn patients. *Crit Care Med.* 2005;33(Suppl 3): S175–S181.

40. Cioffi WG Jr, Rue LW III, Graves TA, et al. Prophylactic use of high-frequency percussive ventilation in patients with inhalation injury. *Ann Surg.* 1991;213(6):575–580; Discussion 580–2.

41. Endorf F, Gamelli RL. Inhalation injury, pulmonary perturbations, and fluid resuscitation. *J Burn Care Res.* 2007;28(1): 80–83.

42. Evidence-based surgery. *J Am Coll Surg.* 2003;196(2):308–312.

43. Moylan JA, Alexander LG Jr. Diagnosis and treatment of inhalation injury. *World J Surg.* 1978;2:185–191.

44. Murakami K, McGuire R, Cox RA, et al. Recombinant antithrombin attenuates pulmonary inflammation following smoke inhalation and pneumonia in sheep. *Crit Care Med.* 2003;31(2):577–583.

45. Enkhbaatar P, Murakami K, Cox R, et al. Aerosolized tissue plasminogen inhibitor improves pulmonary function in sheep with burn and smoke inhalation. *Shock.* 2004;22(1):70–75.

46. Pallua N, Warbanow K, Noah EM, et al. Intrabronchial surfactant application in cases of inhalation injury: First results from patients with severe burns and ARDS. *Burns.* 1998;24(3): 197–206.

47. Sheridan RL, Hurford WE, Kacmarek RM, et al. Inhaled nitric oxide in burn patients with respiratory failure. *J Trauma.* 1997;42:629–634.

48. Crapo RO. Smoke-inhalation injuries. *JAMA.* 1981;246:1694–1696.

49. Sheridan RL, Tompkins RG. What's new in burns and metabolism. *J Am Coll Surg.* 2004;198(2):243–263.

50. Baxter CR, Shires T. Physiological response to crystalloid resuscitation of severe burns. *Ann N Y Acad Sci.* 1968;150(3):874–894.

51. Engrav LH, Colescott PL, Kemalyan N, et al. A biopsy of the use of the Baxter formula to resuscitate burns or do we do it like Charlie did it? *J Burn Care Rehabil.* 2000;21(2):91–95.

52. O'Mara MS, Slater H, Goldfarb IW, et al. A prospective, randomized evaluation of intra-abdominal pressures with crystalloid and colloid resuscitation in burn patients. *J Trauma.* 2005;58(5): 1011–1018.

53. Sullivan SR, Ahmadi AJ, Singh CN, et al. Elevated orbital pressure: Another untoward effect of massive resuscitation after burn injury. *J Trauma.* 2006;60(1):72–76.

54. Pruitt BA Jr. Does hypertonic burn resuscitation make a difference? *Crit Care Med.* 2000;28(1):277–278.

55. Ahrns KS. Trends in burn resuscitation: Shifting the focus from fluids to adequate endpoint monitoring, edema control, and adjuvant therapies. *Crit Care Nurs Clin North Am.* 2004;16(1): 75–98.

56. Arbabi S. Hypovolemic shock. In: Mulholland MW, Doherty GM, eds. *Complications in surgery.* Philadelphia: Lippincott Williams & Wilkins; 2005:136–143.

57. Staudenmayer KL, Maier RV, Jelacic S, et al. Hypertonic saline modulates innate immunity in a model of systemic inflammation. *Shock.* 2005;23(5):459–463.

58. Arbabi S, Rosengart MR, Garcia I, et al. Hypertonic saline solution induces prostacyclin production by increasing cyclooxygenase-2 expression. *Surgery.* 2000;128(2):198–205.

59. Murao Y, Loomis W, Wolf P, et al. Effect of dose of hypertonic saline on its potential to prevent lung tissue damage in a mouse model of hemorrhagic shock. *Shock.* 2003;20(1):29–34.

60. Angle N, Hoyt DB, Cabello-Passini R, et al. Hypertonic saline resuscitation reduces neutrophil margination by suppressing neutrophil L selectin expression. *J Trauma.* 1998;45(1):7–12. Discussion 12–3.

61. Kien ND, Antognini JF, Reilly DA, et al. Small-volume resuscitation using hypertonic saline improves organ perfusion in burned rats. *Anesth Analg.* 1996;83(4):782–788.

62. Murao Y, Hoyt DB, Loomis W, et al. Does the timing of hypertonic saline resuscitation affect its potential to prevent lung damage? *Shock.* 2000;14(1):18–23.

63. Bortolani A, Governa M, Barisoni D. Fluid replacement in burned patients. *Acta Chir Plast.* 1996;38(4):132–136.

64. Griswold JA, Anglin BL, Love RT Jr, et al. Hypertonic saline resuscitation: Efficacy in a community-based burn unit. *South Med J.* 1991;84(6):692–696.

65. Shimazaki S, Yukioka T, Matuda H. Fluid distribution and pulmonary dysfunction following burn shock. *J Trauma.* 1991;31(5):623–626. Discussion 626–8.

66. Huang PP, Stucky FS, Dimick AR, et al. Hypertonic sodium resuscitation is associated with renal failure and death. *Ann Surg.* 1995;221(5):543–554. Discussion 554–7.

67. Elgjo GI, Poli de Figueiredo LF, Schenarts PJ, et al. Hypertonic saline dextran produces early (8–12 hrs) fluid sparing in burn resuscitation: A 24-hr prospective, double-blind study in sheep. *Crit Care Med.* 2000;28(1):163–171.

68. Shimazaki S, Yoshioka T, Tanaka N, et al. Body fluid changes during hypertonic lactated saline solution therapy for burn shock. *J Trauma.* 1977;17(1):38–43.

69. Cooper AB, Cohn SM, Zhang HS, et al. Five percent albumin for adult burn shock resuscitation: Lack of effect on daily multiple organ dysfunction score. *Transfusion.* 2006;46(1):80–89.

70. Finfer S, Bellomo R, Boyce N, et al. A comparison of albumin and saline for fluid resuscitation in the intensive care unit. *N Engl J Med.* 2004;350(22):2247–2256.

71. Palmieri TL, Caruso DM, Foster KN, et al. Effect of blood transfusion on outcome after major burn injury: A multicenter study. *Crit Care Med.* 2006;34(6):1602–1607.

72. Still JM Jr, Belcher K, Law EJ, et al. A double-blinded prospective evaluation of recombinant human erythropoietin in acutely burned patients. *J Trauma.* 1995;38(2):233–236.

73. Hart DW, Wolf SE, Mlcak R, et al. Persistence of muscle catabolism after severe burn. *Surgery.* 2000;128(2):312–319.

74. Hart DW, Wolf SE, Herndon DN, et al. Energy expenditure and caloric balance after burn: Increased feeding leads to fat rather than lean mass accretion. *Ann Surg.* 2002;235(1):152–161.

75. Hart DW, Wolf SE, Chinkes DL, et al. Determinants of skeletal muscle catabolism after severe burn. *Ann Surg.* 2000;232(4): 455–465.

76. Hart DW, Wolf SE, Chinkes DL, et al. Effects of early excision and aggressive enteral feeding on hypermetabolism, catabolism, and sepsis after severe burn. *J Trauma.* 2003;54(4):755–761. Discussion 761–4.

77. Herndon DN, Tompkins RG. Support of the metabolic response to burn injury. *Lancet.* 2004;363(9424):1895–1902.

78. Mochizuki H, Trocki O, Dominioni L, et al. Mechanism of prevention of postburn hypermetabolism and catabolism by early enteral feeding. *Ann Surg.* 1984;200(3):297–310.

79. Herndon DN, Barrow RE, Stein M, et al. Increased mortality with intravenous supplemental feeding in severely burned patients. *J Burn Care Rehabil.* 1989;10(4):309–313.

80. Gore DC, Chinkes D, Heggers J, et al. Association of hyperglycemia with increased mortality after severe burn injury. *J Trauma.* 2001;51(3):540–544.

81. Pham TN, Warren AJ, Phan HH, et al. Impact of tight glycemic control in severely burned children. *J Trauma.* 2005;59(5): 1148–1154.

82. Heyland D, Dhaliwal R. Immunonutrition in the critically ill: From old approaches to new paradigms. *Intensive Care Med.* 2005;31(4):501–503.

83. Ochoa JB, Makarenkova V, Bansal V. A rational use of immune enhancing diets: When should we use dietary arginine supplementation? *Nutr Clin Pract.* 2004;19(3):216–225.

84. Dubick MA, Williams C, Elgjo GI, et al. High-dose vitamin C infusion reduces fluid requirements in the resuscitation of burn-injured sheep. *Shock.* 2005;24(2):139–144.

85. Nathens AB, Neff MJ, Jurkovich GJ, et al. Randomized, prospective trial of antioxidant supplementation in critically ill surgical patients. *Ann Surg.* 2002;236(6):814–822.

86. Bulger EM, Maier RV. Antioxidants in critical illness. *Arch Surg.* 2001;136(10):1201–1207.

87. Demling RH. The burn edema process: Current concepts. *J Burn Care Rehabil.* 2005;26(3):207–227.

88. Herndon DN, Nguyen TT, Wolfe RR, et al. Lipolysis in burned patients is stimulated by the beta 2-receptor for catecholamines. *Arch Surg.* 1994;129(12):1301–1304. Discussion 1304–5.

89. Louis SN, Jackman GP, Nero TL, et al. Role of beta-adrenergic receptor subtypes in lipolysis. *Cardiovasc Drugs Ther.* 2000;14(6):565–577.

90. Prass K, Meisel C, Hoflich C, et al. Stroke-induced immunodeficiency promotes spontaneous bacterial infections and is mediated by sympathetic activation reversal by poststroke T helper cell type 1-like immunostimulation. *J Exp Med.* 2003;198(5):725–736.

91. Herndon DN, Hart DW, Wolf SE, et al. Reversal of catabolism by beta-blockade after severe burns. *N Engl J Med.* 2001;345(17):1223–1229.

92. Arbabi S, Ahrns KS, Wahl WL, et al. Beta-blocker use is associated with improved outcomes in adult burn patients. *J Trauma.* 2004;56(2):265–269. discussion 269–71.

93. Hart DW, Wolf SE, Ramzy PI, et al. Anabolic effects of oxandrolone after severe burn. *Ann Surg.* 2001;233(4):556–564.

94. Demling RH, Orgill DP. The anticatabolic and wound healing effects of the testosterone analog oxandrolone after severe burn injury. *J Crit Care.* 2000;15(1):12–17.

95. Wolf SE, Edelman LS, Kemalyan N, et al. Effects of oxandrolone on outcome measures in the severely burned: A multicenter prospective randomized double-blind trial. *J Burn Care Res.* 2006;27(2):131–139. Discussion 140–1.

96. Schonfeld N. Outpatient management of burns in children. *Pediatr Emerg Care.* 1990;6:249–253.

97. Martinez S. Ambulatory management of burns in children. *J Pediatr Health Care.* 1992;6:32–37.

98. Baxter CR. Management of burn wounds. *Dermatol Clin.* 1993;11:709–714.

99. Rockwell WB, Ehrlich HP. Should burn blister fluid be evacuated? *J Burn Care Rehabil.* 1990;11:93–95.

100. Peate WF. Oupatient management of burns. *Am Fam Physician.* 1992;45:1321–1330.

101. Clayton MC, Solem LD. No ice, no butter. Advice on management of burns for primary care physicians. *Postgrad Med.* 1995;97:151–155, 159–160, 165.

102. Sheridan R. Outpatient burn care in the emergency department. *Pediatr Emerg Care.* 2005;21:449–459.

103. Mertens DM, Jenkins ME, Warden GD. Outpatient burn management. *Nurs Clin North Am.* 1997;32:343–364.

104. Demling RH. Improved survival after massive burns. *J Trauma.* 1983;23(3):179–184.

105. Deitch EA. A policy of early excision and grafting in elderly burn patients shortens the hospital stay and improves survival. *Burns Incl Therm Inj.* 1985;12:109–114.

106. Thompson P, Herndon DN, Abston S, et al. Effect of early excision on patients with major thermal injury. *J Trauma.* 1987;27(2):205–207.

107. Engrav LH, Heimbach DM, Reus JL, et al. Early excision and grafting *vs.* nonoperative treatment of burns of indeterminate depth: A randomized prospective study. *J Trauma.* 1983;23:1001–1004.

108. Sheridan RL, Szyfelbein SK. Staged high dose epinephrine clysis in pediatric burn excisions: Proceedings of the American Burn Association. *J Burn Care Rehabil.* 1998;19:S199.

109. Sheridan RL, Szyfelbein SK. Trends in blood conservation in burn care. *Burns.* 2001;27:272–276.

110. Xiao-Wu W, Herndon DN, Spies M, et al. Effects of delayed wound excision and grafting in severely burned children. *Arch Surg.* 2002;137:1049–1054.

111. Barret JP, Herndon DN. Modulation of inflammatory and catabolic responses in severely burned children by early burn wound excision in the first 24 hours. *Arch Surg.* 2003;138:127–132.

112. Hart DW, Wolf SE, Chinkes DL, et al. Effects of early excision and aggressive enteral feeding on hypermetabolism, catabolism, and sepsis after severe burn. *J Trauma.* 2003;54(4):755–764.

113. Klein MB, Logsetty S, Costa B, et al. Extended time to wound closure is associated with increased risk of heterotopic ossification of the elbow. *J Burn Care Res.* 2007;28:1–4.

114. Klein MB, Hunter S, Heimbach DM, et al. The Versajet water dissector: A new tool for tangential excision. *J Burn Care Rehabil.* 2005;26(6):483–487.

115. Gibran N, Luterman A, Herndon D, et al. Comparison of fibrin sealant and staples for attaching split-thickness autologous sheet grafts in patients with deep partial- or full-thickness burn wounds: A phase $1/2$ clinical study. *J Burn Care Res.* 2007;28:1.

116. Moisidis E, Heath T, Boorer C, et al. A prospective, masked, randomized, controlled clinical trial of topical negative pressure use in skin grafting. *Plast Reconstr Surg.* 2004;114:917–922.

117. Llanos S, Danilla S, Barraza C, et al. Effectiveness of negative pressure closure in the integration of split thickness skin grafts. A randomized, double-masked, controlled trial. *Ann Surg.* 2006;244:700–705.

118. Edgar D, Brereton M. Rehabilitation after burn injury. *Br Med J.* 2004;329:343–345.

119. Greenleaf G, Hansbrough JF. Current trends in the use of allograft skin for patients with burns and reflections on the future of skin banking in the United States. *J Burn Care Rehabil.* 1994;15:428–431.

120. Elliott RA Jr, Hoehn JG. Use of commercial porcine skin for wound dressings. *Plast Reconstr Surg.* 1973;52:401–405.

121. Sawhney CP. Amniotic membrane as a biological dressing in the management of burns. *Burns.* 1989;15:339–342.

122. Yannas IV, Burke JF. Design of an artifical skin. I. Basic design principles. *J Biomed Mater Res.* 1980;14:65–81.

123. Lorenz C, Petracic A, Hohl HP, et al. Early wound closure and early reconstruction. Experience with a dermal substitute in a child with 60 percent surface area burn. *Burns.* 1997;23:505–508.

124. Dantzer E, Queruel P, Salinier L, et al. Dermal regeneration template for deep hand burns: Clinical utility for both early grafting and reconstructive surgery. *Br J Plast Surg.* 2003;56:764–774.

125. Klein MB, Engrav LH, Holmes JH, et al. Management of facial burns with a collagen/glycosaminoglycan skin substitute-prospective experience with 12 consecutive patients with large, deep facial burns. *Burns.* 2005;31:257–261.

126. Jeng JC, Fidler PE, Sokolich JC, et al. Seven years' experience with Integra as a reconstructive tool. *J Burn Care Res.* 2007;28:120–126.

127. Wainwright D, Madden M, Luterman A, et al. Clinical evaluation of an acellular allograft dermal matrix in full-thickness burns. *J Burn Care Rehabil.* 1996;17:124–136.

128. DeLuca M, Albanese E, Bondanza S, et al. Multicentre experience in the treatment of burns with autologous and allogenic cultured epithelium, fresh or preserved in a frozen state. *Burns.* 1989;15:303–309.

129. Boyce ST, Kagan RJ, Meyer NA, et al. The 1999 clinical research award. Cultured skin substitutes combined with Integra artificial skin to replace native skin autograft and allograft for the closure of excised full-thickness burns. *J Burn Care Rehabil.* 1999;20(6):453–461.

130. Boyce ST, Kagan RJ, Yakuboff KP, et al. Cultured skin substitutes reduce donor skin harvesting for closure of excised, full-thickness burns. *Ann Surg.* 2002;235(2):269–279.

131. Kumar RJ, Kimble RM, Boots R, et al. Treatment of partial-thickness burns: A prospective, randomized trail using Transcyte. *ANZ J Surg.* 2004;74(8):622–626.

132. Rakel BA, Bermel MA, Abbott LI, et al. Split-thickness skin graft donor site care: A quantitative synthesis of the research. *Appl Nurs Res.* 1998;11:174–182.

133. Kirker KR, Luo Y, Morris SE, et al. Glycosaminoglycan hydrogels as supplemental wound dressings for donor sites. *J Burn care Rehabil.* 2004;25:276–286.

134. Ho WS, Ying SY, Choi PCL, et al. A prospective controlled clinical study of skin donor sites treated with a 1-4,2-acetamide-deoxy-B-D-glucan polymer: A preliminary report. *Burns.* 2001;27:759–761.

135. Innes ME, Umraw N, Fish JS, et al. The use of silver coated dressings on donor site wounds: A prospective, controlled matched pair study. *Burns.* 2001;27:621–627.

136. Davis KA, Santaniello JM, He LK, et al. Burn injury and pulmonary sepsis: Development of a clinically relevant model. *J Trauma.* 2004;56(2):272–278.

137. Sasaki J, Fujishima S, Iwamura H, et al. Prior burn insult induces lethal acute lung injury in endotoxemic mice: Effects of cytokine inhibition. *Am J Physiol Lung Cell Mol Physiol.* 2003;284(2):L270–L278.

138. Dancey DR, Hayes J, Gomez M, et al. ARDS in patients with thermal injury. *Intensive Care Med.* 1999;25(11):1231–1236.

139. Barie PS, Williams MD, McCollam JS, et al. Benefit/risk profile of drotrecogin alfa (activated) in surgical patients with severe sepsis. *Am J Surg.* 2004;188(3):212–220.

140. Fry DE, Beilman G, Johnson S, et al. Safety of drotrecogin alfa (activated) in surgical patients with severe sepsis. *Surg Infect (Larchmt).* 2004;5(3):253–259.

141. Brunsvold ME, Wahl WL, Arbabi S. Drotecogin Alfa in patients with soft tissue injury. *39th Annual Meeting of American Burn Association.* San Diego, California; 2007.

142. Hansbrough JF, Wikstrom T, Braide M, et al. Neutrophil activation and tissue neutrophil sequestration in a rat model of thermal injury. *J Surg Res.* 1996;61(1):17–22.

143. Piccolo MT, Wang Y, Verbrugge S, et al. Role of chemotactic factors in neutrophil activation after thermal injury in rats. *Inflammation.* 1999;23(4):371–385.

144. Till GO, Johnson KJ, Kunkel R, et al. Intravascular activation of complement and acute lung injury. Dependency on neutrophils and toxic oxygen metabolites. *J Clin Invest.* 1982;69(5):1126–1135.

145. Ipaktchi K, Mattar A, Niederbichler AD, et al. Topical p38MAPK inhibition reduces dermal inflammation and epithelial apoptosis in burn wounds. *Shock.* 2006;26(2):201–209.

146. Ipaktchi K, Mattar A, Niederbichler AD, et al. Attenuating burn wound inflammatory signaling reduces systemic inflammation and acute lung injury. *J Immunol.* 2006;177(11):8065–8071.

147. McLeod BC. Therapeutic apheresis: Use of human serum albumin, fresh frozen plasma and cryosupernatant plasma in therapeutic plasma exchange. *Best Pract Res Clin Haematol.* 2006;19(1):157–167.

148. Kravitz M, Warden GD, Sullivan JJ, et al. A randomized trial of plasma exchange in the treatment of burn shock. *J Burn Care Rehabil.* 1989;10(1):17–26.

149. Ballesteros MF, Jackson ML, Martin MW. Working toward the elimination of residential fire deaths: The Centers for Disease Control and Prevention's Smoke Alarm Installation and Fire Safety Education (SAIFE) Program. *J Burn Care Rehabil.* 2005;26(5):434–439.

150. DiGuiseppi C, Roberts I, Wade A, et al. Incidence of fires and related injuries after giving out free smoke alarms: Cluster randomised controlled trial. *Br Med J.* 2002;325(7371):995–998.

151. Schieber RA, Gilchrist J, Sleet DA. Legislative and regulatory strategies to reduce childhood unintentional injuries. *Future Child.* 2000;10:111–136.

152. Fallat ME, Rengers SJ. The effect of education and safety devices on scald burn prevention. *J Trauma.* 1993;34:560–564.

153. Cagle KM, Davis JW, Dominic W, et al. Results of a focused scald-prevention program. *J Burn Care Res.* 2006;27:859–863.

Management of Traumatic Wounds: Complex Soft Tissue Reconstruction

57

Christopher A. Park   **Joseph A. Molnar**

Open wounds are often the most obvious physical finding on the trauma patient. *Regardless of how dramatic the wound, the treating physician must realize that this may not be the most life-threatening injury.* To avoid the pitfall of being distracted by the most obvious, but perhaps not the most urgent injury, maintaining adherence to the fundamental principles taught in the other chapters of this book are essential.

Initially, the patient must undergo an initial assessment following the Advanced Trauma Life Support (ATLS) principles of primary survey with control of airway, breathing, and circulation; complete secondary survey, and radiographic examinations.[1] In the course of this overall evaluation, all wounds will be identified in a systematic and thorough manner. During this process, prioritization must be determined and constantly reassessed. At this stage, the major role of traumatic wounds is to serve as a locator of sites of major impact. They are usually of lower importance, except for wounds associated with potential exsanguination or life-threatening injuries.

INITIAL MANAGEMENT

In the initial survey, the primary goals of wound management include control of hemorrhage, preventing further injury, and limiting contamination. Pressure should be held to bleeding wounds. *It is rare that direct pressure will not control bleeding.* Tourniquets are not recommended unless bleeding is life threatening and unable to be controlled with direct pressure. One should avoid using clamps in wounds in a nonsurgical setting because one may inadvertently damage nerves or other structures near a bleeding vessel. Bleeding from fractures is best managed by stabilizing the fracture with reduction and splinting or traction. This is true even of open Le Fort facial fractures where bleeding may be controlled with disimpaction, closed reduction, and wrapping with a pressure dressing such as an ace wrap.

To avoid further contamination, a sterile, moist dressing should be applied to all open wounds as soon as other priorities are addressed. In a similar manner, amputated parts should be kept clean and preserved in moist, sterile saline-soaked gauze, placed in an impermeable barrier such as a plastic bag or specimen cup, and submerged in iced water.

As part of the initial survey, one must limit further injury of tissues. For example, compartment syndrome requires immediate operative release with fasciotomies of the involved compartments. Injured limbs should be elevated as feasible to prevent progressive edema and loss of circulation. Fracture reduction will frequently assist to improve vascular inflow to an injured extremity by eliminating vascular stretch or pinching of the vessels.

After the control of hemorrhage and treatment of life-threatening injuries, management of traumatic wounds rises in priority. It must be determined whether the wound can be managed in the primary setting (emergency room, field, clinic, etc) or if the wound requires surgical management. Key factors include amount of contamination, extent of devitalized tissue, proximity to important structures, and comfort of the patient.

Tetanus

Patients with wounds at risk for tetanus who have not had a booster within 5 years, are not sure of immunizations, or cannot provide a history of immunization status, require a tetanus booster. Non–tetanus-prone wounds reduce the cutoff to 10 years since last booster. If a patient with a high-risk wound has never been immunized or has not completed the three-dose tetanus immunization, tetanus immune globulin should be administered.

Antibiotics

The administration of systemic antibiotics in acute trauma patients is controversial. With the rapid proliferation of antibiotic-resistant organisms, prophylactic antibiotics are not indicated except for selected cases, including open fractures, open joints, exposed cartilage, heavy contamination, bite wounds, delayed wound management, and patients with impaired wound healing (immunosuppressed, diabetic, and severe atherosclerosis). Topical antibiotics, including antibiotic ointments, silver impregnated dressings, or saline dressings, are more often appropriate.

Wound Preparation

In wounds amenable to management in the priority setting, the principles are wound preparation, local anesthesia, decontamination, and closure. The area surrounding the wound should be prepared with topical bactericidals such as iodine or chlorhexidine products. These products are cellular toxins in the concentrations used to prepare the skin surrounding the wound and as such are detrimental to wound healing.[2] They are not recommended for open wound application. Shaving the surrounding area is not necessary and has actually been shown to increase wound infections in some cases.[3,4]

Anesthesia

Before wound manipulation, adequate anesthesia must be obtained. This can be accomplished in smaller wounds with local injection or nerve blocks because topical anesthetics are of limited benefit in traumatic wounds. Dosages, durations, and adverse reactions of local anesthetics vary depending on the anesthetic and the physician must be aware of these (see Table 1). Local anesthetic central nervous system (CNS) toxicity begins with tinnitus, tremors, metallic taste in the mouth, numbness, and can progress to seizures. Cardiovascular toxicity is the result of myocardial depression, leading to hypotension, altered heart rate, and ultimately arrhythmias.

Larger areas can be anesthetized with minimal anesthetic with knowledge of the anatomy of sensory nerves. The most common regional blocks performed include digital blocks (radial and ulnar digital nerves), wrist blocks (median nerve, ulnar nerve, and radial sensory nerve), and facial blocks (supraorbital, infraorbital, or mental nerve) (see Fig. 1). Ears, nose, and genitalia are frequently anesthetized with field blocks of anesthetic without epinephrine to avoid vascular compromise.

Finally, the largest wounds will require general anesthetics and must be explored in the operative suite to allow adequate exposure, to control hemorrhage, and to have access to needed operative tools to do the procedure in an optimal manner. Indeed, the test of whether one must

TABLE 1
LOCAL ANESTHETICS

Amino Amides	Onset	Maximum Dose (with Epinephrine)	Duration (with Epinephrine)
Lidocaine	Rapid	4.5 mg/kg (7 mg/kg)	2 hr (4 hr)
Mepivicaine	Rapid	5 mg/kg (7 mg/kg)	3 hr (6 hr)
Prilocaine	Medium	5 mg/kg (7.5 mg/kg)	90 min (6 hr)
Bupivicaine	Slow	2.5 mg/kg (3 mg/kg)	4 hr (8 hr)
Etidocaine	Rapid	2.5 mg/kg (4 mg/kg)	4 hr (8 hr)
Tetracaine	Slow	1.5 mg/kg (2.5 mg/kg)	3 hr (10 hr)
Procaine	Slow	8 mg/kg (10 mg/kg)	45 min (90 min)
Chlorprocaine	Rapid	10 mg/kg (15 mg/kg)	30 min (90 min)
Cocaine	Used topically	1.5 mg/kg (NA)	30 min (NA)

NA, not available.

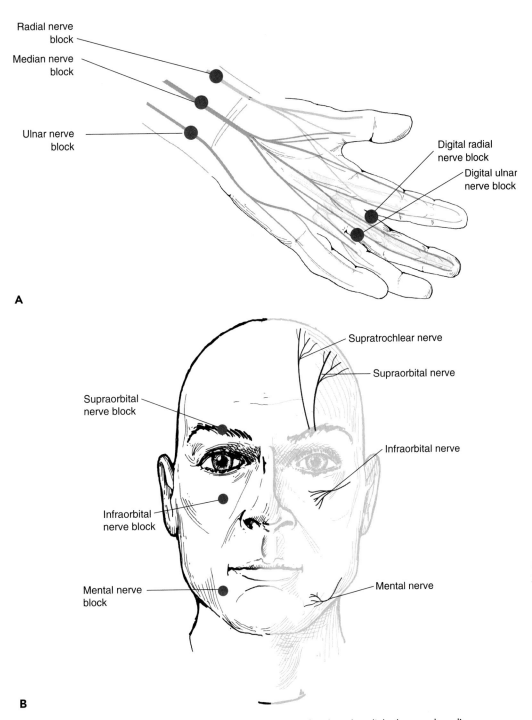

Figure 1 Diagram of peripheral nerve blocks. **A:** Sites for digital, radial, ulnar, and median nerve blocks. **B:** Sites for supraorbital, infraorbital, and mental nerve blocks.

treat the wound in the operative suite must be judged by whether the operative surgeon can do the procedure just as well in the setting of the emergency department (see Fig. 2).

Debridement

After obtaining adequate anesthesia, the open wound requires exploration for additional injuries, removal of contamination and foreign bodies, irrigation, and debridement of nonviable or heavily contaminated tissue. As stated, topical antiseptics impair wound healing unless used in a very dilute solution. Surgical debridement and copious irrigation are necessary and sufficient to decontaminate the open wound. The decision regarding how much to debride requires multifactorial analysis. Obviously, nonviable tissue should be debrided as it impairs

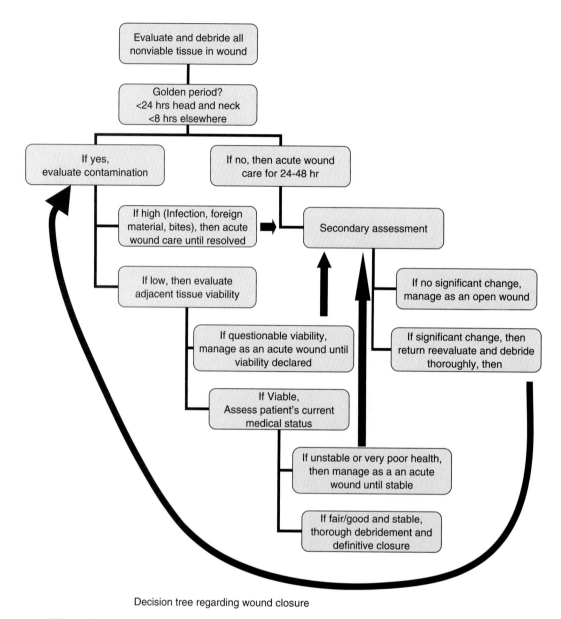

Decision tree regarding wound closure

Figure 2 Wound care decision tree.

healing and increases the risk of infection. Marginal tissue may best be managed by preservation with plans for repeat debridement and delayed closure unless it is of minimal functional benefit. Once the wound has been irrigated and debrided, the physician must determine whether the wound is amenable to closure based on size, available tissue, and level of contamination.

Decision Regarding Closure

The decision to close a wound or to manage it as an open wound requires a determination of the likelihood of success of primary closure. The risk of failure of primary closure can lead to more damage and a worse outcome than open wound care with delayed healing. An important factor to consider in this decision is the length of time since injury. Six to eight hours is considered the "golden period" during which primary closure is possible. After this period of time, bacterial counts are significantly higher. Longer periods of time (typically 24 hours) are acceptable for injuries above the neck as these wounds are cosmetically more apparent and relatively resistant to infection due to better blood supply.

The degree of contamination either based on mechanism, history, or examination is another important variable to weigh. Relative contraindications to primary closure include human bites, nonhuman bites (except for the face), and embedded foreign material.

Systemic factors must also be considered in the decision for wound closure. Associated conditions to consider include patient age, diabetes, immune function, vascular status, immunization history, coagulation status, and associated injuries. For example, a patient with intra-abdominal hemorrhage may be too unstable to undergo wound closure on the face until fluid resuscitation is complete.

Questions of the viability of adjacent tissues should preclude primary closure. This is an important variable in thermal burns, electrical injury, crush injury, and "missile" injury. In each of these situations there is frequently found a zone of nonviable tissue and an area of tissue of questionable viability. This is similar to the zones established in burns, which Jackson referred to as the *zone of coagulation*, the *zone of stasis*, and the *zone of hyperemia*.[5] The zone of coagulation in burns is quite similar to the zone of necrotic tissue found in a crush or avulsion type injury. This tissue is dead at the time of first observation and must be removed from the wound to avoid progressive sepsis or myoglobinuria. Adjacent to this is an area of edema and tissue of questionable viability, which is the zone of stasis. In this tissue, the blood flow is sluggish and depending upon the events of the next few days may go on to survive or die. As a result, in many complicated injuries such as open tibial fractures, serial debridements are necessary before closure. In some cases, this may take several surgeries over a period of 2 weeks or more. It is the authors' experience that in these situations, the temptation is to close the wound sooner than is biologically safe leading to infection, dehiscence, and increased morbidity and hospital stay. As a result, the "rule-of-thumb" is to debride the wound "N + 1" times. That is, it is recommended that in order to minimize the risk of failure of closure that the wound be debrided one more time after the wound appears that it "might" be able be closed safely.

The "N+1" rule

An additional surgical debridement is usually beneficial before closure and rarely harmful

---

THE RECONSTRUCTIVE LADDER

Numerous decisions are made in the management of traumatic wounds. A plethora of options exist for dealing with a particular wound. Each option has its own advantages and disadvantages, requirements and costs, side effects, and complications. Expert management requires a large amount of experience as many options and priorities must be weighed. The principles can be practiced by anyone. In general, the goal is to obtain a clean, closed wound with the lowest physical, emotional, and temporal cost to the patient. It is essential to bear in mind that no method has complete success. It is important to consider and protect options that can be implemented if initial attempts are unsuccessful. The advantage of obtaining early

closure is not only of obvious financial and psychological benefit but also shortens the wound healing process.

The three phases of wound healing are inflammatory, proliferative, and remodeling. The inflammatory phase occurs in the first several days after injury and the major events are hemostasis and recruitment of inflammatory cells. The proliferative phase proceeds until wounds are closed and consists of granulation, contraction, and epithelialization. The remodeling phase can last years and the major event is collagen maturation. The inflammatory and proliferative phases of wound healing are minimized when early closure of clean wounds is obtained. This improves overall medical status because these phases utilize significant metabolic energy and cause considerable pain and disability. Traditional thinking taught that wound reconstruction should occur early before significant inflammation. Subatmospheric pressure has been shown to limit inflammatory mediators and has adjusted this timeline, allowing serial debridements to prepare wounds before definitive reconstruction.[6]

Principles of Traumatic Wound Reconstruction

1. Reduce contamination
2. Expedite phases of wound healing
3. Minimize morbidity
4. Minimize complications
5. Maximize long-term function
6. Preserve future options

Methods of Wound Closure

Increasing Complexity

Wound Closure Techniques
   1. Primary intention (primary closure)
   2. Secondary intention
   3. Tertiary intention (delayed primary closure)
Reconstruction
   4. Autograft
   5. Local flaps
   6. Free tissue transfer

Primary Intention

In healing by primary intention (primary closure), the wound can be reapproximated in one or multiple layers. Deeper wounds require closure of structures of strength. Fascial layers that have been violated should be closed in order to reduce tension on the skin. If necessary, the skin edges can be undermined or fascias can be incised and released remotely from the wound to allow closure of the wound.

The cutaneous edges can be closed in many ways. The strongest closure is closure of the deep dermis with

TABLE 2	
STANDARD SUTURE REMOVAL RECOMMENDATIONS	
Face	3–5 d
Scalp/trunk	7–10 d
Extremities	10–14 d

an absorbable suture (i.e., polyglycolic acid) followed by closure of the epidermis with subcuticular or intercuticular suture. This is called a *layered closure*. The least amount of observable scar is created with a running, nonabsorbable, subcuticular suture with the least inflammatory response (i.e., polypropylene). However, this suture does require removal (see Table 2). An absorbable subcuticular suture (i.e., poliglecaprone 25) can be used but has a prolonged inflammatory phase during suture degradation. Small, clean, simple lacerations with minimal retraction can be managed with noninvasive techniques, including suture strips and cutaneous adhesive (i.e., Dermabond, Ethicon: Cornelia, GA). If external sutures are used in an interrupted, mattress, or running fashion, they should be removed as early as possible to minimize scarring from the suture. Staples can also be used and are preferred in the scalp to expedite closure and reduce pain of application and removal without compromising cosmesis.[7] Vertical mattress sutures are used for extra strength and eversion of wound edges. Horizontal mattress sutures provide additional hemostasis (see Figs. 3 and 4).

Replantation

The most complex form of primary closure occurs when an appendage is amputated in such a way that it can be replanted. This is frequently performed for thumbs, fingers, hands, penises, and scalps. It has also been used for ears, nose, hands, feet, and entire extremities. Replantation requires repair of support structures (bones/tendons/fascia) followed by microvascular arterial and venous anastamoses and nerve repair. The skin is closed last. To be suitable for replantation, the amputated part must meet certain general criteria. Specific criteria are beyond the scope of this chapter. The amputated part must be present, preserved appropriately, recently amputated, minimally contaminated, and presumed to be viable. The patient must be medically stable and informed of the prognosis and need for prolonged postoperative care and therapy. Maximum ischemia time is frequently quoted to be 6 hours based on muscle damage at room temperature beyond 6 hours, but when preserved appropriately, cold ischemia can be extended even beyond 24 hours in amputated parts with minimal muscle (i.e., hands/digits). Preservation should include wrapping the part in sterile gauze moistened with lactated Ringers, sealing the part in a plastic bag, and

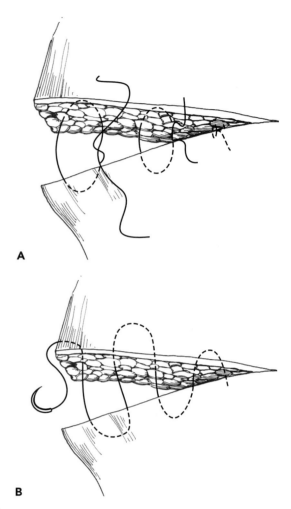

Figure 3 Dermal sutures **(A)** simple buried **(B)** running dermal.

placing the plastic bag in a container of water and ice at 4°C. Viability is compromised by crush injuries, avulsion injuries, and injuries at multiple levels.[8,9]

Secondary Intention

Healing by secondary intention is necessary when wounds are too large and/or too contaminated to close by other means. The wound is debrided and left open to heal secondarily. Healing is by a combination of contraction, proliferation of granulation tissue, and epithelialization. Epithelialization occurs from wound edges and skin appendages if still present. Secondary healing can be dramatically augmented by subatmospheric pressure therapy (see subsequent text).

Tertiary Intention

Healing by third intention is also known as *delayed primary closure* and is typically performed in smaller wounds that are contaminated. The patient undergoes initial debridement followed by open wound care for typically 3 to 5 days, at

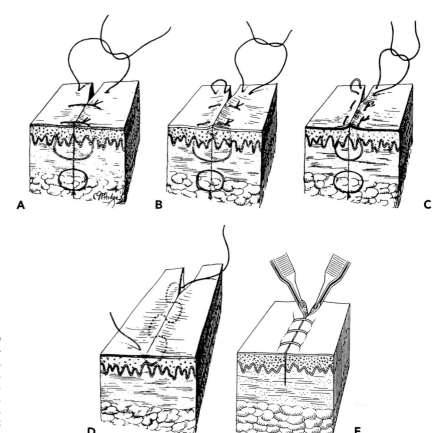

Figure 4   Superficial sutures **(A)** simple interrupted, **(B)** vertical mattress, **(C)** horizontal mattress, **(D)** subcuticular continuous, **(E)** staples. (With permission from Thorne CH. Techniques and principles in plastic surgery. In: Thorne CH, Beasley RW, Asten SJ, et al. eds. *Grabb & Smith's plastic surgery 6e.* Philadelphia: Lippincott Williams & Wilkins; 2007.)

which point the local phagocytic activity is maximized. The wound is then closed. These wounds are typically drained. This technique reduces infection rates in high-risk wounds. Wounds treated initially with wound care followed by skin grafting or flap closure as discussed in the next section could be considered a variation of tertiary intention healing.

AUTOGENOUS TISSUE RECONSTRUCTION

Many wounds require more complex forms of closure due to size of wound, exposed structures, or limited adjacent tissue. The options of reconstruction are best viewed as a ladder of increasing complexity, morbidity, and risks. *The first principle of reconstruction is to start with the simplest approach with a reasonable possibility of success. The best treatment plan for any wound is always the technique with the best outcome with the least amount of sacrifice.* If the simple technique fails, the more complex options are still available. That leads to the second principle of reconstruction; reconstructive efforts should not violate, or at least minimize violations of future reconstructive options. All reconstruction has physical costs in that uninjured tissues are used to cover the existing wound. The final principle of reconstruction is to minimize the harm or morbidity that the reconstruction costs the patient

The Principles of Reconstruction

1. Start simple
2. Do not violate later reconstructive options
3. Minimize the morbidity for the patient

Skin Graft

If a wound is clean, relatively smooth, and well vascularized, it can be covered with autogenous skin. Options include full-thickness skin graft and split-thickness skin graft. The advantages of full-thickness skin graft are improved cosmesis and reduced secondary contraction but full-thickness skin grafts are limited by donor site size. The donor sites require closure or less ideally, healing by split-thickness skin graft or secondary intention. Typical donor sites include the groin crease, inner thigh, inner arm, supraclavicular, preauricular, or postauricular skin.[10] A goal is to use like skin to cover like skin. Grafts for the face are usually harvested above the clavicles. Skin of the upper inner thighs tends to be darker and is used to reconstruct darker areas, such as the nipples. Full-thickness grafts undergo more primary contracture as a result of elastin in the dermis. Secondary contracture, which is the result of wound contracture, is far less in full-thickness grafts.[11]

Split-thickness skin is usually harvested at 10–16/1,000 in. from a remote site, typically the thigh or buttock. This harvests the epidermis but preserves a portion of the dermis and the skin appendages. Split grafts are more prone to secondary contracture. Donor sites heal by epithelialization from skin appendages left in the dermis.[12] The skin can either be used as a sheet graft or meshed. Sheet grafts provide the best cosmetic outcome but reduces the area covered by donor skin and has an increased risk of fluid buildup, namely seromas, hematomas, and abscesses. "Pie crusting" or making drainage slits in the skin graft allows for improved drainage. Skin can be meshed in nearly any ratio but most commonly 1:1, 1:2, or 1:3. The higher ratios cover a larger area but require more secondary intention healing and lead to more scarring. Meshed grafts easily expel fluid and are far less prone to hematomas, seromas, and infection. Sheet grafts are preferred in cosmetically sensitive areas such as the face or in highly functional areas such as hands and joint surfaces.

Skin grafts survive by imbibition for the first 24 to 48 hours. The skin graft is adhered to the wound bed by a fibrin layer and nutrients are absorbed by a capillary action from the recipient bed. Ultimately recipient and donor end capillaries are rejoined in the inosculatory phase and neovascularization occurs. After 72 hours, the adherent fibrin layer is replaced by an ingrowth of fibrous tissue.[13]

To expedite this process of vascularization, skin grafts must be secured with a dressing that performs two functions. It must keep the adherent skin graft moist but not wet in order to prevent desiccation and maceration. It must also provide constant pressure to the skin graft onto the wound bed. This has typically been accomplished with a bolster dressing of petroleum gauze (with or without wrapped sterile cotton balls) sutured in place. This technique works well but does not provide even pressure over the graft and can lead to maceration. The vacuum assisted closure VAC over a protective nonadherent layer has dramatically improved skin graft take by providing constant pressure with an even distribution over the wound and by removing excess fluid.[14]

Skin Substitutes

In the last 3 decades, considerable research has been directed to development of a skin substitute or artificial skin. The definition of an artificial skin varies by the author but for the present discussion it is defined as a product that is biologically accepted by the host organism as part of the skin without rejection and in some way provides a skin that is more like the original skin. Substitution of a physical property of skin is not a sufficient criterion for an artificial skin because many of the dressings listed in the subsequent text substitute physical properties of the skin. On the basis of present techniques, surgeons are able to substitute for the epidermal and dermal layers.

The most widely used artificial dermis at this time is Integra (Integra Life Sciences Inc, Plainsboro, N.J.), which is a porous matrix of fibers of bovine type I collagen that is crosslinked with chondroitin-6-sulfate and glycosaminoglycan (GAG) extracted from shark cartilage. This matrix serves as a template for infiltration of the patient's own vasculature, fibroblasts, macrophages, and lymphocytes. The outer silicone layer of Integra serves as a temporary epidermis, allowing water flux, protecting from microbial invasion, and preventing wound desiccation. The silicone layer must ultimately be removed and replaced with a skin graft. Because an artificial dermis is present, the autogenous skin graft can be thin, typically 6–8/1,000 in., which limits donor morbidity and increases take of skin graft. The end result is a bilaminate skin graft that is believed to improve durability and skin mobility, while reducing contracture formation.[15]

There are other artificial dermis products. Alloderm (Life Cell Corporation, The Woodlands, TX) is an immunologically inert cadaveric dermal graft that can be covered with a thin split-thickness autograft, but its revascularization is limited. Apligraf (Graftskin; Organogenesis Inc, Canton, MA) and Dermagraft (Advanced Tissue Sciences, La Jolla, CA) are composite dermal and epidermal skin replacements derived from bovine collagen and neonatal fibroblasts.

Epidermis can be synthesized *in vitro* by a process referred to as *cultured epithelial autograft* (CEA). By growing the patient's own epithelial cells in tissue culture, the surgeon may expand a small sample of skin potentially 10,000 times. Commercially available as Epicel (Genzyme Tissue Repair Corporation, Cambridge, MA), it is limited by fragility and a high rate of contracture formation. However, it is a viable option in patients with near complete body surface area burns.[16]

Composite Tissue Reconstruction

There are times that wounds not amenable to primary closure are best managed with composite tissue coverage. If vital, poorly vascularized tissue (i.e., bone, tendon, and joint), or nonvascularized tissue (i.e., alloplastic hardware, implants, etc.) are exposed or wound requires significant coverage for cosmesis, function, or durability, composite tissue may be necessary. Composite tissue reconstruction implies that multiple layers/types of tissue are to be used in the reconstruction. This is necessary when the wound cannot be closed and skin graft coverage is inadequate.

Indications for Composite Tissue Reconstruction

1. Require durable coverage
2. Alloplastic materials or vital structures exposed
3. Tissues of limited vascularity (bones/tendons/joints)
4. Cosmetically necessary

Composite tissue can come from nearby tissue or remote tissue. Local tissue reconstruction is indicated in cases where nearby tissue can cover the wound with minimal donor site morbidity. Regional or remote flap coverage is necessary in circumstances when local tissue is inadequate. Flap reconstruction requires extensive knowledge of the relevant anatomy. It is important to try to reconstruct entire aesthetic subunits with flap reconstruction.

Local Flaps

Several techniques exist for using local tissue to cover defects (see Figs. 5 to 8). These are not based on specific blood vessels and are at risk for ischemia. The most common examples are random flaps, rotational flaps, interpolation flaps, transposition flaps (rhombic, bilobed), and advancement flaps (axial advancement, V-Y advancement).

1. Random flaps are not based on vascular supply and are subject to ischemia. They use nearby tissue to close a wound.
2. Rotational flaps are designed to use a nearby semicircular flap of skin and subcutaneous tissue to rotate into a

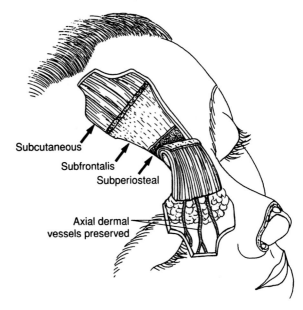

Figure 6   Interpolation: forehead flap. (With permission from Thorne CH. Techniques and principles in plastic surgery. In: Thorne CH, Beasley RW, Asten SJ, et al. eds. *Grabb & Smith's plastic surgery 6e.* Philadelphia: Lippincott Williams & Wilkins; 2007.)

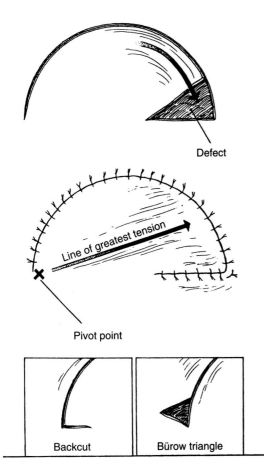

Figure 5   Rotational flap. A backcut or Bürow triangle can be used. (With permission from Thorne CH. Techniques and principles in plastic surgery. In: Thorne CH, Beasley RW, Asten SJ, et al. eds. *Grabb & Smith's plastic surgery 6e.* Philadelphia: Lippincott Williams & Wilkins; 2007.)

defect. The length of the flap is typically four to six times the diameter of the defect. The radius of the arc is the line of greatest tension. The tension is distributed throughout the closure. If tension is excessive, a back-cut from the pivot point or an excision of a Bürow triangle can assist with closure. It is also possible to leave a second defect at the donor site of the rotation that has a vascularized wound bed amenable to skin grafting. Vascular supply of the flap is through the subdermal plexus.
3. Interpolation flaps are rotated into a defect without sacrificing its pedicle. After the flap has been revascularized from the wound bed (typically at 2 to 3 weeks), the pedicle can be divided and the flap inset.
4. Transposition flaps rotate neighboring tissue designed to fill the defect. The donor site is either closed primarily, with a second flap (bilobed flap), or with a skin graft. The idea is to use skin from an area of less tension to close a wound that will not close primarily. Rhombic flaps are designed with angles of 60 and 120 degrees to rotate into a defect, leaving an adjacent linear scar. Bilobed flaps use an initial flap, slightly smaller than the original defect, to rotate into a defect as well as a second flap, approximately half the size of the original flap and from an area of less tension, to close the first donor site. The second donor site should be primarily closed.
5. Advancement flaps are advanced on their subdermal plexus to fill a defect. In a single pedicled axial flap, a rectangular or square flap is advanced forward based on skin elasticity. Excision of the Burow triangles is usually necessary. Bipedicled axial flaps use a pedicled axial flap from each side of a defect to close a larger defect. V-Y

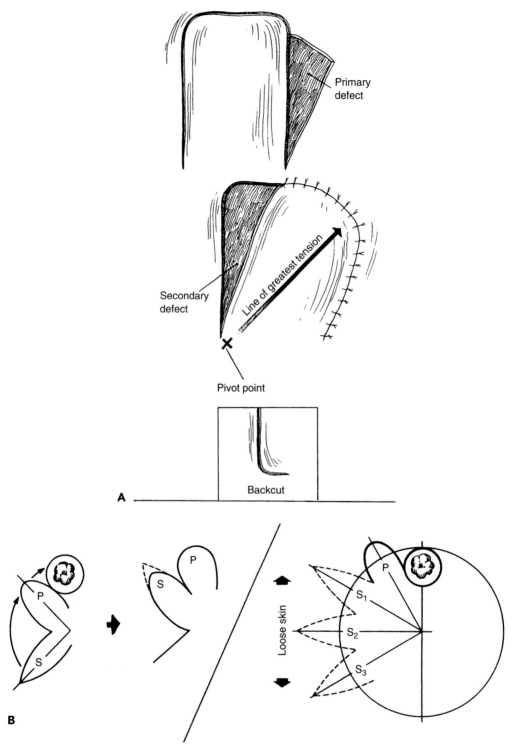

Figure 7 **A:** Transposition flap. **B:** Bilobed transposition flap. After the lesion is excised, the primary flap (*P*) is transposed into the initial defect. The secondary flap (*S*) is then transposed into the defect left after the primary flap has been moved. Three possible choices for the secondary flap (*S₁*, *S₂*, and *S₃*) are depicted. **C:** Rhombic transposition flap. The rhomboid defect must have 60- and 120-degree angles. The flap is planned in an area of loose skin so that direct closure of the wound edges is possible. The short diagonal *BD* (which is the same length as each side) is extended by its own length to point *E*. The line *EF* is drawn parallel to *CD* and is of the same length. After the flap margins have been incised, the flap is transposed into the rhomboid defect. (With permission from Thorne CH. Techniques and principles in plastic surgery. In: Thorne CH, Beasley RW, Asten SJ, et al. eds. *Grabb & Smith's plastic surgery 6e.* Philadelphia: Lippincott Williams & Wilkins; 2007.)

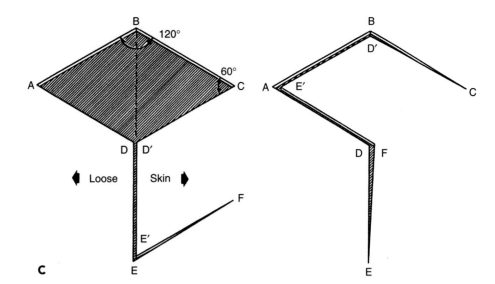

Figure 7   (Continued)   **C**

advancement flaps essentially advance a flap forward as the narrow angle of the V is closed primarily.

Regional/Pedicled Flaps

A thorough knowledge of anatomy is necessary in the use of pedicled flaps to close donor defects. A full discussion of pedicled flaps is beyond the scope of this chapter. The first pedicled flaps were transferred to a recipient bed with delayed sectioning from the donor site after neovascularization had occurred from the recipient bed, usually after 3 weeks. Examples of this include groin flaps, which are frequently used to cover hand defects, the Tagliacozzi flap which use arm tissue to reconstruct the nose, and cross leg flaps which use contralateral leg tissue to reconstruct a leg.

Immediate pedicled flaps are usually based on major arterial and venous channels and these pedicles must be preserved. Pedicled flaps can be transferred as composite skin, muscle flaps, osseous flaps, or any combination of these. The key principles of pedicled flap reconstruction are knowledge of anatomy, preservation of pedicle, avoidance of tension, and reduction of morbidity of donor site. Common pedicled flaps are listed in Table 3.

Distant/Free Flaps

Distant tissue can be used to reconstruct wounds (see Table 4). Many of these flaps are the same flaps that are used as pedicled flaps. The difference is that the flap and its arterial, venous, and sometimes neural supply are transected and transferred to a recipient wound bed, where anastamosis is completed to recipient vessels and nerves near the wound bed. Free tissue transfer requires microvascular skills and equipment. The advantages of these techniques are obvious. Remote tissue can provide larger amounts of tissue, tissue that has been spared the trauma of the wounded area, and tissue that does

not require a vascularized wound bed. Disadvantages include the risk of flap loss, complexity of surgery, and donor site morbidity. Donor sites can be closed primarily, with skin grafts, or with another form of flap closure. Postoperative care includes maintaining a warm environment, vasodilators, anticoagulants, and close observation for vascular compromise with immediate exploration and repair if necessary.

Free flaps can provide skin, soft tissue, muscle, fascia, bone, or any combination of these for reconstructive purposes. The decision to use a free flap in reconstruction requires consideration of all variables including defect, donor site availability, morbidity of donor sites, alternatives, patient status, and anticipated outcome goals. In general, free flaps are necessary when local tissue is not available to reconstruct a wound. Classic indications are inability to cover bone, joint, major vessels, implanted materials, or organs as well as a need for composite reconstruction, that is, mandibular reconstruction with radial forearm free flap including bone, subcutaneous tissue, and skin. Frequent areas with these requirements are head and neck defects, perineal defects, and defects of the lower third of the lower extremity. One area where other options are available, but many favor free flap reconstruction, is breast reconstruction.

A recent trend is toward the use of perforator flaps. These flaps are based on perforating branches to the skin and subcutaneous tissue leaving most muscle behind, with dissection to minimize muscular trauma. This requires more skill, time, and expertise but reduces donor site morbidity.

Digits can also be transferred to replace absent digits with more important functions. Toes are frequently transferred for thumb and index finger reconstructions.

Another area of potential expanse is the use of composite tissue transfers for reconstruction. These are transplanted parts used to replace missing or nonfunctional parts. Hand transplants have already occurred and facial transplantation is being considered.

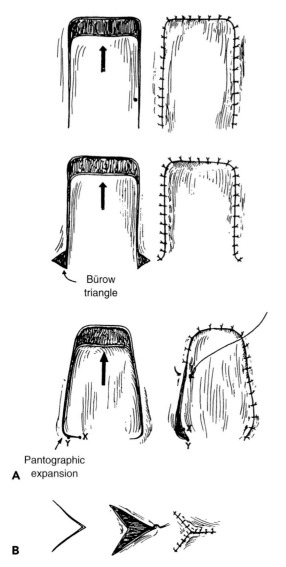

Figure 8 Advancement flaps. **A:** Single pedicle advancement flap using skin elasticity (*top*), Bürow triangles (*middle*) or pantographic expansion (*bottom*). **B:** VY advancement flap (With permission from Thorne CH. Techniques and principles in plastic surgery. In: Thorne CH, Beasley RW, Asten SJ, et al. eds. *Grabb & Smith's plastic surgery 6e.* Philadelphia: Lippincott Williams & Wilkins; 2007.)

Complications of Reconstruction

Infection: Infection is a risk of any surgical management. The possibility of causing infection in a donor site demands rigorous antiseptic technique.

Flap Failure/Necrosis: Advanced, rotated, pedicled, and free flaps can suffer partial or complete flap necrosis from either arterial or venous insufficiency.

Contracture: Contracture is more common with partial-thickness wound coverage, especially split-thickness skin grafts. These are typically treated with composite flap coverage, z-plasties, or re-excision with splinting postreconstruction. A decreased incidence of contracture recurrence after skin grafting has been seen with artificial dermis reconstruction (i.e., Integra) followed by skin grafting.[17]

Dehiscence: Dehiscence, or wound separation, can be either partial or complete. Dehiscence can be managed with open wound care, reclosure primarily, or with reconstruction after wound is clean. The most common causes for dehiscence are tension, suture failure, and infection. If infection is suspected, the wound should not be closed acutely, but rather only after infection has been managed.

Excessive Scarring: Excessive scarring exists in two major forms, hypertrophic scarring and keloids. They both occur more often in pigmented races, in traumatized wound, and in wounds closed under tension or across areas of tension. Thick skin of the chest, back, and shoulder is more susceptible as well as the earlobes.

A thick, inflamed scar confined to the borders of the original scar characterizes hypertrophic scarring. Treatment options include topical or injected steroids, massage therapy, silicone sheeting, or re-excision.

Keloids are benign overgrowths of scar tissue that extend beyond the original scar. Collagen synthesis and collagenase activity are higher in keloids. The collagen that is present is poorly crosslinked and immature (more type III collagen). Keloids tend to recur after treatment but recurrence is less likely if treated with postexcision steroid injections or radiotherapy.[18]

OPEN WOUND CARE

Open wound care is always part of the management of traumatic wounds. Initial wound care is important in preventing sepsis and decontaminating wounds. Unsuccessful wound care prevents closure by tertiary intention. Chronic wound care, as in healing by secondary intention, must promote healing while preventing secondary infection. Wounds that are left open require case specific modification. It is important to maintain a moist, clean wound-healing environment. It should be replaced with saline solution once bacterial infection has been eradicated. Complete description of wound dressings is beyond the scope of this chapter. However, it is important to grasp the different types of dressings (see Table 5).

Supportive dressings attempt to preserve an *in vivo* environment and promote healing by limiting contamination, trauma, and desiccation. The standard wet-to-dry dressing is an isotonic saline solution used on sterile gauze. The wet gauze dressing is changed two to three times per day and allowed to partially dry on the wound. As it is removed, it removes adherent, nonviable debris with the gauze.

Antibacterial dressings are important if the wound is contaminated with bacteria. Most frequently, a sodium hypochlorite solution (Dakin solution) that is bactericidal

TABLE 3
COMMON PEDICLED FLAPS

Use	Flap	Vessels	Sensory Nerve
Nasal, upper face	Forehead	Supratrochlear or supraorbital	Supratrochlear or supraorbital
Scalp, face, and ear	Temporalis	Temporal branch maxillary artery	Auriculotemporal
Scalp	Orticochea	Supraorbital, supratrochlear, superficial temporal, postauricular, and occipital	None
Posterior/lateral scalp, cervical/thoracic spine, and neck	Trapezius	Transverse cervical artery	Cervical plexus
Chest, neck, posterior scalp, and shoulder	Latissimus dorsi	Thoracodorsal	Thoracodorsal
Sternum, shoulder, chest, head, and neck	Pectoralis	Pectoral thoracoacromial branch or internal mammary perforators	None
Chest	Deltopectoral	Internal mammary perforators	None
Abdomen, perineum	Hypogastric	Superficial epigastric	None
Chest, abdomen, and perineum	Rectus	Superior or deep inferior epigastric	Intercostals
Chest/sternum, abdomen, and perineum	Omental	Right gastroepiploic	None
Perineum	Rectus femoris	Lateral circumflex	None
Perineum	Gracilis	Medial femoral circumflex	Obturator
Groin	Sartorius	Profunda femoris perforators	None
Hand	Dorsal radial	Radial	Radial sensory
Hand	Radial forearm	Radial	Superficial radial and antebrachial cutaneous
Hand, forearm	Groin	Superficial circumflex iliac	None
Fingers	Littler	Digital artery	Digital nerve
Trochanter, ischium	TFL	Transverse branch of lateral circumflex	Lateral cutaneous nerve of thigh
Sacrum, ischium,	Gluteal	Superior gluteal	Cutaneous branches
Ischium	Posterior thigh	—	Cutaneous branches
Proximal and midtibia	Gastrocnemius	Sural branches of popliteal	None
Mid and distal tibia, small ankle	Soleus	Popliteal/posterior tibial	Medial popliteal

TFL, tensor fascia lata.

may be used but it also impairs wound healing unless used in the proper concentration. Standard Dakin solution was 0.25%. A 0.025% Dakin solution is toxic to most common bacteria and fungi but not toxic to fibroblasts *in vitro*.[19]

Debriding agents are also available but should not be used to replace surgical debridement.

Promoting agents have been developed with messengers in the healing pathways by recombinant techniques.

Subatmospheric Pressure Treatment

Vacuum-assisted closure (VAC, Kinetic Concepts, Inc, San Antonio, TX) is a wound dressing system consisting of a polyurethane sponge covered with an occlusive dressing. Subatmospheric pressure (topical negative pressure) is applied by means of a vacuum pump, typically at a constant negative 125 mm Hg. The VAC device has become a well-established technique for the treatment of complex wounds. VAC has been shown to promote healing by increasing blood flow, enhancing wound contracture,

removing edema, promoting granulation tissue, and enhancing bacterial clearance. Numerous studies have shown that the VAC increases healing, simplifies dressings, improves patient comfort, and decreases medical costs. It has also been shown to minimize inflammatory response and can keep wounds in an acute phase allowing for continued debridement and wound care before definitive reconstruction.[20-22]

Temporary Coverage

Large wounds are typically unable to be closed primarily and carry the complications of ongoing fluid loss, a continuous acute inflammatory phase, and pain associated with its presence. Early coverage of these large wounds is desirable, even if only temporary, in that it limits fluid losses, reduces the inflammatory response, and removes the morbidity of dressing changes over open wounds. However, a wound must be clean enough to close primarily in order to use these materials. There are organic dressings

TABLE 4

DISTANT/FREE FLAPS

Common Use	Flap	Artery	Sensory Nerve
Scalp, breast, sternum, lower extremity, and perineum	Rectus abdominus	Superior or deep inferior epigastric artery	None
Scalp, breast, sternum, thorax, and lower extremity	Latissimus dorsi	Thoracodorsal	Thoracodorsal
Head and neck	Radial forearm (with or without bone)	Radial	Superficial radial and antebrachial cutaneous
Head and neck, bone	Iliac crest	Deep circumflex iliac	None
Mandible, bone	Free fibula	Peroneal	None
Large defects of thorax, head, and neck	Gluteus maximus	Superior or inferior gluteal artery	None
Small wounds, facial reanimation, and perineal/penile reconstruction	Gracilis	Medial femoral circumflex	Obturator branches
Skull, extremity	Scapular flap (with or without bone)	Circumflex scapular	None
Large wounds, sternum	Omentum	Right gastrepiploic	None
Breast, large defects	Anterolateral thigh	Lateral femoral circumflex	None
Breast	Ruben flap	Deep circumflex iliac	None
Breast	DIEP flap	Deep inferior epigastric perforator	None
Breast	SIEP flap	Superficial inferior epigastric perforator	None
Hand, lower extremity	Lateral arm	Posterior radial collateral	Posterior cutaneous

DIEP, deep inferior epigastric perforator; SIEP, superficial inferior epigastric perforator.

TABLE 5

WOUND DRESSINGS

Dressing	Active Ingredient	Mechanism of Action
Supportive		
Normal saline	Sodium chloride	Atraumatic, keeps wound moist, debrides and removes exudate
Hydrogel	Water	Maintains moisture
Hydrocolloids	Hydrophilic colloid	Absorbs fluid, protects wound, autolysis, and promotes epithelialization
Semiocclusive films	Semipermeable membrane	Limits contamination, minimizes desiccation
Alginates	Calcium alginate	Provides moisture, absorbs exudate
Antibacterial		
Dakin solution	Sodium hypochlorite	Toxic to bacteria and fungi, but impairs fibroblasts/epithelialization
Acetic acid	Acetic acid	Toxic to bacteria and fungi, but impairs fibroblasts/epithelialization
Silver sulfadiazine	Silver sulfadiazine	Broad spectrum antibacterial, moist, accelerates epithelialization
Sulfamylon	Mafenide acetate	Bacteriostatic, penetrates deeply (even into cartilage)
Silver-coated polymers	Silver	Antimicrobial, promotes epithelialization, and debrides at removal
Debriding agents		
Papain/urea	Cysteine protease	Debrides nonviable tissue
Collagenase	Collagenase	Digest collagen of nonviable tissue
Promoting agents		
Regranex (Ethicon: Cornelia, GA)	PDGF	Stimulates fibroblast migration and collagenase production
VAC. (K.C.I., Inc., San Antonio, TX)	Topical negative pressure	Promotes neovascularization, wound contracture, removes edema, promotes granulation, and enhances bacterial clearance

PDGF, platelet derived growth factor; VAC, vacuum-assisted closure.

TABLE 6
IMPORTANT HEALING FACTORS

Protein	Hypoalbuminemia leads to edema and deficiency of essential amino acids, especially arginine and glutamine
Vitamin A	Important for epithelialization and immune function (promotes inflammatory phase and collagen synthesis)
Vitamin C	Cofactor required for hydroxylation of proline and lysine in collagen formation
Vitamin D	Required for calcium metabolism, bone healing
Trace elements	
Zinc	Cofactor for DNA polymerase/reverse transcriptase and proliferation of lymphocytes and NK cells
Copper	Cofactor in collagen formation with vitamin C
Iron	Cofactor in proliferation of DNA (ribonucleotide reductase) and hydroxylation of proline

NK, natural killer.

TABLE 7
SYSTEMIC INHIBITORS OF HEALING

Malnutrition	Impaired immune response and anabolism
Diabetes	Vascular compromise, impaired inflammatory response, lack of insulin as growth factor
Steroids	Suppresses inflammatory response and prolyl hydroxylase, reversed by vitamin A
Sepsis	Impaired inflammatory response, decreased tissue oxygenation
Cytotoxic drugs	Suppress collagen synthesis and fibroblast proliferation
Radiation	Arteriolar fibrosis reduces oxygen delivery, damage to fibroblasts
Smoking	Elevated carboxyhemoglobin reduces oxygen delivery
Ischemia	Compromised tissue oxygenation
Anemia	Compromised tissue oxygenation

available which carry the additional benefit of promoting wound healing. These dressings are harvested from cadavers (allograft) or from animals (xenograft). They are pretreated (i.e., radiation) to prevent viral or bacterial contamination. These grafts will initially adhere to the wound, as would an autografted skin graft. This ends the inflammatory phase of wound healing and promotes regeneration. Ultimately, these organic dressings are rejected by the immune system, typically at 10 to 20 days, at which point reconstruction must be initiated.[23]

Nutrition

Once the decision has been made that a wound is not amenable to primary closure, one must optimize the wound-healing environment. Nutrition plays a critical role. Many nutritional factors are necessary for optimal healing (see Table 6). In addition to ensuring good oral intake, it is important to promote healing by supplementing protein, vitamins (especially vitamin C) and essential elements, especially zinc. Often, the acute trauma patient has other injuries or conditions that impair their ability to support their own nutrition (see Table 7). In those situations, it is necessary to initiate nutritional assistance. Enteric feeding can be initiated with gastric or jejunal feeding tubes. If enteric intake is contraindicated, parenteral nutrition should be initiated.

CONCLUSIONS

The management of traumatic wounds requires acute decisions with short- and long-term implications. Initially, the severity and importance of the wound must be determined in the primary assessment of the patient. Early decisions regarding wound management determine the outcome and course of events. The golden period of acute wounds is typically referred to as 6 hours, after which primary closure is less desirable (24 hours in the face). However, the multitudes of wound care decisions far exceed the question of closure. Decisions must be made regarding dressings, antibiotics, tetanus, setting of management, and consultations. General principles of management include initial debridement, possible serial debridements (N+1 rule), early closure, optimal wound care and wound healing environment, and preservation of future options.

REFERENCES

1. American College of Surgeons Committee on Trauma. Advanced trauma life support program for doctors, 7th ed. Chicago: American College of Surgeons Committee on Trauma; 2004.
2. Hopson WB Jr, Britt LG, Sherman LG, et al. The use of topical antibiotics in the prevention of experimental wound infections. *J Surg Res.* 1968;8:261–266.
3. Alexander JW, Fischer JE, Boyajian M, et al. The influence of hair-removal methods on wound infections. *Arch Surg.* 1983;118(3):347–352.
4. Mishriki SF, Law DJ, Jeffery PJ. Factors affecting the incidence of postoperative wound infection. *J Hosp Infect.* 1990;16:223–230.
5. Jackson DM. The diagnosis of the depth of burning. *Br J Surg.* 1953;40:588–596.
6. Plikaitis CM, Molnar JA. Subatmospheric pressure wound therapy and the vacuum-assisted closure device: Basic science and current clinical successes. *Exp Rev Med Devices.* 2006;3(2):175–184.
7. Ritchie AG, Rocke LG. Staples versus sutures in the closure of scalp wounds: A prospective, double-blind, randomized trial. *Injury.* 1989;20(4):217–218.
8. Axelrod TS, Buchler U. Severe complex injuries to the upper extremity: Revascularization and replantation. *J Hand Surg.* 1991;16A:574.
9. Aston SJ, Beasley RW, Thorne CH, eds. *Grabb and smith's plastic surgery,* 5th ed. Philadelphia: Lippincott-Raven; 1997.
10. Ratner D. Skin grafting. From here to there. *Dermatol Clin.* 1998;16(1):75–79.

11. Smahel J. The healing of skin grafts. *Clin Plast Surg.* 1977;4(3): 409–424.
12. Rudolph R, Fisher JC, Ninnemann JL. *Skin grafting.* Boston: Little, Brown, and Company; 1979.
13. Converse JM, Rapaport FT. The vascularization of skin autografts and homografts: An experimental study in man. *Ann Surg.* 1956;143:306.
14. Schneider AM, Morykwas MJ, Argenta LC. A new and reliable method of securing skin grafts to the difficult recipient bed. *Plast Reconstr Surg.* 1998;102(4):1195–1198.
15. Eisenbud D, Huang N, Luke S, et al. Skin substitutes and wound healing: Current status and challenges. *Wounds.* 2004;16(1): 2–17.
16. Hasen SL, Voigt DW, Wieblehaus P, et al. Using skin replacement products to treat burns and wounds. *Adv Skin Wound Care.* 2001;14(1): 37–46.
17. Frame JD, Stil J, Lakhel-LeCoadou A, et al. Use of dermal regeneration template in contracture release procedures: A multicenter evaluation. *Plast Reconstr Surg.* 2004;113(5):1330–1338.
18. Kelly AP. Medical and surgical therapy of keloids. *Dermatol Ther.* 2004;17(2):212–218.
19. Kozol RA, Gillies C, Elgebaly SA. Effects of sodium hypochlorite (Dakin's solution) on cells of the wound module. *Arch Surg.* 1988;123(4):420–423.
20. Morykwas MJ, Argenta LC, Shelton-Brown EI, et al. Vacuum-assisted closure: A new method for wound control and treatment: Animal studies and basic foundation. *Ann Plast Surg.* 1997;38(6):553–562.
21. Ford CN. Interim analysis of a prospective, randomized trial of vacuum assisted therapy versus the healthpoint system in the management of pressure ulcers. *Ann Plast Surg.* 2002;49(1):55–61.
22. DeFranzo AJ. The use of vacuum assisted closure therapy for the treatment of lower extremity wounds with exposed bone. *Plast Reconstr Surg.* 2001;108(5):1184–1191.
23. Rosenberg AS, Munitz TI, Maniero TG, et al. Cellular basis of skin allograft rejection across a class I major histocompatibility barrier in mice depleted of CD8+ T cells *in vivo. J Exp Med.* 1991;173:1463–1471.

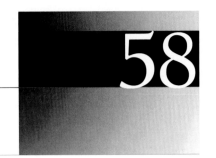

Traumatic Peripheral Nerve Injury

Nicholas Arredondo   *Donald A. Smith*

Managing patients with peripheral nerve injuries (PNIs) in the trauma setting is particularly challenging. Concomitant central nervous system (CNS), orthopaedic, and vascular injuries easily confound the evaluation of limb function. Patients with PNIs also tend to have relatively high mean injury severity scores because of the frequent association with head injury, chest trauma, and spine fractures.[1,2] During convalescence, the patient with PNI has a greater need of posthospitalization rehabilitative and social services than does the general trauma patient population.[3]

PNI is estimated to occur in 2% to 5% of multitrauma victims,[4,5] often being diagnosed in a delayed manner after other more obvious and life-threatening issues have been addressed. Because diagnostic delay can mitigate functional outcomes and may sometimes bear medicolegal consequences, a rapid and reliable protocol for evaluating nerve injuries is important. Despite dramatic advances in soft tissue imaging and electrophysiologic evaluation, the most sensitive and cost-effective diagnostic tool remains a sound and thorough clinical examination. Current management practice for PNI is largely a derivative from experience gained in the treatment of large numbers of 20th century combat wounds.[6] As in many areas of clinical practice currently, there is a dearth of class one evidence upon which to base our treatment decisions.

ANATOMY OF PERIPHERAL NERVES

Peripheral nerves have three principal constituents: axons, the elongated cell processes of neurons which propagate nerve action potentials (NAPs); Schwann cells, which ensheathe axonal processes within a wrapper of myelin;

and a connective tissue matrix, which itself has three components—the epineurium, the perineurium, and the endoneurium (see Fig. 1). The cell bodies of peripheral nerves reside in the ventral horn of the central gray matter of the spinal cord (motor fibers), in the dorsal root ganglia (sensory fibers), and in the paraspinal autonomic ganglia. Both neurotransmitters and structural cytoskeletal elements are manufactured within these neuronal cell bodies and are transferred centrifugally through processes of slow and rapid axoplasmic transport.

The three-layered connective tissue matrix organizes the fibers into small bundles termed *fascicles*. Schwann cells may envelope individual axons in a multilayered protective wrapping of myelin, as in the case of heavily myelinated "Ia fibers" that supply the muscle spindle, or a group of axons such as in unmyelinated "C fibers" responsible for

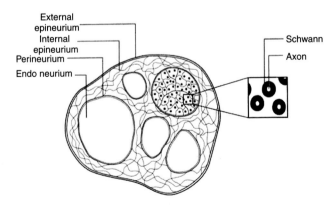

Figure 1 Schematic cross-section of a peripheral nerve. (Grant GA, Goodkin R, Kliot M. Evaluation and surgical management of peripheral nerve problems. *Neurosurgery.* 1999;44:825–840.)

pain sensation. The myelin investment acts as an electrical insulator promoting saltatory conduction jumping between the nodes of Ranvier, thereby considerably accelerating neural conduction velocity. Small unmyelinated pain fibers appear to be more susceptible to injury than are larger myelinated sensory or motor fibers.

Proximally within a peripheral nerve there is an intermingling of motor, sensory, and autonomic fibers. Distally they segregate into separate fascicles grouped by function and target organ. This segregation is reflected in varying fascicular patterns: polyfascicular nerves have many differently sized fascicles; oligofascicular nerves have few fascicles; and monofascicular nerves consist of one large fascicle. As an example, the ulnar nerve is polyfascicular in the upper arm, transitioning to oligofascicular at the elbow, and terminating in monofascicular nerves in the fingers.[7] The blood supply to peripheral nerves is relatively robust and is provided by longitudinally oriented vessels running within the epineurium. This permits telescopic lengthening and shortening of the vasculature associated with joint movement. Small collateral vessels branch obliquely from the parent trunk into the perineurium and endoneurium to give segmental supply to individual fascicles.[8]

CLASSIFICATION OF PERIPHERAL NERVE INJURY

A clinically useful schema for classifying PNI is important for understanding mechanisms of injury and recovery, as well as for predicting clinical outcomes and guiding therapeutic interventions. Although quite simplistic, the well-known Seddon classification retains a high level of utility for these purposes (see Fig. 2).[9] PNI is classified into three broad categories based on an idealized conception of the primary pathophysiology involved.

Neuropraxic injury is the least severe form of injury. It is thought to arise from a transient conduction block resultant from a local perturbation of the ionic balances that sustain normal transmembrane electrical potentials. Because the nerve itself retains its physical integrity, the prognosis for spontaneous recovery is very good, although the myelin sheath can sometimes experience permanent damage. Recovery from neuropraxic injury is usually swift, with marked clinical improvement generally observed within hours to a few days.

Axonotmetic injury is more severe. The axon itself is disrupted with degeneration of the distal stump. However, the surrounding support structures including the endoneurial tubules and perineurial sheaths remain intact to a variable degree, leaving in place a conduit-guiding axonal outgrowth to appropriate reinnervation of target organs. The quality of recovery is dependent on the degree to which this intrinsic architecture has been maintained and the distance which the reparative axonal growth cone must traverse to its target (*vide infra*). Some cases may require surgical intervention if extensive scarring impedes axonal regeneration.

Neurotmetic injury is the most severe form of PNI and results in discontinuity of both the axon and the endoneurial conduits, either from internal scarring or by physical transection. This class of injury has the worst outlook for functional recovery despite optimal management, including surgical intervention.

Although the terminology of the Seddon classification continues to enjoy wide usage, the underlying pathophysiology in most cases of PNI is complex, incorporating several mechanisms of injury at variable locations in the nerve.[10] The Sunderland classification expands the Seddon schema into five different grades of injury according to a more elaborate characterization of the imputed pathophysiolgy.[11] (See Table 1.)

PATHOPHYSIOLOGY OF PERIPHERAL NERVE INJURY AND REGENERATION

Axonotmetic and neurotmetic injury unleash an inflammatory cascade leading to the distal degeneration of the nerve first described by Augustus Waller.[12] Although all the mechanisms underlying Wallerian degeneration are not completely understood, a characteristic process of dissolution of the axoplasm and axolemma of the distal stump commences within 24 to 48 hours postinjury. Calcium ion influx and activation of axonal proteases are the initial signatures of this event. In the days and weeks subsequent to injury cytokine-activated macrophages continue this process.[13]

Recovery from PNI depends on the degree and type of injury. Neuropraxic injuries such as conduction blocks that

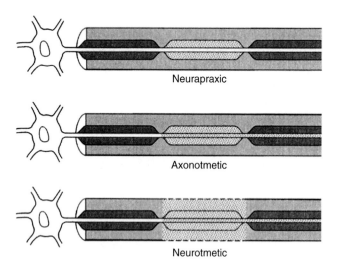

Figure 2 Schematic of Seddon classification of nerve injuries. (Grant GA, Goodkin R, Kliot M. Evaluation and surgical management of peripheral nerve problems. *Neurosurgery.* 1999;44: 825–840.)

TABLE 1

CLASSIFICATION SYSTEMS FOR PERIPHERAL NERVE INJURY

Seddon Classification	Sunderland Classification	Pathology	Prognosis
Neuropraxia	First degree	Myelin injury or ischemia	Excellent recovery in weeks to months
Axonotmesis		Axon loss Various stromal disruption	Good to poor depending on integrity of supporting structures and distance to muscle
	Second degree	Axon loss Endoneurial tubes intact Perineurium intact Epineurium intact	Good depending on distance to muscle
	Third degree	Axon loss Endoneurial tubes disrupted Perineurium intact Epineurium intact	Poor Axonal misdirection Surgery may be required
	Fourth degree	Axon loss Endoneurial tubes disrupted Perineurium disrupted Epineurium intact	Poor Axonal misdirection Surgery usually required
Neurotmesis	Fifth degree	Axon loss Endoneurial tubes severed Perineurium severed Epineurium severed	No spontaneous recovery Surgery required Prognosis after surgery guarded

(Adapted from Dillingham TR. Approach to trauma of peripheral nerves. In: 1998 AAEM Course C: Electrodiagnosis in traumatic conditions. Rochester: American Association of Electrodiagnostic Medicine; 1998:7–12; Robinson LR. Traumatic injury to peripheral nerves. *Muscle Nerve.* 2000;23:863–873.)

are the result of a transient ischemic insult recover most rapidly. These are usually without significant structural disruption to the axon. Following axonotmetic injury, distal axonal sprouting can begin within the first several days. If endoneurial channels are preserved to guide axonal regeneration down preestablished pathways, regrowth can progress at a rate of 1 to 5 mm per day. Laceration injuries seem to recover more slowly than do crush injuries, even after surgical reapproximation.

Much of this delay appears to occur at the site of the transection itself, where the advancing growth cone must bridge a physical gap and then find its way into existing endoneurial sheaths. In neurotmetic and the more severe grades of axonotmetic injury that are associated with endoneurial disruption, axonal regeneration can be slowed, misdirected, or even halted by intraneural scarring. This may ultimately result in neuroma formation. Recovery from demyelinating injuries is even slower and is dependent upon the location, degree, and the length of involvement.

Poor outcomes traditionally associated with more proximal PNI are believed to relate in part to the failure to achieve reinnervation in a timely manner. If target muscles are deprived of the trophic influences of neural input for more than 18 months, they become permanently damaged and are no longer receptive to reinnervation.[14] Given that axonal regrowth proceeds at a rate of approximately 25 mm per month under optimal conditions, this essentially precludes successful reinnervation of muscles more than 40 to 45 cm remote from the site of axonotmetic injury or nerve repair. Besides the distance to target organ, other factors relevant for functional recovery include the degree of intraneural scarring, the proximity of severed nerve ends to one another, patient age, and the amount of misdirected reinnervation that occurs.[15] The latter is especially problematic in proximal injuries to a peripheral nerve where there is extensive intermingling of the sensory and motor components and significant potential for misdirected reinnervation.

MECHANISMS OF INJURY

Common mechanisms of PNI include stretch, compression, ischemia, contusion, and laceration. Thermal, electrical, and injection injuries are less frequently encountered. In a civilian population, stretch and traction mechanisms account for approximately 70% of PNIs.[16] These injuries occur once the nerve has been elongated beyond its elastic limit, imparting both a mechanical trauma and a microvascular insult. The classic case is that of a brachial plexus injury (BPI). According to the severity of the applied forces, injury may range from a very transient neuropraxic deficit to a permanent internal derangement affecting multiple elements of the plexus over an extended length.

The extreme form of this injury culminates in proximal avulsion of the constitutive rootlets of the plexus from the spinal cord itself. Peripheral nerves are also vulnerable to stretch where they travel in close proximity to a dislocated joint or a long bone fracture. Fractures of the midhumeral shaft causing a radial nerve injury are a well-known example of this phenomenon.[17]

Compressive injury is typified by the classic "Saturday night palsy." In this case, the radial nerve is pinched against the underlying humerus by an external force. Although the nerve retains its physical continuity, a profound sensorimotor deficit can ensue. Combinations of mechanical deformation and microcirculatory arrest are implicated as causative factors. PNI is occasionally the result of an internally expanding hematoma (e.g., in the retroperitoneum affecting the lumbar plexus) or an expanding pseudoaneurysm (e.g., of the subclavian artery affecting the brachial plexus). Compartment syndromes in the forearm and calf are examples of injury by a primarily ischemic mechanism. The ischemic tolerance of various peripheral nerves is not fully known, but there is some evidence to indicate that vascular insufficiency in excess of 8 hours can lead to irreversible injury.[18]

The simplest form of penetrating injury is that of the sharp, clean laceration, as would be caused by a shard of glass or a knife wound. Missile wounds may be of low or high energy, and with or without fragmentation. High-energy and fragmentation wounds are associated with bony and ligamentous injury, as well as soft tissue loss. This mechanism is typical of a combat wound, the management of which is often further complicated by gross contamination. Blast effect and shock wave transmission in missile wounds may impart very damaging injury remote from the projectile trajectory, even where physical continuity of the nerve has been maintained. High-energy projectile wounds are often very difficult to repair for these reasons. Thermal and electrical PNIs are frequently associated with other significant soft injuries. Conservative treatment is usually advised, as aggressive management with extensive neural grafting has not improved outcomes for these patients.[19]

CLINICAL EVALUATION OF PERIPHERAL NERVE INJURIES

After identifying and stabilizing any life-threatening injuries, a thorough evaluation of peripheral nerve function should be included in the course of the secondary examination. A high index of suspicion should be adopted for patients with penetrating wounds in proximity to major nerve trunks (e.g., shoulder, volar forearm, buttock, groin, and popliteal fossa), and for those patients with certain joint dislocations and fractures known to be associated with PNI (see Table 2).

Examination should be systematic and standardized, beginning proximally and progressing distally. The existence

TABLE 2

FREQUENCY OF ORTHOPAEDIC INJURIES WITH ASSOCIATED PERIPHERAL NERVE INJURY

Injury	Nerve Injured	Frequency (%)
Humeral fracture	Radial	9.5
	Median	1.4
	Ulnar	3.8
Radius/ulna fracture	Median	1.3
	Ulnar	2.4
Shoulder anterior dislocation	Variable/multiple[a]	48
Femur fracture	Sciatic	1.1
Pelvic fracture	Sciatic	1.7
	Femoral	0.16
Tibia/fibula fracture	Peroneal	2.2
	Tibial	0.5
Hip dislocation	Sciatic	7.1

[a]Axillary 42%, suprascapular 14%, radial 7%, musculocutaneous 12%, median 4%, ulnar 8%.
Inaba K, Sharkey PW, Stephen DJ, et al. The increasing incidence of severe pelvic injury in motor vehicle collisions. *Injury, Int J Care Injured.* 2004;35:759–765.

of PNI is defined by motor and sensory deficits conforming to the anatomic distribution of named peripheral nerves. The limbs should be completely exposed and assessed for symmetry. Muscle tone and bulk and joint range of motion should be evaluated. Atrophy, fasciculation, and contractures all signify a prior injury unrelated to an acute trauma. Nor are spasticity, rigidity, or pathologic movements such as tremor features of PNI. Occasionally, a Tinel phenomenon can be provoked during the acute phase by lightly percussing over a partially injured nerve. This evokes characteristic electric paresthesias distally in the distribution of the affected nerve.

Functionally important muscle groups should be tested individually and throughout the range of motion of the associated joint. A detailed review of individual muscle testing is beyond the scope of this chapter, but the reader is referred to the excellent text, "*Aids to the examination of the peripheral nervous system,*"[20] which includes pictorial demonstrations. Certain key index muscles and autonomous sensory zones can be quickly assessed to screen for a major PNI in patients whose condition precludes detailed examination (see Table 3).

For a workable and comprehensive motor assessment, we recommend the organizational method of Dr. Joseph Miller (personal communication): in the shoulder girdle, there are 7 readily testable muscles innervated by 6 peripheral nerves (see Table 4); there are 25 reliably testable muscles in the upper extremity, reflecting function in 5 major peripheral nerves (see Table 5); and in the lower limb, there are 19 testable muscles that demonstrate function in 8 peripheral nerves and their major branches

TABLE 3

TABLE 3

QUICK EVALUATION OF MOTOR AND SENSORY FUNCTION BY NERVE

Nerve	Unique Muscle	Autonomous Sensory Region
Radial	Extensor pollicis longus	Dorsal first web space
Median	Abductor pollicis brevis	Radial tip of index finger
Ulnar	First dorsal interosseous	Ulnar tip of little finger
Femoral	Quadriceps	—
Tibial	Abductor hallucis	Sole of foot[a]
Superficial peroneal	Peronei longus and brevis	Dorsum of foot[b]
Deep peroneal	Extensor hallucis longus	Dorsal first web space

[a]The central portion of the heel and sole.
[b]Variable.

(see Table 6). (Miller J, personal communication, 2003). The examiner should recognize that even alert and oriented patients might not put forth a full effort in the presence of pain or for reasons of secondary gain.[21] The examiner should also be aware that certain adaptive movements undertaken to compensate for functional deficits could sometimes mask weakness. A common example of this is the substitution of the brachioradialis muscle for the biceps brachii to accomplish elbow flexion while holding the forearm halfway between pronation and supination. Palpation of the muscle belly during motor testing helps clarify these situations.

A full sensory evaluation includes testing of light touch, pinprick sensitivity, vibration, proprioception, two-point discrimination, stereognosis, and graphesthesia. In the acute setting, the circumstances of examination and the patient's own level of consciousness may preclude such exhaustive testing. Light touch and pinprick testing are usually the most informative. Both dermatomal and cutaneous sensory distributions for peripheral nerves are relatively consistent (see Fig. 3).[22] Recognizing the pattern of sensory

TABLE 4

SHOULDER GIRDLE

Nerve	Group	Muscle
Spinal accessory	Back	Trapezius
Long thoracic		Serratus anterior
Thoracodorsal		Latissimus dorsi
Dorsal scapular	Scapular	Rhomboid
Suprascapular		Supraspinatus
Suprascapular		Infraspinatus
Pectoral (medium and lateral)	Odd	Anterior pectoralis

TABLE 5

UPPER EXTREMITY PERIPHERAL NERVES AND MUSCLES TO BE TESTED

Nerve	Group	Muscle
Axillary		Deltoid
Musculocutaneous		Biceps
Radial (extensor)	Odd	Triceps
		Brachioradialis
		Supinator
	Forearm	Extensor carpi radialis longus
		Extensor carpi ulnaris
		Extensor digitorum
	Thumb	Extensor pollicis longus
		Extensor pollicis brevis
		Abductor pollicis longus
Median (flexor)	Odd	Pronator Teres
	Forearm	Flexor carpi radialis
		Flexor digitorum sublimes
		Flexor digitorum profundus I/II
	Thumb	Flexor pollicis longus
		Opponens pollicis
		Abductor pollicis brevis
Ulnar (hand)	Odd	Flexor carpi ulnaris
	Little finger	Abductor digiti minimi
		Opponens digiti minimi
		Flexor digitorum profundus III/IV
	Thumb	First dorsal interosseous
		First volar interosseous
		Adductor pollicis

loss can be extremely helpful in distinguishing a PNI from a radicular (dermatomal) or spinal cord (segmental) injury. However, there is sufficient variability and overlap in the distribution of peripheral nerves to sometimes obscure a clear-cut sensory deficit to correspond with motor findings in some cases of PNI. Additionally, as many nerve injuries are incomplete, different modalities may be differentially affected. It is not uncommon for a patient to experience loss of nociception or two-point discrimination, while maintaining a relatively acute sense of light touch. Despite the inconsistencies and incongruities that sometimes emerge during sensory testing, documentation of the patient's baseline examination and the quality of that examination are important. It will facilitate accurate diagnosis of neurologic injury, enable trending of function, and occasionally has medicolegal relevance.

The most commonly accepted methods of grading strength and sensation are based on the well-known British Medical Research Council (BMRC) 1 to 5 scales (see Tables 7 and 8).[23] Although widely employed, the BMRC motor scale is deficient in its quantification of the frequently encountered condition of a muscle that is weak, but stronger than antigravity (grade 4). The Louisiana State University Medical Center (LSUMC) grading scale

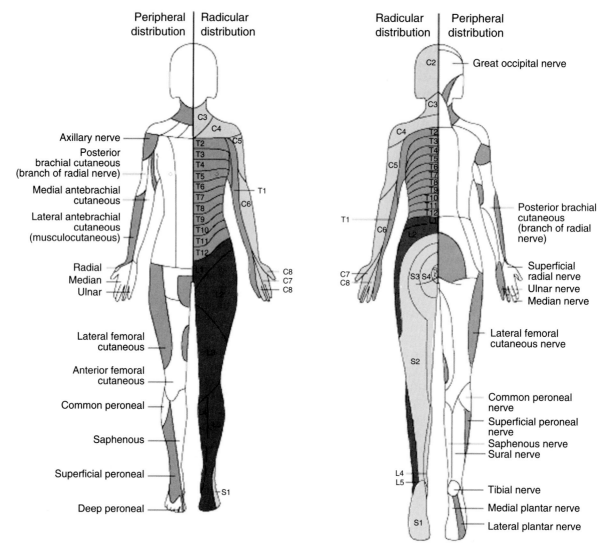

Figure 3 Location of peripheral nerve and radicular sensory regions. (Grant GA, Goodkin R, Kliot M. Evaluation and surgical management of peripheral nerve problems. *Neurosurgery*. 1999; 44:825–840.)

attempts to address this deficiency with a more precise and reproducible characterization of sensorimotor function[24] (see Tables 9 and 10). As we become more sophisticated in our management of PNI, the LSUMC scale will probably find wider currency.

Evaluation of sympathetic function is often neglected, but it can sometimes yield useful clues about the existence of PNI. Sympathetic innervation of skin runs within peripheral nerves and distributes to sweat glands. Careful examination may reveal asymmetric anhidrosis after PNI. Several methods have been described to detect anhidrosis, including dusting with starch or inspection for sweat droplets with an ophthalmoscope in dimmed light. Preserved sweating in the distribution of an injured nerve is evidence for an incomplete injury.

Potentially useful in a comatose patient, performance of the O'Rian wrinkle test may reveal autonomic dysfunction.

In the distribution of an injured nerve, immersion of fingers in tepid water for 5 to 10 minutes will fail to produce wrinkling.[25]

IMAGING AND ELECTROMYOGRAPHIC INVESTIGATIONS

Routine trauma x-rays can be a useful alerting sign for potential nerve injuries. A raised hemidiaphragm on a chest radiograph suggests a phrenic nerve injury. Limb dislocations and fractures that are frequently associated with PNI are listed in Table 2. In the subacute setting, magnetic resonance imaging (MRI) and intrathecally enhanced computed tomography (CT) can be useful in the evaluation of BPI for possible cervical nerve root avulsion. Avulsion injuries may be visualized directly or inferred

TABLE 6
LOWER EXTREMITY

Nerve	Group	Muscle
Femoral	Odd	Iliopsoas
		Sartorius
		Quadriceps
Superior gluteal	Proximal	Gluteus medius and minimus
Inferior gluteal		Gluteus maximus
Obturator		Adductors of the thigh
Sciatic		Hamstrings
Deep peroneal	Anterior	Tibialis anterior
		Extensor hallucis longus
		Extensor digitorum
		Extensor digitorum brevis
Tibial	Posterior	Gastrocnemius
		Flexor hallucis longus
		Flexor digitorum
		Posterior tibialis
Superficial peroneal	Distal	Peroneus longus
Superficial peroneal		Peroneus brevis
Lateral plantar (tibial)		Abductor pollicis

through the demonstration of a pseudomeningocele. Their demonstration precludes any hope of spontaneous recovery at the affected segments (see Fig. 4). With MRI it is also becoming possible to directly image sites of injury in the peripheral nerves themselves (see Fig. 5); with T2 and short T1 inversion recovery (STIR) sequences signal changes in acutely denervated muscle have been demonstrated within 4 days of injury (see Fig. 6).[26] MRI neurography could have a future role to play as an acute prognostic aid, informing the selection of certain injuries for surgical exploration at an earlier stage than would otherwise be possible.

TABLE 7
BRITISH MEDICAL RESEARCH COUNCIL (BMRC) MOTOR FUNCTION GRADING SCALE

Grade	Evaluation	Description
0	None	No palpable muscle contraction
1	Trace	Palpable muscle contraction, detectable by examiner
2	Poor	Active joint motion present with gravity eliminated
3	Fair	Muscle can move joint through full range of motion against gravity
4	Good	Full range of motion against gravity and some resistance
5	Normal	Full range of motion with a maximum force that is normal for that muscle

TABLE 8
BRITISH MEDICAL RESEARCH COUNCIL (BMRC) SENSORY FUNCTION GRADING SCALE

Grade	Evaluation	Description
0	Anesthesia	No sensation
1	Dysesthesia	Pain sensation (deep)
1+	—	Pain sensation (superficial)
2	—	Pain and some touch
2+	—	Pain and some touch, over-response
3	Protective sensation	Pain and touch without over-response
3+	—	Imperfect two point (S2PD 7–15 mm)
4	Normal	Complete recovery (S2PD 2–6 mm)

Electrophysiologic examination plays an important role in the diagnosis of PNI and in tracking recovery. Parameters for testing include nerve conduction velocity (NCV), compound muscle action potentials (CMAP), sensory nerve action potentials (SNAP), F- and H-waves, and electromyographic (EMG) recordings. Electrical changes are not consistently detectable immediately after injury. In most cases, studies should be purposefully delayed 3 to 4 weeks after injury to allow time for the effects of distal Wallerian degeneration to become electrically manifest. Even so, interpretation of electrodiagnostic data is not always clear-cut, especially in cases involving combinations of neuropraxic, axonotmetic, and neurotmetic PNI with primary muscular trauma.[15] Newer technologies incorporating automated neurosensory testing are improving the reliability of these modalities.[27] It is not uncommon for electrophysiologic improvement to precede clinically detectable recovery, and so serial examinations may be particularly helpful in guiding management decisions regarding the timing and advisability of a surgical intervention (*vide infra*).

TABLE 9
LOUISIANA STATE UNIVERSITY MEDICAL CENTER MOTOR FUNCTION GRADING SCALE INDIVIDUAL MUSCLE GRADES

Grade	Evaluation	Description
0	Absent	No contraction
1	Poor	Trace contraction
2	Fair	Movement against gravity only
3	Moderate	Movement against gravity and some (mild) resistance
4	Good	Movement against moderate resistance
5	Excellent	Movement against maximal resistance

TABLE 10

LOUISIANA STATE UNIVERSITY MEDICAL CENTER SENSORY FUNCTION GRADING SCALE SENSORY GRADES

Grades	Evaluation	Description
0	Absent	No response to touch, pin, or pressure
1	Bad	Testing gives hyperesthesia or paresthesia; deep pain recovery in autonomous zones
2	Poor	Sensory response sufficient for grip and slow protection; sensory stimuli mislocalized with overresponse
3	Moderate	Response to touch and pin in autonomous zones; sensation mislocalized and not normal with some overresponse
4	Good	Response to touch and pin in autonomous zones; response localized but sensation not normal; no overresponse
5	Excellent	Near normal response to touch and pin in entire field including autonomous zones

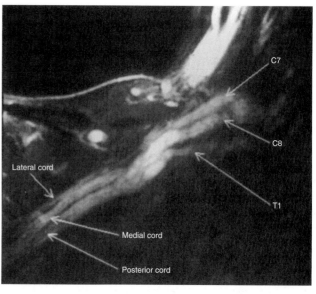

Figure 5 Coronal short T1 inversion recovery (STIR) magnetic resonance neurography (MRN) image of a 49-year-old man who sustained a traumatic brachial plexus injury. Evident is the hyperintense signal involving the C7, C8, and T1 spinal nerves, extending distally into the middle and lower trunks, divisions, and lateral, medial, and posterior cords. (Grant GA, Goodkin R, Kliot M. Evaluation and surgical management of peripheral nerve problems. *Neurosurgery*. 1999;44:825–840.)

CERTAIN COMMON PERIPHERAL NERVE INJURIES

The Brachial Plexus

BPI is a commonly encountered problem in the emergency department. As illustrated in Fig. 7, the brachial plexus

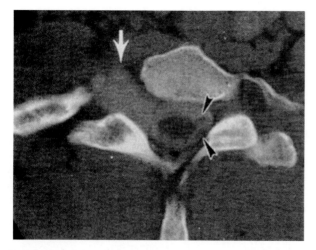

Figure 4 Axial computed tomography (CT) myelogram demonstrating a large meningocele (*white arrow*) and absent spinal nerve roots intradurally on the right side suggesting proximal root avulsion. On the left side, both dorsal and ventral spinal nerve roots (*black arrowheads*) can be seen intradurally. (Grant GA, Goodkin R, Kliot M. Evaluation and surgical management of peripheral nerve problems. *Neurosurgery*. 1999;44:825–840.)

originates in the cervical spine from the C5-T1 roots that then join and resegregate above and below the clavicle in a daunting pattern of trunks, divisions, cords, and branches. The plexus terminates in the five peripheral nerves that supply the upper limb—axillary, musculocutaneous, radial, median, and ulnar nerves. A classic injury scenario is that of the motorcyclist who crashes in a manner such as to cause depression of the shoulder with simultaneous forceful lateral flexion of the neck to the side opposite. If the plexus is overly stretched in this manner, injury may result. This type of injury accounts for approximately half of BPIs. Gunshot wounds and stab wounds are other common mechanisms of injury.[28] Table 11 lists muscles and the branches of the brachial plexus that innervate them.

BPIs are classified as either pre or postganglionic, according to whether or not elements proximal or distal to the dorsal root ganglion (DRG) are involved. Proximal injury has a very poor prognosis and its existence is signified clinically by the presence of a Horner syndrome or phrenic nerve paralysis. Proximal injury often results in avulsion of rootlets from the spinal cord with pseudomeningocele formation, as was previously discussed. Denervative potentials (fibrillations) determined in the paraspinal muscles (supplied by very early branching posterior primary rami) with "paradoxical" preservation of SNAPs (because the sensory cell body in the DRG remains intact) during electrophysiologic investigation are also indicative of proximal injury and poor prognosis.

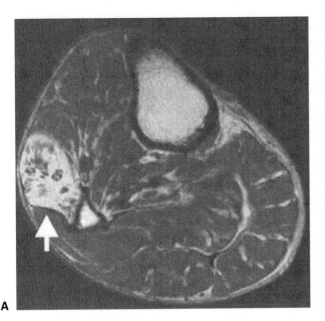
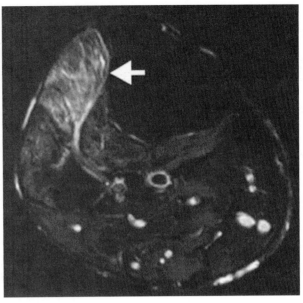

Figure 6 Demonstration of magnetic resonance imaging (MRI) changes in denervated muscle. **A:** T1 axial image of leg showing chronic fatty degeneration of the long peroneal muscle. **B:** Fat suppressed axial T2 demonstrating hyperintense signal in the anterior tibial muscle and extensor digitorum consistent with acute denervation. (Koltzenburg M, Bendszus, M. Imaging of peripheral nerve lesions. *Curr Opin Neurol.* 2004;17:621–626.)

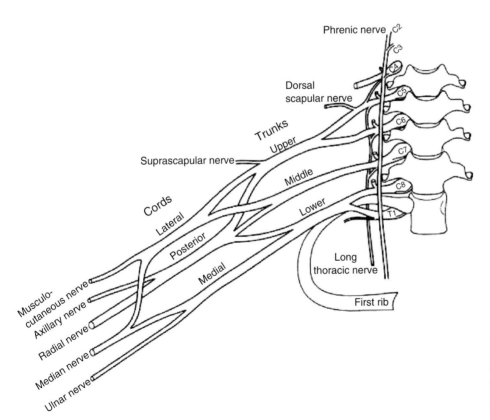

Figure 7 Diagram of brachial plexus and major nerve branches. (Grant GA, Goodkin R, Kliot M: Evaluation and surgical management of peripheral nerve problems. *Neurosurgery.* 1999;44:825–840.)

TABLE 11

BRACHIAL PLEXUS ROOTS, TRUNKS, CORDS, AND INNERVATED MUSCLES

Muscle	Root	Trunk	Cord	Nerve
Trapezius	CN XI			Spinal accessory
Serratus anterior				Long thoracic
Latissimus dorsi				Thoracodorsal
Rhomboid	C5	Upper		Dorsal scapular
Supraspinatus	C5	Upper		Suprascapular
Infraspinatus	C5	Upper		Suprascapular
Pectoralis major	C5, 6, 7		Lateral	Lateral pectoral
Pectoralis minor	C7, 8		Medial	Medial pectoral
Deltoid	C5, 6	Upper	Posterior	Axillary
Biceps	C5, 6	Upper	Lateral	Musculocutaneous
Triceps	C6, 7	Middle	Posterior	Radial
Brachioradialis	C5, 6	Upper	Posterior	Radial
Supinator	C6	Upper	Posterior	Radial
Extensor digitorum	C6, 7, 8	Middle	Posterior	Radial
Pronator teres	C6, 7	Upper	Lateral	Median
Flexor carpi radialis	C7	Middle	Lateral	Median
Abductor pollicis brevis	C8, T1	Lower	Medial	Median
Dorsal interosseous I	C8, T1	Lower	Medial	Ulnar

Suprascapular Nerve

The suprascapular nerve may be injured with resulting shoulder pain and weakness of abduction and external rotation. Most commonly, this is the result of direct trauma to the shoulder and resulting compression and stretch of the suprascapular nerve. This injury has been associated with anterior shoulder dislocation, scapular fractures, traumatic hematomas, midshaft clavicular fractures, and humeral fractures.[29]

Axillary Nerve

Axillary nerve injury occurs in 5% to 25% of shoulder dislocation.[30,31] This results in deltoid weakness and a sensory loss over the lateral humerus. The musculocutaneous nerve that innervates the biceps muscle usually escapes injury in closed trauma. Occasionally, it is subject to compressive injury in body builders and weight lifters.

Radial Nerve

The radial nerve is the direct continuation of the posterior cord of the brachial plexus. It exits the axilla in close association with the profunda brachii artery to wind posteriorly around the midshaft of the humerus in the spiral groove and pierce the lateral intermuscular septum of the upper arm. It continues its descent toward the cubital fossa between the brachioradialis and brachialis muscles, giving branches to the power supinators of the forearm, before dividing into deep and superficial branches at the level of the lateral epicondyle. The deep or posterior interosseous branch gives motor supply to the wrist and finger extensors, whereas the superficial branch is a sensory nerve that distributes to the posterior radial hand, including the relatively autonomous "anatomic snuff box area."

Most radial nerve injuries occur at a humeral level.[31] This can arise as the nerve is compressed between an external object and the proximal humerus as in a "Saturday night palsy," or in association with humeral fractures at the level of the spiral groove. Typical weakness of wrist and finger extensors and forearm supination is the result. Triceps function is preserved since its innervation derives more proximally from the radial nerve.

Median Nerve

The median nerve is formed from terminal branches of the medial and lateral cords. It exits the axilla to enter the anterior compartment of the upper arm, coursing unbranched in close relationship to the brachial artery. At the cubital fossa it gives innervation to the pronator teres, the radial wrist flexors, and the superficial finger flexors. The median nerve continues into the anterior compartment of the forearm between the two heads of the pronator teres where it gives off the important anterior interosseous branch, supplying the flexor pollicis longus and flexor digitorum profundus 1 and 2. The main trunk continues its distal descent in the volar forearm beneath the flexor digitorum superficialis group to enter the carpal tunnel at the wrist. Here it lies radial and superficial to the flexor tendons; it innervates the "LOAF" muscles of the hand: the first and second *lumbricals*, *opponens pollicis*, the *abductor pollicis brevis*, and the *flexor digitorum pollicis*. The latter three muscles comprise the bulk of the thenar eminence. The sensory distribution of the median nerve is to the radial palm through branches emanating proximal to the carpal tunnel and to the radial three and one-half fingers through digital nerves branching distal to the carpal tunnel.

The median nerve is most commonly injured in the forearm or at a humeral level.[31] When injured in the axilla or proximal upper arm, concurrent ulnar nerve injury is sometimes the result owing to the proximity of the two nerves at this level. Median nerve-related deficit depends on the exact level of injury, but at the forearm level impairments would typically include weakness of grip and finger flexion, and loss of distal phalangeal flexion for the thumb and first and second fingers, along with sensory loss in the radial aspect of the hand. The anterior interosseous syndrome causes opponens pollicis weakness with a loss of the deep flexors to the first and second fingers without an associated sensory loss. This can easily be mistaken for a flexor tendon rupture.

Ulnar Nerve

The ulnar nerve originates from the medial cord of the brachial plexus and enters the upper arm on the medial aspect of the brachial artery. At midhumeral level, it pierces the medial intermuscular septum to swing into the posterior compartment and emerge from beneath the medial head of the triceps to pass behind the medial epicondyle into the cubital tunnel on the posteromedial aspect of the elbow. There are no branches in the upper arm. The ulnar nerve continues into the forearm between the two heads of the flexor carpi ulnaris, which it supplies, also giving branches to the deep flexors of the ring and little fingers and descending in companionship with the ulnar artery. It enters the wrist ventral to the flexor retinaculum through the Guyon canal in close association with the ulnar artery and superficial to flexor tendons. The ulnar nerve innervates the intrinsic muscles of the hand except for the four median-supplied "LOAF" muscles: the muscles comprising the hypothenar eminence (abductor digiti minimi, opponens digiti minimi, and flexor digiti minimi), all of the interossei, the third and fourth lumbricals, and the adductor pollicis muscle. Sensory distribution is to the ulnar palm and last one and one-half fingers. The ulnar nerve is most commonly injured through contusive mechanisms at the elbow or by a penetrating trauma anywhere along its course.[31]

Lumbar and Sacral Plexi

Anterior rami from the upper four lumbar roots join within the psoas muscle to form the lumbar plexus. From the lateral border of this muscle emerge the iliohypogastric, ilioinguinal, lateral femoral cutaneous, and femoral nerves;

the genitofemoral nerve exits from its anterior surface; and the obturator nerve and the lumbosacral trunk leave from its medial surface. The ilioinguinal and iliohypogastric nerves enter the lateral and anterior wall of the abdominal cavity, where they provide a sensory distribution (see Fig. 8). The lateral femoral cutaneous nerve travels in the fascia of the iliacus muscle to enter the thigh beneath the lateral edge of the inguinal ligament; it has sensory distribution to the anterolateral thigh. The femoral nerve travels in the iliopsoas crease to enter the thigh beneath the midportion of the inguinal ligament, immediately lateral to the femoral sheath. It ramifies into multiple branches upon entering the upper leg to supply the quadriceps mechanism as well as giving sensory branches to the anterior and medial thigh and the medial calf. The obturator nerve courses anterolaterally over the sacroiliac joint and then onto the pelvic sidewall between the internal and external iliac vessels to enter the obturator canal, where it innervates motor supply to the adductor mechanism of the thigh.

The sacral plexus is formed from the anterior rami of L4 and L5 (through the lumbosacral trunk) and the first three sacral nerves. Its most important branches are the superior and inferior gluteal nerves, the pudendal and pelvic splanchnic nerves, the posterior femoral cutaneous nerve, and its largest branch, the sciatic nerve. The sciatic nerve is the largest peripheral nerve in the body and gives extensive supply to the muscles of the posterior thigh and the entire lower leg through its tibial and peroneal components, as will be discussed in the subsequent text. Figure 9 is a schematic diagram summarizing the innervation of the lower extremity nerves.

Injuries to the lumbar and sacral plexi are less commonly diagnosed than are brachial plexus injuries. Whether this is because of their lesser incidence or because of difficulty in their ascertainment is less clear. They usually occur in the context of major pelvic trauma, and the attendant orthopaedic injuries may confound their recognition. A study of 2,706 motor vehicle collision victims found that 17.7% of those with pelvic fractures had associated injuries to the nerves of the plexus or lower extremities, compared to only 1.9% of those without pelvic fractures.[2] In particular, injuries to the lumbosacral trunk causing weakness of foot and toe dorsiflexion are probably underdiagnosed.[33] As these are primarily closed injuries with preserved anatomic continuity of proximally affected nerves, they are mostly managed nonoperatively. However, a progressive deficit in the association with an expanding retroperitoneal hematoma could warrant surgical exploration. A burning dysesthetic paresthesia caused by genitofemoral neuralgia can be the result of blunt trauma to the abdomen. More often it is seen as an iatrogenic complication of gynecologic or abdominal surgery. It can be difficult to differentiate from ilioinguinal or iliohypogastric neuropathies[34] that are more likely to be associated with a Tinel sign at the point of compression. Most injuries will improve with conservative

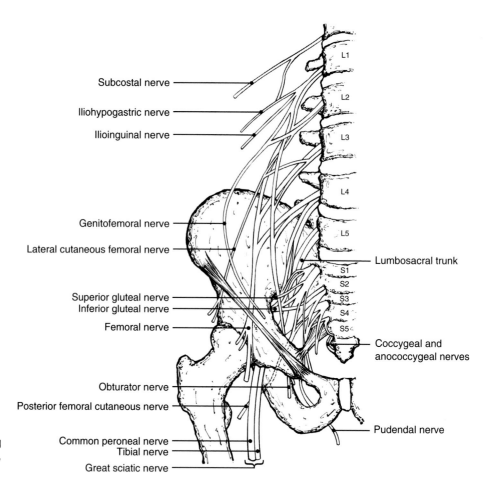

Subcostal nerve

Iliohypogastric nerve

Ilioinguinal nerve

Genitofemoral nerve

Lateral cutaneous femoral nerve

Superior gluteal nerve
Inferior gluteal nerve

Femoral nerve

Obturator nerve

Posterior femoral cutaneous nerve

Common peroneal nerve
Tibial nerve

Great sciatic nerve

L1
L2
L3
L4
L5
S1
S2
S3
S4
S5

Lumbosacral trunk

Coccygeal and anococcygeal nerves

Pudendal nerve

Figure 8   Schematic of lumbosacral plexus. (Christopher Alan Harden, artist.)

management, including selective nerve blocks, which also help confirm the diagnosis.[35]

Sciatic Nerve

The sciatic nerve is the largest and most important branch of the sacral plexus. It contains tibial and peroneal components that exit the pelvis as a single trunk through the greater sciatic foramen to enter the buttock. The sciatic nerve then courses inferolaterally over the gemelli, obturator internus, and quadratus femoris muscles and beneath the pyriformis and gluteal muscles to enter the posterior thigh. There it descends in a plane deep to the biceps femoris and semimembranosus muscles and above the adductor magnus. The tibial component of the sciatic nerve innervates the hamstring muscles of the posterior thigh. The sciatic then divides into its terminal branches, the tibial and common peroneal nerves, at the junction of the middle and distal thirds of the thigh. Sciatic nerve injury is revealed by weakness of knee flexion and the functions sub-served by the tibial and peroneal nerves to be discussed in the subsequent text. It may be injured in hip dislocation and pelvic trauma, by penetrating mechanisms, or iatrogenically as during hip arthroplasty or by poorly placed injections.[36]

Tibial Nerve

The tibial nerve continues its descent into the lower leg through the popliteal fossa to enter the calf deep to the gastrocnemius and soleus muscles, which it also supplies. Its further descent through the posterior compartment of the calf occurs in close relationship to the posterior tibial artery that it accompanies to enter the foot behind the medial malleolus, ultimately terminating in medial and lateral plantar branches. Within the calf, it innervates the long flexors of the toes and the tibialis posterior muscle in addition to the gastrocnemius and soleus. Its main functions are to plantarflex and invert the ankle, and to flex the toes. It is most commonly injured during knee dislocation or by penetrating trauma.

Peroneal Nerve

The common peroneal nerve descends through the popliteal fossa lateral to the posterior tibial nerve. It gives off the lateral sural cutaneous nerve providing sensation to the posterolateral calf. It then enters the lateral compartment of the calf, winding around the lateral head of the gastrocnemius muscle closely applied to the neck of the fibula. It then passes through the peroneus longus muscle,

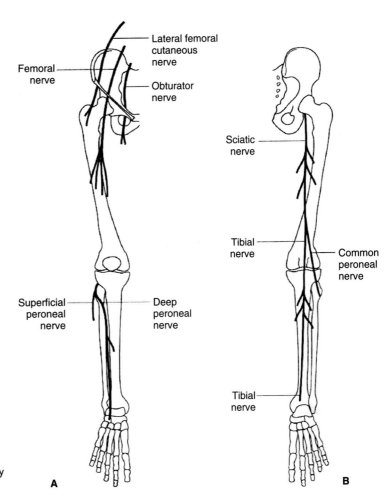

Femoral nerve

Lateral femoral cutaneous nerve

Obturator nerve

Sciatic nerve

Tibial nerve

Common peroneal nerve

Superficial peroneal nerve

Deep peroneal nerve

Tibial nerve

Figure 9 Schematic diagram of major lower extremity nerves. (http://www.medkaau.com/)

A

B

dividing into deep and superficial branches. The deep peroneal nerve continues into the anterior compartment of the calf and supplies the tibialis anterior muscle along with the extensor hallucis longus and extensor digitorum longus, whose main actions are to dorsiflex the ankle and extend the toes. The superficial peroneal nerve remains in the lateral compartment, supplying the peroneus muscles that evert the foot, and giving sensory distribution to the distal shin and foot dorsum.

The common peroneal nerve is relatively vulnerable to injury because of its relatively superficial location and close relationship to the fibula. Fractures of the fibula along with compartment syndromes and pressure injury from ill-applied casts or splints are common mechanisms of injury.[37]

TREATMENT

Treatment considerations for PNI can be complex, taking into account the nature and magnitude of the deficit, the location and mechanism of injury, associated injuries, the condition of the wound, and whether a lesion in continuity is probable. Decision trees adopted from Kliot are included

in Figures 10 and 11. If a sharp clean laceration has occurred for which no significant possibility of spontaneous recovery exists, obviously a surgical exploration and repair is warranted. This can be undertaken on a nonemergent basis, unless other considerations such as a concomitant vascular injury demand otherwise. However, most injuries are less straightforward, and usually a period of surveillance is advised to allow for spontaneous reversal of any neuropraxic component to the deficit. This is also true for missile wounds that include variable degrees of tissue loss as well as remote effects of shock and blast injury. These are best approached with purposeful delay, allowing not only for neurologic recovery in reversibly injured elements but also for demarcation of nonviable tissue margins. If associated injury demands emergent exploration, "tagging" neural tissues with nonresorbable epineural sutures is a helpful strategy to assist in their identification at a subsequent exploration and in orienting them for repair. Table 12 lists the frequencies of surgical intervention for PNIs and the average time to diagnosis for each from a large series in a major trauma center.

Injuries-in-continuity are always approached in a delayed manner. Patients are followed up with serial neurologic examinations and EMGs. Because regeneration

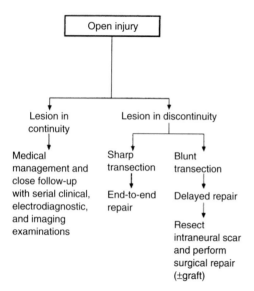

Figure 10   Schematic decision tree for open nerve injuries. (Grant GA, Goodkin R, Kliot M: Evaluation and surgical management of peripheral nerve problems. *Neurosurgery.* 1999;44:825–840.)

TABLE 12

FREQUENCY OF PERIPHERAL NERVE INJURY (PNI), TIME TO DIAGNOSIS, AND FREQUENCY OF SURGICAL REPAIR

Nerve	Percentage of Nerve Injuries	Mean Days to Diagnosis	Percentage Requiring Surgery
Radial	29.0	2.3	56.9
Peroneal	19.5	15.0	15.4
Ulnar	19.0	3.5	63.2
Sciatic	14.0	2.0	17.9
Median	12.5	4.7	60.0
Tibial	4.0	14.1	37.5
Femoral	2.0	51.8	25.0
Total	100.0	6.7	43.5

Midha R. Epidemiology of brachial plexus injuries in a multi-trauma population. *Neurosurgery.* 1997;40:1182–1189.

progresses from proximal to distal, the first signs of recovering function will be evident in reinnervated tissues just distal to the site of injury. An advancing Tinel sign may track the progress of the reparative axonal growth cone and is taken as a favorable sign. EMGs are helpful because the return of polyphasic potentials may signal early evidence of reinnervation that precedes detection by physical examination.

During this period of observation, the patient is enrolled in a physical and occupational therapy program and provided with functional splinting devices as appropriate to the deficit. An active therapy program has many benefits: maintenance of uninjured functions, implementation of adaptive strategies to help overcome acquired functional

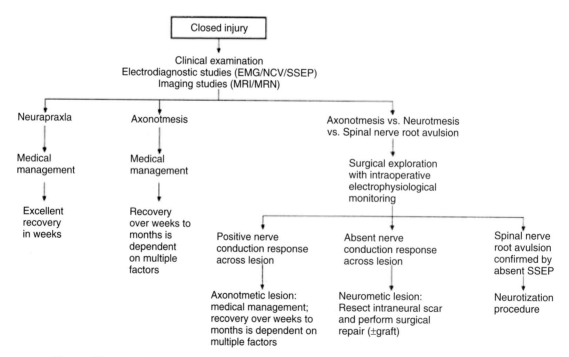

Figure 11   Schematic decision tree for closed nerve injuries. EMG, electromyographic; NCV, nerve conduction velocity; SSEP, secondary structural elements of proteins; MRI, magnetic resonance imaging; MRN, magnetic resonance neurography. (Grant GA, Goodkin R, Kliot M: Evaluation and surgical management of peripheral nerve problems. *Neurosurgery.* 1999;44:825–840.)

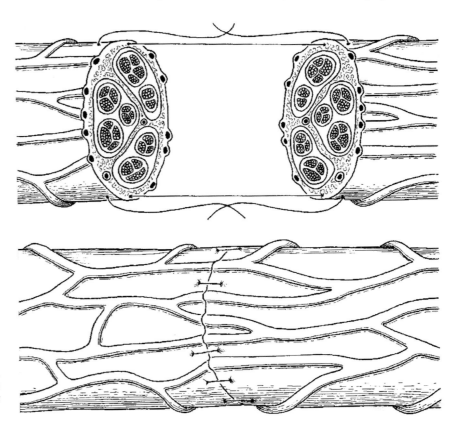

Figure 12 Epineurial neurorrhaphy. (Lee SK & Wolfe SW: Peripheral Nerve Injury and Repair. *Academy of Orthopedic Surgery.* 2000;8:243–252.)

deficits, prevention of joint contractures, and promotion of psychological well-being through institution of a dynamic intervention.

Other adjunctive therapies can be employed to help promote recovery. Neuromuscular electrical stimulation is currently used in the rehabilitation setting and may promote regrowth of motor axons.[38] Transcutaneous ultrasonography also appears to hold some promise of accelerating recovery of neurologic function, although its mechanism of action is not well understood.[39]

In the absence of evidence of significant improvements within 3 to 4 months of injury, strong consideration should be given to surgical exploration and repair.[40] For lesions-in-continuity, the overarching surgical strategy is to identify, isolate, excise, and repair those elements that are incapable of spontaneous recovery. Even in injuries for which spontaneous recovery is possible, it is not always apparent within this 3- to 4-month time frame. However, a more extended delay before exploration risks compromising the success of a neural repair for those lesions incapable of significant spontaneous recovery. As evidenced by a recent survey of peripheral nerve surgeons, there is no consensus as to the ideal timing of surgical intervention or the repair technique.[40,41] Recently, some practitioners have begun advocating earlier exploration and repair in selected cases.[42]

The intraoperative assessment of lesions-in-continuity has been significantly advanced by the use of NAP recording.[43] When a NAP is recordable across the site of injury, only an external or internal neurolysis is performed. If a conduction block is determined to be present, the damaged element is isolated and excised, and then either a primary or secondary repair is affected according to the length of the tissue gap to be overcome. Common to either form of repair is the requirement for a tensionless and accurate anastomosis that will encourage appropriate motor-to-motor and sensory-to-sensory axonal regrowth through the interface with reconstitution of functional fascicles. Techniques for nerve mobilization, transposition, and limb shortening (in the upper extremity) are available to facilitate primary repair. Epineural neurorrhaphy is a reasonable option if the two nerve ends can be accurately oriented to one another to encourage fascicle-to-fascicle contact (see Fig. 12). If not, a grouped fascicular repair is employed. When tissue loss precludes a tensionless reanastomosis, interfascicular cable grafting is utilized to overcome the gap. The sural nerve, postauricular nerves, and the antebrachial cutaneous nerves are the usual donor sources. Even more elaborate reconstructive techniques using vascularized nerve grafts and allografts are available for especially difficult situations.

PROGNOSIS

The extremes of injury are easy to prognosticate: recovery from neuropraxic injuries is usually quite good; cervical nerve root avulsions and complete injuries of the lower cord of the brachial plexus have a dismal prognosis. It is more difficult to generalize about outcomes from other types of PNI. Factors related to recovery include injury severity, patient age, psychosocial status, the length of any secondary repair, and very importantly, the distance between the lesion and the functionally important target tissues to be reinnervated.[44] The timing and quality of any surgical repair are also relevant, but may have a comparatively lesser role to play in the final result than does the nature and extent of the primary injury itself.[45] Overall, only approximately 50% of patients undergoing a nerve repair will recover useful function.[46] Table 13 lists outcomes for PNI in a large trauma population in which PNIs were distributed fairly evenly among the five Seddon grades independent of etiology. It should be noted that in this study the grade of the injury correlated strongly with the outcome. Ninety-seven percent of Seddon grade 1 injuries recovered normal function, whereas 83% of grade 5 injuries were judged poor or nonfunctional outcomes and none of them recovered normal function.

Children are anticipated to experience more robust recoveries than are adults. This may not only relate to greater plasticity of the child's nervous system and the superior recuperative powers of youth but also to the fact that the distances to be overcome by axonal regrowth are accordingly shorter than in the adult.[45] As has been previously discussed, the motor endplate must be reinnervated within 18 months of injury; otherwise the muscles become unreceptive to subsequent reinnervation. The possibility of restoring some protective sensation to the affected body part beyond this time frame may exist, but the overall functional outcome will be significantly compromised. This temporal constraint to reinnervation remains a major unsolved obstacle to recovery of distal limb functions in lower cord injuries of the brachial plexus and in gluteal level injuries of the sciatic nerve. Because of the velocity with which axonal outgrowth proceeds, target muscles must be within 40 to 45 cm of the lesion for

even the possibility of timely reinnervation to exist. In view of this constraint, it is important not to delay a surgical exploration and repair once it is determined that significant spontaneous recovery is unlikely, even for injuries that are well within this spatial domain.

The prognosis for useful recovery of hand functions in complete injuries of the lower cord of the brachial plexus remains extremely poor. Some degree of limb functionality is attainable through indirect restorative procedures such as tendon and muscle transfers, or joint arthrodesis.[47] "Neurotization" is a procedure that attempts to reestablish elbow flexion through anastomosis of supra-capular or intercostal trunks to the musculocutaneous nerve.[48]

Injury to the lumbosacral plexus bears some analogy to BPI, but has only rarely been operated upon in the past. These are usually stretch injuries seen in conjunction with cauda equina syndromes and severe pelvic trauma.[2] These associations make their diagnosis and treatment among the most difficult of all PNIs. Traditionally conservative management has been traditionally advised, but recently some surgeons have attempted direct exploration and repair as for lesions of the brachial plexus. Proximal root avulsions may be relatively more amenable to surgical intervention than in BPI.[49] Even as we gain more experience with the aggressive surgical management of these lesions, time and distance constraints to the reinnervation of the functionally relevant target muscles in the distal lower extremity present a significant impediment to success.

COMPLICATIONS OF PERIPHERAL NERVE INJURY

Besides sensorimotor and autonomic deficits, patients with PNI are also frequently subject to a variety of arthralgias and a cluster of related chronic pain disorders—causalgia, reflex sympathetic dystrophy, and "chronic regional pain syndrome." The variable prognosis of PNI combined with a long recovery time and frequently difficult to treat paresthesias can be trying for both the patient and the physician charged with their care. One of the most important roles of the trauma clinician in this setting is to educate the patient and the family regarding the possible long-term sequelae of PNI.

Causalgia is a painful condition initially described with penetrating wounds of major peripheral nerves. Characterized by severe burning dysesthetic pains and autonomic dysfunction, it is especially associated with injury to the median or sciatic nerves.[50] Vasomotor and sudomotor dysfunction cause the affected hand to be swollen and discolored; it may be either warm or cool, and trophic changes in the skin and nail beds are evident. The hand is exquisitely sensitive to any form of physical manipulation, including exposure to flowing air. It is usually reserved from any form of contact in a protective posture. Variations of this disorder are also encountered in patients with less specific musculoskeletal and PNI lacking a penetrating mechanism. This condition was formerly referred to as *reflex sympathetic dystrophy*, but current practice reclassifies this as *"chronic regional pain syndrome, types 1 and 2,"* and incorporates diagnostic criteria.[51] Up to 5% of patients with PNI may go on to develop this complication, which seems to have a curious predilection for females.[52]

Management of these pain syndromes can be quite vexing, but agents such as gabapentin, topiramate, and pregabulin in conjunction with antidepressants are often effective in attenuating the dysesthetic symptoms. Individuals refractory to these simple pharmacotherapies are best managed in a pain clinic setting with multidisciplinary access to nerve blocks, physiotherapy, desensitization techniques, biofeedback, psychological counseling, and invasive electrical stimulation.

Neuroma formation is another complication of PNI. Painful stump neuromas can be dealt with by excision and then reburial of the proximal remnant nerve more deeply in a protected soft tissue bed. Pain arising in a neuroma in continuity is more problematic. Assuming a failure of symptomatic therapies, it may also lend itself to excision if it can be successfully isolated from functional neural elements as judged by intraoperative NAP monitoring.[53]

CONCLUSION

PNI is frequent in the multitrauma patient and its recognition is often delayed. Although not life threatening in itself, it can have serious functional consequences with significant impact on the patient's subsequent socioeconomic reintegration into the community. A careful physical examination remains the most sensitive tool available for its diagnosis. Neuropraxic and low-grade axonotmetic injuries have a good prognosis for spontaneous recovery. The indications for emergent surgery are few, but sharp nerve lacerations will require surgical repair, and these should be dealt with under controlled conditions within a few days of injury. A period of purposeful delay with serial clinical and electrophysiologic assessment is advisable in most other instances, allowing time for the physical and functional demarcation of the injury. If the deficit is functionally significant and exists at a level amenable to surgery, surgical exploration and either a primary or secondary repair is undertaken within several months of injury. Randomized controlled clinical trials comparing various surgical techniques and nonsurgical therapy in the context of traumatic PNI do not currently exist, nor are any likely forthcoming in the immediately foreseeable future. In this absence, a central registry for PNI using web-based reporting of clinical parameters to a standardized database should be considered.

Despite a heightened technical prowess available since the introduction of the operating microscope and advanced intra and extraoperative electrophysiologic monitoring, the prognosis for severe proximal PNI remains very poor. The problem is much more complicated than the mechanical issue of reestablishing neural continuity. Unresolved are issues of accurate and functionally specific connectivity across the nerve gap; the speed with which the axonal growth cone progresses distally; and the maintained receptivity of muscles for subsequent reinnervation. Basic science has brought significant understanding to these processes and has indicated several novel strategies to answer these challenges. Artificial physical conduits constructed of biomaterials to guide directed axonal outgrowth[54], augmentative neurotrophic, and neurotaxic agents such as brain-derived neurotrophic factor (BDNF), glia-derived neurotrophic factor (GDNF), transforming growth factor-β (TGF-β), and neural reconstruction employing cell grafting techniques are under investigation.[47] Immunosuppressive agents such as FK506 or low-dose radiation show promise as methods of reducing scar formation.[55,56] Other lines of research have focused on the adaptive plasticity of the CNS in response to PNI, substituting additional stimuli through alternative sensory modalities to compensate for the loss of tactile input.[48] As some of these strategies may also be applicable to the repair of CNS injury, they are of extreme interest and importance to the neurosciences community at large.

REFERENCES

1. Noble J, Munro CA, Prasad VS, et al. Analysis of upper and lower extremity peripheral nerve injuries in a population of patients with multiple injuries. *J Trauma*. 1998;45(1):116–122.
2. Inaba K, Sharkey PW, Stephen DJ, et al. The increasing incidence of severe pelvic injury in motor vehicle collisions. *Injury Int J Care Injured*. 2004;35:759–765.
3. Rosberg HE, Steen Carlsson K, Höjgård S, et al. Injury to the human median and ulnar nerves in the forearm – analysis of costs for treatment and rehabilitation of 69 patients in southern Sweden. *J Hand Surg [Am]*. 2005;30B(1):35–39.
4. Selecki BR, Ring IT, Simpson DA, et al. Trauma to the central and peripheral nervous systems: part II. A statistical profile of surgical treatment in New South Wales 1977. *Aust N Z J Surg*. 1982;52:111–116.
5. Midha R. Epidemiology of brachial plexus injuries in a multitrauma population. *Neurosurgery*. 1997;40:1182–1189.
6. Woodhal B, Beebe GW. *Peripheral nerve regeneration, a follow-up study of 3656 World War II injuries, Veterans Administration, Medical Monograph*. Washington, DC: US Government Printing Office; 1956:117–118.
7. Rowshan K, Jones NF, Gupta R. Current surgical techniques of peripheral nerve repair. *Oper Tech Orthop*. 2004;14:163–170.
8. Lee SK, Wolfe SW. Peripheral nerve injury and repair. *J Am Acad Orthop Surg*. 2000;8:243–252.
9. Seddon H. Three types of nerve injury. *Brain*. 1943;66:237–288.
10. Grant GA, Goodkin R, Kliot M. Evaluation and surgical management of peripheral nerve problems. *Neurosurgery*. 1999;44:825–840.
11. Sunderland S. A classification of peripheral nerve injuries producing loss of function. *Brain*. 1951;74:491–516.
12. Waller A. Experiments on the section of the glossopharyngeal and hypoglossal nerves of the frog, and observations of the alterations produced thereby in the structure of their primitive fibers. *Philos Trans R Soc*. 1850;140:423–429.
13. Stoll G, Jander S, Myers RR, et al. Degeneration and regeneration of the peripheral nervous system: From Augustus Waller's observations to neuroinflammation. *J Peripher Nerv Syst*. 2002;7:13–27.

14. Burnett MG, Zager EL. Pathophysiology of peripheral nerve injury: A brief review. *Neurosurg Focus.* 2004;16(5):1–7.

15. Robinson LR. Traumatic injury to peripheral nerves. *Muscle Nerve.* 2000;23:863–873.

16. Kline DG, Hudson AR. *Nerve injuries; operative results for major nerve injuries, entrapments, and tumors.* Philadelphia: WB Saunders; 1995:30.

17. Mazurek MT, Shin AY. Upper extremity peripheral nerve anatomy: Current concepts and applications. *Clin Orthop Relat Res.* 2001;383:7–20.

18. Burnett MD, Zager EL. Pathophysiology of peripheral nerve injury: A brief review. *Neurosurg Focus.* 2004;16(5):1–7.

19. Kline DG, Hudson AR. *Nerve injuries; operative results for major nerve injuries, entrapments, and tumors.* Philadelphia: WB Saunders; 1995:46–47.

20. O'Brien MD. *Aids to the examination of the peripheral nervous system,* 4th ed. WB Saunders; 2000.

21. Kline DG, Hudson AR. *Nerve injuries; operative results for major nerve injuries, entrapments, and tumors.* Philadelphia: WB Saunders; 1995:68.

22. http://www.medkaau.com/album/details.php?image_id=675, 2005.

23. Highet WB. *Grading of motor and sensory recovery in nerve injuries. Report to the Medical Research Council.* London: Her Majesty's Stationary Office; 1954.

24. Kline DG, Hudson AR. *Nerve injuries; operative results for major nerve injuries, entrapments, and tumors.* Philadelphia: WB Saunders; 1995:89.

25. Kline DG, Hudson AR. *Nerve injuries; operative results for major nerve injuries, entrapments, and tumors.* Philadelphia: WB Saunders; 1995:58–59.

26. Koltzenburg M, Bendszus M. Imaging of peripheral nerve lesions. *Curr Opin Neurol.* 2004;17:621–626.

27. Ustun ME, Ogun Tc, Eser O, et al. Use of enhanced stimulation voltage to determine the severity of compressive peripheral nerve injury. *J Trauma Injury Infect Crit Care.* 2001;51:503–507.

28. Kim DH, Murovic JA, Tiel RL, et al. Mechanisms of injury in operative brachial plexus lesions. *Neurosurg Focus.* 2004;16(5):1–8.

29. Kim DH, Murovic JA, Tiel RL, et al. Management and outcomes of 42 surgical suprascapular nerve injuries and entrapments. *Neurosurgery.* 2005;57:120–127.

30. Visser CPJ, Coene NJ, Brand R, et al. The incidence of nerve injury in anterior dislocation of the shoulder and its influence on functional recovery: A prospective clinical and EMG study. *J Bone Joint Surg.* 1999;81(B4):679–685.

31. Noble J, Munro CA, Prasad VS, et al. Analysis of upper and lower extremity peripheral nerve injuries in a population of patients with multiple injuries. *J Trauma.* 1998;45(1):116–122.

32. Inaba K, Sharkey PW, Stephen DJ, et al. The increasing incidence of severe pelvic injury in motor vehicle collisions. *Injury Int J Care Injured.* 2004;35:759–765.

33. Schmidek HH, Smith DA, Kristiansen TK. Sacral fractures. *Neurosurgery.* 1984;15:735–746.

34. Murovic JA, Kim DH, Tiel RL, et al. Surgical management of 10 genitofemoral neuralgias at the Louisiana State University Health Sciences Center. *Neurosurgery.* 2005;56:298–303.

35. Kim DH, Murovic JA, Tiel RL, et al. Surgical management of 33 ilioinguinal and iliohypogastric neuralgias at Louisiana State University Health Sciences Center. *Neurosurgery.* 2005;56:1013–1020.

36. Kim DH, Murovic JA, Tiel RL, et al. Management and outcomes in 353 surgically treated sciatic nerve lesions. *J Neurosurg.* 2004;101:8–17.

37. Kim DH, Murovic JA, Tiel RL, et al. Management and outcomes in 318 operative common peroneal nerve lesions at the Louisiana State University Health Sciences Center. *Neurosurgery.* 2004;54:1421–1429.

38. Brushart TM, Hoffman PN, Royall RM, et al. Electrical stimulation promotes motoneuron regeneration without increasing its speed or conditioning the neuron. *J Neurosci.* 2002;22(15):6631–6638.

39. Mourad PD, Lazar D, Curra FP, et al. Ultrasound accelerates functional recovery after peripheral nerve damage. *Neurosurgery.* 2001;48:1136–1141.

40. Belzberg AJ, Dorsi MJ, Storm PB, et al. Surgical repair of brachial plexus injury: A multinational survey of experienced peripheral nerve surgeons. *Neurosurg Focus.* 2004;16(5):1–11.

41. Midha R. Nerve transfers for severe brachial plexus injuries: A review. *Neurosurg Focus.* 2004;16(5):1–10.

42. Carlstedt T, Anand P, Hallin R, et al. Spinal nerve root repair and reimplantation of avulsed ventral roots into the spinal cord after brachial plexus injury. *J Neurosurg.* 2000;93(Suppl 2):237–247.

43. Tiel RL, Happel LT Jr, Kline DG, et al. Nerve action potential recording method and equipment. *Neurosurgery.* 1996;39(1):103–109.

44. Gordon T, Sulaiman O, Boyd JG, et al. Experimental strategies to promote functional recovery after peripheral nerve injuries. *J Peripher Nerv Syst.* 2003;8:236–250.

45. Lundborg G. Nerve injury and repair – a challenge to the plastic brain. *J Peripher Nerv Syst.* 2003;8:209–226.

46. Lee SK, Wolfe SW. Peripheral nerve injury and repair. *J Am Acad Orthop Surg.* 2000;8:243–252.

47. Barrie KA, Steinmann SP, Shin AY, et al. Gracilis free muscle transfer for restoration of function after complete brachial plexus avulsion. *Neurosurg Focus.* 2004;16(5):1–9.

48. Malessy MJA, De Ruiter GCW, De Boer KS, et al. Evaluation of suprascapular nerve neurotization after nerve grafting or transfer in the treatment of brachial plexus traction lesions. *Neurosurg Focus.* 2004;16(5):1–13.

49. Lang EM, Borges J, Carlstedt T, et al. Surgical treatment of lumbosacral plexus injuries. *J Neurosurg Spine.* 2004;1:64–71.

50. Hassantash SA, Afrakhteh A, Maier RV. Causalgia: A meta-analysis of the literature. *Arch Surg.* 2003;138:1226–1231.

51. Stanton-Hicks M, Janig W, Hassenbusch S, et al. Reflex sympathetic dystrophy: Changing concepts and taxonomy. *Pain.* 1995;63(1):127–133.

52. Veldman PH, Reynen HM, Arntz IE, et al. Signs and symptoms of reflex sympathetic dystrophy: Prospective study of 829 patients. *Lancet.* 1993;342(8878):1012–1016.

53. Kline DG, Hudson AR. *Nerve injuries; operative results for major nerve injuries, entrapments, and tumors.* Philadelphia: WB Saunders; 1995:34.

54. Belkas JS, Shoichet MS, Midha R. Peripheral nerve regeneration through guidance tubes. *Neurol Res.* 2004;26(2):151–160.

55. Sosa I, Reyes O, Kuffler DP. Immunosuppressants: Neuroprotection and promoting neurological recovery following peripheral nerve and spinal cord lesions. *Exp Neurol.* 2005;195:7–15.

56. Gorgulu A, Uzal C, Doganay L, et al. The effect of low-dose external beam radiation on extraneural scarring after peripheral nerve surgery in rats. *Neurosurgery.* 2003;53:1389–1396.

Critical Care
of Injured Patients

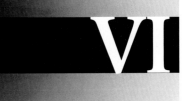

Ventilation and Oxygenation

59

Donald A. Reiff   *L. Christopher DeRosier*   *Loring W. Rue, III*

HISTORY

Mechanical ventilation was first described by Versalius during the 16th century. He conducted experiments by inserting a reed into the trachea of animals and then blowing into the conduit, demonstrated adequate ventilation. The first known device constructed expressly to provide mechanical ventilation was created by Fell O'Dwyer in 1888. The basic design was similar to an accordion that would be intermittently compressed delivering a volume of gas to the patient. During the following 90 years, ventilators have become technically more sophisticated; however, volume-cycled ventilation remains the principal mode by which mechanical ventilation is delivered. Alternate advanced modes of mechanical ventilation became available during the early 1980s when technologically complex microprocessors were incorporated into the design of mechanical ventilators. The addition of minicomputers to ventilators has broadly expanded the capabilities of our invasive monitoring of the pulmonary cycle enabling a more accurate measurement of airway pressures and comprehensive assessment of pulmonary compliance. While no data exists to support the fact that these sophisticated microprocessor ventilators achieve significantly improved results above those rendered by conventional ventilators, microprocessor-controlled ventilators have several intuitive advantages in the management of the critically ill patient. In addition to a more compact design, microprocessor-driven ventilators possess the added advantages of enhanced monitoring capabilities, computer correction capabilities, improved and comprehensive liquid crystal display (LCD) display, and the addition of several new spontaneous and mechanical modes of ventilation not previously available.

RESPIRATORY PHYSIOLOGY

Ventilation is defined as the movement of air from the exterior environment to the alveolus. Although the principal function of the lung is gas exchange within the alveolus, ventilation is solely descriptive of the mechanical function of the lung. Inadequate ventilation due to any number of factors is often an underappreciated cause of respiratory dysfunction and significant morbidity among injured and postoperative patients.

When considering the mechanical process of ventilation, it is helpful to define and understand pulmonary volumes and capacities used to describe all phases of the respiratory cycle (see Fig. 1). *Tidal volume* (VT) describes the volume of air inspired and expired in a normal breath. The extra volume of air that can be inspired beyond a normal VT is termed *inspiratory reserve volume* (IRV). Similarly, at the end of a normal VT the additional volume of air available to exhale is the *expiratory reserve volume* (ERV). The volume of air remaining within the lungs following maximal expiration is referred to as the *residual volume* (RV). The *critical closing volume* (CCV) represents the volume of air required within the pulmonary tree necessary to maintain the patency of small airways.

By combining one or more pulmonary volumes, the four pulmonary capacities are established. *Functional residual capacity* (FRC) represents the amount of air remaining within the lung following normal expiration and is the sum of the ERV and RV. The sum of the IRV, VT, and ERV is termed the *vital capacity* (VC), or the maximal amount of expired air after deepest inspiration. *Total lung capacity* (TLC) is the greatest volume to which the lungs can be expanded and is formed as the sum of the VC and the RV.

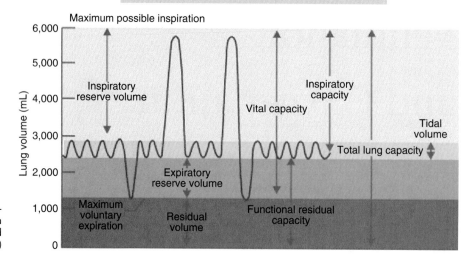

Lung volumes and capacities

Figure 1   Diagram depicting ventilation excursion during normal respiration and maximum effort of inspiration and expiration. (Courtesy of Anesthesia UK.)

The maximal volume of air that can be inspired following a normal expiration is termed the *inspiratory capacity* (IC) and is determined by the sum of VT and IRV. The ability to cycle volumes of air during the phases of respiration is affected by several factors including the mechanical resistance of chest wall and abdomen, airway resistance, and pulmonary compliance of the expanding lung parenchyma.

Airway resistance is the opposition to flow caused by the forces of friction. It is defined as the ratio of driving pressure to the rate of airflow. Resistance to flow in the airways depends on whether the flow is laminar or turbulent, on the dimensions of the airway, and on the viscosity of the gas. The viscosity of gases used during conventional mechanical ventilation remain relatively constant whereas the other two variables are quite dynamic among patients within the intensive care unit (ICU).

Laminar flow resistance is calculated using the Poiseuille Law: $R = 8l\eta/\pi r^4$ where resistance is directly proportional to the length of the conduit and inversely related to the radius of the tubing raised to the fourth power. Therefore, very subtle changes in the radius of the ventilator circuit, particularly the endotracheal tube, will have rather profound effects on the airflow. Whereas the resistance to flow is quite low under laminar conditions such that minute changes in driving pressures will result in substantial changes in flow rates, under turbulent conditions resistance is relatively large necessitating much higher driving pressures for the same flow rate. Common conditions resulting in disturbance of laminar flow include partial obstruction of the endotracheal tube by inspissated secretions, bronchospasm, endotracheal tube abutting the carina and fluid trapped within the ventilator circuit tubing.

Airway resistance decreases throughout inspiration as a consequence of increasing airway distension, wider airways provide less resistance (see Fig. 2). Furthermore, although a single small airway provides more resistance than a

single large airway, resistance to airflow also depends on the number of parallel pathways present. That is, airway resistance initially increases as air travels from the single large trachea to the smaller mainstem bronchi and onward to lobar bronchi. However, as the airways continue to bifurcate, the overall surface area of the channels exponentially expands resulting in drastic reduction in airway resistance (see Fig. 3). Subtle changes in airway diameter at the terminal bronchiolar level, as seen in patients with reactive airway disease, will have profound adverse effect on airway resistance.

A second important factor affecting ventilation is abdominal and chest wall elastic resistance. Increased thoracic stiffness can be caused by chest wall edema, contusion, hematoma associated with rib fractures, circumferential escar formation associated with severe truncal burn wounds,

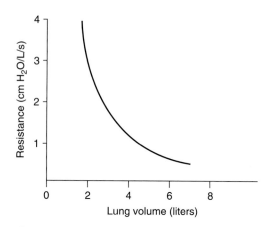

Figure 2   Increases in pulmonary volume result in airway distension and a corresponding fall in airway resistance. (Ball WC. Johns Hopkins School of Medicine's Interactive Respiratory Physiology.)

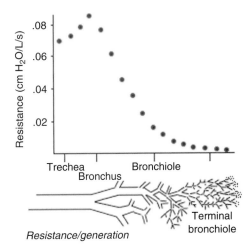

Figure 3 Bifurcation in the tracheobronchiolar tree result in a substantial increase in airway diameter and a profound reduction in airway resistance moving from the mainstem bronchi to the terminal bronchioles. (Ball WC. Johns Hopkins School of Medicine's Interactive Respiratory Physiology.)

morbid obesity and/or thoracic spine fractures. Irrespective of the cause, any reduction in elasticity of the chest wall is correspondingly associated with worsening compliance and loss of ventilation capacity. Among patients sustaining blunt force thoracoabdominal trauma, rib fractures and chest wall contusion is the most common etiology of worsening elastic resistance. The loss of ventilatory capacity as a consequence of four rib fractures has been associated with substantial morbidity and mortality.[1]

The most frequent factor associated with reduction in thoracic and diaphragmatic elasticity among elective surgical patients is abdominal surgery. As a consequence of the laparotomy, intestinal and retroperitoneal edema coupled with bowel distension results in increased abdominal volume. The bony pelvis and strong musculature laterally limit the expansion of the abdominal cavity inferiorly and laterally, the increased abdominal volume is therefore limited to anterior and cephalad expansion. If the rectus and oblique muscles relax, anterior abdominal distension results allowing for downward diaphragmatic excursion and improved ventilation. If however, the abdominal musculature is contracted in response to somatic pain, the diaphragm and anterior abdominal musculature are in direct opposition to one and other during all phases ventilation. The greater strength of the rectus and oblique muscles will overcome the diaphragm, causing cephalad displacement of the abdominal contents toward the thoracic cavity impairing effective ventilation.

Irrespective of whether a patient has sustained trauma or is recovering from elective surgery, VC is reduced in the immediate postinjury period.[2,3] The loss of VC associated with elective abdominal surgery can routinely approach 50%; this coupled with abdominal distension directed toward the thorax can impede ventilation by as much as 70%.

Although the loss of VC is significant, FRC losses are critical. Ventilation capacity loss associated with reduction in FRC is underscored by the concept of CCV. Under normal conditions, the FRC exceeds the CCV and small airways remain open. Elective thoracic and/or abdominal surgery, chest wall trauma, interstitial edema, recumbent position, and acute respiratory deficiency syndrome (ARDS) are medical/surgical conditions that can lead to a reduction in FRC below CCV causing progressive bronchiolar and alveolar collapse, with significant atelectasis resulting in profound alterations in gas exchange and exacerbating the risk of pulmonary infectious complications. The detrimental effect of the lost FRC can be negated and atelectatic lung reclaimed by delivery of positive end-expiratory pressure (PEEP), which enables the rerecruitment of these collapsed alveoli.[4-6]

Under normal circumstances, the elastic recoil of the lung should be considered in conjunction with the chest wall. Although they are mechanically coupled and function inseparably, a number of pathophysiologic conditions can lead to altered pulmonary compliance without an alteration in chest wall elasticity. Pulmonary fibrosis, ARDS, pulmonary hypertension, and pulmonary edema will substantially reduce pulmonary elasticity while chest wall compliance remains relatively unaffected. Pulmonary resistance may exceed that of the chest wall by several fold.[7]

Pulmonary compliance is defined as the ratio of change in lung volume to change in pulmonary pressure ($\Delta V/\Delta P$) and is used to represent the relative stiffness of the pulmonary parenchyma and chest wall. Most modern ventilators now enable physicians to easily and accurately calculate this value at the bedside on a real-time basis thereby permitting changes in ventilator strategies to maximize lung function while limiting barotrauma. When considering pulmonary compliance, it is helpful to quantitate the value without the effect of airflow through the pulmonary conduits, which is defined as static compliance (C_{stat}). During inspiration, pressure is exerted on the pulmonary parenchyma by gases moving through the airways, thereby raising the value of the denominator in the calculation of compliance. When attempting to minimize the barotrauma induced by mechanical ventilation and assess the true elasticity of the alveolar unit, the effect of moving gases within the airway should be eliminated. This is accomplished by measuring the airway pressure at the conclusion of inspiration by performing an inspiratory pause to yield the plateau pressure. The set PEEP is subtracted from the end inspiratory pause pressure, or plateau pressure, for the calculation of the C_{stat} represented in the formula: C_{stat} = V_T/(plateau pressure − PEEP). The pulmonary peak pressure is measured at the end of inspiration and is used to calculate the dynamic compliance (C_{dyn}) wherein C_{dyn} = V_T/(peak pressure − PEEP).

The importance of minimizing high pulmonary pressures throughout the respiratory cycle cannot be overemphasized. Several landmark studies have demonstrated significant survival advantage and reduction in morbidity among patients in whom the peak and plateau pressures were restricted below 25 cm H_2O.[8] Furthermore, other investigators have demonstrated that acute lung injury (ALI) may be induced in patients with physiologically normal lung parenchyma who are ventilated with excessively high V_{TS} (>8 mL per kg ideal body weight).[9,10] Current data suggests that volume-restricted and pressure-limited ventilation is superior. V_{TS} are recommended not to exceed 6 mL per kg ideal body weight with peak pressure limited to <25 cm H_2O.[8,11]

Differences in peak and plateau pressures can be used to evaluate acute deterioration in respiratory function among mechanically ventilated patients. An acute increase in peak pulmonary pressure with concomitant increase in plateau pressure is found among patients with worsening pulmonary compliance. The worsening compliance could result from any number of factors including abdominal distension associated with abdominal compartment syndrome, dysynchronous breathing against the mechanical ventilator, atelectasis and/or lobar collapse, auto-PEEP, ARDS, and pneumothorax. Mechanically ventilated patients with stable plateau pressures in whom peak pressures are progressively increasing should be evaluated for airway obstruction due to aspiration, inspissated pulmonary secretions, bronchospasm, or mainstem bronchial intubation.

Among patients without pulmonary injury and normal lung elasticity, normal C_{stat} values will range from 50 mL per cm H_2O to 80 mL per cm H_2O. As the degree of pulmonary insult worsens as a consequence of trauma and/or inflammatory changes associated with injury, compliance values will fall to the range of 20 mL per cm H_2O to 50 mL per cm H_2O. When compliance is found <40 mL per cm H_2O, ventilation independent of mechanical assistance becomes impossible even among the young and healthy. ARDS is hallmarked by diffuse pulmonary infiltrates, severe hypoxemia (PaO_2/FIO_2 ratio <200), noncardiogenic pulmonary edema, and extraordinarily poor compliance measured <20 mL per cm H_2O. Several studies have documented compliance, and sometimes more importantly changes in compliance, can be used as a predictor of mortality among ICU patients.[12,13]

While establishing an orotracheal or surgical airway should not be taken lightly, instituting mechanical ventilation should not be viewed as failure. All too often, postoperative and injured patients will exert increased work of breathing, worsening hypoxemia, atelectasis, and lobar collapse with acute pulmonary failure whereas the inexperienced introduce often-ineffective measures to improve pulmonary physiology in an effort to avoid orotracheal intubation. The efficacy of noninvasive ventilation (NIV) among a wide spectrum of patient populations including those with chronic obstructive pulmonary disease (COPD) exacerbation, reactive airway disease, obstructive sleep apnea, and cardiogenic pulmonary edema is

well established.[14–16] While exacerbation of many chronic medical conditions are well managed by NIV, the role for noninvasive assistance with ventilation for the acutely injured is less well established and somewhat controversial.[17–19]

MECHANICAL VENTILATION

Continuous Positive Airway Pressure/Bilevel Positive Airway Pressure

Continuous positive airway pressure (CPAP) ventilation and bilevel positive airway pressure (BiPAP) ventilation are similar methods of augmenting the patient's own ventilatory efforts through a tight fitting nasal or facial mask. CPAP ventilation delivers continuous positive airway pressure (usually 5–10 cm H_2O) throughout the respiratory cycle, which aids in increasing FRC and PaO_2 levels with the expansion of atelectatic alveoli. BiPAP provides two different levels of positive pressure. A higher pressure (usually 10 cm H_2O) is delivered during inspiration (inspiratory airway pressure [IPAP]) whereas a lower pressure (usually 5 cm H_2O) is delivered during expiration (expiratory airway pressure [EPAP]) and functions as PEEP in patients with a secure nose/mouth mask. Patients who demonstrate the greatest benefit from noninvasive forms of ventilation are those suffering from COPD exacerbations.[20] Contraindications to these noninvasive forms of ventilation include decreased mental status, suspected facial or airway trauma, suspected gastrointestinal trauma, untreated pneumothorax, and hypotension. Although studies have shown some indications and advantages of noninvasive positive airway ventilation in avoidance of intubation,[21] this does not apply to the multitrauma patient who requires oxygenation and/or ventilation support. It is the practice of our institution to avoid noninvasive modes of ventilation in the acute setting following traumatic injury and for patients with multisystem traumatic injury who demonstrate pulmonary deterioration during their hospitalization. If the decision is made to use noninvasive positive pressure ventilation, a functioning nasogastric tube as well as a tube thoracostomy (if pneumothorax is suspected) is essential in preventing aspiration or tension pneumothorax respectively.

CPAP and BiPAP are tempting alternatives in patients who have recently been extubated and who have deteriorating oxygenation so as to potentially avoid reintubation. A large multicenter randomized clinical trial of extubated patients who demonstrated postextubation respiratory insufficiency compared standard medical therapy to medical therapy that included NIV. They concluded that although NIV did not reduce mortality or need for reintubation, there was a trend to higher mortality rates among those assigned to NIV.[22] Although only a small number of these patients were trauma patients (10% in the NIV group and 7% in the standard medical therapy group), it is reasonable to extrapolate this data to the trauma patient and not rely on CPAP or BiPAP as a mode of avoidance of reintubation in the recently extubated trauma patient with postextubation respiratory insufficiency.

Endotracheal Intubation and Modes of Ventilation

Once the decision has been made to intubate a patient and initiate mechanical ventilation, multiple ventilatory modes are available to the clinician. As technology has advanced, capabilities of mechanical ventilators have increased enormously. These modes generally differ on the basis of volume- versus pressure-cycled modalities and control versus assist modalities. A thorough understanding of the advantages and disadvantages of these strategies are necessary for successful management of the ventilated patient and minimizing the adverse sequelae of mechanical ventilation such as barotrauma. To understand the various modalities, it is essential to understand the different settings available and what variables determine these settings.

Breath Initiation

Trigger is the term used to define the setting on a ventilator that the system uses to initiate a delivered breath. In controlled mechanical ventilation (CMV), the ventilator delivers a preset number of breaths determined by the clinician. This set mandatory rate is independent of those initiated by the patient and is an appropriate mode of ventilation for patients with neuromuscular paralysis, respiratory paralysis from trauma, or with deep sedation. Assist control ventilation (ACV) provides a preset rate of breaths that will be delivered regardless of patient initiation; however, if the patient initiates a spontaneous breath (trigger), the ventilator will deliver the preset breath in either a volume- or pressure-limited manner. ACV will allow a patient to increase respiratory rate because the patient may trigger the ventilator to deliver extra breaths over and above the preset rate. Intermittent mechanical ventilation (IMV), which has largely been replaced with synchronized intermittent mechanical ventilation (SIMV) also allows for a preset rate. However, if the patient initiates a breath during the expiratory phase, the ventilator will allow the patient to pull gas from the circuit. The physician can regulate the extent of assistance for these patient-initiated breaths through pressure support (PS). If the patient initiates a breath in close temporal proximity to the set ventilator breath, the preset breath will be given. The final end of the "trigger" spectrum is pressure support ventilation (PSV), in which a preset amount of assistance is delivered with each patient-initiated breath. PSV does not have a preset rate and all breaths are initiated by the patient with a preset amount of support. Current ventilators will have a backup apnea alarm that will trigger a preset rate if the patient does not initiate a predetermined respiratory rate. These various descriptions relate only to when a breath

is delivered in relation to the patient's inherent breathing cycle and range from full control in ACV to partial control in SIMV and totally patient initiated as in PSV. It is important to realize that ACV and SIMV provide the same form of ventilation in the apneic patient. In terms of how the breath is delivered, the choices are volume limited or pressure limited.

Volume versus Pressure-Limited Ventilation

Ventilators may be set to deliver either a certain V_T (volume control) or to achieve a specific inspiratory pressure (pressure control). The mode selected determines what parameter the ventilator uses to limit the individual-delivered V_T. Volume-limited ventilation requires the clinician to set a desired V_T but consideration must also be given to establishing the inspiratory flow and time. Volume-limited ventilation provides the advantage of ensuring adequate minute ventilation ($V_T \times$ respiratory rate); however, if the patient's pulmonary compliance decreases, escalating airway pressures will result in progressively higher peak airway pressures thereby placing the patient at risk for ventilator-induced pulmonary injury.

In contrast, when a patient is placed on a pressure-limited setting, a volume of air is delivered by the ventilator until the selected airway pressure is achieved. Variables affecting the generated V_T include PEEP, inspiratory time, and gas flow rates. A longer proportion of time spent during the inspiratory phase of respiration allows for a more gradual approach to the peak pressure and delivery of a larger V_T. Consequently the V_T achieved will be determined by the patient's respiratory physiology, largely their pulmonary compliance, and airway resistance. The ventilator will deliver this pressure at a ventilator-determined flow rate to maintain certain inspiratory flow parameters.[23] Pressure-limited ventilation will result in variable minute ventilation as the V_T varies. Pressure-limited ventilation offers the benefit of controlling mean airway pressure (MAP) in the patient with dynamic ever-changing pulmonary mechanics because airway pressure will remain constant as compliance changes, theoretically limiting barotrauma. Because of the variations in compliance, close attention must be paid to ensure that adequate minute ventilation is achieved in these patients.

There have been multiple studies comparing volume-limited ventilation with pressure-limited ventilation, although none are large randomized blinded clinical trials. A 1996 study comparing volume-limited ventilation and pressure-limited ventilation found no difference in short-term parameters of ventilation improvement (PaO_2, required inspiratory pressure) when decelerating flow volume-limited ventilation was compared with pressure-limited ventilation.[24] It is the practice of our institution to initiate mechanical ventilation using a volume-limited mode (assist control, volume control [ACVC] or SIMV), and transition to a pressure-limited mode if MAP is consistently >30 cm H_2O.

Modes of Ventilation

On the basis of the above-mentioned terminology and basic ventilatory principles, it is now possible to understand the commonly used ventilator modalities and describe their differences based on trigger and limit (volume vs. pressure). For the apneic patient or patient requiring deep sedation, ACV should be used. Pure volume control or pressure control is now obsolete and not commonly used because assist control settings provides the same advantages with more patient comfort. On the basis of the descriptions given in the preceding text, ACVC or assist control, pressure control (ACPC) may be used. There are no definitive studies promoting volume- or pressure-limited ventilation over one another. Although ACPC has become particularly useful in the management of ARDS, ACVC allows the clinician to set the V_T and the number of these breaths that will be delivered per minute. Careful attention must be paid to prevent "auto-PEEP" or "breath stacking", a situation that can occur when the rate is so high that there is no time for adequate exhalation between breaths resulting in a buildup of positive pressure in the airway and overall elevation of the MAP to potentially dangerous levels.

SIMV can be applied to both volume- and pressure-limited settings. The advantage of SIMV is that it can be used over a wide range of severity of pulmonary dysfunction. For the critically ill patient who is heavily sedated, chemically paralyzed, or paralyzed from a devastating neurologic injury, SIMV can essentially function as AC. When the patient begins to initiate breaths, the patient may pull gas from the circuit with a variable level of PS provided by the physician and is a useful strategy in weaning from the ventilator because the support can be adjusted in concert with improving lung function. Many weaning strategies employ PS trials interspersed with periods of rest on an SIMV mode of ventilation.

Weaning Mechanical Ventilation and Extubation

Mechanical ventilation is associated with significant morbidity[25,26] and several misconceptions delay physicians from weaning support and extubation. The most important and common myth perpetuated is that the longer the duration of mechanical ventilation the more difficult the wean thought to be related to a weakened diaphragm that develops during assisted ventilation. In reality though, the accessory muscles of respiration, being completely voluntary, will no doubt experience some degree of atrophy during long periods of assisted ventilation; the diaphragm is not a voluntary muscle and continues to contract independently during mechanical ventilation. With the exception of cervical spine or high thoracic spinal cord transection and complex clinical conditions, which require prolonged periods of pharmacologic paralysis, the diaphragm remains active during all forms of mechanical ventilation.[27] Furthermore, investigators have determined that diaphragm strength is not adversely influenced by duration of mechanical ventilation and no evidence exists to prove that diaphragm weakness is the cause of failure to wean from mechanical ventilation.[28]

There are countless methods to initiate the gradual withdrawal of mechanical ventilation and no particular practice has been demonstrated superior to all others. The author's preferred approach allows for a stepwise reduction of support, enabling the patient to slowly increase responsibility of ventilation. Before initiating a ventilatory wean, several clinical and physiologic parameters need assessment with satisfactory findings; several of these parameters are listed in Table 1. The weaning process begins by changing assisted modes of ventilation toward the synchronized ventilation modes. As convalescence within the ICU proceeds and the injured patient's overall minute ventilation improves, the ventilation mode should be changed to synchronized intermittent ventilation. In making the transition to the less invasive support mode, the surgeon must ensure that enough PS is provided to enable the patient to achieve independent V_Ts of 4 to 6 mL per kg ideal body weight. Failure to reach this goal could result in progressive tachypnea to maintain adequate minute ventilation, ultimately resulting in pulmonary failure and the need for escalation of ventilatory support. Once adequate independent V_Ts are achieved, the physician should gradually reduce the number of machine-driven V_T-delivered breaths toward six breaths per minute. Next, short durations of 4 to 6 hours of PS only may be attempted. As these durations of PSV ventilation are tolerated, hallmarked by acceptable respiratory rate, their length should be extended. Concurrently, while the duration of the PS trials are lengthened, the magnitude of the PS should be reduced 2 cm per H_2O every 8 to 12 hours. Progress may continue so long as the respiratory rate remains below 24 to 26 breaths a minute and V_Ts remain acceptable (4 to 6 mL per kg) (see Fig. 4).

TABLE 1

PHYSIOLOGIC PARAMETERS PREDICTIVE OF SUCCESSFUL EXTUBATION FOR PATIENTS REQUIRING MECHANICAL VENTILATION

Parameter	Threshold Value Predicting Successful Extubation
Minute ventilation	<12 L/min
Negative inspiratory force	>20–30 cm H_2O
Forced vital capacity	10 mL/kg
Respiratory rate	<26/min
Spontaneous tidal volume	4–6 mL/kg
f/V_T ratio	60–105

f/V_T ratio, frequency to tidal volume ratio.

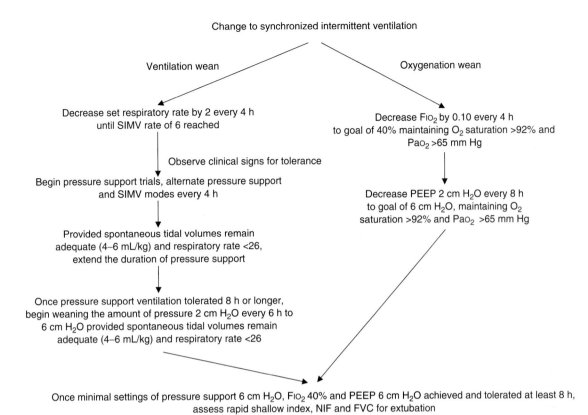

Change to synchronized intermittent ventilation

Ventilation wean

Oxygenation wean

Decrease set respiratory rate by 2 every 4 h
until SIMV rate of 6 reached

Decrease FIO_2 by 0.10 every 4 h
to goal of 40% maintaining O_2 saturation >92% and
PaO_2 >65 mm Hg

Observe clinical signs for tolerance

Begin pressure support trials, alternate pressure support
and SIMV modes every 4 h

Decrease PEEP 2 cm H_2O every 8 h
to goal of 6 cm H_2O, maintaining O_2
saturation >92% and PaO_2 >65 mm Hg

Provided spontaneous tidal volumes remain
adequate (4–6 mL/kg) and respiratory rate <26,
extend the duration of pressure support

Once pressure support ventilation tolerated 8 h or longer,
begin weaning the amount of pressure 2 cm H_2O every 6 h to
6 cm H_2O provided spontaneous tidal volumes remain
adequate (4–6 mL/kg) and respiratory rate <26

Once minimal settings of pressure support 6 cm H_2O, FIO_2 40% and PEEP 6 cm H_2O achieved and tolerated at least 8 h,
assess rapid shallow index, NIF and FVC for extubation

Figure 4   Author's strategy to an uncomplicated ventilatory wean. SIMV, synchronized intermittent mandatory ventilation; PEEP, positive end-expiratory pressure; NIF, negative inspiratory force; FVC, forced vital capacity.

Once mechanical support is reduced to minimal assistance so as to account for resistance of airflow caused by the endotracheal tube, several parameters can be used to predict the success of extubation. The frequency to V_T ratio (f/V_T), minute ventilation, negative inspiratory force, spontaneous V_T, and forced vital capacity are measures that have been shown useful in determining success of extubation (see Table 2). Extubation failure should be avoided wherever possible because the need for reintubation is associated with a significant risk of nosocomial pneumonia and mortality.[29,30] While no single parameter or combination of parameters is absolute in predicting success of extubation, maintenance of unnecessary mechanical ventilation is clearly associated with risk of infection and iatrogenic complications.[31] Once intubated patients start tolerating spontaneous breathing trials with minimal ventilatory support and have no superseding clinical variables preventing extubation, the endotracheal tube should be removed.

OXYGENATION

Whereas ventilation refers to the mechanical function of moving air from the environment into the alveolar components of the lung, oxygenation is often referred to as the parenchymal function of the lung. Oxygenation

of the pulmonary capillaries begins with diffusion, a passive process driven by the gas partial pressure differences from the alveolus and the capillary bed. Carbon dioxide and oxygen gas diffusion across the alveolar membrane is dependent on their solubility within fluid and the pressure gradient between the alveolus and the capillary

TABLE 2	
FINDINGS CONSISTENT WITH ENTRY INTO MECHANICAL VENTILATION WEAN	
Parameter	**Threshold Allowing for Consideration of Weaning Mechanical Ventilation**
Adequate oxygenation	PaO_2 >60 mm Hg, PaO_2/FIO_2 >300
Satisfactory hemodynamics	HR <130, MAP >70 without vasoactive and/or inotropic support
Adequate ventilation	$PaCO_2$ <50 mm Hg
Adequate mental status	Arousable with independent respiratory drive
Satisfactory metabolic profile	7.25 < pH <7.50, acceptable electrolytes
Subjective assessment	Resolution of acute phase of injury/illness

HR, heart rate; MAP, mean arterial pressure.

bed. Both oxygen and carbon dioxide are highly soluble in the lipid membranes of the alveolus; however the diffusion coefficient of carbon dioxide is 20-fold that of oxygen in water. Therefore, the rate-limiting step in the exchange of the by-product of metabolism, carbon dioxide, is the pressure differential between the alveolar and pulmonary capillary carbon dioxide tensions. Under normal physiologic conditions with adequate ventilation and pulmonary perfusion, oxygen exchange is not limited. During conditions where the total surface area of the respiratory membrane is reduced and/or the $\dot{V}/\dot{Q}$ ratio of the lung is altered, the diffusion capacity of oxygen is diminished and hypoxemia results.

Among patients without pulmonary insult there exists a healthy matching of alveolar ventilation ($\dot{V}$) and pulmonary capillary perfusion ($\dot{Q}$), which is essential to efficient gas exchange.[32,33] The pulmonary parenchyma is composed of more than 300 million alveolar-capillary units each receiving various degrees of $\dot{V}$ and $\dot{Q}$. The ratio of ventilation and perfusion is dependent upon the posture of the patient and relative airflow into the different zones of the lung. Although the entire cardiac output is managed by the pulmonary circulation, at any given time approximately 100 mL of the blood volume can be found within the pulmonary capillaries.[34] The relative distribution of the blood with the pulmonary capillaries divided between the zones of the pulmonary parenchyma will be influenced by several forces including local vasoconstriction, microembolization caused by ALI and/or ARDS, macroembolization as a consequence of deep venous thrombosis (DVT), alveolar ventilation, and the hydrostatic forces within the lung caused by gravity. In a standing person, the near 30 cm of height of lung tissue will represent a >20 mm Hg pressure gradient between

the base and apex. With average normal pulmonary artery systolic pressures measured 15 to 25 mm Hg, the right ventricle is just able to overcome the hydrostatic pressure within the parenchyma and perfuse the apex and as a consequence, flow is 18 times greater in the bases than the apices.[34] Alveolar distension associated with ventilation also affects pulmonary blood flow. When the pressure within the alveolar unit exceeds the pulmonary capillary pressure, the capillary collapses the pulmonary blood flow locally ceases. These relationships are best depicted in Fig. 5.

The $\dot{V}/\dot{Q}$ relationships within the lung can be summarized into one of three general categories: normal $\dot{V}/\dot{Q}$ matching, dead space ventilation, and shunting. When alveolar ventilation and perfusion match, $\dot{V}/\dot{Q} = 1$, normal exchange of oxygen and carbon dioxide will occur. Under circumstances resulting in a $\dot{V}/\dot{Q} > 1$, alveolar ventilation is excessive relative to pulmonary capillary blood flow. This clinical condition is referred to as *dead space ventilation* and is considered wasted ventilation where alveolar gas cannot equilibrate with capillary blood. As a consequence, minute ventilation must increase to allow for the adequately perfused segments of lung to ensure adequate removal of carbon dioxide. Among injured patients, worsening dead space ventilation is often associated with pulmonary thromboembolism (PTE). Quantification of dead space ventilation can be useful in making this diagnosis.[35-37] Among normal patients, dead space ventilation should account for 20% to 30% of total ventilation, whereas a calculation resulting in >30% is suggestive of a PTE.

$$\text{Dead space ventilation} = (\text{Pa}_{CO_2} - \text{end tidal } CO_2)/\text{Pa}_{CO_2}$$

A $\dot{V}/\dot{Q}$ relationship <1.0 describes conditions where capillary blood flow is excessive relative to ventilation.

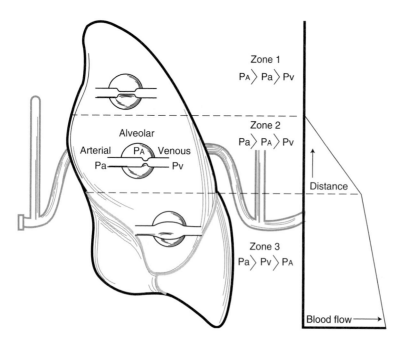

Zone 1
$P_A > Pa > Pv$

Alveolar

Arterial $\boxed{P_A}$ Venous
Pa —— Pv

Zone 2
$Pa > P_A > Pv$

Distance

Zone 3
$Pa > Pv > P_A$

Blood flow →

Figure 5 Depiction of the three zones of ventilation/perfusion of the upright lung. As a consequence of hydrostatic pressure, alveolar pressure (P_A) exceeds arterial pressure (Pa) in zone 1 and blood flow ($\dot{Q}$) is poorly matched to satisfactory ventilation ($\dot{V}$). In zone 2, Pa is > P_A and the alveolar pressure remains higher than the venous pressure (Pv). Flow through the pulmonary capillary beds is governed by the arterial–alveolar pressure gradient, which gradually increases down the zone allowing for superior $\dot{V}/\dot{Q}$ matching. Transitioning into zone 3, the Pv now exceeds the alveolar pressure and flow through the capillaries is governed by the Pa–Pv gradient. Gravitational effects on the lung in conjunction with the elevated venous pressure render this segment of lung the poorest ventilation contributing the $\dot{V}/\dot{Q}$ mismatch. (Adapted from West JB. *Ventilation/blood flow and gas exchange*, 2nd ed. Oxford: Blackwell Science; 1970.)

The clinical condition is termed *intrapulmonary shunt* and is associated with alveolar collapse, pulmonary edema, and regions of lung parenchyma not affected by PTE. The fraction of cardiac output that represents the shunt is referred to as the *shunt fraction*. The shunt fraction, or excess blood flow, will not participate in gas exchange and therefore will have a profound effect on arterial oxygenation. Among healthy individuals, the shunt fraction is <10% and as the magnitude of the shunt fraction increases as a consequence of pulmonary pathophysiology, the measured arterial oxygen tension will correspondingly fall. Correction of the hypoxemia can be accomplished by either increasing the PEEP and/or the FiO_2. As the ratio of the shunt fraction increases >30%, only very large changes in the FiO_2 will affect arterial oxygen concentration.

HYPOXEMIA

Hypoxemia can result from one of three principal disorders: hypoventilation, primary pulmonary disorder, and/or oxygen delivery-consumption imbalance. To evaluate and determine the source of the hypoxemia, begin by determining the alveolar to arterial oxygen gradient (A–a Po_2 gradient). Under circumstances where the gradient is normal, generalized hypoventilation is the cause of the hypoxemia and is frequently associated with traumatic brain injury, oversedation with opioid analgesics or benzodiazepines. When the A–a Po_2 gradient is increased, mixed venous oxygen tension will help differentiate between oxygen delivery/consumption abnormalities and $\dot{V}/\dot{Q}$ mismatching. Normal mixed venous Po_2 indicates that the hypoxemia is solely a consequence of $\dot{V}/\dot{Q}$ abnormalities, whereas a low value would suggest either an oxygen delivery problem (low cardiac index and/or anemia) or a higher rate of oxygen consumption (hypermetabolism associated with the systemic inflammatory response).

Oxygenation can be improved through several measures including increasing the fraction of inspired oxygen (FiO_2), increasing the PEEP, altering the inspiration-to-expiration ratio (I/E ratio) and kinetic therapy and/or prone positioning. The use of any one or combination of these approaches should improve arterial oxygenation; however, each intervention is associated with potential morbidity. Higher FiO_2 levels can be used to increase plasma dissolved oxygen and improve saturation of hemoglobin. Within the alveolus, approximately 5% of oxygen is partially reduced to a free radical state instead of harmlessly being combined with hydrogen to form water. As the partial pressure of oxygen in the alveolus rises while the FiO_2 fraction is increased >50%, antioxidant defense systems are overwhelmed and oxygenfree radicals can cause substantial cellular injury.[38] Free radical damage as a consequence of high FiO_2 levels can be observed in several organ systems; however, the lungs receive the brunt of the injury. Increases in inflammatory mediators are first observed within the alveolar complexes followed by development of worsening pulmonary edema. Next, the inflammatory cascade will cause accumulation of platelets and neutrophils within the pulmonary capillaries ultimately resulting in capillary thrombosis and pulmonary fibrosis.[39–41] The primary means of managing oxygen toxicity is to prevent it because no therapeutic intervention is currently available to reverse the pulmonary fibrosis associated with prolonged exposure to high levels of FiO_2. The author's approach to avoiding oxygen toxicity is to maintain higher levels of PEEP while preferentially reducing FiO_2 below 50%.

PEEP improves oxygenation by restoring the FRC and increasing the MAP, thereby improving $\dot{V}/\dot{Q}$ mismatching. Injured patients requiring mechanical ventilation frequently have multiple reasons for worsening pulmonary compliance and as a consequence will develop dependent pulmonary atelectasis and a worsening shunt fraction. PEEP reduces the shunt fraction by increasing the FRC and preventing alveolar collapse, encouraging alveolar recruitment and discouraging interstitial pulmonary edema all together substantially, improves arterial oxygenation, and permits rapid reduction in FiO_2. PEEP may be accompanied by adverse sequelae including fall in cardiac output and barotrauma-induced ALI or ARDS. As PEEP is increased, the rising thoracic pressures are transmitted to the mediastinum affecting venous return to the heart. Particularly in pathophysiologic states where the central venous pressures are low, the increased mediastinal pressures as a consequence of high levels of PEEP can significantly affect cardiac filling, stroke volumes, and the cardiac output. Separately, high levels of PEEP will generate higher peak airway pressures causing alveolar overdistension and barotrauma. Pulmonary barotrauma is a clinically important phenomenon that may delay the healing of injured lungs and lead to the development, or the exacerbation, of ARDS.[42]

As conventional measures to provide oxygenation for hypoxemic patient who are mechanically ventilated are exhausted, less traditional interventions need be considered. There exists a wide body of literature addressing several different options at the disposal of the clinician in dealing with severe and refractory hypoxemia; however, the most commonly employed interventions include inverse ratio pressure controlled ventilation (IRV) and kinetic therapy. IRV differs from other ventilation techniques in that the inspiration time is prolonged beyond that allotted for expiration rendering an I/E ratio of <1:1. IRV achieves higher levels of oxygenation at lower peak airway pressures particularly among patients with ARDS not responding to high levels of PEEP.[43,44] IRV is best suited for patients with poor pulmonary compliance, diffuse microatelectasis, and increased intrapulmonary shunt.[45] While helpful in improving oxygenation, IRV is associated with decreases in venous return to the right of the heart, higher pulmonary artery pressures, and reduction in cardiac output. Before instituting IRV, clinicians should assess central venous pressure and/or pulmonary artery wedge pressures to ensure adequate cardiac preload.[46] A second measure to improve $\dot{V}/\dot{Q}$ matching and enhance oxygenation is kinetic therapy. Kinetic therapy is defined as the use of a bed that rotates continuously >40 degrees along its longitudinal axis. Advantages of kinetic therapy include lower incidence of pneumonia and atelectasis and improved $\dot{V}/\dot{Q}$ matching. Use of the continuous lateral rotational therapy has been demonstrated to improve PaO_2/FIO_2 ratio among mechanically ventilated patients with ARDS.[47]

ARDS is accompanied by profound cardiopulmonary changes severely impairing the ability to oxygenate and ventilate. ARDS is characterized by diffuse bilateral infiltrates radiographically, decreased respiratory compliance, and severe hypoxemia (PaO_2/FIO_2 ratio <200) without evidence of cardiogenic shock. The basic pathophysiologic change associated with ARDS is the disruption of the normal alveolar-capillary barrier. The consequence of lung edema includes a decrease in lung volumes, compliance, and large intrapulmonary shunts. A fall in the FRC is uniformly present and contributes to $\dot{V}/\dot{Q}$ inequality. Patients who die of respiratory failure usually show a progressive decrease in lung compliance, worsening hypoxemia, and progressive increase in dead space with hypercapnia. Correcting the life-threatening hypoxemia and providing adequate mechanical ventilation remain the mainstay goals of therapy. The manner by which critical care physicians have provided support for ARDS has evolved considerably over a short period of time. Current data supports that restricting barotrauma and limiting peak airway pressures below 25 cm H_2O is associated with improved morbidity, fewer days of mechanical ventilation and decreased mortality.[8] Current strategies approaching ventilation emphasize low VTs (4 to 6 mL per kg ideal body weight) with a higher respiratory rate accepting degrees of hypercapnea provided arterial pH is >7.25. Providing support for adequate oxygenation is equally as challenging among those with ARDS. Microvascular changes and alveolar collapse are general so profound creating a severe $\dot{V}/\dot{Q}$ mismatch such that maximizing any single intervention in an effort to improve oxygenation is uniformly inadequate. As a consequence, a multifaceted approach to managing oxygenation is required including high levels of PEEP and FIO_2, kinetic therapy and/or prone ventilation and pharmacologic paralysis reducing the work of breathing and enabling IRV.[8,48,49]

SUMMARY

Management of acutely injured trauma patients with multisystem injury requires physician-directed assistance with ventilation and/or oxygenation oftentimes requiring orotracheal intubation and the use of a mechanical ventilator. A thorough knowledge base of respiratory physiology is critical in appropriately managing mechanically ventilated patients so as to minimize the risk of iatrogenic injury.

Although the use of mechanical ventilation is necessary, the invasive nature of the device exposes the patient to a broad array of new pulmonary pathogens. Only by understanding contemporary approaches to ventilatory management can the surgeon charged with the responsibility of the injured patient provide the acceptable risk associated with mechanical ventilation by limiting barotrauma and optimizing oxygenation appropriately using PEEP and lower FIO_2 concentration.

REFERENCES

1. Holcomb JB, McMullin NR, Kozar RA, et al. Morbidity from rib fractures increases after age 45. *J Am Coll Surg.* 2003;196(4): 549–555.
2. Meyers JR, Limbeck L, O'Kane H, et al. Changes in functional residual capacity of the lung after operation. *Arch Surg.* 1975;110: 576–583.
3. Ali J, Weisel RD, Layug AB, et al. Consequences of postoperative alterations in respiratory mechanics. *Am J Surg.* 1974;128: 376–382.
4. Girgis K, Hamed H, Khater Y, et al. A decremental PEEP trial identifies the PEEP level that maintains oxygenation after lung recruitment. *Respir Care.* 2006;51(10):1132–1139.
5. Marini JJ. How to recruit the injured lung. *Minerva Anestesiol.* 2003; 69(4):193–200.
6. Jardin F, Genevray B, Brun–Ney D, et al. Influence of lung and chest wall compliance on transmission of airway pressure to the pleural space in critically ill patients. *Chest.* 1985;88(5):653–658.
7. The ARDS Network. Ventilation with lower tidal volumes as compared with traditional tidal volumes for acute lung injury and the acute respiratory distress syndrome. *N Engl J Med.* 2000;342: 1301–1308.
8. Gajic O, Mendez JL, Dara SI, et al. Ventilator associated lung injury in patients without acute lung injury at the onset of mechanical ventilation. *Crit Care Med.* 2004;32(9):1817–1824.
9. Ramnath VR, Hess DR, Thompson BT. Conventional mechanical ventilation in acute lung injury and acute respiratory distress syndrome. *Clin Chest Med.* 2006;27(4):601–613.
10. Gillis RC, Weireter LJ, Britt RC, et al. Lung protective ventilation strategies: Have we applied them in trauma patients at risk for acute lung injury and acute respiratory distress syndrome?. *Am Surg.* 2007;73(4):347–350.
11. Barbas CS, De Matos GF, Pincelli MP, et al. Mechanical ventilation in acute respiratory failure: Recruitment and high positive end-expiratory pressure are necessary. *Curr Opin Crit Care.* 2005; 11(1):18–28.
12. Weinacker AB, Vaszar LT. Acute respiratory distress syndrome: Physiology and new management strategies. *Annu Rev Med.* 2001; 52:221–237.
13. Rouby JJ, Puybasset L, Cluzel P, et al. Regional distribution of gas and tissue in acute respiratory distress syndrome. Physiological correlations and definition of an ARDS severity score. *Intensive Care Med.* 2000;26(8):1046–1056.
14. Brochard L, Mancebo J, Wysocki M, et al. Noninvasive ventilation for acute exacerbations of chronic obstructive pulmonary disease. *N Engl J Med.* 1995;333:817–822.
15. Hilbert G, Gruson D, Vargas F, et al. Noninvasive ventilation in immunosuppressed patients with pulmonary infiltrates, fever and acute respiratory failure. *N Engl J Med.* 2001;344:481–487.
16. Pang D, Keenan SP, Cook DJ, et al. The effect of positive pressure airway support on mortality and the need for intubation in cardiogenic pulmonary edema: A systematic review. *Chest.* 1998;114: 1185–1192.
17. Bollinger CT, Van Eeden SF. Treatment of multiple rib fractures. Randomized controlled trial comparing ventilatory with nonventilatory management. *Chest.* 1990;97:943–948.
18. Rana S, Jenad H, Gay PC, et. al. Failure of non-invasive ventilation in patients with acute lung injury: Observational cohort study. *Crit Care.* 2006;10(3):R79.

19. Nava S, Ceriana P. Causes of failure of noninvasive mechanical ventilation. *Respir Care.* 2004;49(3):295–303.

20. Keenan S, Kernerman P, Cook DJ, et al. Effect of noninvasive positive pressure ventilation on mortality in patients admitted with acute respiratory failure: A meta-analysis. *Crit Care Med.* 1997;25(10):1685–1692.

21. Hurst J, DeHaven C, Branson R. Use of CPAP mask as the sole mode of ventilatory support in trauma patients with mild to moderate respiratory insufficiency. *J Trauma.* 1985;25(11):1065–1068.

22. Esteban A, Frutos-Vivar F, Ferguson ND, et al. Noninvasive positive-pressure ventilation for respiratory failure after extubation. *N Engl J Med.* 2004;350(24):2452–2260.

23. Campbell R, Davis B. Pressure-controlled versus volume-controlled ventilation: Does it matter? *Respir Care.* 2002;47(4):416–424.

24. Davis K, Branson R, Campbell RS, et al. Comparison of volume control and pressure control ventilation: Is flow waveform the difference? *J Trauma.* 1996;41(5):808–814.

25. Kollef MH. The prevention of ventilator-associated pneumonia. *N Engl J Med.* 1999;340:627–634.

26. Stauffer JL, Olson DE, Petty TL. Complications and consequences of endotracheal intubation and tracheotomy. *Am J Med.* 1981;70:65–76.

27. Marini JJ. Strategies to minimize breathing effort during mechanical ventilation. *Crit Care Clin.* 1990;6:635–661.

28. Swartz MA, Marino PL. Diaphragm strength during weaning from mechanical ventilation. *Chest.* 1985;88:736–739.

29. Torres A, Serra-Batlles J, Ros E, et al. Pulmonary aspiration of gastric contents in patients receiving mechanical ventilation. *Ann Intern Med.* 1992;116:540–543.

30. Epstein SK, Ciubotaru RL, Wong JB. Effect of failed extubation on the outcome of mechanical ventilation. *Chest.* 1997;112:186–192.

31. Fagon JY, Chastre J, Hance AJ, et al. Nosocomial pneumonia in ventilated patients: A cohort study evaluating attributable mortality and hospital stay. *Am J Med.* 1993;94:281–288.

32. Dantzker DR. Ventilation-perfusion inequality in lung disease. *Chest.* 1987;91:749–754.

33. Wagner PD. Ventilation-perfusion relationships. *Ann Rev Physiol.* 1980;42:235–247.

34. West JB. Regional differences in gas exchange in the lung of erect man. *J Appl Physiol.* 1963;17:893.

35. Tang Y, Turner MJ, Baker AB. Effects of alveolar dead-space, shunt and V/Q distribution on respiratory dead-space measurements. *Br J Anaesth.* 2005;95(4):538–548.

36. Verschuren F, Liistro G, Coffeng R, et al. Volumetric capnography as a screening test for pulmonary embolism in the emergency department. *Chest.* 2004;125:841–850.

37. Kline JA, Israel EG, Michelson EA, et al. Diagnostic accuracy of a bedside D-dimer assay and alveolar dead-space measurement for rapid exclusion of pulmonary embolism: A multicenter study. *JAMA.* 2001;285:761–768.

38. Kleen M, Messmer K. Toxicity of high PaO_2. *Minerva Anestesiol.* 1999;65(6):393–396.

39. Suratt BT, Parsons PE. Mechanism of acute lung injury/acute respiratory distress syndrome. *Clin Chest Med.* 2006;27(4):579–589.

40. Navarrete-Navarro P, Rivera-Fernandez R, Rincon MD, et al. Early markers of acute respiratory distress syndrome development in severe trauma patients. *J Crit Care.* 2006;21(3):253–258.

41. Ware LB. Pathophysiology of acute lung injury and the acute respiratory distress syndrome. *Semin Respir Crit Care Med.* 2006;27(4):337–349.

42. Meade MO, Cook DJ. The aetiology, consequences and prevention of barotraumas: A critical review of the literature. *Clin Intensive Care.* 1995;6(4):166–173.

43. Gurevitch MJ, Vandyke J, Young ES, et al. Improved oxygenation and lower peak airway pressures in severe acute respiratory distress syndrome with inverse ratio ventilation. *Chest.* 1986;89:211–213.

44. Tharratt RS, Allen RP, Albertson TE. Pressure controlled inverse ratio ventilation in severe acute respiratory distress. *Chest.* 1988;94:755–762.

45. Johnson M, Cane RD. The technique of inverse ration ventilation. Steps to improve oxygenation and decrease dead space ventilation. *J Crit Illn.* 1992;7(6):969–973.

46. Jardin F, Vieellard-Baron A. Is there a safe plateau pressure in ARDS? the right heart only knows. *Intensive Care Med.* 2007;33(3):444–447.

47. Raoof S, Chowdhrey N, Raoof S, et al. Effect of combined kinetic therapy and percussion therapy on the resolution of atelectasis in critically ill patients. *Chest.* 1999;115:1658–1666.

48. Verbrugge SJ, Lachmann B, Kesecioglu J. Lung protective strategies in acute lung injury and acute respiratory distress syndrome: From experimental findings to clinical application. *Clin Physiol Funct Imaging.* 2007;27(2):67–90.

49. Donahoe M. Basic ventilator management: Lung protective strategies. *Surg Clin North Am.* 2006;86(6):1389–1408.

60

Hemodynamic Management and Shock

Lucas P. Neff   *Michael C. Chang*

Shock is defined as a functional uncoupling between the cardiovascular system and the peripheral tissues which leads to inadequate delivery of oxygen, energy, and other vital nutrients to the cells of the body. This uncoupling can be due to one or more of several different mechanisms, ranging from primary cardiac failure to inadequate red blood cell mass and subsequent failure of oxygen delivery. A thorough knowledge of the causes and progression of this disorder is essential to treating patients with shock, as management of the shock state is directly determined by a careful and comprehensive knowledge of the etiology of shock in any given patient. Failure to identify and treat the stimulus for shock, coupled with inadequate resuscitation, leads to multiple organ failure (MOF), the leading cause of delayed mortality in the surgical intensive care unit (ICU). Shock is much more than simply a process marked by hemodynamic dysfunction. It has a very latent, yet dangerous inflammatory component as well. Prolonged periods of uncompensated shock are an important stimulus for dysregulated systemic inflammation, and failure to downregulate this inflammatory response leads to persistent hypermetabolism, functional malnutrition, and MOF. This delayed organ failure and mortality can be minimized by detecting shock in its early stages and aggressively resuscitating the patient while addressing the underlying causes.

The conceptual outline of this chapter encompasses the various causes and classifications of shock, clinical findings in the shock patient, and the pathophysiology

of shock on both the hemodynamic level and the biochemical level. The chapter focus then turns to methods of hemodynamic monitoring with respect to treatment strategies and resuscitation endpoints.

CAUSES AND CLASSIFICATION OF SHOCK

There are many ways to classify shock. Although classification schemes may vary, all share a common pattern. There is an initial period of compensation which, lacking adequate stimulus control and resuscitation, will give way to decompensated shock. Although both are reversible to a point, failure to address either compensated or decompensated shock leads to an irreversible condition, which eventually leads to MOF and death.

Cardiogenic

Cardiogenic shock can be defined as failure of the heart to generate enough power to deliver oxygen, energy, and nutrients to meet the demand of the peripheral tissues. This failure is attributable to inadequate myocardial contractility. Myocardial contractility is defined as intrinsic ventricular function that is independent of preload and afterload. Inadequate contractility can be due to a number of causes, including myocardial ischemia, infection, and hypertrophy or atrophy of myocardial tissue. Cardiogenic shock can also result from the diastolic dysfunction of a stiff, noncompliant ventricle that cannot adequately relax to allow ventricular filling to occur.

Regardless of the underlying cause, increased strain is put on the already taxed heart as its own metabolic demands increase in the context of the entire body needing more perfusion and greater effort from the heart. This vicious cycle can lead to rapid decline in already compromised cardiac performance and worsening of the patient's condition.

Other "cardiac-related" causes of shock include constrictive and obstructive shock. Although these two categories differ in name, the pathology is similar. The underlying issue is that the venous return to the heart is impeded, thereby reducing cardiac preload and leading to reduced cardiac output. Constrictive shock generally relates to processes that prevent ventricular filling, such as cardiac tamponade. Obstructive shock, on the other hand, encompasses situations like tension pneuthoraces in which the blood never even returns to the right atrium.

Hypovolemic Shock

Inadequate preload leads to suboptimal ventricular performance, independent of afterload and myocardial contractility. Decreased intravascular volume results in inadequate stretching of the myocardial fibers before contraction. Regardless of the reason, low intravascular volume leads to decreased transport of oxygen, energy, and nutrients to end organs. The intravascular depletion can be due to any pathologic state that causes blood loss, increased capillary permeability, or loss of venous capacitance.

Neurogenic Shock

Neurogenic shock typically occurs in the setting of a high spinal cord injury that also includes the sympathetic chain. Loss of the sympathetic tone on the highly compliant venous system leads to an increase in unstressed venous capacitance, which in turn leads to decreased preload and subsequent functional cardiac failure.

Septic Shock (Distributive Shock)

Septic shock differs little from the previously mentioned types with respect to what is ultimately occurring at the vascular level. In fact, it is very similar to anaphylactic shock in that the real causative agent is the body's immune response to a threat, whether real (sepsis from bactremia and inflammation) or perceived (the benign antigens that evoke the activation of innate immunologic systems in anaphylaxis). Essentially, massive immunologic activation from bacterial toxins and dying or injured tissues evokes the same pathophysiologic process of vascular leakage and subsequent loss of intravascular volume. Although there are various subsets of septic shock, endotoxic shock is

one of the more common types. Endotoxin is actually lipopolysaccharide (LPS), an integral protein embedded in the cell wall of gram-negative organisms. As the bacteria are destroyed by antibiotics and the body's own defense mechanisms, LPS is elaborated and free to circulate in the blood. The massive inflammatory response comes as LPS interacts with immune cell surface receptors (toll-like receptors) that can recognize a wide array of primitive antigens that humans have encountered for eons. Therefore, in an attempt to eliminate invading pathogens, the host receives one final blow from the dying bacteria as the immune system undergoes the devastating consequences of unregulated activation.

Although several etiologies of shock are mentioned previously, the causes of shock are even more varied than the types. Although it is important to know the many causes for shock in patients, there is also a simple principle that unifies them. Different types of shock and their particular causes can overlap and exist simultaneously. This may not be intuitive, but quickly makes sense as one plays out the various scenarios of a patient's course. For example, a patient in septic shock may put such a demand on the heart to maintain cardiac output in the face of low systemic pressure that the myocardium cannot meet that demand and begin to fail. This will lead to cardiogenic shock and a rapid downward decline. For trauma patients it may be a different situation. Perhaps the hypovolemia of hemorrhagic shock leads to decreased gastrointestinal (GI) mucosal blood flow and eventual bowel ischemia. The clinical picture and resuscitation are further complicated by the dying tissue. Therefore, a patient can be in shock for more than one reason. It is imperative that all the data is correlated with the clinical picture and good judgment to ensure that one key component of shock is not overlooked.

CLINICAL FINDINGS

A thorough physical examination and collection of all the clinical and laboratory data can help establish a diagnosis of shock and the degree of severity. Furthermore, physical and clinical findings should always be taken in context, as multiple pathophysiologic states can exist simultaneously. Important clinical signs include abnormal vital signs, changes in neurologic status, decreased urine output, and changes in extremity temperature (see Table 1). These clinical signs can be either a direct result of the source of shock (tachycardia, bradycardia, hypotension) or a clinical finding resulting from functional hypoperfusion (oliguria, agitiation).

Other Markers of Shock Severity

Measurement of blood lactate levels can be useful in determining shock status, both as a marker of adequacy of ongoing resuscitation and as a predictor of occult shock

TABLE 1

CLINICAL FINDINGS OF SHOCK

Shock Type	Physical Examination	PAOP	Systemic Vascular Resistance	Cardiac Output
Cardiogenic	Cool, clammy skin, with or without tachycardia	↑	↑	↓
Distributive	Warm skin, tachycardia	↑	↑	↓
Hypovolemic	Cool, clammy skin, tachycardia	↓	↑	↑
Constrictive/obstructive	Cool, clammy skin, tachycardia	↑ or ↓	↑	↓
Neurogenic	Warm skin, bradycardia	↓	↓	↓

PAOP, pulmonary artery occlusion pressure; ↑, increase; ↓, decrease.

not manifest by clinical findings. Produced by cells that have converted to anaerobic metabolism to sustain cellular function, elevated lactate levels are an indicator that tissues are not supplied with adequate oxygen to meet their metabolic demands. The sole source of lactate is pyruvate, the end product of glycolysis. This transformation takes place in the cytoplasm of cells during periods of hypoxia and results in grossly inefficient production of adenosine triphosphate (ATP) when compared to ATP production during aerobic conditions. This anaerobic process can occur in any of the body's tissues, but most lactate production takes place in skeletal muscle, the brain, red blood cells, and the renal medulla. Lactate is cleared both by renal elimination and by the conversion back to pyruvate in the liver. The elevation of lactate occurs when production exceeds normal clearance mechanisms. This is especially true in terms of hepatic metabolism of lactate. During periods of hypoperfusion and hypoxia, the inability of the liver to metabolize lactate through lactate dehydrogenase is juxtaposed with its own increased production of the anaerobic by-product.

Rapid clearance of lactate has been associated with a decreased incidence of MOF and death. Elevated lactate levels at admission and the inability to normalize these levels after 48 hours have been correlated with much higher mortality levels. In a prospective resuscitation study of trauma victims, there was an 86% mortality rate for patients who were unable to clear their elevated lactate levels within the first 48 hours. This is a stark contrast to the 100% survival of all patients in the study who normalized lactate values in the first 24 hours and 25% mortality of those who normalized within the 24- to 48-hour period. Therefore, lactate levels provide a fair prognostic indicator and can be used as one of the many variables to assess resuscitation efficacy. Although this observation does not conclude that lactate is the direct cause of mortality, it should be noted that lactate itself has deleterious effects of physiologic function. The acidosis caused by increased levels of lactate can decrease cardiac performance, increase

sympathetic discharge of catecholamines, and increase protein catabolism and many other counterproductive processes.

Arterial base deficit (BD) is another readily available marker of widespread metabolic acidosis. Used as a marker of lactate levels, it is easily calculated from the pH and $Paco_2$ values in arterial blood gases and is a powerful predictor of survival in critically ill patients. Furthermore, the utility of BD extends longer than just the initial resuscitative period. Elevated levels of BD over long periods of time (up to 96 hours) can indicate ongoing oxygen debt and herald adverse outcomes, especially given the fact that acid–base homeostasis is usually achieved rapidly. Persistent elevation of BD is a good indicator of ongoing and cumulative dysoxia throughout the resuscitation of the critically ill patient.

SHOCK AT THE MACRO AND MICRO LEVEL

As with many diseases, shock is not a static process. Rather, a fairly dynamic progression of events takes place. Hemodynamic compromise and subsequent decrease in delivery of oxygen to the tissues (regardless of the etiology) leads to a progressive inflammatory response that leads to MOF. Moreover, this progression can cycle back on itself to exacerbate any step in this continuum. Aggressive resuscitation and removal of the underlying stimulus are the cornerstones of attenuating this damaging inflammatory response. Surgeons in generations past understood that shock lead to death, but they often missed the key phenomenon of inflammation now observed because their patients simply did not survive past the initial resuscitative efforts. As medicine advanced and new technologies developed, better resuscitation and the technical ability to support or replace the physiologic function of organs with machines gave clinicians a chance to see beyond the initial encounter in very sick patients to witness an entirely new obstacle—systemic inflammatory response syndrome (SIRS). SIRS came to the forefront in Vietnam as battle-wounded GIs started to fall victim to "Da Nang lung," the condition now known as *acute respiratory distress syndrome* (ARDS), the pulmonary manifestation of SIRS. This "new" inflammatory phenomenon was actually an uncovering of the natural progression of a pathologic process, which was not seen until the 1960s because those that would have gone on to develop SIRS never survived long enough.

Conceptually, shock is first a disorder of the bulk transport of oxygen to the body's tissues. To achieve the goal of adequate tissue perfusion the body must have oxygen available and must be able to carry it in the blood. The first requirement is ensured by a secure airway, sufficient ventilation and oxygenation, and lung parenchyma that will allow the diffusion of oxygen across the *alveoli*. The second requirement of tissue perfusion is that oxygen gets to the end organ. A blood pressure sufficient to ensure flow to all tissues commensurate to their oxygen needs and an adequate hemoglobin concentration and composition to facilitate the delivery of oxygen are essential. Although seemingly simplistic, a thorough grasp of this concept allows systematic identification of the underlying source of shock. This is the typical cardiopulmonary understanding of shock. Yet, recent scientific advances make it clear that shock is no longer simply concerned with the bulk transport of oxygen, fluid status, and gas exchange. The biochemical component of systemic inflammation is just as important, and needs to be taken into consideration in clinical settings. As with many other systems in the body, the immune system relies on complex regulatory mechanisms to ensure proper function. The destructive nature of the body's defenses must be harnessed to protect against autoimmune reactions and destruction of healthy tissue, while still maintaining the ability to eliminate foreign pathogens. For example, proinflammatory cytokines interleukin (IL)-1, IL-2, and IL-6 must be held in check by IL-10 and other anti-inflammatory molecules. It is this very balance of stimulation and inhibition that is thought to be lost in shock and its massive inflammatory component. The activation of endothelial cells, macrophages, T lymphocytes, neutrophils, and other immune cells by these cytokines leads to massive immunologic stimulation. The resulting inflammation then leads to coagulation abnormalities, increased endothelial permeability, and enzymatic tissue destruction.

Physiologic Derangements of Shock

Scientists and clinicians have long realized that health is linked to the body's ability to maintain physiologic homeostasis in the face of a stressor. Whether that stressor is infection, organ failure, trauma and so on, it is the interconnectedness of organ systems that makes homeostasis possible. In other words, organs systems communicate and cooperate with each other (e.g., the cardiovascular system

and the kidneys in blood pressure regulation). Intrinsic to this very complex web of communication and function sharing is a variability that is the hallmark of normal physiologic function. Consider the beat to beat variation of the heart or respirations or any other normal function of the body. In fact, several recent studies have suggested that decreased heart rate variability (HRV) in the first 24 hours after trauma correlates well with declining physiologic reserve. This "cardiac uncoupling," or lack of communication with higher regulatory centers (autonomic nervous system) has the potential to be a new noninvasive biomarker that can herald the trauma victim's physiologic exhaustion and impending death. Further study is necessary to determine if HRV will emerge as a new "vital sign" for the 21st century, but there is potential.

Owing to the influence of the other organ systems none of these functions are entirely regular. Interestingly, it is this homeostatic interconnectedness of organ systems that is lost as inflammation progresses in the shock patient. Inflammation in its simplest form is the coordinated stimulation of various cells types (not just the cells of immunity) by various signals to kill nonself organisms in the face of a perceived threat to the body through oxidative damage and cytotoxic chemicals elaborated by the inflammatory cells. Yet, even with the noblest of intentions, the immune system can wreak havoc on the body when unregulated activation occurs and tissue destruction takes place. The activation and amplification of the immune system is good up to a point, allowing a quick and sufficient response to an invader in the attempt to restore homeostasis. In shock, this amplification is massively charged by some intense stimulus or loss of counterregulatory mechanisms and the deleterious effects of inflammation result. Not only is there systemic tissue destruction, but the interconnectedness of organ systems begins to crumble and physiologic variation that marked normal function is replaced with more predictable, ordered processes. In essence, each organ system reverts to a self-preservation mode and the usual cooperation and interconnectedness is lost. This ordering and seeming "loss of randomness" is not only seen on the macro level, but all the way down to gene expression. Therefore, in some ways, the "rude unhinging of the machinery of life" is actually the "orderly and predictable decline towards death."

HEMODYNAMIC MONITORING AND MANAGEMENT OF THE TRAUMA PATIENT

Identification and treatment of the source is the cornerstone of management for all shock states. There is a need to manage fluid status, optimize cardiac performance, and ensure adequate blood pressures, but the most important step toward reversing the effects of shock is treating the inciting event quickly. If it is sepsis, the source of the infection must be sought out and removed using antimicrobial therapy and surgery (when warranted). If it is necrotic tissue that is stimulating an inflammatory response, then the tissue must be excised. This principle of addressing the root cause is never truer than in hypovolemic shock due to uncontrolled hemorrhage. Bleeding must be stopped. Some studies have postulated that aggressive fluid resuscitation to maintain blood pressure and perfusion before the source of bleeding is controlled actually does more harm than good. Fluid resuscitation in hemorrhage is vital, but must never take precedence over surgical control of the bleeding. Several theories have been proposed to support this finding. One thought is that increased fluid results in a predictable rise in mean arterial pressures, which can disrupt clotting and other attempts by the body to control the hemorrhage. Or, with uncontrolled bleeding, the increased cardiovascular pressures simply cause the rate of hemorrhage to increase. Whatever the real reason, bleeding must be controlled and no amount of crystalloid or colloid or pressor will adequately manage the problem for very long.

Along with identifying and correcting the inciting event comes the need to optimize cardiac performance to its fullest. Patients whose resuscitation is dictated by markers of cardiac function in a goal-directed manner (e.g., end-diastolic volume index, mixed venous oxygen saturation, ventricular stroke work, and power output) have better outcomes than those patients whose resuscitation is specifically guided by simple clinical endpoints (urine output, mental status, skin turgor, blood pressure, and heart rate). Whether specific "endpoints of resuscitation" may or may not be useful, optimizing cardiovascular performance has long been recognized as a vital step in resuscitation and assisting the body's attempt to return to homeostasis. Therefore, the twofold goal of the clinician should be to (i) identify and treat the underlying cause and (ii) determine if global cardiac function is adequate. If the cardiovascular system is functioning properly and compensating well, then addressing the root cause should be sufficient. If there is an evidence of compromised global cardiac function, then a systematic evaluation of the independent determinants of cardiac function (preload, afterload, myocardial contractility, and heart rate) should be undertaken in a timely manner in order to optimize the heart's performance.

Improving global cardiac function requires a working knowledge of cardiac physiology, both theoretically and at the bedside. In addition to understanding the basic tenets of preload, afterload, and contractility, clinicians should understand the variables that describe each determinant. Additionally, the clinician must have a functional knowledge of monitoring techniques describing each of these variables and accurately interpret recorded values to determine appropriate therapeutic interventions. The following discussion of cardiac physiology and monitoring will attempt to lay a foundation for a novel approach to the resuscitation and treatment of the patient in shock with respect to optimizing cardiac performance: the ventricular pressure–volume diagram.

Delivery of optimal care to critically ill trauma patients during resuscitation requires rapid, accurate, and comprehensive monitoring of several major subsystems. Since 1970, with the introduction of the flotation pulmonary artery catheter (PAC), right-heart catheterization has been the accepted method of monitoring cardiac preload and myocardial performance in the ICU. The information from the PAC is used to assess the independent determinants of ventricular function (preload, contractility, and afterload). Ventricular preload has been estimated indirectly by transducing central venous pressure (CVP) and pulmonary artery occlusion pressure (PAOP). Afterload has been assessed by calculating systemic and pulmonary vascular resistance from other directly measured variables. Estimates of contractility have been inferred by changes in ventricular stroke work. Unfortunately, there are several common situations encountered in the critical ill trauma patient that render the PAC values inaccurate. Increased airway and pleural pressure secondary to increased positive end-expiratory pressure (PEEP) therapy for ARDS can increase transduced values of CVP and PAOP, leading the unsuspecting clinician to think that intravascular volume status is adequate when it is not. Intra-abdominal hypertension (intra-abdominal pressure >25 mm Hg) arising from a number of causes (retained packing material, bowel edema, retroperitoneal swelling) can also affect CVP and PAOP in a similar manner. Moreover, the process to obtain values using a thermodilution PAC is labor intensive and does not give real-time information on a continuous basis.

Fortunately, the advent of more powerful PACs that are able to continuously measure cardiac output and oxygen transport status represents an advance in tramatic shock care. The volumetric PACs provide useful information regarding preload, contractility, and afterload that was not previously available. This monitoring is helpful in patients with multisystem involvement, and the extrinsic forces that rendered information derived from the traditional thermodilutional PAC unreliable can now be accounted for with newer PAC models. The volumetric PAC directly measures right ventricular volumes, the oxygen saturation of mixed venous blood, body temperature, and estimates a host of other physiologic variables with minimal mathematical coupling errors. The temperature and right ventricular volume measurements are then used to calculate the right ventricular ejection fraction (RVEF). This RVEF is combined with the directly measured stroke volume index (SVI) to derive the right ventricular end-diastolic volume index (EDVI) (RVEDVI = SVI/RVEF). This right ventricular end-diastolic volume index (RVEDVI) is an easily identified value on the PAC computer interface and provides valuable information on cardiac preload and is useful in deriving estimations of contractility and afterload as well.

Assessing the Independent Determinants of Ventricular Function

Measuring Preload

Cardiac preload is defined physiologically as myocardial fiber length; in the intact heart, this is represented by ventricular volume at end-diastole. As it is a measure of ventriclar volume, the RVEDVI, by definition, is a better estimate of preload than indirect estimates based on transduced pressures. Furthermore, extrinsic forces acting upon the ventricle and pulmonary artery, such as pleural pressure and abdominal pressure, do not artificially affect volumetric measurements. Therefore, RVEDVI should theoretically be more closely related to preload then either CVP or PAOP. Clinical studies by several authors have confirmed that RVEDVI is more accurate than CVP or PAOP not only in theory, but also in multiple different types of trauma patients, including those who received large volume fluid resuscitations, those exposed to high levels of PEEP, and those who developed intra-abdominal hypertension. Estimating preload and intravascular volume status with the RVEDVI is not merely of physiologic interest, but actually provides useful information that affects patient-centered interventions. Studies examining the relationship between cardiac preload and gastrointestinal perfusion have utilized RVEDVI as the gauge of preload in trauma patients. The results demonstrated that occult hypovolemia (indicated by lower RVEDVI) was associated with decreased intestinal perfusion. Patients with a lower RVEDVI and gastric intramucosal pH (a surrogate marker for decreased GI perfusion) had a higher rate of death and MOF. Systemic perfusion, indicated by cardiac index (CI) and oxygen delivery, was not different between the occult hypovolemia and control groups. A subsequent, randomized prospective evaluation of the effects of maintaining various levels of RVEDVI on pulmonary function and GI perfusion was also performed. The patients maintained at an RVEDVI of ≥ 120 mL per m^2 had a significantly better intestinal perfusion than those patients maintained at lower levels of RVEDVI (90 to 100 mL per m^2) who were supported with various inotropic agents. Furthermore, these higher levels of preload were not associated with any differences in oxygenation function, ventilator days, or an increased incidence of ARDS.

Therefore, the ability to measure ventricular volumes has led to a new definition of adequate levels of preload. Although preload has traditionally been defined in terms of its relationship with cardiac function and the Frank-Starling curve, increasing preload beyond levels that result in increased cardiac output may replenish blood flow to regional tissue beds, such as the GI tract (see Figs. 1 and 2). This resuscitation may occur due to either replenishing occult intravascular volume deficits, or by ameliorating the need for the shunting of blood away from the gut through other mechanisms.

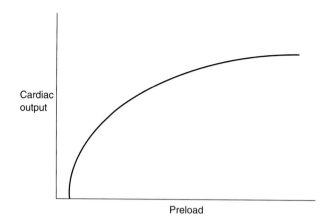

Figure 1   The Starling ventricular function curve.

Assessing Contractility and Afterload

Myocardial contractility is the determinant of intrinsic ventricular performance that is independent of preload and afterload. Afterload is the impedance to ejection of blood by the ventricle. Commonly used variables describing these independent determinants of ventricular function have several potential shortcomings. Variables such as ejection fraction and stroke work have been used as clinical estimates of contractility, but they are preload- and afterload- dependent (due to their mathematical derivations), and therefore do not represent contractility *per se*. Vascular resistance indices, based on mean systemic and pulmonary arterial pressure, are also less than ideal. They do not account for oscillatory pressure, pulsatile load, or reflected pulse waves. Ignoring pulsatile load may be a problem in older patients where oscillatory pressure proportionally accounts for a greater amount of afterload. Furthermore, each of these clinical indices of contractility and afterload are expressed in different units, or have no

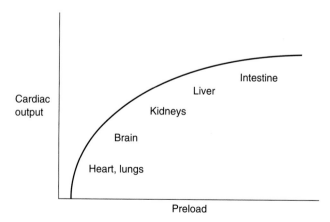

Figure 2   Representative Starling ventricular function curve illustrating the effects of various levels of preload on cardiac output and regional perfusion.

units at all; the relationship of each of these variables with each other and how these relationships affect each other are unclear, at best. Yet, there is a way to incorporate more accurate variables into a cohesive framework that aids in determining the best course of action at the bedside for the trauma patient in shock.

The Ventricular Pressure–Volume Diagram

Ideally, the clinician would only have to manipulate the familiar parameters of preload, afterload, and contractility to optimize cardiac performance. But, as stated in the preceding text these variables are difficult to accurately assess at the bedside with current monitoring equipment. Moreover, the traditional surrogates for these parameters (PAOP, systemic vascular resistance index [SVRI], and ejection fraction) are interdependent and it becomes difficult to accurately predict how changes in one variable affect the other two. For example, studies have demonstrated just how poor PAOP is at predicting cardiac output. Instead, the surgeon can use the equations provided to derive new variables (EDVI, E_{es}, and E_a) that better represent preload, afterload, and contractility separately and independently. These new values can then be plotted onto ventricular pressure–volume diagrams and used to identify problems with cardiac performance. Given current monitoring techniques, the ventricular pressure–volume diagram, as described by Suga et al. in the 1980s, is a potential monitoring tool that is free of many of the above limitations. Figure 3 shows a hypothetical ventricular pressure–volume diagram. Preload is represented on the diagram by the EDVI. The slope of the ventricular end-systolic pressure–volume relationship, or end-systolic elastance (E_{es}), represents myocardial contractility. The parameter has long been used as a load-independent measure of contractility in the cardiovascular laboratory, and a clinical adaptation of this variable has recently been described and tested in trauma patients.

Afterload can also be estimated within the pressure–volume framework. Effective arterial elastance (E_a), calculated as end-systolic pressure divided by SVI, is represented by the slope of a line drawn through the end-systolic point. As the slope of this line increases, impedance to ventricular ejection increases, and as the slope decreases afterload decreases. There are several theoretic reasons why this term is a better measure of afterload than vascular resistance. First, E_a is rate independent, whereas systemic vascular resistance is not. Second, E_a accounts for oscillatory pressure. This is important when estimating afterload in older patients, in whom pulsatile load had an increasing effect on both myocardial performance and the development of subsequent cardiac complications. (Recall that impedance to ventricular ejection may be quite marked in older patients with decreased compliance in their large arteries.) Finally, E_a can be examined in conjunction

with E_{es} on the pressure–volume diagram to evaluate the relationship between the heart and the arterial system, or ventricular–vascular coupling.

Ventricular–Vascular Coupling

The interactions between any physical energy source and its output environment are critical in determining the amount of useful work and power output the system is able to generate. In cardiovascular physiology, the efficacy of circulation is closely related to the coupling of the heart and the arterial system. Because cardiac contractility is represented by E_{es} and afterload by E_a, the relationships between E_{es} and E_a on the ventricular pressure–volume diagram can be used to estimate the ventricular–vascular coupling status, and the effects of each of these variables on resultant stroke work and power output can be examined. Relationships between E_{es} and E_a have been studied in various patient populations, including trauma patients. One study found that survivors of posttraumatic shock have better ventricular–vascular coupling than nonsurvivors, and described the effects that the better ventricular–vascular coupling in survivors had on stroke work and power output.

Ventricular Stroke Work and Power

Referring again to Fig. 3, end-diastolic volume, E_{es}, and E_a define the boundries of ventricular stroke work, a term classically described by both Starling and Sarnoff as the most appropriate measure of ventricular energy output. Stroke work and ventricular power output (stroke work performed over time) are both more closely related to cardiovascular performance and perfusion in trauma patients than CI, oxygen delivery, or oxygen consumption. Using the ventricular pressure–volume diagram, preload, contractility and afterload can be evaluated in a common, integrated framework, and the effects of changes in any one variable on stroke work and power output can be predicted. Furthermore, by constructing pressure–volume diagrams at the bedside with measurements obtained from the PAC, inadequate perfusion resulting from cardiovascular dysfunction can be evaluated in terms of the independent determinants of ventricular function (preload, contractility, afterload) and specific therapy can be applied in a goal-directed manner.

Ideally, the clinician would only have to manipulate the familiar parameters of preload, afterload, and contractility to optimize cardiac performance. But, as shown in the preceding text, these variables are difficult to accurately assess at the bedside with current monitoring equipment. Moreover, conventional surrogates for these parameters (PAOP, SVRI, and ejection fraction) are all intertwined and it becomes difficult to accurately predict how changes in one variable affect the other two. For example, studies have demonstrated

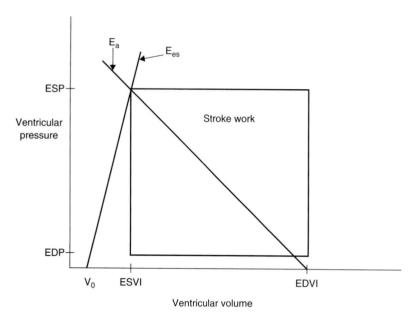

Figure 3 Ventricular pressure–volume diagram E_{es} represents ventricular end-systolic elastance, a load-independent measure of ventricular contractility; E_a, effective arterial elastance, a rate-independent measure of afterload that accounts for oscillatory pressure and steady-flow pressure; ESP, end-systolic ventricular pressure, derived from peak systolic pressure; EDP, ventricular end-diastolic pressure; V_0, ventricular volume at zero pressure; ESVI, ventricular end-systolic volume index; EDVI, ventricular end-diastolic volume index.

just how poor PAOP is at predicting cardiac output. Instead, the surgeon can use the equations provided to derive new variables (EDVI, E_{es}, and E_a) that better represent preload, afterload, and contractility separately and independently. These new values are then plotted onto ventricular pressure–volume diagrams and used to identify problems with cardiac performance. These diagrams enable the clinician to seek out and correct these problems is a goal-oriented manner. Ideally, one would be able to assess each of the primary determinants of cardiac function independently and in relation to each other. The problem with this has already been discussed. However, EDVI, arterial elastance, and end-systolic ventricular elastance can all be plotted on a ventricular pressure–volume diagram and manipulated to achieve the maximum amount of cardiac work (the area inside the box created in the ventricular pressure–volume diagrams). At the bedside, the clinician can determine how to best maximize cardiovascular performance by graphing the changes to E_a that would result from afterload increases (vasopressors), and/or increasing E_{es} with inotropic agents (see Figs. 4 and 5). A recent analysis of this goal-directed therapy using the ventricular pressure–volume diagram

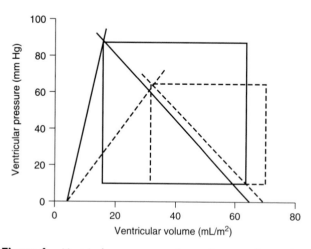

Figure 4 Ventricular pressure–volume diagram of a patient with hypotension due to inadequate contractility after initial fluid resuscitation (*dashed lines*). Blood pressure and stroke work increased after administration of 5 μg/kg/minute of dobutamine (*solid lines*). Increase in contractility represented by the increase in the slope of ventricular end-systolic elastance (E_{es}). Note that effective arterial elastance (E_a) did not change.

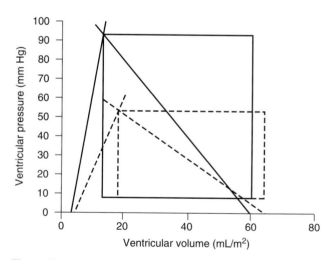

Figure 5 Ventricular pressure–volume diagram of a patient with inadequate perfusion and hypotension due to both inadequate afterload and inadequate contractility after initial fluid resuscitation (*dashed lines*). Blood pressure and stroke work increased after administration of 10 μg/kg/minute of dopatine (*solid lines*). The increase in contractility is represented by increase in slope of ventricular end-systolic elastance (E_{es}), the increase in afterload represented by increase in slope of effective arterial elastance (E_a).

was conducted in a trauma ICU. After resuscitating all study subjects to a set RVEDVI to standardize the preload aspect of cardiovascular performance, the contractile ability of the heart and afterload were assessed. On the basis of data obtained from volumetric PACs, specific goal-directed interventions were undertaken to optimize cardiac performance. If the patient's underlying hemodynamic dysfunction was decreased intrinsic cardiac performance then inotropes such as dobutamine were used in the resuscitation. If the problem was decreased afterload, then agents such as norepinephrine were started. For mixed clinical pictures with both cardiac dysfunction and decreased afterload, epinephrine and dopamine were used. This identification of the cardiovascular abnormality is critical to avoiding ischemia in underperfused tissue beds in the effort to simply increase the mean arterial pressure of the entire system. A false sense of security may arise from normalization of common hemodynamic parameters by using certain vasoactive drugs that are actually exacerbating the overall problem of shock, underperfusion of tissues.

ENDPOINTS

What determines the resolution of shock and its sequelae? This question has become a highly debatable topic as our understanding of shock has evolved. As mentioned previously, the inflammatory aspects of shock can linger far beyond the initial resuscitation leaving the resolution of the disease process a much more nebulous issue. Despite the many advances made in the field of shock, still no solid clinical study points to any one particular marker as the indicator that shock has resolved. Therefore, it is essential to evaluate all the information at the physician's disposal to ensure that the treatment strategy is appropriate and make changes as necessary. Laboratory values such as arterial BD and lactate can be used in conjunction with real-time physiologic monitoring to help determine where the shock victim falls on the clinical spectrum. In addition, the physician must consider the patient's overall clinical appearance and physical examination in completing the assessment and seeking new therapeutic interventions. Above all it is important to quickly recognize shock and aggressively treat it, thereby avoiding the progression to MOF that will result if not adequately treated.

SUGGESTED READINGS

Argenta LC, ed. *Basic science for surgeons: a review*. Philadelphia: WB Saunders; 2004.

Buchman TG. Physiologic stability and physiologic state. *J Trauma.* 1996;41(4):599–605.

Buchman TG. The community of the self (review). *Nature.* 2002;420(6912):246–251.

Chang MC. Monitoring of the critically injured patient. *Soc Crit Care Med: New Horizon.* 1999;7(1):35–45.

Chang MC, Blinman TA, Rutherford EJ, et al. Preload assessment in trauma patients during large-volume shock resuscitation. *Arch Surg.* 1996;131(7):728–731.

Chang MC, Meredith JW. Cardiac preload, splanchnic perfusion, and their relationship during resuscitation in trauma patients. *J Trauma.* 1997;42(4):577–582; discussion 582–584.

Chang MC, Meredith JW, Kincaid EH, et al. Maintaining survivors' values of left ventricular power output during shock resuscitation: A prospective pilot study. *J Trauma.* 2000;49(1):26–33; discussion 34–37.

Chang MC, Miller PR, D'Agostino R Jr, et al. Effects of abdominal decompression on cardiopulmonary function and visceral perfusion in patients with intra-abdominal hypertension. *J Trauma.* 1998;44(3):440–445.

Chang MC, Mondy JS III, Meredith JW, et al. Clinical application of ventricular end-systolic elastance and the ventricular pressure-volume diagram. *Shock.* 1997;7(6):413–419.

Diebel LN, Myers T, Dulchavsky S. Effects of increasing airway pressure and PEEP on the assessment of cardiac preload. *J Trauma.* 1997;42(4):585–590; discussion 590–591.

Fall PJ, Szerlip HM. Lactic acidosis: From sour milk to septic shock (review). *J Intensive Care Med.* 2005;20(5):255–271.

Kincaid EH, Miller PR, Meredith JW, et al. Elevated arterial base deficit in trauma patients: A marker of impaired oxygen utilization. *J Am Coll Surg.* 1998;187(4):384–392.

Martin RS, Kincaid EH, Russell HM, et al. Selective management of cardiovascular dysfunction in posttraumatic SIRS and sepsis. *Shock.* 2005;23(3):202–208.

Martin RS, Norris PR, Kilgo PD, et al. Validation of stroke work and ventricular arterial coupling as markers of cardiovascular performance during resuscitation. *J Trauma.* 2006;60(5):930–934; discussion 934–935.

Miller PR, Kincaid EH, Meredith JW, et al. Threshold values of intramucosal pH and mucosal-arterial CO2 gap during shock resuscitation. *J Trauma.* 1998;45(5):868–872.

Miller PR, Meredith JW, Chang MC. Randomized, prospective comparison of increased preload versus inotropes in the resuscitation of trauma patients: Effects on cardiopulmonary function and visceral perfusion. *J Trauma.* 1998;44(1):107–113.

Moore EE, Feliciano DV, Mattox KL, eds. *Trauma,* 5th ed. New York: McGraw-Hill; 2004.

Morris JA Jr, Norris PR, Ozdas A, et al. Reduced heart rate variability: An indicator of cardiac uncoupling and diminished physiologic reserve in 1,425 trauma patients. *J Trauma.* 2006;60(6):1165–1173; discussion 1173–1174.

Norris PR, Morris JA Jr, Ozdas A, et al. Heart rate variability predicts trauma patient outcome as early as 12 h: Implications for military and civilian triage. *J Surg Res.* 2005;129(1):122–128.

Wiel E, Vallet B, ten Cate H. The endothelium in intensive care (review). *Crit Care Clin.* 2005;21(3):403–416.

SIRS, Sepsis, and Multi-system Organ Dysfunction and Failure

61

Wendy L. Wahl

Sepsis is the body's systemic inflammatory and coagulation response to infection. It is a life-threatening syndrome which affects tissue remote from the site of initial infection and can lead to multiple system organ failure (MSOF) and death. It is estimated that there are more than 750,000 new cases of sepsis in the United States each year with as many as 215,000 deaths annually.[1] The Centers for Disease Control and Prevention ranks septicemia as the tenth leading cause of death in the United States,[2] with a severe sepsis mortality estimated at 28% to 50%[3] (see Fig. 1).

Before 1992, the reporting of deaths or even the incidence of sepsis was clouded by a lack of clear definitions for sepsis and associated conditions. The American College of Chest Physicians (ACCP) and the Society of Critical Care Medicine (SCCM) established standard definitions for systemic inflammatory response syndrome (SIRS) and sepsis.[4] Despite this, mortality from severe sepsis is often coded as a complication of some other disease process, rather than a primary discharge diagnosis leaving the true incidence underreported.[3] A sepsis consensus conference in 2001 reviewed the diagnostic criteria for sepsis to include the concept of predisposition, insult (infection), response, and organ dysfunction (P'RO).[5] The four categories are summarized by the following terms:

SYSTEMIC INFLAMMATORY RESPONSE SYNDROME

SIRS is a bodily response to a wide variety of clinical insults such as tissue injury from pancreatitis, trauma, burns, blood product infusion, malignancy, endocrine disease, or infection. It is manifested by two or more of the following signs or symptoms: (a) heart rate >90 beats per minute, (b) respiratory rate >20 breaths per minute or $PaCO_2$ <32 mm Hg, (c) temperature >38°C or <36°C, and (d) a white blood cell count >12,000 cells per mm^3 or <4,000 cells per mm^3 or immature (band) forms accounting for >10% of the neutrophils present. SIRS does not imply the presence of an infectious organism but is a sign of systemic inflammation.

SEPSIS

The clinical syndrome is defined by the presence of both a systemic inflammatory response and infection. In addition to the signs of SIRS, the 2001 consensus conference added mental status changes, significant edema, hypotension, acute oliguria, and tissue hypoperfusion as nonspecific signs to aid clinicians in the diagnosis of sepsis (see Table 1).

Severe Sepsis

The development of multisystem organ dysfunction (MSOD) accompanying sepsis was added for use in various sepsis assessment tools. This category includes MSOF and MSOD (to be discussed later in the chapter).

Septic Shock

The onset of acute circulatory failure with persistent arterial hypotension despite adequate fluid resuscitation

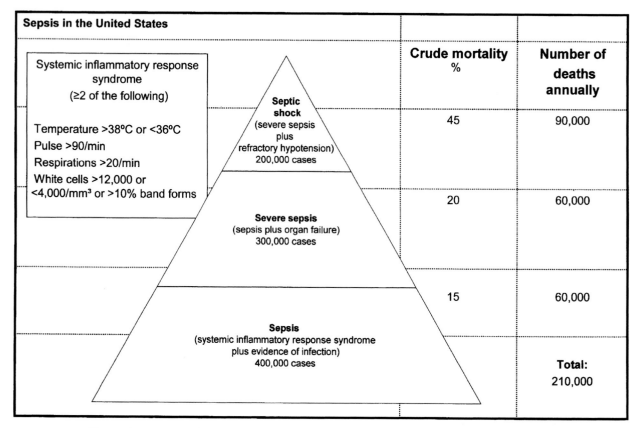

Figure 1   Sepsis in the United States. (Adapted from Manns BJ, Lee H, Doig CJ, et al. An Economic Evaluation of Activated Protein C Treatment for Severe Sepsis. *N Engl J Med.* 2002; 347(13):993–1000.)

and with no other cause of hypotension characterizes septic shock. For adults, a systolic arterial pressure of <90 mm Hg or a drop of >40 mm Hg from baseline defines hypotension. For children, septic shock includes tachycardia, decreased peripheral pulses compared to central pulses, and diminished urine output.

Even with proper definitions in place, the diagnosis of whether or which infection is present in sepsis can still be difficult for the clinician. One or two of every three septic patients will have no growth on blood cultures or have no definite site of infection identified.[3,6] Yet, the term *sepsis* indicates infection, and studies show that SIRS may persist even after treatment of the infectious source.[7] The presence of SIRS alone does not increase the risk of death, but the deterioration of organ dysfunction seen in severe sepsis does worsen outcome.[8] In a large study that followed the natural history of SIRS patients, 48% were diagnosed with an infection. Twenty-six percent of patients had uncomplicated sepsis, 18% developed severe sepsis with organ dysfunction, and 4% had septic shock. Bacteremia was more common in those with increased symptom severity, with positive blood cultures in 17% of septic patients and 69% of patients with septic shock.[9]

EVALUATION AND DIAGNOSIS

Physical Examination

Fever is the most common presenting symptom of sepsis and should be a signal for further clinical evaluation of infection in the patient. Elderly patients with sepsis or those with thermoregulatory dysfunction may present with hypothermia.[10] Physical examination should include a rapid, global review of the patient's condition with continuous monitoring. Patients in shock should have arterial catheters placed for blood pressure monitoring. Signs of SIRS may suggest infection or ongoing inflammation. Other clinical evidence of poor perfusion such as change in mental status, low urine output, mottling, and poor capillary refill should be evaluated in addition to blood pressure (Table 1). Sites of potential infection such as the chest, abdomen, wounds, or skin and existing catheters should be examined for obvious signs of infection. The lung, abdominal cavity, and urinary tract are the three most common sites of infection causing severe sepsis.[11,12] Infections leading to sepsis can also arise in surgical sites from the skin to the deep muscle layers. Other nosocomial causes of sepsis are intravenous catheter infections, ventilator-associated pneumonia, and

TABLE 1

SIGNS AND SYMPTOMS SUGGESTIVE OF SEPSIS

Documented or suspected infection with some of the following:

General physiologic variables

Temperature $>38.3°C$ or $<36°C$

Heart rate >90 beats/min or 2 SD above the mean for age

Tachypnea

Altered mental status

Significant edema or positive fluid balance (>20 mL/kg/24 hr)

In the absence of diabetes, plasma glucose >120 mg/dL

Inflammatory variables

WBC count $<4,000/\mu L$ or $>12,000/\mu L$

Normal WBC with $>10\%$ immature forms

Plasma C-reactive protein >2 SD above normal value

Plasma procalcitonin >2 SD above normal value

Hemodynamic variables

Hypotension: SBP <90 mm Hg, MAP <70 mm Hg or SBP decrease of 40 mm Hg

$S\bar{V}O_2 >70\%$

Cardiac index >3.5 L/min/M^2

Organ dysfunction variables

Arterial hypoxemia: $PaO_2/FIO_2 <300$

Acute oliguria: urine output <0.5 mL/kg/hr for at least 2 hr

Creatinine increase >0.5 mg/dL

Abnormal coagulation: INR >1.5 or aPTT >60 s

Ileus (absent bowel sounds)

Thrombocytopenia: platelet count $<100,000/\mu L$

Hyperbilirubinemia: plasma total bilirubin >4 mg/dL

Tissue perfusion variables

Elevated lactate: >1 mmol/L

Decreased capillary refill or mottling

SD, standard deviation; WBC, white blood cells; SBP, systolic blood pressure; MAP, mean arterial pressure; $S\bar{V}O_2$, mixed venous oxygenation; PaO_2, partial pressure of arterial oxygen; FIO_2, fraction of inspired oxygen; INR, international normalized ratio.

---

sinusitis. For 20% to 30% of patients, the site of infection may not be identified.[3] In patients undergoing more specialized procedures such as maxillofacial reconstruction, spine fixation or craniotomies, closed space infections of the sinuses, or intracranial space should be considered if other, more common sources are not identified as the infectious source.

Laboratory Data

Laboratory studies should include a complete blood count with differential, chemistry profile, arterial blood gas with lactate level, prothrombin time and partial thromboplastin time, and urinalysis.[13] Monitoring lactate levels for guiding resuscitation has been shown to be helpful in septic patients for prognostication.[14,15] Clearance of lactic acidosis with fluid resuscitation is associated with improved outcomes.

A major response to inflammatory or infectious insults is the release of cytokines. Although not routinely monitored

in the clinical setting, plasma levels of tumor necrosis factor alpha (TNF)-α, interleukin (IL)-1, IL-6, IL-8, IL-10 and their soluble receptors are elevated in both infections and noninfectious SIRS. The degree of elevation correlates with the severity of disease.[12] After the release of TNF-α, IL-1, and IL-6, acute phase reactant proteins, C-reactive protein (CRP), and procalcitonin (PCT) levels rise. A 10- to 100-fold increase in CRP is common in SIRS patients. Patients with systemic infections have been found to have a rise in levels of PCT, which can be predictive of sepsis and multiorgan dysfunction. Elevated PCT levels have been shown to be a better marker of sepsis than temperature, leukocyte count, TNF-α, IL-6, or CRP levels.[16–19]

By definition, sepsis is a response to infection. Consideration of noninfectious etiologies for SIRS should be considered including surgery, trauma, burns, hematoma, subarachnoid hemorrhage, venous thrombosis, pancreatitis, myocardial infarction, transplant rejection, thyroid storm, acute renal insufficiency, lymphoma, tumor lysis syndrome, blood products, opiates, benzodiazepines, anesthetic-related malignant hyperpyrexia, neuroleptic malignant syndrome, and erythroderma.[11,20] After a thorough physical examination and consideration of noninfectious causes of SIRS, cultures and diagnostic studies should be performed to identify causative agents.

Site of Infection

Despite the problems in making the diagnosis of infection, it is important to continually examine the patient for changes. Thirty percent of septic patients may never have a causative organism identified. In some cases, it may be difficult to differentiate colonization from infection. In others, previous use of antibiotics may affect culture results. The Surviving Sepsis Campaign guidelines recommend prompt diagnostic testing. Blood cultures are indicated in patients who appear septic with fever or hypothermia, chills, leukocytosis or neutropenia, left shift of neutrophils, suspected infection, hemodynamic instability, or new renal insufficiency. The SCCM guidelines recommend that one pair of blood cultures be obtained at the onset of symptoms and once again at 24 hours.[20] Subsequent blood cultures should be based on the clinician's suspicion for ongoing bacteremia or fungemia. Two sets of blood cultures should be drawn from peripheral sites. If this is not possible, then one set should be drawn peripherally and the other from a recently inserted central catheter after careful cleansing of the port site.

Diagnosis of pulmonary infections should be based on clinical examination, chest radiographs, and inspection of the patient's respiratory secretions. Positive findings in conjunction with alteration in leukocyte counts and changes in oxygenation are fairly suggestive of a respiratory tract infection. If the patient is intubated, we prefer diagnosis of ventilator-associated pneumonia using bronchoalveolar lavage (BAL) and quantitative cultures to decrease the chance of treating colonization.[21-23] Use of "mini-BAL," where a catheter is passed deep into the airway and blindly lavaged, has been used by some, but comparison to regular BAL is recommended to ensure reliability in one's own practice. Also, in patients with infiltrates on one side of the chest radiograph, a mini-BAL may not accurately diagnose the infectious process because it may not sample the affected side.

For hospitalized patients with central venous catheters, the catheter exit site and tunnel should be inspected for evidence of erythema or purulence. In the face of thrombosis of the catheter, purulence, embolic phenomenon, or sepsis, the catheter should be removed and cultures from the tip sent. Blood cultures from the catheter and a peripheral site are useful to determine if the infection was primarily from the catheter or related to another site of bacteremia or whether the catheter was colonized versus infected.[24]

Urinary tract infections are common in hospitalized patients, and urine samples should be sent for culture, microscopy, and Gram stain in febrile patients. Presence of pyuria is easily detected with leukocyte esterase testing. For patients with an indwelling Foley catheter, specimens should be taken from the urine port and not from the collection bag.[24]

Recent surgery adds the risk of surgical site infections as a cause of sepsis. Consideration of both superficial infection of the skin and soft tissue, as well as of the deeper layers of muscle and fascia should be made. For intracavitary infection such as intra-abdominal abscess or fascial infection, abdominal computed tomography (CT) may be necessary for detection.[24] In cases of clean-contaminated or contaminated procedures, the organisms common to the organ involved in the surgery should be considered as the potential infectious flora. For clean surgical procedures, *Staphylococcus aureus* is the most common causative organism.[18]

Central nervous system infections should be considered in patients who have unexplained alterations in consciousness or focal neurologic signs or in recent trauma patients who have had intracranial pressure monitors or other neurosurgical interventions. A noncontrast head CT should be performed to detect contraindications to lumbar puncture (signs of high pressure). Otherwise, lumbar puncture should be performed.

For a summary of the evaluation for sepsis see Fig. 2.

TREATMENT

Antibiotics

Identification of the site of infection is a major determinant in antimicrobial therapy. Pneumonia, urinary tract infection, and bloodstream infections comprise 75% of medical nosocomial infections, and of these, 90% are related to indwelling tubes such as endotracheal tubes, Foley catheters, and central venous lines.[11] These devices should be removed as soon as possible to decrease the risk of infection. However in the face of sepsis, the clinician must make the best educated guess as to the source of infection and likely pathogens. Delays in administering antibiotic therapy in septic patients have been associated with

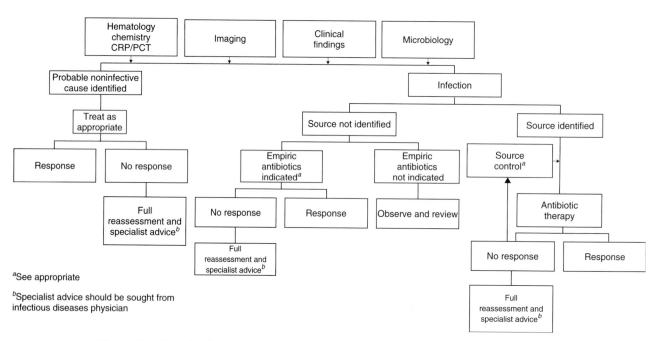

^{a}See appropriate

^{b}Specialist advice should be sought from infectious diseases physician

Figure 2   Algorithm for evaluation of suspected sepsis. (Adapted from Llewelyn M, Cohen J. Diagnosis of infection in sepsis. *Intensive Care Med.* 2001;27:S10–S32.)

increased mortality.[25] In addition, inappropriate antibiotic therapy has also been shown to increase morbidity and mortality from survival rates of 63% to 92% for correct antibiotic therapy down to 10% to 50% for ineffective antibiotic regimens.[26–28] When selecting empiric antibiotic therapy, clinicians should take into account the following factors: likely site of infection, likely organisms, history of recent antibiotic use (which may increase resistance), culture data if known, drug penetration into the suspected site of infection, dose, and frequency of dosing.[28,29] Because the speed of delivery and the appropriateness of antibiotics affect patient outcomes, broad-spectrum coverage of likely pathogens should be empirically started. When culture and sensitivity data become available, the antibiotic regimen can then be adjusted. Lack of correct initial antibiotic coverage for offending pathogens is a primary risk for increased mortality. Even with the correct antibiotics in the face of septic shock, delays in antibiotic administration increase mortality. In 2,154 septic shock patients who received correct antibiotic therapy after onset of hypotension, each hour of delay was associated with a decrease in survival of 7.6%. Septic shock patients receiving antibiotics in the first hour after onset of hypotension had a survival rate of 79.9%, but only 50% of patients received effective antimicrobial therapy within the first 6 hours.[25]

To assist in choosing the correct antibiotic regimen, the clinician should categorize the likely pathogen into the following categories: (i) Gram positives, with or without *Enterococcus* and with or without methicillin-resistant *Staphyloccus aureus* (MRSA), (ii) Gram negatives, with or without *Pseudomonas, Acinetobacter,* or *Enterobacter,* (iii) atypical organisms, including *Legionella,* and (iv) anaerobic organisms, including *Bacteroides.* Prolonged hospitalization, recent exposure to antibiotics, immune status, and age contribute to the likelihood of having an infection with a nosocomial pathogen such as MRSA, *Enterococcus* species, resistant Gram negatives, *Clostridium difficile,* and *Candida* species.[30] Knowledge of the likely pathogens in one's own intensive care unit (ICU) is instrumental to choosing the correct antibiotic regimen because there is wide variability across ICUs even in the same institution.[31]

Fluids and Resuscitation

Hypotension associated with septic shock has many contributing factors. There may be large decreases of plasma volume from fluid loss into the interstitial space causing hypovolemia.[32] There can be myocardial depression and decreased vasomotor tone. Despite the etiology, outcomes are improved with early fluid resuscitation. In patients randomized to early fluid boluses guided by either central venous or pulmonary artery catheter monitoring, Rivers et al. found a decrease in mortality when patients were aggressively resuscitated with fluid within the first 6 hours of presentation to the emergency department in septic shock.[33] "Early goal-directed therapy" targeted a mean arterial pressure of 65 mm Hg. If after fluid administration the goal pressure was not obtained, vasopressors were added. Central venous oxyhemoglobin saturations (CvO_2 sat) were followed in an attempt to achieve CvO_2 of 70%. The mortality of the early goal-directed therapy group was 30.5% compared to the observed mortality of the standard therapy group of 46.5%.[33] The type of fluid infused for resuscitation was not predetermined for the early goal-directed study but was left to clinician preference with the recommendation that a hematocrit <30 mg per dL be treated with red blood cell transfusion.

The debate over whether colloid or crystalloid is the best fluid for sepsis remains controversial. In an almost 7,000-patient, randomized study in Australia and New Zealand comparing use of 4% albumin to normal saline solution in patients admitted to the ICU, there was no difference in mortality, hospital or ICU days, onset of new organ failure, or mechanical ventilation for those receiving albumin compared to normal saline.[34] For trauma patients, there was a trend toward improved survival with normal saline ($p = 0.06$), whereas in patients with severe sepsis there was a trend toward improved survival with albumin use ($p = 0.09$).[34] In other meta-analyses, there have been mixed results where morbidity may be decreased but mortality remained unaffected with albumin use.[35] However, other meta-analysis revealed no apparent difference in pulmonary edema, mortality, or length of stay between colloid and crystalloid resuscitation.[36,37]

A second part to the fluid resuscitation piece is the question of the need for pulmonary artery catheter monitoring. Rivers did not mandate the use during early, goal-directed therapy, but left it to the discretion of the clinician, although central venous catheters were used for CvO_2 monitoring.[33] In patients with a history of congestive heart failure or who do not respond to aggressive fluid administration, information on cardiac function such as cardiac output, may be helpful. Data on central filling pressures may also aid in managing patients who require pressure-controlled ventilation or high positive end-expiratory pressures (PEEP) for ventilator management. However, in a randomized controlled trial assessing the risk and benefits of pulmonary artery catheters in high-risk surgical patients, there was no detected benefit in 1,994 patients studied.[38] Other investigators have shown increased mortality in ICU patients randomized to use of pulmonary artery catheter monitoring,[39] whereas other researchers attributed worsened outcomes to development of organ dysfunction and higher acuity of illness rather than to the catheter use.[40]

Vasopressors

In the face of adequate volume expansion, ongoing hypotension in sepsis indicates the need for vasopressors and inotropes. Expansion of the intravascular volume with fluid is the first-line treatment for hypotension. If cardiac output does not improve or hypotension continues, a vasopressor may be needed for adequate perfusion during periods of severe or life-threatening hypotension. Vasopressors can improve perfusion by counteracting the decreased vasomotor tone, which often occurs in sepsis. Some of the hypotension seen in septic shock may be due to vasopressin deficiency[41] and downregulation of vasopressin receptors.[42] Vasopressin has been reported to increase blood pressure to allow weaning of other pressor agents. However, vasopressin therapy may cause intestinal ischemia, decreased cardiac output, skin necrosis and even cardiac arrest, especially at doses >0.04 U per minute.[43] Most of the studies in septic patients using vasopressin have been small, with data collected during the first few hours and not long term. Most of the advantages of vasopressin therapy were in weaning down other pressor agents, but did not translate into improved survival rates.[44,45]

There are many vasopressors available, but recent recommendations from the SCCM Surviving Sepsis Campaign support the use of norepinephrine for septic shock.[46] Studies comparing norepinephrine to dopamine found that norepinephrine was more effective in restoring blood pressure in septic shock.[47-49] Patients treated with norepinephrine for hemodynamic support during sepsis had a mortality rate of 62% compared to an 82% mortality rate in those treated with vasopressors other than norepinephrine.[49] Some of the advantages of norepinephrine may be due to the lower incidence of tachycardia compared to dopamine,[48] and the diminished endocrine effect on the hypothalamic pituitary axis seen with norepinephrine compared to dopamine.[50,51] For a summary of the cardiovascular management of sepsis see Fig. 3.

Corticosteroids

Although the SCCM Surviving Sepsis Campaign supports the use of corticosteroids in the use of septic patients, the utilization of steroids has been recommended for patients who are only vasopressor dependent. There is no role for high-dose corticosteroids or steroids in patients who are not vasopressor dependent. Earlier, randomized controlled trials that evaluated the early use of high-dose corticosteroids did not show a survival benefit in severe sepsis.[52,53] With the recognition that adrenal insufficiency may be a confounding variable in septic shock, new studies have revived interest in the use of steroids in sepsis. Only two of five small, randomized studies have demonstrated decreased vasopressor support in septic patients,[53,54] but only one trial was adequately powered to reveal a survival benefit for septic patients who had no response to corticotrophin stimulation testing.[55] In this trial, ventilated, oliguric patients who were vasopressor dependent underwent a 250 μg corticotrophin stimulation test and were

then assigned to receive placebo or hydrocortisone plus fludrocortisone for 7 days. Nonresponders to the stimulation test were defined as those whose cortisol level rose <10 μg per dL. Those who were nonresponders and received steroids had a lower mortality rate than those who received placebo, but the overall mortality was not significant at $p = 0.09$.[55]

The definition for what constitutes adrenal insufficiency is also extremely complex for critically ill patients who often have low albumin levels. Serum total cortisol is a sum of both protein-bound cortisol and free cortisol. Patients with low albumin levels may have falsely low serum total cortisol levels, despite normal or even increased levels of free cortisol.[56,57] Therefore, the use of corticosteroids and the diagnosis of adrenal insufficiency in patients with sepsis remains complex and warrants further randomized controlled trials to fully evaluate the effects of early short-course corticosteroids. Currently in severe sepsis, high-dose corticosteroids do not improve survival and are not warranted.[57,58]

Activated Protein C Therapy

After initiation of goal-directed therapy and antibiotic therapy, the use of activated protein C (APC) should be considered for patients who have severe sepsis and an increased risk of death with Acute Physiology and Chronic Health Evaluation (APACHE) II scores of >24 or organ dysfunction of two or more organ systems. Administration of APC was approved by U.S. Food and Drug Administration (FDA) at the dose of 24 μg/kg/minute for 96 hours. Patients with one or both of the inclusion criteria showed an absolute decrease in mortality of 13% in the Recombinant Human Activated Protein C Worldwide Evaluation in Severe Sepsis (PROWESS) trial.[59-61] Contraindications to the use of APC in the initial trial included recent trauma or surgery in the 12 hours before use, active hemorrhage, ongoing use of other anticoagulants, thrombocytopenia with a platelet count <30,000 per μL^3, and recent stroke.[59]

The PROWESS trial revealed a trend toward an increased rate of serious bleeding, defined as the need for either three units of packed red blood cells transfused over 2 days or intracranial hemorrhage, compared to those in the placebo group (3.5% compared to 2%, $p = 0.06$).[59] Recently, two subsequent trials looking at APC in sepsis were terminated early (Administration of Drotrecogin Alfa in Early Stage Severe Sepsis [ADDRESS] trial, and the Resolution of Organ Failure in Pediatric Patients with Severe Sepsis trial [RESOLVE],) because of failure to show significant differences, and a warning was issued to the FDA that there may be an increased risk of bleeding.[62] The Extended Evaluation of Recombinant Human Activated Protein C United States trial (ENHANCE U.S.) reported a 6.5% risk of serious bleeding, compared to the PROWESS trial bleeding incidence of 3.5%.[57,62]

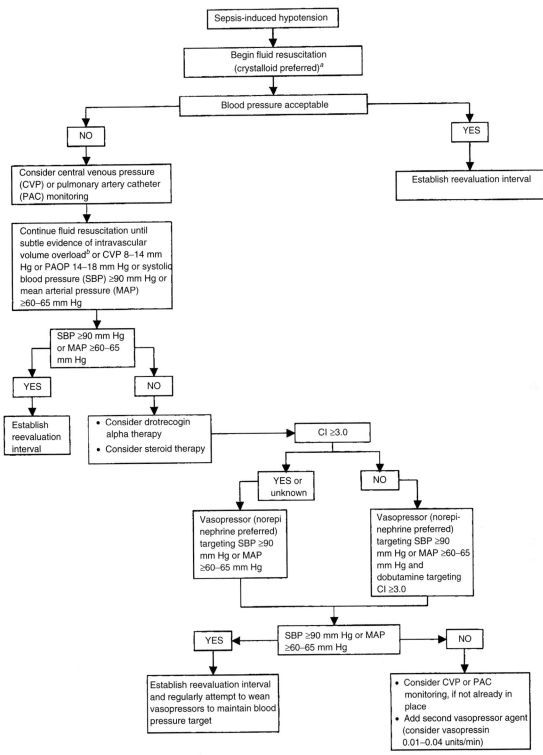

^{a}250–1000 mL boluses of crystalloid, each over 5-15 min
^{b}Basilar crackles on lung anscultation or increase in pulse oximetry O$_5$ saturation

Figure 3 Flow diagram for guidance in management decisions in septic shock. PAOP, pulmonary artery occlusion pressure; SBP, systolic blood pressure; CI, confidence interval. (Adapted from Shapiro NI, Wolfe RE, Moore RB, et al. *Crit Care Med.* 2003;31(3):670–675.)

SUPPORTIVE THERAPY/ORGAN SUPPORT

Respiratory System

The lung is the organ most prone to injury during sepsis. Pulmonary support implementing lung-protective ventilator strategies improves survival (acute respiratory distress syndrome [ARDS]). Lung-protective mechanical ventilation with relatively low tidal volumes of 4 to 6 mL per kg of ideal body weight compared to 12 mL per kg decreased mortality from 40% to 31% and improved organ dysfunction.[63,64] Overdistension and repetitive opening and closing of alveoli during mechanical ventilation appear injurious. PEEP can decrease oxygen requirements, but did not appear to influence mortality in patients treated with higher versus lower levels of PEEP in the Acute Respiratory Distress Syndrome Clinical Trials Network.[63] Permissive hypercapnia down to pH >7.20 to 7.25 should be allowed in ARDS patients if required to minimize plateau pressures and tidal volumes.[65] This strategy may not be possible in some patients, such as those with severe neurologic injury where increased P_{CO_2} may worsen edema or pregnancy where increased P_{CO_2} and acidosis may not be tolerated by the fetus. Appropriate, but not excessive, sedation is important for ventilator support, with care to awaken patients daily for assessment of weaning and extubation potential to avoid infectious complications.[66] Minimization of neuromuscular paralytic agents is important to avoid potential complications of polyneuropathy, particularly in patients treated with corticosteroids.[67]

Renal Dysfunction and Renal Replacement Therapy

Acute renal failure in sepsis is an independent risk factor for mortality in sepsis, and when accompanied by other organ dysfunction it can have mortality rates as high as 53% to 73%. For patients who develop acute renal failure during an episode of severe sepsis, renal replacement therapy is required in up to 70% of patients.[68,69] There is ongoing debate over the renal replacement therapy dose and modality. In septic shock, there may be a benefit to hemofiltration, which can decrease the sepsis-induced inflammatory response.[70] There is one prospective, randomized study, which demonstrates a survival benefit for higher doses of hemofiltration in critical illnesses including sepsis. On the basis of this study, a target dose of at least 35 mL/kg/hour for the ultrafiltration rate during dialysis sessions is recommended.[71,72] Studies that assess daily doses and intermittent doses of dialysis are difficult to compare because the reported survival benefits may be related to the higher overall dialysis dose and not to the timing of the dialysis.[71,73] In acute renal failure, the outcomes associated with intermittent hemodialysis

are considered equivalent to continuous venovenous hemofiltration; however, continuous hemofiltration may be easier to deliver in hemodynamically unstable patients. Many of the studies addressing this issue are retrospective or have not been randomized.[72] A meta-analysis comparing the two modes of renal replacement therapy found no difference in hospital mortality.[74]

GLYCEMIC CONTROL

Hyperglycemia and insulin resistance are common in critically ill patients. In the only large, randomized study showing improved outcomes for glucose control in surgical patients, tight glycemic control geared at maintenance of glucose values <110 g per dL was compared to conventional treatment of values >180 mg per dL. There was a decrease in mortality from 8% to 4.6%. Most of those in this study were surgical patients, and more than half had undergone cardiothoracic surgery.[75] Other studies in the surgical population have been small or not randomized, and have shown lower rates of bacteremia, catheter-related infections, and wound infections.[76,77] The question remains about which is important, whether it is glycemic control or insulin. Van den Berghe et al., who have studied this most intensively, advocate that it is glycemic control,[72] although insulin has been shown to inhibit TNF-α and favorably effect coagulation and macrophage function.[78–80]

On the basis of current data and the need to avoid hypoglycemia, which has been shown to decrease survival in any affected population studied, maintenance of blood glucose <150 mg per dL with insulin infusion, and frequent monitoring of blood sugars should be instituted in septic patients.[72]

ANEMIA AND BLOOD TRANSFUSION

Anemia and red blood cell transfusion are common in critically ill and septic patients.[81] The risks of red blood cell transfusion are well described and range from immunosuppression to increased nosocomial infections and death.[82] On the basis of relative risks compared to the benefits, red blood cell transfusion is recommended for hemoglobin levels <7.0 g per dL (target 7 to 9.0 g per dL) unless there are potential contraindications to withholding transfusion such as ongoing hemorrhage or significant coronary artery disease.[81,83] The rationale for red blood cell transfusion has been to increase oxygen delivery, which does occur, but improved oxygen delivery does not change oxygen consumption in sepsis. Conditions that may require higher hemoglobin levels, in addition to bleeding and severe cardiovascular disease, are severe arterial hypoxemia or evidence of tissue ischemia manifested by low mixed venous saturations or elevated lactate levels.[82]

Currently, there are no studies which report improved patient outcomes with the use of erythropoietin in sepsis. Some clinical trials have shown a decreased need for red cell transfusion, but this did not improve clinical outcomes. Erythropoietin is reasonable when there are other accepted indications for administration such as renal failure–induced deficits in red cell production.[81,82,84,85]

SCORING SYSTEMS FOR MULTISYSTEM ORGAN DYSFUNCTION AND FAILURE

The only organ dysfunction scoring system that has been validated for use in patients over time is the Sequential Organ Failure Assessment (SOFA) score.[86] SOFA scores assess respiratory function, coagulation parameters, liver, cardiovascular, central nervous system, and renal function (see Table 2). Initial, highest, and mean SOFA scores correlate well with mortality. Initial or highest SOFA scores which total more than 11 or average over 5 for the different organ system scores correlated with a mortality of >80%. At 96 hours after onset of organ dysfunction, mortality rates were at least 50% if the score was increasing, 27% to 35% if the score was unchanged, and <27% if the score was decreasing. Other than initial scores of >11, a decreasing score during the first 48 hours corresponded to a mortality rate of <6%.[86]

SUMMARY

Sepsis remains a common problem with a high mortality rate. Rapid diagnosis and treatment of the infectious source are paramount to success. Broad-spectrum antibiotics should be started empirically based on the likely site of infection and pathogens. Knowledge of one's own unit flora is important for appropriate antibiotic selection. Delays in the appropriate antibiotic regimen or initiation of antibiotics increase mortality and morbidity. Aggressive and early fluid resuscitation using "early, goal-directed" therapy does improve outcomes. Vasopressors should be added after fluid resuscitation has been attempted, if possible. Support of other failing organs, such as the lungs or kidneys should be instituted as needed, and lung-protective strategies used for ventilator management. Indications for APC and low-dose corticosteroids should be reviewed for each patient and therapy initiated accordingly. Minimization of other complications should be attempted by early mechanical ventilation weaning, maintaining sedation holidays, minimizing the use of paralytic medications, and providing adequate glycemic control.

TABLE 2
THE SEQUENTIAL ORGAN FAILURE ASSESSMENT (SOFA) SCORE[a]

Variables	SOFA Sub-Scores				
	0	1	2	3	4
Respiratory					
PaO$_2$/FIO$_2$, mm Hg	>400	≤400	≤300	≤200[b]	≤100[b]
Coagulation					
Platelets × 10^{37}L[b]	>150	≤150	≤100	≤50	≤20
Liver					
Bilirubin, mg/dL[c]	<1.2	1.2–1.9	2.0–5.9	6.0–11.9	>12.0
Cardiovascular					
Hypotension	No hypotension	Mean arterial pressure <70 mm Hg	Dop ≤5 or dob (any dose)[d] Dop >5, epi ≤0.1, or norepi ≤0.1[d]	Dop >15, epi >0.1, or norepi >0.1[d]	
Central nervous system					
Glasgow Coma Score scale	15	13–14	10–12	6–9	<6
Renal					
Creatinine, mg/dL or urine output, mL/d[e]	<1.2	1.2–1.9	2.0–3.4	3.5–4.9 or <500	>5.0 or <200

[a]Norepi, norepinephrine; dob, dobuatmine; dop, dopamine; epi, epinephrine; and FIO$_2$, fraction of inspired oxygen.
[b]Values are with respiratory support.
[c]To convert bilirubin from mg/dL to μmol/L, multiply by 17.1.
[d]Adrenergic agents administered for at least 1 hr (doses given are in μg/kg per min).
[e]To convert creatinine from mg/dL to μmol/L, multiply by 88.4.
(Table 2 adapted from JAMA, October 10, 2001— Vol 286, No. 14)

REFERENCES

1. Angus DC, Linde-Zwirble WT, Lidicker J, et al. Epidemiology of severe sepsis in the United States: Analysis of incidence outcome, and associated costs of care. *Crit Care Med.* 2001;29:1303–1310.
2. Hoyert DL, Heron MP, Murphy SL, et al. Deaths: Final data for 2003. Updated death statistics are available at the National Center for Health Statistics Web site, http://www.cdc.gov/nchs.. *Natl Vital Stat Rep.* 2006;54:1–120.
3. Ely EW, Bernard GR. The scope of the problem. *Contemporary diagnosis and management of sepsis*, 1st ed. Newton: Handbooks in Health Care; 2005:5–14.
4. Bone RC, Balk RA, Cerra FB, et al. Definitions for sepsis and organ failure and guidelines for the use of innovative therapies in sepsis. The ACCP/SCCM Consensus Conference. American College of Chest Physicians/Society of Critical Care Medicine. *Chest.* 1992;101:1664–1655.
5. Levy MM, Fink MP, Marshall JC, et al. 2001 SCCM/ESICM/ACCP/ATS/SIS International Sepsis Definitions Conference. *Crit Care Med.* 2003;31:1250–1256.
6. Nystrom PO. The systemic inflammatory response syndrome: Definitions and aetiology. *J Antimicrob Chemother.* 1998;41(Suppl A):1–7.
7. Bone RC, Fisher CJ, Clemmer TP, et al. The Methylprednisolone Severe Sepsis Study Group. Sepsis syndrome: A valid clinical entity. *Crit Care Med.* 1989;17:389–393.
8. Wenzel RP. Treating sepsis. *N Engl J Med.* 2002;347:966–967.
9. Brun-Buisson C, Doyon F, Carlet J. French Bacteremia-Sepsis Study Group. Bacteremia and severe sepsis in adults: a multicenter prospective survey in ICUs and ward of 24 hospitals. *Am J Respir Crit Care Med.* 1996;154(3 part 1):617–624.
10. Krieger BP. Sepsis in the geriatric age group. In Fein AM, Abraham EM, Balk RA, et al. eds. *Sepsis and mutliorgan failure.* Baltimore: Williams & Wilkins; 1997:373–380.
11. Llewelyn M, Cohen J. Diagnosis of infection in sepsis. *Intensive Care Med.* 2001;27(Suppl 1):S10–S214.
12. Bernard GR, Wheeler AP, Russell JA, et al. The effects of ibuprofen on the physiology and survival of patients with sepsis. *N Engl J Med.* 1997;336:912–918.
13. Balk RA, Ely EW, Goyette RE. General principles of sepsis therapy. Sepsis Handbook: National Initiative in Sepsis Education. 2001. Available at: http://www.nise.cc.
14. Friedman G, Berlot G, Kahn RJ, et al. Combined measurements of blood lactate and gastric intramucosal pH in patients with severe sepsis. *Crit Care Med.* 1995;23(7):1184–1193.
15. Vincent JL, Dufaye P, Berre J, et al. Serial lactate determinations during circulatory shock. *Crit Care Med.* 1983;11(6):449–451.
16. Shaw AC. Serum C-reactive protein and neopterin concentrations in patients with viral or bacterial infections. *J Clin Pathol.* 1991;44:596–599.
17. Yentis SM, Soni N, Sheldon J. C-reactive protein as an indicator of resolution of sepsis in the intensive care unit. *Intensive Care Med.* 1995;21:602–605.
18. Assicot M, Gendrel D, Carsin H, et al. High serum procalcitonin concentration in patients with sepsis and infections. *Lancet.* 1993;341:515–518.
19. Wanner GA, Keel M, Steckholzer U, et al. Relationship between procalcitonin plasma levels and severity of injury, sepsis, organ failure, and mortality in injured patients. *Crit Care Med.* 2000;28:950–957.
20. O'Grady NP, Barie PS, Bartlett JG, et al. Practice guidelines for evaluating new fever in critically ill adult patients. Task Force of the Society of Critical Care Medicine and the Infectious Disease Society of America. *Clin Infect Dis.* 1998;26:392–408.
21. Fagon JY, Chastre J, Hance AJ, et al. Detection of nosocomial lung infection in ventilated patients: Use of a protected specimen brush and quantitative culture techniques in 147 patients. *Am Rev Respir Dis.* 1989;139:110–116.
22. Croce MA, Fabian TC, Schurr MJ, et al. Using bronchoalveolar lavage to distinguish nosocomial pneumonia from systemic inflammatory response syndrome. *J Trauma.* 1995;39:1134–1140.
23. Wahl WL, Franklin GA, Brandt MM, et al. Does bronchoalveolar lavage enhance our ability to treat ventilator-associated pneumonia in a trauma-burn intensive care unit? *J Trauma.* 2003;54:633–639.
24. Richards MJ, Edwards JR, Culver DH, et al. Nosocomial infections in medical-surgical intensive care units in the United States. *Infect Control Hosp Epidemiol.* 2000;21:510–515.
25. Kumar A, Roberts D, Wood KE, et al. Duration of hypotension before initiation of effective antimicrobial therapy is the critical determinant of survival in human septic shock. *Crit Care Med.* 2006;34:1589–1896.
26. Luna CM, Vujacich P, Niederman MS, et al. Impact of BAL data on the therapy and outcome of ventilator-associated pneumonia. *Chest.* 1997;111:676–685.
27. Ibrahim EH, Sherman G, Ward S, et al. The influence of inadequate antimicrobial treatment of bloodstream infections on patient outcomes in the ICU setting. *Chest.* 2000;118:146–155.
28. Kollef MH, Sherman G, Ward S, et al. Inadequate antimicrobial treatment of infections: A risk factor for hospital mortality among critically ill patients. *Chest.* 1999;115:462–474.
29. Trouillet JL, Chastre J, Vuagnat A, et al. Ventilator-associated pneumonia caused by potentially drug-resistant bacteria. *Am J Respir Crit Care Med.* 1998;157:531–539.
30. Safdar N, Maki DG. The commonality of risk factors for nosocomial colonization and infection with antimicrobial-resistant *Staphylococcus aureus*, *Enterococcus*, Gram-negative bacilli, *Clostridium difficile*, and *Candida*. *Ann Intern Med.* 2002;136:834–844.
31. Namias N, Samiian L, Nino D, et al. Incidence and susceptibility of pathogenic bacteria vary between intensive care units within a single hospital: Implications for empiric antibiotic strategies. *J Trauma.* 2000;49:638–645.
32. Wang SW. Septic shock. Mulholland MW, Doherty GM, eds. *Complications in surgery.* Philadelphia: Lippincott Williams & Wilkins; 2006:126–135.
33. Rivers E, Nguyen B, Havstad S, et al. Early goal-directed therapy in the treatment of severe sepsis and septic shock. *N Engl J Med.* 2001;344:699–709.
34. The SAFE Study Investigators. A comparison of albumin and saline for fluid resuscitation in the intensive care unit. *N Engl J Med.* 2004;350:2247–2256.
35. Vincent JL, Navickis RJ, Wilkes MM. Morbidity in hospitalized patients receiving human albumin: A meta-analysis of randomized, controlled trials. *Crit Care Med.* 2004;32:2029–2038.
36. Choi PT, Yip G, Quinonez LG, et al. Crystalloids *vs* colloids in fluid resuscitation: A systemic review. *Crit Care Med.* 1999;27:200–210.
37. Schierhout G, Roberts I. Fluid resuscitation with colloids or crystalloids solutions in critically ill patients: A systematic review of randomised trials. *Br Med J.* 1998;316:916–964.
38. Sandham JD, Hull RD, Brant RF, et al. A randomized, controlled trial of the use of pulmonary-artery catheters in high-risk surgical patients. *N Engl J Med.* 2003;348:5–14.
39. Connors AF, Speroff T, Dawson NV, et al. The effectiveness of right heart catheterization in the initial care of critically ill patients. SUPPORT Investigators. *JAMA.* 1996;276:889–897.
40. Afessa B, Spencer S, Khan W, et al. Association of pulmonary artery catheter use in-hospital mortality. *Crit Care Med.* 2001;29:1145–1149.
41. Patel BM, Chittock DR, Russell JA, et al. Beneficial effects of short-term vasopressin infusion during severe septic shock. *Anesthesiology.* 2002;96:576–582.
42. Grinvech V, Knepper MA, Verbalis J, et al. Acute endotoxemia in rats induces down-regulation of V2 vasopressin receptors and aquaporin-2 content in the kidney medulla. *Kidney Int.* 2004;65:54–62.
43. Holmes CL, Walley KR, Chittock DR, et al. The effects of vasopressin on hemodynamics and renal function in severe septic shock, a case series. *Intensive Care Med.* 2001;27:1416–1421.
44. Dunser MW, Mayr AJ, Ulmer H, et al. Arginine vasopressin in advanced vasodilatory shock, a prospective, randomized, controlled study. *Circulation.* 2003;107:2313–2319.

45. Tsuneyoshi I, Yamada H, Kakihana Y, et al. Hemodynamic and metabolic effects of low-dose vasopressin infusions in vasodilatory septic shock. *Crit Care Med.* 2001;29:487–493.

46. Dellinger RP, Carlet JM, Masur H, et al. Surviving Sepsis Campaign guidelines for management of severe sepsis and septic shock. *Crit Care Med.* 2004;32:858–873.

47. Martin C, Papazian L, Perrin G, et al. Norepinephrine or dopamine for the treatment of hyperdynamic septic shock? *Chest.* 1993;103: 1826–1831.

48. Meadows D, Edwards JD, Wilkins RG, et al. Reversal of intractable septic shock with norepinephrine therapy. *Crit Care Med.* 1988; 16:663–666.

49. Martin C, Vivian X, Leone M, et al. Effect of norepinephrine on the outcome of septic shock. *Crit Care Med.* 2000;28:2758–2765.

50. LeDoux D, Astiz ME, Carpati CM, et al. Effects of perfusion pressure on tissue perfusion in septic shock. *Crit Care Med.* 2000;28:2729–2732.

51. Van den Berghe G, de Zegher F. Anterior pituitary function during critical illness and dopamine treatment. *Crit Care Med* 1996;24: 1580–1590.

52. Sprung CL, Caralis PV, Marcial EH, et al. The effects of high-dose corticosteroids in patients with septic shock: A prospective, controlled study. *N Engl J Med.* 1984;311:1137–1143.

53. Annane D, Bellisant E, Bollaert PE, et al. Corticosteroids for severe sepsis and septic shock: A systematic review and meta-analysis. *Br Med J.* 2004;329:480.

54. Briegel J, Forst H, Haller M, et al. Stress doses of hydrocortisone reverse hyperdynamic septic shock: A prospective, randomized double-blind, single-center study. *Crit Care Med.* 1999;27: 723–732.

55. Annane D, Sebille V, Charpentier D, et al. Effect of treatment with low doses of hydrocortisone and fludrocortisone on mortality in patients with septic shock. *JAMA.* 2002;288:862–871.

56. Hamrahian AH, Oseni TS, Arafah BM. Measurements of serum free cortisol in critically ill patients. *N Engl J Med.* 2004;350:1629–1638.

57. Russell JA. Management of sepsis. *N Engl J Med.* 2006;355:1699–1713.

58. Keh D, sprung CL. Use of corticosteroid therapy in patients with sepsis and septic shock: An evidence-based review. *Crit Care Med.* 2004;32:S527–S533.

59. Bernard GR, Vincent JL, Laterre PF, et al. Efficacy and safety of recombinant human activated protein C for severe sepsis. *N Engl J Med.* 2001;344:699–709.

60. Vincent JL, Angus DC, Artigas A, et al. Effects of drotrecogin alfa (activated) on organ dysfunction in the PROWESS trial. *Crit Care Med.* 2003;31:834–840.

61. Ely EW, Laterre PF, Angus DC, et al. Drotrecogin alfa (activated) administration across clinically important subgroups of patients with severe sepsis. *Crit Care Med.* 2003;31:12–19.

62. Eichacker PQ, Natnson C, Danner RL. Surviving sepsis-practice guidelines, marketing campaigns, and Eli Lilly. *N Engl J Med.* 2006; 355:1640–1642.

63. The Acute Respiratory Distress Syndrome Network. Ventilation with lower tidal volumes for acute lung injury and the acute respiratory distress syndrome. *N Engl J Med.* 2000;342:1301–1308.

64. Ranieri VM, Sutter PM, Tortorella C, et al. Effect of mechanical ventilation on inflammatory mediators in patients with acute respiratory distress syndrome; a randomized controlled trial. *JAMA.* 1999;282:54–61.

65. Brower RG, Lanken PN, MacIntyre N, et al. Higher versus lower positive end-expiratory pressures in patients with the acute respiratory distress syndrome. *N Engl J Med.* 2004;351: 327–336.

66. Kress JP, Pohlman AS, O'Connor MF, et al. Daily interruption of sedative infusions in critically ill patients undergoing mechanical ventilation. *N Engl J Med.* 2000;342:1471–1477.

67. Segredo V, Caldwell JE, Mathay MA, et al. Persistent paralysis in critically ill patients after long-term administration of vecuronium. *N Engl J Med.* 1992;327:524–528.

68. Brivet FG, Kleinknecht DJ, Loirat P, et al. Acute renal failure in the intensive care unit: Causes, outcome and prognostic factors of hospital mortality. A prospective, multicenter study. *Crit Care Med.* 1996;24:192–198.

69. Hoste EAJ, Lamiere NH, Vanholder RC, et al. Acute renal failure in patients with sepsis in a surgical ICU: Predictive factors, incidence, comorbidity, and outcome. *J Am Soc Nephrol.* 2003;14: 1022–1030.

70. Hoffman JN, Hartl WH, Deppsich R, et al. Effect of hemofiltration on hemodynamics and systemic concentration of anaphylatoxins and cytokines in human sepsis. *Intensive Care Med.* 1996;22: 1360–1367.

71. Ronco C, Bellomo R, Homal P, et al. Effects of different dose in continuous veno-venous haemofiltration on outcomes of acute renal failure: A prospective randomized trial. *Lancet.* 2000;356: 26–30.

72. Cariou A, Vinsonneau C, Dhainaut JF. Adjunctive therapies in sepsis: An evidence-based review. *Crit Care Med.* 2004;32:S562–S570.

73. Schiffl H, Lang S, Fischer R. Daily hemodialysis and the outcome of acute renal failure. *N Engl J Med.* 2002;346:306–310.

74. Kellum J, Angus DC, Johnson JP, et al. Continuous versus intermittent renal replacement therapy: A meta-analysis. *Intensive Care Med.* 2002;28:29–37.

75. Van den Berghe G, Wouters P, Weekers F, et al. Intensive insulin therapy in critically ill patients. *N Engl J Med.* 2001;345:1359–1367.

76. Wahl WL, Talsma AN, Dawson C, et al. Use of computerized ICU documentation to capture ICU core measures. *Surgery.* 2006;140: 684–690.

77. Zerr KJ, Furnary Ap, Grunkemeier GL, et al. *Ann Thorac Surg.* 1997; 63:356–361.

78. Satomi N, Sakurai A, haranaka K. Relationship of hypoglycemia to tumor necrosis factor production and antitumor activity; role of glucose, insulin, and macrophages. *J Natl Cancer Inst.* 1985;74: 1255–1260.

79. Carr ME. Diabetes mellitus: A hypercoagulable state. *J Diabetes Complications.* 2001;15:44–54.

80. Kwoun MO, Ling PR, Lydon E, et al. Immunologic effects of acute hyperglycemia in nondiabetic rats. *J Parenter Enteral Nutr.* 1997; 21:91–95.

81. Corwin HL, Gettinger A, Pearl RG, et al. The CRIT study: Anemia and blood transfusion in the critically ill-current clinical practice in the United States. *Crit Care Med.* 2004;32:39–52.

82. Zimmerman JL. Use of blood products in sepsis: An evidence-based review. *Crit Care Med.* 2004;32:S542–S547.

83. Hebert PC, Wells G, Blajchman MA, et al. A multicenter, randomized, controlled clinical trial of transfusion in critical care. *N Engl J Med.* 1999;340:409–417.

84. Corwin HL, Gettinger A, Rodriguez RM, et al. Efficacy of recombinant human erythropoietin in critically ill patients; a randomized double-blind, placebo-controlled trial. *Crit Care Med.* 1999;27: 2346–2350.

85. Corwin HL, Gettinger A, Pearl RG, et al. Efficacy of recombinant human erythropoietin in critically ill patients. *JAMA.* 2002;28: 2827–2835.

86. Ferreira FL, Bota DP, Bross A, et al. Serial evaluation of the SOFA score to predict outcome in critically ill patients. *JAMA.* 2001; 286:1754–1758.

Infection Control in the Intensive Care Unit

62

Rodney M. Durham   *Shawn Larson*

Hospital-acquired infections, or nosocomial infections (NIs), have received much attention in the mainstream media and represent a growing area of concern to patients and health care workers alike. These conditions pose a serious risk to all hospitalized patients but are particularly serious threats to critically ill patients in the intensive care unit (ICU). NIs, reported to affect approximately 2 million patients each year, are associated with longer hospital stays, higher hospital costs, and increased mortality.[1] A recent report from Institute of Medicine stated that preventable adverse health events, including NIs, were responsible for 44,000 to 98,000 deaths per year and a cost of $17 to $29 billion.[2] There is also growing concern that with increasing rates of antibiotic resistance, NIs will become an even greater threat to hospitalized patients. Therefore, the importance of infection control in the ICU cannot be stressed strongly enough.

Patients in the ICU are 5 to 10 times more likely to acquire NIs compared to other hospitalized patients.[3] Recent trends in health care have shifted the emphasis to outpatient medical management, thereby resulting in a decreased number of hospital beds and fewer patient admissions. Conversely, during the same time period, data from the Centers for Disease Control and Prevention (CDC) has shown an increase in the number of ICU beds by 17% reflecting a greater severity of illness in hospitalized patients.[4]

According to CDC data, at least one third of NIs are preventable by the implementation of infection control programs.[1,5,6] Understanding risk factors and paying careful attention to preventative measures, including hand hygiene and restriction of antibiotic use, have been demonstrated to be effective in reducing NIs.[7-12] Because NIs are a growing risk, all health care workers, especially those participating in the care of ICU patients, must have an understanding of NIs and measures to prevent them.

DEFINITIONS/EPIDEMIOLOGY/RISK FACTORS

Although NIs are broadly defined as any infection that is not present on hospital admission, the CDC has proposed precise definitions of NIs, which are now generally considered the gold standard (a detailed list is available online at www.cdc.gov/ncidod/dhqp/nnis-pubs.html).[13,14] In general, an infection is considered nosocomial if it develops 48 hours after hospital admission with no evidence of prior incubation. Additionally, infections that develop up to 3 days after the patient is discharged from the hospital or within 30 days of a surgical procedure are attributed to the hospital or surgical procedure, respectively.

The CDC National Nosocomial Infection Surveillance (NNIS) system[15] collects data from numerous hospitals around the country for epidemiologic purposes. This data has demonstrated that infection rates vary widely depending on the type of ICU and the population of patients served (e.g., medical, surgical, or pediatric). These variations in infection rates suggest that the epidemiology for NIs differs with the type of units. Because of such demographic and geographic variations in infection rates, it is therefore recommended that each type of unit compare its own locally collected data with that collected by the NNIS for units of similar patient populations and alter infection control measures accordingly.

Pneumonia, urinary tract infections (UTIs), and bloodstream infections (BSIs) make up most of the reported

NIs.[16,17] A report that looked at NIs from 205 combine medical-surgical ICUs from 1992 to 1998 found that infections from these three sites represented 68% of all reported infections with nosocomial pneumonia being the most frequently reported (31%), followed by UTIs (23%), and bloodstream infections (14%).[17] Most infections were associated with medical devices: 83% of episodes of nosocomial pneumonia were associated with mechanical ventilation, 97% of UTIs occurred in patients with urinary catheters, and 87% of BSIs occurred with central line usage.[17]

Independent risk factors for the development of NIs have been identified. These include the severity of the underlying illness as assessed by the Applied Physiology and Chronic Health Evaluation (APACHE) score, prolonged hospitalization, mechanical ventilation, vascular access catheterization, and use of parenteral nutrition.[18] Changes in hospital economics may also contribute to the risk of developing NIs. Understaffing of ICUs, as well as patient overcrowding, has been reported to be a risk factor for the development of NIs.[19,20] Patient-to-nurse ratios were found to be a major independent risk factor with significantly increased relative risks associated with higher ratios.[21] Reduced numbers of nursing and hospital staff with increasingly greater patient-care responsibilities for care givers not only has the potential to increase the risk of NIs, but also potentially impacts medical error rates and mortality. Risk factors for site-specific infections are discussed in each individual section given in the subsequent text.

PATHOPHYSIOLOGY

The pathophysiology of NIs is believed to be dependent on two key factors: colonization of the host by potentially pathogenic microorganisms and impaired host defenses.[22] Critically ill patients often have impaired host defenses due to the underlying disease process. The release of various cytokines and anti-inflammatory mediators can suppress the patient's immune system, thereby increasing the risk of infection. Patients' local immune defense mechanisms can also be impaired by invasive medical devices. For example, coughing and sneezing are impaired by endotracheal intubation and sedation leading to increased risk of respiratory infections. These devices can also act as a nidus for infection.

Colonization of the host can arise from endogenous or exogenous sources. Patients in the ICU are susceptible to bacterial colonization due to decreased host defense mechanisms, prolonged hospital stays, the use of indwelling medical devices, and the use of antibiotics. Antibiotics can exert selective pressure on the patient's endogenous flora, potentially leading to colonization by pathogenic microorganisms. Common host reservoirs for NIs include the skin, oropharynx, urinary tract, and the gastrointestinal (GI) tract.[22] The hands of health care workers are a well-documented and common source of exogenous colonization. Other sources include droplet or aerosol spread or contaminated medical equipment. Understanding potential sources of colonization is important to help identify routes of transmission and to assist in taking preventative infection control measures.

MICROORGANISMS

Any microorganism can be responsible for NIs in critically ill patients. Many infections in this subset of patients are polymicrobial in nature. There has been a recent change in the pattern of organisms with increased gram-positive infections.[21] Recent evidence suggests that fungal infections are increasing in prevalence as well.[16] The European Prevalence of Infection in Intensive Care (EPIC) study[23] identified the most common reported pathogens responsible for NIs. *Staphylococcus aureus* and *Pseudomonas aeruginosa* were identified most frequently (30% and 29%, respectively), with the remaining microorganisms including coagulase-negative *staphylococci* (19%), yeast (17%), *Escherichia coli* (13%), *enterococci* spp (12%), *Acinetobacter* spp (9%), and *Klebsiella* spp.[23,24]

It is important to understand that the exact patterns of microorganisms responsible for NIs vary by patient population, local infection control policies, antibiotic usage, type of ICU, and even geographic locations. Once again, the physician caring for critically ill patients must have a solid knowledge of local microorganisms and resistance patterns to best institute infection control practices and appropriate antibiotic usage. This is best achieved by careful coordination between health care workers, ICU pharmacists, the infection control team, and microbiology.

GENERAL PREVENTATIVE STRATEGIES

One of the most effective strategies against NIs is prevention. The simplest and most effective preventative strategy appears to be basic hygiene and care with the insertion and maintenance of indwelling medical devices (i.e., central lines). The transmission of microorganisms from the hands of health care workers is well documented in the literature. Hand washing before and after patient contact remains one of the simplest and most effective infection control procedures, but compliance is often poor.[25–28] Numerous factors may play a role in the low compliance with hand washing including lack of time and inconvenient placement of hand washing facilities. Additionally, health care workers who participate in frequent hand washing run the risk of skin damage including allergy and intolerance to hand cleaning solutions. Skin damage results in potential shedding of more organisms into the surrounding environment, thereby increasing the risk of infection.[29]

There is growing evidence that hand washing with alcohol-based gel solutions not only reduces hand contamination more than hand washing alone but may also in fact improve compliance.[30,31] Updated guidelines for hand hygiene in the health care setting are available from the CDC website (www.cdc.gov/handhygiene/). The use of universal precautions should also be stressed. Gloves should be worn in all situations where contact with blood, mucous membranes, secretions, or a wound is anticipated. Hand washing must be undertaken after glove removal because hands may be contaminated during the procedure or after glove removal. Masks should be worn when contamination from splashes or sprays may occur.

Contact Precautions

NIs that are transmitted by direct and indirect physical contact with an infected patient or the surrounding environment are best prevented by contact precautions. Patients with infections from microorganisms such as methicillin-resistant *Staphylococcus aureus* (MRSA), vancomycin-resistant *enterococci* (VRE), and *Clostridium difficile* should be placed in a private room or with another patient harboring the same infection. Health care workers should use gloves and impervious gowns for all patient contact. The gowns and gloves should be removed before exiting the room and followed by hand washing. Patients on contact isolation should have dedicated medical devices in their rooms (e.g., stethoscopes) that are not used on other patients. Where this is not feasible, medical devices must be thoroughly disinfected before using them on other patients.

Patients with immunosuppression (e.g., transplant or chemotherapy patients) should, in addition to contact precautions, have private rooms with positive pressure air flow systems. Previously hospitalized patients are at a high risk for carrying resistant organisms and can transmit them to uninfected patients upon readmission. Such patients should be identified at the time of admission and placed in appropriate rooms (e.g., private or with patient having similar infections).

Airborne and Droplet Precautions

Airborne precautions prevent the transmission of small, aerosolized infected organisms (<5 μm in size) whereas droplet precautions are for larger particles ($\geq$5 μm). Airborne transmission is by inhalation of these small particles that can remain in the air for extended periods of time. They are also capable of traveling longer distances compared to droplets, which usually do not remain in the air as long nor travel long distances due to their size. Droplets are produced by activities such as coughing and sneezing or during invasive procedures such as endotracheal tube suctioning and bronchoscopy.

In addition to standard infection control procedures, patients with infections and a risk of airborne transmission, such as pulmonary tuberculosis, need to be placed in a private room with a negative air filtration system. Airborne precautions also require respiratory protection with the use of high efficiency masks approved by the National Institute for Occupations Safety and Health.[32,33] Patients with *Haemophilus influenzae* type B infection, multidrug-resistant pneumococcal infection, or any multidrug-resistant respiratory infection should be placed on droplet precaution. These patients require private rooms, but do not require special air filtration systems. Health care workers should utilize masks with a shield during close contact (<1 m) or during all invasive procedures.

Antibiotic Use

The use of antibiotics in the ICU is commonplace. Patients may be prescribed antibiotics for known infections or empirically started when an infection is suspected. However, overuse of antibiotics is a major factor in the development of resistant organisms.[34] Recently, strategies have been published to help control the emergence of resistant strains.[8] These strategies include optimal use of antibiotics and cycling, or using antibiotic rotations. Restricting antibiotic use has been shown to not only reduce costs but also to reduce the excessive use of broad-spectrum agents.[34] One large study showed a 32% decrease in associated costs with a reciprocal increase in susceptibility of bacterial isolates.[35] Additionally, there were no adverse clinical outcomes noted, particularly survival.

One challenge facing clinicians is when to start antibiotics. Commencing antibiotics without sufficient evidence of infection only compounds the problems of resistance. However, waiting for infection to become clinically evident in critically ill patients leads to increased morbidity and mortality. The Society of Critical Care Medicine and the Infectious Disease Society of America have published practice guidelines for the evaluation of fever in critically ill patients.[36] Once the decision is made to start empiric antibiotics, a definite time period should be determined. Patients should be reevaluated after 48 to 72 hours. A decision to continue antibiotics must be made on the basis of the patient's clinical progress and the results of the initial microbiology cultures. Antibiotics should be discontinued if no evidence of infection is determined and the patient's clinical course improves. Additionally, the antibiotic regimen should be narrowed to focus on specific organisms. Most hospital ICUs have a dedicated pharmacist and their expertise should be sought to further improve antibiotic usage.

Antibiotic cycling has received much attention in the literature and is advocated as one strategy to limit antimicrobial resistance.[8,34,37,38] The scheduled change of ceftazidime to ciprofloxacin for the empiric treatment of septic patients after cardiac surgery showed a decrease in the incidence of ventilator-associated pneumonia (VAP) including VAP attributed to resistant gram-negative bacteria.[11] Another report demonstrated a reduction in VAP due to resistant gram-negative bacteria after the implementation of a strategy combining rotation and restriction of the use of antibiotics.[39] During this study, a schedule consisting of four different β-lactams combined with four different aminoglycosides were used for 4-month intervals over a 2-year period. A significant reduction in GI tract VRE colonization was observed after cefotaxime, vancomycin, and clindamycin were replaced by β-lactam/β-lactamase inhibitors.[40]

Antibiotic rotation is thought to be most effective for limited periods of time and requires careful monitoring of microorganisms to prevent resistance to unrelated classes of antimicrobials.[34] Additionally, a good knowledge of the local epidemiology of hospital flora and resistance patterns is required. A multidisciplinary approach including the ICU pharmacist, microbiology laboratory, health care workers, and infection control specialist is needed for such a strategy to be maximally effective.

INFECTION SITE AND PREVENTIVE MEASURES

Respiratory Tract

The most common site of NIs in the ICU is the respiratory tract. Nosocomial pneumonia accounted for 31% of all NIs according to NNIS data and it is the leading cause of death from NIs in the ICU.[17,41] In addition to general risk factors for the development of NIs, nosocomial pneumonia is also associated with certain predisposing risk factors such as endotracheal intubation, prolonged mechanical ventilation, and the continued aspiration of contaminated oropharyngeal secretions. Endotracheal intubation impairs host defense mechanisms such as mucociliary clearance and coughing. The duration of mechanical ventilation has been identified as a key risk factor with the highest rates of infection within the first 8 to 10 days.[22] Upper airway colonization by pathogenic organisms occurs frequently with critically ill patients. Patients with altered mental status seem to be particularly at risk. Noninvasive mechanical ventilation has been recommended wherever appropriate because it has been shown to reduce the risk of nosocomial pneumonia.[42–44] The reduced risk may be in part due to decreased amounts of sedation and less invasive monitoring. Kollef[10] reviewed a number of preventive strategies for nosocomial pneumonia. These recommendations include semirecumbent positioning of patients (i.e., head of the bed to 45 degrees), avoidance of large gastric volumes, routine maintenance of ventilatory circuits, the use of chlorhexidine oral rinse, and the use of sucralfate for stress-ulcer prophylaxis. The use of prophylactic antibiotics for longer than 24 hours or long-term empiric antibiotics (>3 days

or until culture results are available) is to be avoided for the reasons previously discussed.

Catheter-Related Bloodstream Infections

Patients in the ICU often have multiple indwelling catheters for the administration of medications and monitoring purposes. Every type of intravascular catheter has been associated with NIs. The incidence appears highest with central venous catheters used for monitoring purposes. A number of measures can be utilized to reduce the incidence of bloodstream infections.

Rigorous sterile insertion practices should always be utilized when inserting a central venous catheter. The skin site should be carefully selected and cleansed with antiseptic solution. The physician should, without exception, wear a gown, gloves, mask, and hat for the procedure. Extra care should always be taken during the insertion procedure especially if the catheter is going to be placed in a central location, utilized long term, the patient is critically ill, or total parenteral nutrition is to be used through the catheter (view the CDC guidelines for prevention of intravascular catheter infection at www.cdc.gov/mmwr/preview/mmwrhtml/rr5110a1.htm). The type of catheter to be placed should also be considered. Multiple-lumen catheters may be associated with higher rates of bloodstream infection compared to single-lumen catheters.[45,46] A catheter with the minimum number of required lumens should be inserted to avoid this potential risk of infection.

The site of insertion has been shown to be a risk factor. Jugular vein sites have been shown to be more frequently colonized when compared to subclavian sites. This may be due to difficulties in securing a sterile dressing and the proximity to oropharyngeal secretions. The femoral route, although not reported to have higher infection rates, is associated with a higher risk of deep vein thrombosis (as high as 21% vs. 2% in one study when compared to subclavian vascular access).[47] Other factors have been shown to reduce catheter-related infections including the use of tunneled central venous catheters (particularly if the catheter is going to be utilized for long periods of time), the use of gauze and tape dressing instead of transparent dressings, and the use of antimicrobial impregnated catheters (i.e., chlorhexidine-silver-sulfadiazine catheters and minocycline-rifampicin coated catheters).[48,49] Both chlorhexidine-silver-sulfadiazine and minocycline-rifampicin-impregnated catheters are commercially available. Various studies have been conducted demonstrating that they do reduce the risk rate of catheter-related infections.[50] When the two catheters were compared in a clinical trial, minocycline-rifampicin–coated catheters were associated with a lower incidence of infection.[51] Minocycline-rifampicin catheters are impregnated on the extraluminal and intraluminal surfaces, whereas the chlorhexidine-silver-sulfadiazine catheters were coated only on the extraluminal surface. This factor may account for the difference in infection rates between the two. Additionally, there is some concern regarding the chlorhexidine-silver-sulfadiazine catheters being responsible for anaphylactoid reactions.[50] There is also concern that the antimicrobial effect of these catheters diminishes with time (i.e., greater effectiveness in the first week of use). Another drawback of antibiotic-impregnated catheters is that they may promote antimicrobial resistance.[50]

Historically, it was commonly accepted practice to change central venous catheters either completely or over a guide wire at fixed time intervals. This practice was believed to decrease the rate of infection with indwelling central venous catheters; however, multiple trials have not demonstrated this practice to be advantageous.[52] Catheters should be changed when infection is suspected or is no longer working properly (e.g., occlusion or a leak at the exit site). Additionally, they should be removed promptly when they are no longer required. The technique of changing a venous catheter over a guide wire is thought to not only be safe, but more comfortable for the patient as well. This practice can be utilized when a catheter change is warranted (i.e., when infection is suspected). If a catheter is changed for suspected infection, the tip should be sent to the microbiology laboratory for quantitative culture. Should the culture return positive, the catheter should be removed immediately and an alternative vascular access site should be utilized for central venous catheterization if needed. Antibiotics are not warranted unless the patient shows signs of systemic infection.

As previously alluded to, one potential mechanism for decreasing catheter-related infections is the use of tunneled or implantable devices for vascular access (e.g., Hickman or Medi-port, respectively). Both devices utilize a Silastic catheter, which is more pliable than traditional polyethylene central catheters, possibly reducing the risk of thrombotic complications. Tunneled devices have a subcutaneous cuff (usually made of Darcon), which potentially helps to reduce catheter colonization. Implantable subclavian devices have the added advantage of requiring no special dressings (they are covered by skin) and do not restrict patient movement. They can be accessed repeatedly with a special needle (Huber needle) and have the lowest infection rates.[53] One disadvantage to both catheters is that they require placement in the operating room. However, tunneled catheters and implantable ports should be considered in all patients who will require long-term or permanent access.

Urinary Tract Infections

UTIs are the second most common site of NIs among hospitalized patients and they are almost always related to urinary catheters or to urinary tract procedures.[22] Colonic flora such as *Enterococcus* and *Klebsiella* spp are the predominant microorganisms. Because of these high rates

of infection, it is suggested that catheterization should only take place when absolutely necessary and be discontinued promptly when no longer required. Suprapubic catheters may in fact be superior to traditional urethral catheters as they appear to be associated with lower rates of infection, have a higher rate of patient satisfaction, and may reduce local complications such as urethral stricture and prostatitis.[18]

Bladder irrigation with antibiotic solutions has not shown to decrease the rate of NIs and may actually increase the incidence of resistant microorganisms.[54,55] The use of such systems is not supported by the literature. There is much debate about the use of bladder irrigation for fungal infections. A large prospective, multicenter surveillance study conducted on behalf of the National Institute for Allergy and Infectious Diseases (NIAID) Mycoses Study group did not show a clear benefit in using antifungal bladder irrigation.[56] Of the patients who received no antifungal treatment, 75% had documented resolution of funguria (vs. 50.2% for all patients receiving either fluconazole or amphotericin-B). Few patients in this study were found to have documented candidemia (1.7%). One drawback to this study is that treatment regimens were not consistent between centers. Additionally, only fluconazole and amphotericin-B were utilized for treatment and patients were not randomized. Another concern with bladder irrigation for fungal infections, such as antibiotic bladder irrigation, is that they may promote antifungal resistance.

Surgical Site Infections

Surgical site infections (SSIs), a common surgical problem, are best prevented by sound surgical technique and proper antibiotic prophylaxis. Risk factors for the development of SSIs include an American Society of Anesthesiologist (ASA) preoperative assessment score of III or greater, a surgery classified as either contaminated or dirty-infected and prolonged surgical procedures.[13,57] Additional perioperative factors that have been shown to reduce the rate of SSIs include close attention to patient temperature levels, arterial oxygen content, and blood glucose levels. Hypothermia, in the ICU or during the perioperative period, may increase a patient's risk for SSIs by causing vasoconstriction and impaired immune function. Recent evidence has suggested that supplemental oxygen may lower SSIs by increasing subcutaneous tissue oxygen levels. A recent study of patients undergoing elective colorectal surgery showed a 50% decrease (5.2% vs. 11.2%) in SSIs in patients who received 80% supplemental oxygen for 2 hours after surgery.[58] High glucose levels are known to impair immune cell function and delay healing. A recent study of strict glucose control in patients undergoing cardiac surgery showed not only a decreased complication rate but also improved survival at 30 days and 1 year.[59]

One of the most important factors for reducing the risk of SSIs involves the proper use of prophylactic antibiotics. Prophylactic antibiotics are indicated for all clean-contaminated or contaminated procedures as well as clean procedures that involve the insertion of prosthetic materials (e.g., arthroplasty or vascular graft material). Consideration should also be given to patients with specific risk factors (e.g., valvular heart disease, diabetes and patients who have undergone transplantation). The timing of administration of antibiotics is important to ensure adequate tissue levels before the surgical incision. There is no evidence to support continuing prophylactic antibiotics beyond the perioperative period. Most procedures require only one preoperative dose, which may be repeated for longer procedures (i.e., procedures exceeding 4 hours in length). Continuing prophylactic antibiotics beyond the perioperative period (12 to 24 hours) does not decrease the rate of SSIs and may contribute to resistance.

If an SSI develops, the wound in most cases should be opened. If the infection is superficial (i.e., above the fascia), limited to the incision, and there are no signs of systemic infection or cellulitis, drainage is likely all that is necessary. Antibiotics should be reserved for patients with local inflammation or signs of systemic infection. Necrotizing infections require prompt recognition and treatment because they can be life threatening. These infections require surgical debridement and adjunctive antibiotic therapy without delay.

Other Site-Specific Infections

Hospital-acquired diarrhea is a common problem. The etiology may be either infectious or noninfectious. The most potentially serious cause of infectious diarrhea is antibiotic-associated diarrhea. In most of the adults this infection is due to *Clostridium difficile*.[60] It may present as a mild case of diarrhea with watery stools to a severe diarrhea and life-threatening pseudomembranous enterocolitis.[61] *C. difficile*-related diarrhea is most commonly associated with the prior administration of antibiotics, particularly clindamycin and third-generation cephalosporins. However, all commonly used antibiotics have been implicated. Diagnosis requires either positive stool cultures or stool enzyme immunoassay. Evidence of pseudomembranes by sigmoidoscopy is also sufficient for diagnosis. Once diagnosed, infection control measures are extremely important to prevent cross contamination to other patients especially by health care workers. Alcohol hand rubs alone are not sufficient to kill the spore-forming organism and hand washing with soap and water must be utilized. Care to disinfect all medical equipment should be undertaken before use on noninfected patients. The most beneficial infection control policy to reduce the incidence of *C. difficile* is careful use and restriction of antibiotics.

An important and likely underreported infection in critically ill patients is nosocomial sinusitis. The presence of sinusitis is in itself a significant risk factor for nosocomial pneumonia, particularly in patients who are mechanically ventilated. The presence of medical devices in the nose (e.g., nasogastric tubes, nasal endotracheal tubes) is a major risk factor for the development of sinusitis.[18] Sinusitis should be suspected in any postoperative patient or patient with facial fractures who develops a fever with nasal tubes in place.[62,63] Purulent drainage from the nose may or may not be present. Plain films can be used to make the diagnosis, but can be difficult to interpret in the ICU setting. Better results are likely to be obtained from computed tomography, which can show air-fluid levels and mucosal thickening. Tapping the sinus at the bedside may be used in patients in whom transport to radiology is hazardous and provides a definitive diagnosis. White blood cells and bacteria are ultimately required for a definitive diagnosis. Once diagnosed, all nasal tubes should be removed and decongestants can be administered. Antibiotics should be used if an organism is identified or the patient has signs and symptoms of systemic infection.

SUMMARY

Hospital-acquired infections or NIs are a serious problem and a risk to all hospitalized patients. Critically ill patients in the ICU are particularly at risk due to impaired host defense mechanisms and colonization with microorganisms. Patients' immune defense mechanisms may be impaired not only by their underlying disease process but by medical interventions (e.g., endotracheal intubation) as well. Patients may be colonized by endogenous sources (e.g., skin, oral cavity, and GI tract) or from exogenous sources (e.g., the hospital environment, health care workers). Any microorganism can infect the critically ill patient. *Staphylococcus aureus* and *Pseudomonas aeruginosa* remain the most commonly identified pathogens. There has been a documented increase in gram-positive and fungal organisms. The clinician should be familiar, however, with local flora and infection patterns as there are numerous variations amongst the type of unit and patient populations.

The CDC estimates that approximately one third of the reported 2 million NIs can be prevented by the implementation of infection control procedures. Hand hygiene remains one of the simplest and most effective measures to prevent NIs. However, compliance is often poor amongst health care workers. Alcohol gel solutions are effective in most cases and may help improve compliance. Universal precautions should always be adhered to when dealing with situations where the potential for infection exists. Other precautions such as contact or airborne/droplet precautions should be utilized.

Antibiotics are frequently utilized in critically ill patients. However, the overusage of these agents leads to increasingly resistant organisms and the potential for NIs. Starting empiric antibiotic therapy should always be followed by a reevaluation of the patient after 48 to 72 hours to assess the clinical effectiveness and to narrow the antibiotic spectrum. The use of antibiotic cycling has been shown to be an effective practice. Such rotations require a multidisciplinary approach to ensure the maximal effectiveness and to prevent unwanted consequences to other antimicrobial classes.

The three most commonly reported NIs in the ICU are pneumonia, UTIs, and BSIs. Most NIs are associated with the use of indwelling medical devices such as endotracheal intubation, urinary catheters, and central venous catheters, all of which can act as a nidus for infection. Care must be taken when inserting and maintaining these devices. Understanding site-specific risk factors can assist the health care worker in helping to prevent NIs.

NIs are a growing concern to patients and health care workers alike. Prevention remains one of the most effective measures in protecting the critically ill patient from NIs and their potentially life-threatening consequences. All health care workers share a responsibility to understand risk factors and patterns of transmission and to adhere to infection control policies to protect patients.

REFERENCES

1. Haley RW, Culver DH, White JW, et al. The efficacy of infection surveillance and control programs in preventing nosocomial infections in US hospitals. *Am J Epidemiol.* 1985;121:182–205.
2. Kohn L, Corrigan J, Donaldson M. *To err is human: building a safer health system.* Washington, D.C.: National Academy Press; 1999.
3. Weber DJ, Raasch R, Rutala WA. Nosocomial infections in the ICU: The growing importance of antibiotic-resistant pathogens. *Chest.* 1999;115:34S–41S.
4. Archibald L, Phillips L, Monnet D, et al. Antimicrobial resistance in isolates from inpatients and outpatients in the United States: Increasing importance of the intensive care unit. *Clin Infect Dis.* 1997;24:211–215.
5. Centers for Disease Control and Prevention. Public health focus: Surveillance, prevention, and control of nosocomial infections. *MMWR Morb Mortal Wkly Rep.* 1992;41:783–787.
6. Widmer AF, Sax H, Pittet D. Infection control and hospital epidemiology outside the United States. *Infect Control Hosp Epidemiol.* 1999;20:17–21.
7. Cook DJ, Kollef MH. Risk factors for ICU-acquired pneumonia. *JAMA.* 1998;279:1605–1606.
8. Gerding DN. Antimicrobial cycling: Lessons learned from the aminoglycoside experience. *Infect Control Hosp Epidemiol.* 2000;21:S12–S17.
9. Gerding DN, Martone WJ. SHEA conference on antimicrobial resistance. Society for Health Care Epidemiology of America. *Infect Control Hosp Epidemiol.* 2000;21:347–351.
10. Kollef MH. The prevention of ventilator-associated pneumonia. *N Engl J Med.* 1999;340:627–634.
11. Kollef MH, Vlasnik J, Sharpless L, et al. Scheduled change of antibiotic classes: A strategy to decrease the incidence of ventilator-associated pneumonia. *Am J Respir Crit Care Med.* 1997;156:1040–1048.
12. Pittet D, Hugonnet S, Harbarth S, et al. Effectiveness of a hospital-wide programme to improve compliance with hand hygiene. Infection Control Programme. *Lancet.* 2000;356:1307–1312.
13. Consensus paper on the surveillance of surgical wound infections. The Society for Hospital Epidemiology of America; The Association for Practitioners in Infection Control; The Centers for Disease Control; The Surgical Infection Society. *Infect Control Hosp Epidemiol.* 1992;13:599–605.
14. Garner JS, Jarvis WR, Emori TG, et al. CDC definitions for nosocomial infections, 1988. *Am J Infect Control.* 1988;16:128–140.
15. Emori TG, Culver DH, Horan TC, et al. National nosocomial infections surveillance system (NNIS): Description of surveillance methods. *Am J Infect Control.* 1991;19:19–35.
16. Richards MJ, Edwards JR, Culver DH, et al. Nosocomial infections in medical intensive care units in the United States. National Nosocomial Infections Surveillance System. *Crit Care Med.* 1999;27:887–892.
17. Richards MJ, Edwards JR, Culver DH, et al. Nosocomial infections in combined medical-surgical intensive care units in the United States. *Infect Control Hosp Epidemiol.* 2000;21:510–515.
18. Eggimann P, Pittet D. Infection control in the ICU. *Chest.* 2001;120:2059–2093.
19. Haley RW, Bregman DA. The role of understaffing and overcrowding in recurrent outbreaks of staphylococcal infection in a neonatal special-care unit. *J Infect Dis.* 1982;145:875–885.
20. Tarnow-Mordi WO, Hau C, Warden A, et al. Hospital mortality in relation to staff workload: A 4-year study in an adult intensive-care unit. *Lancet.* 2000;356:185–189.
21. Friedman G, Silva E, Vincent JL. Has the mortality of septic shock changed with time. *Crit Care Med.* 1998;26:2078–2086.
22. Vincent JL. Nosocomial infections in adult intensive-care units. *Lancet.* 2003;361:2068–2077.
23. Vincent JL, Bihari DJ, Suter PM, et al. The prevalence of nosocomial infection in intensive care units in Europe. Results of the European Prevalence of Infection in Intensive Care (EPIC) Study. EPIC International Advisory Committee. *JAMA.* 1995;274:639–644.
24. Spencer RC. Predominant pathogens found in the European Prevalence of Infection in Intensive Care Study. *Eur J Clin Microbiol Infect Dis.* 1996;15:281–285.
25. Goldmann D, Larson E. Hand-washing and nosocomial infections. *N Engl J Med.* 1992;327:120–122.
26. Maury E, Alzieu M, Baudel JL, et al. Availability of an alcohol solution can improve hand disinfection compliance in an intensive care unit. *Am J Respir Crit Care Med.* 2000;162:324–327.
27. Rubinovitch B, Pittet D. Screening for methicillin-resistant Staphylococcus aureus in the endemic hospital: What have we learned? *J Hosp Infect.* 2001;47:9–18.
28. Sproat LJ, Inglis TJ. A multicentre survey of hand hygiene practice in intensive care units. *J Hosp Infect.* 1994;26:137–148.
29. Larson E. Skin hygiene and infection prevention: More of the same or different approaches? *Clin Infect Dis.* 1999;29:1287–1294.
30. Doebbeling BN, Stanley GL, Sheetz CT, et al. Comparative efficacy of alternative hand-washing agents in reducing nosocomial infections in intensive care units. *N Engl J Med.* 1992;327:88–93.
31. Voss A, Widmer AF. No time for handwashing! Handwashing versus alcoholic rub: Can we afford 100% compliance? *Infect Control Hosp Epidemiol.* 1997;18:205–208.
32. Edmond M. Isolation. *Infect Control Hosp Epidemiol.* 1997;18:58–64.
33. Jarvis WR, Bolyard EA, Bozzi CJ, et al. Respirators, recommendations, and regulations: The controversy surrounding protection of health care workers from tuberculosis. *Ann Intern Med.* 1995;122:142–146.
34. Weinstein RA. Controlling antimicrobial resistance in hospitals: Infection control and use of antibiotics. *Emerg Infect Dis.* 2001;7:188–192.
35. White AC Jr, Atmar RL, Wilson J, et al. Effects of requiring prior authorization for selected antimicrobials: Expenditures, susceptibilities, and clinical outcomes. *Clin Infect Dis.* 1997;25:230–239.
36. O'Grady NP, Barie PS, Bartlett JG, et al. Practice guidelines for evaluating new fever in critically ill adult patients. Task Force of the Society of Critical Care Medicine and the Infectious Diseases Society of America. *Clin Infect Dis.* 1998;26:1042–1059.
37. Goldmann DA, Weinstein RA, Wenzel RP, et al. Strategies to prevent and control the emergence and spread of antimicrobial-resistant microorganisms in hospitals. A challenge to hospital leadership. *JAMA.* 1996;275:234–240.
38. Niederman MS. Is "crop rotation" of antibiotics the solution to a "resistant" problem in the ICU? *Am J Respir Crit Care Med.* 1997;156:1029–1031.
39. Gruson D, Hilbert G, Vargas F, et al. Rotation and restricted use of antibiotics in a medical intensive care unit. Impact

on the incidence of ventilator-associated pneumonia caused by antibiotic-resistant gram-negative bacteria. *Am J Respir Crit Care Med.* 2000;162:837–843.

40. Quale J, Landman D, Saurina G, et al. Manipulation of a hospital antimicrobial formulary to control an outbreak of vancomycin-resistant enterococci. *Clin Infect Dis.* 1996;23:1020–1025.

41. Peters M, Petros A, Dixon G, et al. Acquired immunoparalysis in paediatric intensive care: Prospective observational study. *Br Med J.* 1999;319:609–610.

42. Antonelli M, Conti G, Rocco M, et al. A comparison of noninvasive positive-pressure ventilation and conventional mechanical ventilation in patients with acute respiratory failure. *N Engl J Med.* 1998;339:429–435.

43. Girou E, Schortgen F, Delclaux C, et al. Association of noninvasive ventilation with nosocomial infections and survival in critically ill patients. *JAMA.* 2000;284:2361–2367.

44. Nourdine K, Combes P, Carton MJ, et al. Does noninvasive ventilation reduce the ICU nosocomial infection risk? A prospective clinical survey. *Intensive Care Med.* 1999;25:567–573.

45. Hilton E, Haslett TM, Borenstein MT, et al. Central catheter infections: Single- versus triple-lumen catheters. Influence of guide wires on infection rates when used for replacement of catheters. *Am J Med.* 1988;84:667–672.

46. Pemberton LB, Lyman B, Lander V, et al. Sepsis from triple- vs single-lumen catheters during total parenteral nutrition in surgical or critically ill patients. *Arch Surg.* 1986;121:591–594.

47. Merrer J, De Jonghe B, Golliot F, et al. Complications of femoral and subclavian venous catheterization in critically ill patients: A randomized controlled trial. *JAMA.* 2001;286:700–707.

48. Hoffmann KK, Weber DJ, Samsa GP, et al. Transparent polyurethane film as an intravenous catheter dressing. A meta-analysis of the infection risks. *JAMA.* 1992;267:2072–2076.

49. Veenstra DL, Saint S, Saha S, et al. Efficacy of antiseptic-impregnated central venous catheters in preventing catheter-related bloodstream infection: A meta-analysis. *JAMA.* 1999;281:261–267.

50. Mermel LA. New technologies to prevent intravascular catheter-related bloodstream infections. *Emerg Infect Dis.* 2001;7:197–199.

51. Darouiche RO, Raad II, Heard SO, et al. A comparison of two antimicrobial-impregnated central venous catheters. Catheter Study Group. *N Engl J Med.* 1999;340:1–8.

52. Caplan ES, Hoyt NJ, Rodriguez A, et al. Empyema occurring in the multiply traumatized patient. *J Trauma.* 1984;24:785–789.

53. Groeger JS, Lucas AB, Thaler HT, et al. Infectious morbidity associated with long-term use of venous access devices in patients with cancer. *Ann Intern Med.* 1993;119:1168–1174.

54. Thompson RL, Haley CE, Searcy MA, et al. Catheter-associated bacteriuria. Failure to reduce attack rates using periodic instillations of a disinfectant into urinary drainage systems. *JAMA.* 1984;251:747–751.

55. Warren JW, Platt R, Thomas RJ, et al. Antibiotic irrigation and catheter-associated urinary-tract infections. *N Engl J Med.* 1978;299:570–573.

56. Kauffman CA, Vazquez JA, Sobel JD, et al. Prospective multicenter surveillance study of funguria in hospitalized patients. The National Institute for Allergy and Infectious Diseases (NIAID) Mycoses Study Group. *Clin Infect Dis.* 2000; 30:14–18.

57. Culver DH, Horan TC, Gaynes RP, et al. Surgical wound infection rates by wound class, operative procedure, and patient risk index. National Nosocomial Infections Surveillance System. *Am J Med.* 1991;91:152S–157S.

58. Greif R, Akca O, Horn EP, et al. Supplemental perioperative oxygen to reduce the incidence of surgical-wound infection. Outcomes Research Group. *N Engl J Med.* 2000;342:161–167.

59. van den Berghe G, Wouters P, Weekers F, et al. Intensive insulin therapy in the critically ill patients. *N Engl J Med.* 2001;345:1359–1367.

60. Barbut F, Corthier G, Charpak Y, et al. Prevalence and pathogenicity of Clostridium difficile in hospitalized patients. A French multicenter study. *Arch Intern Med.* 1996;156:1449–1454.

61. Kelly CP, Pothoulakis C, LaMont JT. Clostridium difficile colitis. *N Engl J Med.* 1994;330:257–262.

62. Deutschman CS, Wilton P, Sinow J, et al. Paranasal sinusitis associated with nasotracheal intubation: A frequently unrecognized and treatable source of sepsis. *Crit Care Med.* 1986;14:111–114.

63. Grindlinger GA, Niehoff J, Hughes SL, et al. Acute paranasal sinusitis related to nasotracheal intubation of head-injured patients. *Crit Care Med.* 1987;15:214–217.

Nutritional Support of the Injured

63

Ernest F.J. Block   *Matthew W. Lube*

The important role of nutritional support in surgical patients is widely recognized. It is now becoming increasingly clear that this role goes far beyond simply providing the patient with adequate amounts of protein and calories. One must not only be concerned with the calories supplied but must also take into consideration the timing, route of administration, and individual components of a nutritional regimen. The gastrointestinal (GI) tract is the largest immune organ in the body and contains 65% of the body's overall immune tissue and up to 80% of the immunoglobulin producing cells. It is a rich source of lymphocytes, plasma cells, and macrophages and has a pivotal role in modulating the patients' response to injury. Providing the GI tract with nutrients directly in the form of enteral nutrition can help prevent mucosal atrophy and increased permeability with resultant bacterial translocation and priming of neutrophils and macrophages. Early aggressive nutritional support within 12 to 24 hours of injury is important to decrease the incidence of the systemic inflammatory response syndrome and organ dysfunction. The goals of nutritional support have spread beyond providing the injured host with energy to actually modifying an individual's response to the insult at the cellular and biochemical level. A basic understanding of these biochemical principles will help the surgeon better understand the rationale behind the evidence practiced.

ENDOCRINE AND METABOLIC RESPONSE TO TRAUMA

Acutely traumatized patients have a well-characterized orchestrated response to injury, which eventually leads to the activation of the hypothalamus-pituitary-adrenal axis,

the renin-angiotensin system, and the autonomic nervous system. The end result is generalized catabolism leading to protein wasting, negative nitrogen balance, and erosion of lean body mass and circulating proteins such as albumin and prealbumin.

Initial activation is multifactorial and is the result of mediators produced both systemically and locally at the site of injury. The inciting events are intravascular and extracellular fluid volume losses, tissue hypoperfusion, tissue damage, pain, fear, and emotion. Tissue damage, either as a direct result of trauma or secondary to hypoperfusion or infection, is perhaps the most potent stimulus. Changes in pH, partial pressures of oxygen and carbon dioxide, temperature, and blood pressure are detected through various central and peripheral receptors, which ultimately lead to the activation of these biochemical pathways. The mediators that regulate one's response to injury and sepsis have been well characterized. With acute injury, we see a rapid rise in the serum concentrations of adrenocorticotropin (ACTH), cortisol, epinephrine, norepinephrine, glucagon, vasopressin (antidiuretic hormone), and aldosterone. Various proinflammatory cytokines, primarily tumor necrosis factor and interleukin 1, are also elevated.

Hepatic glycogen is rapidly utilized and the goal is to provide substrates for hepatic gluconeogenesis to support the massive energy needs of acute injury. The counter-regulatory hormones previously mentioned lead to proteolysis and amino acid production as well as lipolysis with the generation of glycerol and free fatty acids. Amino acids (namely, glutamine and alanine), lactate, and glycerol serve as carbon skeletons for the hepatic production of glucose for use by erythrocytes, leukocytes, and cells of the central nervous system that do not require insulin for glucose transport and utilization. Release of these substances also leads to decreased levels of insulin produced from the pancreas as well as a state of peripheral insulin resistance and hyperglycemia. Insulin is normally a dominant anabolic stimulus and its absence in times of injury and stress is not without consequence. Normally, insulin stimulates amino acid transport into muscle. Low levels of insulin stimulate protein degradation, adding to the state of negative nitrogen balance and catabolism. In contrast to starvation, suppression of proteolysis does not occur and gluconeogenesis continues at an accelerated rate at the expense of lean body mass (mainly skeletal muscle). Low levels of insulin further promote lipolysis and the production of free fatty acids, which will also serve as an important fuel source to support hypermetabolism. Early and aggressive nutritional therapy is necessary to minimize the insults put forth by the neurohumoral axis.

In the absence of preexisting nutritional defects, the goal of nutritional support in the critically ill patient is to support the hypermetabolic state and preserve as much lean body mass as possible. It is important to realize that nutritional support is an *adjunct* to the overall care of these critically injured patients. The underlying disease process is the cause of the malnutrition. One cannot expect to convert a hypermetabolic, catabolic individual to a state of positive nitrogen balance with nutrition alone. It is impossible to completely halt amino acid degradation, and some degree of muscle wasting is inevitable. Depending on the severity of the illness, it may take weeks to months to achieve anabolism and one must be patient enough to avoid the complications associated with overfeeding. It is equally important to concentrate on the initial cause of the hypermetabolic illness by eliminating ongoing blood loss, sources of sepsis, and other secondary insults that can prolong the catabolic state.

FORMULATION AND COMPOSITION

Caloric Requirements

The fundamental goal in nutritional supplementation is to meet the energy requirements for metabolic processes, to support hypermetabolism, and to minimize protein catabolism. Nutritional support begins with an estimation of the patient's caloric requirements. The Harris Benedict equation is one of the most commonly used methods for estimating caloric needs or basal energy expenditure (BEE):

Males: BEE = 66.5 + 13.8(weight in kg)
            +5 (height in cm) − 6.8 (age)
Females: BEE = 65.5 + 9.6(weight in kg)
            +1.7 (height in cm) − 4.7 (age)

(Stress factors: minor surgery 1.2, trauma 1.35, sepsis 1.6, major burns 2.1)

These equations yield basal energy requirements that are frequently multiplied by various activity and/or stress factors to generate a resting energy expenditure (REE), although this may lead to an overestimation of the patient's actual caloric needs which could lead to unnecessary administration of nutrients and overfeeding. Another important consideration is the patient's weight that is used for these calculations. One must avoid using the patient's actual body weight (ABW), which could be quite elevated after a period of aggressive volume resuscitation. Ideally an admission weight before interventions should be obtained. In practice, this assessment is impractical and not normally part of the primary and secondary surveys in the acutely injured patient. An accurate measurement of body weight (BW) is an arduous task in critically ill patients with bulky dressings, catheters, monitoring wires, tubes, and drains. The ideal body weight (IBW) could prove useful in such circumstances and is calculated as follows:

$$IBW = 2.3 \text{ (height in inches over ft)} + (45.5 \text{ [females] or } 50 \text{ [males]})$$

Obesity poses another scenario where overfeeding may result if one uses the patient's ABW. In such circumstances (Obesity = ABW 20% over IBW or a body mass index [BMI] >30), we typically use the adjusted BW for energy calculations and requirements:

$$\text{Adjusted BW} = (ABW - IBW)\,0.25 + IBW$$

A more specific method frequently used to determine caloric needs in ventilated patients is to perform indirect calorimetry. A metabolic cart is used to collect expired gases to determine CO_2 production and O_2 consumption which are used to calculate the REE using the Weir equation:

$$REE = (V_{O_2}[3.941] + V_{CO_2}[1.11])\,1,440 \text{ minutes/day}$$

Indirect calorimetry also provides the respiratory quotient (RQ) (RQ = CO_2 production divided by O_2 consumption), which can be further used to monitor the adequacy of nutritional support. An RQ of >1 suggests overfeeding and lipogenesis. An RQ of 1 indicates pure carbohydrate utilization. Unlike glucose metabolism, oxidation of fatty acids requires less oxygen and produces less carbon dioxide. Pure fat utilization produces an RQ of 7 and a value of <7 suggests underfeeding and ketogenesis. Mixed substrate utilization is suggested when the RQ value falls within the 0.8 and 0.9 range.

There are several limitations to indirect calorimetry including the need for dedicated equipment and staff. Such measurements are costly and are for the most part limited to those patients on the ventilator. Measurements may be inaccurate in patients with conditions often encountered in the critically ill. These include patients on high levels of oxygen ($F_{IO_2} > 0.6$), high positive-end expiratory pressure, air leaks that may limit the ability to adequately collect and analyze expired gases, and peritoneal and hemodialysis due to removal across the membrane of CO_2 that is not measured by the indirect calorimeter. One must also consider the fact that these measurements are only a reflection of the short window of time that the patient is being studied. In general, the patient selected for this study should be in a stable, steady state. The patient should be protected from noise or other stimulation as permitted.

Despite these limitations, indirect calorimetry serves several roles. Underestimation of the stress factor in the formulas given in the preceding text could lead to inadequate caloric delivery which may be detected. Equally troubling would be overfeeding; the metabolic cart should be considered a diagnostic study in patients who fail attempts at liberation from mechanical ventilation to measure the O_2 cost of breathing and the components of or to determine the cause of increased ventilatory requirements.

Specific literature addressing the optimal method for nutritional assessment is lacking. It should be remembered that no specific formula has been proved to be superior to the others and these should be considered to provide at best an estimate of the patient's initial protein and caloric needs. Currently, recommendations for most surgical patients are to provide approximately 25 to 30 kcal/kg/day through the administration of carbohydrates (70%) and lipids (30%). Protein should not be included in these energy calculations. Oxidation of 1 g of fat yields approximately 9 kcal of energy and 1 g of carbohydrate yields approximately 4 kcal of energy. It should be noted, however, that those sugars found in enteral formulas and total parenteral nutrition (TPN) typically yield 3.4 kcal per g. We typically start out with 30 kcal/kg/day based on the patient's admission weight, if available. As previously mentioned, in obese individuals we will use the adjusted ABW.

Carbohydrate and Lipid Requirements

The exogenous administration of glucose (50 to 100 g per day) favors fat entry into the TCA cycle and avoids the formation of ketone bodies, and in the absence of severe illness limits amino acid degradation and urinary urea production. In the absence of severe hyperglycemia or brain injury, it is therefore important to consider adding dextrose to the patient's maintenance intravenous fluids. Once formal nutritional support is begun, the exact percentage of the caloric source is predetermined by the enteral formulation one chooses (see Table 1). If one is receiving TPN, the amount of carbohydrate infusion should not exceed the maximum rate of glucose utilization, which is approximately 5 mg/kg/minute. This is rarely a problem when adequate amounts of lipids are given as an additional caloric source.

Protein Requirements

Protein is the building block of life. Once hepatic glycogen stores are depleted, muscle protein is degraded to provide three carbon backbones for hepatic gluconeogenesis. Initially protein catabolism is resistant to the administration of exogenous amino acids and it takes weeks until a critically ill patient is found to be in a state of positive nitrogen balance. In addition to protein catabolism, exogenous protein is required for wound healing and to replace that lost in wounds and fistulae. The goal is to minimize the loss of lean body mass and as a general rule this requires anywhere from 1.0 to 1.5 g/kg/day of protein depending on the degree of illness and injury. A severely burned patient may require in excess of 2.0 g/kg/day to replace the large quantities of protein lost through their wounds. Another circumstance that one must consider is the patient with an open abdomen who may lose additional amounts of nitrogen through the temporary dressing.

TABLE 1
ENTERAL FORMULATIONS

	Nutren 1.5	Replete with Fiber	Glytrol	Nutren 2.0	Nutren Renal	Nutren Pulmonary
Kcal/mL	1.5	1.0	1.0	2.0	2.0	1.5
Protein (g/L)	60 (20%)	62.4 (30%)	45.2 (23%)	80 (21%)	70 (19%)	68 (26%)
Carbohydrates (g/L)	169.2 (57%)	113 (54%)	100 (52%)	196 (52%)	204 (54%)	100 (38%)
Fat (g/L)	67.6 (23%)	34 (16%)	47.6 (25%)	104 (27%)	104 (27%)	94.8 (36%)
Osmolality (mOsm/L)	430	310	280	745	650	330
Fiber (soluble/insoluble) (g/L)	None	0.8/13.2	10/5	None	None	None
Sodium (mEq/L)	50.78	38.1	32.2	56.5	32.17	50/78
Potassium (mEq/L)	48	38.5	35.9	49.2	32.17	50.78
Zinc (mg/L)	20	24	15.2	28	20	21.2
Vitamin C (mg/L)	212	340	140	280	90	210
Vitamin K (mg/L)	75	50	50	100	75	75

There are several ways to estimate protein requirements. One simple method is to look at the ratio of nonprotein calories to grams of nitrogen. A typical postoperative patient requires a ratio of 150 carbohydrate calories to 1 g of nitrogen to prevent the use of protein as an energy source. Critically ill subjects and burn victims may require values <100. Another method is to calculate the nitrogen balance following collection of a 24-hour urine specimen:

$$\frac{\text{Total protein intake (grams) per day}}{6.25\text{g protein/g nitrogen}}$$
$$- \text{UUN} + 4\text{g (insensible losses)}$$
$$+ (1.9 \text{ [liters of abdominal fluid]})$$

where UUN is urine urea nitrogen in grams of nitrogen excreted in the urine over the 24-hour period. Four grams is typically used to estimate insensible nitrogenous losses through the skin and GI tract. This is a very crude estimate of nitrogen balance and may not be valid in the patient with large burns or wounds. Cheatham et al. showed that patients with an open abdomen lose on average 1.9 g nitrogen per L of abdominal fluid. In patients with temporary abdominal dressings, this needs to be added to the insensible losses to avoid overestimating nitrogen balance, which would in turn lead to underfeeding and inadequate nutritional support.[1] A patient in positive nitrogen balance excretes less nitrogen than is being consumed and is incorporating nitrogen into newly formed protein. A patient in negative nitrogen balance excretes more nitrogen than they consume and continues to degrade muscle protein for gluconeogenic precursors.

Overfeeding

It is often difficult to estimate a patient's energy requirements and excess caloric administration can lead to overfeeding. The importance of estimating one's premorbid dry weight was previously discussed. The Harris Benedict equation and indirect calorimetry can both overestimate caloric needs. An RQ >1.0 suggests overfeeding. Excess carbohydrate administration can lead to lipogenesis, hepatic steatosis, glycogen deposition, hypercarbia, and respiratory insufficiency. Although usually not a problem in the typical young, previously healthy trauma victim, problems may occur in patients with chronic obstructive pulmonary disorder (COPD) and preexisting pulmonary insufficiency. Excess carbohydrate intake also results in hyperglycemia, which can lead to immunosuppression and leukocyte dysfunction, increased infectious complications, glycosuria, and dehydration. Choosing a formulation with a greater proportion of lipids may be necessary to avoid these complications. Lipid overfeeding is not benign, however, and may be associated with hyperlipidemia, cholestasis, increased risk of infection, immunosuppression, and inhibition of the reticuloendothelial system. In patients receiving intravenous lipids, one must periodically check serum triglyceride levels and withhold further infusions when the concentrations rise above 400 to 500 mg per dL.

Special Circumstances

Renal Failure

The goal of feeding patients with renal insufficiency is to prevent further accumulation of nitrogenous wastes, volume, electrolytes, and minerals. Many critically ill patients exhibit varying degrees of renal impairment. In the patient with renal failure and a worsening blood urea nitrogen concentration, it is important to avoid the overzealous administration of protein. This is less of a concern in dialyzed patients and those on continuous forms of dialysis may even require more protein due to the considerable losses in the dialysate. Many different formulas exist for the patient with worsening renal function or acute renal failure. These formulations have lower concentrations of potassium and phosphate and a higher ratio of nonprotein calories to gram of nitrogen. These products are also more concentrated, hyperosmolar, and calorically rich. Adequate collaboration between the nephrologist and the surgical nutritionist should accomplish these goals with intensive dialysis and careful metabolic monitoring and supplementation.

Hepatic Failure

Critically ill patients may develop hepatic failure as a part of the multiple organ dysfunction syndrome (MODS). These individuals may have jaundice, elevated transaminase levels, encephalopathy, and an elevated ammonia level. The initial stress hyperglycemia may progress to hypoglycemia. The liver is responsible for the metabolism of aromatic amino acids (AAAs). In patients with acute injury, branched chain amino acids (BCAA) are used by the muscle, and in the presence of hepatic failure the ratio of AAA to BCAA is disturbed. AAAs have been postulated to become false neurotransmitters and worsen encephalopathy in patients with liver failure. Various formulations exist for the patient with liver failure and encephalopathy. These formulations contain more BCAAs (leucine, isoleucine, and valine) and less AAAs. This is a theoretic option that rarely alters the ultimate clinical outcome in the critically ill patient with severe hepatic derangement.

Pulmonary Failure

Many critically ill patients remain in the intensive care unit (ICU) for prolonged periods of time on the ventilator for a variety of reasons. Whether the patient has acute lung injury or preexisting obstructive pulmonary disease, disorders of oxygenation and carbon dioxide elimination may exist. Patients with pulmonary compromise may have difficulty with formulations that contain high amounts of carbohydrate that in turn produce large amounts of carbon dioxide when oxidized. A rising end-tidal carbon dioxide level in ventilated patients requiring an escalating minute ventilation may be the first clue of carbohydrate overfeeding. It is important to consider, however, that the respiratory failure in traumatically injured patients is infrequently due to overfeeding and usually secondary to the chest trauma itself and the sequelae that follow. If one is truly concerned, indirect calorimetry can be performed. An RQ >1 further strengthens the diagnosis. These individuals may theoretically benefit from having their carbohydrate:lipid ratio adjusted, so lipids that produce less carbon dioxide and have a lower RQ provide a greater proportion of the caloric source. Various enteral formulations exist with a larger proportion of fat for the caloric source. However, there has not been a consistent clear benefit seen with the routine use of such formulations, and their routine application has not been supported by the literature.

ELECTROLYTE AND TRACE ELEMENTS

Sodium and Water

Disorders of sodium and water balance are commonplace in surgical, trauma, and critically ill patients. Water constitutes 50% to 70% of total BW. The appropriate choice of intravenous fluids and enteral formulations is very important to minimize the chance of electrolyte abnormalities and the risks associated with them. Several mechanisms are responsible for the regulation of osmolality including the ability of the hypothalamus to allow us to experience and respond to thirst. Osmoreceptors and baroreceptors respond to changes in osmolality and blood pressure, respectively, and restore homeostasis by altering the levels of vasopressin (antidiuretic hormone) secreted by the posterior pituitary gland. Vasopressin results in the reabsorption of free water in the distal tubule and collecting ducts. It has many other vasoactive and metabolic properties as well.

Human beings consume several liters of water each day. Much of this is contained in the food we eat. Measuring a patient's intake of fluid over a 24-hour period is relatively easy. Quantifying losses can be much more difficult. Many of our traumatically injured patients lose massive quantities of fluid and electrolytes in their nasogastric aspirate and stool. Massive losses can also occur in patients with open abdomens and fistulae. Insensible losses through the skin and respiratory tract are even more difficult to quantify especially in febrile, hypermetabolic individuals. Abnormalities of sodium and water balance are frequently characterized by varying losses of sodium and water in relation to one another and whether the losses are renal or nonrenal in nature.

Hyponatremia

Hyponatremia is a common electrolyte disorder seen in clinical practice. Hyponatremic patients may be hypertonic (P_{osm} >285 mEq per L) or hypotonic (P_{osm}

<280 mOsm per L). Hypertonic forms are frequently secondary to the presence of excess solute such as glucose. This is a dilutional form of hyponatremia. For a 100 mg per dL rise in the serum glucose concentration, one should expect to see a 2 mEq per L decrease in the serum sodium concentration. Therapy is aimed at correcting the glucose concentration.

The most common form of hyponatremia is that of hypotonic hyponatremia. It is frequently the result of the inappropriate administration of hypotonic intravenous fluids to postoperative patients. These patients already have elevated levels of antidiuretic hormone, are resorbing free water, and are prone to this electrolyte disorder without the added insult of receiving additional hypotonic fluid. Another relatively common condition is the syndrome of inappropriate secretion of antidiuretic hormone (SIADH). This is characterized by low urinary output, urinary sodium levels of >20 mEq per L, and hyponatremia. The plasma is hypoosmolar (240 to 250 mOsm per L). The treatment of this condition is fluid restriction and sodium replacement with isotonic or less frequently hypertonic intravenous solutions.

Hyponatremia may also be due to the loss of sodium in contrast to the previously mentioned conditions that are the result of free water excess. The urinary sodium level allows one to differentiate renal from nonrenal causes. Causes of excess renal losses of sodium (U_{Na} >20 mEq per L) include diuretics, acute tubular necrosis, and adrenal (mineralocorticoid) insufficiency. Extrarenal losses (U_{Na} <10 mEq per L) may be common in surgical patients and include vomiting and prolonged nasogastric suction, small bowel, and pancreatic fistulae as well as insensible losses through the skin and lungs. Appropriate treatment is accomplished with the replacement of losses with isotonic saline.

Proper administration of intravenous solutions is the first step in avoiding problematic hyponatremia. Surgical patients, at least initially, should rarely be given hypotonic saline. This is especially true in patients with head injuries. One must also consider the amount of salt in the enteral formula given to the patient (Table 1). Most of these formulations are quite hypotonic with regard to sodium, and in the event of hyponatremia it is frequently necessary to add salt to these formulas. Our department has protocols for creating isotonic or hypertonic formulas that become helpful in reducing free water administration, treating hyponatremia, and raising serum osmolarity. Nutren 1.5 has a sodium content of 51 mEq per L. To make that solution isotonic (0.9% NaCl), it would be necessary to add 1.25 teaspoons of NaCl per liter, and to make that solution hypertonic (1.5% NaCl) it would be necessary to add 2.5 teaspoons of NaCl to a liter of tube feeding. In the rare event of a patient receiving parenteral nutrition, it is frequently necessary to increase the sodium content of the solution to correct a hyponatremic state.

Hypernatremia

Hypernatremia is usually secondary to a loss of free water and is frequently associated with a hyperosmolar state. Diabetes insipidus (DI), in contrast to SIADH, is a condition related to low levels of circulating vasopressin and is frequently seen in patients with severe traumatic brain injury. This syndrome is characterized by large volumes of dilute urine, hypernatremia, hypovolemia, and shock. Treatment is aimed at replacing the free water deficit and administering exogenous vasopressin. Hypovolemic hypernatremia is a result of water loss that exceeds sodium loss. The urinary sodium level can help differentiate renal losses: (urinary sodium >20 mEq per L: diuretics, glycosuria, urea diuresis, and renal failure) from nonrenal losses (urinary sodium <10 mEq per L: sweating, hypotonic GI losses, and respiratory losses). Hypernatremia in the ICU is most often iatrogenic. Hypertonic intravenous solutions, sodium bicarbonate and many medications, especially antibiotics, contain large amounts of sodium that can result in hypernatremia. The primary goal is to identify and treat the underlying cause. Sodium restriction and free water administration are the backbones of treatment. Free water can be administered parenterally or through the feeding tube.

Phosphorus and Magnesium

Hypophosphatemia and hypomagnesemia are common metabolic derangements seen in critically ill patients. Requirements for these electrolytes increase as the body becomes anabolic and synthesizes new cells. Adequate levels of these electrolytes are important in respiratory processes and muscle contraction. These cations are necessary cofactors for enzymatic processes and fuel for cellular machinery. It is necessary to periodically check the levels of these electrolytes and replace them accordingly. Our department has adult electrolyte replacement protocols (see Table 2). A prerequisite is that the patient has adequate urinary output and renal function.

Hypophosphatemia and hypomagnesemia may be part of a refeeding syndrome. Refeeding malnourished patients may result in These electrolyte abnormalities along with hypokalemia, cardiac arrhythmias, glucose intolerance, and GI dysfunction.

Vitamins and Trace Minerals

Vitamins and minerals also serve as important cofactors for a variety of enzymatic reactions. Although rare in the standard surgical patient, several patient populations are at increased risk for micronutrient deficiency, especially those with preexisting malnutrition. Most vitamin and trace mineral deficiencies have been described in patients on long-term TPN with little or no oral intake.

Virtually all nutritionally complete enteral preparations contain adequate levels of vitamins and minerals when

TABLE 2

PROTOCOLS FOR MAGNESIUM AND PHOSPHORUS REPLACEMENT

Current Serum Magnesium Level	Total Magnesium Replacement
1.5–2.0 mg/dL	2 g magnesium sulfate IV over 1 hr
0.9–1.4 mg/dL	4 g magnesium sulfate over 2 hr
<0.9 mg/dL	Call physician
Current Serum Phosphorus Level	**Total Phosphorus Replacement**
2.0–2.5 mg/dL	15 mmol potassium phosphate IV over 4 hr
1.0–1.9 mg/dL	21 mmol potassium phosphate IV over 4 hr
<1.0 mg/dL	30 mmol potassium phosphate IV over 4 hr

sufficient amounts of the formula are given to meet one's caloric needs. On the other hand, patients receiving parenteral nutrition require complete vitamin and mineral supplementation. Parenteral formulations created in most hospitals contain a commercially available product containing the 12 essential vitamins. It is necessary, however, to add vitamin K, either daily or weekly, to those patients receiving parenteral nutrition alone. It is also prudent to supplement parenteral solutions with zinc, copper, manganese, chromium, as well as selenium. Trace mineral deficiencies can occur as a result of increased utilization, malabsorption syndromes, and elevated urinary excretion.

Specific disease processes may warrant a disease-specific formulation or additional/restricted amounts of various supplements. Patients with fat malabsorption, as seen in those with pancreatic insufficiency, may require supplementation of the fat-soluble vitamins A, D, E, and K. For patients receiving oral anticoagulant therapy with warfarin, one may choose to have vitamin K withheld. Manganese and copper are excreted in the bile and care must be given when supplementing these trace minerals in patients with cholestasis. Patients who are extremely catabolic and those with persistent diarrhea or high-output stomas or fistulae will have elevated zinc requirements. Chronic malnourished and alcoholic patients benefit from the administration of thiamine. Many vitamins and minerals are also subject to poor absorption in patients with short bowel syndrome and those having had extensive ileal resections and parenteral supplementation may be necessary.

IMMUNOMODULATION

It was previously mentioned that the gut is an important immunologic organ. Over the last several decades much attention has been given to the supplementation of parenteral and enteral formulations with various substances, namely glutamine, arginine, Omega-3 fatty acids, β carotene, and nucleotides. Several enteral formula manufacturers are now producing products that contain varying combinations of these immunonutrients. Many animal and human studies have been undertaken to determine whether the addition of these nutrients either alone or in combination could potentially change the pathophysiology of traumatic injury, sepsis, and other forms of critical illness. Unfortunately, many of the findings identified in the preclinical trials have not been replicated in the counterpart human trials.

Glutamine

Amino acids are classified as either being essential or nonessential, depending on the organism's ability to synthesize the amino acid *de novo* from other amino acids and precursors. Recently, the concept of the "conditionally essential" amino acid has come into existence. Several amino acids are nonessential under normal conditions, but in times of a major catabolic illness, the body's ability to synthesize adequate amounts becomes overwhelmed, demand is greater than supply, and supplementation may be necessary. Glutamine is a prime example of a conditionally essential amino acid.

The importance of the GI tract as an immune organ and the significant benefits of early nutritional support are widely recognized. Glutamine has received much attention over the last several years in the surgical literature and its importance in improving gut barrier function is well known. It is the most abundant amino acid in the body and is considered a nonessential amino acid under normal circumstances. This important amino acid has several roles. Most notably, it is the preferred fuel source for rapidly dividing cells such as enterocytes and immunocytes. It is a precursor for many other substances such as nucleotides and the antioxidant glutathione. It is also a precursor to urinary ammonia and thereby regulates acid–base balance. It is a major substrate for renal gluconeogenesis. Glutamine is one of the "conditionally essential" amino acids and during critical illness glutamine stores become depleted and a state of glutamine deficiency exists.

Preclinical studies of glutamine supplementation have consistently demonstrated decreased mucosal atrophy, decreased intestinal permeability, and increased resistance to the effects of gut ischemia and reperfusion. A meta-analysis of 14 randomized trials evaluating human enteral glutamine therapy demonstrated fewer infectious complications and a shorter hospital stay.[2] The greatest benefit was in those patients receiving high-dose, parenteral glutamine.

Arginine

Arginine is a dibasic amino acid with many important roles in the transport, storage, and excretion of nitrogen. Like glutamine, arginine is conditionally essential and the ability to synthesize adequate levels of this important nutrient in times of stress may be exceeded. Arginine is a precursor to nitric oxide, stimulates the secretion of growth hormone and other anabolic agents such as insulin and insulin-like growth factor. It is important in wound healing and is essential to the proper functioning of the immune system through the stimulation of T lymphocytes. Through ornithine, which is a polyamine precursor, arginine also plays a pivotal role in DNA synthesis.

Omega 3 Fatty Acids

Major injury, sepsis, and critical illness all result in significant alterations in immune function. Omega-6 polyunsaturated fatty acids (linoleic acid) are a major constituent of cell membranes. These cannot be synthesized *de novo* and are therefore considered to be essential. Linoleic acid is a precursor for the synthesis of various immunosuppressive prostaglandins and leukotrienes. The detrimental effects of lipids in general have been previously described. Of the long-chain fatty acids, the Omega-3 polyunsaturated fatty acids appear to have the greatest potential for clinical benefit in modulating immune response and improving patient outcome. Omega-3 fatty acids (fish and canola oils) have been found to be more immunostimulatory and have the potential to modulate the catabolic response to injury. The ratio of Omega-3 to Omega-6 fatty acids appears to be important in optimizing immune function. The difference lies in their more favorable prostanoid and leukotriene end products. The Omega-3 family of fatty acids has been shown to reduce the development of atherosclerosis and incidence of myocardial infarction, reduce hypertension, and improve outcome from various proinflammatory states.

Summary

Several of the previously mentioned nutrients have been shown in experimental animal models to favorably modulate the immune system. Clinical trials have also been conducted to examine the clinical efficacy of many of these specialized formulations with immunostimulatory activity. It is difficult to draw conclusions due to the heterogeneity of both the product formulations tested and the patient populations studied. Many of these publications suggested a benefit; however, the findings have not been consistently corroborated. A recently published large randomized controlled trial showed no benefit to immunonutrition on outcome parameters in a general ICU population.[3] Because of these varying results, several meta-analyses have been conducted. Although subject to the limitations inherent to meta-analyses, it was suggested that these products lead to shorter lengths of hospital stay and a decrease in the numbers of infectious complications seen. Other meta-analyses drew differing conclusions. The topic of immunonutrition in critically ill patients obviously continues to be subject to much debate and remains very controversial. As suggested in a recent editorial by Heyland et al.,[4] perhaps it will be necessary to individually evaluate specific nutrients in homogeneous patient populations to draw any sound conclusions on this topic. It is important to realize that in any given critically ill patient, a hyper- and hypoinflammatory state may coexist in differing arms of the complex inflammatory response.

It appears that supplementing enteral formulations with glutamine confers a benefit to patients with trauma and burns. Such a benefit seems to be absent with regard to arginine, and in septic patients this may even be harmful. Arginine supplementation is not recommended at this time. It is unclear at this time whether additional benefit is gained from the addition of Omega-3 fatty acids. A benefit in patients with acute respiratory distress syndrome (ARDS) has been suggested. When evaluating the risk–benefit ratio of these formulations, one must also consider that some of these products are quite expensive.

ENTERAL VERSUS PARENTERAL NUTRITION

Although parenteral nutrition can be lifesaving and has been recognized as one of the great medical accomplishments of the 20th century,[5] indiscriminant use is associated with poor wound healing, increased infectious complications and higher septic morbidity,[6] increased mucosal permeability, gut flora alterations, as well as increased costs. The landmark Veterans Affairs (VA) Cooperative Study demonstrated that the risks of parenteral nutritional therapy exceeded the benefits when TPN was administered to borderline or mildly malnourished patients undergoing elective general surgery procedures.[7] Enteral nutrition is more physiologic, preserves immune and gut barrier function, and by blunting the release of counter-regulatory stimuli may help diminish the hypermetabolic response to injury. It results in decreased activation of the gut-associated lymphoid tissue (GALT) with decreased activation of proteolytic cytokines. The theory of immunoglobulin A (IgA)-mediated maintenance of other organ systems' mucosa is yet another potential benefit. With the use of the enteral route the liver is not bypassed and hepatic function is maintained, thereby preserving acute phase protein synthesis and adequate biliary secretion. Enteral administration of nutrition is also associated with better glycemic control for insulin-independent uptake of glucose from the portal vein occurs. Less hyperglycemia and hyperinsulinemia is seen, the benefits of which have been discussed.

It is important to remember that the small bowel can tolerate enteral nutrition in the recovery room! The presence of bowel sounds or the passage of flatus or stool is not a prerequisite for the initiation of enteral nutritional support. There is a generalized misconception across several medical specialties that in many disease states the gut will not work. In contrast to these beliefs, contraindications are few and include complete bowel obstruction and severe hemodynamic instability. Enteral nutrition should be delayed until mesenteric perfusion is restored. Relative contraindications include high-output intestinal fistula, severe acute inflammatory bowel disease and/or diarrhea, marked ileus, and massive upper or lower GI hemorrhage. It has been shown that the enteral route is safe even in patients with sever pancreatitis.

Patients with a nonfunctioning GI tract or those with limited absorptive capacity (short bowel syndrome) may benefit from parenteral modalities. One should always consider low-rate trophic enteral nutrition as an adjunct to parenteral nutritional therapy to preserve gut mucosal integrity. If at all possible, at least 20% of the caloric intake should be provided enterally. Parenteral nutrition is certainly an option when the enteral route is contraindicated. It has also been used to augment inadequate oral intake, although a properly placed feeding tube can certainly accomplish this. Outside of the absolute contraindications previously listed, our group rarely uses parenteral nutrition in our daily surgical critical care practice.[10,11]

Patients with open abdomens and "enteroatmospheric" fistulae pose a specific problem. Decisions on how to feed these patients depend on the location and number of fistulae, as well as the amount and character of the output. The importance of some type of enteral sustenance in these fragile and malnourished individuals cannot be overstated. Combinations of low-rate tube feedings and parenteral nutrition may be necessary. Nutritional formulations can be delivered proximal to, distal to, or directly into fistulas that are present. Although feeding such individuals can increase the output volume, we have found that the integrity of the bowel wall involved in such fistulae is strengthened with direct enteral support, allowing easier surgical or at times even spontaneous closure.

ENTERAL ACCESS APPROACHES

It is our practice to begin enteral nutritional support within 12 to 24 hours on our severely burned and traumatically injured patients. Several studies have suggested that patients who are likely to need nutritional support (i.e., access) include ICU disposition, Injury Severity Score, Abdominal Trauma Index, and the need for early surgical intervention.

Many options are available for the delivery of enteral nutrition including nasogastric, nasoenteric, gastrostomy, and jejunostomy tubes. Surgically or endoscopically created transgastric jejunostomy feeding tubes are yet another option. Frequently we will use the simplest and most physiologic option, the nasogastric tube that was placed in the trauma room, to initiate gastric feedings. If initiated early, tolerance is acceptable. Gastric secretions help dilute the hyperosmolar formulations, thereby decreasing problematic diarrhea. The small bowel is less able to tolerate hyperosmotic loads. Gastric feedings stimulate the liver and pancreas with resultant positive effects on the small bowel. In the event of gastric hypomotility and elevated residuals (>200 mL per 4 hours), a post pyloric feeding tube should be placed. It may be necessary to simultaneously feed the jejunum and drain the stomach through two separate tubes.

We will routinely change our nasogastric tubes to smaller bore feeding tubes if it appears that the patient will receive tube feedings for a prolonged time. Several methods of placement include blind insertion, fluoroscopic guidance, or endoscopic placement. Many other insertion adjuncts are now commercially available. Smaller tubes improve patient comfort, are less erosive to the pharynx and esophagus, decrease the risk of reflux, and help avoid the complications associated with prolonged placement of large nasal tubes such as sinusitis. In patients undergoing laparotomy, transpyloric feeding tubes are placed at the time of surgery unless the patient is found to have a minor isolated injury.

It is also important to avoid routine orders for the discontinuation of enteral feedings after midnight in intubated patients undergoing surgical procedures the following day. This is especially important in burned individuals who have massive energy needs and require frequent trips back and forth to the operating room. It is usually safe to continue feedings up to the time of surgery and some burn centers even continue feeding through the surgical procedure. Other options include increasing the rate or concentration of the formula in the hours leading up to the NPO period to maintain adequate nutritional intake.

For patients requiring enteral nutrition for longer periods (>1 month) with oropharyngeal dysfunction or other conditions that preclude resumption of adequate oral intake, we place a percutaneous endoscopic gastrostomy (PEG) tube. This may need to be done earlier in patients with massive craniofacial trauma. Placement can be done under local anesthesia and intravenous sedation either in the endoscopy suite or in the ICU. Laparoscopic and radiologic methods have also been described. Complications include wound problems and necrotizing soft tissue infections, dislodgement with separation of the stomach from the abdominal wall and resultant peritonitis, bleeding and injury to the colon. Proper insufflation of the stomach and adequate transillumination of the abdominal wall helps ensure adequate placement. Meticulous care and hygiene of the tube site and avoidance of excessive tension against the gastric wall will help prevent gastric necrosis at the PEG insertion site. It is prudent to protect against inadvertent removal and we have found the use of binders helpful in patients with traumatic brain injury. When checking residuals in patients with poor tolerance to gastric feedings it is important to remember that the dependant portions of the stomach are not adequately drained by the anteriorly positioned button of the tube, and in such circumstances

the placement of a nasogastric tube may be necessary to accomplish adequate drainage.

In patients requiring a laparotomy for other reasons, thought should be given during surgery toward the creation of a Stamm type of gastrostomy. We rarely create a surgical jejunostomy.

COMPLICATIONS OF NUTRITION

Gastric Dysmotility and Aspiration

Mortality secondary to enteral nutrition is mostly due to aspiration, especially in septic patients who may exhibit abrupt changes in gastric motility. It is important to maintain the patient with the head of the bed elevated in the 30-degree reverse Trendelenburg position to decrease the risk of aspiration. Fatal aspiration can occur even in the presence of a cuffed endotracheal or tracheostomy tube. The evidence that gastric versus postpyloric feeding is associated with differences in the rate of aspiration pneumonitis is controversial. Heyland et al., using radioisotope-labeled enteral feeds, showed that feeding beyond the pylorus was associated with a significant reduction in gastroesophageal regurgitation and a trend toward less microaspiration.[8] It may be that many critically ill patients are at risk for aspiration regardless of which part of the gut is fed.

The benefits of feeding the stomach as opposed to the small bowel have been discussed. Early initiation of gastric feedings, especially in burned patients, helps to improve gastric tolerance. Nevertheless, several patients exhibit varying forms of gastric atony and will simply need to be fed more distally. Patients tolerating gastric administration of enteral solutions may have abrupt changes in motility thereby increasing their risk for aspiration. Heightened suspicion for a cause of the dysmotility is warranted, because it may be a sign of developing sepsis or acute stress ulceration. More prolonged gastric atony may be seen in up to 30% of critically ill patients.

We will frequently check gastric residuals in patients being fed into the stomach and if they are >200 mL, the infusion will be held for 4 hours and the residuals rechecked. If gastroparesis persists, the patient is placed on a prokinetic agent. Metoclopramide is a dopamine agonist that has effects on the esophagus, stomach, and small intestine. It can be given intravenously or as a syrup into the feeding tube. Erythromycin is reserved for continued gastroparesis resistant to metoclopramide. Erythromycin can be given intravenously or as a suspension into the feeding tube and increases motilin release from the duodenum, thereby improving gastric motility.

Although the concept of postpyloric feeding is controversial, it is probably wise to feed beyond the pylorus and perhaps even beyond the ligament of Treitz if gastric residuals remain high. Initially, it is important to simultaneously drain the stomach and continue to monitor the daily nasogastric output. Persistent large volume drainage from the stomach may warrant endoscopy or a radiographic study to rule out a gastric outlet obstruction and/or ulceration. It is also important in such individuals to carefully monitor their overall intake and output because significant amounts of volume, chloride and acid can be lost, and metabolic derangements can occur. Pure gastric volume loss leads to the development of a hypochloremic, hypokalemic metabolic alkalosis, which is preventable with adequate fluid and electrolyte replacement. In the event of reflux of feedings into the stomach, consideration must be given to the possibility of a more distal obstruction.

Diarrhea

Diarrhea is yet another cumbersome "complication" of enteral nutrition. It results in significant loss of volume and electrolytes and makes nursing care very difficult. Diarrhea may or may not be related to the delivery of the enteral solution itself. Osmolalities of enteral products are normally between 200 and 500 mOsm per L. More concentrated solutions with osmolalities that approach 700 mOsm per L, when delivered directly into the small bowel have the potential to cause an osmotic type of diarrhea. Initiating these formulas gradually may limit this problem. It is frequently necessary to slow the rate of the formula, decrease its strength by adding free water, or to switch to a less concentrated solution altogether.

Other causes of diarrhea must be excluded. Antibiotic-associated diarrhea (pseudomembranous colitis) is a form of secretory diarrhea that is becoming commonplace in ICUs, sometimes with life-threatening complications. Persistent high volume, foul smelling diarrhea warrants a workup for antibiotic-associated causes. Several pharmacologic agents can also cause diarrhea including the use of metoclopramide instituted for gastroparesis. Oral magnesium replacement or other medications containing large amounts of sorbitol may be the culprit.

Shortly after admission to our ICU, patients are initially placed on a regimen to decrease problems associated with *constipation*. When a patient begins to have problematic diarrhea, our first intervention is to discontinue the docusate sodium and bisacodyl that these patients are frequently receiving. It is prudent to review the medications' sorbitol content, and consideration toward switching to an intravenous form must be given. Metoclopramide should be discontinued. It is frequently necessary to use loperamide (Kaopectate) and/or opioids to slow the diarrhea. As with any condition associated with the loss of volume and electrolytes, meticulous observation with respect to the patient's fluid balance, electrolyte, and acid–base status needs to be carried out. Choosing a fiber-containing formula is yet another strategy to consider.

Many tube-feeding preparations now contain a combination of soluble and insoluble fiber. Fiber-based solutions may delay intestinal transit time and reduce the incidence of diarrhea compared to nonfiber solutions. Soluble fiber is provided in the form of pectins. Soluble fiber may serve as a substrate for the formation of short chain fatty acids (SCFAs) by luminal bacterial fermentation. These SCFAs (namely, butyrate) are not synthesized endogenously but are important nevertheless because they are the primary respiratory fuel for the colonocyte. Indirectly fiber can help in the ability of the cell to increase sodium, potassium, and water absorption, thereby benefiting patients with diarrhea. Fiber has a myriad other benefits. By slowing down the gastric emptying process, rapid peaks of glucose concentrations are minimized. Fiber also binds bile acids and dietary cholesterol and lowers serum cholesterol.

Hyperglycemia

The subject of hyperglycemia in the critically ill has become a popular topic in peer-reviewed journals dealing with patients across many medical and surgical subspecialties. It is becoming increasingly clear that avoidance of hyperglycemia improves clinical outcome and frequent blood glucose determinations are warranted at the initiation of nutritional therapy. Van Den Berghe et al. showed that intensive insulin therapy to maintain blood glucose levels at or <110 mg per dL reduces morbidity and mortality among critically ill patients in the surgical ICU.[9] It should be mentioned, however, that the subpopulation of patients that benefited from intensive glucose control were mostly patients recovering from cardiac surgery and in the group of patients with multiple trauma or severe burns, mortality was actually higher when the glucose levels were kept <110 mg per dL (12.1 vs. 8.6%). Our practice is to maintain blood glucose levels <150 mg per dL with the use of an aggressive sliding scale regimen and neutral protamine hagedorn (NPH) insulin. On occasion, especially in diabetic patients, a diabetic enteral formulation is useful. Continuous insulin infusions are typically reserved for patients with glucose levels resistant to such therapy that remain >200 mg per dL.

REFERENCES

1. Cheatham ML, Safcsak K, Brzezinski SJ, et al. Ensuring adequate nutritional support: Nitrogen balance, protein loss, and the open abdomen. *ANZ J Surg.* 2005;75(4):a17–a18.
2. Novak F, Heyland DK, Avenell A, et al. Glutamine supplementation in serious illness: A systematic review of the evidence. *Crit Care Med.* 2002;30:2022–2029.
3. Kieft H, Roos AN, van Drunen JDE, et al. Clinical outcome of immunonutrition in a heterogenous intensive care population. *Intensive Care Med.* 2005;31:524–532.
4. Heyland D, Dhaliwal R. Immunonutrition in the critically ill: From old approaches to new paradigms. *Intensive Care Med.* 2005;31:501–503.
5. Dudrick SJ, Wilmore DW, Vars HM, et al. Long-term total parenteral nutrition with growh, development, and positive nitrogen balance. *Surgery.* 1968;64:134.
6. Moore FA, Feliciano DV, Andrassy FJ, et al. Early enteral feeding, compared with parenteral, reduced postoperative septic complications. *Ann Surg.* 1992;216:172–183.

7. The Veteran Affairs TPN Cooperative Study Group. Perioperatrive TPN in surgical patients. *N Engl J Med.* 1991;325:525–532.
8. Heyland DK, Drover JW, MacDonald S, et al. Effect of feeding on gastroesophageal regurgitation and pulmonary microaspiration: Results of a randomized controlled trial. *Crit Care Med.* 2001;29:1495–1501.
9. Van Den Berghe G, Wouters P, Weekers F, et al. Intensive insulin therapy in critically ill patients. *N Engl J Med.* 2001;345:1359–1367.
10. Mainous MR, Block EFJ, Deitch EA. Nutritional support of the gut: how and why. *New Horiz.* 1994;2(2):193–201.
11. Byers PM, Block EJ, Albornoz JC, et al. Critical pathways in trauma: The need for aggressive nutritional interventional support in the injured patient – a predictive model. *J Trauma.* 1995;39(6):1103–1109.

SUGGESTED READINGS

Dabrowski GP, Rombeau JL. Practical nutritional management in the trauma intensive care unit. *Surg Clin North Am.* 2000;80:921–932.
Heyland DK, Dhaliwal R, Drover JW, et al. Canadian Critical Care Clinical Practice Guidelines Committee. Canadian clinical practice guidelines for nutrition support in mechanically ventilated, critically ill adult patients. *J Parenter Enteral Nutr.* 2003;27: 355–373.
Jacobs DG, Jacobs DO, Kudsk KA, et al. EAST Practice Management Guidelines Work Group. Practice management guidelines for nutritional support of the trauma patient. *J Trauma.* 2004;57:660–679.

Renal Failure

64

Glen H. Tinkoff

Posttraumatic acute renal failure is an infrequent occurrence. Less than 1% of all trauma admissions sustain acute renal failure severe enough to warrant dialysis.[1] This relatively small number of patients progressing to dialysis likely reflects the demographics of the trauma population and improvements in transport, resuscitation, and critical care that have evolved over the last 50 years. However, for those patients requiring dialysis and intensive care, the mortality rate is 50% to 70%.

In the injured patient, primary risk factors for the development of acute renal failure is more related to the severity and duration of renal hypoperfusion, exposure to nephrotoxins, and the preexistence of renal insufficiency or comorbidities associated with renal compromise rather than direct injury to the kidneys. Three quarters of renal injuries are minor and incur almost no risk of renal compromise. However, after major renovascular injury the incidence of dialysis-dependent renal failure has been reported to be as high as 6.4%.[2]

DEFINITIONS

Acute renal failure is an abrupt decline in kidney function resulting in an inability to clear and excrete metabolic waste and maintain proper fluid balance. There is not a universal laboratory or clinical definition for acute renal failure. Most commonly used definitions include the following:

(A) An absolute increase in serum creatinine of 0.5 mg per dL or greater from baseline
(B) A 50% increase in serum creatinine
(C) A 50% reduction in calculated creatinine clearance
(D) A decrease in renal function that warrants dialysis

Acute renal failure is marked by azotemia, an increase (>50% over baseline) in serum blood urea nitrogen (BUN) and other nitrogenous substances. Azotemia is associated with oliguria defined as urine output <400 mL per 24 hours and on occasion, anuria defined as urine output <100 mL per 24 hours.

CLASSIFICATIONS

Azotemia resulting from decreased renal perfusion without cellular injury is known as *prerenal azotemia*. The injured patient is subject to many factors that can lead to diminished renal blood flow including loss of intravascular volume, decreased effective intravascular volume, diminished cardiac output, or exposure to vasoconstrictive medications. Prerenal azotemia accounts for most of the azotemia found in trauma patients and can be usually remedied by addressing the primary etiology (e.g., correction of the volume deficit).

Azotemia related to obstruction of urinary out flow can be termed *obstructive uropathy*. Common trauma-related causes are urethral disruption associated with a pelvic fracture, ureteral or cystic compression from pelvic retroperitoneal hemorrhage, clotted blood within the genitourinary tract, neurogenic bladder associated with a spinal cord injury, or an obstructed urinary catheter. Timely sonographic assessment and correction or diversion of the obstruction is essential because duration of obstruction is inversely related to recovery of renal function.

Intrinsic causes for acute renal failure can be categorized according to the primary anatomic sites of injury. These are the renal interstitium, the glomeruli, and the renal tubules. The renal interstitium is subject to a diffuse inflammatory process known as *interstitial nephritis*. Interstitial nephritis is most often caused by an allergic reaction to medication. Other causes include autoimmune disease, malignancy, and/or infectious agents. Renal failure due to interstitial nephritis is often reversible after withdrawal of the offending agent. Corticosteroids may hasten the recovery of renal function; however, their role remains controversial in the absence of controlled clinical trials.

The glomeruli can also be affected and glomerulonephritis can present as a subacute or acute renal failure. Histopathologic examination of the kidney is often necessary to make a diagnosis of etiology. Prompt use of appropriate immunosuppressive agents and plasma exchange may be indicated to reduce the occurrence of end-stage renal failure.

Injury to the tubules, acute tubular necrosis (ATN), is the most common etiology of acute renal failure in the trauma patient. The cause of this injury is usually due to ischemic insult to the tubules. Prerenal azotemia is a common precursor to this ischemia. If renal perfusion is not corrected in a timely manner, ATN will arise. Nephrotoxins such as myoglobin, contrast media, aminoglycosides, or amphotericin can also play a role in the development of ATN.

ANATOMY

The functional unit of the kidney is the nephron. It is estimated that the human kidney contains 1 to 1.5×10^6 nephrons. The nephron consists of a glomerulus, a capillary complex with afferent and efferent arterioles, and the Bowman capsule that receives the filtrate from the glomerulus and a tubule. The nephron's tubule consists of a proximal convoluted tubule, a loop of Henle, a thick ascending tubule, and a distal convoluted tubule which empties into the collecting duct. These collecting ducts coalesce into the calyces and pelvis of the kidney. The renal cortex contains the glomeruli and proximal and distal convoluted tubules, whereas the loop of Henle and thick ascending tubules extend into the renal medulla along with a distal capillary bed known as the *vasa recta*.

PHYSIOLOGY

The major elements of renal function are glomerular filtration, and tubular excretion and reabsorption. The kidneys receive 20% of the cardiac output with the majority of that flow directed at the renal cortex to support glomerular filtration. Renal blood flow including glomerular blood flow is subject to autoregulation and is maintained within a narrow range (<10% variation) over a wide range of perfusion pressures (80 to 180 mm Hg). Renal blood flow autoregulation is governed by neural, hormonal, and local paracrine mediators.

The afferent arteriole of the glomerulus empties into a porous capillary bed contained within the Bowman capsule. Effluent glomerular blood empties into a high-resistance efferent arteriole, which enters a peritubular capillary network (vasa recta). Virtually all plasma without proteins passes into the Bowman capsule due to the relatively high hydrostatic pressure to which the glomerulus is subjected. This proteinfree plasma ultrafiltrate is produced at a well-controlled rate known as the *glomerular filtration rate* (GFR). Naturally occurring substances such as creatinine can be utilized to measure GFR by the following equation:

$$\text{Creatinine clearance} = \frac{\frac{\text{urine volume (mL/minute)}}{\text{collection time}}}{\times \frac{\text{urine creatinine}}{\text{plasma creatinine}}}$$

This dilute ultrafiltrate enters the nephron's tubule where it is concentrated by reabsorption of sodium and water. Within the renal medulla, the surrounding vasa recta allows for countercurrent exchange. Active reabsorption of sodium occurs at the water-impermeable thick ascending limb while water is extracted from the relatively solute impermeable loop of Henle. Glucose, potassium, chloride, and phosphate are also actively reabsorbed in the tubule. Urea is passively reabsorbed with the amount inversely proportional to tubular flow rate. During high flow, up to 70% of urea is excreted; urea excretion drops to only 10% to 20% in low flow situations. Hydrogen and ammonium ions are both secreted in the tubule in response to the surrounding pH.

PATHOPHYSIOLOGY OF TRAUMATIC ACUTE TUBULAR NECROSIS

Regardless of the inciting event, ATN arises from two major factors, renal ischemia and direct toxic insult to the nephron tubule. Renal ischemia occurs from diminished absolute effective circulating volume. This ischemia leads to renal vasoconstriction with reduction in renal blood flow and loss of autoregulation. The consequent reduction in glomerular blood flow decreases glomerular filtration. Furthermore, the medullary thick ascending tubule due to its high oxygen demands is exquisitely sensitive to an ischemic insult. This insult leads to early impairment of the countercurrent exchange mechanism and the loss of the concentration ability of the kidney. As decreased intrarenal blood flow persists, adherent neutrophils and platelets obstruct capillaries and cause persistence of the ischemia with collapse of normal feedback mechanisms.

In response to the ischemic insult, morphologic changes occur in tubule cells, including loss of their brush border, loss of polarity, and loss of integrity of the tight junctions between cells. Dead and dying cells along the tubule obstruct the lumen contributing to cast formation and increase intratubular pressure, further reducing GFR. Loss of these tubular epithelial cells and the tight junctions between viable cells lead to leakage of glomerular filtrate into the interstitial space causing medullary congestion. Nephrotoxins can harm tubular epithelial cells in a similar manner and cause ATN despite the presence of adequate circulating renal blood volume.

Following ischemic or toxic injury, the renal tubule cells can progress onto apoptosis, necrosis, or dedifferentiation and proliferation. With timely and adequate supportive measures, the latter response predominates and leads to recovery of tubular function. The kidney can completely regenerate normal structure and restore full function after injury.

ETIOLOGY

The most common cause of traumatic ATN is due to prolonged volume deficit without sufficient resuscitation. However, a variety of other conditions commonly experienced in the management of the injured patient significantly contribute to the development of ATN.

Myoglobin and Hemoglobin

Rhabdomyolysis is the release of myoglobin after muscle necrosis and occurs with major crush injuries, limb ischemia often associated with compartment syndrome, and thermal or electrical injuries. Massive hemoglobinuria occurs in settings of extensive hemolysis from transfusion reactions. Both these pigments, hemoglobin and myoglobin, are not nephrotoxic, but are converted to ferrihemate in the presence of acid urine (pH <5.6), which is directly toxic to renal tubular cells. Furthermore, heme and myoglobin pigments may precipitate and coalesce with accompanying tubular cellular debris to form obstructing luminal casts. Finally, both agents induce nitric oxide–mediated renal juxtamedullary vasoconstriction, which further diminishes medullary oxygenation.

Radiologic Contrast Media

The iodinated contrast material utilized for intravascular imaging in trauma patients is nephrotoxic. These agents are potent renal vasoconstrictors and are toxic to the proximal tubule in a dose-dependent manner. The risk of contrast-induced acute renal failure is higher when associated with preexisting renal insufficiency, diabetes mellitus, or volume depletion. Fortunately, the clinical course is usually self-limited so that most patients return to baseline renal function by 7 to 10 days.

Abdominal Compartment Syndrome

Increased abdominal pressure (>25 mm Hg) in the trauma patient is a well-recognized phenomenon that may be caused by hemorrhage, ascites, bowel edema, bowel dilation, or intra-abdominal packing. Elevated intra-abdominal pressure can induce renal impairment by decreasing venous blood return to the heart, thereby compromising cardiac output, and more importantly, by local pressure exceeding renal arteriolar pressure and impairing GFR. Both processes

set the stage for ATN unless recognition of the abdominal compartment syndrome and abdominal decompression ensue in a timely manner.

Sepsis

Sepsis is the most common cause of late-onset ATN in the trauma patient. A major factor in sepsis-induced ATN is the induction of nitric oxide–mediated systemic vasodilation with compensatory intrarenal vasoconstriction and ischemia. Renal failure can also occur without systemic hypotension in the septic patient because decreased effective intravascular volume from these systemic hemodynamic derangements may cause intrarenal perfusion deficits. The combination of sepsis and real failure is associated with 70% mortality.

Aminoglycosides

An estimated 10% to 25% of patients receiving aminoglycosides develop some element of renal insufficiency, making these agents the most common cause of drug toxicity–induced ATN. Similar to many other nephrotoxins, aminoglycosides are directly injurious to the cells of the proximal tubule and are associated with vasoconstriction of the renal microcirculation. Nephrotoxicity is related to duration of therapy and trough serum concentrations. ATN seldom occurs if duration of therapy is <5 days. Once-a-day dosing may be less nephrotoxic by allowing a lower nadir in trough serum concentrations.

Amphotericin B

Polyene macrolides such as amphotericin B are particularly nephrotoxic agents that directly damage cell membranes and produce profound renal vasoconstriction. Amphotericin B can also cause a renal tubular acidosis with resultant metabolic acidosis and potassium and magnesium wasting. The renal insufficiency produced is dependent on total dose administered because doses <600 mg are rarely associated with renal toxicity. Cumulative doses exceeding 3 g cause ATN in 80% of patients.

PREVENTION

Preventing acute renal failure in the critically ill trauma patient is challenging. Prior medical history and exposure to nephrotoxins may not be readily available, nor can the patient be properly prepared to reduce their risk. Renal ischemia or nephrotoxin exposure may be unavoidable if hemorrhagic shock or rhabdomyolysis is present or if computed tomography (CT) scan or angiography is necessary. Whenever possible, efforts should be made to limit exposure of the patient to factors that increase the risk of developing acute renal failure. High-risk patients for development of acute renal failure should be identified. Age, in itself, is an important risk factor and is inversely related to the creatinine clearance as calculated by the Cockcroft-Gault equation:

$$\frac{(140 - age) \times \text{lean body weight (kg)}}{\text{Serum creatinine (mg/dL)} \times 72} \times 0.85 \text{ (for females)}$$

Lean body weight = the lesser of actual body weight or

$$50 \text{ kg (male) or } 45.5 \text{ kg (female)}$$
$$+2.3 \text{ kg/in. of height over 5 ft}$$

Other factors such as history of chronic renal insufficiency or diabetes mellitus should be sought during the secondary survey. Crush injuries or prehospital hypotension should alert caregivers about potential of renal compromise. Nephrotoxic antibiotics should be avoided unless specifically indicated and there are no better alternatives available.

Although frequently used, low-dose dopamine, loop diuretics such as furosemide, or mannitol have not been shown to be protective against the development of acute renal failure. For patients at risk for rhabdomyolysis (e.g., crush injuries, high-energy extremity fractures, electrical injuries, etc.) prevention of acute renal failure can be addressed through aggressive volume resuscitation, careful hemodynamic monitoring, and maintaining an adequate urine output of ≥1 mL/kg/hour. Alkalization of the urine should be considered in these patients to prevent pigment precipitation. An appropriate sodium bicarbonate solution, typically 150 mEq (three ampules) of sodium bicarbonate in a liter of 5% dextrose solution, can be administered and titrated to urine pH. Mannitol can be also infused at 10 mL per hour to 20 mL per hour to maintain diuresis as needed.

Recently, several prophylactic measures have arisen to mitigate the risk of contrast-induced nephropathy. These regimens that include the use of sodium bicarbonate solution, acetylcysteine, and fenoldopam are listed in Table 1. Although each regimen has been validated to some extent in the literature, none has been shown to be effective specifically in the acute management of the trauma patient.

DIAGNOSIS

The most common presentation of renal dysfunction in the trauma patient is an abrupt decrease in urine output (oliguria) with a commensurate rise in serum creatinine. Additional associated clinical findings are listed in Table 2. Nonoliguric renal failure can also occur and is most commonly associated with toxic renal insults such as rhabdomyolysis, hemolysis, or contrast-induced nephropathy.

In patients suspected of posttraumatic acute renal failure, diagnostic efforts should be directed at assuring

TABLE 1

REGIMENS FOR PREVENTION OF CONTRAST-INDUCED ACUTE RENAL FAILURE

Sodium bicarbonate solution[3]	154 mEq/L Na bicarbonate solution; 3 mL/kg/hr for 1 hr immediately before contrast administration, then 1 mL/kg/hr during and for 6 hr post contrast
Acetylcysteine[4]	600 mg b.i.d; day prior and day of contrast administration 0.45% or 0.9% saline at 1 mL/kg/hr for 12 hr precontrast and 6–12 hr postcontrast
Fenoldopam mesylate[5]	Fenoldopam 0.1–0.3 μg/kg/min 30 min to 2 hr before contrast administration 0.45% or 0.9% saline at 1 mL/kg/hr for 12 hr precontrast and 6–12 hr postcontrast

normovolemia, ruling out urinary obstruction, and early detection of renal parenchymal dysfunction. Any vascular volume deficit must be addressed promptly to optimize renal blood flow. Repletion should be guided by central venous pressure or pulmonary capillary wedge pressure monitoring. The urinary bladder should be catheterized and position and patency confirmed with irrigation and aspiration of the irrigant. If obstructive uropathy is suspected, renal ultrasonography or CT of the urinary tract should be undertaken to confirm or exclude the diagnosis.

Intrinsic renal function can be assessed through urinalysis. The fractional excretion of sodium (FE_{Na^+}) is considered to be the most reliable laboratory discriminator between prerenal azotemia and intrinsic renal failure. The fractional excretion of sodium (FE_{Na^+}) is calculated as shown:

$$FE_{Na^+} = (U_{Na}/Pl_{Na}) \div (U_{Cr}/Pl_{Cr}) \times 100$$

TABLE 2

CLINICAL FINDINGS ASSOCIATED WITH ACUTE RENAL FAILURE

Progressive azotemia
Hyperkalemia, hyperphosphatemia, hypocalcemia, hypermagnesemia
Metabolic acidosis
Congestive heart failure, hypertension, pericarditis, arrhythmias
Neurologic abnormalities—lethargy, confusion, seizures
Hematologic abnormalities—anemia, platelet dysfunction
Gastrointestinal—ileus, anorexia, nausea, vomiting, bleeding
Infections—impaired cellular immune defenses
Impaired wound healing
Drug toxicity due to impaired drug clearance

TABLE 3

COMPARISON OF PRERENAL AZOTEMIA AND ACUTE RENAL FAILURE

Test	Prerenal Azotemia	Intrinsic Renal Failure
Urine specific gravity	>1.020	<1.010
Urine osmolality (mOsm/L)	>500	<300–500
Urine sodium (mEq/L)	<20	>40
FE_{Na^+} (%)	<1%	≥2%
Urine sediment	Normal, occasional granular casts	Brown, granular casts, cellular debris

TABLE 4

TEMPORIZING TREATMENT OF HYPERKALEMIA

- Calcium gluconate (10%)—10 mL over 3–5 min (may repeat)
- 50 mL $D_{50}W$ administered with 10 units regular insulin IV
- Albuterol 5 mg nebulized or 400 μg subcutaneously
- If acidotic <pH 7.2, sodium bicarbonate 50–100 mEq IV
- Sodium polystyrene sulfonate (kayexalate)
  Oral—15 g in 50 mL of 20% sorbitol
  Rectal—30–50 g in 200 mL of 20% sorbitol as a retention enema

where U_{Na} = urea sodium, Pl_{Na} = plasma sodium, U_{Cr} = urea creatinine, and Pl_{Cr} = plasma creatinine.

Urine specific gravity, sodium, osmolality, and sediment may also be helpful (see Table 3).

MANAGEMENT

The initial management of the trauma patient with acute renal failure includes reversal or mitigation of the underlying etiology, limiting any further insults to the kidneys, and correcting acidosis and electrolyte imbalances. Any volume deficit should be corrected preferably with the guidance of a central venous pressure monitor or a pulmonary artery (PA) catheter. Once normovolemia is achieved, further administration of intravenous fluids should be judiciously administered on the basis of maintenance needs (≈10 mL/kg/day) and existing fluid losses. Associated anemia or coagulopathy should be corrected and nephrotoxins should be identified and discontinued if possible or adjusted appropriately.

Although conversion of oliguric renal failure to nonoliguric renal failure is an attractive therapeutic option given the reduced mortality and morbidity of the latter, attempts at doing so utilizing low-dose dopamine, high doses of furosemide, and mannitol infusions have not been supported by the evidence in the literature. In fact, the presence of nonoliguric renal failure is more related to the degree of the ischemic or toxic insult and is not an attribute of renal injury that is readily manipulated.

Hyperkalemia associated with renal failure can induce electrocardiographic abnormalities including life-threatening arrhythmias when serum concentrations exceed 6 mEq per dL. The rapidity of the rise in serum potassium is more important in cardiotoxicity than the absolute concentration. The electrocardiogram (ECG) changes associated with hyperkalemia are peaked T waves, PR interval prolongation, ST depression, and widened QRS complex leading ultimately to ventricular fibrillation. Cardiotoxic hyperkalemia should be treated with renal replacement therapy. However, temporizing measures can be initiated to avert life-threatening arrhythmias as outlined in Table 4.

Metabolic acidosis (pH <7.1) can also be temporized with bicarbonate administration. However, in most instances profound metabolic acidosis associated with renal failure is an indication for renal replacement therapy. Finally, because the most common cause of mortality in posttraumatic acute renal failure is sepsis, efforts should be directed at preventing and treating any infectious complications.

In trauma patients with their increased demands for wound healing and infection control, administration of sufficient protein and substrate are necessary for wound healing and immunocompetence. This effort is especially difficult in the fluid restricted patient with renal failure. Therefore, in most instances in the catabolic trauma patient with renal failure, renal replacement therapy should be initiated promptly. However, if the patient is noncatabolic, protein administration requirements should be limited to 0.8 to 1 g/kg/day of protein with an intake of 20 to 25 cal/kg/day of mixed substrate. Enteral feeding is the preferred route because it is associated with a reduced incidence of septic morbidity.

RENAL REPLACEMENT THERAPY

In most instances, the management of acute renal failure in the critically ill trauma patient will require renal replacement therapy. Although there are no absolute indications, common indications for initiating renal replacement therapy include volume overload, hyperkalemia, metabolic acidosis, and symptoms and signs of severe azotemia. While the technical aspects are beyond the scope of this chapter, the trauma surgeon should be knowledgeable as to the basic concepts and various modalities of this therapeutic option.

The goals of renal replacement therapy are straightforward: to remove accumulated fluid and toxins. All methods employ extracorporeal vascular access to deliver the patient's blood into a chamber, which contains a semipermeable membrane. Clearance of fluid and toxins results from convection (ultrafiltration or hemofiltration) and diffusion (dialysis) across this membrane. Convection techniques depend on the bulk movement of both the solutes and solvents across the membrane. Volume losses must be at least partially replaced with a fluid whose composition is similar to plasma. Diffusion techniques use the movement of solute across the membrane based on the concentration gradient across the membrane in countercurrent to a dialysate fluid.

In recent years, continuously administered venovenous and arteriovenous therapies have emerged as the preferred approach in critically ill trauma patients. These techniques include the following:

- Slow continuous ultrafiltration (SCUF)
- Continuous arteriovenous hemofiltration (CAVH) or continuous venovenous hemofiltration (CVVH)
- Continuous arteriovenous hemodialysis (CAVHD) or continuous venovenous hemodialysis (CVVHD)
- Continuous arteriovenous hemodiafiltration (CAVHDF) or continuous venovenous hemodiafiltration (CVVHDF)

The advantage of continuous renal replacement therapies over intermittent hemodialysis includes more precise fluid and metabolic control, decreased hemodynamic instability, the possibility of removing injurious cytokines, and the ability to administer adequate nutrition. These advantages must be weighed against the need for prolonged anticoagulation and nearly constant surveillance necessary for this continuous modality.

REFERENCES

1. Morris JM, Mucha P, Ross SE, et al. Acute post traumatic renal failure: A multicenter experience. *J Trauma.* 1991;31:1584–1590.
2. Knudson MM, Harrison PB, Hoyt DB, et al. Outcome after major resuscitation injuries: A Western Trauma Association multicenter report. *J Trauma.* 2000;49:1116–1122.
3. Merteu GJ, Burgess WP, Gray LV, et al. Prevention of contrast-induced nephropathy with sodium bicarbonate: A randomized controlled trail. *JAMA.* 2004;291:2328–2334.
4. Kay J, Chow WH, Chan TK, et al. Acetylcysteine for prevention of acute deterioration of renal function following elective coronary angiography and intervention: A randomized controlled trial. *JAMA.* 2003;289:553–558.
5. Stone GW, McCullough PA, Tumlin JA, et al. Fenoldopam Mesylate for the prevention of contrast-induced nephropathy: A randomized controlled trial. *JAMA.* 2003;290:2284–2291.

SUGGESTED READINGS

Clynne PA, Lightstone L. Acute renal failure. *Clin Med (Northfield Il).* 2001;1:263–273.

Chandler CF, Blinman T, Cryer HG. Acute renal failure. In: Feliciano DV, Moore EE, Mattox KL, eds. *Trauma,* 5th ed. New York: McGraw-Hill; 2004:1323–1550.

Fischer RP, Reed RL, Yatsu JS. Renal failure. In: Mattox KL, ed. *Complications of trauma,* 1st ed. New York: Churchill Livingstone; 1994:41–80.

Meyer AA. Renal failure. In: Souba WW, Fink MP, Jurkovich, GJ, et al. eds. *ACS Surgery principles and practice,* 2nd ed. New York: WebMD; 2002: 1441–1453.

Sangri N, Shubhada NA, Levin ML. Acute renal failure. *JAMA.* 2003;289:747–751.

Thadhani R, Marvel P, Bouvantre JV. Medical progress: Acute renal failure. *N Engl J Med.* 1996;334:1448–1460.

Vuchino S, Kellum JA, Bellomo R, et al. Acute renal failure in critically ill patients: A multinational, multicenter study. *JAMA.* 2005;294:813–818.

Transfusion and Coagulation in Trauma

Babak Sarani   **Patrick Reilly**

Hemorrhage remains the second leading cause of death from injury (brain injury being the first).[1] Approximately 33% of trauma-related deaths are due to hemorrhage, and of the 12 million units of blood that are transfused annually in the United States, 1.8 million units (15%) are used in trauma patients.[2] Early mortality in bleeding patients who do not die at the scene is due to acidosis, hypothermia, and coagulopathy—the lethal triad of trauma. Appropriate and aggressive blood and factor replacement is a vital part of the overall resuscitation of these patients and may be as important as the strategy for stopping the bleeding. Recent research on this issue has focused both on novel approaches to resuscitation and novel techniques and adjuncts for preventing or treating coagulopathy.

Blood transfusion was first used to support bleeding patients during the United States Civil War and was accepted into medical practice during World War I.[1] More recently, the military's experiences continue to provide new insights into how aggressive transfusion practices and novel hemostatic agents may improve outcome in exsanguinating patients. However, these practices must be balanced against increasing evidence that transfusion is an independent risk factor for morbidity and mortality in critically ill and injured patients. This chapter discusses the need to balance the short-term benefits of blood and blood component transfusion with the long-term risks in trauma patients. This chapter will describe indications where allogenic transfusion may be lifesaving, when it may be detrimental, and how blood component therapy should be used in trauma patients.

RED BLOOD CELL TRANSFUSION

Transfusion of red blood cells (RBCs) can help restore both oxygen-carrying capacity and circulating blood volume. The normal blood volume is 7% to 8% of ideal body weight. This corresponds to a hemoglobin level of 14 to 16 g per dL and a hematocrit of 40% to 45%. It is generally accepted that patients do not need to be transfused to a *normal* hemoglobin or hematocrit value; however, the exact hemoglobin or hematocrit that should serve as a trigger for transfusion remains ill defined, especially in acutely anemic or injured patients. Indications, or triggers, for transfusion in trauma patients are discussed further in the subsequent text.

Ideally, the patient should receive blood that has been typed and crossmatched. Blood typing involves identifying the patient's blood type based on ABO and Rh antigens and crossmatching involves mixing the patient's blood with donated blood to ensure that there is no cross-reaction from minor antigen or undetected antibody. A correctly performed type and crossmatch minimizes the chances of the patient developing a transfusion reaction resulting from antigen–antibody interactions (the most common reason for a transfusion reaction is clerical error in dispensing or administering blood). A patient's blood type can be determined and type-specific blood dispensed within 10 to 20 minutes, but a complete crossmatch takes 30 to 45 minutes.

Because of the time required to determine and dispense either type-specific or crossmatched blood, other options must be readily available for hemorrhaging patients. All trauma patients should have a "type and hold" or "type and crossmatch" specimen sent to the blood bank on arrival, but transfusion should be instituted immediately in those who present with ongoing hemorrhage or shock. Type "O" blood can be used in these instances because this blood type does not express A or B antigen and therefore is the "universal donor." Furthermore, type O− blood can be used in women of childbearing age to prevent sensitization to the Rh antigen and possible complications in future pregnancy. All trauma centers should either have several units of type O blood available in the ED area or immediately dispensed by the blood bank at the time of trauma-system activation.

Packed red blood cells (PRBCs) can be reconstituted using warmed normal saline at the time of infusion to promote warming, decrease viscosity, and enhance flow. A rapid infusion, in-line blood warmer system should be used in all instances where patients are being emergently transfused with nonreconstituted PRBC to prevent worsening hypothermia from administration of a large volume of cold blood. As discussed elsewhere, hypothermia is both a marker for mortality in trauma patients and also a known cause of coagulopathy.

Indications for and Benefits of Red Blood Cell Transfusion

The ultimate goal of PRBC transfusion is to increase oxygen delivery. Oxygen delivery is described by the formula: O_2 delivery = cardiac output $\times$ O_2 content where O_2 content = $1.34 \times$ hemoglobin $\times$ O_2 saturation + 0.003 $\times$ PaO_2. On the basis of this equation, oxygen delivery can be increased only by increasing cardiac output or the oxygen content of blood. Most often, attempts are made to increase O_2 delivery by increasing the oxygen saturation or hemoglobin. Increasing cardiac output beyond that seen in injured patients may result in increased myocardial oxygen consumption, which can cause demand ischemia in patients with coronary artery disease.

Indications for PRBC transfusion can be based on signs/symptoms of severe hemorrhagic shock or anemia, physiologic endpoints of hypoperfusion, or blood count. The need for transfusion can also be predicted using several scoring systems, although this is less useful during the actual resuscitation. Signs and symptoms of severe shock or anemia include ongoing bleeding, tachycardia, hypotension, oliguria, or altered mental status. Physiologic endpoints of hypoperfusion include lactic acidosis, base deficit, or decreased central/mixed venous oxygen saturation (SvO_2).

The Advanced Trauma Life Support manual of the American College of Surgeons categorizes severity of hemorrhage into four classes. Class I and II hemorrhage can be treated with crystalloid resuscitation alone and do not require PRBC transfusion; whereas, class III and IV hemorrhage (>30% loss of total blood volume or >1,500 mL) require PRBC as a key component of resuscitation. Such patients will be tachycardic (pulse >120 beats per minute), hypotensive, tachypneic, anxious, or confused.[3] Crystalloid resuscitation of severely anemic patients will not improve oxygen delivery and may actually worsen it by further diluting the RBC concentration. Furthermore, stored RBCs rapidly deplete 2,3 diphosphoglycerate (DPG) and can require up to 24 hours to replete their stores following transfusion.[4] During this time, there is a left shift of the oxyhemoglobin disassociation curve resulting in impaired offloading of oxygen from hemoglobin to the tissues. Therefore, transfusion should be used liberally during initial resuscitation and the physician should not wait for symptoms to develop before the start of transfusion in patients who may be bleeding because the benefit of restoring oxygen content may not be realized for many hours. Criteria for transfusion should be more stringent once the patient has been resuscitated and hemorrhage either excluded or controlled. Indications and techniques of massive transfusion will be discussed separately.

Physiologic criteria for transfusion are based on laboratory indices of end-organ ischemia and include lactic acidosis, base deficit, and decreased SvO_2. These tests are needed because they are more sensitive markers of hemorrhage and impaired oxygen delivery than vital signs alone.[5] In a series of studies, Davis et al. showed a dose–response curve between the magnitude of base deficit on admission and blood volume needed for resuscitation.[6,7] More recently, elevated lactate levels have been shown to be as reliable as the base deficit for predicting the need for transfusion with the added advantage of being more predictive of mortality than base deficit alone.[8-10] There have been few studies evaluating the role of SvO_2 in predicting the need for transfusion, and these studies have had conflicting results.[8,11] Whereas the role of SvO_2 in monitoring the cardiovascular status of patients in the intensive care unit has been validated, its role in resuscitation of acutely injured patients remains uncertain. Moreover, various single center studies have yielded conflicting results regarding the efficacy of blood transfusion in increasing tissue oxygen delivery in various trauma populations.[12-15] Because of the many detrimental effects of transfusion (discussed in the subsequent text), a consistent increase in tissue oxygen delivery has not been demonstrated in trauma patients, and SvO_2 alone is not an indication for transfusion following hemorrhage.

Historically, the transfusion trigger based *solely* on hemoglobin value was a level of 10 g per dL or a hematocrit of 30%. This was the value at which the blood was felt to have the highest oxygen-carrying capacity while also having the lowest viscosity, thereby decreasing cardiac work while maintaining peripheral oxygen delivery.[16] This practice was validated, in part, by studies on Jehovah's Witnesses showing that perioperative mortality increases significantly for each gram of hemoglobin <8 and lessens if the preoperative hemoglobin is >12.[17,18] However, more recently, several well-designed multicenter studies have shown either no benefit or an increase in morbidity and mortality when asymptomatic, *nonbleeding*, critically ill patients are transfused above a hemoglobin value of 7 g per dL.[19-21] This finding was corroborated through multiple single-center studies in various types of trauma patients, where blood transfusion was shown to be an independent predictor of increased length of stay, infection, morbidity, and mortality.[13,15,22-28] On the basis of these studies, the current recommendation in asymptomatic, nonbleeding, anemic patients who have been resuscitated and are hemodynamically stable is to transfuse to maintain a hemoglobin concentration >7 g per dL unless there is evidence of ongoing end-organ ischemia.

Multiple scoring systems, such as the prehospital index, trauma score, revised trauma score, and injury severity score can be used to assess severity of injury and predict the need for blood transfusion. Although exact calculation of these scores is often cumbersome during the actual resuscitation, knowledge of the approximate degree of severity of injury and score can help the trauma surgeon predict the need for transfusion and mobilize necessary resources. Table 1 shows the various scoring systems and their variables. West et al. showed that 70% of patients with a trauma score ≤14 required a blood transfusion and 90% of patients with a score >14 did not.[29] Starr et al. showed that both the revised trauma score and the injury severity score predict

TABLE 2

BENEFITS AND RISKS OF BLOOD TRANSFUSION

Benefits	Risks
Restoration of intravascular volume and systemic perfusion	Transfusion reaction
Restoration of oxygen-carrying capacity	Transmission of blood-borne pathogen
Treatment of end-organ ischemia	Transfusion-related acute lung injury
Overall lower transfusion need (applies to use of whole blood in those requiring massive transfusion)	Transfusion-related immunomodulation
	Volume overload
	Coagulopathy (due to anticoagulant used when storing RBC)
	Multisystem organ failure and death

RBC, red blood cells.

the need for transfusion in patients with severe pelvic fractures.[30] The relationship between injury severity score and blood transfusion was further validated by Como[31] and more recently by Holcomb et al.[2] in a study of soldiers in Iraq.

In most reports, early transfusion of severely injured and bleeding patients is lifesaving and a standard of emergency care. Ultimately, the trauma surgeon must combine the mechanism of injury, probability of hemorrhage, vital signs, and laboratory tests in deciding whether to initiate transfusion. Although transfusion of blood is beneficial in bleeding patients and in those with severe anemia (hemoglobin <7 g per dL), as discussed in the subsequent text, it is also associated with late complications. Table 2 lists the possible benefits and detrimental effects of RBC transfusion. The trauma surgeon must weigh these risks and benefits in deciding if the patient meets indications for transfusion.

Detrimental Effects of Transfusion

As previously noted, blood transfusion carries risk and has been shown to increase morbidity and mortality independent of other factors in various patient populations, including trauma patients. Although transfusion reaction and transmission of blood-borne pathogen are rare, the cumulative risk of transmission of blood-borne pathogen can be significant following massive transfusion. Table 3 lists the incidence of blood-borne disease transmission following transfusion of 1 unit of PRBC. In addition, other adverse events are now being reported with increasing

TABLE 1

TRAUMA SCORING SYSTEMS

Trauma Score	Physiologic score based on the sum of scores for respiratory rate, respiratory effort, capillary refill, systolic blood pressure, and Glasgow Coma Score. A higher value is associated with *less* severe injury. Maximum score is 16, minimum score is 1.
Revised Trauma Score	Physiologic score based on the sum of scores for respiratory rate, systolic blood pressure, and Glasgow Coma Score. A higher value is associated with *less* severe injury. Maximum score is 12, minimum score is 0.
Injury Severity Score	Anatomic score based on the square of the sum of the three most injured regions: general, head/neck, chest, abdomen, extremity, and pelvis. Each region can have a score of 1–5, with 5 being life-threatening injury. A higher value is associated with *more* severe injury. Maximum score is 75, minimum score is 0.

TABLE 3

INCIDENCE OF BLOOD-BORNE PATHOGEN TRANSMISSION FOLLOWING RED BLOOD CELL TRANSFUSION

- Hepatitis A 1:1 million
- Hepatitis B 1:250,000
- Hepatitis C 1:150,000
- HIV 1:2 million
- Cytomegalovirus
- Prion/Creutzfeldt-Jakob disease unknown

---

frequency and include transfusion-related immunomodulation (TRIM), transfusion-associated volume overload, transfusion-related acute lung injury (TRALI), and possibly end-organ ischemia due to sludging. To date, the exact cause underlying these observations has not been elucidated, although many hypotheses are proposed. It is known, however, that the risks of transfusion are cumulative and may be related to cotransfusion of leukocytes and/or to storage time of the blood before transfusion. Furthermore, it has been suggested that cotransfusion of other soluble proteins, such as human leukocyte antigen (HLA) or antibody in blood or blood products may be responsible for some of the detrimental effects noted, especially TRIM and TRALI. It is possible that recipient leukocytes are activated through the interaction between the donor's antibody and the recipient's tissue resulting in a potent inflammatory response, particularly in the lung.

Immunomodulation following transfusion was first described more than 25 years ago when recipients of cadaveric renal transplants were noted to have a lower incidence of rejection if they received a unit of random donor PRBC in the perioperative period.[33–35] Most likely this immunosuppressive effect also accounts for the reason that transfused patients are also more likely to develop wound infection and pneumonia in the perioperative period.[19,25,36,37] In a meta-analysis by Hill et al., the odds ratio of infection following transfusion in the trauma cohort was 5.2 (confidence interval 5.03–5.43). The immunosuppressive effects of blood transfusion were further described in trauma patients with the observation that donor leukocytes can be found in the peripheral blood of transfused patients years after the transfusion itself.[27] Although the clinical significance of this finding is still unknown, this suggests that engraftment of donor stem cells and tolerance of donor leukocytes is occurring because of immunomodulation resulting from transfusion. This phenomenon has not been reported in transfused medical patients or those undergoing elective surgery. It is possible that the immunomodulatory effects of the trauma itself predispose some patients to develop this chimeric state. Lastly, increasing age of the blood transfused has also been

shown to cause derangement of the immune system by both causing the generation of inflammatory mediators and also increasing the incidence of wound infection.[26] This is especially relevant to trauma centers which tend to transfuse blood that is older than that in low-volume, nontrauma hospitals.

Transfusion-associated volume overload can occur in patients with preexisting cardiomyopathy or depressed cardiac function due to trauma or medications. Because blood products are colloids, they are able to draw fluid from the interstitial space into the intravascular space and are therefore very potent expanders of intravascular volume. It is generally taught that the ratio of the volume of colloid infused to the volume of colloid retained in the intravascular space is approximately 1:1 whereas this ratio is 3:1 for crystalloid. This means that patients with impaired cardiac function are at risk of developing cardiogenic pulmonary edema following robust colloid-based resuscitation. Similarly, patients may also develop anasarca without pulmonary edema, impeding healing of surgical wounds as well as efforts to mobilize the patient.[38–40] Complications related to massive transfusion are discussed separately in the subsequent text and are also listed in Table 4.

TRALI is increasingly diagnosed, although its true incidence is probably still underreported because of lack of consensus on its definition and overlap of signs and symptoms with adult respiratory distress syndrome (ARDS). TRALI is defined as noncardiogenic pulmonary edema occurring <4 hours after the start of transfusion. It is distinguished from ARDS by its temporal association with transfusion, but can be difficult to diagnose in patients with preexisting cardiac or pulmonary failure, such as those

---

TABLE 4

COMPLICATIONS OF MASSIVE TRANSFUSION[a]

- Hypothermia from transfusion and also from the injury/environment
- Coagulopathy from hemorrhage, dilution, tissue destruction, citrate toxicity
- Thrombocytopenia from hemorrhage and consumption
- Citrate toxicity that can cause hypocalcemia, coagulopathy, myocardial depression
- Hyperkalemia from hemolysis and tissue destruction
- Compartment syndrome (either abdominal or extremity) from volume resuscitation or crush/blast injury
- Leukopenia from dilution and hemorrhage
- Metabolic acidosis from generation of lactate and poor clearance of citrate

---

[a]Many of these complications do not result from the massive transfusion *per se* but from the associated physiologic changes that occur because of massive injury and the need for transfusion.

with significant pulmonary contusion or ARDS. As with TRIM, the mechanism underlying this disorder has not yet been described but current hypotheses under consideration include transfusion of leukocytes (even with leukoreduced blood), transfusion of HLA protein or other soluble foreign proteins, and/or transfusion of cellular or fatty debris.[41] It is possible that TRALI may be a localized manifestation of TRIM with acute, localized inflammation of the lung due to emboli of foreign antigen. Treatment involves supportive care only and most cases resolve quickly.

Most concerning in the trauma population is the independent association between blood transfusion and development of multisystem organ failure and death. A dose-dependent increase in the odds ratio of developing multisystem failure has been described.[24,42,43] As with the other side effects of transfusion, the cause of this observation is not known but may be related to the age of the blood transfused.[44] PRBCs undergo substantial changes during storage, many of which are irreversible. Depletion of adenosine triphosphate (ATP) and oxidation of spectrin results in a conformational change in the cytoskeleton that is irreversible (see Fig. 1).[45,46] Because the cell, which is 7 μm in diameter, is now deformed and "stiff," it is less able to maneuver through the capillary, which is 3 μm in diameter. This may result in sludging and paradoxical end-organ ischemia following transfusion. This hypothesis has been validated in animal models, but there is conflicting human data on the actual occurrence and clinical significance of this proposed mechanism.[47,48] Another proposed mechanism to account for end-organ ischemia states that depletion of nitric oxide causes localized vasospasm with resultant sludging. Transfused RBCs have variable lifespan depending, in part, on the storage time, and the hemoglobin liberated from lysed cells is a potent nitric oxide scavenger. The concentration of nitric oxide, a smooth muscle relaxant and vasodilator, has been shown to decrease following transfusion, resulting in vasoconstriction.[49,50] On the basis of these observations,

fresh blood (<14 days old) may be better than aged blood transfusion in trauma patients who are elderly and/or have limited physiologic reserve due to their severe injury.

Leukoreduced Red Blood Cell Transfusion

The need to leukoreduce PRBCs remains controversial. Whereas European and Canadian studies have shown reduction in morbidity with leukoreduction of transfused PRBC, studies in the United States have not substantiated these findings. Those opposed to universal leukoreduction point out the cost associated with the procedure. Proponents argue that the potential benefits justify the cost. The potential benefits include reduction in febrile reaction, reduction in transmission of cytomegalovirus, reduction in the risk of HLA alloimmunization, and *possible* reduction in TRIM and infectious complications resulting from immunosuppression.[51]

Utter et al. have shown in trauma patients that leukoreduced blood does not decrease the risk of developing microchimerism despite removal of 99.9% of white blood cells, and that patients have decreased response to antigen challenge following transfusion.[52,53] Conversely, others have shown that leukoreduction decreases the relative risk of developing HLA alloimmunization by 70%.[54] The reason for the conflicting results remains unknown.

Especially relevant to the trauma patient are the contradictory findings on the effect of leukoreduction on TRIM and infectious complications resulting from transfusion. Whereas many studies in surgical patients showed that infectious complications and/or mortality are higher following transfusion of nonleukoreduced blood, others have shown no difference. Two meta-analyses showed a decrease in postoperative infection following transfusion of leukoreduced blood relative to nonleukoreduced blood but no impact on mortality, but each individual study had a small sample size.[55] It has been suggested that at least 10,000 patients are needed to

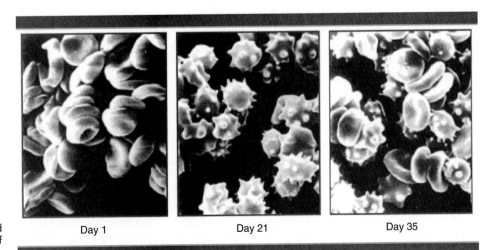

Day 1   Day 21   Day 35

Figure 1 Changes in red blood cell morphology as a function of storage time.

perform an adequately powered prospective, randomized study to evaluate the impact that leukoreduction might have on subsequent infection or mortality.[56]

Alternatives to Allogenic Transfusion

Autotransfusion

Autotransfusion can significantly decrease the need for allogenic PRBC transfusion. Blood can be salvaged and reinfused from the pleural and abdominal cavities. Of note, blood that has been suction collected intraoperatively from the abdominal cavity must be heparinized and washed before reinfusion. The resultant transfused blood is void of clotting factors and platelets and therefore represents an RBC transfusion only. Previous study has validated the safety of using this type of blood salvage even in patients with perforated viscus, although its use in patients with gross contamination of the abdomen is not advocated.[57,58] Blood collected from the pleural cavity using thoracostomy tubes can be reinfused within 6 hours of the time of collection. In this case, the blood is not washed and therefore contains all clotting factors and platelets. There is a theoretic concern that the activated leukocytes and platelets may increase the risk for development of disseminated intravascular coagulation (DIC) after transfusion of 2 L of blood.

Blood Substitutes

Despite many years of research and initially promising trials, currently there are no blood substitutes approved for use outside of clinical trials. The possibility of a synthetic blood substitute is very appealing due to the chronic shortage of allogenic blood and the previously described detrimental effects associated with transfusion of allogenic blood. However, all products tested to date have been found to be toxic or ineffective.

COAGULATION

The incidence of clinically significant coagulopathy increases with severity of injury independent of crystalloid resuscitation such that 25% to 50% of seriously injured patients are coagulopathic on arrival at the hospital.[59,60] In a 2-year review, Cosgriff et al. found that pH <7.1, temperature $<34°C$, injury severity score >25, or systolic blood pressure <70 mm Hg independently predicted severe coagulopathy.[61] The risk for each variable was additive such that patients with all four variables had a 98% risk of being coagulopathic. This has been termed the *coagulopathy of trauma* and is due to hypothermia, acidosis, consumption of clotting factors, and, at times, DIC. Dilutional coagulopathy can be a cause of persistent or recurrent coagulopathy and bleeding after admission, but is rarely the problem on arrival at the hospital.

Specific injuries can trigger DIC. Classically, this has been associated with severe traumatic brain injury, fat embolism from long bone fracture, and amniotic fluid embolism. These emboli contain thromboplastin, which activates intravascular thrombin, thereby causing a consumptive coagulopathy. Treatment is supportive care, which frequently necessitates blood component transfusion due to concurrent hemorrhage.

Factor Repletion in Trauma—Plasma, Cryoprecipitate, and Recombinant Factor VII

The plasma portion of donated whole blood contains most of the necessary clotting factors of the coagulation cascade, although it has decreased concentrations of factors V, VII, and VIII due to degradation and fibrinogen due to dilution. It is dosed as 15 mL per kg (ideal body weight) and generally 4 units will result in 40% factor recovery.[62] It is vital to know this dosing regimen because plasma is frequently underdosed—most patients require *at least* 4 units of plasma to treat coagulopathy effectively.

Plasma is commonly frozen to prevent degradation of the clotting factors. It has a shelf life of 5 to 7 days at room temperature, but this will result in further degradation of factors V and VIII during storage. It takes approximately 30 minutes to thaw plasma because it must be thawed slowly in a water bath to prevent degradation of protein. It has been shown that each 30-minute delay in administration of the first unit of plasma decreases the odds of correction of warfarin-induced coagulopathy by 20% in patients with intracerebral bleeding.[63] Because of this, centers that use fresh frozen plasma (FFP) frequently store several units at room temperature for use in emergencies. The units can be dispensed for nonemergent needs after 3 to 4 days if their shelf life is about to expire.

The main indication for transfusion of plasma in trauma patients is bleeding or massive RBC transfusion. This is different from the indication in elective surgery, where the reason for transfusion is known coagulopathy and risk of bleeding. Aggressive use of plasma in bleeding trauma patients may result in a higher incidence of transfusion and total units transfused relative to elective patients, but it may also result in a net lower need for transfusion of PRBC and other blood products by reversing coagulopathy.[64,65] Approximately 70% of patients have an elevated prothrombin time/international normalized ratio (PT/INR) after transfusion of 10 units of PRBC and 100% are coagulopathic after transfusion of 12 units of PRBC. As discussed further in the section " Massive and Fresh Whole Blood Transfusion," these patients benefit from early, aggressive transfusion of both PRBC and plasma.

Transfusion of plasma has the same risks as described for transfusion of RBCs, but the incidence of adverse events is higher for all possible complications. The most frequent adverse event associated with plasma transfusion is TRALI due to the variable plasma proteins (and presumably antibody) being transfused.[66] Furthermore, some studies suggest that this risk is higher in plasma obtained from multiparous women, although further research is needed to validate this assertion. The other major risk associated with transfusion of plasma is prion transmission, although its exact incidence is unknown and most likely variable depending on the donor pool. This risk is mostly germane in countries, such as England, that have had an epidemic of bovine spongiform encephalopathy and may be mitigated, although not abolished, through use of leukodepleted blood.[66] The true incidence of prion transmission may never be known because its symptoms manifest many years to decades after transfusion. Finally, hemolytic transfusion reaction is also possible following transfusion of plasma because plasma contains variable titers of anti-A and anti-B antibody.

Cryoprecipitate is the precipitated fraction obtained from thawing FFP at $4°C$. Because of this, it is pooled from the FFP obtained from multiple donors. Cryoprecipitate is rich in factor VIII, von Willebrand factor, factor XIII, and fibronectin. Most importantly, it is the only blood component that contains concentrated fibrinogen and therefore its main indication is for treatment of coagulopathy in hypofibrinogenemic patients, such as DIC or exsanguinating hemorrhage/massive transfusion.[67] Dosed adequately, plasma can be used to replete all coagulation factors, including fibrinogen, but hypofibrinogenemia can be better treated using cryoprecipitate. Cryoprecipitate is recommended in patients with a fibrinogen level <1 g per L, and is dosed as a 10-pack transfusion—each pack raises the fibrinogen level to 75%.[62] Also, bleeding patients with known von Willebrand deficiency should receive cryoprecipitate to optimize platelet function; whereas, nonbleeding patients with this disorder can be treated with desamino-D-arginine vasopressin (DDAVP).

Risks associated with transfusion of cryoprecipitate are the same as those reported for the other blood components; however, the incidence of TRALI and TRIM is lower than that associated with transfusion of plasma. The reason for the lower incidence is that the total volume of cryoprecipitate transfused is much less than plasma and therefore the recipient's exposure to foreign protein antigen is lower. The risk of transmission of blood-borne pathogen, however, may be higher due to the pooled nature of this product.

Recombinant activated factor VII is approved for the treatment of hemophilia and those with factor VII deficiency, but its use in trauma remains off-label. Its mechanism of action involves binding exposed tissue factor on the endothelial surface of damaged blood vessels, thereby rendering it a "smart bomb" with ability to activate the coagulation cascade where it is needed most. The first reported use of factor VIIa involved a soldier with a high-velocity gunshot to the vena cava, whereas the first use in the United States was in a patient who had received more than 100 units of PRBC following multiple stab wounds.[68,69]

Bleeding stopped immediately in both patients. Numerous studies have now confirmed these initial observations and factor VIIa has been shown to be a potent procoagulant agent in various surgical patients (including trauma) and to significantly reduce the need for PRBC transfusion, particularly in those who require massive transfusion.[70] The efficacy of factor VIIa is limited by severe acidosis, thrombocytopenia, and profound coagulopathy. Dutton et al. reported that use of the drug with an arterial pH <7.0 or platelet count $<50,000$ cells per μL is futile, and Stein et al. reported that an admission PT >17.6 seconds, lactate >13 mg per dL, or revised trauma score <4.1 also predict failure to respond.[71,72]

Concerns regarding off-label use of factor VIIa currently center on issues of cost and safety. Depending on the dosage and number of doses given, the direct cost can be as much as $20,000 per course, although the cost savings in terms of reduction of PRBC needed and possible reduction in length of stay and infectious/pulmonary complications resulting from lesser overall transfusion are unknown. On the basis of recommended dose for hemophilia, the most commonly used dose in trauma is 90 μg per kg, although there are reports that 40 μg per kg is equally efficacious.[73] The serum half-life of the drug is 2.7 hours, and repeated dosing may be necessary. There are varying studies on the thromboembolic risk associated with administration of factor VII. The arterial risk relates to exposed endothelium on preexisting ulcerated plaque most commonly due to atherosclerosis. Multiple single-center studies have shown no increase in risk in surgical patients, but a review of all adverse events resulting from off-label use of factor VIIa reported to the U.S. Food and Drug Administration (FDA) revealed a 7% to 9% incidence of ischemic stroke, heart attack, or pulmonary embolism.[74] This compares to a complication rate of 0.02% when the drug is administered to hemophiliac patients.[70] Most of the complications from off-label use occurred in patients older than 50 years and within 24 hours of dosing. Because reporting adverse events to this database is voluntary, the true incidence of adverse events may be higher. Therefore, the recommendations for use of factor VIIa in trauma patients currently restrict it to massive transfusion and exsanguination of those with significant intracranial bleeding and coagulopathy.

Platelet Repletion

Platelet transfusion is less common in trauma than RBC or plasma transfusion. Despite the fact that the platelet count can be determined easily and quickly, there is no reliable method to test platelet function. The sole possible exception is thrombelastography (TEG), discussed in the subsequent text. The minimum recommended platelet count is 50,000 cells per μL for nonbleeding trauma patients and 100,000 cells per μL for patients who are bleeding. However, the absolute cell count may be falsely reassuring because it may not correlate with function.

As previously stated, there are no good studies in trauma patients that can be used to recommend timing and volume of platelet transfusion. Furthermore, although there are no good studies to determine the impact that use of aspirin or nonsteroidal anti-inflammatory agents has on hemorrhage following injury, a review of the literature suggests that use of aspirin may worsen intracranial hemorrhage following traumatic brain injury.[75] It has been shown that platelet transfusion can reverse the platelet dysfunction caused by clopidogrel,[76] and many trauma centers utilize platelet transfusion in patients with traumatic brain injury who were prescribed antiplatelet medications, including nonsteroidal anti-inflammatory agents. Other than this indication, based on expert opinion, platelets should be routinely used only as a part of a massive transfusion protocol (discussed in the subsequent text) and for proven thrombocytopenia.

Role of Coagulation Tests

Although a coagulation panel consisting of the PT, partial thromboplastin time (PTT), and platelet count should be ordered for every patient, the decision to transfuse plasma or platelets should not be delayed pending these results in bleeding patients. Experience and anticipation should be used to prevent coagulopathy rather than relying on tests to treat it because testing can both delay the onset of transfusion and may not accurately reflect degree of coagulopathy present.[77] As discussed in the subsequent text, this is especially true in patients who require massive transfusion because these patients are all coagulopathic to varying degrees on arrival at the hospital. Of the tests mentioned, PT is the most sensitive test for detecting coagulation derangement, whereas the platelet count is the least sensitive.[65]

TEG was first described in 1948 to measure the clotting properties of whole blood. The test can be performed at the bedside and requires <20 minutes to measure clotting ability and strength. A pin that is attached to a wire is placed in a specimen of whole blood. The blood rotates slowly, and, as clot forms, the pin begins to move with the specimen. The wire is attached to a transducer, which records this motion as a tracing. The image generated depicts the interaction from initial platelet aggregation and clot formation to clot stabilization and strength to clot dissolution. As shown in Fig. 2, the R time reflects the function of the intrinsic pathway and is the time to initial detection of clot in the specimen. The K time, also called the *thrombin constant*, reflects platelet–coagulation factor interaction. An abnormally long K time is treated with platelet transfusion and plasma. The R+K time represents time to form the initial platelet plug that stops hemorrhage. This is equivalent to the bleeding time but is more consistent and objective. The α angle represents fibrinogen activity and differentiates hypo- from hypercoagulability. An abnormally shallow angle is treated

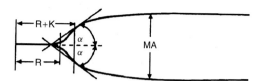

Figure 2 Normal thrombelastogram (TEG) tracing. R = reaction time — interaction between platelets and fibrin. Reflects the function of the intrinsic pathway (factors XII, XI, IX, VIII). (Normal 5 to 7 minutes). K = clot time — time to a fixed clot firmness, which is defined as the point at which the amplitude of the tracing is +20 mm. Reflects platelet–coagulation factor interaction. (Normal 3 to 7 minutes). R+K = time to fibrin cross-linking. (Normal 10 to 12 minutes). α = slope of TEG tracing — rate of clot formation. Reflects function of fibrinogen, factor VIII, and platelets. (Normal 55 to 66 degrees). MA = maximal amplitude — strength of the clot formed. Reflects mainly platelet activity. The point at which the MA begins to decrease denotes clot lysis.

with cryoprecipitate. The MA represents maximal clot strength and is mainly associated with platelet number and function; therefore, decreased MA is treated with platelet transfusion. Finally, the tracing can be continued until such time that the MA is noted to decrease. This represents time to clot dissolution and will be shortened in fibrinolytic states such as DIC.

TEG has been shown to correlate with traditional tests of coagulation, such as the PT/PTT.[78,79] The biggest difference between TEG and traditional coagulation panel tests is that TEG measures clot formation, strength, and dissolution whereas the other tests only measure clot formation. Moreover, TEG can also be used to detect hypercoagulable states.[80] As such, TEG represents a more physiologic measure of the patient's coagulation status. Figure 3 depicts various abnormal tracings and their causes.

TEG has been used extensively in cardiac and transplant surgery, but there are limited reports of its use in trauma. Two studies in trauma patients reported that TEG not only correlated with other tests of coagulation but also had value both in predicting the need for transfusion and in diagnosing a hypercoagulable state.[79,80] The authors suggested that TEG can also be helpful in guiding which blood components are needed during resuscitation as well as determining which patients are hypercoagulable and need to be anticoagulated after they have been resuscitated. Other studies in liver transplant and cardiac surgery patients have shown that utilization of TEG results in a net decrease in amount of blood products transfused due to the ability to replete only the missing components.[81,82] Despite these promising studies, TEG is not readily available in most hospitals and has not gained wide acceptance for use by the trauma community.

Massive and Fresh Whole Blood Transfusion

There are variable definitions of massive transfusion, but the one most commonly used refers to transfusion of one blood volume (or 10 units PRBC in an average-sized adult)

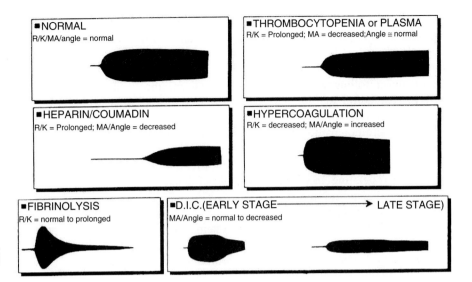

Figure 3 Various abnormal thrombelastogram tracings. DIC, disseminated intravascular coagulation.

in 24 hours. The shortcoming of this definition is that it does not include or draw attention to the concomitant coagulopathy that nearly all of these severely injured patients have on arrival. Because of the effects of hemodilution, transfusion of one whole blood volume only repletes 75% of the original blood volume. Furthermore, such patients are at increased risk for many complications, some of which are due to the severity of the injuries sustained and some of which are a result of the massive PRBC transfusion itself. Complications include development of compartment syndrome, thrombocytopenia, coagulopathy, hyperkalemia, hypocalcemia, hypothermia, leukopenia, and acidosis, to name a few (Table 4). Finally, it is critical to beware of the lethal triad of trauma—coagulopathy, acidosis, and hypothermia—in such patients and to work aggressively to prevent or reverse it. Whereas acidosis and hypothermia are effectively treated in most cases, current algorithm and practice patterns may not address coagulopathy adequately.[83,84]

Coagulopathy is frequently viewed as an inevitable consequence of hemodilution and massive bleeding, but recent reports from the military in Iraq suggest that this view is erroneous and that most severely injured patients arrive at the care facility in a coagulopathic condition.[84] In addition to loss of RBCs, these patients have also lost a significant amount of platelets and clotting factors, and the activity of the remaining platelets and factors is reduced because of the concomitant acidosis and hypothermia.

Early, emperic transfusion of plasma and platelets is advocated in exsanguinating patients, not for prophylaxis but for treatment of coagulopathy and volume resuscitation.[65,84] Anecdotal evidence from the military suggests that this regimen significantly decreases coagulopathic bleeding in the operating room, prevents edema and further dilutional coagulopathy from excessive crystalloid resuscitation, minimizes hypothermia, and may improve mortality.[84] The ratio of units of PRBC to units of plasma

transfused should be at least 1:2 and preferably 1:1 in exsanguinating patients.[64] Furthermore, cryoprecipitate may be needed to prevent hypofibrinogenemia. There are currently no good studies that can be used to recommend a transfusion strategy for platelet repletion, although maintaining a level >100,000 cells per μL in exsanguinating patients appears appropriate.[85] On the basis of expert opinion, empiric platelet transfusion as a part of a massive transfusion protocol should be started after 7 to 10 units of PRBC have been transfused and should continue at a ratio of 1:1:1 for each unit of PRBC and plasma transfused until hemorrhage is controlled.[65] Although the prescribed course of therapy may result in higher use of blood products, it is not possible to predict a particular patient's exact transfusion needs prospectively and coagulopathy due to underutilization of transfusion being far more common than overutilization in exsanguinating patients.[64]

Whole blood transfusion was the norm until the 1960s when transfusion of blood components was adopted as a means to utilize donated blood more efficiently. However, the overall military experience with whole blood is significant and was best exemplified during World War II when 2,000 units of whole blood were being sent to Europe daily.[86] More recently, the war in Iraq has renewed interest in transfusion of whole, fresh (<24 hours after donation) blood due to constraints on the stored blood supply in forward military hospitals and reports that such transfusions are safe and associated with faster resolution of coagulopathy in hemorrhaging patients.[87] The proposed benefits of whole blood relative to each unit of stored component are that it contains both a higher number of platelets (~200,000 to 350,000 cells per μL vs. 60,000 cells per μL), higher hematocrit after transfusion (33% to 43% vs. 30%), and better coagulation activity (86% vs. 65%).[88,89] In addition, the transfused fresh RBCs and platelets function normally as opposed to their stored counterparts, which require hours to become fully active. The biggest concern regarding transfusion of fresh, whole blood is safety. However, clinically significant transfusion reaction is rare during massive transfusion. Moreover, because the net transfusion needs of the patient will be lower following whole blood transfusion, the risk of transmission of blood-borne pathogen is lower using single-donor whole blood that has been rapidly screened for common pathogens than it is when transfusing components from multiple donors.[89]

Protocols must be established between the trauma service, the operating room, and the blood bank to facilitate mobilization of blood for massive resuscitation. The critical nature of these patients and their need for ongoing resuscitation preclude having a system whereby each component has to be ordered separately by the treating surgeon or anesthesiologist, both of whom will be occupied treating the patient. The trauma exsanguination protocol utilized at the Hospital of the University of Pennsylvania releases 10 units of PRBC (uncrossmatched if necessary), 4 units of platelets, and 4 units of thawed plasma. Factor VII is also released at the discretion of the surgeon after 10 units of blood have been transfused, if the arterial pH is >7.1 and surgical bleeding has been controlled. Furthermore, although component transfusion satisfies the transfusion needs of isolated or multiple trauma patient scenario, mass casualty events, such as war or terrorist-related events, can quickly overwhelm local and regional blood banking resources. In these situations, transfusion of whole, fresh blood that is rapidly screened for communicable disease may be needed to meet patients' needs. Blood banks and trauma protocols need to be established in the civilian arena to account for this possibility.

CONCLUSION

Transfusion is a vital part of the treatment of the injured patient. However, whereas transfusion can be lifesaving and pivotal in the initial resuscitation of the injured patient, it can also be detrimental if utilized inappropriately. Recent studies of outcomes from early and aggressive transfusion from the military suggest that mortality is improved when crystalloid resuscitation is minimized and very severely injured, hemorrhaging patients are transfused aggressively. As noted, a 1:1:1 transfusion strategy (RBC:plasma:platelets) may be beneficial in this select group. This is different for patients who have asymptomatic anemia and have been resuscitated, in whom a restrictive transfusion policy is preferred. The trauma surgeon must be familiar with the risks and benefits associated with transfusion to maximize its benefits while minimizing its liabilities.

Future studies are now needed to validate the military's experience in Iraq with scenarios encountered in the civilian setting. In addition, expanded use of topical hemostatic agents, perhaps by paramedics, in addition to novel medications to enhance coagulation may allow earlier arrest of hemorrhage and more efficient reversal of shock and coagulopathy. Furthermore, continued efforts are needed to develop blood substitutes that have a long shelf life and minimal adverse effects.

REFERENCES

1. Kauvar DS, Lefering R, Wade CE. Impact of hemorrhage on trauma outcome: An overview of epidemiology, clinical presentations, and therapeutic considerations. *J Trauma.* 2006;60(Suppl 6):S3–S11.
2. Eastridge BJ, Malone D, Holcomb JB. Early predictors of transfusion and mortality after injury: A review of the data-based literature. *J Trauma.* 2006;60(Suppl 6):S20–S25.
3. The Committee on Trauma of the American College of Surgeons. Shock. *Advanced trauma life support for doctors student manual.* 7th ed. Chicago: American College of Surgeons; 2004:69–85.
4. Valeri CR, Hirsch NM. Restoration *in vivo* of erythrocyte adenosine triphosphate, 2,3-diphosphoglycerate, potassium ion, and sodium ion concentrations following the transfusion of acid-citrate-dextrose-stored human red blood cells. *J Lab Clin Med.* 1969;73(5):722–733.
5. Baron BJ, Scalea TM. Acute blood loss. *Emerg Med Clin North Am.* 1996;14(1):35–55.
6. Davis JW, Shackford SR, Mackersie RC, et al. Base deficit as a guide to volume resuscitation. *J Trauma.* 1988;28(10):1464–1467.
7. Davis JW, Parks SN, Kaups KL, et al. Admission base deficit predicts transfusion requirements and risk of complications. *J Trauma.* 1996;41(5):769–774.
8. Bannon MP, O'Neill CM, Martin M, et al. Central venous oxygen saturation, arterial base deficit, and lactate concentration in trauma patients. *Am Surg.* 1995;61(8):738–745.
9. Martin MJ, FitzSullivan E, Salim A, et al. Discordance between lactate and base deficit in the surgical intensive care unit: Which one do you trust? *Am J Surg.* 2006;191(5):625–630.
10. Husain FA, Martin MJ, Mullenix PS, et al. Serum lactate and base deficit as predictors of mortality and morbidity. *Am J Surg.* 2003;185(5):485–491.
11. Scalea TM, Hartnett RW, Duncan AO, et al. Central venous oxygen saturation: A useful clinical tool in trauma patients. *J Trauma.* 1990;30(12):1539–1543.
12. Leal-Noval SR, Rincon-Ferrari MD, Marin-Niebla A, et al. Transfusion of erythrocyte concentrates produces a variable increment on cerebral oxygenation in patients with severe traumatic brain injury: A preliminary study. *Intensive Care Med.* 2006;32(11):1733–1740. [Epub 2006 Sep 22.]
13. McIntyre LA, Fergusson DA, Hutchison JS, et al. Effect of a liberal versus restrictive transfusion strategy on mortality in patients with moderate to severe head injury. *Neurocrit Care.* 2006;5(1):4–9.
14. Smith MJ, Stiefel MF, Magge S, et al. Packed red blood cell transfusion increases local cerebral oxygenation. *Crit Care Med.* 2005;33(5):1104–1108.
15. McIntyre LA, Hebert PC. Can we safely restrict transfusion in trauma patients? *Curr Opin Crit Care.* 2006;12(6):575–583.
16. Messmer K. Hemodilution. *Surg Clin North Am.* 1975;55(3):659–678.
17. Carson JL, Duff A, Poses RM, et al. Effect of anaemia and cardiovascular disease on surgical mortality and morbidity. *Lancet.* 1996;348(9034):1055–1060.
18. Carson JL, Noveck H, Berlin JA, et al. Mortality and morbidity in patients with very low postoperative Hb levels who decline blood transfusion. *Transfusion.* 2002;42(7):812–818.
19. Corwin HL, Gettinger A, Pearl RG, et al. The CRIT Study: Anemia and blood transfusion in the critically ill – current clinical practice in the United States. *Crit Care Med.* 2004;32(1):39–52.
20. Hebert PC, Wells G, Blajchman MA, et al. A multicenter, randomized, controlled clinical trial of transfusion requirements in critical care. Transfusion Requirements in Critical Care Investigators, Canadian Critical Care Trials Group. *N Engl J Med.* 1999;340(6):409–417.

21. Vincent JL, Baron JF, Reinhart K, et al. Anemia and blood transfusion in critically ill patients. *JAMA.* 2002;288(12):1499–1507.

22. Beale E, Zhu J, Chan L, et al. Blood transfusion in critically injured patients: A prospective study. *Injury.* 2006;37(5):455–465. [Epub 2006 Feb 14.]

23. Carlson AP, Schermer CR, Lu SW. Retrospective evaluation of anemia and transfusion in traumatic brain injury. *J Trauma.* 2006;61(3):567–571.

24. Charles A, Shaikh AA, Walters M, et al. Blood transfusion is an independent predictor of mortality after blunt trauma. *Am Surg.* 2007;73(1):1–5.

25. Dunne JR, Riddle MS, Danko J, et al. Blood transfusion is associated with infection and increased resource utilization in combat casualties. *Am Surg.* 2006;72(7):619–625. Discussion 25–6.

26. Napolitano L. Cumulative risks of early red blood cell transfusion. *J Trauma.* 2006;60(Suppl 6):S26–S34.

27. Reed W, Lee TH, Norris PJ, et al. Transfusion-associated microchimerism: A new complication of blood transfusions in severely injured patients. *Semin Hematol.* 2007;44(1):24–31.

28. Silverboard H, Aisiku I, Martin GS, et al. The role of acute blood transfusion in the development of acute respiratory distress syndrome in patients with severe trauma. *J Trauma.* 2005;59(3):717–723.

29. West HC, Jurkovich G, Donnell C, et al. Immediate prediction of blood requirements in trauma victims. *South Med J.* 1989;82(2):186–189.

30. Starr AJ, Griffin DR, Reinert CM, et al. Pelvic ring disruptions: Prediction of associated injuries, transfusion requirement, pelvic arteriography, complications, and mortality. *J Orthop Trauma.* 2002;16(8):553–561.

31. Como JJ, Dutton RP, Scalea TM, et al. Blood transfusion rates in the care of acute trauma. *Transfusion.* 2004;44(6):809–813.

32. Goodnough LT, Brecher ME, Kanter MH, et al. Transfusion medicine. First of two parts – blood transfusion. *N Engl J Med.* 1999;340(6):438–447.

33. Opelz G, Sengar DP, Mickey MR, et al. Effect of blood transfusions on subsequent kidney transplants. *Transplant Proc.* 1973;5(1):253–259.

34. Opelz G, Vanrenterghem Y, Kirste G, et al. Prospective evaluation of pretransplant blood transfusions in cadaver kidney recipients. *Transplantation.* 1997;63(7):964–967.

35. Williams KA, Ting A, French ME, et al. Perioperative blood-transfusion improve cadaveric renal-allograft survival in non-transfused recipients. A prospective controlled clinical trial. *Lancet.* 1980;1(8178):1104–1106.

36. Claridge JA, Sawyer RG, Schulman AM, et al. Blood transfusions correlate with infections in trauma patients in a dose-dependent manner. *Am Surg.* 2002;68(7):566–572.

37. Hill GE, Frawley WH, Griffith KE, et al. Allogeneic blood transfusion increases the risk of postoperative bacterial infection: A meta-analysis. *J Trauma.* 2003;54(5):908–914.

38. Lee MR, Hong CW, Yoon SN, et al. Risk factors for anastomotic leakage after resection for rectal cancer. *Hepatogastroenterology.* 2006;53(71):682–686.

39. Joshi GP. Intraoperative fluid restriction improves outcome after major elective gastrointestinal surgery. *Anesth Analg.* 2005;101(2):601–605.

40. Brandstrup B, Tonnesen H, Beier-Holgersen R, et al. Effects of intravenous fluid restriction on postoperative complications: Comparison of two perioperative fluid regimens: A randomized assessor-blinded multicenter trial. *Ann Surg.* 2003;238(5):641–648.

41. Looney MR, Gropper MA, Matthay MA. Transfusion-related acute lung injury: A review. *Chest.* 2004;126(1):249–258.

42. Malone DL, Dunne J, Tracy JK, et al. Blood transfusion, independent of shock severity, is associated with worse outcome in trauma. *J Trauma.* 2003;54(5):898–905. Discussion -7.

43. Moore FA, Moore EE, Sauaia A. Blood transfusion. An independent risk factor for postinjury multiple organ failure. *Arch Surg.* 1997;132(6):620–624. Discussion 4–5.

44. Zallen G, Offner PJ, Moore EE, et al. Age of transfused blood is an independent risk factor for postinjury multiple organ failure. *Am J Surg.* 1999;178(6):570–572.

45. Berezina TL, Zaets SB, Morgan C, et al. Influence of storage on red blood cell rheological properties. *J Surg Res.* 2002;102(1):6–12.

46. Nagaprasad V, Singh M. Sequential analysis of the influence of blood storage on aggregation, deformability and shape parameters of erythrocytes. *Clin Hemorheol Microcirc.* 1998;18(4):273–284.

47. Marik PE, Sibbald WJ. Effect of stored-blood transfusion on oxygen delivery in patients with sepsis. *JAMA.* 1993;269:3024.

48. Walsh TS, McArdle F, McLellan SA, et al. Does the storage time of transfused red blood cells influence regional or global indexes of tissue oxygenation in anemic critically ill patients? *Crit Care Med.* 2004;32(2):364–371.

49. Napolitano LM, Corwin HL. Efficacy of red blood cell transfusion in the critically ill. *Crit Care Clin.* 2004;20(2):255–268.

50. Schechter AN, Gladwin MT. Hemoglobin and the paracrine and endocrine functions of nitric oxide. *N Engl J Med.* 2003;348(15):1483–1485.

51. Blajchman MA. The clinical benefits of the leukoreduction of blood products. *J Trauma.* 2006;60(Suppl 6):S83–S90.

52. Utter GH, Owings JT, Lee TH, et al. Microchimerism in transfused trauma patients is associated with diminished donor-specific lymphocyte response. *J Trauma.* 2005;58(5):925–931. Discussion 31–2.

53. Utter GH, Nathens AB, Lee TH, et al. Leukoreduction of blood transfusions does not diminish transfusion-associated microchimerism in trauma patients. *Transfusion.* 2006;46(11):1863–1869.

54. Slichter S. Leukocyte reduction and ultraviolet B irradiation of platelets to prevent alloimmunization and refractoriness to platelet transfusions. The Trial to Reduce Alloimmunization to Platelets Study Group. *N Engl J Med.* 1997;337(26):1861–1869.

55. Fergusson D, Khanna MP, Tinmouth A, et al. Transfusion of leukoreduced red blood cells may decrease postoperative infections: Two meta-analyses of randomized controlled trials. *Can J Anaesth.* 2004;51(5):417–424.

56. Vamvakas EC, Blajchman MA. Deleterious clinical effects of transfusion-associated immunomodulation: Fact or fiction? *Blood.* 2001;97(5):1180–1195.

57. Ozmen V, McSwain NE Jr, Nichols RL, et al. Autotransfusion of potentially culture-positive blood (CPB) in abdominal trauma: Preliminary data from a prospective study. *J Trauma.* 1992;32(1):36–39.

58. Bowley DM, Barker P, Boffard KD. Intraoperative blood salvage in penetrating abdominal trauma: A randomised, controlled trial. *World J Surg.* 2006;30(6):1074–1080.

59. Brohi K, Singh J, Heron M, et al. Acute traumatic coagulopathy. *J Trauma.* 2003;54(6):1127–1130.

60. MacLeod JB, Lynn M, McKenney MG, et al. Early coagulopathy predicts mortality in trauma. *J Trauma.* 2003;55(1):39–44.

61. Cosgriff N, Moore EE, Sauaia A, et al. Predicting life-threatening coagulopathy in the massively transfused trauma patient: Hypothermia and acidoses revisited. *J Trauma.* 1997;42(5):857–861. Discussion 61–2.

62. Pugent Sound Blood Center 2006, accessed at http://www.psbc.org/therapy/ffp.htm. Accessed April 2007.

63. Goldstein JN, Thomas SH, Frontiero V, et al. Timing of fresh frozen plasma administration and rapid correction of coagulopathy in warfarin-related intracerebral hemorrhage. *Stroke.* 2006;37(1):151–155. Epub 2005 Nov 23.

64. Hirshberg A, Dugas M, Banez EI, et al. Minimizing dilutional coagulopathy in exsanguinating hemorrhage: A computer simulation. *J Trauma.* 2003;54(3):454–463.

65. Ketchum L, Hess JR, Hiippala S. Indications for early fresh frozen plasma, cryoprecipitate, and platelet transfusion in trauma. *J Trauma.* 2006;60(Suppl 6):S51–S58.

66. MacLennan S, Williamson LM. Risks of fresh frozen plasma and platelets. *J Trauma.* 2006;60(Suppl 6):S46–S50.

67. O'Shaughnessy DF, Atterbury C, Bolton Maggs P, et al. Guidelines for the use of fresh-frozen plasma, cryoprecipitate and cryosupernatant. *Br J Haematol.* 2004;126(1):11–28.

68. Kenet G, Walden R, Eldad A, et al. Treatment of traumatic bleeding with recombinant factor VIIa. *Lancet.* 1999;354(9193):1879.

69. O'Neill PA, Bluth M, Gloster ES, et al. Successful use of recombinant activated factor VII for trauma-associated hemorrhage in a patient without preexisting coagulopathy. *J Trauma.* 2002;52(2): 400–405.

70. Mohr AM, Holcomb JB, Dutton RP, et al. Recombinant activated factor VIIa and hemostasis in critical care: A focus on trauma. *Crit Care.* 2005;9(Suppl 5):S37–S42. Epub 2005 Oct 7.

71. Stein DM, Dutton RP, O'Connor J, et al. Determinants of futility of administration of recombinant factor VIIa in trauma. *J Trauma.* 2005;59(3):609–615.

72. Dutton RP, McCunn M, Hyder M, et al. Factor VIIa for correction of traumatic coagulopathy. *J Trauma.* 2004;57(4):709–718. Discussion 18–9.

73. Harrison TD, Laskosky J, Jazaeri O, et al. "Low-dose" recombinant activated factor VII results in less blood and blood product use in traumatic hemorrhage. *J Trauma.* 2005;59(1):150–154.

74. O'Connell KA, Wood JJ, Wise RP. et al. Thromboembolic adverse events after use of recombinant human coagulation factor VIIa. *JAMA.* 2006;295(3):293–298.

75. Sakr M, Wilson L. Best evidence topic report. Aspirin and the risk of intracranial complications following head injury. *Emerg Med J.* 2005;22(12):891–892.

76. Vilahur G, Choi BG, Zafar MU, et al. Normalization of platelet reactivity in clopidogrel-treated subjects. *J Thromb Haemost.* 2007;5(1):82–90.

77. Schreiber MA. Coagulopathy in the trauma patient. *Curr Opin Crit Care.* 2005;11(6):590–597.

78. Zuckerman L, Cohen E, Vagher JP, et al. Comparison of thrombelastography with common coagulation tests. *Thromb Haemost.* 1981;46(4):752–756.

79. Rugeri L, Levrat A, David JS, et al. Diagnosis of early coagulation abnormalities in trauma patients by rotation thrombelastography. *J Thromb Haemost.* 2007;5(2):289–295. Epub 2006 Nov 16.

80. Kaufmann CR, Dwyer KM, Crews JD, et al. Usefulness of thrombelastography in assessment of trauma patient coagulation. *J Trauma.* 1997;42(4):716–720. Discussion 20–2.

81. Shore-Lesserson L, Manspeizer HE, DePerio M, et al. Thromboelastography-guided transfusion algorithm reduces transfusions in complex cardiac surgery. *Anesth Analg.* 1999;88(2):312–319.

82. Coakley M, Reddy K, Mackie I, et al. Transfusion triggers in orthotopic liver transplantation: A comparison of the thromboelastometry analyzer, the thromboelastogram, and conventional coagulation tests. *J Cardiothorac Vasc Anesth.* 2006;20(4):548–553. Epub 2006 Apr 19.

83. Gonzalez EA, Moore FA, Holcomb JB, et al. Fresh frozen plasma should be given earlier to patients requiring massive transfusion. *J Trauma.* 2007;62(1):112–119.

84. Holcomb JB, Jenkins D, Rhee P, et al. Damage control resuscitation: Directly addressing the early coagulopathy of trauma. *J Trauma.* 2007;62(2):307–310.

85. Moore EE, Dunn EL, Breslich DJ, et al. Platelet abnormalities associated with massive autotransfusion. *J Trauma.* 1980;20(12):1052–1056.

86. Hess JR, Thomas MJ. Blood use in war and disaster: Lessons from the past century. *Transfusion.* 2003;43(11):1622–1633.

87. Kauvar DS, Holcomb JB, Norris GC, et al. Fresh whole blood transfusion: A controversial military practice. *J Trauma.* 2006;61(1):181–184.

88. Hardy JF, De Moerloose P, Samama M. Massive transfusion and coagulopathy: Pathophysiology and implications for clinical management. *Can J Anaesth.* 2004;51(4):293–310.

89. Repine TB, Perkins JG, Kauvar DS, et al. The use of fresh whole blood in massive transfusion. *J Trauma.* 2006;60(Suppl 6):S59–S69.

Pain Control and Sedation

66

John D. Lang, Jr.   *Onuma Chaiwat*

Trauma is a major cause of morbidity and mortality worldwide. Injuries and complications due to motor vehicle accidents, gunshots, stabbings, and burns are frequently associated with both short- and long-term physical suffering and mental anguish. In 2000, more than 50 million Americans suffered injuries requiring medical treatment, with approximately 150,000 injuries being fatal. This resulted in projected lifetime costs of approximately $406 billion; $80 billion for medical treatment, and $326 billion for lost productivity.[1] In recent years, pain control has been of particular concern because improving pain management has not only shown to improve comfort but has also been demonstrated to reduce morbidity and improve short- and long-term outcomes.[2-4] According to Whipple et al.,[5] 74% of polytrauma patients in intensive care unit (ICU) rated their pain intensity by a verbal pain intensity scale as either moderate or severe, whereas 95% of house staff and 81% of nurses reported analgesia to be "adequate." Additionally, Choiniere et al.,[6] demonstrated that approximately 50% of burn patients studied reported little or no analgesia from the doses of medication administered before and during dressing changes. There are multiple reasons for inadequate pain control in trauma patients including excessive concern about hemodynamic instability, fear of inducing addiction, and respiratory depression. However, the effect of inadequate pain control in trauma patients can result in remarkable physiologic stress responses that may potentiate disability and prolong the healing process. Consequently, it is essential to treat pain aggressively because the ramifications of inadequate pain control are more than psychological. However, most pain research involving trauma patients is based on so called *iatrogenic* trauma, also referred to as *elective surgery*. Hence, care must be limited by extrapolating these studies to the nonelective trauma patient.

Apart from pain control, sedation in the critically ill trauma patient also plays a vital role. Administration of sedatives is a common adjunct for the treatment of anxiety, delirium, and agitation in those critically ill patients especially in the ICU. Although the frequency of delirium varies from 15% to 50% among general medical or surgical patients,[7-9] these statistics did not apply to the critically ill trauma patient and few data exist concerning delirium in patients admitted in ICU.[10-13] Most previous studies have been focused on patients with hip fractures, in which the incidence of delirium varied from 4% to 53.3%.[14] Additionally, the causes of anxiety in critically ill trauma patients are multifactorial including an inability to communicate, excessive stimulation, and sleep deprivation. The attempt to reduce the anxiety and delirium including frequent reorientation, maintenance of patient comfort, and optimization of environment may be supplemented with sedatives. To review the necessity and value of pain and sedation control in the trauma patients, the author will discuss the following:

- The stress response of critical illness
- Physiologic impact of trauma
- Evaluation of pain and sedation in critically ill trauma patients
- Analgesia and sedation for trauma patients
- Pain management in outpatients.

THE STRESS RESPONSE OF CRITICAL ILLNESS

The effect of severe trauma, disease, infection, and surgery can cause remarkable metabolic stress on the human body. The ability of the body to cope with stress is known as *physiologic reserve*. Critical illness is a state in which this reserve is inadequate to maintain life, and exogenous organ support is needed. Tissue injuries elicit marked neuroendocrine changes that result in predictable alterations. These neuroendocrine responses to critical illness have been discussed and characterized for decades and are recognized as appropriate mechanisms of adaptation.[15] There is also alteration in the autonomic nervous system, which is accompanied by diffuse changes in endocrine function. In addition to changes in the autonomic nervous system and endocrine function, other alterations occur such as the pattern of protein synthesis within the liver increasing coagulation pathways. Recently, it has been found that traumatic injuries are associated with increased plasma concentrations of select cytokines that may contribute to adverse outcomes.[16,17]

The Neuroendocrine Response to Critical Illness

In acute illness, the mean levels of growth hormone (GH) become elevated. There is an increase in both peak and trough levels; however, the response may be variable.[18–20] The rising levels lead to lipolysis and inhibit lipid uptake. In addition, GH also has direct insulin antagonizing effects. In normal people, the overall hormonal effect of GH is for protein anabolism as opposed to critically ill patients in whom acute protein degradation, liberation of amino acids, glucose, and free fatty acid occur instead of anabolism.

Active thyroid hormones (T3 and T4) are essential for regulation of cardiac, pulmonary, and neurologic function. In acute phase of critical illness, T3 levels decrease as a result of a drop in peripheral conversion of T4 to T3.[21] This drop in T3 levels tends to persist during critical illness. There are studies that report the magnitude of the decrease in T3 levels correlates well with patient mortality.[22,23] On the other hand, T4 levels may remain in the normal range although there may be an early transient rise during the illness. Under normal circumstances, a drop in T3/T4 levels would inhibit the feedback loops that results in an increase in thyroid-stimulating hormone (TSH) level. However, TSH tends to remain in a normal or low range during stress.[24–26] This fact has been attributed to a change in thyroid hormone set point.[27] Interestingly, such seriously ill patients generally do not show evidence of thyroid illness. This condition (low T3/T4 and normal TSH level) has been termed *sick euthyroid syndrome, low-T3 syndrome,* or *nonthyroidal illness.*

A state of hypercortisolism is generally known to occur during acute critical illness. Cortisol shifts energy production and substrates to vital organs and delays anabolic process.[18,28] This creates the immediate source of energy during the initial phase response ("fight or flight"). At the same time, there is an increase in catecholamine levels. The major functions of epinephrine and norepinephrine are stimulation of heart rate; increased myocardial contractility; and vasoconstriction of gut, skin, and skeletal muscle vascular beds. These actions

maintain perfusion to vital organs in the setting of acute critical illness. In addition to an increase in both cortisol and catecolamines, the renin–angiotensin system is stimulated and aldosterone is produced, which results in fluid retention, hypokalemia, sodium retention, and vasoconstriction. With regard to other axes, testosterone levels are acutely reduced during the stress stage state, resulting in a decrease in anabolism.[29,30] If the critical illness is protracted, hypogonadism is frequently the result of this hormone change.[31] Prolactin levels also fluctuate during the acute and critical illness, rising acutely[32] followed by demonstrating a blunted pulsatile secretion in the chronic phase. It may play a role in the stimulation of inflammatory cascade.[28]

Another important physiologic alteration of critical illness involves renal function. There is a significant increase in plasma vasopressin (ADH) concentration especially in patients undergoing surgery[33] and it remains elevated for approximately 7 days postoperatively. The consequence of rising of plasma ADH is retention of free water. Other electrolyte changes include an increase in sodium retention mediated by sympathetic outflow to the kidney.

Regarding the hematologic system, there appears to be a tendency toward hypercoagulability. In surgical patients, plasma fibrinogen concentrations are increased as a result of augmented synthesis of this protein by the liver. There is also an increase in platelet aggregation and a decrease in fibrinolysis. The latter occurs as a result of increased plasma concentration of plasminogen activator inhibitor-1.[34] In addition, traumatic injuries also alter the pattern of protein synthesis in the liver. There is an increase in production and release of the so-called *acute phase reactants,* whereas synthesis of albumin and other hepatic products is decreased. Finally, recent data demonstrated that cytokines can be a component of stress response. In the setting of tissue inflammation, macrophages produce many different cytokines including tumor necrosis factor α (TNF-α), interleukin (IL)-1, IL-6, and IL-8. High circulating levels of IL-1 and TNF-α can induce and stimulate the release of classic stress hormones. They can also contribute to the synthesis of acute phase reactants and lead to the upregulation of nitric oxide synthase that ultimately yields the biomolecule, nitric oxide. However, it has been found that traumatic injury is associated with increased plasma concentration of IL-6. On the contrary, TNF-α rises only slightly and IL-1 concentrations do not appear to alter with isolated trauma.[16,17]

PHYSIOLOGIC IMPACT OF TRAUMA

The stress response after major trauma is much greater than that after elective surgery. If moderate to severe, it may lead to catabolic and thromboembolic stages that are associated with decreased survivability, increased morbidity, and slow recovery of function. Although the initial process of stress response is neurohormonal, the secondary effects involve multiple organ systems including cardiovascular, pulmonary, gastrointestinal (GI), musculoskeletal, immunologic, renal, and even central nervous system (CNS). A previous study reviewed the components of the stress response and determined that analgesic interventions that do not adversely modify the stress response will have minimal impact on patient outcome.[35] Untreated pain can potentiate the adverse effects on normal physiology. For instance, trauma-related pain primarily caused by chest and upper abdomen injuries can lead to impaired pulmonary function from chest splinting and reflex-activated diaphragmatic dysfunction. Functional residual capacity, cough, and vital capacity are all decreased, resulting in serious complications such as atelectasis and ventilator-associated pneumonia. In addition to adverse pulmonary effects, GI tract motility might be adversely affected due to an increase in sympathetic tone from pain, producing an ileus, which impedes early enteral nutritional absorption. Over the last 2 decades, several studies have reported that the persistence of severe and inadequately treated pain can lead to anatomic and physiologic changes in nervous system.[36] The phenomenon is described as "neuroplasticity" and defined as the ability of neuronal tissue to change in response to repeated incoming stimuli. This can lead to the development of chronic, disabling neuropathic pain. In addition, neuroma formation, complex regional pain syndromes associated with sympathetic dysfunction, and neuralgia can also occur following traumatic injuries. Nevertheless, there has been an effort to interrupt the stress response by both skilled surgical and anesthetic management such as using high doses of intravenous narcotic technique to blunt the cardiovascular stress response in patients undergoing cardiac surgery or implementing regional anesthetic techniques to attenuate the stress response.

EVALUATION OF PAIN AND SEDATION IN CRITICALLY ILL TRAUMA PATIENTS

Pain Assessment

There are a limited number of studies that address pain assessment in the critically ill patient. Although it has been publicized that methodic documentation and pain evaluation lead to the improvement in the quality of pain management,[37] pain control in these patients, especially when they are admitted in ICUs with hemodynamic instability, is not often considered a priority. However, accurate evaluation of pain in the critical care setting is very challenging for a number of reasons. Patients frequently have impaired cognitive function and may be unable to communicate because of having sedation and/or neuromuscular blockage agents on board. It has also been found that a high percentage of health care

extenders in this setting are not able to evaluate the pain correctly.

Sources of Pain for Critically Ill Patients

There are many sources of pain for these patients. The sources can be from either acute or chronic pain conditions or both. Nevertheless, acute pain is more prevalent due to direct traumatic injuries, surgical wounds, and invasive procedures conducted in the acute care setting. In addition, one should keep in mind that immobility can lead to remarkable discomfort or "frozen" joints from prolonged bed rest or extremity stabilizers. Finally, pain originating from occult infections such as sinusitis in nasotracheally intubated patients, otitis media, perianal abscesses, and diabetic ulcers should not be overlooked. With regard to the chronic pain conditions, a careful history of prior pain medication useand dosage before the injury is important. If significant doses of narcotics were used on a chronic basis, one must consider tolerance when administering opioids. In this setting, if the doses of opioids given in the acute setting are inadequate, withdrawal syndromes, which can contribute to agitation and altered mental status, can occur. A similar situation can occur with benzodiazepines, tricyclic antidepressants (TCA), and selective serotonin reuptake inhibitors (SSRI) as well.[38,39]

Pain Evaluation Methods in the Fully Conscious Patients

"All critically ill patients have the right to adequate analgesia and management of their pain."[40] The most reliable and valid indicator of pain is the patient's self-report.[41] There are a variety of existing tools to assess pain. It is essential to use those that are brief, simple, reliable, and sensitive in their ability to accurately detect the changes in pain severity, and reflect the effect of analgesic intervention.

Present and Past History

As mentioned in the preceding text, the patient's report of pain is the ideal way for assessing pain. Moreover, it should include the characteristics of pain such as burning, stabbing, aching and stinging, the frequency and duration, the distribution of the pain, and which factors those make it worse or better. For critically ill adults who are unable to communicate effectively, it would be very useful to receive this information from their relatives. A prior pain history may be helpful in interpreting patient's reaction to the current pain management being utilized. In addition, a past history of previous hospital or ICU admission, pertinent psychiatry, and alcohol or recreation drug usage are important for health care providers to obtain. Finally, the patient's ethnic[42–44] and cultural background[45,46] is vitally important in understanding how pain control implementation and assessment are to be interpreted.

Unidirectional Tools

- A visual analog scale (VAS) is a reliable and valid tool for many patient populations[47] and is considered the gold standard for pain assessment. It comprises a 10 cm horizontal line with the one end labeled "no pain" and the other end labeled "severe pain or worst pain ever." Patients are asked to make marks along the line in the areas that best represent their pain. There are also a vertical VAS or pain thermometer versions that might be easier to understand by younger children. Although there are no specific tests for the ICU, VAS is often used in this setting.[48-51] VAS performance may suffer when applied to elderly patients because of the impairment of their visual and cognitive function. Moreover, postoperative patients and especially the elderly require sedation and sleep at night, which might be an obstacle to perform VAS.[48]

- Numeric rating scale (NRS) is a scale of 11 points ranging from 0 to 10. Patients choose a number that describes the pain in which 0 corresponds to no pain and 10 represents the worst pain. NRS correlates with VAS and can be used with patients of different ages. In addition, patients are able to complete the NRS by either writing or speaking. Consequently, it is the preferred tool of ICU staff.

- Verbal descriptor scales (VDS) is a word(s) scale that represents the intensity of patients' pain from a vertical list of words or from words evenly spaced along a horizontal line.[52] Although this scale can be used effectively in chronic pain patients, it requires the ability of patients to understand the words. Not surprisingly, it is not frequently used for critically ill patients.

- The verbal graphic scale (VGS), originated from the emergency department, was subsequently adapted for the ICU for the continuity of treatment. It consists of a numeric scale from 1 to 10 (0 = no pain; 1 to 3 = mild pain; 2 to 4 = moderate pain; 5 to 7 = severe pain and 8 to 10 = really severe pain).[53] Previous studies have demonstrated strong intercorrelation among VGS, VAS, NRS, and VDS.[54,55]

Pain Evaluation Methods in Patients Unable to Communicate

- The evaluation of the physiologic parameters such as heart rate, blood pressure, and respiration rate may be reproducible;[56] however, the confounding factors found in critical illness make the use of a single set of these parameters questionable.

- Physical examination is as important as the informational history. In addition to the routine examination, emphasis should be placed on the injuries where the pain may have originated. Also, the presence of agitation, lacrimation, papillary dilation, and perspiration may be helpful.

- The behavioral-physiologic scale is a tool that assesses pain-related behaviors (movement, facial expression, and posturing) and physiologic indicators (heart rate, blood pressure, and respiration rate). The behavioral-physiologic scales have been compared with an NRS and a moderate-to-strong correlation was found between them.[57]

All in all, it is essential to insert pain among the parameters routinely assessed in critically ill patients and the response to pain treatment should be controlled utilizing appropriate scales for individual patients. In fact, The Joint Commission on Accreditation of Health Care Organizations declared pain level to be the "fifth vital sign." This has led to increased efforts to reduce patients' pain scores. The level of pain reported by the patient must be considered the current standard for pain assessment and response to analgesia whenever possible. In ICUs, the NRS is recommended for pain assessment. Finally, patients who are unable to communicate should be assessed through both subjective observation of pain-related behaviors and physiologic indicators.[40]

Sedation Evaluation

Agitation is frequently seen in critically ill patients. According to Fraser et al., it occurred at least once in 71% of patients in a medical-surgical ICU.[58] Agitation can be caused by many factors, for example, extreme anxiety, delirium, adverse drug effects, and pain.[58] Nevertheless, when patients develop signs of agitation or anxiety, the first priority is to identify and treat the underlying physiologic abnormality such as hypoxemia, hypercarbia, hypoglycemia, hypotension, and pain. In addition, the patient population that incurs trauma has a high prevalence of drug and alcohol abuse, so withdrawal syndromes particularly from alcohol is high.[59-61] As with pain control, assessment of sedation should be evaluated as part of the comprehensive assessment of the critically ill patient at the time of admission, and should be recorded with particular attention to detail. An ideal scale should provide simple and recordable data and accurately describe the degree of sedation and agitation within well-defined categories. The scales should also be able to guide the titration of therapy, and more importantly should have validity and reliability in critically ill patients. Although many scoring systems are available, a true gold standard has not existed.[62,63] The major methodological problems encountered with these scales were that they were, for the most part, studied in patients who had undergone anesthesia and were recovering in the postanesthesia care units, and not among patients admitted to the ICU with injuries resulting from trauma.

The methods to evaluate the depth of sedation and agitation can be divided into two groups:

Subjective Assessment

These methods are on the basis of clinical observation. The data are recorded after the direct observation by the observers. The Riker Sedation-Agitation Scale (SAS) was the first scale proved to be reliable and valid in critically ill patients.[64,65] There are several items listed describing patient consciousness, agitation, and behavior (see Table 1). The Motor Activity Assessment Scale (MAAS) was adapted from SAS. It comprises seven items to describe patient behavior in response to noxious stimuli (Table 1) MAAS also has demonstrated validity and reliability in critically ill patients.[66] In addition to SAS and MAAS, the Ramsay scale assesses three levels of awake and asleep states (Table 1).[67] Although it has been used in many sedation trials and clinical practices, it has been criticized for lack of clear explanations and discrimination between categories (Table 1).[65,68] Another scale, the COMFORT scale, has been widely used in

the ICUs but is limited to children.[69] Although in a systemic review by De Jonghe et al.,[63] this group showed high reliability and satisfactory correlation among other scales with the Ramsey scale and the COMFORT scale. Many previous sedation assessment instruments have focused exclusively on the level of consciousness alone or with another dimension such as agitation. Furthermore, in these instruments, the assessment of both consciousness and agitation have been minimized in a single scale containing multiple dimensions resulting in unclearly defined levels of sedation leading to loss of useful clinical information. Recently, De Jonghe et al.[62] established a new instrument, the Adaptation to the Intensive Care Environment (ATICE), which is highly reproducible for patients in the ICU who are

TABLE 1

SCALES USED TO ASSESS SEDATION AND AGITATION

Score	Description	Definition
		Riker Sedation-Agitation Scale (SAS)
7	Dangerous agitation	Pulling at endotracheal tube (ETT), trying to remove catheters, climbing over bedrail, striking staff, thrashing side to side
6	Very agitated	Does not calm despite frequent verbal reminding of limits, requires physical restraints, biting ETT
5	Agitated	Anxious or mildly agitated, attempting to sit up, calm down to verbal instructions
4	Calm and cooperative	Calm, awakens easily, follows commands
3	Sedated	Difficult to arouse, awakens to verbal stimuli or gentle shaking but drifts off again, follows simple commands
2	Very sedated	Arouse to physical stimuli but does not communicate or follow commands, may move spontaneously
1	Unarousable	Minimal or no response to noxious stimuli, does not communicate or follow commands
		Motor Activity Assessment Scale (MAAS)
6	Dangerous agitation	No external stimulus is required to elicit movement and patient is uncooperative pulling at tubes or catheters or thrashing side to side or striking at staff or trying to climb out of bed and does not calm down when sedated
5	Agitated	No external stimuli is required to elicit movement and attemping to sit up or move limbs out of bed and does not consistently follow commands (e.g., will lie down when asked but soon reverts to attempts to sit up or move limbs out of bed)
4	Restless and cooperative	No external stimuli is required to elicit movement and patient is picking at sheets or tubes or uncovering self and follows commands
3	Calm and cooperative	No external stimuli is required to elicit movement and patient is adjusting sheets or clothes purposefully and follows commands
2	Responsive to touch or name	Open eyes or raises eyebrows or turns head toward stimulus or moves limbs when touched or name is loudly spoken
1	Responsive only to noxious stimulus[a]	Opens eyes or raises eyebrows or turns head toward stimulus or moves limbs with noxious stimuli
0	Unresponsive	Does not move with noxious stimuli
		Ramsay Scale
1	Awake	Patient anxious and agitated or restless or both
2	—	Patient cooperative, oriented, and tranquil
3	—	Patient responds to commands only
4	Asleep	A brisk response to a light glabellar tap or loud auditory stimulus
5	—	A sluggish response to light glabellar tap or loud auditory stimulus
6	—	No response to a light glabellar tap or loud auditory stimulus

[a]Noxious stimuli = suctioning or 5 seconds of vigorous orbital, sterna, or nail bed pressure
Riker RR, Picard JT, Fraser GL. Prospective evaluation of the Sedation-Agitation Scale for adult critically ill patients. *Crit Care Med.* 1999;27:1325–1329; Devlin JW, Boleski G, Mlynarek M, et al. Motor activity assessment scale: A valid and reliable sedation scale for use with mechanically ventilated patients in an adult surgical intensive care unit. *Crit Care Med.* 1999;27:1271–1275; Ramsay MA, Savege TM, Simpson BR, et al. Controlled sedation with alphaxalone-alphadolone. *Br Med J.* 1974;2:656–659.

receiving mechanical ventilation. ATICE consists of five items, awakeness and comprehension combined in a consciousness domain, calmness, ventilator synchrony, and face relaxation combined in a tolerance domain. However this instrument did not include the assessment of delirium, which is the major contributing factor to ICU agitation.

In ICUs, delirium negatively affects 6-month survival and weaning from mechanical ventilation and contributes to the development of nosocomial pneumonia and prolonged lengths of stay.[13,70] Delirium has also been associated with higher hospital and ICU costs.[71] Delirium is best evaluated using a specific and validated instrument by Ely et al.,[13] the Confusion Assessment Method for the Intensive Care Unit (CAM-ICU). It is used to assess nonverbal but arousable mechanical ventilated patients performed by two critical care nurses compared with using the Diagnostic and Statistical Manual of Mental Disorders (DSM-IV)-based evaluation by two delirium experts. The sensitivity and specificity of the CAM-ICU is >89% for all measurements when compared with DSM-IV–based evaluations, and the interrater reliability for the CAM-ICU is very good to excellent. Consequently, the CAM-ICU may represent a significant advance in the ability to monitor delirium and also enable deterrence of the serious sequelae of delirium including increased mortality, higher costs, longer lengths of hospital and ICU stays, failure to extubate, and long-term cognitive impairment.[72]

Objective Assessment of Sedation

Objective measurements of a patient's level of sedation may be helpful during very deep sedation or when therapeutic neuromuscular blockade may mask observational behavior. This is a similar situation to pain assessment, as vital signs are not specific and sensitive parameters. The most objective assessment is based on a specific patient's electroencephalogram (EEG). The raw EEG is a complex waveform that can be difficult to interpret. In the effort to simplify and quantify the EEG, several devices have been used to improve the interpretation and reliability. For example, the bispectral index (BIS) that consists of a digital scale from 100 (completely awake) to 0 (isoelectric EEG).[73] This technology has been studied extensively in the field of anesthesiology, but to a lesser degree in the ICU setting. It does have limitations in the ICU environment.[74–76] Patients at the same subjective level of sedation may have different BIS scores and subjective scales may be more reproducible during light sedation.[74,75] Essentially, additional confirmatory studies involving critically ill patients are required before the BIS or other objective monitoring tools can be recommended without reservation.

ANALGESIA AND SEDATION FOR TRAUMA PATIENTS

To promote patient comfort after trauma, therapy should involve both pharmacologic and nonpharmacologic limbs.

Nonpharmacologic intervention includes stabilization of fracture sites, appropriate patient positioning, and elimination of irritating physical stimulation. Application of heat and cold therapy might be useful to alleviate pain in particular areas. In addition, more nontraditional interventions may be offered such as environment modification, back massage, and music therapy as they had been demonstrated to benefit the anxious critically ill patient.[77–79]

Pharmacologic intervention consists of opioid and nonopioid analgesics. The characteristics of commonly used opioids and nonopioids are reviewed in Table 2. Opioids have been utilized for pain relief through the centuries and have to be considered the gold standard for treatment of severe pain. Opioids mediate analgesia by interacting with both multiple central and peripheral opioid receptors. The μ and κ receptors are the most important receptors for analgesia. However, the predominant analgesic sites are believed to reside in the CNS including the brainstem, thalamus, forebrain, and spinal cord. There are many routes of opioid administration including parenteral, oral, neuraxial, rectally, transdermally, and transmucosally. In addition to a variety of choices of administration, the other advantages of opioids include rapid onset, lack of the accumulation of the parent drugs, ease to titration, and relatively low cost. In critically ill patients, the agents most commonly used are fentanyl, morphine, and hydromorphone. Fentanyl has the most rapid onset and shortest duration of action. Morphine has a longer duration of action, and an active metabolite, morphine-6-glucuronide contributes to prolonged sedation in patients with renal insufficiency. Unfortunately, hypotension from direct vasodilation may result from administration of moderate to high doses of morphine. In contrast, hydromorphone lacks clinically significant active metabolites and histamine release. Another opioid, meperidine, also has an active metabolite, normeperidine, which can cause neuroexcitation and may interact with antidepressant (it is contraindicated with monoamine oxidase inhibitors (MAOIs) and should be avoided with SSRIs as well). Consequently, intravenous infusion and repetitive use are not recommended.[80,81] In critically ill patients, adverse effects of opioids can occur more frequently including respiratory depression, hemodynamic instability resulting from hypotension, depression of level of consciousness, and gastric hypomotility. In addition, patients with renal and/or hepatic insufficiency, which are common amongst polytrauma critically ill patients, may alter opioids and their metabolites' elimination resulting in the higher frequency of untoward effects. Titration to the desired response and assessment of their adverse effects should be performed routinely.

Patient-controlled analgesia (PCA) is a popular opioid delivery system in patients with acute trauma. It provides basal rate of opioids infusion. The patient is allowed to initiate a bolus dose of medication by pushing a button or foot pedal, which is limited by locked out mechanism. Previous studies have demonstrated mixed outcomes when comparing the use of PCA and intermittent intravenous or

TABLE 2

PHARMACOLOGY OF COMMONLY USED OPIOIDS AND NONOPIOIDS ANALGESICS

Agent	Onset (IV)	Half-life	Active Metabolites	Adverse Effects	Intermittent Dose[a]	Infusion Dose Range
Fentanyl	1–2 min	1.5–6 hr	No metabolite, parent accumulates	Rigidity with high doses	0.35–1.5 μg/kg IV q 0.5–1 hr	0.7–10 μg/kg/hr
Hydromorphone	5 min	2–3 hr	None	—	10–30 μg/kg IV q 1–2 hr	7–15 μg/kg/hr
Morphine	5 min	3–7 hr	Yes (sedation, especially in renal insufficiency)	Histamine release	0.01–0.15 mg/kg IV q 1–2 hr	0.07–0.5 mg/kg/hr
Meperidine	5–10 min	3–4 hr	Yes (neuroexcitation, especially in renal insufficiency or high doses)	Avoid with MAOIs[b] and SSRIs[c]	—	Not recommended
Remifentanil	1–3 min	3–10 min	None	—	—	0.6–15 μg/kg/hr
Ketorolac	3–5 min	2.4–8.6 hr	None	Risk of bleeding, GI, and renal adverse effects	15–30 mg IV q 6 hr, decrease if age >65 yr or wt <50 kg or renal impairment, avoid >5 days use	—
Ibuprofen	30 min (oral)	1.8–2.5 hr	None	Risk of bleeding, GI, and renal adverse effects	400 mg PO q 4–6 hr	
Acetaminophen	30 min (oral)	2 hr			325–650 mg PO q 4–6 hr, avoid >4 g/day	—
Codeine	10–30 min (IM and SC)[e]	3 hr	Yes (analgesia, sedation)	Lacks potency, histamine release	Not recommended 15–60 mg q 4–6 hr (IM and SC)[e]	Not recommended
Dexmedetomidine	—	2 hr[d]	None	Hypotension, hypertension, and bradycardia	—	Loading dose 1 μg/kg over 10 min followed by 0.2–0.7 μg/kg/hr, not to exceed 24 hr
Ketamine	1–2 min	4–5 hr	Yes	Tachycardia and increased blood pressure, increased ICP	0.5–1 mg/kg	0.05–0.25 mg/kg/hr

[a]More frequent doses may be needed for acute pain management in mechanically ventilated patients.
[b]MAOIs = monoamine oxidase inhibitors.
[c]SSRIs = selective serotonin-reuptake inhibitors.
[d]Following infusion, dexmedetromidine exhibits a rapid distribution phase with a half-life of approximately 6 minutes.
[e]Intramuscular and subcutaneous.
GI, gastrointestinal; ICP, intracranial pressure.
Jacobi J, Fraser GL, Coursin DB, et al. Clinical practice guidelines for the sustained use of sedatives and analgesics in the critically ill adult. *Crit Care Med.* 2002;30:119–141; *Clin Pharm.* Acute pain management: Operative or medical procedures and trauma. Agency for Health Care Policy and Research. 1992;11:309–331; Duke P, Maze M, Morrison P. Dexmedetomidine: A general overview. *Int Congr Symp Ser Redefin Sedat.* 1998;221:11–22; Smythe M. Patient-controlled analgesia: A review. *Pharmacotherapy.* 1992;12:132–143; Barr J, Donner A. Optimal intravenous dosing strategies for sedatives and analgesics in the intensive care unit. *Crit Care Clin.* 1995;11(4):827–847; Webster LR, Walker MJ. Safety and efficacy of prolonged outpatient ketamine infusions for neuropathic pain. *Am J Ther.* 2006;13(4):300–305.
Smythe M. Patient-controlled analgesia: A review. *Pharmacotherapy.* 1992;12:132–143.

intramuscular narcotic boluses; however, the majority tends to support the use of PCA in terms of improved analgesia and decreased opioid consumption.[84] Furthermore, most studies demonstrated no improvement in pain relief but increased the narcotic consumption with the use of basal rate.[85,86] Therefore, it may be preferred to initiate a PCA with demand doses in patients, especially in the opioid-naïve patient.

There have been many adjuvant drugs using nonopioid analgesics for pain management in traumatic patients. Nonsteroidal anti-inflammatory drugs (NSAIDs) are frequently a first-line treatment for many painful conditions in this group of patients. NSAIDs provide analgesia through the nonselective, competitive inhibition of cyclooxygenase (COX), a critical enzyme in the inflammatory cascade. Administration of NSAIDs may reduce opioid requirements. Many oral forms are available. Ibuprofen and naproxen are available in liquid form. Ketorolac is the only parenterally available NSAID. The drawbacks of NSAIDs include inhibition of platelet function, GI bleeding, and the development of renal insufficiency. There have been several studies demonstrating that prolonged use (>5 days) of ketorolac has been associated with a twofold increase in the risk of GI and operative-site bleeding.[87,88] In the late 1990s, a new generation of NSAIDs, which selectively inhibits the COX-2 isoenzyme, was introduced into clinical practice. Selective COX-2 inhibiting agents provide all the beneficial effects of the previous generation NSAIDs and demonstrate less GI bleeding and ulcer formation with long-term use compared to traditional NSAIDs.[89] In addition to oral COX-2 inhibiting agents, there is an injectable COX-2 inhibitor, paracoxib, which has analgesic properties equivalent to ketorolac.[90] This medication has multiple advantages, including administration intraoperatively and immediately postoperatively before oral medications would be tolerated. Nevertheless, the risk for cardiovascular events may be increased when COX-2 inhibitors are used.[91] Regarding this adverse effect, one of COX-2 inhibitors (rofecoxib) has been withdrawn from the market since 2004 because of increased arterial thrombosis risk including myocardial infarction and cerebrovascular accident after prolonged administration (>18 months).[92]

Acetaminophen also exerts its analgesic effects by the inhibition of COX, which is the rate-limiting enzyme in prostaglandin synthesis. Acetaminophen is used to treat mild to moderate pain. It also produces antipyresis with minimal anti-inflammatory effects. Although acetaminophen may not be sufficient to treat severe pain, in combination with opioids, it demonstrates greater analgesia than using higher doses of opioids alone.[93] In addition, with regard to its safety profile in proper doses, it becomes valuable adjunct medication in trauma patients. Acetaminophen can be administered by both oral and rectal routes with the maximal dose of 65 mg/kg/day in order to avoid hepatotoxicity.

Ketamine is an arylcyclohexamine congener of phencyclidine. Ketamine competitively blocks *N*-methyl-D-aspartate (NMDA) receptors that contribute to the analgesic effect. The major advantages of ketamine include stimulation of cardiovascular system, preservation of spontaneous breathing, and airway protective reflex. It is commonly used as an induction agent in general anesthesia for patients with hemodynamic instability and/or severe bronchospastic airway disease. However, there are some adverse effects, which include increased secretion and hallucination that can be alleviated by concomitant use of benzodiazepines. In the trauma patient, ketamine has a role for painful procedures such as closed reduction and wound debridements. In adult patients with musculoskeletal trauma, compared to intermittent intravenous morphine, ketamine provided more intense analgesia, lower drowsiness scores, and improved peak expiratory flow rates.[94]

Originally, anticonvulsants were only able to suppress spontaneous neuronal firing in the brain. However, new generation drugs such as gabapentin, topiramate, and lamotrigine can also exhibit suppression of peripheral nociceptive neuronal firing. These agents are sometimes useful in trauma patients for the treatment of neuropathic pain, especially among burn patients. Antidepressants such as TCA also have a role in the management of neuropathic pain. They also contribute to reducing pain, treating depression, and facilitating sleep in trauma patients.

Local anesthetics (LAs) have been shown to have a variety of positive effects including analgesic, broncodilatory, antiarrhythmic, and antithrombotic properties, if given or absorbed in nontoxic doses. On the other hand, LAs have the potential for adverse effects such as neurotoxicity (dose-dependent), cardiotoxicity (dose-dependent), and excitation or depression of CNS (dose-dependent).[95] It is recommended to administer a test dose (local anesthetic or saline with 1:200,000 epinephrine) with catheter placement in order to prevent LA intoxication from accidental intravascular injection. Rare cases of systemic toxicity have been observed with topical application to mucosal membranes, and topical lidocaine provides useful analgesia in traumatic conditions such as burns.[96] Intravenous lidocaine also has a role in trauma pain. Jonsson et al. reported that it was safe and effective to use lidocaine intravenously in treating pain resulting from burns.[97] There was no systemic toxicity observed during the infusion period of lidocaine.

REGIONAL ANALGESIA IN TRAUMA PATIENTS

Regional analgesia approaches with LA or the selective neuraxial delivery of opioids offer significant advantages over systemic opioids in terms of lower side effects, especially with respect to respiratory depression, altered mental status, and reduced bowel motility. Among regional techniques, epidural analgesia is the most frequently employed procedure in trauma patients. Chest trauma, trauma of lower extremities, and thoracic and abdominal surgery are all common indications for this technique, but must be individualized based on the individual patient. Though epidural analgesia has not been definitively shown to improve mortality rates, in many cases, postoperative management is improved by avoiding the side effect of general anesthesia and the need for moderate to high systemic opioid doses, thereby resulting in superior pain scores. Opioids or LAs alone or some combinations of these are able to be administered into the epidural space. The technique may range from single-dose injection to continuous infusion with patient-controlled epidural-analgesia (PCEA). PCEA is similar to PCA in that the patient can press a button to deliver the bolus dose in addition to basal rates infusion. Dose suggestions for bolus regimen are 5 to 10 mL of 0.125% to 0.25% bupivacaine or 0.1% to 0.2% ropivacaine every 8 to 12 hours and 0.0625% bupivacaine or 0.1% ropivacaine at 5 mL per hour for continuous infusion.[98] Opioids (fentanyl, sufentanil, and hydromorphone) or clonidine at doses of

1 to 2 μg per kg in hemodynamic stable patients can be considered for addition.[98] However, epidural analgesia technique is not without risks. The most common side effects are bradycardia and hypotension from sympathetic blockade, which can be aggravated by intermittent bolus dosing. In addition, one should be alerted to the patient's coagulation status, infectious-related risk, the potential for local anesthesia toxicity and the masking effect of analgesia that may delay the diagnosis of compartment syndromes, compressive cast or with life-threatening conditions such as ruptured spleen.[99] Regarding the patient's coagulation and the use of regional anesthetic techniques, due to the scant clinical evidence that exists, the current recommendations provided by the American Society of Regional Anesthesia should be followed.[100,101]

Peripheral Nerve Blocks for the Extremities

Severe trauma to the shoulder, arm, and hand is frequently a component of the multiple injuries sustained in association with brain injuries in the polytrauma patient. Usage of systemic opioids might mask the neurologic status and lead to difficulties in performing serial neurologic examinations, especially if mechanical ventilation is necessitated. Neural blockade of the brachial plexus with various approaches including continuous interscalene,[102,103] continuous cervical paravertebral,[102,104] supraclavicular, infraclavicular,[105] and axillary can be viable alternative techniques. The continuous infraclavicular and axillary[103,106] approaches provide good analgesia for most of the arm, elbow, and hand. In patients who require surgical anesthesia, debridements for burns, or painful dressing changes, intermittent bolus injection through the catheters should be considered. Nevertheless, in critically ill sedated patients, there should be concern regarding nerve and spinal cord injuries related to particular approaches such as interscalene technique. A combination of ultrasound and nerve stimulation for placement of catheters should help to reduce the risk of these complications.[107] In addition to nerve and spinal cord injuries, pneumothorax is another complication of which one should be aware although the incidence is quite low (the incidence of pneumothorax ranges from 0.5% to 6% with the classic supraclavicular technique)[108,109] this is obviously even a lesser issue in the presence of a pre-existing chest tube which is common in these patients. With regard to unilateral lower limb pain, those patients who are not candidates for epidural analgesia may benefit from particularly those with femoral neck fractures. Three-in-one (femoral, obturator, and lateral femoral cutaneous) and lumbar plexus block also effectively address pain emanating from the anterior thigh. Furthermore, sciatic nerve blockade provides good analgesia to posterior thigh and most of the lower leg. Continuous femoral catheters in combination with a sciatic block results in excellent pain relief for the whole leg and can even be utilized to provide surgical anesthesia.[110]

Other Regional Analgesic Techniques

In patients with severe chest trauma who are not candidates for epidural blockade, intrapleural analgesia has a valuable role for an alternative analgesic technique, although the outcomes have been mixed.[111,112] The main complication of this method is pneumothorax. Although it can be minimized in patients who have preexisting chest tubes, this technique has less value due to the chest tubes drainage of the pleura space. Intercostal nerve blocks are another form of analgesia for treating somatic chest pain. One study demonstrated a significant improvement in respiratory function 1 hour after placement of the nerve block, but this effect had completely subsided 6 hours later.[113] There are other problems relating to this technique including the risk of pneumothorax, anesthetic toxicity, the requirement for multiple levels to be blocked, and the relative short duration of action.

SEDATION THERAPY

Benzodiazepines

This class of medication promotes sedation, anxiolysis, and muscle relaxation but lacks analgesic properties (see Table 3). It also produces anterograde amnesia that can benefit a patient's perception of traumatic pain. When benzodiazepines are used in combination with opioids, reduced analgesic doses are required.[115] Compromised hepatic or renal function may slow the clearance of benzodiazepines or their active metabolites. In addition, induction or inhibition of hepatic or intestinal enzyme activity can alter the oxidative metabolism of most benzodiazepines.[116] Midazolam and diazepam have been used as first-line drugs for systemic sedation. Midazolam has a rapid onset and short duration with single doses.[117] Consequently, it is preferable for treating acutely agitated patients. Accumulation of an active metabolite, α-hydroxymidazolam, can prolong the sedative effects especially in patients with renal insufficiency. Diazepam also has a rapid onset and awakening after single doses.[117] Because of its long-acting metabolites, a prolonged duration of sedative effect may occur with repeated dose. Although lorazepam has a slower onset, it provides fewer potential drug interactions. Similar to midazolam, the usual therapeutic dosages of lorazepam have minimal effect on cardiovascular and respiratory function in healthy subjects but may produce mild respiratory depression in patients with chronic pulmonary disease.[118] As a consequence of its slow onset, lorazepam is not a drug of choice for treating acutely-agitated patients. On the other hand, lorazepam is a useful alternative to midazolam for the long-term sedation of patients in the ICU and provides easier management of the sedation level. Also, sedation with lorazepam offers significant cost savings.[119]

TABLE 3

PHARMACOLOGY OF SEDATIVE DRUGS

Agent	Onset	Half-life of Parent Compound	Active Metabolite	Adverse Effects	Intermittent IV Dose[a]	Infusion Dose Range
Diazepam	2–5 min	20–120 hr	Yes (prolonged sedation)	Phlebitis	0.03–0.1 mg/kg q 0.5–6 hr	—
Lorazepam	5–20 min	8–15 hr	None	Solvent-related acidosis/renal failure in high doses	0.02–0.06 mg/kg q 2–6 hr	0.01–0.1 mg/kg/hr
Midazolam	2–5 min	3–11 hr	Yes (prolonged sedation, especially with renal failure)	—	0.02–0.08 mg/kg q 0.5–2 hr	0.04–0.2 mg/kg/hr
Propofol	1–2 min	26–32 hr	None	Elevated triglycerides, pain on injection	—	5–80 μg/kg/min
Haloperidol	3–20 min	18–54 hr	Yes (EPS[b])	QT interval prolongation	0.03–0.15 mg/kg q 0.5–6 hr	0.04–0.15 mg/kg/hr

[a]More frequent doses may be needed for acute pain management in mechanically ventilated patients.
[b]Extrapyramidal symptoms.
Jacobi J, Fraser GL, Coursin DB, et al. Clinical practice guidelines for the sustained use of sedatives and analgesics in the critically ill adult. *Crit Care Med.* 2002;30:119–141; Smythe M. Patient-controlled analgesia: A review. *Pharmacotherapy.* 1992;12:132–143. Barr J, Donner A. Optimal intravenous dosing strategies for sedatives and analgesics in the intensive care unit. *Crit Care Clin.* 1995;11(4):827–847; Shapiro BA, Warren J, Egol AB, et al. Practice parameters for intravenous analgesia and sedation for adult patients in the intensive care unit: An executive summary. Society of Critical Care Medicine. *Crit Care Med.* 1995;23(9):1596–1600.

Propofol

Propofol (Table 3) was originally an intravenous general anesthetic agent. It demonstrated sedative and hypnotic properties at lower doses. As with benzodiazepines, propofol does not possess any analgesic effects. Propofol has a rapid onset and short duration of sedation upon discontinuation; however, prolonged recovery has been reported after more than 12 hours of infusion.[120] For patients with head injuries, propofol has been used to reduce elevated intracranial pressure (ICP) and the rapid reversal after discontinuation makes it feasible for regular neurologic assessment.[121]

Adverse effects of propofol include hypotension, bradycardia, pain following peripheral venous injection, and hypertriglyceridemia which resulted from long-term or high-dose infusion.[122] In addition, prolonged use (>48 hours) of high doses of propofol (>66 μg/kg/minute) has been associated with lactic acidosis, bradycardia, and lipidemia in pediatric patients and doses >83 μg/kg/minute have been associated with an increased risk of cardiac arrest in adults.[123,124] Consequently, it is recommended to monitor for unexplained metabolic acidosis and/or arrhythmias in patients who are given prolonged propofol infusion.

Central Acting α-Agonists

Clonidine has both analgesic and sedative properties that are useful in trauma pain management. Studies have demonstrated good outcomes with clonidine in terms of reduced perioperative analgesic requirements, prolonged effects of LAs, and enhanced opioid analgesia.[125] The more selective α-2 agonist, dexmedetomidine, was recently approved for use as a sedative with analgesic sparing activity of short-term duration for initially intubated and ventilated patients in intensive care setting. Its properties include decreased norepinephrine levels and sympathetic activity resulting in decreased blood pressure and heart rate.[126] Dexmedetomidine also reduces the need for concurrent analgesic and sedative administration.[127] Furthermore, patients remain sedated when undisturbed, but arouse readily with gentle stimulation. Additionally, dexmedetomidine has found to have neuroprotective properties in various experimental designs, involving cerebral ischemia in adult animals.[128] A recent study investigated the neuroprotective properties of α_2-adrenoceptor agonists in developing brains that are highly susceptible to neuronal damage and the result suggested that neuroprotective properties of dexmedetomidine are mediated by the α_{2A}-adrenoceptor subtype.[129] Patients may develop bradycardia and hypotension during dexmedetomidine infusion, especially in volume-depleted and high sympathetic tone status. Although not specifically studied, if dexmedetomidine is administered chronically and stopped abruptly, withdrawal syndrome may occur. As a result, it is not recommended to administer dexmedetomidine for >24 hours.

Neuroleptic Agents

Neuroleptic agents (chlorpromazine and haloperidol) are the most frequently used drugs to treat patients with delirium. Their effects are to antagonize dopamine-mediated neurotransmission at the level of cerebral synapse and basal ganglia. Chlorpromazine is not commonly used in critically ill patients because it has a pronounced anticholinergic effect, is very sedative, and possesses α-adrenergic antagonist effects. On the other hand, haloperidol has a more tolerative sedative effect and a lower risk of inducing hypotension. Haloperidol has a long half-life and a loading dose is recommended to achieve a rapid response in acute derilium. Neuroleptic agents can cause a dose-dependent QT-interval prolongation resulting in an increased risk of ventricular dysrhythmias, including torsades de pointes.[130] Other important side effects include the development of extrapyramidal symptoms (EPS) and neuroleptic malignant syndrome. A slowly eliminated active metabolite of haloperidol contributes to cause EPS.[131] Treatment of EPS includes discontinuing the neuroleptic agents and a clinical trial of diphenhydramine or benztropine mesylate. Neuroleptic malignant syndrome is a rare and potentially lethal side effect. Successful treatment of neuroleptic malignant syndrome depends on early clinical recognition and prompt supportive care. Dantrolene sodium, bromocriptine, and pancuronium have been reported to be beneficial in the treatment of neuroleptic malignant syndrome.[132]

PAIN MANAGEMENT OF THE TRAUMA PATIENT AS AN OUTPATIENT

Choices of Analgesia after Discharge

Oral analgesia is still the major mode of administration for continuing pain management at home. It is essential to start oral analgesia before the effects of LAs have ceased.[133] It might be sufficient to use only acetaminophen for patients with mild pain. For mild to moderate pain, the combinations of NSAIDs and "weak" opioids such as codeine, hydrocodone, and tramadol in addition to regional anesthesia may benefit the patient. According to patient feedback, rescue drugs for postoperative pain may be required depending on the pain scores and previous preoperative

narcotic history. COX-2 selective drugs (celeroxib) may also have a role in posthospitalization analgesia. Further ongoing trials looking at the newer coxibs as well as the older agents are being awaited because the previous studies did not answer the question of the risk–benefit ratio of short-term use of these drugs in patients at little or no risk for adverse cardiac events.[134,135] In addition to oral analgesia, Rawal N et al. have introduced a concept of patient-controlled regional anesthesia (PCRA) using an elastrometric balloon pump which allows the patient to self-administer local anesthetic analgesia at home.[136] Although new equipment has been developed to minimize the concern of LA toxicity, further studies are necessary to establish the efficacy and safety of this promising new technique at home after ambulatory surgery.

CONCLUSION

The management of pain and sedation plays a crucial and essential part in the overall treatment of the trauma patient. Inadequate pain management can adversely affect patient morbidity and mortality. It has been observed that trauma impacts the patient not only physiologically but also psychologically. Multimodal analgesia with combinations of both systemic and regional anesthesia benefit the quality of pain control, thereby enhancing ambulation and reducing days to discharge. It is recommended that frequent pain and sedation assessments occur, and the necessary adjustments in medications, dosages, and techniques are implemented based on the feed back. Although in recent years, the health care community has better understood both the mechanisms and consequences of pain, much more research is still needed. Regardless of outcomes, the treatment of pain is fundamental to compassionate patient care.

REFERENCES

1. Corso P, Finkelstein E, Miller T, et al. Incidence and lifetime costs of injuries in the United States. *Inj Prev.* 2006;12:212–218.
2. Bulger EM, Edwards T, Klotz P, et al. Epidural analgesia improves outcome after multiple rib fractures. *Surgery.* 2004;136:426–430.
3. Davidson EM, Ginosar Y, Avidan A. Pain management and regional anaesthesia in the trauma patient. *Curr Opin in Anaesthesiol.* 2005;18:169–174.
4. Cohen SP, Christo PJ, Moroz L. Pain management in trauma patients. *Am J Phys Med Rehabil.* 2004;83:142–161.
5. Whipple JK, Lewis KS, Quebbeman EJ, et al. Analysis of pain management in critically ill patients. *Pharmacotherapy.* 1995;15:592–599.
6. Choiniere M, Amsel R. A visual analog thermometer for measuring pain intensity. *J Pain Symptom Manage.* 1996;11:299–311.
7. Francis J, Martin D, Kapoor WN. A prospective study of delirium in hospitalized elderly. *JAMA.* 1990;263:1097–1101.
8. Inouye SK, Bogardus ST, Charpentier PA, et al. A multicomponent intervention to prevent delirium in hospitalized older patients. *N Engl J Med.* 1999;340:669–676.

9. Levkoff SE, Evans DA, Liptzin B, et al. Delirium. The occurrence and persistence of symptoms among elderly hospitalized patients. *Arch Int Med.* 1992;152.2:334–340.

10. Granberg A, Engberg IB, Lundberg D. Acute confusion and unreal experiences in intensive care patients in relation to the ICU syndrome. Part II. *Intensive Crit Care Nurs.* 1999;15:19–33.

11. Granberg A, Engberg IB, Lundberg D. Intensive care syndrome: A literature review. *Intensive Crit Care Nurs.* 1996;12:173–182.

12. Bergeron N, Dubois MJ, Dumont M, et al. Intensive care delirium screening checklist: Evaluation of a new screening tool. *Intensive Care Med.* 2001;27:859–864.

13. Ely EW, Siegel MD, Inouye SK. Delirium in the intensive care unit: An under-recognized syndrome of organ dysfunction. *Semin Respir Crit Care Med.* 2001;22:115–126.

14. Bruce A.J, et al. The incidence of delirium associated with orthopedic surgery: a meta-analytic review. *Int Psychogeriatr.* 2007:197–214.

15. Chernow B, Alexander R, Smallridge RC, et al. Hormonal responses to graded surgical stress. *Arch Int Med.* 1987;147:1273–1278.

16. Naito Y, Tamai S, Shingu K, et al. Responses of plasma adreno-corticotropic hormone, cortisol, and cytokines during and after upper abdominal surgery. *Anesthesiology.* 1992;77:426–431.

17. Pullicino EA, Carli F, Poole S, et al. The relationship between the circulating concentrations of interleukin 6 (IL-6), tumor necrosis factor (TNF) and the acute phase response to elective surgery and accidental injury. *Lymphokine Res.* 1990;9:231–238.

18. Van den Berghe G, de Zegher F, Bouillon R. Clinical review 95: Acute and prolonged critical illness as different neuroendocrine paradigms. *J Clin Endocrinol Metab.* 1998;83:1827–1834.

19. Ross R, Miell J, Freeman E, et al. Critically ill patients have high basal growth hormone levels with attenuated oscillatory activity associated with low levels of insulin-like growth factor-I. *Clin Endocrinol (Oxf).* 1991;35.1:47–54.

20. Voerman HJ, Strack van Schijndel RJ, de Boer H, et al. Growth hormone: Secretion and administration in catabolic adult patients, with emphasis on the critically ill patient. *Neth J Med.* 1992;41:229–244.

21. Chopra IJ, Huang TS, Beredo A, et al. Evidence for an inhibitor of extrathyroidal conversion of thyroxine to 3,5,3′-triiodothyronine in sera of patients with non-thyroidal illnesses. *J Clin Endocrinol Metab.* 1985;60:666–672.

22. Chow CC, Mak TW, Chan CH, et al. Euthyroid sick syndrome in pulmonary tuberculosis before and after treatment. *Ann Clin Biochem.* 1995;32(Pt 4):385–391.

23. Jarek MJ, Legare EJ, McDermott MT, et al. Endocrine profiles for outcome prediction from the intensive care unit. *Crit Care Med.* 1993;21:543–550.

24. Van den Berghe G. Novel insights into the neuroendocrinology of critical illness. *Eur J Endocrinol.* 2000;143:1–13.

25. Van den Berghe G. Dynamic neuroendocrine responses to critical illness. *Front Neuroendocrinol.* 2002;23:370–391.

26. Van den Berghe G, de Zegher F, Veldhius JD, et al. Thyrotrophin and prolactin release in prolonged critical illness: Dynamics of spontaneous secretion and effects of growth hormone-secretagogues. *Clin Endocrinol (Oxf).* 1997;47:599–612.

27. Fliers E, Alkemade A, Wiersinga WM. The hypothalamic-pituitary-thyroid axis in critical illness. *Best Pract Res Clin Endocrinol Metab.* 2001;15:453–464.

28. Van den Berghe G. Endocrine evaluation of patients with critical illness. *Endocrinol Metab Clin North Am.* 2003;32:385–410.

29. Van den Berghe G, de Zegher F, Lauwers P, et al. Luteinizing hormone secretion and hypoandrogenaemia in critically ill men: Effect of dopamine. *Clin Endocrinol (Oxf).* 1994;41:563–569.

30. Spratt DI, Cox P, Orav J, et al. Reproductive axis suppression in acute illness is related to disease severity. *J Clin Endocrinol Metab.* 1993;76.6:1548–1554.

31. Woolf PD, Hamill RW, McDonald JV, et al. Transient hypogonadotropic hypogonadism caused by critical illness. *J Clin Endocrinol Metab.* 1985;60:444–450.

32. Noel GL, Sub HK, Stone JG, et al. Human prolactin and growth hormone release during surgery and other conditions of stress. *J Clin Endocrinol Metab.* 1972;35:840–851.

33. Bormann B, Weidler B, Dennhardt R, et al. Influence of epidural fentanyl on stress-induced elevation of plasma vasopressin (ADH) after surgery. *Anesth Analg.* 1983;62:727–732.

34. Rosenfeld BA, Beattie C, Christopherson R, et al. The effects of different anesthetic regimens on fibrinolysis and the development of postoperative arterial thrombosis. Perioperative Ischemia Randomized Anesthesia Trial Study Group. *Anesthesiology.* 1993;79.3:435–443.

35. Kehlet H. Surgical stress: The role of pain and analgesia. *Br J Anaesth.* 1989;63:189–195.

36. Woolf CJ, Salter MW. Neuronal plasticity: Increasing the gain in pain. *Science.* 2000;288:1765–1769.

37. Gould TH, Crosby DL, Harmer M, et al. Policy for controlling pain after surgery: Effect of sequential changes in management. *Br Med J.* 1992;305:1187–1193.

38. Lejoyeux M, Ades J. Antidepressant discontinuation: A review of the literature. *J Clin Psychiatry.* 1997;58(Suppl 7):11–15.

39. Schatzberg AF, Haddad P, Kaplan EM, et al. Serotonin reuptake inhibitor discontinuation syndrome: A hypothetical definition. Discontinuation Consensus panel. *J Clin Psychiatry.* 1997;58(Suppl 7):5–10.

40. Jacobi J, Fraser GL, Coursin DB, et al. Clinical practice guidelines for the sustained use of sedatives and analgesics in the critically ill adult. *Crit Care Med.* 2002;30:119–141.

41. *Clin Pharm.* Acute pain management: Operative or medical procedures and trauma. Agency for Health Care Policy and Research. 1992;11:309–331.

42. Moore R. Combining qualitative and quantitative research approaches in understanding pain. *J Dent Educ.* 1996;60:709–715.

43. Neill KM. Ethnic pain styles in acute myocardial infarction. *West J Nurs Res.* 1993;15:531–543.

44. Zborowski M. *People in pain.* San Francisco: Jossey-Bass; 1969:14–48.

45. Harkins SW, Price DD. Aessessment of pain in the elderly. In: Melzack R, Turk DC, eds. *Handbook of pain aessessment.* New York: Guilford Press; 1992:315–331.

46. Zola IK. Culture and symptoms – an analysis of patients' presenting complaints. *Am Sociol Rev.* 1966;31:615–630.

47. Ho K, Spence J, Murphy MF. Review of pain-measurement tools. *Ann Emerg Med.* 1996;27:427–432.

48. Terai T, Yukioka H, Asada A. Pain evaluation in the intensive care unit: Observer-reported faces scale compared with self-reported visual analog scale. *Reg Anesth Pain Med.* 1998;23:147–151.

49. Puntillo KA. Dimensions of procedural pain and its analgesic management in critically ill surgical patients. *Am J Crit Care.* 1994;3:116–122.

50. Meehan DA, McRae ME, Rourke DA, et al. Analgesic administration, pain intensity, and patient satisfaction in cardiac surgical patients. *Am J Crit Care.* 1995;4:435–442.

51. Melzack R, Katz J. Pain measurement in persons in pain. In: Wall PD, Melzack R, eds. *Textbook of pain.* Edinburgh, Scotland: Churchill Livingstone; 1994:337–351.

52. McGrath PA, Johnson G, Goddman JT. CHEOPS: a behavioral scale for rating postoperative pain in children. In: Csrzero F, Field HL, Dubner R, eds. *Advance in pain research and therapy.* New York: Raven Press; 1985:395–402.

53. Noback CR, Demarest RJ. *The human nervous system: basic principlas of neurobiology.* New York: McGraw-Hill; 1981.

54. Bergh I, Sjostrom B, Oden A, et al. An aplication of pain rating scales in geriatic patients. *Aging (Milano).* 2000;12:380–387.

55. Ten Klooster PM, Vlaar APJ, Taal E, et al. The validity and reliability of the graphic rating scale and verbal rating scale for measuring pain across cultures: A study in Egyptian and Dutch women with rheumatoid arthritis. *Clin J Pain.* 2003;22:827–830.

56. Payen JF, Bru O, Bosson JL, et al. Assessing pain in critically ill sedated patients by using a behavioral pain scale. *Crit Care Med.* 2001;29:2258–2263.

57. Puntillo KA, Miaskowski C, Kehrle K, et al. Relationship between behavioral and physiological indicators of pain, critical care patients' self-reports of pain, and opioid administration. *Crit Care Med.* 1997;25:1159–1166.

58. Fraser GL, Prato BS, Riker RR, et al. Frequency, severity, and treatment of agitation in young versus elderly patients in the ICU. *Pharmacotherapy*. 2000;20:75–82.

59. Jenkins DH. Substance abuse and withdrawal in the intensive care unit. Contemporary issues. *Surg Oncol Clin N Am*. 2000; 80:1033–1053.

60. Cornwell EE III, Belzberg H, Velmahos G, et al. The prevalence and effect of alcohol and drug abuse on cohort-matched critically injured patients. *Am Surg*. 1998;64:461–465.

61. Spies CD, Rommelspacher H. Alcohol withdrawal in the surgical patient: Prevention and treatment. *Anesth Analg*. 1999;88: 946–954.

62. De Jonghe B, Bastuji-Garin S, Fangio P, et al. Adaptation to the intensive care environment (ATICE): Development and validation of a new sedation assessment instrument. *Crit Care Med*. 2003;31:2344–2354.

63. De Jonghe B, Bastuji-Garin S, Fangio P, et al. Using and understanding sedation scoring systems: A systematic review. *Intensive Care Med*. 2000;26:275–285.

64. Riker RR, Fraser GL, Cox PM. Continuous infusion of haloperidol controls agitation in critically ill patients. *Crit Care Med*. 1994;22:433–440.

65. Riker RR, Picard JT, Fraser GL. Prospective evaluation of the Sedation-Agitation Scale for adult critically ill patients. *Crit Care Med*. 1999;27:1325–1329.

66. Devlin JW, Boleski G, Mlynarek M, et al. Motor activity assessment scale: A valid and reliable sedation scale for use with mechanically ventilated patients in an adult surgical intensive care unit. *Crit Care Med*. 1999;27:1271–1275.

67. Ramsay MA, Savege TM, Simpson BR, et al. Controlled sedation with alphaxalone-alphadolone. *Bras Med*. 1974;2:656–659.

68. Hansen-Flaschen J, Cowen J, Polomano RC. Beyond the ramsay scale: Need for a validated measure of sedating drug efficacy in the intensive care unit. *Crit Care Med*. 1994;22:732–733.

69. Ambuel B, Hamlett KW, Marx CM, et al. Assessing distress in pediatric intensive care environments: The COMFORT scale. *J Pediatr Psychol*. 1992;17:95–109.

70. Ely EW, Shintani A, Truman B, et al. Delirium as a predictor of mortality in mechanically ventilated patients in the intensive care unit. *JAMA*. 2004;291:1753–1762.

71. Milbrandt EB, Deppen S, Harrison PL, et al. Costs associated with delirium in mechanically ventilated patients. *Crit Care Med*. 2004;32:955–962.

72. Miller RR III, Ely EW. Delirium and cognitive dysfunction in the intensive care unit. *Curr Psychiatry Rep*. 2007;9:26–34.

73. Rosow C, Manberg PJ. Bispectral index monitoring. *Anesthesiol Clin North America*. 2001;19:947–966, xi.

74. Simmons LE, Riker RR, Prato BS, et al. Assessing sedation during intensive care unit mechanical ventilation with the bispectral index and the Sedation-Agitation Scale. *Crit Care Med*. 1999;27:1499–1504.

75. Riker RR, Fraser GL, Simmons LE, et al. Validating the Sedation-Agitation Scale with the bispectral index and visual analog scale in adult ICU patients after cardiac surgery. *Intensive Care Med*. 2001;27:853–858.

76. De Deyne C, Struys M, Decruyenaere J, et al. Use of continuous bispectral EEG monitoring to assess depth of sedation in ICU patients. *Intensive Care Med*. 1998;24:1294–1298.

77. Byers JF, Smyth KA. Effect of a music intervention on noise annoyance, heart rate, and blood pressure in cardiac surgery patients. *Am J Crit Care*. 1997;6:183–191.

78. Chlan L. Effectiveness of a music therapy intervention on relaxation and anxiety for patients receiving ventilatory assistance. *Heart Lung*. 1998:169–176.

79. Chlan L. Effectiveness of a music therapy intervention on relaxation and anxiety for patients receiving ventilatory assistance. *Heart Lung*. 1998;27:169–176.

80. Richards KC. Effect of a back massage and relaxation intervention on sleep in critically ill patients. *Am J Crit Care*. 1998;7:288–299.

81. Danziger LH, Martin SJ, Blum RA. Central nervous system toxicity associated with meperidine use in hepatic disease. *Pharmacotherapy*. 1994;14:235–238.

82. Barr J, Donner A. Optimal intravenous dosing strategies for sedatives and analgesics in the intensive care unit. *Crit Care Clin*. 1995;11(4):827–847.

83. Webster LR, Walker MJ. Safety and efficacy of prolonged outpatient ketamine infusions for neuropathic pain. *Am J Ther*. 2006;13(4):300–305.

84. Hagmeyer KO, Mauro LS, Mauro VF. Meperidine-related seizures associated with patient-controlled analgesia pumps. *Ann Pharmacother*. 1993;27:29–32.

85. Owen H, Szekely SM, Plummer JL, et al. Variables of patient-controlled analgesia. 2. Concurrent infusion. *Anaesthesia*. 1989;44:11–13.

86. Krenn H, Oczenski W, Jellinek H, et al. Nalbuphine by PCA-pump for analgesia following hysterectomy: Bolus application versus continuous infusion with bolus application. *Eur J Pain*. 2001;5:219–226.

87. Feldman HI, Kinman JL, Berlin JA, et al. Parenteral ketorolac: The risk for acute renal failure. *Ann Int Med*. 1997;126:193–199.

88. Strom BL, Berlin JA, Kinman JL, et al. Parenteral ketorolac and risk of gastrointestinal and operative site bleeding. A postmarketing surveillance study. *JAMA*. 1996;275:376–382.

89. Bombardier C, Laine L, Reicin A, et al. Comparison of upper gastrointestinal toxicity of rofecoxib and naproxen in patients with rheumatoid arthritis. VIGOR Study Group. *N Engl J Med*. 2000;343:1520–1528.

90. Camu F, Beecher T, Recker DP, et al. Valdecoxib, a COX-2-specific inhibitor, is an efficacious, opioid-sparing analgesic in patients undergoing hip arthroplasty. *Am J Ther*. 2002;9:43–51.

91. Solomon SD, McMurray JJ, Pfeffer MA, et al. Cardiovascular risk associated with celecoxib in a clinical trial for colorectal adenoma prevention. *N Engl J Med*. 2005;352:1071–1080.

92. Topol EJ. Failing the public health—rofecoxib, Merck, and the FDA. *N Engl J Med*. 2004;351:1707–1709.

93. Peduto VA, Ballabio M, Stefanini S. Efficacy of propacetamol in the treatment of postoperative pain. Morphine-sparing effect in orthopedic surgery. Italian Collaborative Group on Propacetamol. *Acta Anaesthesiol Scand*. 1998;42:293–298.

94. Gurnani A, Sharma PK, Rautela RS, et al. Analgesia for acute musculoskeletal trauma: Low-dose subcutaneous infusion of ketamine. *Anaesth Intensive Care*. 1996;24:32–36.

95. Zink W, Graf BM. Toxicology of local anesthetics. Clinical, therapeutic and pathologicl mechanisms. *Anaesthesist*. 2003;52: 1102–1123.

96. Brofeldt BT, Cornwell P, Doherty D, et al. Topical lidocaine in the treatment of partial-thickness burns. *J Burn Care Rehabil*. 1989; 10:63–68.

97. Jonsson A, Cassuto J, Hanson B. Inhibition of burn pain by intravenous lignocaine infusion. *Lancet*. 1991;338:151–152.

98. Schulz-Stubner S, Boezaart A, Hata JS. Regional analgesia in the critically ill. *Crit Care Med*. 2005;33:1400–1407.

99. Hedderich R, Ness TJ. Analgesia for trauma and burns. *Crit Care Clin*. 1999;15:167–184.

100. Kaplan R. ASRA consensus statements for anticoagulated patients. American Society of Regional Anesthesia. *Reg Anesth Pain Med*. 1999;24:477–478.

101. Horlocker TT, Wedel DJ, Benzon H, et al. Regional anesthesia in the anticoagulated patient: defining the risks (the second ASRA Consensus Conference on Neuraxial Anesthesia and Anticoagulation). *Reg Anesth Pain Med*. 2003;28:172–197.

102. Boezaart AP, de Beer J, du Toit C, et al. A new technique of continuous interscalene nerve block. *Can J Anaesth*. 1999;46: 275–281.

103. Schulz-Stubner S. Brachial plexus. Anesthesia and analgesia. *Anaesthesist*. 2003;52:643–656.

104. Boezaart AP, Koorn R, Rosenquist RW. Paravertebral approach to the brachial plexus: An anatomic improvement in technique. *Reg Anesth Pain Med*. 2003;28:241–244.

105. Ilfeld BM, Enneking FK. Brachial plexus infraclavicular block success rate and appropriate endpoints. *Anesth Analg*. 2002;95: 784.

106. Sia S, Lepri A, Campolo MC, et al. Four-injection brachial plexus block using peripheral nerve stimulator: A comparison between axillary and humeral approaches. *Anesth Analg*. 2002;95:1075–1079, table.

107. Meier G, Bauereis C, Maurer H, et al. Interscalene plexus block. Anatomic requirements–anesthesiologic and operative aspects. *Anaesthesist.* 2001;50:333–341.

108. Brown DL, Cahill DR, Bridenbaugh LD. Supraclavicular nerve block: Anatomic analysis of a method to prevent pneumothorax. *Anesth Analg.* 1993;76:530–534.

109. Bridenbaugh LD. The upper extremity: Somatic blockade. In: Cousins MJ, Bridenbaugh PO, eds. *Neural blockade.* Philadelphia: JB Lippincott Co; 1988:387–416.

110. Kaden V, Wolfel H, Kirsch W. Experiences with a combined sciatic and femoral block in surgery of injuries of the lower leg. *Anaesthesiol Reanim.* 1989;14:299–303.

111. Gabram SG, Schwartz RJ, Jacobs LM, et al. Clinical management of blunt trauma patients with unilateral rib fractures: A randomized trial. *World J Surg.* 1995;19:388–393.

112. Schneider RF, Villamena PC, Harvey J, et al. Lack of efficacy of intrapleural bupivacaine for postoperative analgesia following thoracotomy. *Chest.* 1993;103:414–416.

113. Pedersen VM, Schultze S, Hoier-Madsen K, et al. Air-flow meter assessment of the effect of intercostal nerve blockade on respiratory function in rib fractures. *Acta Chir Scand.* 1983;149:119–120.

114. Shapiro BA, Warren J, Egol AB, et al. Practice parameters for intravenous analgesia and sedation for adult patients in the intensive care unit: An executive summary. Society of Critical Care Medicine. *Crit Care Med.* 1995;23(9):1596–1600.

115. Patterson DR, Ptacek JT, Carrougher GJ, et al. Lorazepam as an adjunct to opioid analgesics in the treatment of burn pain. *Pain.* 1997;72:367–374.

116. Michalets EL. Update: Clinically significant cytochrome P-450 drug interactions. *Pharmacotherapy.* 1998;18:84–112.

117. Ariano RE, Kassum DA, Aronson KJ. Comparison of sedative recovery time after midazolam versus diazepam administration. *Crit Care Med.* 1994;22:1492–1496.

118. Cernaianu AC, DelRossi AJ, Flum DR, et al. Lorazepam and midazolam in the intensive care unit: A randomized, prospective, multicenter study of hemodynamics, oxygen transport, efficacy, and cost. *Crit Care Med.* 1996;24:222–228.

119. Swart EL, van Schijndel RJ, van Loenen AC, et al. Continuous infusion of lorazepam versus medazolam in patients in the intensive care unit: Sedation with lorazepam is easier to manage and is more cost-effective. *Crit Care Med.* 1993;27:1461–1465.

120. Kowalski SD, Rayfield CA. A post hoc descriptive study of patients receiving propofol. *Am J Crit Care.* 1999;8:507–513.

121. Kelly DF, Goodale DB, Williams J, et al. Propofol in the treatment of moderate and severe head injury: A randomized, prospective double-blinded pilot trial. *J Neurosurg.* 1999;90:1042–1052.

122. Sanchez-Izquierdo-Riera JA, Caballero-Cubedo RE, Perez-Vela JL, et al. Propofol versus midazolam: Safety and efficacy for sedating the severe trauma patient. *Anesth Analg.* 1998;86:1219–1224.

123. Bray RJ. Propofol-infusion syndrome in children. *Lancet.* 1999;353:2074–2075.

124. Cremer OL, Moons KGM, Bouman EAC, et al. Long-term propofol infusion and cardiac failure in adult head-injured patients. *Lancet.* 2001;357:117–118.

125. Sanderson PM, Eltringham R. The role of clonidine in anaesthesia. *Hosp Med.* 1998;59:221–223.

126. Duke P, Maze M, Morrison P. Dexmedetomidine: A general overview. *Int Congr Symp Ser Redefin Sedat.* 1998;221;11–22.

127. Martin E, Ramsay G, Mantz J, et al. The role of the alpha2-adrenoceptor agonist dexmedetomidine in postsurgical sedation in the intensive care unit. *J Intensive Care Med.* 2003;18:29–41.

128. Hoffman WE, Kochs E, Werner C, et al. Dexmedetomidine improves neurologic outcome from incomplete ischemia in the rat. Reversal by the alpha 2-adrenergic antagonist atipamezole. *Anesthesiology.* 1991;75:328–332.

129. Paris A, Mantz J, Tonner PH, et al. The effects of dexmedetomidine on perinatal excitotoxic brain injury are mediated by the alpha2A-adrenoceptor subtype. *Anesth Analg.* 2006;102:456–461.

130. Sharma ND, Rosman HS, Padhi ID, et al. Torsades de pointes associated with intravenous haloperidol in critically ill patients. *Am J Cardiol.* 1998;81:238–240.

131. Fang J, Baker GB, Silverstone PH, et al. Involvement of CYP3A4 and CYP2D6 in the metabolism of haloperidol. *Cell Mol Neurobiol.* 1997;17:227–233.

132. Burke C, Fulda GJ, Castellano J. Neuroleptic malignant syndrome in a trauma patient. *J Trauma.* 1995;39:796–798.

133. Rudkin GE. Local and regional anesthesia in the adults day surgery patients. *Practical anaethesia and analgesia for day surgery.* Oxford: BIOS Scientific Publishers; 1997:207–210.

134. Walsh K. Are COX-2 inhibitors really more likely to cause heart attacks and strokes than conventional NSAIDs. *BMA News.* 2005;3:76.

135. Savage R. Cyclo-oxygenase-2 inhibitors: When should they be used in the elderly? *Drugs Aging.* 2005;22:185–200.

136. Rawal N, Axelsson K, Hylander J, et al. Postoperative patient-controlled local anesthetic administration at home. *Anesth Analg.* 1998;86:86–89.

137. Smythe M. Patient-controlled analgesia: A review. *Pharmacotherapy.* 1992;12:132–143.

Ethics and Compassionate Care

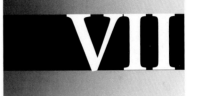

67

Ethical Issues in Trauma Care

James Forrest Calland   C. William Schwab

Caring for a patient during what is often the greatest crisis of their lifetime often leads to ethical and moral dilemmas. As life changing as these major trauma events are for our patients, they have at least as great an impact on their families.

The clinician must have a strong moral and philosophic grounding to successfully navigate through these risk-laden, complex situations. It is certainly beyond the capacity of this chapter to fundamentally change how a clinician practices. Rather, this chapter will likely serve to describe the moral and philosophic foundation that underlies the bioethics or trauma care, and the way that ethical decisions are made after injury.

HISTORICAL PERSPECTIVE

Biomedical ethics are often traced all the way back to the Hippocratic Code, which admonishes us, "...to help, or at least do no harm." The first great work of the modern era, written by Thomas Percival in 1803, provided the first wide-ranging and inclusive treatise on the topic. Percival argued that beneficence and nonmaleficence (the physician mandates to help others and to do no harm) were the two most important ethical principles in medicine, and that the drive to optimize these two factors may supersede the need to preserve autonomy.[1]

In 1979, Beauchamp and Childress published their first edition of their landmark work, *Principles of Biomedical Ethics*, which fully delineated and justified the principles of respect for patient autonomy and justice as sharing equal importance to the principles of beneficence and nonmaleficence, is central to any discussion of modern medical ethics, and required reading for anyone with more than a passing interest in the field.[2]

RESPECT FOR AUTONOMY

First and foremost, the trauma practitioner has the responsibility to seek out the wishes of injured patients and to honor them whenever possible. The challenges associated with fulfilling this responsibility are countless, and are found in every phase of the process: ascertainment of such wishes, determination of relevance and practicality, and implementation.

To claim that we are doing something, "...for an individual's own good" when such an action would directly violate a patient's express wishes, is rarely a defensible or reasonable course of action. The key to this principle is an understanding of what it means to be autonomous, and acquiescence to the idea that few individuals want to be cut out of life-altering decisions or the process of self-determination.

Central to the concept of autonomy, as it is described by Beauchamp and Childress, is the notion that to be autonomous an individual must have: (a) liberty, that is, freedom from controlling influences and (b) agency, or the capacity to act with intention and understanding.[3] Therefore, an individual who is befuddled by mental illness, ignorance, incapacitation, immaturity, or addiction cannot be said to be fully autonomous, and therefore, each patient request in such circumstances must be weighed against what is the standard of what is safe and practical. More controversial is the idea that autonomy calls for an individual to be able to subvert certain basic desires in order to promote higher order ideals, that is, be capable of reasoning beyond the primary desires for thirst, hunger, and comfort, but this standard is more stringent, and as a result, more controversial.[1]

Patients have a right to autonomy, but not a duty to exercise it. Therefore, a patient may reasonably confer medical decision-making power to friends, spouse and family, or even in some rare circumstances to a physician. The responsibility of the physician is to promote autonomy through education, relief from suffering, and support, to optimize the patient's capacity for self-determination.[4] Finally, even when it is unsafe or unwise to allow for patient self-determination because of mental illness, ignorance, or irrationality, patient wishes and preferences should be weighed individually and implemented wherever possible if such wishes are not overly disruptive to the delivery of care and are reasonably safe.

DO NO HARM: NONMALEFICENCE

To address the need to minimize harm to others seems superfluous, however, the practice of medicine, including treatment of the sick and injured, is full of mitigable opportunities for harm. Indeed, there are probably at least 100,000 potentially preventable deaths from medical misadventures each year in the United States.[5] The moral duty of the clinician is to minimize risk to the patient, and to prevent iatrogenic harm wherever possible.

A more challenging area of nonmaleficence, on the other hand, involves withholding and withdrawal of treatments. Treatments that are ineffective in treating a patient's condition, including such interventions as mechanical ventilation, dialysis, and surgical procedures, can be reasonably not offered (or even withdrawn) when such treatments promote suffering or offer minimal hope of cure or palliation. For example, a patient with brain death cannot benefit in any way from initiation of dialysis—the treatment cannot cure or palliate the patient, and as such, should be withdrawn or not offered. Most examples in the daily practice of medicine are not this clear-cut, although the same principles apply in weighing whether to offer or withdraw aggressive medical interventions: Each must be considered in light of its capacity to cure the patient's primary disease process or palliate their symptoms, and not in the light of whether it will merely replace a failing organ system.

A more difficult distinction can be found in the discernment as to whether intravenous and enteral feeding constitutes medical interventions, or basic human care, and, whether such treatments prolong dying rather than promote living. In a landmark case in 1976, the Supreme Court of New Jersey allowed the guardians of a patient in a persistent vegetative state from anoxic brain injury to disconnect the ventilator with the express intention of preventing the suffering induced by the mechanical intervention, and allowing the patient to die.[6] When the patient subsequently survived for several years thereafter receiving tube feeds, the guardians reasoned that the ventilator had contributed to suffering, whereas the tube feeds did not.[7] The boundaries between basic sustenance and medical interventions are indistinct and certainly shaped by an individual's philosophic and spiritual beliefs, experiences, and convictions. However, medical nutrition and hydration is reasonable to administer when, at least according to one prominent author, they offer, reasonable hope of benefit and are attainable without excessive expense, pain, or inconvenience.[8]

A discussion of physician-assisted suicide probably has no place in a textbook related to care of the injured patients. However, very often we are called on to administer treatments that cause harm as a secondary effect to their intended primary clinical benefit. Examples of this are easy to find, but none perhaps more controversial than the use of narcotics during withdrawal of care from fatally injured and terminally ill patients. Minor alterations in the dose of an intravenous narcotic can determine the difference between humane care and active euthanasia. Safe moral ground can be attained in such circumstances when an intended action is at least morally neutral and the clinician, although understanding and anticipating the bad effect, intends only the desired effect. For example, when giving narcotics to reduce pain and suffering, a clinician may realize this action has the capacity to hasten death, but just so long as the physician does not administer the medication for this purpose, but instead doses them to provide for relief from suffering, the "rule of double effect" renders the action ethically justifiable. Coexistent with these requirements is the need for the good (desired) effect to not come about *as a result of* the *bad (undesired)* effect, that is, halting suffering with death.[9]

BENEFICENCE AND PATERNALISM

Beneficence refers to our duty to take action for the benefit of others. We are morally responsible to protect and defend others from abrogation of their rights and harm, to assist those in need, and to rescue those in danger, but with what limitations?

Morally, where one finds conflicting duties to beneficence, one must discern which one takes precedence, and also weigh the potential for benefit against the collective physical, financial, emotional costs of the action under consideration. Where giving to others unreasonably lessens the future capacity of the healer or the institution to help others and to fulfill prior and competing obligations to aid, continuation or escalation of intervention ought not to be undertaken. In the end, the total potential for good must be weighed against the sum potential for harm.

Where some individuals are unable to care for themselves, cannot participate meaningfully in decision making, and have not provided the means for advanced directive or substituted decision making, then (and only then) should the clinician knowingly override the patients' expressed wishes. For example, when treating patients with purposeful self-induced injuries or those who irrationally (not out of moral or philosophic conviction) refuse low-risk life-saving interventions, the clinician has the responsibility to act in the best interest of the patient until capacity is restored.

Paternalism, as such, is defensible where the potential harm to the individual is great without intervention, only a paternalistic action will abrogate this risk, the benefit of the proposed action outweighs the risks, and the restriction of the patient's autonomy is minimized as much as possible.[10]

Occasionally, the trauma physician is called upon to participate in analyses related to rationing of care, or more subtly, to design plans of care seeking to balance cost with potential health benefit—a measure that often incorporates quantification not just of survival or freedom from morbidity, but also, quality of life-adjusted outcomes. Put simply, it is very difficult to simultaneously seek two goals, and best to segregate one's role so as to minimize the conflict between the objectives. When seriously and inextricably conflicted, it is best to rescue oneself from any role that has the actual or perceptual capacity to be in opposition to the well-being of the patient. An example of this is the involvement of the trauma surgeon in the care of patients with potentially unsurvivable brain injury where the clinician has the obligation to avoid counseling the family toward organ donation—it is nearly impossible to simultaneously advocate for the patient and the organ procurement agency.[11]

JUSTICE

Consideration of justice as a moral and ethical principle often defaults to discussion of criminal justice to the neglect of distributive and rectificatory justice. The latter two forms of justice apply respectively to the distribution of rights, responsibilities, and benefits in society and the compensation of individuals and groups for breaches of contracts.

In our society health care access is allocated primarily to those who are employed as a fringe benefit of holding a job. A major theoretic benefit of a physician devoting his or her career to the care of injured patients is dispensation of the need to ascertain insurance status before initiating care, and therefore avoidance having to deny care on the basis of financial concerns. But, are there times when individuals give up their right to medical care either through willful neglect of health or risk-taking?[12] Such a conclusion is nearly impossible to defend as nearly all health disorders have some aspect of personal choice that plays into the pathophysiology whether it be choice in diet, neglect of physical activity, failure to participate in preventative medicine efforts, or even willful commitment to a life of poverty.

ASSESSING COMPETENCE

The capacity to participate in medical decision making in a meaningful way involves more than the capacity

to answer in the affirmative or negative when posed a question. The individual must have agency—that is, the capacity for informed decisions unencumbered by controlling influences, and to understand the consequences of the decision being made. Therefore, competence can be deemed sufficient (or not) for decision making minute-to-minute depending on the gravity of the individual decisions being made. In the care of a nonautonomous patient, where the risk, cost, and inconvenience of the decision are small, the patient may at all times be considered in the process. If, on the other hand, the decision has considerable gravity, it may become necessary to rely on a health care proxy or surrogate, or even, reference to advanced directives.

Proxies (individuals assigned to make medical decisions in the setting of incapacity) and living wills play little or no role in the care of alert patients who are of sound mind and have the ability to express their wishes. Living wills have the potential weakness of being incorrectly invoked as "Do-Not-Resuscitate" orders even when they lack of relevant language in the document to describe the actual health care decision being made—as such, they must be activated only after they are read in their entirety and judged for the relevance and applicability to the decision being made.

INFORMED CONSENT

Of course, complete and perfect informed consent is nearly impossible, as it would require that patients have all the same information as their physicians as they make decisions as to whether or not to undergo a procedure. The issue is one of preservation of autonomy by ensuring patient understanding before giving permission for an intervention that carries risk for morbidity or mortality. But, understanding is only part of the equation. The decision must also be voluntary, and be made in the context of possible alternative treatments. Inevitably, the issue of informed consent is rendered yet more complicated when the patient is consenting to participation in research—especially when such research carries little or no possible benefit for the participant.

The standard for what constitutes adequate disclosure in the delivery of care varies considerably by locality. Some jurisdictions favor the *reasonable doctor (or professional practice) standard* whereby physicians are held to the standard of what other local physicians disclose for a given consent process.[13,14] This becomes problematic when one considers the possibility that a large group can potentially legitimize poor disclosure by institutionalizing it. Alternatives to the *reasonable doctor standard* include the *reasonable person standard* and the subjective standard. In these two examples, physicians are of help to the standard of disclosing what a reasonable hypothetical patient would want disclosed to them, or what each individual patient would hypothetically want disclosed as determined by their individual circumstances and needs. Therapeutic privilege, when invoked, theoretically allows a clinician to avoid informed consent on the principle that the information disclosed to the patient would be harmful to them. Fortunately, this process is rarely invoked because it is quite difficult to counter and carries substantial risk by abrogation of individual autonomy.[3]

When an individual has limited capacity to understand or simple refusal to accept factual information, the provider has the responsibility to ascertain the perceptual reasons that underlie the individual's inability to address reality, and to augment the patient's capacity to make an *informed* consent or refusal. In the absence of this, surrogate opinion will have to be solicited and implemented. Even in this circumstance, coercion by way of threatening to withdraw therapies or care until compliance is attained must be avoided. Likewise, dangling privileges or pandering to a person's vulnerabilities must be avoided wherever it may be perceived as coercive.

BREAKING BAD NEWS

Although not purely a topic of medical ethics, this topic is not covered well elsewhere, and is central to the practice of the trauma surgeon. Oncologist Robert Buckman has laid out a six-step process for disclosing bad news as follows:

1. Get started: Find a private place to talk and begin by asking the person receiving information an open-ended question such as "How are you doing?"
2. Determine what the recipient already knows: "What have you already learned?"
3. Find out what they want to know: "Please let me know what level of detail you want—some want every detail, others want only the big picture—which would you prefer now?"
4. Share information: diagnosis, treatment, prognosis, and support. Ascertain understanding between chunks of data.
5. Acknowledge patient/family feelings.
6. Planning and follow through: synthesize situation with integration of patient concerns, and plans for the next stage of care and follow-up.

Whereas such a structured discussion is not always possible or practical, the six-step process mentioned in the preceding text serves as a template or guide, not a strict mandate.[15] The disclosure process is yet another activity that is central to promoting autonomy.

Frequently, in the presumed best interest of their loved one, families will ask for nondisclosure of information to protect the patient from the harm of receiving bad news. In such circumstances it is important that patient and family alike realize that the physician's primary duty is to the

patient, and that all disclosure will occur in the context of the patient's stated desire to receive such information, and the capacity to understand it. If the patient is to not receive health care information, he or she must consent to not only the process of skipping over such disclosure *and* substituted disclosure to a proxy, power of attorney, or family member. A power of attorney court order does not necessarily remove the need to primarily disclose vital health care information to the patient, but in context, often includes the involvement of the individual assigned by the court to make decisions for the patient when he or she is unable to do so.

RIGHT TO PRIVACY AND CONFIDENTIALITY

Another form of preservation of autonomy is found in the right to privacy. Central to this concept is the idea that physicians have the obligation to preserve the individual's autonomous right to reasonable freedom from the scrutiny of the government and others. Patients further have the right to reasonably refuse to be observed, touched, or intruded upon. Patients must be provided the right to be seen by only those they want to involved in their care, such care may be accommodated for personal or religious reasons, but must be not be accommodated if it is preferred simply because of racial or gender bias, or likewise if it is unduly disruptive to the process of clinical care delivery to other patients.

As for disclosure of protected health information, patients have the right to maintain dominion of their clinical record, and to protection from disclosure of facts about them to third parties. Some disclosure is absolutely necessary to the care delivery process (i.e., communication with a patient's insurer, etc.) whereas other forms, such as disclosure to family members without the consent of the patient must be closely monitored, controlled, and limited to only the necessary information given only to the people who need it.[16]

FUTILITY

Futility is generally a collective agreement of several clinicians, using all the available data in combination with a thorough understanding of the patient, to render a judgment as to whether a proposed course of action has any reasonable hope of helping the afflicted patient.[17]

Futile interventions may increase patient discomfort in the final days of life and therefore violate the principle of nonmaleficence. Promoting respect for autonomy often leads to honoring the wishes of a competent patient, but does not entitle patients to receive treatments that physicians do not believe conform to professional standards of care. Dialysis, for example, might not to be offered to the elderly patient with extensive full-thickness thermal injuries who is intubated and in multisystem organ failure as it may only serve to improve alertness (with clearance of uremia) so that the patient suffers more from the injuries.

When finding it difficult to care for a patient because of a physician's own perception of futility, it may be best to offer to the patient and family the assurance that one will perform all available interventions to promote the patient's dignity and well-being, and to reduce the potential for unnecessary suffering. In fact, after adequate time is given for an emotional adjustment to be made, it is best to inform the patient and family of what interventions one is withholding or withdrawing, and the reasons for doing so.[18] If the family disagrees with the assessment of futility for a given intervention, it may be best to involve other clinicians to render their opinion regarding what is, and what is not possible to achieve.

ADVANCED DIRECTIVES

The federal government passed the *Patient Self-Determination Act* in 1991—a law that for the first time mandated that patients be informed of their participation in health care decisions, including their right to state in writing ahead of time what their wishes are should they fall victim to a cardiac arrest.[19]

Advanced directives are, in general, divided into two broad categories, those that are instructive and those that are proxy. Examples of instructive advanced directives include statements made in documents such as *living wills* and *do-not-intubate* or *do not dialyze* orders. Unfortunately, instructive advanced directive orders often fail to be relevant to address temporary heroic life-saving or sustaining therapies intended to push the patient back toward independence. As such, instructive advanced directives must often be set aside, with decisions (instead of *do-not-resuscitate)* being made according to the unique condition of the patient, and a communication with the patient and family regarding prognosis.

Proxy-based advance directives in general amount to Durable Power of Attorney for Health Care. For these orders, the appointed individual carries no innate power to determine or participate in care unless the patient becomes incapacitated. The need to appoint a proxy is less relevant for patients with large extended families and a spouse—in these cases, according to state laws, the spouse automatically becomes the surrogate decision maker when the patient is incapacitated, with succession by various first-degree family members should the spouse become unable to fulfill his or her duties.

CONCLUSIONS

The principles of respect for autonomy, beneficence, nonmaleficence, and justice provide us with an ethical framework to examine and implement sound, ethical practice to the care of injured patients. These principles do not make us more moral, virtuous, or ethical, but do provide us with a lexicon we can use to describe ethical practice and to better understand the moral and ethical basis for the modern delivery of trauma care.

REFERENCES

1. Percival T. *Medical Ethics: A Code of Institutes and Precepts Adapted to the Professional Conduct of Physicians and Surgeons.* 1803.
2. Beauchamp TL, Childress JF. *Principles of Biomedical Ethics,* 5th ed. New York: Oxford University Press; 2001.
3. Beauchamp TL, Childress JF. *Principles of biomedical ethics,* 5th ed. New York: Oxford University Press; 2001:57–112.
4. Blackhall LJ, Murphy ST, Frank G, et al. Ethnicity and attitudes toward patient autonomy. *JAMA.* 1995;274:820–825.
5. Leape LL, Berwick DM. Five years after to err is human: What have we learned? *JAMA.* 2005;293:2384–2390.
6. In re Quinlan, 70 N.J. 10, 355 A2d 647, cert. denied sub nom. Garger v. New Jersey, 429 U.S. 922. 1976.
7. Armstrong PW, Colen BD. From Quinlan to Jobes: The courts and the PVS patient. *Hastings Cent Rep.* 1988;18:37–40.
8. Kelly G. *The Duty to Preserve Life, Theological Studies.* 1950:218.
9. Boyle JM Jr. Toward understanding the principle of double effect. *Ethics.* 1980;90(4):527–538.
10. Pellegrino ED, Thomasma DC. *For the patient's good: the restoration of beneficence in health care.* New York: Oxford University Press; 1988:29.
11. Roth BJ, Sher L, Murray JA, et al. Cadaveric organ recruitment at Los Angeles County Hospital: Improvement after formation of a structured clinical educational and administrative service. *Clin Transplant.* 2003;17(Suppl 9):52–57.
12. Sturm R. The effects of obesity, smoking, and drinking on medical problems and costs. *Health Aff.* 2002;21(2):245–253.
13. Barry MJ. Involving patients in medical decisions: How can physicians do better? *JAMA.* 1999;282:2356–2357.
14. Briguglio J, Cardella JF, Fox PS, et al. Development of a model angiography informed consent form based on a multiinstitutional survey of current forms. *J Vasc Interv Radiol.* 1995;6(6):971–978.
15. Baile WF, Buckman R, Lenzi R, et al. SPIKES: A six-step protocol for delivery bad news. *Oncologist.* 2000;5:302–311.
16. Surbonne A, Zwitter M, eds. *Communication with the cancer patient: information and truth.* Annals of the New York Academy of Sciences; 1997:809.
17. Kasman DL. When is medical treatment futile? *J Gen Intern Med.* 2004;19(10):1053–1056.
18. Leonard CT, Doyle RL, Raffin TA. Do-not-resuscitate orders in the face of patient and family opposition. *Crit Care Med.* 1999;27(6):1045–1047.
19. Emanuel EJ, Weinberg DS, Gonin R, et al. How well is the Patient Self-Determination Act working?: An early assessment. *Am J Med.* 1993;95:619–628.

End-of-Life Care

68

Robert M. Nelson, Jr.

> *"Nothing could stop you.*
> *Not the best day. Not the quiet. Not the ocean rocking.*
> *You went on with your dying."*
>
> –Elegy for My Father (1970). 3.Your Dying.
> Mark Strand

As is noted in the excerpt from this poem, there will always be patients who, despite the attempts of the patient, physicians, and other health care workers, reach a point where their decisions no longer focus on a cure, but rather, on how best to accomplish their final journey.

End-of-life care issues have become increasingly complex as new technologies and medications have expanded the options available to sustain life. Patients have also become more involved in all aspects of their medical care, as religious and cultural influences are increasingly recognized. The greater number of medical specialists involved in patient care further complicates end-of-life care issues. For the severely injured trauma patient, the time available to address end-of-life issues may be as short as hours, or it may extend over weeks or months.

This chapter will review end-of-life care issues that practitioners should be aware of, and it will provide a framework to assist practitioners in dealing with this important aspect of patient care. The chapter is divided into two sections. The first section addresses the issues surrounding the arrival at the decision that life-sustaining efforts will cease, and that end-of-life care issues need to be addressed. The second section addresses various aspects of end-of-life care.

BARRIERS TO EFFECTIVE END-OF-LIFE CARE

Clinicians with experience in caring for critically ill injured patients have recognized the large gap between the intended quality of end-of-life care and the product that is actually delivered for patients, their families, and the medical professionals who deliver the care.[1] National recognition of the importance of this issue resulted in a decision by the Institute of Medicine to designate improved end-of-life care as a national health priority. This gap was confirmed in a recent report by Nelson et al.[2] of a national survey of critical care providers. The survey disclosed important barriers pertinent to the practices and beliefs of physicians, features of patient and family attitudes toward death, lack of institutional preparedness, and physical characteristics of critical care units. Patients may unknowingly create a barrier by failing to have an advance directive in place when it is needed. A frequent, more frustrating problem is family certainty that an advance directive exists but cannot be located. Unrealistic expectations by family members contribute as well. Physician factors that were identified included insufficient training in end-of-life practices and too little time devoted to discussions of this problem with patients and families. Institutional factors included lack of space for private family consultations and the lack of a formally organized palliative care service.

ARRIVING AT THE DECISION

The initial step in the decision-making process is to correctly identify the patients who, due to their clinical condition, are unlikely to survive beyond a relatively short, yet undefined, period of time. Studies that have investigated the ability of physicians to predict when the end-of-life will occur have reported that only 70% of physicians can predict survival time within 33% of actual length of survival.[3] Overall, physicians overestimate survival, and the more familiar they are with the patient, the more inaccurate their predictions. This inability to accurately predict survival time applies to many clinical conditions, including advanced cancer—a disease for which one might expect better predictive ability due to 3 decades of accumulated data. For patients who have experienced significant life-threatening trauma, often with multiple system involvement, there are frequently even less data available to assist the physician in answering the question, "Doctor, how much time do I have left?"

The patient may have his or her own personal views regarding the type of life they want to live, and these views will influence the end-of-life decisions. Recently, the process known as Decision Analysis was outlined at a session on Clinical Palliative Care in the Trenches at the American College of Surgeons.[4] Decision Analysis attempts to illustrate how the differences in the patient's view of the importance of a given set of symptoms influences what they consent to. For example, some patients place greater value on having painfree time than on a longer survival time. It has been speculated that in the future, software programs will be available that will provide end-of-life plans that are based on the patient's or surrogate's individual preferences.[5,6] Most likely such computer programs will only assist in plan development by helping quantify the effect of potential competing personal preferences. It would seem unlikely that these types of decisions could or should be a computer model rather than individual values.

LEGAL/INSTITUTIONAL POLICIES

Practitioners should be aware of the variety of institutional policies and procedures that all hospitals have in place to address end-of-life care issues. This section will briefly review the most pertinent of these policies. These policies vary from state to state, and they may also vary within a given hospital, especially if the hospital is sponsored by a religious organization.

Advance Directives

There are two types of advance directives—durable power of attorney and living wills. Durable power of attorney for health care is the easiest to interpret. It gives an individual the power to act as a decision maker for the patient. The most commonly used durable power of attorney directives are between spouses, or between parents and an adult child. A living will directs treatment in accordance with a patient's personal preferences. Living wills have been criticized as being inadequate because it is not possible to anticipate all of the potential end-of-life scenarios,[7] just as it is not possible to predict when death will occur.

There are three other policies that should be well understood by practitioners: (i) do-not-resuscitate orders, (ii) withholding or withdrawing life-prolonging procedures, and (iii) brain death. Brain death policies are usually written according to specific guidelines that are designated

by state legislators. The policies address the conditions that constitute brain death, and what procedures must have been performed for brain death to be diagnosed. Once the diagnosis is made, the patient should be pronounced promptly, and the family should be informed immediately. Occasionally, conflicts arise due to a poor understanding of the issues surrounding the diagnosis of brain death. Once the diagnosis has been made, families should not be told that continuation of life-prolonging procedures remains an option. A do-not-resuscitate order implies that the patient has a terminal condition caused by injury, disease, or illness; that there is no reasonable probability of recovery; and that, without treatment, the condition can be expected to cause death. Usually, these conditions must be documented in the chart by the attending physician and by one additional consulting physician. A life-prolonging procedure is a mechanical or other artificial means of restoring, sustaining, or supplanting a spontaneous vital function. When applied to a patient in a terminal condition, life-prolonging procedures serve only to prolong the process of dying. For both do-not-resuscitate orders and for withholding or withdrawing life-prolonging treatment, a note should be placed in the chart that documents the discussions that the attending physician had with the patient and the family.

Do-not-resuscitate orders must be written by a licensed physician. Ideally, they specify precisely what the order implies. For example, the orders may specify that intubations and chest compressions are not to be performed. Issuing do-not-resuscitate orders may be complicated in patients who require a palliative procedure. Under these conditions, the implications of the do-not-resuscitate order must be clarified for the patient and caregivers, as well as the surgical and anesthesiology team, if applicable. The decision may be made to remove the do-not-resuscitate order during the procedure, and to reinstate it once the patient is awake.

Most institutions have separate versions of these policies for pediatric patients. The policies identify the decision maker, and they are appropriately modified for the population. For example, the diagnosis of brain death in a newborn or young child requires a different diagnosis, and different diagnostic considerations compared with older patients. In the pediatric population, the diagnosis of brain death is much more difficult to verify with standard testing.

For the patient who is not competent to make a decision, most states have proxy lists that identify, in order, the persons or entities that are responsible for making end-of-life decisions for the patient. The list for the State of Florida is in Table 1. Surrogate decision makers fall under the legal standard of substituted judgment, and therefore they must comply with durable power of attorney or other advanced directives. When these documents are not available, the "best interest" standard should be followed, in which the designated decision maker makes a decision that he or she believes is in the best interest of the patient.

TABLE 1
WHO IS THE DECISION MAKER?

- Competent patient
- Patient-appointed surrogate (when decisional capacity is impaired)

- Proxy list:
  1. Court appointed guardian
  2. Spouse
  3. Adult child or majority
  4. Parent
  5. Adult sibling or majority
  6. Relatives
  7. Close friend of the patient
  8. Licensed clinical social worker (LCSW) not employed by the provider

Florida Statute 765 – Health Care Advance Directives

TABLE 2
CURRENT LEGAL MYTHS AND REALITIES

Myth	Reality
Forgoing life-sustaining treatment for patients without decision-making capacity requires evidence of the patient's actual wish.	Such treatment may be forgone if the patient's surrogate relates that this was the patient's wish.
Withholding of artificial fluids and nutrition from terminally ill patient is illegal.	Like any other medical treatment, fluids and nutrition may be withheld if the patient refuses them.
Risk management personnel must be consulted before life-sustaining medical treatment may be terminated.	There is no such legal requirement.
Advance directives must comply with specific forms, are not transferable between states, and govern all future treatment decisions. Oral advance directives are unenforceable.	Advance directives, often the best indication of an incapacitated patient's wishes, may guide end-of-life decision making even if legal formalities are not completely met.
If a physician prescribes high doses of medication to relieve pain in a terminally ill patient, resulting in death, he or she will be criminally prosecuted.	If a patient inadvertently dies from the use of high doses of medication intended to treat pain, the physician has not committed murder or assisted suicide.
When a terminally ill patient's suffering is overwhelming despite palliative care, and he or she requests a hastened death, there are no legally permissible options to ease suffering.	Although physician-assisted suicide is illegal in most states, terminal sedation is a legal option to treat otherwise intractable symptoms in the imminently dying.

(From Meisel A, Snyder L, Quill T. Seven legal barriers to end-of-life care. Myths, realities, and grains of truth. *JAMA.* 2000;284:2495–2501.)

A brief mention should be made of the concept of medical futility. It is difficult, if not impossible, to codify a definition of medical futility into a policy. As with art, people know what they mean when they use the term medical futility. However, since individuals' definitions will vary widely, it is probably best to use the term in concert with the patient's identified preferences. For one individual it may be a 10% chance of success and for another 1%. The concept is an ever-changing target as medicine advances. Today's futility is tomorrow's standard of care, literally.

As with other areas of health care ethics, there are a number of myths associated with the making of end-of-life decisions. Meisel et al.[8] discussed the legal myths versus the realities of end-of-life issues (see Table 2). As with all legal issues, practitioners should review policies annually to ensure that they are aware of any changes in state laws.

END-OF-LIFE CONFLICTS

As with all important crossroads of life, the recognition that life is ending provides fertile ground for conflict to develop among family members. Although the recent events surrounding the death of Terri Schiavo are extreme examples of a family in crisis, these end-of-life conflicts undoubtedly occur nearly daily across the country. Each individual brings to these conflicts his or her own beliefs that have been gathered over a lifetime. Such episodes always bring out all of the complexities of families' interactions, both spoken and unspoken, and family conflicts unrelated to the end-of-life decision process.

The religious background or ethical belief framework of the patient and the family should also be recognized as a potential for conflict.[9] This is especially important in American society currently, which increasingly includes patients and caregivers whose backgrounds may not encompass the Judeo-Christian faith and traditions. Individuals with different religious and/or ethical backgrounds likely have different expectations about the end of life. Similarly,

studies have shown that physicians' own religious beliefs affect their attitude or behavior regarding end-of-life care. Wenger and Carmel[10] demonstrated that very religious physicians were the least likely to "ever stop life-sustaining treatment provided to the suffering, terminally ill patient." The authors encourage physicians to recognize their religious perspective to ensure that it does not interfere with the patient's own desires and beliefs.

In addition, cultural differences and attitudes toward decision making are changing with the curtailing of the health care professional's dominance in the decision-making process and with the increasing use of life-prolonging technology. These changes further add to the load of conflicts that the caregiver needs to understand.[9,11]

Caregivers may also contribute to conflict when end-of-life decisions are being made. The nurse who spends

10 to 12 hours a day at the patient's bedside likely has a different perspective than the physician who may intermittently spend a total of 1 or 2 hours at the bedside. In modern hospitals, there are also caregivers from other disciplines, such as respiratory therapists, pharmacists, and social workers, who, in addition to their expertise, bring their own set of biases to the end-of-life issues.

Changes in the health care system have added further complexity to dealing with end-of-life issues. Many hospitals now use a hospitalist system, in which the physician providing direct care provides only that care within the hospital. However, the primary care physician is the individual who has the longest and closest relationship with the patient and the family. The increasing number of other specialists who may care for the patient may result in a superb level of health care; however, each specialist may contribute his or her own interests and end-of-life concerns. These issues emphasize the importance of communication at all levels in order to avoid conflicts when possible.

A further possible complication arose with the Pain Relief Promotion Act of 1999. This law and subsequent Department of Justice directives would allow the federal government to step in and investigate deaths where opioids or barbiturates were used as possible violations of the Controlled Substance Act by "assisting in a suicide." The issue currently is being reviewed at the U.S. Supreme Court.[12]

It would be inappropriate not to mention financial issues. Although many would argue that financial concerns should not shape debates about end-of-life care, they likely play some role for many patients and their families. In a recent article, Bloche[13] argues from the societal standpoint that patients and their families are not expected to deal with financially based contradictions when the country is unable to resolve the issue of health care expenditures versus an individual desire to have "everything" done. The Terri Schiavo episode clearly demonstrated the wide range of beliefs that various members of society have regarding end-of-life issues.

Health care providers also need to be aware that they may be inadvertently, but steadily, withdrawing from patient involvement. Physicians need to guard against avoiding the patient who represents "failure," and need to recognize when colleagues and trainees withdraw from patient involvement. An approach that can help physicians deal with personal conflicts is discussed in a subsequent section of the chapter.

Depression in a patient may also impact end-of-life issues. Increasingly, evidence from medical literature supports the contention that depression should be actively diagnosed and treated in patients before consideration of any end-of-life issues.[14–17] Untreated depression may result in a patient's wishes being influenced by this condition, which is treatable and often reversible.

In view of the numerous conflicts that may occur related to end-of-life care, what options are there to assist the patients, their families, and the health care team at this critical time? Bloche[13] describes the role of a mediator—a person who has suggestions that may ease reactions when tension appears to be increasing. The physicians, nurses, and social workers should become active listeners to the spoken and unspoken concerns so that they may diagnose and ameliorate potential conflict.

In many hospitals, an Ethics Committee can assist in addressing end-of-life issues. Ethics Committees generally comprise a multidisciplinary group that includes physicians, nurses, and social workers, in addition to clergy, attorneys, and community members. Risk managers who serve on Ethics Committees should only serve in an *ex officio* position. A hospital's policy regarding who can request an ethics consult may vary. In our hospital, any professional who is part of the health care team, the patient, or the family can request such a consult. If the consulting individual is other than the attending physician, the attending physician is notified of the consult and the findings. The goal of the ethics consult may include assisting with the thought processes regarding identification of the decision maker, clarifying the decisions that need to be made, and facilitating discussions to elucidate the facts of the case. Ethics Committees can also offer expert advice on ethical problems. The role of the Ethics Committee is advisory, in general, and the health care team and the family are under no obligation to comply with the consults. Ultimate responsibility for the case always rests with the attending physician. Any legal ramifications that could impact the Ethics Committee recommendations are the purview of the legal counsel of the health care facility.

An important role of the Ethics Committee is to provide ongoing education. It should educate each member of the health care team regarding his or her specific role in a particular case. In this writer's experience, individuals requesting an Ethics Committee consult are occasionally motivated by the expectation that it will take decisions. In reality, the role of an Ethics Committee is one of looking at the data and the process leading to a decision, not making one. The Ethics Committee is to help identify the sources of conflicts, clarify ethics policies or legal issues, and provide a forum for communication among all interested parties.

END-OF-LIFE CARE ISSUES

The performance of a surgical procedure of quality is accomplished by organized and preplanned preparation, and by an organized approach to the procedure. When confronted with providing end-of-life care, a similar approach ensures quality to this "procedure." Being prepared to recognize that we are now switching from life-prolonging mode to palliative approaches, although difficult, ensures that quality patient care is provided. The goal is to develop and organize an approach to providing care to the terminal patient.[18]

An important step in understanding end-of-life care is to consider the factors that are important to patients, families, and caregivers. Steinhauser et al.[14] reported that issues important to patients and caregivers included managing pain and symptoms, preparing for death, achieving a sense of completion, deciding about treatment preference, and being considered "a whole person." However, other priorities of patients and caregivers differed significantly. For example, issues that are very important to patients include planning their funeral, being sure they are not a burden to others, and coming to peace with their God. These issues are less important to physicians. In this study, freedom from pain ranked highest for both patients and caregivers. A simple checklist of possible concerns to consider when beginning discussions with the patient and family member will assist the health care team in achieving quality care (see Table 3). Language and cultural mores require specific attention. If English is not the customary language of the patient and/or family, communication in the native language is necessary. Similarly, patients whose cultural and religious beliefs are different from those encountered commonly in the hospital's service population should be recognized early. Consultation with cultural and religious experts may be necessary.

Most items in Table 3 are self-explanatory, and are noted as important variables to consider before reaching end-of-life care in a patient's course. With some trepidation, the authors included financial cost. Personally, I consider financial cost to be an important variable to consider with the family. This is not to suggest that financial consideration is important for an individual case; however, it is a consideration that is frequently focused on by families, and it may be of concern to the patient as well.

Hall et al. in Canada[18] demonstrated relatively simple initiatives that may improve end-of-life care. The authors began by having focus groups with patients, families, and caregivers, and then developed an *aide memoiré* and a checklist to be used during end-of-life processes. A similar approach can assist each specialized care unit in providing end-of-life care.

Other investigators have similarly illustrated activities that can assist both the patient and the caregiver in providing support as needed. Indeed, all studies emphasize the importance of listening carefully to both the patient and the family to discern what information they are asking for, and providing that information in an understandable manner.[11,19] At times, family members may respond with anger; the anger is usually aimed randomly, and it should be anticipated.

The families should be assisted in communicating their desires and their loved one's desires with all members of the health care team including the nurses, social workers, pharmacists, clergy, and hospice workers as appropriate. The difficulty for most physicians involved in providing intensive care at the end of a patient's life is their anger at having failed the patient. Discussions with patients and families should never be hurried, and it should be expected that the same questions might be asked multiple times. Not infrequently, a number of other issues surface during this phase of patient care. Surgical or other palliative procedures require full understanding of the goals to be achieved by the procedure and the variables that may be encountered. This process will result in varied decisions from patient to patient. Steinhauser et al.[14] note that one of the challenges physicians face is to design flexible health care systems that allow for variable expression of a "good" death.

Several other considerations arise as part of end-of-life care decision making. If there is technology supporting one or more vital functions, then electing to withdraw such technology requires a separate approach. Cohen et al.[15,20,21] have reviewed considerations regarding the withdrawal of renal dialysis.

The use of artificial nutrition and hydration frequently raises additional concerns. Is this a medical treatment that should be subject to guidelines similar to those for renal dialysis, or is it something closer to providing shelter and pain relief? If it is the latter, it should require a higher standard of consideration before being discontinued. Casarett et al.[22] have argued that because artificial nutrition and hydration require the use of devices that must be placed by trained individuals, they should be held to the same standards as other medical treatments. The authors make a strong case that the health care team should provide more detailed risk–benefit data for this therapy. They also note that the published data only support the use of this therapy for a few clinical situations. State laws in some cases have turned to a "reasonable person" standard rather than the more difficult to interpret "best interest" standard. On the other hand, the Catholic Church has recently issued a statement that strongly discourages withdrawal of artificial nutrition and hydration. Adoption of this doctrine may affect individual state laws.

Once a decision has been made to withdraw life-sustaining treatment, a plan needs to be outlined for the

TABLE 3

VARIABLES TO BE CONSIDERED BEFORE REACHING END-OF-LIFE CARE

End-of-life patient goals
Treatment risk vs. benefit
Symptom burden
Treatment burden to caregiver
Age and life stage
Treatment financial cost
Psychological variables—hope, denial, anticipatory grief, and
   depression
Personal and family culture

(From Weissman DE. Decision making at a time of crisis near the end of life. *JAMA.* 2004;292(14):1738–1743.)

patient and family that will allow refinements of care, including do-not-resuscitate orders. The health care team needs to ensure that there are no treatable conditions or symptoms motivating the decision to withdraw life-sustaining therapy. This includes treatable depression, as well as any social or family pressures. Decisions regarding the site at which the death will occur have implications that should be reviewed with the patient and family. The events that will occur after the patient has expired are important to families, whether death occurs in a hospital, hospice, or in the patient's home. One should review what to expect in the final hours; this will help relieve the family's anxiety. In general, palliative medications should be stopped and additional palliative medications ordered if needed for ongoing symptoms or new symptoms. The family needs to know that some part of the health care team will continue to be available to them. It should be recognized that religious or spiritual support will be important for some patients and families. If a family seems especially vulnerable, grief counselor referral should be considered.

Currently, there are an increasing number of resources on the worldwide web that are of use to families and health care providers. These are listed in the reference section.[3,23]

REFERENCES

1. Asch DA, Hansen-Flaschen J, Lanken PN. Decisions to limit or continue life-sustaining treatment by critical care physicians in the United States: conflicts between physicians' practices and patients' wishes. *Am J Respir Crit Care Med.* 1995;151:288–292.
2. Nelson, Angus DC, Weissfeld LA, et al. End-of-life care for the critically ill: A national intensive care unit survey. *Crit Care Med.* 2006;34:2547–2553.
3. *Fast facts and concepts.* www.mcw.edu/pallmed. (Accessed 2005).
4. Lamont EB, Christakis NA. Complexities in prognostication in advanced cancer "To help them live their lives the way they want to." *JAMA.* 2003;290(1):98–104.
5. Lee KF, Purcell GP, Hinshaw DB, et al. Clinical palliative care for surgeons: Part 1. *J Am Coll Surg.* 2004;198:303–319.s
6. Lee KF, Johnson DL, Purcell GP, et al. Clinical palliative care for surgeons: Part 2. *J Am Coll Surg.* 2004;198:477–491.
7. Fagerlin A, Schneider CE. Enough – the failure of the living will. *Hastings Cent Rep.* 2004;34(2):30–42.
8. Meisel A, Snyder L, Quill T. Seven legal barriers to end-of-life care. Myths, realities, and grains of truth. *JAMA.* 2000;284:2495–2501.
9. Kagawa-Singer M, Blackhall LJ. Negotiating cross-cultural issues at the end of life. "You Got to Go Where He Lives." *JAMA.* 2001; 286:2993–3001.
10. Wenger NS, Carmel S. Physicians' religiosity and end-of-life care attitudes and behaviors. *Mt Sinai J Med.* 2004;71:335–343.
11. Weissman DE. Decision making at a time of crisis near the end of life. *JAMA.* 2004;292(14):1738–1743.
12. Quill TE, Meier DE. The big chill – inserting the DEA into end-of-life care. *N Engl J Med.* 2006;354(1):1–3.
13. Bloche MG. Managing conflict at the end of life. *N Engl J Med.* 2005;352(23):2371–2373.
14. Steinhauser KE, Christakis NA, Clipp EC, et al. Factors considered important at the end of life by patients, family, physicians, and other car providers. *JAMA.* 2000;284:2476–2482.
15. Cohen LM, Germain MJ, Poppel DM. Practical considerations in dialysis withdrawal. "To Have That Option Is a Blessing." *JAMA.* 2003;289:2113–2119.
16. Drazen JM. Decisions at the end of life. *N Engl J Med.* 2005; 352(23):1109–1110.
17. Quill TE. Dying and decision making – evolution of end-of-life options. *N Engl J Med.* 2005;350(20):2029–2032.
18. Hall RI, Rocker GM, Murray D. Simple changes can improve conduct of end-of-life care in the intensive care unit. *Can J Anaesth.* 2004;51(6):631–636.
19. Kissane DW. The contribution of demoralization to end of life decisionmaking. *Hastings Cent Rep.* 2004;34(4):21–31.
20. Prendergast TJ, Puntillo KA. Withdrawal of life support. Intensive caring at the end of life. *JAMA.* 2002;288:2732–2740.
21. Prendergast TJ, Puntillo KA. Withdrawal of life support. Intensive caring at the end of life. *JAMA.* 2002;288(21):2732–2740.
22. Casarett D, Kapo J, Caplan A. Appropriate use of artificial nutrition and hydration – fundamental principles and recommendations. *N Engl J Med.* 2005;353(24):2607–2612.
23. *Harvard medical school program in palliative care education and practice.* http://www.hms.harvard.edu/cdi/pallcare. Accessed 2007.

Pastoral Care

69

William Baugh   *C. Wayne Maberry*

Medical doctors as a group and trauma surgeons in particular are unprepared to deal with multiple issues of faith and religion as these are important areas pertaining to the care of the injured patient and the critically ill. Groopman[1] provides an eloquent description of the patient encounter, where there was an expectation on the part of the patient that the physician would participate in an exercise of faith. The author emphasized the sense of helplessness that he felt at the time because he was unprepared to provide the participation that the patient desired. The wrenching effect that an injury has on the patient, the patient's family, and loved ones is an intensely stressful experience for those touched by the injury event. Surgeons and other caregivers are not immune to these effects. Because there is increasing recognition of the importance of these issues in surgical practice,[2,3] the need and potential benefit of pastoral care services as a component of the trauma center caregiver team has rapidly become recognized.

A few years ago, the decision was made to give the chaplain members of the pastoral care service at our trauma center the responsibility for identifying all trauma patients, notifying their next of kin, and greeting friends and relatives as they hurried to the emergency room (ER). Chaplains had proved themselves to be professionals who were trained or being trained to deal with people in crises and grief. In addition to being in house 24/7, chaplains also had a unique access to patients, families, and staff because of their role in the hospital. The chaplains immediately recognized the stress and, sometimes, anguish felt by the medical professionals who carry the heavy responsibility for life and death decisions. They needed the desired care, which they readily received from the chaplains.

The role of chaplain means many different things to different people. Most people understand the role of the military chaplain. The chaplain supports troops in a time of war and informs families of the death of their loved one. The prison chaplain brings a religious message to the inmates and attempts to help them change their way of living. The chaplain in a modern trauma center brings hope and perhaps a prayer for a brighter future in the midst of a dark, life-altering experience.

Chaplains support people who are in crisis, as well as staff members who care for them. The medical staff is often under extreme pressure due to the urgency of a patient's condition. At any point of time they are responsible for treating a number of people who needs medical care. The clinically trained chaplain understands the importance of responding to people at the point of their need and uncertainty. The chaplain encourages people to relate their experiences, to tell the story of what happened, and to explore what they are losing or can realistically expect from life. Chaplains draw on insights about people and relationships relying on their experience in caring for others, their insights about the nature of people, awareness about how family systems work, and how people from many faith traditions call on God to cope with their crisis.

The text enclosed in the box describes some of the emotions experienced by a chaplain responding to a trauma team activation. The descriptions provide insight into the types of responses these talented individuals bring to the trauma team organization. Once the chaplain arrives at the trauma activation and assesses the situation, the initial intake begins.

INITIAL INTAKE

The chaplain's next assessment is, "*At what point do I insert myself into the frantic activity surrounding the care of the newly received trauma patient?*" As the trauma surgeons and nurses focus intently on their examination, maintaining vital signs and airways, the chaplain seeks out the prehospital rescue and transport team. Very often the emergency medical services (EMS) crew can provide a tentative name, address, date of birth, social security number, and, possibly, other essential information that might help the chaplain to locate family members. When they have no information, the chaplain and security personnel examine the patient's personal effects searching for information about the patient's identity. We have found that this task gives chaplains an automatic connection to the patient and his/her family. The chaplain quickly becomes familiar with the situation and gaining this familiarity is a critical element in the intake process. It is important to be accurate when notifying next of kin. When the patient cannot speak, this process becomes more difficult but no less important. The chaplain receives vital information from the family that might be critical to the urgent care and treatment of the patient. Our trauma medical staff recognized, early on, the value of this information and rapidly came to appreciate the input from the trauma chaplain.

LOCATING NEXT OF KIN

The task of locating next of kin can be taxing, tricky and demands patience and a willingness to follow sometimes obscure leads. Obviously, the conscious patient can give the name and telephone contact information for the person to be notified. Often the patient is unconscious or in a life-threatening situation and the chaplain must rely on other sources or techniques to identify and locate next of kin. Each case is very different. In one instance our records showed that we made 55 phone calls trying to locate the father of a trauma victim and finally, after a few days found him at a resort in another state.

The Internet provides a number of resources that are useful in efforts to contact family members. An address from a driver's license or other identification permits location of the next-door neighbor. The neighbors can often help locate a family member. For example, several years ago we received a patient who was involved in an accident. She lived on the east coast of Florida. Unfortunately the patient lived alone. We contacted the neighbor who let us know that the patient was *en route* to her son's wedding on the west coast of Florida. The neighbor also provided the name of the church where the wedding was to take place. These facts enabled the chaplain to contact the patient's family ensuring their timely arrival at the hospital. In addition, we have found that police agencies around the country are incredibly helpful. When asked they will send an officer to a person's home or to an address in order to facilitate the search.

MAKING THE CALL

Once the chaplain positively identifies the patient he or she places telephone calls to the patient's next of kin. The chaplain must resolve some important questions before the call is made. "How shall I introduce myself?" Introducing oneself as the chaplain can frighten family members. Many

perceive the hospital chaplain to be like the military chaplain who brings news of death. The family reaction, "My loved one has died because the chaplain is calling" is most often inaccurate. This perception demands yet another self-assessment from the chaplain. How am I being heard? Am I being too abrupt? Do they hear the concern in my voice? What happens to people when I introduce myself to them as a chaplain? Does it make them want to shy away and avoid contact with me? Does it help them to immediately share intimate concerns because they see me as a caring representative of a loving God? Does it raise fear immediately? These and many other more subtle questions are raised by the call from the chaplain.

Chaplains in trauma centers identify themselves as the chaplain at some point during the initial phone call. Reassuring families that the chaplain is responsible for contacting all families during a traumatic situation eases some of the fear accompanying the news that a loved one has been injured. When fear is eased, family members are able to realize that the chaplain's call is a normal part of the hospital protocol. It also helps the loved one to relax enough to hear the content of what the chaplain has to communicate.

A third and critical assessment during the initial call to the patient's family is "how much should be divulged?" As a general rule chaplains do not give out medical information. An attempt is made to summarize the patient's condition in one word. The chaplain is able to add more detail when the patient is stable and survival is assured. In cases of death we let family members know the patient is critical and urge them to come to the hospital as quickly and safely as possible. The chaplain's initial assessment evaluates the frame of mind and the coping resources of the family. Every effort is made to avoid giving a message of patient death by telephone. An exception is made when family members live at a distance. In those cases we ask the trauma surgeon to speak with the family on the phone. In that conversation the surgeon provides information about the medical circumstances as well as how the trauma occurred. Some surgeons are very good at giving this information over the phone or in person. Others have less comfort in delivering bad news or dealing with the emotions of grieving people. In the latter case, the surgeon is usually relieved to inform the patient of the death and leave the rest to the chaplain. It certainly underlines the importance of having a well-integrated chaplaincy staff capable of assuming this function at critical moments.

THE FAMILY ARRIVES

When family members arrive at the hospital they are ushered into a consultation room. The optimal combination of quiet, privacy, and proximity to the patient care area is sought. Physical structure barriers are frequently cited as causes for failure of communication between grieving families and caregivers.[4] The chaplain meets the family in the consultation area. This can be a difficult moment for the chaplain. He or she has information that the family wants and yet the chaplain knows it would be professionally inappropriate to share the information at the time of the initial interview. At this time, the chaplain tries to work with the anxiety of the family and assure them that a surgeon will speak with them as soon as possible. As the chaplain sits with the family he/she builds on their initial telephone assessment of the family and possible dynamics present in the family.

The chaplain delivers the assessment of the family to the surgeon before the first contact between surgeon and family. The chaplain then introduces and connects the surgeon to the family. The surgeon is able to enter the interview more completely informed as a result of the chaplain's assessment. The chaplain often provides critical information about the family or family dynamics that shape the approach to this critical early encounter. As the surgeon talks with the family, the chaplain continues to assess whether and how much the family understands from the information that has been given. Occasionally, when the chaplain believes the family has missed information, he/she may simply raise the question in a new way. At other times the chaplain will assist the surgeon to hear and understand the question or concerns of the family. In these ways the chaplain helps ensure clear communication. A number of factors, including the family's anxiety for the well-being of their loved one and the surgeon's primary concern for the medical condition of the patient, can combine to lead to poor communication.[5]

As the surgeon leaves the consultation room the family members face a world turned upside down. Their various reactions to news can range from the extreme expression of rage to numbness. The chaplain responds to the family at the point of their emotion. All along the way, the chaplain assesses how to build on the family strengths or to address family weaknesses.

ACQUAINTANCE WITH GRIEF

This, perhaps, is the most crucial moment for the family and for the chaplain. The chaplain helps family members recognize the reality of their loss when the message conveyed involves the death of a loved one. The chaplain seeks to help the family build on coping skills they have used in the past when faced with traumatic circumstances. When the family is clearly unfamiliar with loss and grief, the chaplain models a way of dealing honestly with feelings. How effectively people move through the grief process is often determined by how effectively and how soon they are able to implement critical coping skills. Experiencing and processing the grief is vital to the newly bereaved family member(s).

The chaplain must know the normal grief process well. People naturally tend to move away from grief rather than toward it. In contrast, the chaplain seeks to move toward the grief. This requires one to be comfortable with and value the expression of deep feelings. Dealing with the feelings of others requires familiarity and facility with the difficult experiences in one's own life. This is a major part of the clinical training and development that certified chaplains receive.

We view the role of the chaplain as "coming alongside" the family. This, in turn, enables them to have a sense that someone understands the pain and anxiety they are experiencing with this terrible news they have just received. The chaplain also has a sense that he/she is fulfilling a vital mission by carrying the other person's burden for a little while. The capacity to listen, to respond empathetically, and to be present to the other person's grief and pain is the essence of the art of pastoral care. This is also a primary focus of the clinical training that student chaplains receive. It is not easy to respond in these ways nor even possible for some. Some student chaplains take to it like a duck to water; others avoid approaching grief like the plague.

MOVEMENT FROM THE EMERGENCY ROOM TO THE FLOORS AND AN ALTERED LIFE

The trauma ministry of chaplains may begin in the ER, but it continues in the intensive care units (ICUs), waiting rooms, and in the other patient care units of the trauma center. It is not only imperative but also a condition of their work at Toronto General Hospital (TGH) that chaplains honor the faith traditions and struggles that are unique to each patient and family. Chaplains provide opportunities for patients, families, and staff members, including physicians, to talk about the interplay between one's life experiences, faith, and the universal search for meaning. In the emergency resuscitation area, that journey can become confusing and uncertain. Once the patient has moved to other patient care areas of the hospital the reality begins to set in. For the patient it involves the realization that this tragic incident affects the way he or she will live the rest of their life. For families it means living without their loved one or reshaping their life to care for their loved one.

Although trauma patients enter a very complex medical setting, the movement of patients generally follows a pattern. The pattern begins with an initial physical examination and assessment by the trauma team followed by imaging studies and one or more surgical procedures. The largest exception to this pattern would be patients who die or whose physical examination requires them to undergo immediate surgery. The pastoral care of families continues after a patient dies as well as when the patient moves to the ICU.

DISCUSSING BAD NEWS

Caregivers often find it difficult to be truthful with patients and families when we expect the difficult news we might impart will provoke emotion-filled responses. When we encounter a family filled with fear we often attempt to soften the news they are receiving. We do this because we do not want to hurt them or add to the hurt they are already experiencing. At the same time, we sometimes avoid the people we perceive to be angry. Dealing with someone's anger often reminds us just how powerless we are. The chaplain needs to counter the normal response of people to grief and tragedy. By moving toward people in painful situations of grief and trauma, the chaplain expresses care and concern.

Surgeons sometimes find it difficult to deal directly with family members. This is particularly true when the feeling exists that their job is to rescue people from situations in which they suddenly, and often through no fault of their own, find themselves. The surgeon may feel he/she has failed. Physicians also need to acknowledge the limits of medicine and medical care and be realistic with their own expectations. In these instances it is important for the surgeon to seek support for himself/herself. No less than nurses and other members of the medical staff, and perhaps precisely because the medical staff look so much to the surgeons for direction, they can benefit from a chaplain who can also extend compassion and empathy to them. Gentleness with oneself is a lesson everyone benefits from.

Learning how to talk to people about tragedy, anticipated poor outcomes, and even death requires a person to be honest and communicate sensitively with another human being. It is a tremendous shift for the surgeon or nurse to move from the intensity of attempting to resuscitate a patient to the different, sometimes more stressful intensity of dealing with a family's anxiety or grief. The required sensitivity comes from one's development as a person and acquaintance with one's own grief. We teach our students to journey alongside the patient or family. This requires them to deal with their anxiety or grief and be responsive in the midst of anxiety producing situations.

Talking to people honestly means respecting their ability to deal with whatever they are facing. The more people are respected, the more they can grow through a situation. In the not so distant past, physicians often prescribed medicine for grieving family members. The desire was to ease the suffering of families, and perhaps also to ease the suffering of the medical team. It is not easy to watch people grieve. Fortunately this has changed in recent years. Seeing others grieve can create feelings of failure in medical professionals although it need not be so. Understanding that grief is a natural and necessary process can help alleviate those feelings. At the same time, seeing others grieve often reminds us of our mortality. When this happens the impact of someone else's tragedy surprises us. The artistry, and it is art, of pastoral care and medicine

lies in helping people address the feelings present around traumatic and tragic situations. This is the first step toward wholeness and healing. As chaplains work with families they model a way of dealing directly with people at the point of their pain. This, in turn, helps physicians and staff members observe the value of dealing openly with people, valuing their feelings, and in this way validating their response to a tragic event.

SPIRITUALITY AT THE TIME OF CRISES

The question "What role does faith and spirituality hold for them?" is an important question at this moment. Over the last 10 years, the use of the term *spirituality* has increased many times. Bidwell[6] has discussed the lack of complete consensus among psychologists and the clergy regarding the role of spirituality in reducing postinjury complications such as post-traumatic stress disorder. He emphasized the frequent rejection of faith in trauma victims and families as similar to the "wilderness experience" described in both the old and new testaments. We have found that people often have the foundations of their faith challenged by traumatic events. Chaplains approach spirituality as the "life" and "liveliness" of patients and family members as well as a connection to faith in a deity. The evolving English word "enthusiasm" contains both meanings. This word, which literally began as, "filled with God," has come to mean a strong liking or excitement for anything. When people receive bad news, their countenances fall and they become lifeless or lethargic. Similarly, when they receive good news their faces brighten. Responding to people on a "spiritual" level also requires a chaplain to pay attention and respond to body language. In a very real way chaplains listen to what they see. The pastoral acknowledgment may lift what is seen, "You are tearful" or provide an interpretation, "You are broken hearted." Family members almost always appreciate an honest and frank acknowledgment of their loss or struggle around a loss.

Chaplains realize that life and theology are dynamic and require a dialogue. The tidiest theologic frameworks are challenged by the messiness of life. Crisis challenges people to the core because it destroys or at least upsets their worldview. Very often religious people struggle to make sense of tragedy in the light of their deeply held convictions and faith. Those who discover a way to process about the crisis generally do better than those who internalize their feelings and isolate themselves. In the end, people who honestly face the situation and openly explore their religious beliefs tend to come out with a new belief system that makes room for bad things happening to good people. They lose theological naiveté and usually value day-to-day life more highly.

Understanding the responses trauma victims and families have to the injury event can be facilitated by drawing on experience in working with people who have mental illness. Sudden and unexpected death or crisis often leads to mental struggles. A variety of feelings surround the inability of any particular family member(s) to cope. An estranged son or daughter may feel guilt. An overly close spouse may feel abandoned. A religious person may be confused and an irreligious person may become overly religious. The ability to include tragedy and crisis in one's faith perspective develops as feelings and thoughts are processed openly. At one point the character Tevye from *Fiddler on the Roof*, the musical drawn from Sholom Aleichem's collection of stories[7] laments a crisis in his life. His horse has gone lame and he is pulling the milk cart to make his deliveries. Tevye addresses a question to God, "I know we are your chosen people, but couldn't you pick someone else once in a while?" Experiencing one's feelings and talking about them with other people helps prevent isolation from others and from oneself.

Very often people respond from their faith and quickly adopt a deterministic posture which allows them to accept whatever may come.[6] They are responding from a tradition that says, in effect, "God is in control," and they may believe this tragedy is an instance where "God will work something good from a bad situation." People who face crisis in this manner often have their feelings go underground. These suppressed feelings of anger and grief may come out sideways and be turned toward a family member, a surgeon, a nurse, or the chaplain. It is important for people to deal with their feelings close to the event that birthed the feelings. Feelings like anger often cover another and deeper feeling like hurt or grief.

A churchgoing woman's husband died 5 years ago in a motor vehicle accident. He spent time in an ICU before dying. She said, "That was the hardest time of my life. I am still having a hard time dealing with it. The Bible said, 'If you have faith you can move a mountain.' I had faith. I never doubted he would get better." As we talked it became clear that her husband's death raised ongoing theologic questions. She was caught between her received religion and the feelings of anger drawn from her experience. In the play JB, Archibald MacLeish[8], has a line, "If God is God he is not good and if God is good he is not God." The phrases catch the dilemma that religious people often find themselves in. Either the "goodness" or the "Godness" of God is at stake for them when either they or people they love are critically injured.

Knowing how and when to address people in crisis, particularly at the point of their "faith," is difficult for all of us. We think this is especially true for medical professionals who may have little to do with religion or who work very hard not to impose their religious views on a patient and family in the midst of a difficult situation. We can all think of an occasion when someone pressured us with religious viewpoints that seemed more connected to musty old scrolls than with present day concerns or troubles. Looking back, religious debates once thought so important are often seen as fairly pointless and certainly fruitless. Impressing one's religious view on another person is neither convincing nor helpful. A hospital setting, particularly an acute setting such as a trauma center, is no place for religious debate. It is, however, a place to address feelings and to walk with people who are facing life-changing events.

As people grow up, they acquire certain images of themselves and the world. For religious people, these images give shape to what should and should not happen. Some of these images make it very difficult to face trauma or tragedy.

- Faithful people have good things happen to them. Because I serve God faithfully, my life should turn out okay.
- Because God is in control, everything will turn out all right. At stake is the person's image of God, and it is very difficult to let go of that image.
- If I cry or show emotion, then it shows a lack of faith and I would be terribly embarrassed.
- If I get into a difficult situation, God or somebody else will rescue me. All I have to do is follow the rules and everything will work out well.

These kinds of images are unconsciously created as people attend church or read or watch television programs. Traumatic events often challenge religious images that give shape to people's worldview. These same traumatic events allow people to examine even their most precious beliefs. Discovering the limitations of one's images is the first step in finding some more useful images to live by. Faith is more than a set of beliefs, it is a way of living often birthed as one factors in tragedy.

Helping people to be in touch with themselves and to verbalize unspeakable thoughts and feelings can be very beneficial. Helping someone move through the period of numbness that follows receipt of bad news is vital to the person's future ability to reconnect in relationships. It is this period that is so critical in the ER. Very often people wait too long to experience their emotions or they never talk about them with others. In our experience with people who are suffering from mental illness, many of them have suffered traumatic losses but had no one to talk with about the losses. They were alone. Trauma does not cause mental illness, but not dealing with one's feelings and thoughts can and often does lead to mental illness, because feelings of sadness and anger are suppressed. Sometimes people overreact to unrelated situations because they have not reacted to the underlying traumatic situation.

Very often trauma pushes people toward strangers, creating an intimacy that begins in a moment but which can have life-sustaining ability. The privilege of being there with people at such a critical time sustains the chaplain by providing meaning and purpose. The chaplain gives up long-term involvement with people in a parish for the intense, deep involvement during a crisis. When someone dies, the loss is immediate and long lasting. Establishing ties with a chaplain or other medical professional can be very significant. In a traumatic time, people discover that there are many sources of comfort and learn to avail themselves of what others can offer because a chaplain has helped them experience receiving support. In a very real although perhaps unstated way, people realize others can be sources of support. Although sources of support are available, they are not always recognized. Very often anger, fear, guilt, or some other strong emotion blinds the patient or family. It is the task of the chaplain to help the patient or family recognize and access their sources of support.

INTENSIVE CARE UNIT—A PLACE OF HIDDEN FEELINGS

When patients move to the ICU the stakes for the patient and family continue to be very high. Surgeons and nurses who work on these units tend to be caring and realistic. They are familiar with death and, at the same time, aware that a point can come where medical treatments are futile. The most sensitive and caring medical personnel communicate the truth as best as they know it. At times it is difficult to be truthful with people. It is also essential to effective caregiving and to the patient or family's successful processing about their situation. It is painful for caregivers to reach out to those who have had multiple losses or for those whose loss corresponds to their own experiences of grief and loss.

Although it may seem counterintuitive, staying engaged with angry family members is very important. In our experience anger is a presenting symptom. The actual issue is whatever lies beneath the anger.. Anger is often a secondary emotion. Anger can be fueled by feelings of grief, guilt, and helplessness. The following example illustrates how anger is fueled by guilt. A 12-year-old patient had been participating in a soccer tournament, which was delayed midway because of rain. The boy's father, who was a devoted religious man, decided to take him out for some lunch while they waited. On the way they were involved in a motor vehicle crash that resulted in the boy's traumatic injuries and subsequent hospitalization. After the initial workup he was placed in the pediatric ICU. After a few days, he was transferred from the trauma service to the pediatric service. It was clear to all the medical staff involved that the patient would not recover. The father could not face the medical facts because his self-imposed guilt for going to lunch and being involved in the accident was too great. In this instance, the pediatrician stayed engaged with the father in spite of the presenting anger. He kept the chaplain involved, and the chaplain helped the parent to look beyond his anger and process his feelings of guilt. A very important aspect in the care of this family was the decision of the medical staff to give the parents time to process through their feelings. It was not possible to preserve the life of the 12-year-old but it was possible to help the family to move into a more forgiving stance.

In this instance the father had to forgive himself, a lifelong process to be sure.

Stories like the one given in the preceding text affect more than the patient and family. They also impact staff members, including surgeons. Staff members, particularly nurses, are sometimes placed in the role of providing ongoing care to patients whose condition is futile. That is a very difficult role for any person to fill. It is painful for staff members to provide care that is usually beneficial when they know it has no value. Because providing such care is so emotionally difficult, chaplains pay attention to staff members, including physicians, nurses, and other health care workers. Chaplains realize providing futile care can quickly drain the caregivers' spirit.

The poet John Donne wrote, "No man is an island" and "Any man's death diminishes me, because I am involved in mankind."[9] Very often staff members are deeply touched by the outcome of a patient. Several years ago a man in his mid-20s was involved in a motor vehicle crash. The trauma surgeon offered little hope of survival to the family, let alone hope of recovery. The patient did survive and was transferred after several months of stay in ICU and inpatient rehabilitation to another state and a rehabilitation unit closer to his family. A year later, he returned to thank his trauma surgeon, other doctors, his nurses, and the chaplain. Everyone felt deep satisfaction for his outcome. Involvement can also lead to sadness, as for example, a 42-year-old man who received a liver transplant 8 years ago returned unexpectedly to the hospital and was admitted to ICU where he subsequently died. The nurse assigned to him happened to be a primary nurse who cared for him when he received his transplant. Their reunion was short-lived. He was talking in the morning and died in the afternoon. The chaplain assessed it was important to give the nurse a forum to talk about her feelings. The chaplain, nurse, and other staff members sat together as the nurse grieved. Her grief was very present as she talked about their interaction periodically throughout the day. She described telling the patient she "should kick his butt for not taking better care of himself" and indicated he chided her for "putting on weight." The chaplain's invitation to tell her story let her know someone understood how his death impacted her. It is hard to quantify the enormous benefit this nurse received through the opportunity to grieve in an atmosphere of permission and acceptance. Allowing people to tell their story gives them greater freedom to grieve their loss and begin to accept the reality of the situation. Making a team of professionals familiar with palliative and/or end-of-life care is important for staff as well as for patients and families.[10]

PALLIATIVE CARE—PART OF THE TEAM

Unfortunately, long-term care and planning must become a major priority in some trauma cases. The palliative care team may become involved through a consult order from the trauma surgeon. The team comprises a board-certified palliative care physician, a nurse, and a chaplain.

Palliative care has two critical functions: (i) to improve communication with the patient and family and (ii) to develop relationships with them in order to make plans for long-term care and end-of-life decisions. Developing a relationship is important because it helps patients and families face difficult issues and make difficult decisions. Clearly, the problem of time management and brief passing relationships has changed the nature of modern medicine. No longer does the physician know the patient and family over many years and numerous visits. The trauma surgeon meets the patient soon after the injury event and is, almost always, unknown to the victim. The patient's placement in an alien environment produces great anxiety or even threat.

The palliative care team seeks to provide care to the patient at the point of the life-threatening diagnosis. That is much earlier than traditional end-of-life care such as hospice. The goal is to have the team get to know each patient well, leading to a 90-minute meeting with the patient and/or family to determine an end-of-life plan.

Many trauma centers have participated in the University Health Consortium's Benchmark Study on Palliative Care programs.[11] The study determined that an extensive interview with the patient and family leads to greater satisfaction, more adequate and complete communication about the patient's situation, and more sensitive and supportive planning for critical care decisions.

The assigned chaplain has played a more significant role on the care team than first projected. The chaplain makes a visit to the patient after the physician. In that initial visit the chaplain makes a pastoral assessment noting the sources of hope, meaning, comfort, strength, and peace along with his/her source of love and connection. Recent studies demonstrate the value of religion in the lives of people in terms of longer life and a need for smaller doses of medications while in ICU. The one constant in these studies seems to be the value of belonging to a group who are concerned for the patient. The chaplain also notes the value organized religion or spirituality has played in his/her life. When patients and families belong to a religious community, efforts are made to connect the patient to the community if requested. The chaplain inquires as to the patient's spiritual practices and aspects of those practices that have had significant meaning in the past. The chaplain spends considerable time looking into the meaning the patient receives from his/her relationship with God and with others. Finally, the chaplain will note the effect of his/her present situation on his/her relationship with God.

A major conflict is often created for the patient as he/she considers the part God might have played in all of this. Questions of theodicy, the place of God in the suffering creates struggle, ambivalence, and frequently intense feelings such as anger or grief. The chaplain spends considerable time and effort getting to know patients by actively listening to their story. Very often the stories of patients contain pain and tragedy as well as joy and successes. Their physical condition may contain emotional or spiritual pain as well as physical pain. The pastoral relationship helps the patient feel cared for and understood. This, in turn, frequently facilitates difficult decisions that need to be made. The relationships built by the palliative care team often lead to a more appropriate and holistic level of care that is provided in a more timely manner.

CARE AT THE TIME OF DEATH

To be able to relate bad news to others requires an ability to say "no" to the impulse to run away from the pain. Even while helping people process through feelings and face life-shaking questions, there is a part in the chaplain that resists, too. As anyone else, chaplains become ill at ease because it is easier to focus on living and avoid thinking about death. Understanding in advance that one's anxiety may rise while sitting with those who are suffering and dying can make identifying and managing one's own anxiety somewhat easier.

It is also important to understand that people resist change, particularly the change that comes when a loved one is dying or dies. Knowing this can help chaplains, physicians, nurses, and other team members to be patient with families who are grieving the death of a loved one. Very often intense feelings are produced at the time of death. Guilt or betrayal, fear or anger, or a general anxiety as well as a profound sadness rise up. The representative questions, "How will I make it?" "Why did he have to die?" "He told me we would live until he was 99," point to these strong feelings. At times the appreciative reflection of a family or family member about the deceased loved one demonstrates that the wonder of their relationship far outweighs the grief. Although people sometimes resist change, they often demonstrate a wonderful and life-affirming resilience, even in the face of death.

After death, the chaplain has the family sign the release of body form thereby making the transition from hospital to funeral home more fluid. The family is given a bereavement folder containing a book on grief, a list of normal grief reactions, and a list of community resources for help with continuing grief. The staff also signs a condolence note, which is mailed to the family 5 days later.

Health care providers work in an environment where people die everyday. In many ways the experience of chaplains is 180 degrees from the experience of others. Chaplains are familiar with death and grief and it is precisely that familiarity which frees them to come alongside people who are grieving. The danger with this kind of familiarity is that the chaplain, as with other health care providers, may forget how personal this death is to this person or family. We constantly find ourselves, as chaplains, wondering what difference this death makes to this person at this time in their lives. Touching the hurt and pain is important so that the individual or family will realize that someone understands, on some level, what they are experiencing. Although loss is always something experienced alone, having someone who understands is very helpful and removes the feeling of being isolated from others. The central image of the 23rd psalm is that someone walks with people in the deepest darkness. The darkness is deep, but the fact that someone walks with us helps immeasurably.

Some of the most powerful actions appear to be too simple when responding to people facing loss. To sit, establish eye contact, acknowledge loss and to speak clearly in a gentle tone of voice, or to place a gentle hand on a shoulder can impact people powerfully. The art of pastoral care is seen in honoring, rather than minimizing, the grief. By honoring the grief, chaplains truly join with the person or family. The physicians who learn this art are deeply appreciated by patients before death and by families following death. The surgeon or chaplain who *sits* 5 minutes with a family creates a stronger bond and deeper appreciation than a surgeon or chaplain who *stands* 5 minutes. Sitting creates the perception that the caregiver really made time for the patient or family. He or she took the time to listen to and answer my questions. On the other hand, minimizing the depth of someone's loss can easily produce explosive anger. When that happens it is easy to be somewhat indignant toward the family member for not realizing an attempt to make them feel better. The truth is that the doctor, chaplain, or health care worker was probably trying to make themselves feel better. It is important to understand that minimizing the depth of someone's grief has roots in our discomfort. This is an issue that is addressed in the clinical training of pastoral care interns and residents. Much of our work with staff members involves helping them to support people who face loss.

EVER-PRESENT ETHICAL CONCERNS

Chaplains and other health care professionals practice amid a sea of ethical concerns. Chaplains frequently serve on trauma center ethics committees and provide valuable consultative services.[12]

Along with the medical staff, chaplains are involved in an increasing number of situations where the limits of medicine have been reached. Decisions regarding futile care cause the most consternation and wrestling for everyone. In this day of the respirator and modern medicine, patients can be kept alive for a very long time although the quality of their life is permanently diminished or nonexistent. The question of what happens, and what decisions are made at the end of life when all medical measures have been exhausted, is the central medical dilemma that needs attention in our modern society.[13]

The chaplains attempt to get close to the trauma surgeon who bears, and often feels, the heavy weight of making the medical decisions. A trauma surgeon must struggle like few other physicians to determine their personal responses to end-of-life questions. These are more than philosophic pondering because they are questions that deal with life-and-death issues. Some questions and dilemmas the trauma surgeon faces are, "What stance should I take when I have lost hope? How can I be faithful to my own responsibility yet care for the family as they also struggle with questions of life and death?"

The following case example illustrates the struggle with the issue of futility in a modern ICU. An 18-year-old boy was involved in a motor vehicle crash. His condition worsened to the point that the nurses were having great difficulty caring for him because it was clear there was no hope. His death was a particularly gruesome one. The medical staff members were very clear with the family about the hopelessness of the situation. The family did not want to take the responsibility of making the decision to "pull the plug." The family distanced themselves from the details of his illness; therefore, they were not as close as the direct care nurses. The nurses were angry because of the length of time taken to make a decision regarding discontinuing care that they judged "futile." The Ethics Committee laid out alternatives for the physicians to consider. The family was disconnected from one another; family members deferred to the father, who had a serious alcohol problem and refused to participate in family conferences. Eventually, the boy died but after almost a month of agony and struggle on everyone's part. Dealing with the futility of care led to great travail for everyone involved.

A number of chaplains were involved in this patient's care. Numerous attempts were made to reach out to all members of the health care team and the family. What eventually happened and helped immensely was the decision to have all caregivers come together to discuss the situation. It provided a wonderful opportunity to vent, to express feelings, to discover unknown facts, and separate those from opinions. The staff members involved came away from this debriefing with renewed appreciation for the value of case conferences in the midst of the turmoil. Nurses heard and understood more deeply the agony of the surgeon. Several staff members realized, for the first time, that the Ethics Committee functions as an advisory body. They had done their work by stating clearly that the hospital had the option of seeking guardianship. They could not, however, dictate a decision even if they had one that would have been helpful.

A dilemma faced by trauma surgeons relates to the determination of how to express and share feelings of inadequacy. Communication among all members of the caregiver team has become increasingly important[14]. It is equally important that the staff hear the struggle of the doctor. In the end the doctor needs to wrestle with his or her own ethical principles. Such an examination will serve him or her very well in the heat of the moment. It is also good to know that the chaplain is equipped and ready to explore the dilemma and the pain involved in these difficult decisions. Clear communication among all members of the health care team is worth the considerable time and effort it demands. When the team is together, when the chaplain is deeply involved, when open and frank discussions are regularly held, then patient satisfaction is high, lawsuits are few, and the health care team functions more effectively.

CULTURAL DIVERSITY

Our society comprises people from many cultures. The diversity requires health care workers to develop cultural sensitivity in order to care for patients and families.[15] Trauma centers need to increase the knowledge of health care workers, particularly in regard to the relationship between belief systems and health care. Pastoral care services, in collaboration with nursing, can develop a series of didactic presentations dealing with cultural diversity and health care. The content may include Hispanic, African-American, Scandinavian, Filipino, Muslim, and Jewish perspectives on culture and health care. The series can furnish information and highlight the fact that the trauma center itself is a culturally diverse institution. By virtue of their training and sensitivity, chaplains often play a significant role in helping other health care providers bridge cultural differences.

Chaplains are trained to honor cultural differences as they minister. This is particularly important when people are suddenly placed into sensitive and critical situations as a result of trauma. Culture plays a major role in health care delivery. Insensitivity or lack of awareness can significantly impact response to treatment and length of recovery. In addition to the injuries sustained by the patient, an injury event creates a great deal of anxiety for a family, for any family. This anxiety is heightened automatically when cultural differences are present and again heightened when a physician, nurse, chaplain, or other staff member unknowingly transgresses a cultural boundary. For example, a male chaplain, and indeed, a physician, needs to be alert to the meaning of his presence with a female Muslim patient. Where possible, a female chaplain or physician should be enlisted to provide care. Because Muslim laws separate men and women in many areas of life, having a man provide health care to a man or a woman provide health care to a woman, respects the customs and practices that give shape to their life. Respecting the values and beliefs of others is the single best way to be respected by others.

Pastoral care training emphasizes the role of cultural differences in several ways. In addition to seeking diversity in the mix of our students we look for ways to help them learn from the patients and families they minister to. In addition to this we ask Rabbis, Imams, and other religious leaders talk to our students about culture, religion, and medicine. There are a number of resources designed for chaplains but available to others that provide an introduction to a rich variety of traditions. One of the best is a learning module created by Sue Wintz and Earl Cooper titled, "*Cultural and Spiritual Sensitivity, A Quick Guide to Cultures and Spiritual Traditions.*" It can be found on the Association of Professional Chaplains website, www .professionalchaplains.org.[16]

The importance of developing one's cultural awareness can be seen in the consideration of end-of-life decisions. These decisions are dramatically affected by the patient's culture and family. One example is seen in patient autonomy, which is generally more important for Europeans than for Hispanics. Hispanic elders are more likely than European Americans to want family members to make end-of-life decisions.[15]

Recognizing this sort of cultural difference enables caregivers to widen the circle and make themselves available to the family rather than to individuals within the family. Issues inherent in suffering, sanctity of life, allowing natural death, and pharmacology are all dramatically impacted by one's own history and culture. Failure to understand the importance of a patient's culture on health care decisions can lead to great conflict. In our experience, people from different cultures quickly recognize when someone wants to understand them. That recognition leads to warm appreciation on the part of the patient and family toward the chaplain, doctor, or nurse.

Chaplains are taught not to impose their religious beliefs or perspectives on a patient or family. A traumatic event is not the time for a patient or family to have to deal with the personal perspectives of the caregiver. Instead chaplains seek to help patients find the strength and resources located within their culture and faith.

CONCLUSION

Pastoral care is an integral part of the trauma team. The team functions as primary caregivers to the family as the patient receives medical care from the highly trained trauma surgeons. Chaplains struggle alongside other team members to make effective and ethical decisions in this era of high technology in medicine. They agonize with the entire staff when faced with care that is clearly futile. They participate with the palliative care team in creating effective relationships that can lead to better medical decisions. They work with patients around issues of *faith and religion as they surface for patients and their families.* With compassion and empathy chaplains seek to complement the work of the trauma surgeons and trauma team, all of whom are working to help patients and their families rebuild their lives following traumatic events.

REFERENCES

1. Groopman J. God at the bedside. *N Engl J Med.* 2004;350(12): 1176–1178.
2. Tarpley JL, Tarpley MJ. Spirituality in surgical practice. *J Am Coll Surg.* 2002;194(5):642–647.

3. Hinshaw DB. The spiritual needs of the dying patient. *J Am Coll Surg*. 2002;195(4):565–568; discussion 568–569.
4. Nelson J. Identifying and overcoming barriers to high-quality palliative care in the intensive care unit. *Crit Care Med*. 2006; 34(Suppl):s324–s331.
5. Lautrette A, Ciroldi M, Ksibi H, et al. End-of-life family conferences: Rooted in the evidence. *Crit Care Med*. 2006;34(Suppl): s364–s372.
6. Bidwell DR. Developing an adequate "pneumatraumatology": Understanding the spiritual impacts of traumatic injury. *J Pastoral Care Counsel*. 2002;56(2):135–143.
7. Aleichem S. *Tevye's daughters*. Moscow: Sholom Aleichem Family Publications; 1999.
8. Macleish A. *J.B. A play in verse*. Boston: Mariner Books (Houghton-Mifflin Publishers); 1989.
9. Donne J, Coffin CM. Modern Library pbk. *The complete poetry and selected prose of John Donne*. New York: Modern Library; 2001.
10. Levy M, Mcbride D. End-of-life care in the intensive care unit: State of the art in 2006. *Crit Care Med*. 2006;34(Suppl):s306–s308.
11. Twaddle ML, Maxwell TL, Cassel JB, et al. Palliative care benchmarks from academic medical centers. *J Palliat Med*. 2007;10(1): 86–98.
12. Schneiderman LJ. Effect of ethics consultations in the intensive care unit. *Crit Care Med*. 2006;34(Suppl):s359–s363.
13. Cook D, Rocker G, Giacomini M, et al. Understanding and changing attitudes toward withdrawal and withholding of life support in the intensive care unit. *Crit Care Med*. 2006;34(suppl): s317–s323.
14. Puntillo KA, McAdam JL. Communication between physicians and nurses as a target for improving end-of-life care in the intensive care unit: Challenges and opportunities for moving forward. *Crit Care Med*. 2006;34(suppl):s332–s340.
15. Blackhall LJ, Murphy ST, Frank G, et al. Ethnicity and attitudes toward patient autonomy. *JAMA*. 1995;274(10):820–825.
16. Wintz S, Cooper, E. *Learning module: cultural and spiritual sensitivity and a quick guide for cultures and spiritual traditions*. 2000.

Index